CELLULOSE-BASED GRAFT COPOLYMERS

Structure and Chemistry

CELLULOSE-BASED GRAFT COPOLYMERS

Structure and Chemistry

Edited by

Vijay Kumar Thakur

CRC Press
Taylor & Francis Group
Boca Raton London New York

CRC Press is an imprint of the
Taylor & Francis Group, an **informa** business

CRC Press
Taylor & Francis Group
6000 Broken Sound Parkway NW, Suite 300
Boca Raton, FL 33487-2742

First issued in paperback 2017

ISBN-13: 978-1-4822-4246-1 (hbk)
ISBN-13: 978-1-138-82719-6 (pbk)

Library of Congress Cataloging-in-Publication Data

Cellulose-based graft copolymers : structure and chemistry / edited by Vijay Kumar Thakur.
pages cm
Includes bibliographical references and index.
ISBN 978-1-4822-4246-1 (hardcover : alk. paper) 1. Graft copolymers. 2. Cellulose. I. Thakur, Vijay Kumar, 1981-

QD382.G7C45 2015
668.9--dc23 2015001497

Visit the Taylor & Francis Web site at
http://www.taylorandfrancis.com

and the CRC Press Web site at
http://www.crcpress.com

To my parents and teachers, who helped me become what I am today.

Vijay Kumar Thakur

Contents

Preface

With the gradual reduction of nonrenewable resources and increasing demand for novel materials, non-oil commodities, catalysts, and photoelectric devices, the development of natural biorenewable polymer–based materials has caught the world's attention. Among various biorenewable polymers, cellulose (a linear polysaccharide of β-(1→4)-linked D-glucose) is one of the most abundant biomacromolecules in nature and has drawn much attention in recent years due to its inherent properties such as renewability, biocompatibility, biodegradability, nontoxicity, and easy availability, to name a few. Cellulose is also the most lavish natural polymeric material that is widely distributed in every corner of the world. It is even more significant that cellulose is renewable by direct fixation of solar energy by plants. Because of the recent soar in prices of petroleum products, cellulosic raw materials have gained special importance since they are available in large amounts all over the world. The history of cellulose was known as cotton in the valley of the Indus River as early as 3000 BC. Since then, there has been a tremendous growth of its use in the whole range of polymers, which has led to the development of a new family of polymers and which, with appropriate modification, can display different promising properties.

In the past century, scientists have paid a great deal of attention in studying the physical and chemical properties of cellulose. But it seems that the current applications of cellulose are still not able to meet the growing needs of the community. Over the years, researchers from both academia and industry have made great efforts to modify the structure of cellulose and strengthen its physical or chemical properties, such as dimension stability, resistance to abrasion and wear, and oil repellency, but it is still insufficient. The reports of extending far beyond the traditional application areas of cellulosic materials, such as ion detectors, biosensors, and electronic devices, are quite limited. This book is a great opportunity to pay attention to value-added cellulose materials for multifunctional applications. There is great potential for these applications to be realized in the near future if we keep a research eye on functional polymer-grafted cellulose, and all those applications would easily benefit from the advantages of cheaper, lighter, flexible, and green cellulose substrates. Cellulose-based materials have the potential as raw materials if the desired functional groups could be effectively coupled onto them.

Different kinds of modifications are intended to impute different desired properties to the modified materials. Modification of the properties of cellulosics according to tailor-made specifications is an important criterion for various applications. The spectrum of its uses may be still more widened considerably by taking recourse to "grafting," a popular route to modify the properties of various high-molecular-weight compounds. Grafting is a tailor-made art. Of the various polymers on which grafting of suitable monomers can be made, cellulose appears to be very interesting and promising. The approaches can be of "grafting from," "grafting to," and "grafting through." Depending on the chemical structure of the monomer grafted onto cellulose, graft copolymers gain new properties such as water absorption, improved elasticity, hydrophilic or hydrophobic character, ion exchange, dye-absorption capabilities, heat resistance, thermosensitivity, pH sensitivity, and resistance to microbiological attack, to name a few.

Keeping in mind the immense advantages of natural cellulosic polymers, this book primarily focuses on the synthesis, characterization, and properties of multifunctional cellulose-based graft copolymers. Several critical issues and suggestions for future work are comprehensively discussed in this book with the hope that it will provide a deep insight into the state of the art of advanced cellulose-based graft copolymers. I thank Allison Shatkin (senior editor) and her colleagues at CRC Press for the invaluable help in the organization of the editing process.

Finally, I thank my parents and my wife, Manju, for their continuous encouragement and support.

Vijay Kumar Thakur, PhD
Washington State University
Pullman, Washington

Editor

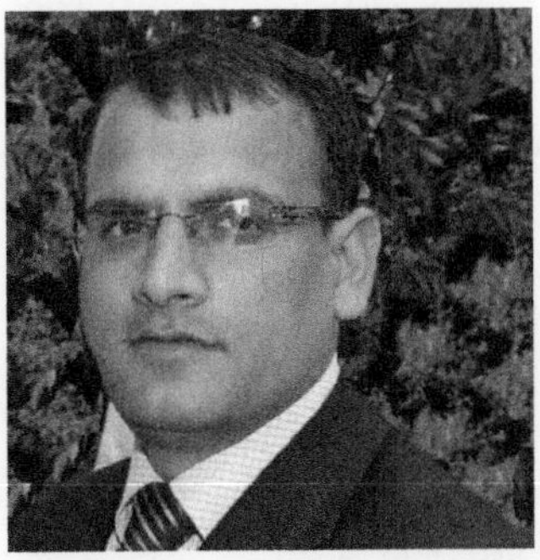

Vijay Kumar Thakur, PhD, has been working as research faculty (staff scientist) in the School of Mechanical and Materials Engineering at Washington State University, Pullman, Washington, since September 2013. His former appointments include a research scientist in Temasek Laboratories at Nanyang Technological University, Singapore, and a visiting research fellow in the Department of Chemical and Materials Engineering at Lunghwa University of Science and Technology, Taiwan. His research interests include the synthesis and processing of biobased polymers, nanomaterials, polymer micro-/nanocomposites, nanoelectronic materials, novel high dielectric constant materials, electrochromic materials for energy storage, green synthesis of nanomaterials, and surface functionalization of polymers/nanomaterials. He completed his postdoctorate in materials science at Iowa State University and his PhD in polymer science (2009) at the National Institute of Technology. In his academic career, he has published more than 75 SCI journal research articles in the field of polymers/materials science and holds one U.S. patent. He has also published 11 books and 30 book chapters on the advanced state of the art of polymers/materials science with numerous publishers. He is an editorial board member of several international journals including *Advanced Chemistry Letters*, *Lignocelluloses*, *Drug Inventions Today*, *International Journal of Energy Engineering*, and *Journal of Textile Science and Engineering*, to name a few. He is also a member of several scientific bodies around the world. In addition to being on the editorial board of journals, he also serves as the guest editor of the *International Journal of Polymer Science* and *Journal of Chemistry*.

Contributors

Faten Hassan Hassan Abdellatif
Laboratory of Macromolecular Physical Chemistry
Chemical Engineering National School
University of Lorraine
Nancy, France

Alex Alfieri
Department of Neurosurgery and Spinal Surgery
Ruppiner Kliniken GmbH
Neuruppin, Germany

T.S. Anirudhan
Department of Chemistry
School of Physical and Mathematical Sciences
University of Kerala
Kariavattom, Trivandrum, India

Marcos Antônio Araujo-Silva
Department of Physics
Federal University of Ceará
Fortaleza, Brazil

Carole Arnal-Herault
Laboratory of Macromolecular Physical Chemistry
Chemical Engineering National School
University of Lorraine
Nancy, France

Mohammad Hossein Babaabbasi
Faculty of Science
Department of Chemistry
Lorestan University
Khoramabad, Iran

Jérôme Babin
Laboratory of Macromolecular Physical Chemistry
Chemical Engineering National School
University of Lorraine
Nancy, France

Massoumeh Bagheri
Faculty of Science
Department of Chemistry
Azarbaijan Shahid Madani University
Tabriz, Iran

S.K. Bajpai
Polymer Research Laboratory
Department of Chemistry
Government Model Science College
Jabalpur, India

Nursel Pekel Bayramgil
Faculty of Science
Department of Chemistry
Hacettepe University
Ankara, Turkey

A. Bhattacharya
Central Salt and Marine Chemicals Research Institute
Council of Scientific and Industrial Research
Bhavnagar, India

Birendra Kumar Bindhani
School of Biotechnology
KIIT University
Bhubaneswar, India

Susanta Kumar Biswal
Department of Chemistry
Centurion University of Technology and Management
Jatni, India

R. Bongiovanni
Department of Applied Science and Technology
Politecnico di Torino
Torino, Italy

Montu Moni Bora
Department of Chemistry
Gauhati University
Guwahati, India

Peter R. Chang
BioProducts and Bioprocesses National Science Program
Agriculture and Agri-Food Canada
Saskatoon, Saskatchewan, Canada

Meiwan Chen
State Key Laboratory of Quality Research in Chinese Medicine
Institute of Chinese Medical Sciences
University of Macau
Macau, People's Republic of China

Xiuli Chen
College of Life Science and Technology
National Engineering Research Center for Nano-Medicine
Huazhong University of Science and Technology
Wuhan, Hubei, People's Republic of China

A. Chiappone
Istituto Italiano di Tecnologia
Torino, Italy

Raghunath Das
Polymer Chemistry Laboratory
Department of Applied Chemistry
Indian School of Mines
Dhanbad, India

Chayanika Deka
Department of Chemistry
Gauhati University
Guwahati, India

Kartick Prasad Dey
Department of Applied Chemistry
Birla Institute of Technology
Ranchi, India

P.L. Divya
Department of Chemistry
School of Physical and Mathematical Sciences
University of Kerala
Kariavattom, Trivandrum, India

Paulo de Tarso C. Freire
Department of Physics
Federal University of Ceará
Fortaleza, Brazil

Marcelo Galarza
Department of Neurosurgery
University Hospital Virgen de la Arrixaca
Murcia, Spain

Mario Gauthier
Department of Chemistry
University of Waterloo
Waterloo, Ontario, Canada

Roberto Gazzeri
Department of Neurosurgery
San Giovanni Addolorata Hospital
Rome, Italy

Soumitra Ghorai
Polymer Chemistry Laboratory
Department of Applied Chemistry
Indian School of Mines
Dhanbad, India

Yanzhu Guo
Liaoning Key Laboratory of Pulp and Paper Engineering
Dalian Polytechnic University
Dalian, People's Republic of China

Jin Huang
College of Chemistry, Chemical Engineering and Life Science
Wuhan University of Technology
Wuhan, Hubei, People's Republic of China

Yajia Huang
College of Life Science and Technology
National Engineering Research Center for Nano-Medicine
Huazhong University of Science and Technology
Wuhan, Hubei, People's Republic of China

Meng Huo
Key Lab of Organic Optoelectronic and Molecular Engineering of Ministry of Education
Department of Chemistry
Tsinghua University
Beijing, People's Republic of China

Jahid M.M. Islam
Institute of Radiation and Polymer Technology
Bangladesh Atomic Energy Commission
Dhaka, Bangladesh

Chunmei Jian
Key Lab of Organic Optoelectronic and Molecular Engineering of Ministry of Education
Department of Chemistry
Tsinghua University
Beijing, People's Republic of China

Anne Jonquieres
Laboratory of Macromolecular Physical Chemistry
Chemical Engineering National School
University of Lorraine
Nancy, France

Abdullah-Al-Jubayer
Institute of Radiation and Polymer Technology
Bangladesh Atomic Energy Commission
Dhaka, Bangladesh

Dilip Kumar Kakati
Department of Chemistry
Gauhati University
Guwahati, India

Mubarak A. Khan
Institute of Radiation and Polymer Technology
Bangladesh Atomic Energy Commission
Dhaka, Bangladesh

Jalel Labidi
Department of Chemical and Environmental Engineering
University of the Basque Country
Donostia-San Sebastián, Spain

Jusha Ma
School of Materials Science and Engineering
Beijing Institute of Technology
Beijing, People's Republic of China

R. Meena
Scale-Up and Process Engineering Unit
Council of Scientific and Industrial Research
Bhavnagar, India

Sumit Mishra
Department of Applied Chemistry
Birla Institute of Technology
Ranchi, India

Marika Morabito
Department of Neurosurgery
San Giovanni Addolorata Hospital
Rome, Italy

Ronaldo Ferreira do Nascimento
Department of Analytical Chemistry and Physical Chemistry
Federal University of Ceará
Fortaleza, Brazil

Padmalochan Nayak
P.L. Nayak Research Foundation
Synergy Institute of Technology
Bhubaneswar, India

J. Nima
Department of Chemistry
School of Physical and Mathematical Sciences
University of Kerala
Kariavattom, Trivandrum, India

Qinyuan Niu
School of Materials Science and Engineering
Beijing Institute of Technology
Beijing, People's Republic of China

and

School of Material and Chemical Engineering
Zhengzhou University of Light Industry
Zhengzhou, Henan, People's Republic of China

Vicente de Oliveira Sousa Neto
Department of Chemistry
State University of Ceará
Fortaleza, Brazil

Sagar Pal
Polymer Chemistry Laboratory
Department of Applied Chemistry
Indian School of Mines
Dhanbad, India

Umesh Kumar Parida
School of Biotechnology
KIIT University
Bhubaneswar, India

Mehlika Pulat
Department of Chemistry
Gazi University
Ankara Turkey

Diego de Quadros Melo
Department of Chemistry
State University of Ceará
Fortaleza, Brazil

Md. Saifur Rahaman
Institute of Radiation and Polymer Technology
Bangladesh Atomic Energy Commission
Dhaka, Bangladesh

Ashvinder Kumar Rana
Department of Chemistry
Sri Sai University
Palampur, India

Eduardo Robles
Department of Chemical and Environmental Engineering
University of the Basque Country
Donostia-San Sebastián, Spain

Luis Serrano
Department of Chemical and Environmental Engineering
University of the Basque Country
San Sebastián, Spain

Gautam Sen
Department of Applied Chemistry
Birla Institute of Technology
Ranchi, India

Surinder Pal Singh
Polymer Research Laboratory
Department of Chemistry
Government Model Science College
Jabalpur, India

Amar Singh Singha
Department of Chemistry
National Institute of Technology
Hamirpur, India

Bhawna Soni
Polymer Research Laboratory
Department of Chemistry
Government Model Science College
Jabalpur, India

Runcang Sun
State Key Laboratory of Pulp and Paper Engineering
South China University of Technology
Guangzhou, People's Republic of China

and

Institute of Biomass Chemistry and Technology
Beijing Forestry University
Beijing, People's Republic of China

Abbas Dadkhah Tehrani
Faculty of Science
Department of Chemistry
Lorestan University
Khoramabad, Iran

Manju Kumari Thakur
Division of Chemistry
Government Degree College, Sarkaghat
Himachal Pradesh University
Shimla, India

Vijay Kumar Thakur
Faculty of College of Engineering and Architecture
School of Mechanical and Materials Engineering
Washington State University
Pullman, Washington

Biranchinarayan Tosh
Department of Chemistry
Orissa Engineering College
Bhubaneswar, India

Iñaki Urruzola
Department of Chemical and Environmental Engineering
University of the Basque Country
Donostia-San Sebastián, Spain

G. Usha Rani
Department of Applied Chemistry
Birla Institute of Technology
Ranchi, India

Xiaohui Wang
State Key Laboratory of Pulp and Paper Engineering
South China University of Technology
Guangzhou, People's Republic of China

Wenhui Wu
School of Materials Science and Engineering
Beijing Institute of Technology
Beijing, People's Republic of China

Guang Yang
College of Life Science and Technology
National Engineering Research Center for Nano-Medicine
Huazhong University of Science and Technology
Wuhan, Hubei, People's Republic of China

Qiquan Ye
Key Lab of Organic Optoelectronic and Molecular Engineering of Ministry of Education
Department of Chemistry
Tsinghua University
Beijing, People's Republic of China

and

Key Laboratory of Cigarette Smoke of State Tobacco Monopoly Administration
Technical Center of Shanghai Tobacco Corporation
Shanghai, People's Republic of China

Hou-Yong Yu
College of Materials and Textile
Zhejiang Sci-Tech University
Hangzhou, Zhejiang, People's Republic of China

Jinying Yuan
Key Lab of Organic Optoelectronic and Molecular Engineering of Ministry of Education
Department of Chemistry
Tsinghua University
Beijing, People's Republic of China

and

Key Laboratory of Cigarette Smoke of State Tobacco Monopoly Administration
Technical Center of Shanghai Tobacco Corporation
Shanghai, People's Republic of China

E. Zeno
Centre Technique du Papier
Domaine Universitaire
Grenoble, France

Haixiang Zhang
College of Life Science and Technology
National Engineering Research Center for Nano-Medicine
Huazhong University of Science and Technology
Wuhan, Hubei, People's Republic of China

Haoquan Zhong
State Key Laboratory of Pulp and Paper Engineering
South China University of Technology
Guangzhou, People's Republic of China

1 Cellulose-Based Graft Copolymers

An Overview

Vijay Kumar Thakur, Manju Kumari Thakur, Ashvinder Kumar Rana, and Amar Singh Singha

CONTENTS

1.1 INTRODUCTION

During the last few years, the utilization of raw materials from different biorenewable resources has seen a rapid increase for different applications (Thakur et al., 2013b). One of the greatest reasons for this increase is the quest for sustainable development (Santos et al., 2013; Thakur et al., 2014b). The effective utilization of materials from biorenewable resources results in a significant reduction in the amount of waste hoarded in our environment (Santos et al., 2013). Furthermore, to obtain a higher profit and make our environment green, an efficient reuse of these biorenewable materials is of great importance. The materials obtained from biorenewable resources also exhibit biodegradability, biocompatibility, and antibacterial activity, which are highly desired for several applications (Thakur and Thakur, 2014). Among various biorenewable materials, natural cellulosic polymers are of prime interest as these are abundantly available all around the globe (Thakur et al., 2013d). In each country, depending upon the geographic conditions, different kinds of natural cellulosic polymers are available, which are sometimes used while most of the times are considered as waste product of the biorenewable plants (Thakur et al., 2013c). The effective utilization of these natural cellulosic polymers such as natural cellulosic fibers in different industrial processes may result in low-cost environmental friendly value-added products (Thakur and Thakur, 2014). Figure 1.1a and b depicts the classification of bio-based polymers and natural fibers (Thakur and Thakur, 2014).

Some of the most commonly used natural cellulosic fibers are *Grewia optiva*, flax, *Hibiscus sabdariffa*, bamboo, sisal, hemp, agave, pine needles, pineapple leaf, *Saccaharum cilliare*, etc. These cellulosic fibers are obtained from different parts of plants through different techniques. Figures 1.2 and 1.3 show the photographic images of *Grewia optiva* fibers and pine apple leaf fibers prior to and after extraction from their parental plants (Santos et al., 2013; Thakur et al., 2014a).

Different kinds of natural cellulosic fibers are used in different forms for a number of applications. Most frequently, natural cellulosic fibers are used as the reinforcing materials for composite applications. These composites vary from partially biodegradable to fully biodegradable composites depending upon the matrix used (Majeed et al., 2013). Different types of fibers (micro/nano) can be obtained from different cellulosic polymers using different extraction techniques (Phong et al., 2013). Figure 1.4 shows the different kinds of cellulosic fiber procured from different resources.

Figure 1.5 shows the extraction of micro/nano-sized bamboo fibrils (MBFs) from raw bamboo, while Figure 1.6 shows the SEM image of these fibers.

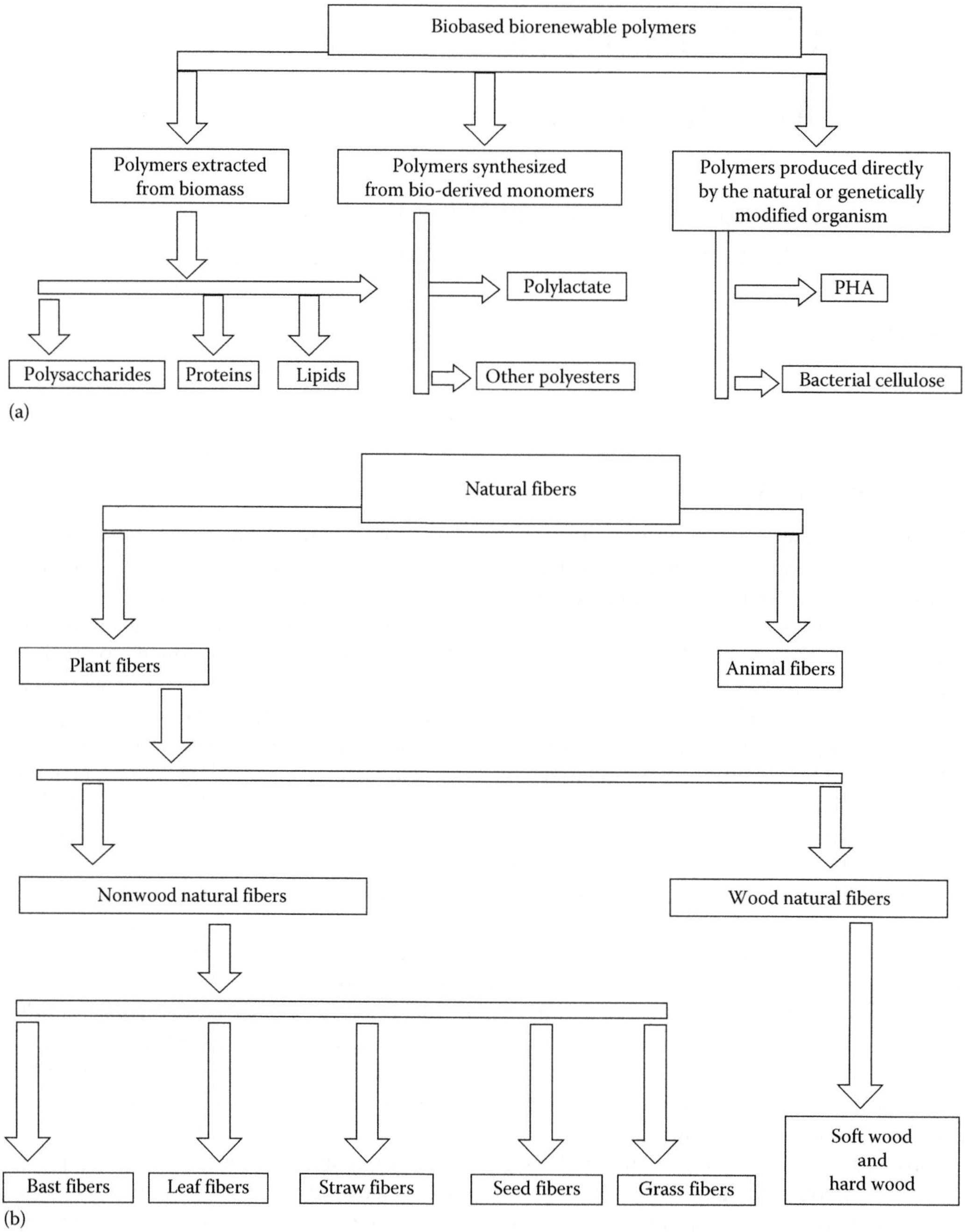

FIGURE 1.1 (a) Classification of biobased polymers and (b) classification of natural fibers. (Reprinted from *Carbohydrate Polymers*, 109, Thakur, V.K. and Thakur, M.K., Processing and characterization of natural cellulose fibers/thermoset polymer composites, 102–117, Copyright 2014, with permission from Elsevier.)

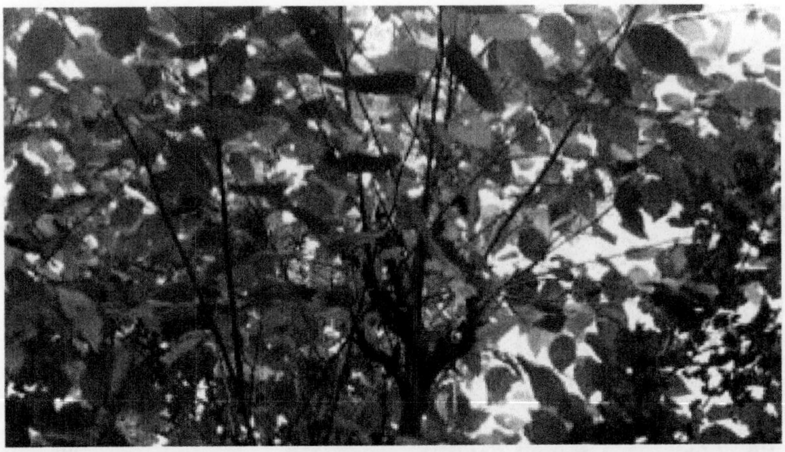

(a)

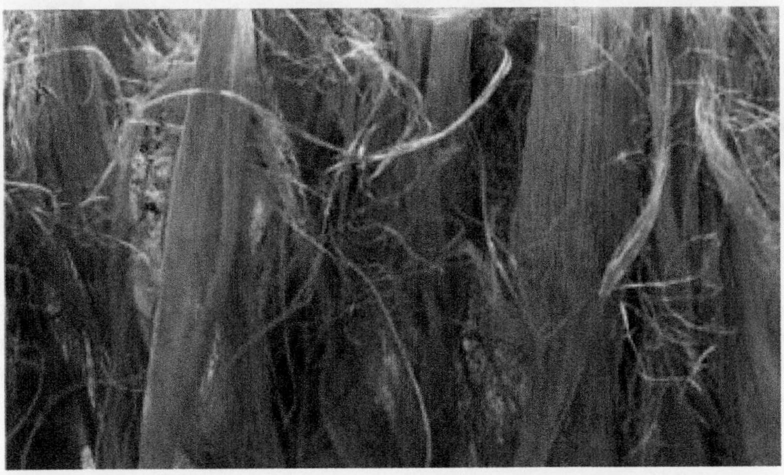

(b)

FIGURE 1.2 Photographic images of (a) *Grewia optiva* plant and (b) fibers derived from *Grewia optiva* plant. (Reprinted from *Carbohydrate Polymers*, 104, Thakur, V.K., Thakur, M.K., and Gupta, R.K., Graft copolymers of natural fibers for green composites, 87–93, Copyright 2014, with permission from Elsevier.)

All natural fibers are composed of different constituents, namely, cellulose, hemicellulose, and lignin. Each of these components plays an imperative role in determining the overall properties of the fibers. Among these three components, cellulose is considered as the major framework component of the fiber structure (Kabir et al., 2012). The prime role of the cellulose is to provide strength, stiffness, and structural stability to the fiber. Cellulose is a non-branched macromolecule that contains a chain of variable length of 1–4 linked β-D-anhydroglucopyranose units. Depending upon the source from which cellulose is extracted, the length of its chains varies. Figure 1.7 shows the chemical structure of different constituents of natural fibers.

Figures 1.8 and 1.9 show a schematic structure of a natural fiber and the model of the structural organization of the three major structural constituents of the fiber cell wall, respectively.

Figure 1.10 summarizes how cellulose is present in nature and its structure (Lavoine et al., 2012).

The physical and chemical aspects of different types of cellulose have been intensively studied by a number of researchers (Thakur and Singha, 2010d). Different functional groups and their ability to form strong hydrogen bonds confer upon cellulose its most important properties such as (1) multi-scale microfibrillated structure, (2) highly cohesive nature (with a glass transition temperature

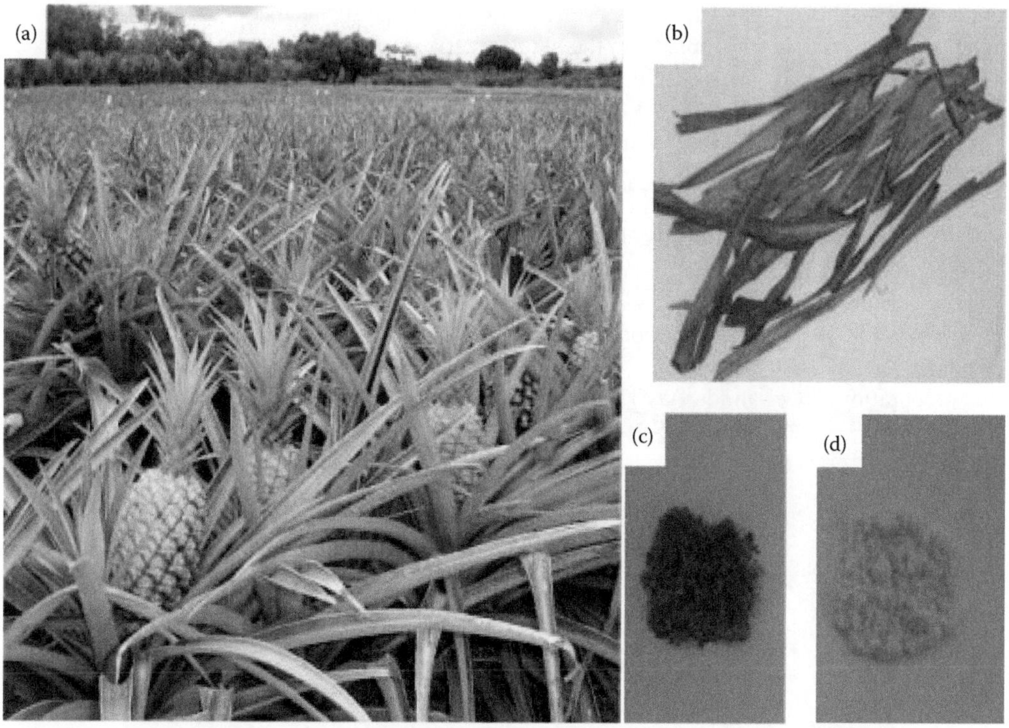

FIGURE 1.3 Photographs of (a) the pineapple cultivation, (b) untreated pineapple leaves, (c) ground pineapple leaves, and (d) treated pineapple leaves. (Reprinted from *Industrial Crops and Products*, 50, Santos, R.M. dos, Flauzino Neto, W.P., Silvério, H.A., Martins, D.F., Dantas, N.O., and Pasquini, D., Cellulose nanocrystals from pineapple leaf, a new approach for the reuse of this agro-waste, 707–714, Copyright 2013, with permission from Elsevier.)

higher than its degradation temperature), and (3) hierarchical organization (crystalline vs. amorphous regions) (Lavoine et al., 2012). Cellulose has been found to exhibit four different kinds of polymorphs (Figure 1.11).

In addition to their inherent properties, these cellulose fibers also suffer from a few disadvantages (Thakur et al., 2010a). Some of the disadvantages include sensitive to moisture absorption, less chemical resistance, and low thermal stability (Thakur and Singha, 2010e; Thakur et al., 2010b). For some applications, cellulose is solely extracted from these cellulose fibers and is used for different applications ranging from automotive to biomedical applications (Thakur and Singha, 2010a,b). The cellulose extracted is also converted into different forms depending upon the targeted applications (Thakur and Singha, 2010c). Very recently cellulose is being used in nanoform for different applications (Kamel, 2007). It has been reported that the structure of native cellulosic fibers during their treatment/extraction to nanoforms consequently results in two families of cellulosic nanoparticles, and these are named differently by the researchers (Roy et al., 2009; Missoum et al., 2013). Figure 1.12 represents the main steps involved in the preparation of cellulose nanocrystals and microfibrillated celluloses (Lavoine et al., 2012).

In addition to conversion into nanoforms, the cellulose is also converted into different derivatives. Figure 1.13 shows the chemical structure of some cellulose derivatives (Fernandes et al., 2013).

To overcome the disadvantages associated with the cellulosic fibers/nanocellulose, their surface is modified with different techniques (Roy, 2006; Thakur and Thakur, 2014; Thakur et al., 2014a). One of the most common techniques to alter the surface characteristics is the graft copolymerization (Kang et al., 2013; Thakur et al., 2013a). It is an attractive method to impart a variety

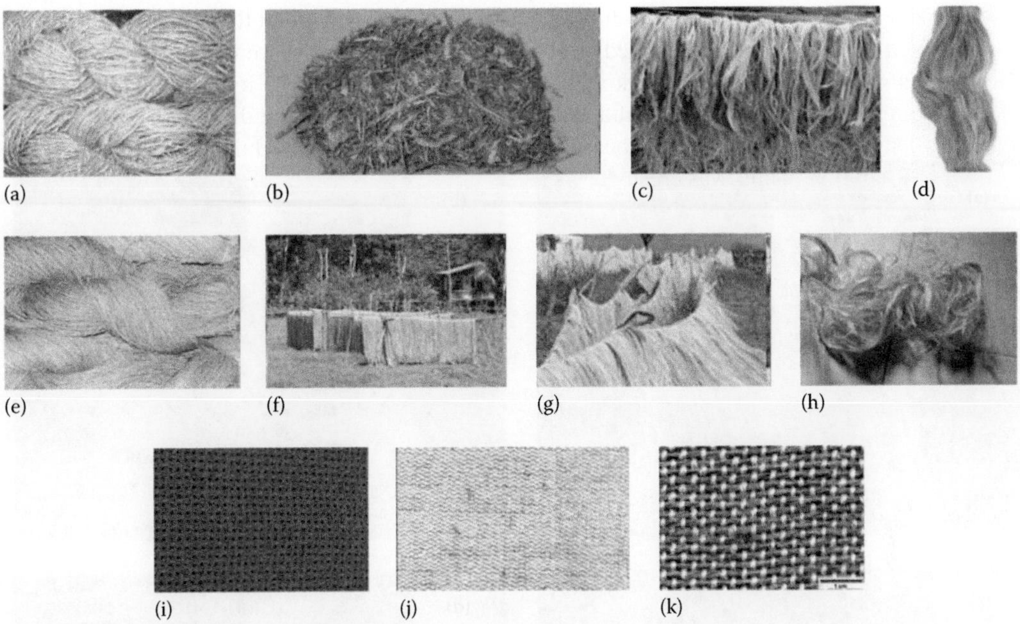

FIGURE 1.4 Lignocellulosic reinforcements. (a) Banana, (b) sugarcane bagasse, (c) curaua, (d) flax, (e) hemp, (f) jute, (g) sisal, and (h) kenaf. Typical pattern of reinforcements used in the hybrid LC-based biodegradable composite synthesis. (i) Jute fabric, (j) ramie–cotton fabric, and (k) jute–cotton fabric. (Reprinted from *Materials and Design*, 46, Majeed, K., Jawaid, M., Hassan, A., Abu Bakar, A., Khalil, H.P.S.A., Salema, A.A., and Inuwa, I., Potential materials for food packaging from nanoclay/natural fibres filled hybrid composites, 391–410, Copyright 2013, with permission from Elsevier.)

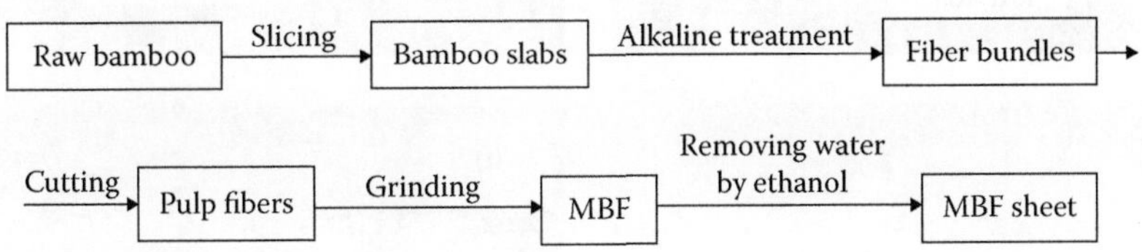

FIGURE 1.5 The extraction process of MBFs from raw bamboo. (Reprinted from *Materials and Design*, 47, Phong, N.T., Gabr, M.H., Okubo, K., Chuong, B., and Fujii, T., Enhancement of mechanical properties of carbon fabric/epoxy composites using micro/nano-sized bamboo fibrils, 624–632, Copyright 2013, with permission from Elsevier.)

of functional groups to a polymer (Bhattacharya and Misra, 2004; Carlmark et al., 2012). The graft copolymerization of cellulosic polymers can be accomplished using different techniques that include free radical—induced graft copolymerization, atom transfer radical polymerization, reversible addition fragmentation chain-transfer polymerization, ring-opening polymerization, photo-irradiation, and high-energy radiation technique (Roy et al., 2009; Wojnarovits et al., 2010). The cellulose-based graft copolymers obtained using these different techniques demonstrate a bright future for advanced applications (Roy, 2006; Tizzotti et al., 2010; Shah et al., 2013).

Chapters 2 through 25 of this book provide in-depth analysis of different types of cellulose-based graft copolymers and their applications. Chapters 2 through 12 discuss the progress in different grafting techniques and the role of different parameters that control the overall grafting. Chapters 13 through 25 discuss in detail the different applications of cellulose-based graft copolymers synthesized using different graft copolymerization techniques.

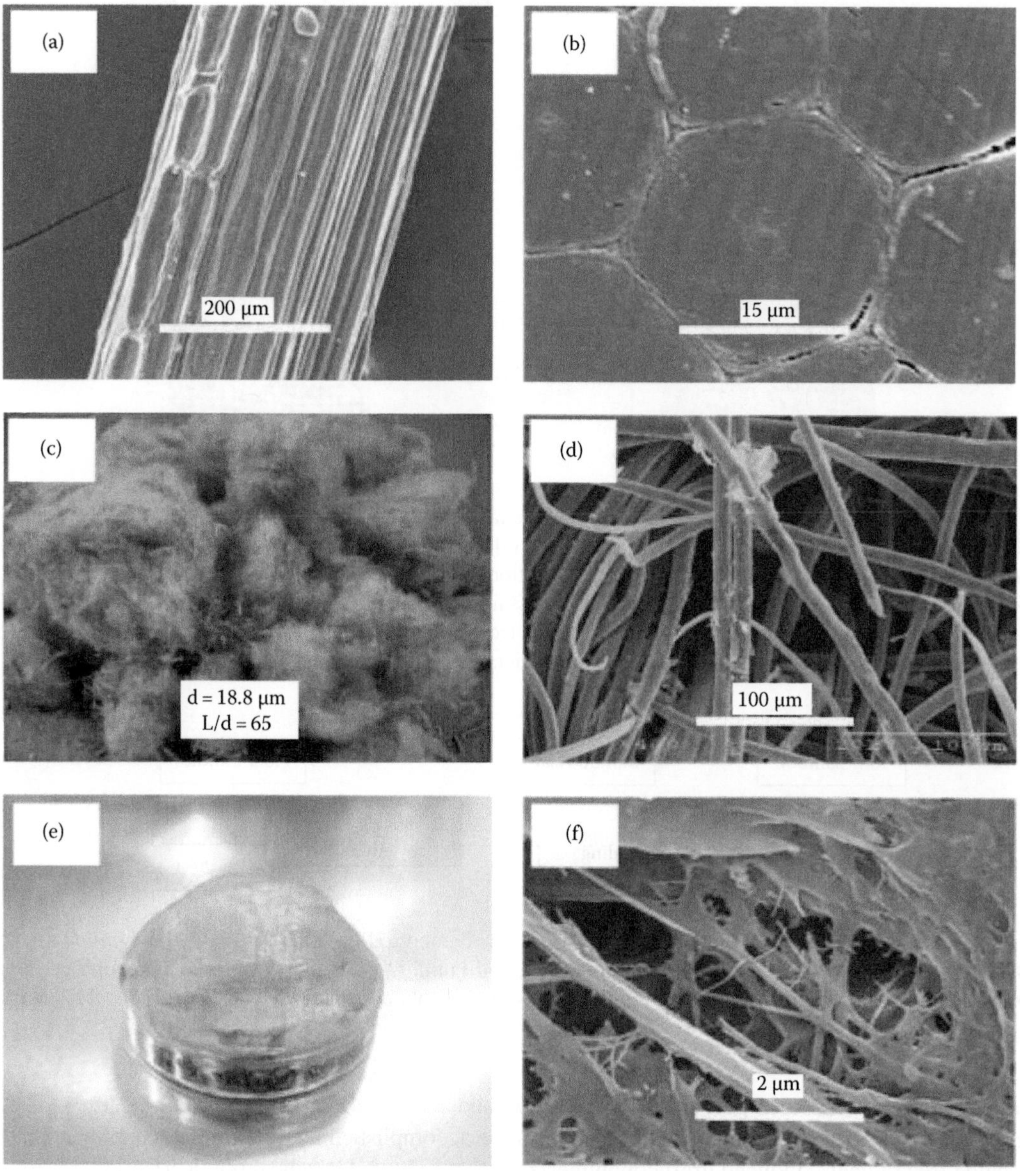

FIGURE 1.6 SEM images for (a, b) bamboo fiber bundle, (c, d) pulp fibers, and (e, f) MBF. (Reprinted from *Materials and Design*, 47, Phong, N.T., Gabr, M.H., Okubo, K., Chuong, B., and Fujii, T., Enhancement of mechanical properties of carbon fabric/epoxy composites using micro/nano-sized bamboo fibrils, 624–632, Copyright 2013, with permission from Elsevier.)

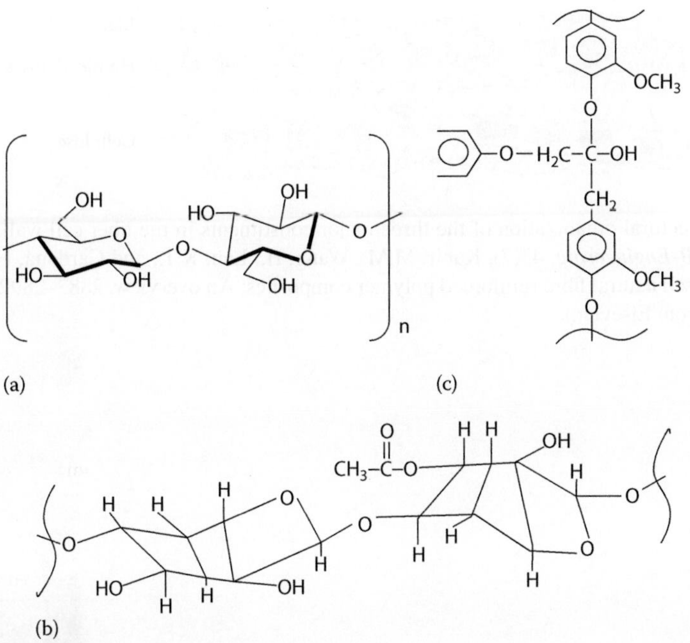

FIGURE 1.7 Chemical structure of (a) cellulose, (b) hemicelluloses, and (c) lignin. (Reprinted from *Composites Part B-Engineering*, 43(7), Kabir, M.M., Wang, H., Lau, K.T., and Cardona, F., Chemical treatments on plant-based natural fibre reinforced polymer composites: An overview, 2883–2892, Copyright 2012, with permission from Elsevier.)

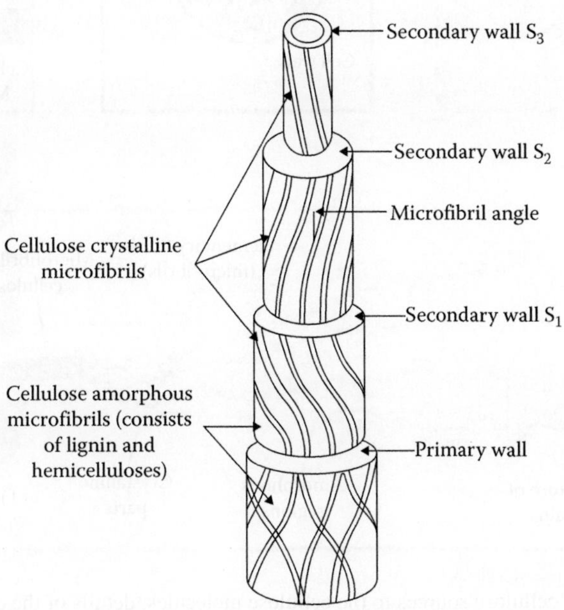

FIGURE 1.8 Structure of natural fiber. (Reprinted from *Composites Part B-Engineering*, 43(7), Kabir, M.M., Wang, H., Lau, K.T., and Cardona, F., Chemical treatments on plant-based natural fibre reinforced polymer composites: An overview, 2883–2892, Copyright 2012, with permission from Elsevier.)

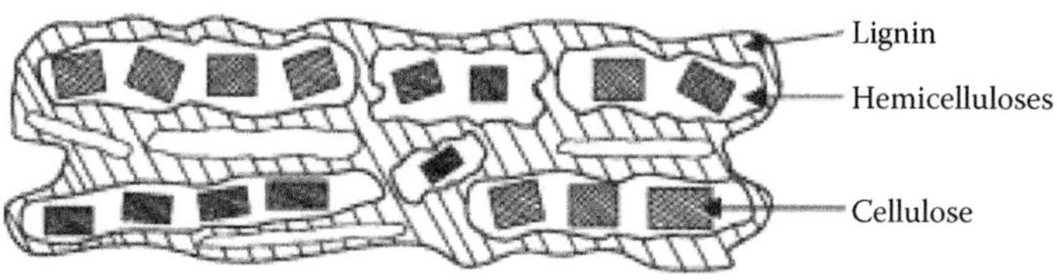

FIGURE 1.9 Structural organization of the three major constituents in the fiber cell wall. (Reprinted from *Composites Part B-Engineering*, 43(7), Kabir, M.M., Wang, H., Lau, K.T., and Cardona, F., Chemical treatments on plant-based natural fibre reinforced polymer composites: An overview, 2883–2892, Copyright 2012, with permission from Elsevier.)

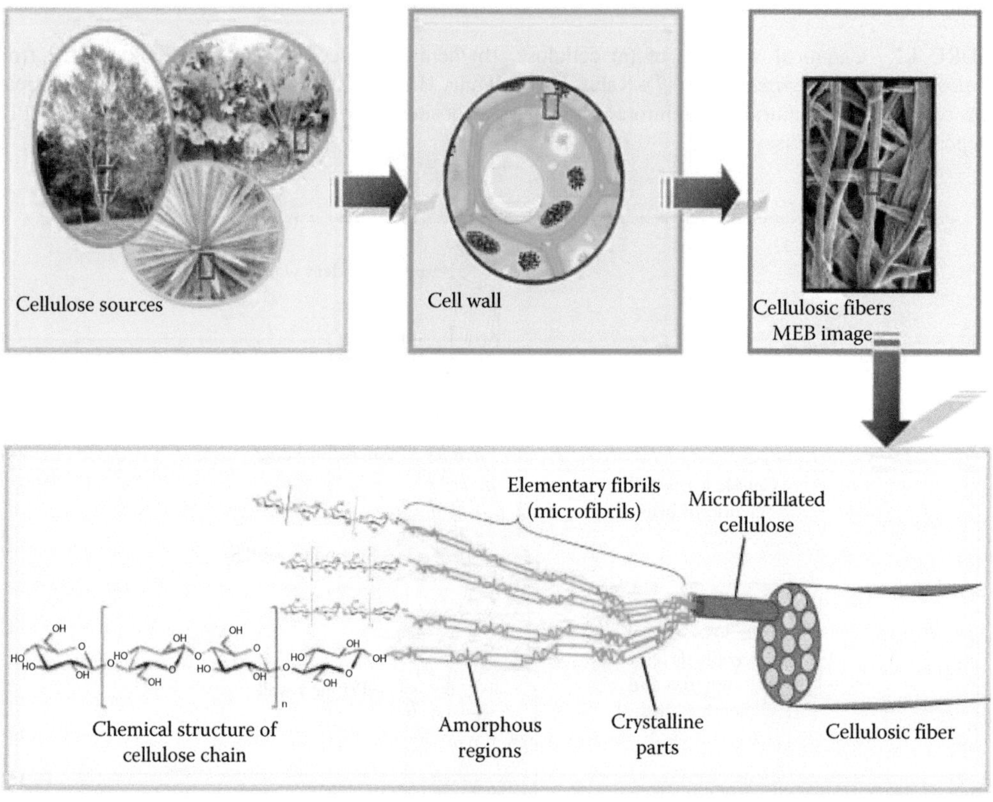

FIGURE 1.10 From the cellulose sources to the cellulose molecules: details of the cellulosic fiber structure with emphasis on the cellulose microfibrils. (Reprinted from *Carbohydrate Polymers*, 90(2), Lavoine, N., Desloges, I., Dufresne, A., and Bras, J., Microfibrillated cellulose—Its barrier properties and applications in cellulosic materials: A review, 735–764, Copyright 2012, with permission from Elsevier.)

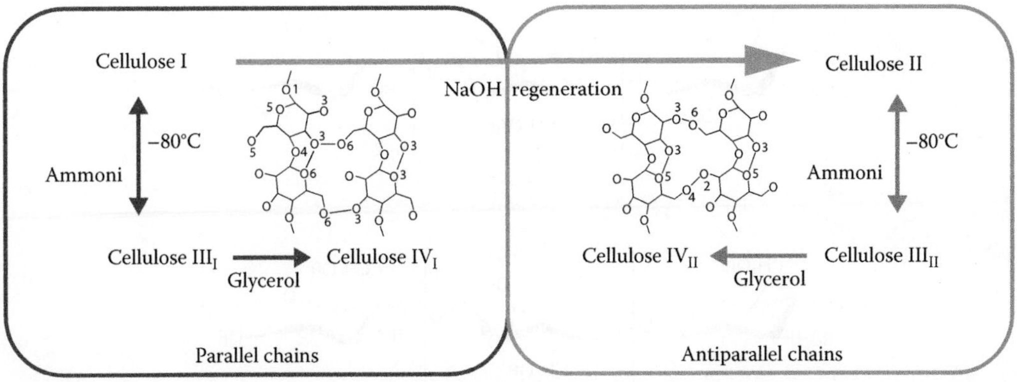

FIGURE 1.11 Polymorphs of cellulose and the main steps to obtain them. (Reprinted from *Carbohydrate Polymers*, 90(2), Lavoine, N., Desloges, I., Dufresne, A., and Bras, J., Microfibrillated cellulose—Its barrier properties and applications in cellulosic materials: A review, 735–764, Copyright 2012, with permission from Elsevier.)

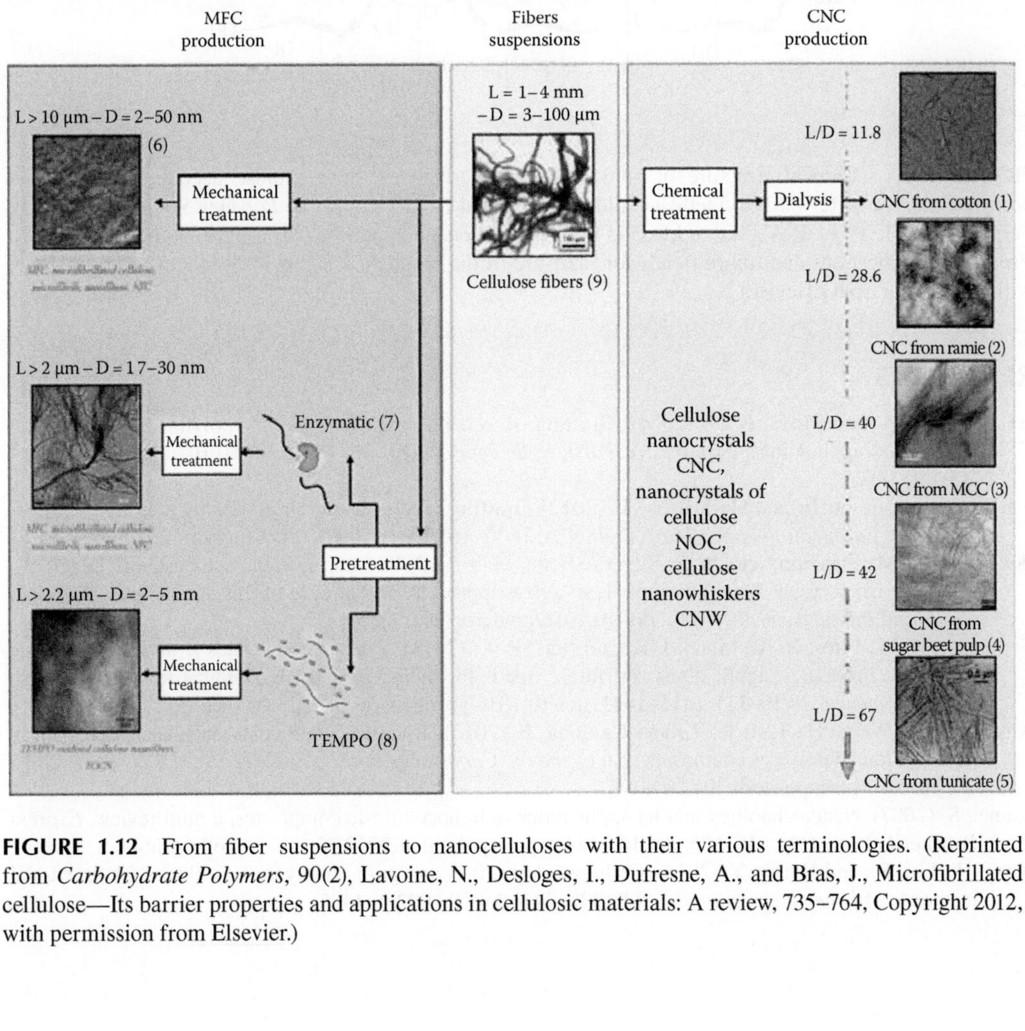

FIGURE 1.12 From fiber suspensions to nanocelluloses with their various terminologies. (Reprinted from *Carbohydrate Polymers*, 90(2), Lavoine, N., Desloges, I., Dufresne, A., and Bras, J., Microfibrillated cellulose—Its barrier properties and applications in cellulosic materials: A review, 735–764, Copyright 2012, with permission from Elsevier.)

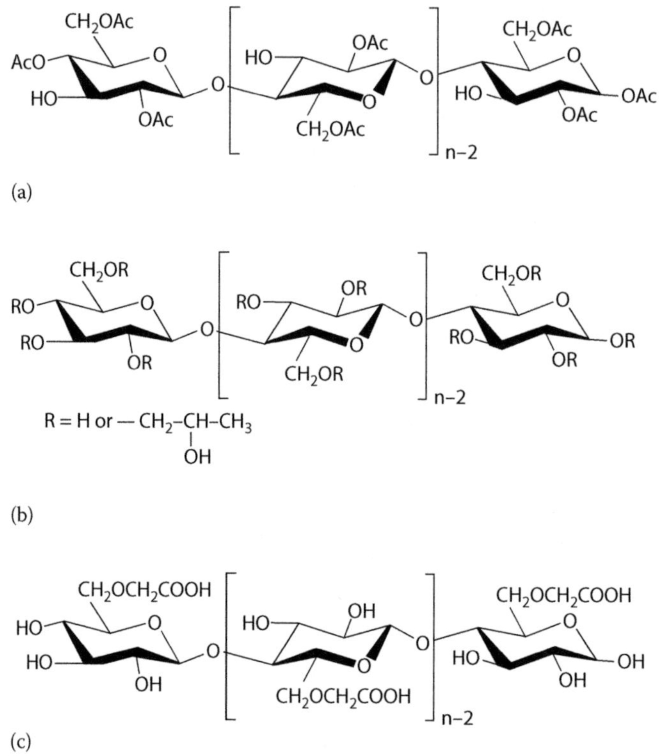

FIGURE 1.13 Chemical structure of some cellulose derivatives. (a) Cellulose acetate, (b) Hydroxypropylcellulose, and (c) Carboxymethylcellulose. (Reprinted from *Progress in Polymer Science*, 38(10–11), Fernandes, E.M., Pires, R.A., Mano, J.F., and Reis, R.L., Bionanocomposites from lignocellulosic resources: Properties, applications and future trends for their use in the biomedical field, 1415–1441, Copyright 2013, with permission from Elsevier.)

REFERENCES

Bhattacharya, A. and Misra, B. N. (2004). Grafting: A versatile means to modify polymers—Techniques, factors and applications. *Progress in Polymer Science*, *29*(8), 767–814. doi:10.1016/j.progpolymsci.2004.05.002.

Carlmark, A., Larsson, E., and Malmstrom, E. (2012). Grafting of cellulose by ring-opening polymerisation—A review. *European Polymer Journal*, *48*(10), 1646–1659. doi:10.1016/j.eurpolymj.2012.06.013.

dos Santos, R. M., Flauzino Neto, W. P., Silvério, H. A., Martins, D. F., Dantas, N. O., and Pasquini, D. (2013). Cellulose nanocrystals from pineapple leaf, a new approach for the reuse of this agro-waste. *Industrial Crops and Products*, *50*, 707–714. doi:10.1016/j.indcrop.2013.08.049.

Fernandes, E. M., Pires, R. A., Mano, J. F., and Reis, R. L. (2013). Bionanocomposites from lignocellulosic resources: Properties, applications and future trends for their use in the biomedical field. *Progress in Polymer Science*, *38*(10–11), 1415–1441. doi:10.1016/j.progpolymsci.2013.05.013.

Kabir, M. M., Wang, H., Lau, K. T., and Cardona, F. (2012). Chemical treatments on plant-based natural fibre reinforced polymer composites: An overview. *Composites Part B: Engineering*, *43*(7), 2883–2892. doi:10.1016/j.compositesb.2012.04.053.

Kamel, S. (2007). Nanotechnology and its applications in lignocellulosic composites, a mini review. *Express Polymer Letters*, *1*(9), 546–575. doi:10.3144/expresspolymlett.2007.78.

Kang, H., Liu, R., and Huang, Y. (2013). Cellulose derivatives and graft copolymers as blocks for functional materials. *Polymer International*, *62*(3), 338–344. doi:10.1002/pi.4455.

Lavoine, N., Desloges, I., Dufresne, A., and Bras, J. (2012). Microfibrillated cellulose—Its barrier properties and applications in cellulosic materials: A review. *Carbohydrate Polymers*, *90*(2), 735–764. doi:10.1016/j.carbpol.2012.05.026.

Majeed, K., Jawaid, M., Hassan, A., Abu Bakar, A., Khalil, H. P. S. A., Salema, A. A., and Inuwa, I. (2013). Potential materials for food packaging from nanoclay/natural fibres filled hybrid composites. *Materials and Design*, *46*, 391–410. doi:10.1016/j.matdes.2012.10.044.

Missoum, K., Belgacem, M. N., and Bras, J. (2013). Nanofibrillated cellulose surface modification: A review. *Materials*, *6*(5), 1745–1766. doi:10.3390/ma6051745.

Phong, N. T., Gabr, M. H., Okubo, K., Chuong, B., and Fujii, T. (2013). Enhancement of mechanical properties of carbon fabric/epoxy composites using micro/nano-sized bamboo fibrils. *Materials and Design*, *47*, 624–632. doi:10.1016/j.matdes.2012.12.057.

Roy, D. (2006). Controlled modification of cellulosic surfaces via the reversible addition—Fragmentation chain transfer (RAFT) graft polymerization process. *Australian Journal of Chemistry*, *59*(3), 229–229. doi:10.1071/CH06012.

Roy, D., Semsarilar, M., Guthrie, J. T., and Perrier, S. (2009). Cellulose modification by polymer grafting: A review. *Chemical Society Reviews*, *38*(7), 2046–2064. doi:10.1039/b808639g.

Shah, N., Ul-Islam, M., Khattak, W. A., and Park, J. K. (2013). Overview of bacterial cellulose composites: A multipurpose advanced material. *Carbohydrate Polymers*, *98*(2), 1585–1598. doi: 10.1016/j.carbpol.2013.08.018.

Thakur, V. K. and Singha, A. S. (2010a). Evaluation of GREWIA OPTIVA fibers as reinforcement in polymer biocomposites. *Polymer-Plastics Technology and Engineering*, *49*(11), 1101–1107. doi:10.1080/03602559.2010.496390.

Thakur, V. K. and Singha, A. S. (2010b). KPS-initiated graft copolymerization onto modified cellulosic biofibers. *International Journal of Polymer Analysis and Characterization*, *15*(8), 471–485. doi:10.1080/1023666X.2010.510294.

Thakur, V. K. and Singha, A. S. (2010c). Mechanical and water absorption properties of natural fibers/polymer biocomposites. *Polymer-Plastics Technology and Engineering*, *49*(7), 694–700. doi:10.1080/03602551003682067.

Thakur, V. K. and Singha, A. S. (2010d). Natural fibres-based polymers: Part I—Mechanical analysis of pine needles reinforced biocomposites. *Bulletin of Materials Science*, *33*(3), 257–264. doi:10.1007/s12034-010-0040-x.

Thakur, V. K. and Singha, A. S. (2010e). Physico-chemical and mechanical characterization of natural fibre reinforced polymer composites. *Iranian Polymer Journal*, *19*(1), 3–16.

Thakur, V. K., Singha, A. S., Kaur, I., Nagarajarao, R. P., and Liping, Y. (2010a). Silane functionalization of *Saccaharum cilliare* fibers: Thermal, morphological, and physicochemical study. *International Journal of Polymer Analysis and Characterization*, *15*(7), 397–414. doi:10.1080/1023666X.2010.510106.

Thakur, V. K., Singha, A. S., and Mehta, I. K. (2010b). Renewable resource-based green polymer composites: Analysis and characterization. *International Journal of Polymer Analysis and Characterization*, *15*(3), 137–146. doi:10.1080/10236660903582233.

Thakur, V. K. and Thakur, M. K. (2014). Processing and characterization of natural cellulose fibers/thermoset polymer composites. *Carbohydrate Polymers*, *109*, 102–117. doi:10.1016/j.carbpol.2014.03.039.

Thakur, V. K., Thakur, M. K., and Gupta, R. K. (2013a). Development of functionalized cellulosic biopolymers by graft copolymerization. *International Journal of Biological Macromolecules*, *62*, 44–51. doi:10.1016/j.ijbiomac.2013.08.026.

Thakur, V. K., Thakur, M. K., and Gupta, R. K. (2013b). Graft copolymers from cellulose: Synthesis, characterization and evaluation. *Carbohydrate Polymers*, *97*(1), 18–25. doi:10.1016/j.carbpol.2013.04.069.

Thakur, V. K., Thakur, M. K., and Gupta, R. K. (2013c). Rapid synthesis of graft copolymers from natural cellulose fibers. *Carbohydrate Polymers*, *98*(1), 820–828. doi:10.1016/j.carbpol.2013.06.072.

Thakur, V. K., Thakur, M. K., and Gupta, R. K. (2013d). Synthesis of lignocellulosic polymer with improved chemical resistance through free radical polymerization. *International Journal of Biological Macromolecules*, *61*, 121–126. doi:10.1016/j.ijbiomac.2013.06.045.

Thakur, V. K., Thakur, M. K., and Gupta, R. K. (2014a). Graft copolymers of natural fibers for green composites. *Carbohydrate Polymers*, *104*, 87–93. doi:10.1016/j.carbpol.2014.01.016.

Thakur, V. K., Thakur, M. K., and Gupta, R. K. (2014b). Review: Raw natural fiber–based polymer composites. *International Journal of Polymer Analysis and Characterization*, *19*(3), 256–271. doi:10.1080/1023666X.2014.880016.

Tizzotti, M., Charlot, A., Fleury, E., Stenzel, M., and Bernard, J. (2010). Modification of polysaccharides through controlled/living radical polymerization grafting—Towards the generation of high performance hybrids. *Macromolecular Rapid Communications*, *31*(20), 1751–1772. doi:10.1002/marc.201000072.

Wojnarovits, L., Foldvary, C. M., and Takacs, E. (2010). Radiation-induced grafting of cellulose for adsorption of hazardous water pollutants: A review. *Radiation Physics and Chemistry*, *79*(8), 848–862. doi:10.1016/j.radphyschem.2010.02.006.

2 Grafting on Cellulosics
Progress toward Purpose

R. Meena and A. Bhattacharya

CONTENTS

2.1 INTRODUCTION

History says cellulose was known as cotton in the valley of the Indus River as early as 3000 BC. Since then, there has been growth in the use into the whole range of polymers, which has led to the development of a new family of polymers that, with appropriate modification, can display different promising properties. Moreover, cellulose is the most abundant material in our living world, and it is even more significant that cellulose is renewable by direct fixation of solar energy by plants. Because of the recent sore prices of petroleum products, cellulosic raw materials have gained special importance since they are available in plenty.

It is no doubt finding new cellulosics as per requirement is not quite an easy task. Thus, the new generation is always intended to modifications. The modifications are intended to impute different typically desired properties to the new modified materials. Modification of the properties of cellulosics according to tailor-made specification is an important criterion for various applications. The spectrum of its uses may be still more widened considerably by taking recourse to "grafting," a popular route to modify the properties of various high-molecular-weight compounds. The grafting is a tailor-made art. Of the various polymers on which grafting of suitable monomers can be made, cellulose appears to be very interesting and promising.

The approaches can be of "grafting from" and "grafting to." The "grafting from" technique involves the polymerization that is initiated at the polymeric substrate (cellulosics) surface by covalent attached initiating groups. On the other hand, "grafting to" technique involves reaction of active part of the functionalized monomer/polymer molecules with the complementary active part located on the polymer (cellulose) surface, resulting in the formation of tethered chains.

In this chapter, attempts have been made to discuss initially the techniques of graft copolymers. Knowledge of the mechanisms involved in grafting is important for further optimization of cellulose grafting procedures. This chapter also covers the characterization and current state of affairs in some applications, viz., wastewater treatment, biomedical, stimuli responsive, and packaging.

2.2 GRAFTING TECHNIQUES

For improving the status of cellulose in comparison with other natural polymers, various specific grafting techniques have been established. Of them, chemical, radiation, and photochemical are most used techniques.

2.2.1 Chemical Grafting

In conventional free radical grafting polymerization (CFRP), redox systems are extensively used. Generally, it comprises the transition metal ion with chain transfer agent (CTA; viz., Fe^{2+}/H_2O_2, Fe^{2+}/persulfate, and Fe^{2+}/*t*-butyl hydroperoxide). Persulfate and reducing agent (viz., $S_2O_8^{=}/Ag^+$, $S_2O_8^{=}/S_2O_3^{=}$, and $S_2O_8^{=}/HSO_3^{-}$) are also used (Bhattacharya and Misra 2004). The schematic reaction is as follows (Scheme 2.1). The main drawback of CFRP is that molecular weight distribution of graft polymers is broad, and formations of homopolymer even predominate.

Different novel chemical grafting techniques are also developed. In this regard, controlled/living free radical polymerization (CRP) and ring-opening polymerization (ROP) methods are important (Roy et al. 2009).

The CRP method has the main advantage over other graft copolymerization techniques in terms of narrow molecular weight distributions. In these reactions, $R_p \gg R_i$ (where R_p and R_i are the rate of propagation and initiation, respectively) contrary to CFRP reactions. The CRP reactions are of atom transfer radical polymerization (ATRP) (Kamigaito et al. 2001; Matyjaszewski and Xia 2001), nitroxide-mediated polymerization (NMP) (Hawker et al. 2001), and reversible addition fragmentation chain transfer (RAFT) (Moad et al. 2008; Gregory and Stenzel 2012).

ATRP technique is based on reversible cleavage of terminal carbon–halide bond in the dormant species. This redox process is catalyzed by transition metal complex. A variety of metals, including ruthenium (Ru), copper (Cu), iron (Fe), and other transition metals in combination with various types of ligands (viz., amines and phosphines) are used (Kamigaito et al. 2001; Matyjaszewski and Xia 2001; Braunecker and Matyjaszewski 2007). Actually atom transfer occurs between the growing chains and catalyst (Matyjaszewski 2000). A general mechanism of ATRP is shown in Scheme 2.2.

ATRP is the most used CRP to prepare cellulose-*g*-copolymers since the first report by Carlmark and Malmström in 2002. Scheme 2.3 presents cellulose-*g*-copolymer via ATRP or SET-LRP (single-electron transfer-living radical polymerization), using cellulose-based macroinitiator. Esterification of cellulosic hydroxyl groups with commercially available reagents (viz., 2-bromoisobutyryl bromide (BiB) or 2-chloropropionyl chloride) forms the macroinitiator (Tizzotti et al. 2010). This macroinitiator forms grafted copolymer with the monomer.

NMP is one of the stable free radical polymerization processes in which a stable nitroxide radical (viz., 2,2,6,6-tetramethyl-1-piperidinyloxy (TEMPO)) is used (Hawker et al. 2001; Braunecker and Matyjaszewski 2007). The dynamic equilibrium among dormant alkoxyamines

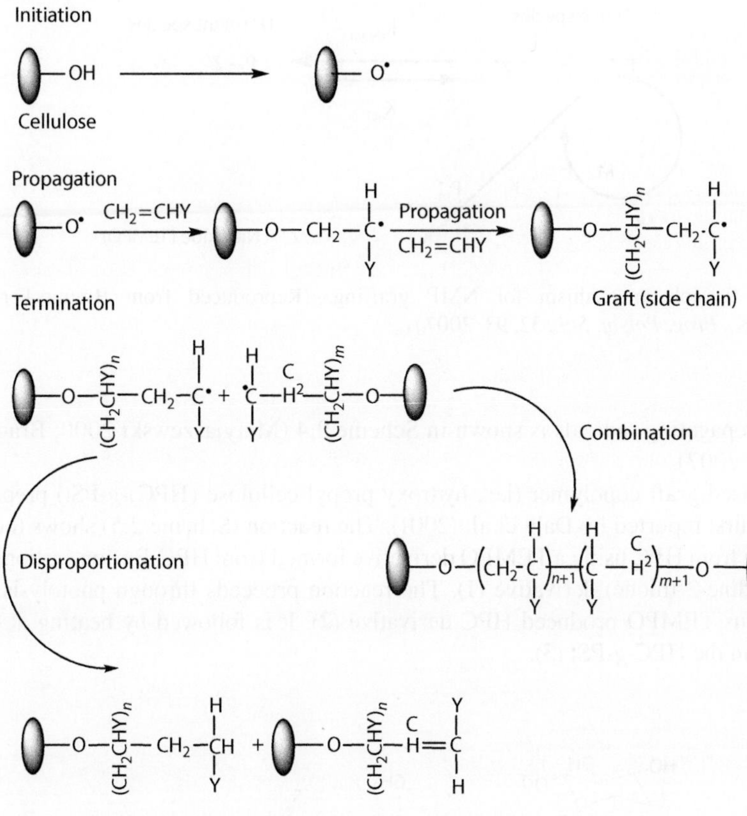

SCHEME 2.1 General reaction steps of grafting.

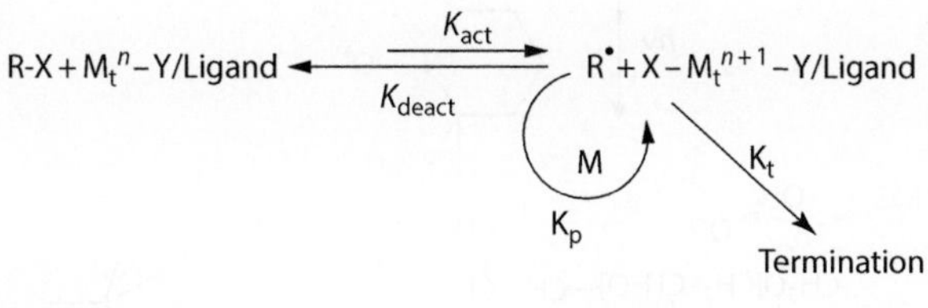

SCHEME 2.2 Mechanism of ATRP.

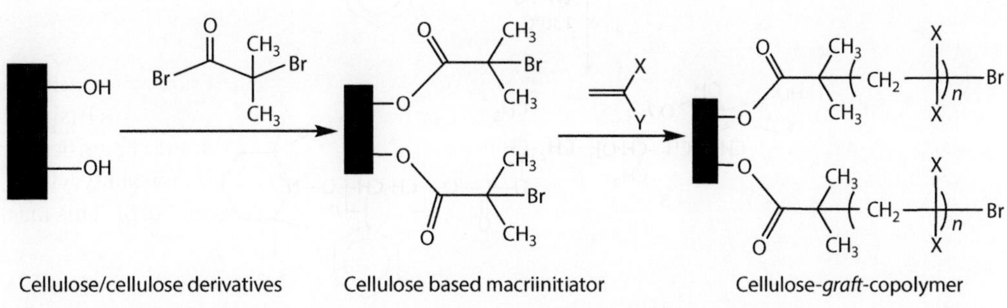

SCHEME 2.3 Synthetic route to cellulose-g-copolymer via ATRP or SET-LRP.

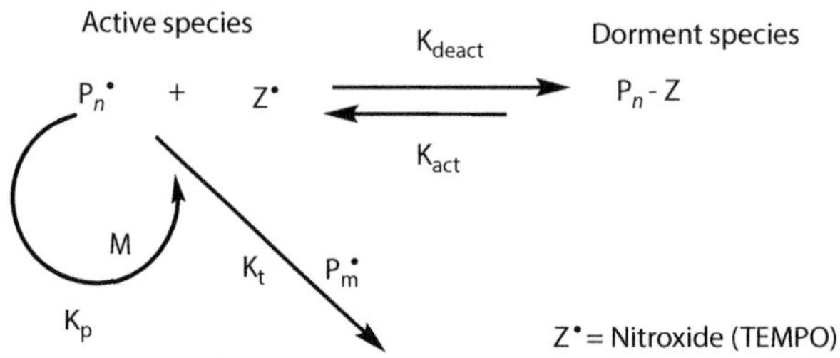

SCHEME 2.4 Possible mechanism for NMP grafting. (Reproduced from Braunecker, W.A. and Matyjaszewski, K., *Prog. Polym. Sci.*, 32, 93, 2007.)

and actively propagating radicals is shown in Scheme 2.4 (Matyjaszewski 2000; Braunecker and Matyjaszewski 2007).

Cellulose-based graft copolymer (i.e., hydroxy propyl cellulose (HPC)-*g*-PSt) prepared in this technique was first reported by Daly et al. (2001). The reaction (Scheme 2.5) shows the controlled radical grafting from HPC using a TEMPO derivative formed from HPC-Barton carbonate (Barton: *N*-hydroxypyridine-2-thione) derivative (**1**). The reaction proceeds through photolysis of (**1**) with styrene, and thus TEMPO produced HPC derivative (**2**). It is followed by heating at 130°C with styrene to obtain the HPC-*g*-PSt (**3**).

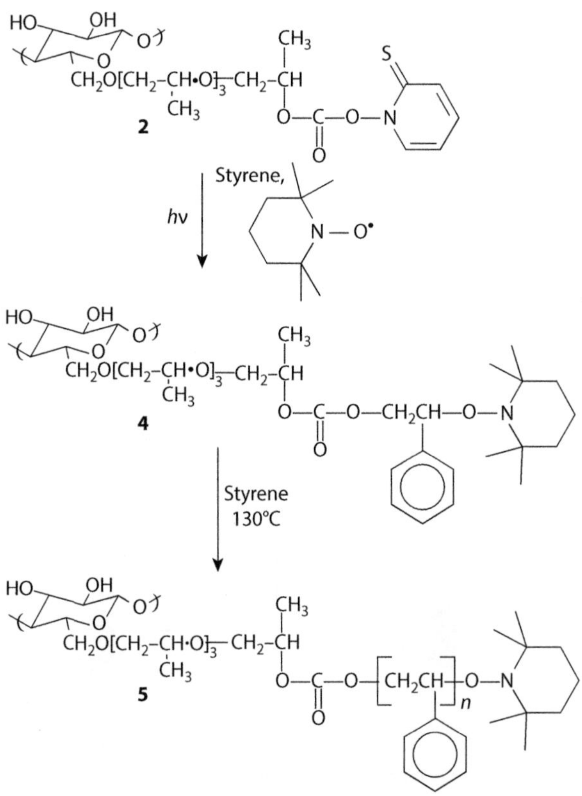

SCHEME 2.5 Nitroxide radical grafting from HPC via NMP. (Reproduced from Daly, W.H. et al., *Macromol. Symp.*, 174, 155, 2001.)

RAFT polymerization is basically a degenerative transfer between low amount of growing radicals and dormant species present at higher concentrations (Braunecker and Matyjaszewski 2007; Barner-Kowollik 2008; Moad et al. 2008; Gregory and Stenzel 2012). The reaction can proceed under similar conditions in CFRP. Use of CTAs (viz., dithioesters, dithiocarbamates, trithiocarbonates, and xanthates) is well accepted. Scheme 2.6 represents the simple addition–fragmentation chemistry. It is termed as the most versatile and successful CRP method.

Two different approaches (R-group, i.e., reinitiating group) and (Z-group, i.e., stabilizing group) (Hernandez-Guerrero et al. 2005) are employed to attach macro CTA to cellulose backbone (Scheme 2.7). The growing macroradical after initiation undergoes transfer to CTA connected to the backbone in both approaches. It leads to the radical located on the backbone after the first addition–fragmentation step, and graft chains are grown directly from the backbone in R-group approach. This may lead to termination combining two growing radicals, whereas the Z-group approach proceeds through propagation results extrinsic to the graft copolymer. The side chain length around CTA controls the shielding effect of the grafts as well as polymerization in Z-group approach (Stenzel and Davis 2002; Hernandez-Guerrero et al. 2005).

HPC-*g*-PSt, HPC-*g*-PVAc, and methyl cellulose (MC)-*g*-PVAc copolymer was prepared utilizing the Z-group approach through trithiocarbonate and thiocarbonylthio (xanthate) CTAs, respectively (Stenzel et al. 2003; Hernandez-Guerrero et al. 2005; Fleet et al. 2008) (Schemes 2.8 and 2.9).

HPC-*g*-PEA and HPC-*g*-PNIPAAM copolymer was prepared utilizing the R-group approach through trithiocarbonate-based HPC-acroCTA (Semsarilar et al. 2010) (Scheme 2.10). The grafted polymer chains show relatively broad molecular weight distribution, due to potential termination reaction between radical's presence in solution and in the HPC.

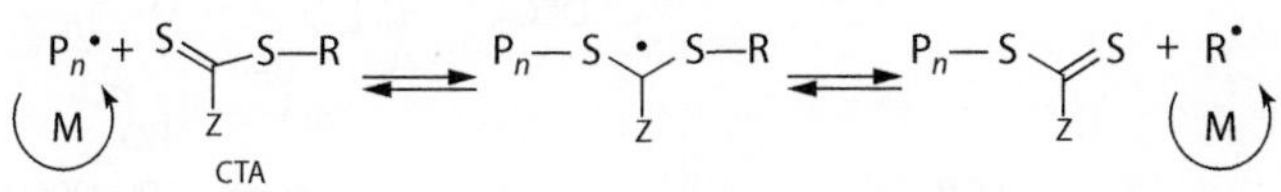

SCHEME 2.6 Mechanism of RAFT polymerization. (Reproduced from Moad, G. et al., *Polymer*, 49, 1079, 2008.)

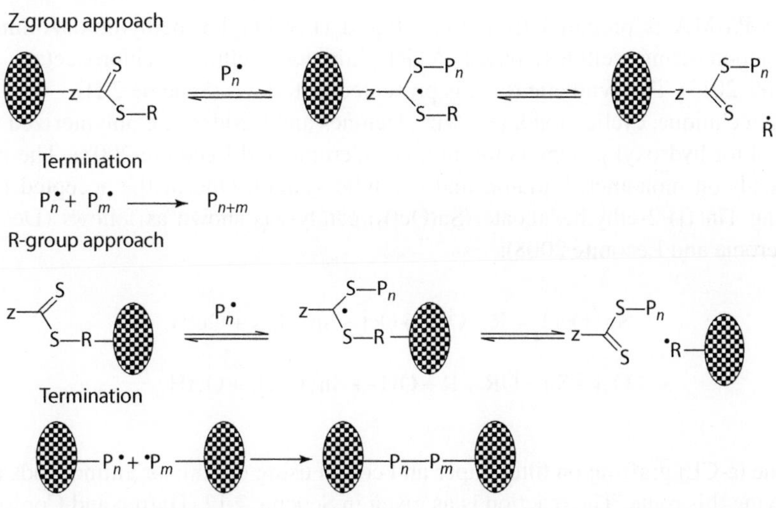

SCHEME 2.7 Graft polymerization through the Z- and R-approaches via RAFT polymerization. (Reproduced from Hernandez-Guerrero, M. et al., *Eur. Polym. J.*, 41, 2264, 2005.)

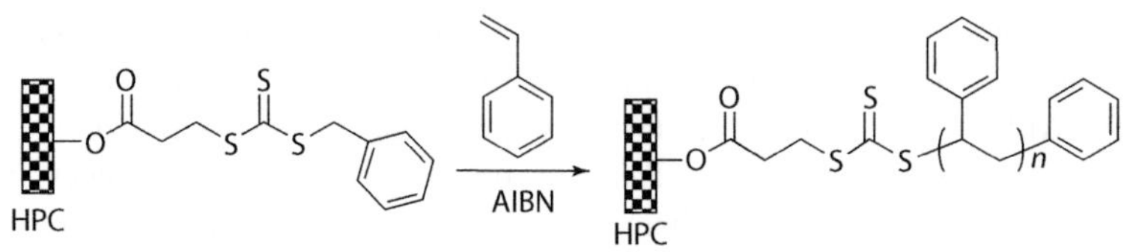

SCHEME 2.8 Synthetic route to HPC-g-PSt via the soluble cellulose-based macro CTA (Z-group approach). (Reproduced from Stenzel, M.H. et al., *J. Mater. Chem.*, 13, 2090, 2003.)

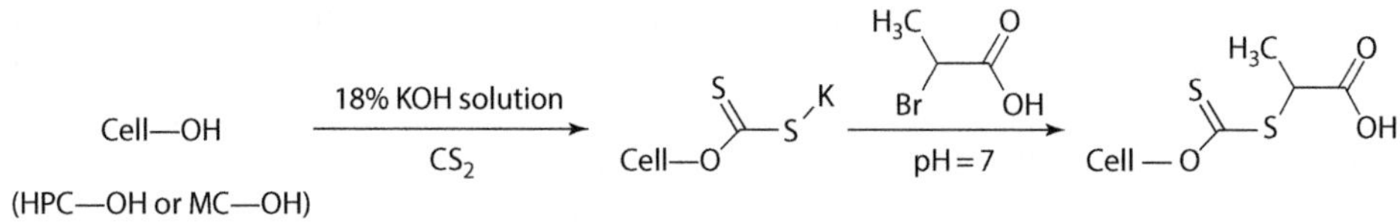

SCHEME 2.9 Synthetic route to xanthate-functionalized cellulose. (Reproduced from Fleet, R. et al., *Eur. Polym. J.*, 44, 2899, 2008.)

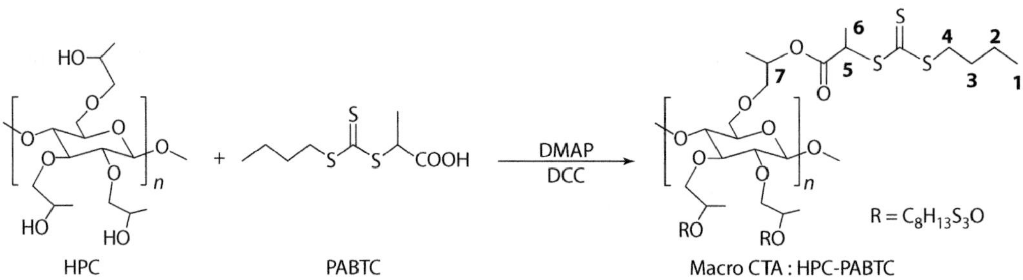

SCHEME 2.10 Synthetic route to cellulose-based macroCTA via the R-group approach. (Reproduced from Semsarilar, M. et al., *J. Polym. Sci. A: Polym. Chem.*, 48, 4361, 2010.)

Cellulose-*g*-PMMA is prepared from ionic liquid (1-*N* butyl-3-methylimidazolium chloride, BMIMCl) solution using cellulose-based ATRP initiator (cellulose chloroacetate, cell-ClAc) (Lin et al. 2009, 2013). The synthetic route is presented as follows (Scheme 2.11).

In the ROP technique, cyclic monomers (viz., lactones and lactides) are polymerized in the presence of alcohol (or hydroxyl group) as the initiator (Jerome and Lecomte 2008). The mechanistic pathway depends on monomer, initiator, and catalytic system. One of the accepted mechanistic pathways using Tin(II) 2-ethylhexanoate ($Sn(Oct)_2$) catalyst is shown as follows (Dechy-Cabaret et al. 2004; Jerome and Lecomte 2008):

$$\mathrm{Sn(Oct)_2 + R-OH \rightarrow Oct-Sn-OR + OctH}$$

$$\mathrm{Oct-Sn-OR + R-OH \rightarrow Sn(OR)_2 + OctH}$$

ε-Caprolactone (ε-CL) grafting on filter paper and cotton using organic or amino acids as catalysts is done following this route. The reaction is as given in Scheme 2.12 (Hafren and Cordova 2005).

Grafting of 2-methyloxazoline on tosylated cellulose is also following this technique. The reaction scheme is shown in Scheme 2.13 (Kahovec et al. 1986).

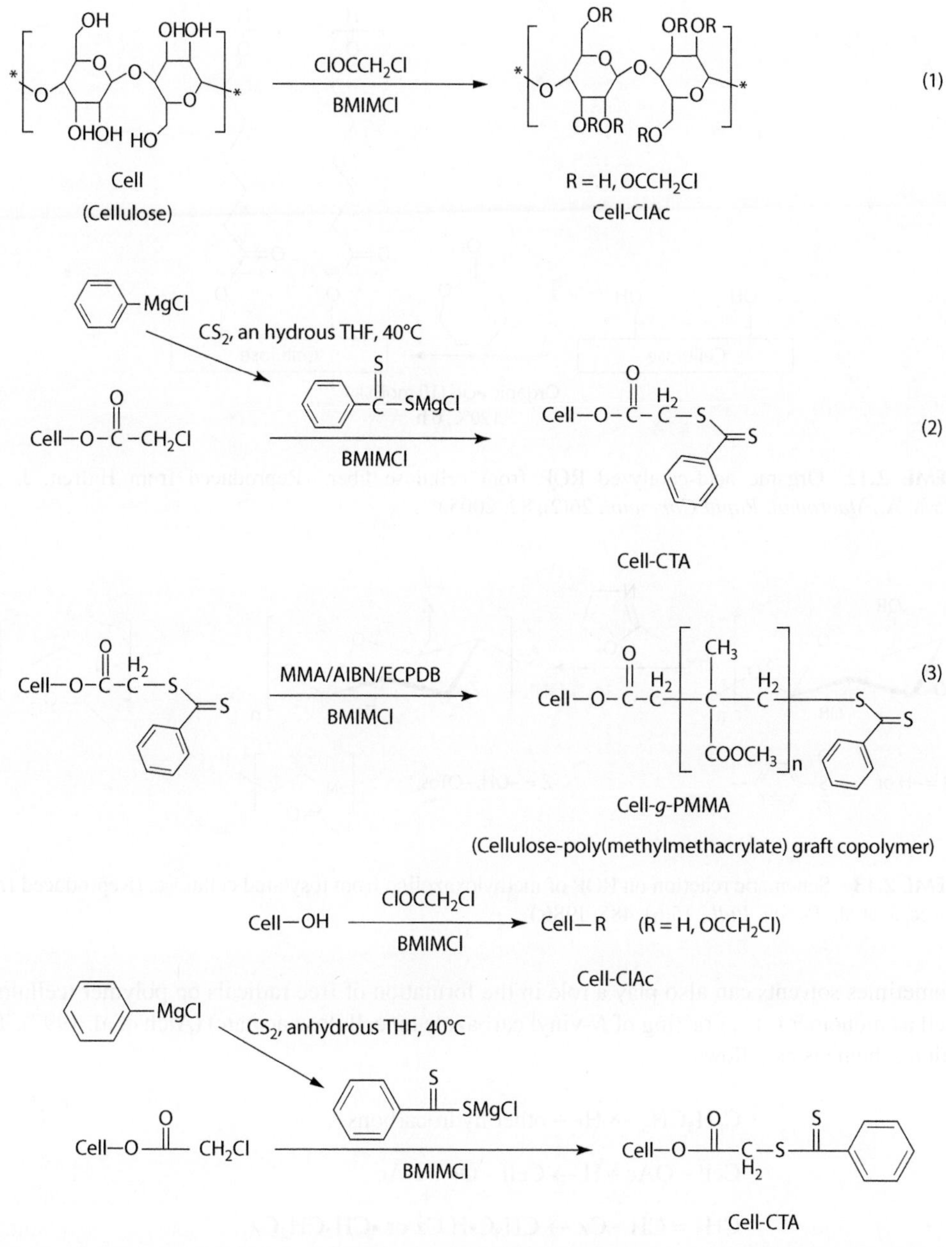

SCHEME 2.11 Synthetic route to cellulose-based macroCTA (cell-CTA) via cellulose-based ATRP initiator (Cell-ClAc) and preparation of graft copolymer. (Reproduced from Lin, C. et al., *J. Appl. Polym. Sci.*, 127, 4840, 2013.)

2.2.2 Radiation Grafting

The formation of free radicals, peroxides, and hydroperoxides formed or trapped in polymeric substrates upon irradiation is used to initiate grafting steps. The formation of free radicals from γ radiation on cellulose can be of three ways by (1) hydrogen and hydroxyl abstraction (Scheme 2.14a), (2) breaking carbon–carbon bonds (Scheme 2.14b), and (3) chain scission (Scheme 2.14c) (Khan and Ahmad 1997; Wang and Yongshen 2006).

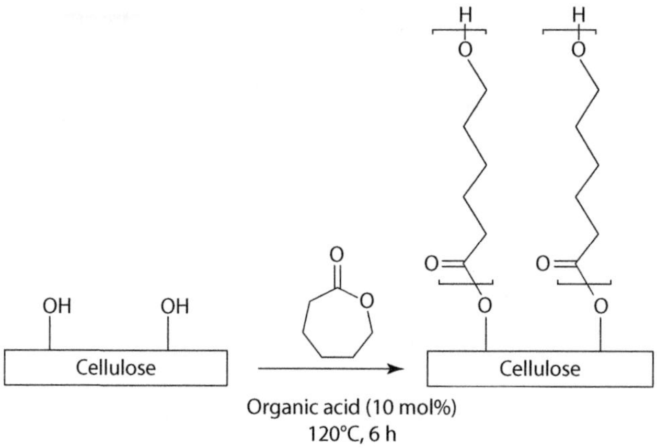

SCHEME 2.12 Organic acid-catalyzed ROP from cellulose fiber. (Reproduced from Hafren, J. and Cordova, A., *Macromol. Rapid Commun.*, 26(2), 82, 2005.)

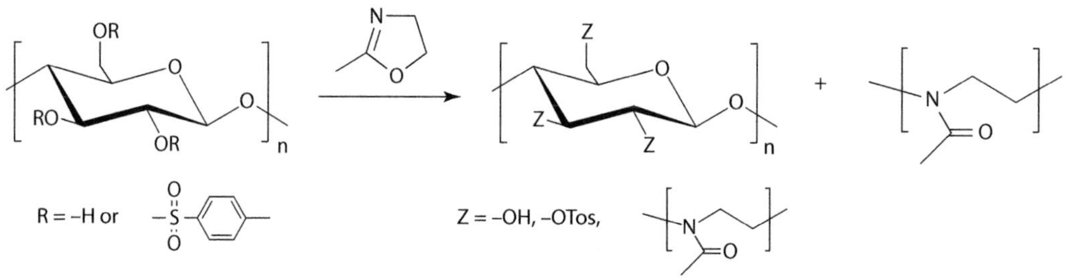

SCHEME 2.13 Schematic reaction on ROP of methyloxazoline from tosylated cellulose. (Reproduced from Kahovec, J. et al., *Polym. Bull.*, 15(6), 485, 1986.)

Sometimes solvents can also play a role in the formation of free radicals on polymer (cellulose) as well as monomer (viz., grafting of *N*-vinyl carbazole on cellulose acetate) (Aich et al. 1997). The reaction scheme is as follows:

$$C_6H_5CH_3 \rightarrow H\bullet + \text{other hydrocarbons}$$

$$\text{Cell} - \text{OAc} + \text{H} \rightarrow \text{Cell} - \text{O}\bullet + \text{HAc}$$

$$CH_2 = CH - Cz \rightarrow CH_3C\bullet H\ Cz \text{ or } \bullet CH_2CH_2Cz$$

$$\text{Cell} - \text{O}\bullet + \bullet CH_2CH_2Cz \rightarrow \text{Cell} - \text{O} - CH_2CH_2Cz$$

Three general methods are used, viz., mutual or simultaneous, pre-irradiation, and peroxidation (Bhattacharya 2000). In simultaneous method, the polymer is subjected to irradiation along with the monomer, where as in pre-irradiation, the polymeric substrate is irradiated in vacuo or in the presence of an inert gas and then treated with the monomer as either liquid, vapor, or solution in a suitable solvent. In the peroxidation method, polymer is subjected to radiation in the presence of air or oxygen. This leads to the formation of hydroperoxides or peroxides.

Considering the peroxidation method, cellulosic material produces cellulose diperoxides (CellOOCell) and hydroperoxides (CellOOH) species by a radical chain reaction process (Khan 1997). The steps are presented as follows:

Step I: Activation

$$\text{Cell} \xrightarrow{\sim} \text{Cell}^{\bullet}$$

Where Cell represents HPMC cellulose substrate and
Cell$^{\bullet}$ corresponds to all possible radical formations

Step II: Propagation

$$\text{Cell} + O_2 \xrightarrow{\sim} \text{CellO}_2^{\bullet}$$

$$\text{Cell} + \text{CellO}_2^{\bullet} \longrightarrow \text{CellOOH} + \text{Cell}^{\bullet}$$

The propagation step is also in competition with the
recombinant reaction

Step III: Termination

$$\text{Cell}^{\bullet} + \text{Cell}^{\bullet} \longrightarrow \text{Cell}_2$$

$$\text{Cell}^{\bullet} + \text{CellO}_2^{\bullet} \longrightarrow \text{CellOOCell}$$

$$\text{CellO}_2^{\bullet} + \text{CellO}_2^{\bullet} \longrightarrow \text{CellOOCell} + O_2$$

$$\text{CellO}_2^{\bullet} + \text{HO}_2^{\bullet} \longrightarrow \text{CellOOH} + O_2$$

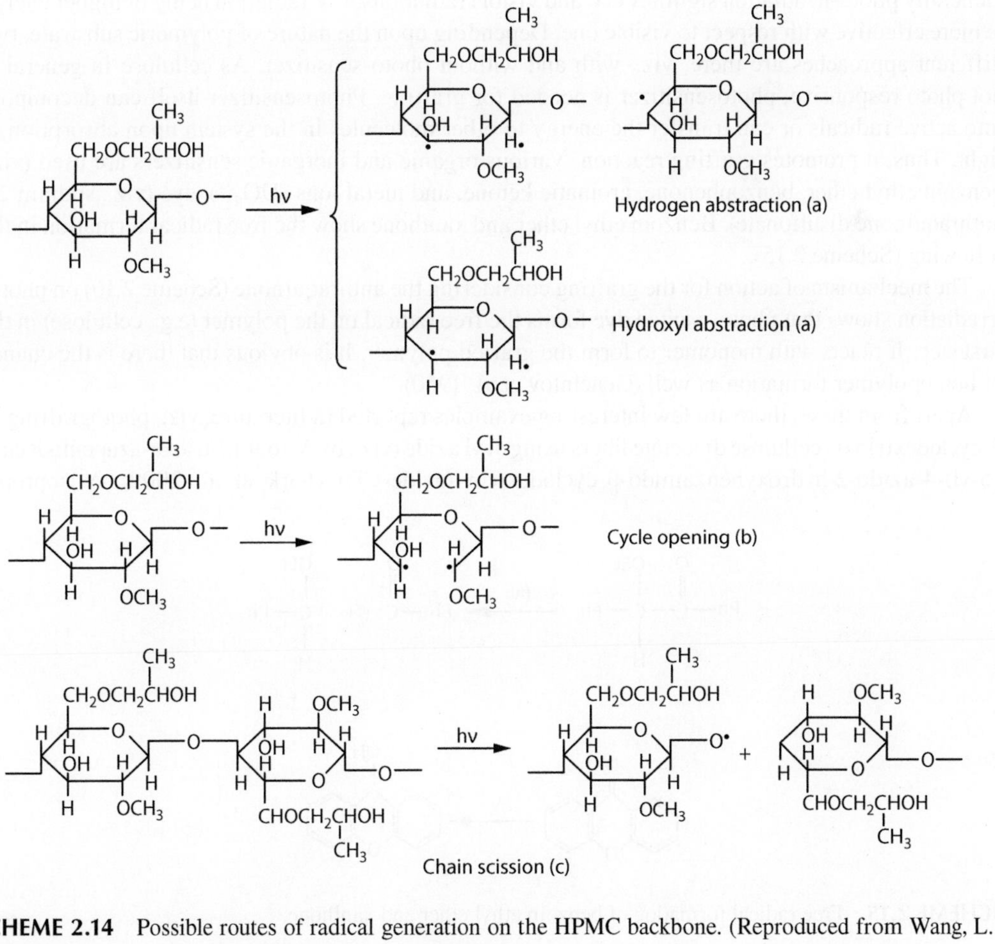

SCHEME 2.14 Possible routes of radical generation on the HPMC backbone. (Reproduced from Wang, L. and Yongshen, X., *Macromol. Mater. Eng.*, 291, 950, 2006.)

The diperoxides and hydroperoxides subsequently decompose at an elevated temperature and initiate a grafted side chain in the presence of monomer. It is seen that diperoxides (CellOOCell) are in general more stable and usually do not lead to homopolymer. On the other hand, hydroperoxides (CellOOH) result in undesirable homopolymerization. The reaction scheme is as follows:

$$\text{CellOOCell} \rightsquigarrow 2\text{CellO}^{\bullet}$$

$$2\text{CellO}^{\bullet} + M_n \longrightarrow \underset{\text{Grafted copolymer}}{2\text{CellOM}_n}$$

$$\text{CellOOH} \rightsquigarrow \text{CellO}^{\bullet} + \text{HO}^{\bullet}$$

$$\text{CellO}^{\bullet} + \text{HO}^{\bullet} + M_n \longrightarrow \text{CellOM}_n + \underset{\text{Homopolymer}}{\text{HOM}_n}$$

All the reaction steps are similar for the simultaneous irradiation technique considering that steps proceeded simultaneously.

2.2.3 Photo Grafting

Generally photo-irradiation signifies UV and visible radiations. UV radiation being of higher energy is more effective with respect to visible one. Depending upon the nature of polymeric substrate, two different approaches are there, viz., with and without photo-sensitizer. As cellulose in general is not photo responsive, photosensitizer is needed for grafting. Photosensitizer itself can decompose into active radicals or can transfer the energy to other molecules in the system upon absorption of light. Thus, it promotes grafting reaction. Various organic and inorganic sensitizers are used (viz., benzoin ethyl ether, benzophenone, aromatic ketone, and metal ions (UO_2^{2+}), dye (viz., sodium 2,7 anthraquinone disulfonate). Benzoin ethyl ether and xanthone show the free radical formation in the following (Scheme 2.15).

The mechanism of action for the grafting considering the anthraquinone (Scheme 2.16) on photo-irradiation shows that photo-excited dye forms the free radical on the polymer (e.g., cellulose) in the first step. It reacts with monomer to form the grafted polymer. It is obvious that there is the chance of homopolymer formation as well (Gcaclntov et al. 1960).

Apart from these, there are few interesting examples reported in literature, viz., photografting of β-cyclodextrin on cellulose diacetate fibers using aryl azide (viz., by *N*-(6,9,12-trioxa-azapentadecan-15-yl)-4-azido-2-hydroxybenzamido-β-cyclodextrin (azide-CD) (Park et al. 2009), *N*-isopropyl

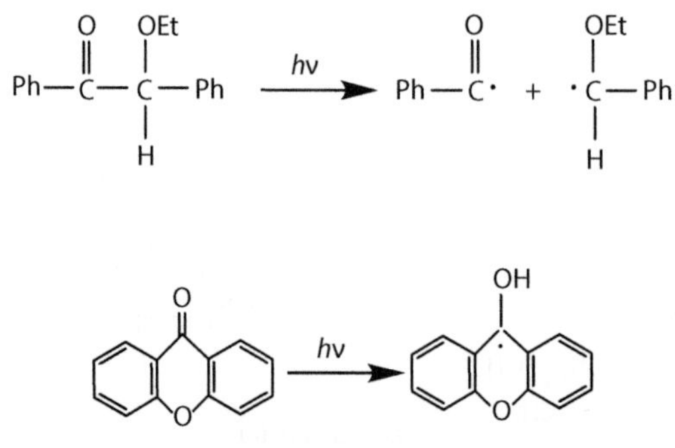

SCHEME 2.15 Free radical formation of benzoin ethyl ether and xanthone.

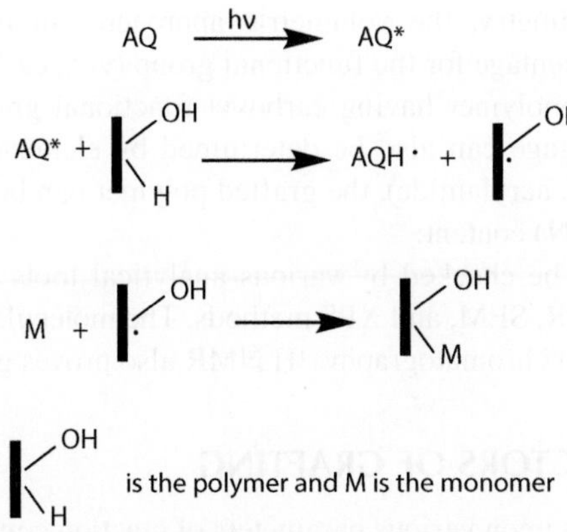

SCHEME 2.16 Photografting mechanism using anthraquinone.

acrylamide on cellulose after oxidizing it by aqueous periodic acid (Kubota and Shiobara 1998). In the former case, first aryl azide is converted into the highly reactive aryl nitrene upon photo-irradiation. Cellulose acetate (CA)-*g*-HEMA, CA-*g*- styrene show salt rejection and ethanol separation from ethanol and water respectively (Worthley 2012; Chowdhury 1988).

2.3 CONFIRMATION OF GRAFTING

The mathematical formulation for the evidence of grafting can be presented by different parameters (viz., grafting percentage (GP), grafting efficiency (GE), and the number of grafts per cellulose chain (N_g)).

$$\text{Grafting percentage}\left(\text{GP}\right)\left(\%\right)=\frac{\text{Wt. of polymer grafted}}{\text{Initial wt. of backbone}}\times 100$$

$$=\frac{W_1-W_0}{W_0}\times 100$$

where W_1 and W_0 are the weights of the graft copolymer of cellulose and cellulose polymer, respectively.

$$\text{Grafting efficency}\left(\text{GE}\right)\left(\%\right)=\frac{\text{Wt. of polymer grafted}}{\text{Wt. of polymer grafted}+\text{wt. of homopolymer}}$$

$$=\frac{W_1-W_0}{W_1-W_0+W_2}\times 100$$

where W_1, W_0, and W_2 are the weights of the cellulose graft copolymer, the original cellulose, and the homopolymer, respectively. The weight of homopolymer (W_2) can be calculated by subtracting the amount of grafted polymer plus the amount of unreacted monomer from the initial amount of monomer.

$$\text{Number of grafts per cellulose chain}\left(N_g\right)=\frac{\text{Mol. wt. of cellulose}}{\text{Mol. wt. of graft copolymer}}\times\frac{\text{Grafting percentage}}{100}$$

Apart from the simple gravimetry, the volumetric approach can be used for the proof and determination of grafting percentage for the functional group (viz., carboxyl) (Gurdag et al. 1997). In this approach, the graft copolymer having carboxyl functional groups is titrated with a base solution. The grafting percentage can also be determined by elemental analysis. In the case of nitrogen-based monomer (viz., acrylamide), the grafted polymer can be qualitatively and quantitatively monitored by nitrogen (N) content.

The proof of grafting can be checked by various analytical tools like FTIR, thermal (DTA/TGA), mechanical, XRD, NMR, SEM, and XPS methods. The molecular weight of the graft chains by viscometric, gel permeation chromatography, ^{1}H NMR also proves grafting.

2.4 CONTROLLING FACTORS OF GRAFTING

The extent of grafting depends upon various parameters of reaction conditions, for example, nature of monomer and concentration, nature of substrate, nature of initiator and concentration, nature of solvent, and reaction temperature. The effects of these factors influencing grafting process have been discussed briefly in the following.

2.4.1 Effect of Monomers

The kind and concentration of monomers are important controlling parameters for the grafting reaction. The reactivity of the monomers depends upon their nature, viz., polarity and steric nature, the power to swell the graft substrate (Bhattacharya and Misra 2004).

The difference in the grafting of monomers (viz., AA, AM, MAA, MA, MMA, and VA) onto amine-treated cotton depends upon their water solubility (Ibrahim et al. 2008). The graft polymerization of hydrophobic monomers among the monomers is preferential. The difference in graft yields between the monomers seems to be attributed to monomer affinity toward cellulose and the copolymerization efficiency of monomers. In another study, it is reported that grafting percentage of AN was 12%–20% higher than that of AA (Dahoua et al. 2010). Structural difference also influences grafting. The grafting order on cellulose acetate AM > MeAM > NN dimethyl acrylamide can be explained in terms of the stability of radical (Bhattacharya et al. 1998).

The grafting depends on the monomer concentration (Nishioka et al. 1986; Abdel-Razik 1990; Gupta and Khandekar 2002, 2006; Goyal 2008). It increases up to a certain concentration, and beyond a certain level, it decreases as homopolymer formation dominates over the grafting reaction. Of course, the optimum monomer concentration depends on the kind of monomers, substrates, and reaction conditions.

Synergistic effects between the comonomers in case of the grafting of binary monomer mixture are also reflected in case of AAM–MA, AAM–EA onto cellulose (Gupta and Khandekar 2002, 2006a). The grafting of binary mixture onto cellulose follows a second-order reaction, that is, depends on both monomer concentrations. The presence of acrylamide in the binary monomer mixture increased the graft yields because of its synergistic effect. The graft copolymerization of acrylic acid (AA) onto cellulose is a first-order reaction, whereas by the addition of $AASO_3H$ (2-acrylamido-2-methylpropane sulfonic acid), synergistic effect is observed (Gurdag et al. 1997, 2001).

2.4.2 Effect of Substrates

The effect of nature of substrates (viz., chemical and physical) is an important point to consider in grafting. The form of cellulose (powder, fiber, and film) influences the grafting. The grafting extent is always higher compared to fiber form. The thickness of the film also influences grafting because of the differences in diffusional restriction of the monomer. It is already reported that the extent of grafting decreases with the increase in the thickness of the film (Stannett 1981; Bhattacharya and Maldas 1984).

Influences of chemical nature of the substrates are also reflected in various reports. The grafting efficiency depends upon the chemical composition of industrial cellulose pulp. The pulping time influences the surface of the pulp and thus grafting. With the increase in specific surface of cellulose, grafting percentage increases, but after reaching maxima, it decreases. The decreasing trend is explained by the fall in the amount of radicals formed on the same surface at a fixed initiator concentration (Borbély and Erdélyi 2004).

The peroxide bleaching of cellulose facilitates grafting as the treatment decreases the crystallinity of the cellulose. It is obvious that the decrease in crystallization results in the expansion of amorphous region, and grafting facilitates (Gupta and Khandekar 2006). The pretreatment with amines also shows the similar behavior. It increases the viscosity in the amorphous region of cellulose. Thus, it causes inter- and intra-crystalline swelling and improves monomer accessibility and thus grafting (Mondal et al. 2008).

The lignin content of the cellulose also influences the grafting percentage. The increase in lignin content of cellulose decrease grafting. It is seen that >12% lignin content decreases the grafting percentage because of its inhibition tendency in the grafting reaction. The industrial cellulose with <2% lignin is preferable for grafting reaction (Borbély and Erdélyi 2004). The bleaching treatment reduces the lignin content in rice straw and thus improves the grafting of vinyl monomers on cellulose. Peroxide reaction with lignin in alkali effectively increases the hydrophilicity of cellulose and allows the monomer to diffuse easily in the cellulosic structure. This phenomenon has also been observed in Sisal fiber-*g*-EA. When NaOH is applied as a lignin remover, the grafting rate is higher (Gao 2003). The hemicellulose content of the cellulose pulp also influences grafting, but not as significant as the effect of lignin content.

2.4.3 Effect of Initiators

All chemical grafting reactions need initiator(s). The nature, concentration, as well as radical creation mechanism of the initiator influence grafting (Bhattacharya and Misra 2004). There are various kinds of initiators for grafting reactions, viz., (Fe^{2+}–H_2O_2), azobisisobutyronitrile (AIBN), $K_2S_2O_8$, Ce^{4+}, Co^{3+}, V^{5+}, and Cr^{6+}.

The choosing of metal ions in grafting depends on their low oxidation potential. The low oxidation potential is preferred as grafting reaction is to proceed with the radical pathway in general. It is seen that APS is a suitable initiator (among APS, KPS, and BPO) for the grafting of AAM onto EC because it leads no degradation in EC chains (Abdel-Razik 1990). The dependence of the concentration profiles with grafting is also different between APS and KPS. The reverse effects of initiators are caused because of the difference in their decomposition rates (Nishioka 1986). On the other hand degradation of EC causes BPO's elimination from the rank. It is seen that APS is a better initiator (among AIBN and APS) for the grafting of MMA on cellulose as AIBN is known to show resonance stabilization, but no such resonance exists in the peroxide initiators (Nishioka and Kosai 1981). The grafting of MA onto cellulose proceeds with APS (the highest number of grafts per cellulose chain was 1.5), but hardly at all with BPO and AIBN initiators.

The initiator concentration influences grafting. It can be the number of grafts per cellulose chain and/or the molecular weights of graft chains. In case of NVP grafting onto cellulose with $Co(acac)_3$-$HClO_4$ initiator, it is seen that the amount of grafted NVP and the conversion of cellulose to graft copolymer increased up to a certain level, but beyond that level it is decreased (Gupta and Sahoo 2001). It also influences the number of grafts per cellulose chains and the number average molecular weights (M_n) of graft chains. The similar findings are also reported in case of CAN–HNO_3 (Gupta and Khandekar 2002, 2006; Sharma et al. 2003; Dhiman et al. 2008; Goyal et al. 2008; Kim and

Mun 2009), ceric ammonium sulfate (Ibrahim et al. 2002), persulfates (Nishioka et al. 1983a,b), and $KHSO_3$–$CoSO_4$ (Sahoo et al. 1986).

The increase in CAN concentration up to a certain level leads to a decrease in the grafting yield because of the increase in homopolymer formation. Although CAN prefers to form complex with cellulose over the monomer, Ce^{4+} ions form complex with the monomer in addition to cellulose, and homopolymer formation can also occur at higher concentrations of CAN. The termination of growing polymer radicals is also accelerated with Ce^{4+} concentration and leads to the decrease in grafting yield (Gupta and Khandekar 2006; Dhiman et al. 2008).

Gupta et al. have shown the relationship between the rates of grafting and CAN concentration for AAM–EA and AAM–MA comonomers onto cellulose (Gupta and Khandekar 2002, 2006). The rate of grafting onto cellulose is found to be dependent on the square root of CAN concentration.

2.4.4 Effect of Solvent

Though graft polymerization can occur in different phases (e.g., solid, vapor, emulsion, and solution), solution phase grafting is the most widely used process. The solvent criteria for the grafting are as follows: (1) better solubility of monomer, (2) requisite swelling property of cellulose, and (3) no/less affinity to react the cellulose radicals with the solvent.

It is seen that grafting of *N*-isopropylacrylamide (NIPAAM) onto cotton cellulose decreases continuously from pure water to pure organic solvents (viz., ethanol, propanol, isopropanol, and acetone), where the grafting yields are almost zero. Though alcohols in general are good swelling agents for cellulose, they show different degrees of inhibiting effects on the grafting of NIPAAM, but acetone shows inertness. The grafting in the alcohol series order is methanol > ethanol > propanol > isopropanol as the swelling power. One interesting point to note is that methanol at low concentration shows lower activity as CTA compared to swelling power for cellulose, whereas at high concentrations, chain transfer activity is higher compared to swelling power (Jun et al. 2001).

The grafting of MMA onto ethyl cellulose shows the dependence on dielectric constants of the solvents. The increasing trend on grafting yield is in the order: chloroform > toluene > benzene (Abdel-Razik 1997).

2.4.5 Effect of Temperature

The temperature is one of the important reaction parameters that control the extent of grafting. Increase in temperature led to several effects, viz., better swelling of the substrate, better monomer swell ability, better diffusion of the monomer to the grafting active site, ease in initiation to decompose redox system, enhancement of rate of initiation, propagation, and termination of the grafting steps.

The temperature effect in terms of grafting yield shows its increasing trend up to a certain temperature and then decreases. The trend is observed in many systems, viz., ethyl cellulose-g-MA, cellulose-*g*-AA, cellulose-*g*-AN/MA, and cellulose-*g*-MA (Nishioka and Kosai 1981; Nishioka et al. 1983b; Abdel-Razik 1997; Gurdag et al. 1997). It also shows that with the increase in temperature, molecular weight of graft chains decreases, but the number of grafts increases up to a certain amount and then leveled off. One interesting observation is that the optimum temperature for highest grafting depends on the initiator used. In cellulose-*g*-HEMA system, optimum temperatures are 40°C for APS, 50°C for KPS, and 60°C for both AIBN and BPO (Nishioka 1986).

The rate constants for AA grafting increase with the increase in temperature, and it also favors the formation of homopolymer poly (acrylic acid) (PAA) (Gurdag et al. 1997). It is also seen that in case of NVP grafting onto salt form of carboxy methyl cellulose/hydroxyethyl cellulose (CMCNa/HEC), a graft copolymer with shorter graft chains results with the increase in temperature, and the number of polymer chain end increases (Ibrahim et al. 2002).

2.5 APPLICATIONS

Cellulose is the most abundant biomass material in nature and possesses some promising properties, such as hydrophilicity, biocompatibility, biodegradability, and mechanical robustness. Cellulose-based materials have great advantages, and they can be applied to many fields. Modifications of cellulose materials by grafting open up various directions. Grafting can be linked to surface as well as bulk property as the side chains may be located at the surface or may be deeply penetrating. Their applications in wastewater treatment, biomedical, stimuli-responsive, and packaging fields are discussed.

2.5.1 Wastewater Treatment

Water contamination is a big threat to mankind. These may be geological or anthropogenic (man-made), that is, contamination can occur through natural processes like weathering of soils and rocks, volcanic eruptions, as well as a variety of human activities involving the use of metals/or metal contaminates (Cd, Cu, Ni, Cr, Co, Zn, and Pb, etc.), industrial discharge through different industries like petroleum refining, chemical manufacturing, metal finishing, printed circuit manufacturing, electroplating, leather, dye industries, and mining processes. Therefore, it is necessary to treat wastewater through some process to recycle it.

There has been subject of interest to evaluate the competency of natural materials regarding the heavy metal removal. In particular, considerable work has been carried out in the use of both natural materials and their modifications. In this arena, cellulose is preferred as it is relatively cheap, abundant in supply, and has significant potential for modification and ultimately enhancement of their adsorption capabilities. Grafting of selected monomers to the cellulose backbone with subsequent functionalization has made the material promising in this area. The heavy metal adsorption capacities for these cellulose-based materials are found to be significant, and levels of uptake are comparable, in many instances, to both other naturally occurring adsorbent materials and commercial ion exchange-type resins. Many of the modified cellulose adsorbents show regenerable and reusable over number cycles (O'Connell et al. 2008).

Adsorption is one of the physical processes in which dissolved contaminants adhere to the porous surface of the solid particles. The cellulose graft copolymers, viz., cellulose-*g*-(AM), cellulose-*g*-(AA), cellulose-*g*-(AN), and cellulose-*g*-(acrylamidomethylpropane sulfonic acid), have been used in the adsorption of hazardous contaminants such as heavy metal ions or dyes from aqueous solutions (Biçak et al. 1999; Wen et al. 2001; Guclu et al. 2003; Coskun and Temuz 2005; Cavus et al. 2006; O'Connell 2006a–c; Liu and Sun 2008; Lin et al. 2010).

Cellulose-*g*-AN treated with triethylenetetramine shows Cu(II) adsorption to the extent of 30 mg g^{-1} (Kubota and Shigehisa 1995). Graft copolymers of AA and acrylamide onto cellulose show its potential in the adsorption capacity for Cu(II) from wastewater; a maximum adsorption capacity for Cu(II) of 49.6 mg g^{-1} is achieved under optimum conditions (Bao-Xiu et al. 2006). Cellulosic materials grafted with poly(acrylonitrile) and poly(AA) molecules are used to remove Cd(II) and Cu(II) ions from the water (Okieimen et al. 2005). Cellulosic wastes-*g*-methacrylic acid treated with sodium chlorite/potassium permanganate shows potentiality of adsorbent for divalent metal ions (Cu^{2+}, Co^{2+}, and Ni^{2+}). It shows the removal efficiency of metal ions 250 mg g^{-1} under optimum conditions (Wojnárovits 2010; Abdel-Halim and Al-Deyab 2012). Densified cellulose-*g*-glycidylmethacrylate functionalized with quaternary ammonium groups shows selective adsorption of chromium (VI) and Zn(II) ions from aqueous solutions (Eromosele and Bayero 2000; Anirudhan et al. 2013).

Wood pulp grafted with AA is useful for removing Fe(III), Cr(III), Pb(II), and Cd(II) from aqueous solutions (Abdel-Aal et al. 2006). The maximum uptake capacity for Fe(III) and Cr(III) is 7 mg g^{-1}, and for Pb(II) and Cd(II), it is 4 and 6 mg g^{-1}, respectively. Cellulose-*g*-glycidyl methacrylate functionalized with imidazole ligand shows that adsorption levels on the resultant materials for Cu(II), Ni(II), and Pb(II) are 68.5, 48.5, and 75.8 mg g^{-1}, respectively (O'Connell 2006a–c). Cellulose-*g*-glycidyl methacrylate functionalized with reactive epoxy groups with polyethyleneimine shows adsorption capacity for Cu(II), Co(II), and Zn(II) of 60, 20, 27 mg g^{-1} from aqueous wastewater, respectively (Navarro et al. 1999).

Cellulose-*g*-(AM) (Biçak et al. 1999) shows the potential to remove of Hg(II) from aqueous solution. The Hg(II) uptake level is of 12.5 mg g^{-1}. Cellulose-*g*-(AN) on saponification shows chromium adsorption up to 73.5 mg g^{-1}, whereas Cu(II) uptake on the carboxylate-functionalized compound is up to 70.5 mg g^{-1} (Liu et al. 2001, 2002). Grafted cellulose powder with AA, *N,N′*-methylene bisacrylamide (NMBA), 2-acrylamido-2-methylpropane sulfonic acid ($AASO_3H$), and a mixture of AA and $AASO_3H$ has been reported by Guclu et al. (2003). These (four) grafted materials of cellulose are compared in the adsorption of Pb(II), Cu(II), and Cd(II) under similar conditions. Uptakes are 0.27, 0.24, and 0.02 mmol g^{-1} for cellulose grafted with AA, AA–NMBA, and $AASO_3H$, respectively. Cellulose-*g*-(AA) shows maximum adsorption of divalent metal ions. The potential of some cellulose graft copolymers (viz. cell-*g*-poly(sty), cell-*g*-poly(sty-*co*-AN), cell-*g*-poly(sty-*co*-MAAc), and cell-*g*-poly(sty-*co*-MAnh)) especially with respect to the structural aspects of graft copolymer chains as new membrane materials are studied for sorption of Cu^{2+} ions from aqueous solution (Chauhan et al. 2000).

Cellulosic Luffa cylindrical fiber-*g*-AA shows its potentiality for the removal of methylene blue and metal ions from the water (Gupta et al. 2013). The maximum adsorption of dye onto the grafted cellulosic material was 62.15 mg g^{-1} after 175 min, while maximum removal of 45.8% is observed for Mg^{2+} as compared to other metal ions. Hyper-branched aliphatic polyester-grafted cellulose (HAPE-cell) having smooth surfaces or the surfaces of porous particles for numerous applications, including separation of the metal ions (viz., Cu(II), Hg(II), Zn(II), and Cd(II)) are exploited (Peng 2007).

Cellulose graft copolymers with thermosensitive graft chains, viz., poly(*N*-isopropylacrylamide) or poly(*N,N*-diethylacrylamide) have been used in the removal of heavy metal ions from aqueous solutions by temperature swing adsorption, which is different from the removal of metal ions by complexation or ion exchange (Chauhan et al. 2000; Bokias et al. 2001; Xie and Hsieh 2003; Csoka et al. 2005; Ifuku and Kadla 2008; Li et al. 2008; Nada et al. 2008; Esen et al. 2011). Multiwalled carbon nanotubes (MWCNTs) grafted on carboxymethyl cellulose (CMC) possess very high sorption ability in the removal of UO_2^{2+} compared to control MWCNT. They have the potential to remove heavy metal ions from large volume of aqueous solutions (Shao et al. 2009).

Flocculation is one of the chemical approaches for water purification. The principle behind this is the enhancement of particle size through aggregation. Numerous studies on the synthesis of flocculants based on cellulosic materials have been discussed in the literature (Singh et al. 2001; Bharti et al. 2013; Das et al. 2013; Rani et al. 2013). Among these, CMC-*g*-PAA and CMC-*g*-PAAM are prominent. CMC-*g*-PAA shows flocculant property for river water clarification toward augmentation of drinking water supply (Mishra et al. 2012). CMC-*g*-PAAM exhibits distinguished flocculation characteristics in various suspensions and effluents (Biswal and Singh 2004). It has also seen that their flocculation and viscosifying characteristics can be enhanced drastically on hydrolysis.

Cellulose-based membranes (viz., cellulose acetate), though largely been replaced by thin film composite membrane shows tremendous potential not only its eco-friendly nature, modification is feasible through grafting for requisite applications. Various reports are there in literature. Cellulose acetate (CA)-*g*-HEMA and CA-*g*-styrene show salt rejection and ethanol separation from ethanol and water respectively (Chowdhury et al. 1988; Worthley 2012). CA-*g*-PAN membranes have excellent oil-fouling-resistance ability in oil/water emulsion (Chen et al. 2009). CA-*g*-PEG, being hydrophilic, shows decreased flux decline during operation of the membrane for desalination activities and had a marginal effect of organic matter rejection (Gullinkala and Escobar 2008).

2.5.2 Biomedical

The fulfillment of basic criteria (viz., biocompatibility, appropriate nature to intend function, and no toxicity) presents several grafted cellulose material fit for biomedical applications. In designing grafted cellulose for the particular applications, it is necessary to design these with desired tunable properties.

Drug delivery is one of the important applications of grafted cellulose. Release of drugs depends on diffusion of drugs, swelling, and degradation of the grafted matrix. Drug release can also be tuned by environment stimuli, viz., temperature and pH. The pH-responsive ethyl cellulose graft poly(2-(diethylamino) ethyl methacrylate) (EC-*g*-PDEAEMA) copolymers show their ability in controlled release of drugs using rifampicin (RIF) as the model drug. It is found that the cumulant release of RIF in the buffer solution at pH 6.6 is higher than that at pH 7.4 (Wang et al. 2011). CMC modified through grafting of poly (hydroxyethyl acrylate) or polyacrylamide shows different drug release behavior for cephalexin antibiotic in three different media (buffer solutions with pH equal to 3, 6.1, and 8) (Moghaddam et al. 2014). The drug-loaded biodegradable cellulose-*g*-poly(L-lactide) micelles formed by the copolymer in aqueous media show sustained drug release, which indicates their potential applicability in drug carrier (Dong et al. 2008). Well-defined cellulose-based dual graft molecular brushes, composed of ethyl cellulose-*g*-poly(*N*,*N*-dimethylaminoethyl methacrylate)-*g*-poly(ε-caprolactone) (EC-*g*-PDMAEMA-PCL) (Yan et al. 2009), show their potentiality in drug nanocarriers (e.g., chlorambucil) for controlled drug release. The behavior of this brush is strongly pH dependent. 2-Hydroxyethyl cellulose-*g*-methoxy poly(ethylene glycol)-poly(ε-caprolactone) HEC-*g*-mPEG-PCL (Hsieh et al. 2008; Chen et al. 2011a) shows its potential for antitumor drug (doxorubicin) delivery.

One of the interesting applications in this regard is the delivery of antioxidative/anti-inflammatory catechins (viz., (−)-epigallocatechin gallate). HEC-*g*-mPEG-PCL porous membrane is used as a penetration matrix for the skin delivery of catechins (Chen et al. 2011b). A Franz diffusion cell (Scheme 2.17) system was used for in vitro permeation test. It is shown HEC-*g*-mPEG-PCL membrane (loading catechin content 1.5 mg cm^{-2}) significantly enhanced the permeation up to 0.84 mg mL^{-1}, whereas the permeated catechin through HEC membrane is only 0.04 mg mL^{-1} in the receptor of Franz cell for a period of 48 h.

Antiadhesive property to proteins for the material is useful in biomedical applications. Surface modification is an effective method to improve the blood compatibility by keeping bulk properties same. The required cellulose material can be developed by grafting. In most of the cases, zwitterionic molecules are used for modification. There are different examples: cellulose-*g*-poly(*N*,*N*-dimethyl-*N*-(p-vinylbenyl)-*N*-(3-sulfopropyl) ammonium) (PDMVSA), cellulose-*g*-poly(2-(methacryloyloxyethyl) ethyl-dimethyl-(3-sulfopropyl)-ammonium) (PDMMSA), and

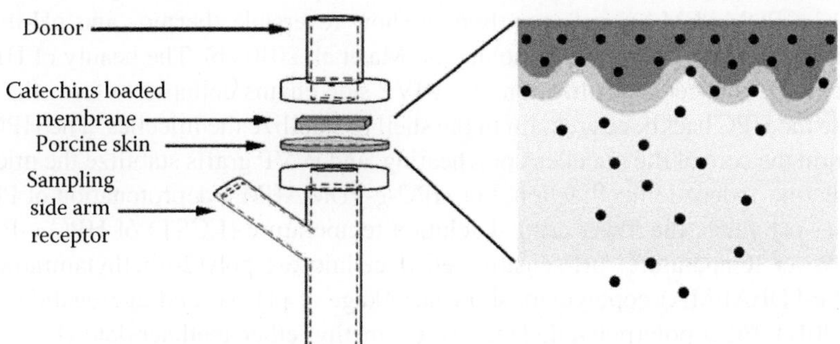

SCHEME 2.17 Schematic diagram of transdermal delivery of catechin. Catechin-loaded membrane and porcine skin sandwiched together to produce a whole transdermal delivery system in a Franz cell (incubated in a water bath at 37°C, refers to the catechin) (Reproduced from Chen, C.H. et al., *J. Membr. Sci.*, 371(1–2), 134, 2011b.)

cellulose-*g*-poly(2-methacryloyloxyethyl phosphorylcholine) (PMPC) (Liu et al. 2010), cellulose-*g*-*N*,*N*-dimethyl-*N*-methacryloxyethyl-*N*-(3-sulfopropyl) ammonium (DMMSA) (Zhang et al. 2003), cellulose-*g*-carboxybetaine-*g*-cellulose sulfobetaine (Yuan et al. 2003), hydroxypropylcellulose-*g*-sulfobetaine (Gaweł et al. 2010), cellulose-*g*-*p*-vinylbenzyl sulfobetaine (Liu et al. 2009a). The zwitterionic polymer-modified surfaces are more hydrophilic than the original cellulose surface. Evaluation by protein adsorption and platelet adhesion tests in vitro is checked for blood compatibility of cellulose substrates. Apart from zwitterion molecules, some examples are also there, viz., cellulose-*g*-poly *N*,*N*-dimethyl acrylamide (DMA) (Yan and Tao 2008a), cellulose-*g*-2-methacryloyloxyethyl-*g*-phosphorylcholine (Ishihara et al. 1992; Yan and Ishihara 2008b), and cellulose-*g*-*O*-butyrylchitosan (OBCS) (Mao et al. 2004), where good protein adsorption resistance is developed.

Antimicrobial property of cellulose and its derivatives can be achieved by grafting of appropriate monomers onto them. Examples in this regard include ethylene diamine-modified cellulose-*g*-polyacrylonitrile (EDA MC-*g*-PAN) (El-Khouly et al. 2011), cellulose-*g*-PDMAEM (2-(dimethylamino) ethyl methacrylate (Roy et al. 2008), CMC-*g*-AA (El-Sherbiny et al. 2009), cellulose thiocarbamates-*g*-AN, and cellulose thiocarbamates-*g*-EA (Nagieb and El-Gammal 1986). EDA MC-*g*-PAN shows its promising behavior toward *Bacillus subtilis*. The cellulose-*g*-PDMAEM (2-(dimethylamino) ethyl methacrylate) fiber with quaternization has found to exhibit particularly high activity against *Escherichia coli* (Roy et al. 2008). CMC-*g*-AA, cellulose thiocarbamates-*g*-AN, and cellulose thiocarbamates-*g*-EA show promising behavior in terms of antifungal activity.

In the proteomic applications and separation science, grafted cellulose shows its potential. Silica capillaries coated with hydroxyethyl cellulose-*g*-poly (dimethyl acrylamide) (HEC-*g*-PDMAAM) or with hydroxyethyl cellulose-*g*-poly (ethyl glycol) (HEC-*g*-PEG) are used in capillary electrophoresis (Yang et al. 2010; Shi et al. 2013). HEC-*g*-PAM graft copolymer shows improvement in the separation of double-stranded DNA fragments by capillary electrophoresis (Yang et al. 2007).

2.5.3 Stimuli Responsive

"Self-assembly" represents a promising strategy for creating structures with well-controlled tailor-made properties. The forces that drive self-assembly are typically relatively weak for the scale of the components, that is, van der Waals, electrostatic, H-bonds, hydrophobic/-phallic interactions, capillary, gravitational. Numerous cellulose-*g*-copolymers have self-assembling properties that can be altered by modifying the length, density, and composition of the graft copolymers. These grafted polymers show stimuli responsive toward, viz., pH, temperature, and solvent. These graft copolymers have the potential in terms of sensor applications.

HPC-*g*-poly (4-vinyl pyridine) (HPC-*g*-P4VP), HPC-*g*-poly (*N*,*N*-dimethyl amino ethyl methacrylate) (HPC-*g*-PDMAEMA) graft copolymers show reversible thermo- and pH-induced core shell micellization properties in aqueous solutions (Ma et al. 2010a,b). The beauty of HPC-*g*-P4VP is that in case of pH-induced micellization, the P4VP side chains collapse to form the core of the micelles, while the HPC backbones remain in the shell to stabilize the micelles. The HPC backbone collapses to form the core of the micelles upon heating, and P4VP grafts stabilize the micelles as the shell during thermo-induced micellization. For HPC-*g*-PDMAEMA deprotonation of PDMAEMA grafts at higher pH value, the lower critical solution temperature (LCST) of HPC-*g*-PDMAEMA shifts to the lower temperature. pH-sensitive ethyl cellulose-*g*-poly(2-(diethylamino)ethyl methacrylate) (EC-*g*-PDEAEMA) copolymers show shrinkage at pH 6.0 and aggregation at pH > 6.9 (Wang et al. 2011). EC-*g*-poly(poly(ethylene glycol) methyl ether methacrylate (EC-*g*-PPEGMA) copolymers also formed spherical micelles in water, show thermo-responsive properties with an LCST of approximately 65°C, which is almost independent of grafting density and side chain length (Çaykara et al. 2006).

Apart from thermo- and pH-sensitive properties, graft polymers also show self-assembling properties in selective organic solvent/s. Ethyl cellulose-*g*-polystyrene (EC-*g*-PSt) copolymer forms

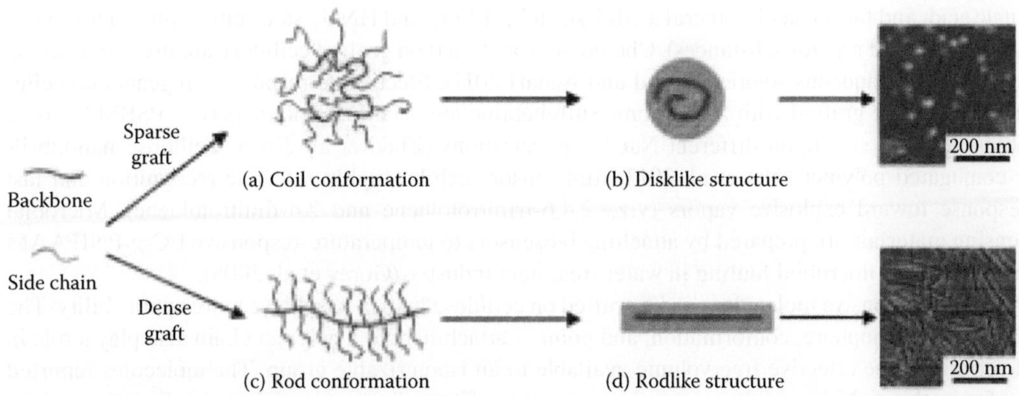

SCHEME 2.18 Schematic presentation of micelle (disk- and rodlike) structure. (Reproduced from Liu, W. et al., *Polymer*, 53, 1005, 2012b.)

spherical core–shell micelles in acetone with the EC backbone in the shell and PSt grafts in the core of the micelles (Shen et al. 2005, 2006; Liu 2009b). Aggregation and self-assemble nature also depend on the nature of solvents. Cellulose-*g*-PMMA copolymer also tends to aggregate and self-assemble into spherical particles in solvent dimethyl formamide (with a diameter range of 100–500 nm) and in acetone (with a diameter range of 50–100 nm) (Lin et al. 2009; Meng et al. 2009; Xin et al. 2011). Amphiphilic EC-*g*-PAA with longer side chains shows intramolecular self-assembly to form unimolecular small spherical structures that may further form larger network structures and those with short side chains form multimolecular large spherical aggregates by intermolecular association in THF/H_2O systems. No micelles (only single-chain disk- and rodlike) are formed in MeOH/H_2O and DMF/H_2O systems (Kang et al. 2006; Liu et al. 2012a,b). Single-chain disk- and rodlike structures are presented as follows (Scheme 2.18).

Apart from self-assembly, different hydrogels (viz., polyacrylamide-*g*-CMC, CMC-*g*-polyacrylonitrile, and cellulose-*g*-PDMAEMA) show pH-responsive properties (Pourjavadi et al. 2007; Sui et al. 2008). It is useful to absorb large quantities of solvents, mainly water, in addition to small solutes in the systems of macromolecules, viz., proteins (Eldin et al. 2011). Thus, it is useful to separate water from protein systems. Some grafted polymers (viz., HEC-*g*-2-hydroxyethyl methacrylate (Peng and Chen 2010), CMC-*g*-PEPO (amino-terminated) (Karakasyan et al. 2008), HPC-*g*-NIPAM (Marsano et al. 2004), and HPC-*g*-poly (*N-tert*-butylacrylamide)-*co*-acrylamide (Çavkara et al. 2006) are thermo-responsive systems. Some materials (viz., HPC-*g*-polyacid (Chen et al. 2008; Liao et al. 2012), HPC-*g*-poly (*N,N*-dimethyl amino ethyl methacrylate), HPC-*g*-poly (4-vinyl pyridine)) show response to both (viz., temperature and pH). Ethyl cellulose-*g*-PNIPAAM microparticles show thermosensitive property in case of drug release delivery system (Shen et al. 2006). The model drug allopurinol release rate shows dependent behavior in different temperatures. It is slower at 40°C compared to 25°C, probably due to collapse of PNIPAAM chains at higher temperature (Kim et al. 2002). Designs of stimuli-responsive bio-based nanocomposite materials are also developed. Cellulose nanocrystals (CNCs)-*g*-poly (*N*-isopropylacrylamide) also show stimuli-responsive nature (Zoppe et al. 2010). Grafting with thermosensitive amine-terminated CNCs (Azzam et al. 2010) leads to unusual properties like colloidal stability at high ionic strength, surface activity, and thermo-reversible aggregation.

Apart from these, humidity sensing (Cellu-*g*-PPy) (Shukla 2013), (Cellu-*g*-PANI) (Shukla 2012), chemical sensing (Cellu-*g*-AM), (Cellu-*g*-AA) (Majumdar and Adhikari 2006a; Majumdar et al. 2006a,b) materials offer promising perspective in this regard. The mentioned humidity sensing material has good behavior in the range of 5%–95%. The chemical sensing material shows distinct response patterns for different taste substances in terms of membrane potential (like acetic acid, citric acid, and formic acid, mineral acids like HCl, H_2SO_4, and HNO_3, salts, bitter substances, sweet substances, and umami substances). Chemo-sensors based on grafted cellulose are used for cyanide ion sensors in aqueous solution (Isaad and Achari 2011). Electrolyte-responsive regenerated cellulose membrane grafted with zwitterionic sulfobetaine methacrylate polymers (i.e., PSBMA) could adjust its pore size upon different NaCl concentrations (Zhao et al. 2010). Cellulose nanofibril-*g*-conjugated polymer (Niu et al. 2013) film sensors exhibit highly selective recognition and fast response toward explosive vapors (viz., 2,4,6-trinitrotoluene and 2,4-dinitrotoluene). Microbial sensing materials are prepared by attaching biosensors to temperature-responsive EC-*g*-PNIPAAM films to detect microbial fouling in water-treatment industry (Gorey et al. 2008).

Photo-responsive molecules can be grafted on cellulose matrix to achieve more applicability. The size of a chromophore, conformation, and point of attachment to a polymer chain also play a role in determining the effective free volume available to an isomerizable group. The molecules reported so far in this field are azobenzene, spiropyran, etc. These have potential applications in sensors and optical materials, viz., EC-*g*-MMAzo (Tang et al. 2007). Cellulose grafted with alkenyloxy-substituted cinnamoyl chloride develops the potential as LCD materials with photosensitive aligning property (Kurioz et al. 2008). In dye-sensitized solar cell application, grafted cellulose gel electrolyte in an ionic liquid ([Bmim]I) is used (Li et al. 2011).

2.5.4 Packaging

Considering the property of cellulose, it is useful as packaging material. In this aspect, few reports are available. Cellulose-*g*-AM loaded with silver nanoparticle material is developed (Tankhiwale and Bajpai 2009). It possesses antimicrobial properties against *E. coli* (Elegir et al. 2008). They showed that the grafting of laccase polymerized oligomeric phenolic structures onto the unbleached kraft liner fiber surface enhanced the antibacterial activity of handsheet paper. Considering this property, they can be used as antibacterial food-packaging material. Transparent EA-*g*-cellulose *Hibiscus sabdariffa* (*Hs*) fiber graft ethyl acrylate (EA) (Takashi et al. 1972), for example, *Hs*-*g*-poly (EA), *Hs*-*g*-poly(EA-*co*-AM), and *Hs*-*g*-poly(EA-*co*-2-VP) (Chauhan and Kaith 2012), showed its potentiality as a packaging material.

2.6 CONCLUSIONS AND FUTURE DIRECTIONS

In conclusion, great achievements have been acquired in the current developments of grafting especially in cellulose. Cellulose is an important natural polymer in which grafting finds more applications. As an effective approach to realize modification, grafting can be used to achieve surface as well as bulk modification. Here we presented an overview of recent study in the area of grafting on cellulose. It demonstrated the growing activity on this research front. The application of grafted cellulosics is not limited to only those fields mentioned earlier. Grafted cellulosics can be applied in many aspects. Thus, grafted cellulosics have a bright future, and their development is practically boundless.

It is advantageous and showed versatility in many aspects, but it has so far not attracted very much attention in commercial scale. It needs proper thought. The laboratory research has also been important for bridging enormous gap between the present-day capabilities for cellulose required for market introduction.

REFERENCES

Abdel-Aal, S.E., Gad, Y., Dessouki, A.M. 2006. The use of wood pulp and radiation modified starch in wastewater treatment. *J. Appl. Polym. Sci.* 99: 2460–2469.

Abdel-Halim, E.S., Al-Deyab, S.S. 2012. Chemically modified cellulosic adsorbent for divalent cations removal from aqueous solutions. *Carbohydr. Polym.* 87: 1863–1868.

Abdel-Razik, E.A. 1990. Homogeneous graft copolymerization of acrylamide onto ethylcellulose. *Polymer* 31: 1739–1744.

Abdel-Razik, E.A. 1997. Aspects of thermal graft copolymerization of methyl ethacrylate onto ethyl cellulose in homogeneous media. *Polym. Plast. Technol. Eng.* 36: 891–903.

Aich, S., Bhattacharya, A., Basu, S. 1997. Fluorescence polarisation of *N*-vinyl carbazole on cellulose acetate film and electron transfer with 1,4 dicyanobenzene. *Radiat. Phys. Chem.* 50(4): 347–354.

Anirudhan, T.S., Nima, J., Divya, P.L. 2013. Adsorption of chromium (VI) from aqueous solutions by glycidylmethacrylate-grafted-densified cellulose with quaternary ammonium groups. *Appl. Surf. Sci.* 279: 441–449.

Azzam, F., Heux, L., Putaux, J.-L., Jean, B. 2010. Preparation by grafting onto, characterization, and properties of thermally responsive polymer-decorated cellulose nanocrystals. *Biomacromolecules* 11: 3652–3659.

Bao-Xiu, Z., Peng, W., Tong, Z., Chun-yun, C., Jing, S. 2006. Preparation and adsorption performance of a cellulosic adsorbent resin for copper(II). *J. Appl. Polym. Sci.* 99: 2951–2956.

Barner-Kowollik, C. (ed.) 2008. *The Handbook of RAFT Polymerization*, Wiley-VCH, Weinheim, Germany.

Bharti, S., Mishra, S., Sen, G. 2013. Ceric ion initiated synthesis of polyacrylamide grafted oatmeal: Its application as flocculant for wastewater treatment. *Carbohydr. Polym.* 93: 528–536.

Bhattacharya, A. 2000. Radiation and industrial polymers. *Prog. Polym. Sci.* 25: 371–401.

Bhattacharya, A., Das, A., De, A. 1998. Structural influence on grafting of acrylamide based monomers on cellulose acetate. *Ind. J. Chem. Tech.* 5: 135–138.

Bhattacharya, A., Misra, B.N. 2004. Grafting: A versatile means to modify polymers techniques, factors and applications. *Prog. Polym. Sci.* 29: 767–814.

Bhattacharya, S.N., Maldas, D. 1984. Graft copolymerization onto cellulosics. *Prog. Polym. Sci.* 10: 171–270.

Biçak, N., Sherrington, D.C., Senkal, B.F. 1999. Graft copolymer of acrylamide onto cellulose as mercury selective sorbent. *React. Funct. Polym.* 41: 69–76.

Biswal, D.R., Singh, R.P. 2004. Characterisation of carboxymethyl cellulose and polyacrylamide graft copolymer. *Carbohydr. Polym.* 57: 379–387.

Bokias, G., Mylonas, Y., Staikos, G., Bumbu, G.G., Vasile, C. 2001. Synthesis and aqueous solution properties of novel thermoresponsive graft copolymers based on a carboxymethyl cellulose backbone. *Macromolecules* 34: 4958–4964.

Borbély, É., Erdélyi, J. 2004. Grafting of industrial cellulose pulp with vinyl acetate monomer by ceric ion redox system as initiator. *Acta. Polytech. Hung.* 1: 86–95.

Braunecker, W.A., Matyjaszewski, K. 2007. Controlled/living radical polymerization: Features, developments, and perspectives. *Prog. Polym. Sci.* 32: 93–146.

Carlmark, A., Malmström, E. 2002. Atom transfer radical polymerization from cellulose fibersat ambient temperature. *J. Am. Chem. Soc.* 124: 900–901.

Cavus, S., Gurdag, G., Yasar, M., Guclu, K., Gurkaynak, M.A. 2006. The competitive heavy metal removal by hydroxyethyl cellulose-g-poly(acrylic acid) copolymer and its sodium salt: The effect of copper content on the adsorption capacity. *Polym. Bull.* 57: 445–456.

Çaykara, T., Şengül, G., Birlik, G. 2006. Preparation and swelling properties of temperature-sensitive semi-interpenetrating polymer networks composed of poly[(*N*-tert-butylacrylamide)-*co*-acrylamide] and hydroxypropyl cellulose. *Macromol. Mater. Eng.* 291: 1044–1051.

Chauhan, A., Kaith, B. 2012. Using the advanced analytical techniques to investigating the versatile cellulosic graft copolymers. *J. Anal. Bioanal. Tech.* 3: 146–153.

Chauhan, G.S., Mahajan, S., Guleria, K.L. 2000. Polymers from renewable resources: Sorption of Cu^{2+} ions by cellulose graft copolymers. *Desalination* 130: 85–88.

Chen, C.H., Cuong, N.V., Chen, Y.-T., So, R.C., Liau, I., Hsieh, M.F. 2011a. Overcoming multidrug resistance of breast cancer cells by the micellar doxorubicin nanoparticles of mPEG-PCL-graft-cellulose. *J. Nanosci. Nanotechnol.* 11: 53–60.

Chen, C.H., Hsieh, M.F., Ho, Y.N. et al. 2011b. Enhancement of catechin skin permeation via a newly fabricated mPEG-PCL-graft-2-hydroxy cellulose membrane. *J. Membr. Sci.* 371(1–2): 134–140.

Chen, W., Su, Y., Zheng, L., Wang, L., Jiang, Z. 2009. The improved oil/water separation performance of cellulose acetate-graft-polyacrylonitrile membranes. *J. Membr. Sci.* 337(1–2): 98–105.

Chen, Y., Ding, D., Mao, Z. et al. 2008. Synthesis of hydroxypropylcellulose-poly(acrylic acid) particles with semi-interpenetrating polymer network structure. *Biomacromolecules* 9: 2609–2614.

Chowdhury, J.P., Ghosh, P., Guha, B.K. 1988. Styrene-grafted cellulose acetate reverse osmosis membrane for ethanol separation. *J. Membr. Sci.* 35(3): 301–310.

Coskun, M., Temuz, M.M. 2005. Grafting studies onto cellulose by atom-transfer radical polymerization. *Polym. Int.* 54: 342–347.

Csoka, G., Marton, S., Gelencser, A., Klebovich, I. 2005. Thermoresponsive properties of different cellulose derivatives. *Eur. J. Pharm. Sci.* 25: S74–S75.

Dahoua, W., Ghemati, D., Oudia, A., Aliouche, D. 2010. Preparation and biological characterization of cellulose graft copolymers. *Biochem. Eng. J.* 48: 187–194.

Daly, W.H., Evenson, T.S., Iacono, S.T., Jones, R.W. 2001. Recent developments in cellulose grafting chemistry utilizing barton ester intermediates and nitroxide mediation. *Macromol. Symp.* 174: 155–163.

Das, R., Ghorai, S., Pal, S. 2013. Flocculation characteristics of polyacrylamide grafted hydroxypropyl methyl cellulose: An efficient biodegradable flocculant. *Chem. Eng. J.* 229: 144–152.

Dechy-Cabaret, O., Martin-Vaca, B., Bourissou, D. 2004. Controlled ring opening polymerization of lactide and glycolide. *Chem. Rev.* 104(12): 6147–6176.

Dhiman, P.K., Kaur, I., Mahajan, R.K. 2008. Synthesis of a cellulose-grafted polymeric support and its application in the reductions of some carbonyl compounds. *J. Appl. Polym. Sci.* 108: 99–111.

Dong, H., Xu, Q., Li, Y., Mo, S., Cai, S., Liu, L. 2008. The synthesis of biodegradable graft copolymer cellulose-graft-poly(L-lactide) and the study of its controlled drug release. *Colloids Surf. B: Biointerfaces* 66: 26–33.

Eldin, M.S.M., El-Sherif, H.M., Soliman, E.A., Elzatahry, A.A., Omer, A.M. 2011. Polyacrylamide-grafted carboxymethyl cellulose: Smart pH-sensitive hydrogel for protein concentration. *J. Appl. Polym. Sci.* 122: 469–479.

Elegir, G., Kindl, A., Sadocco, P., Orlandi, M. 2008. Development of antimicrobial cellulose packaging through laccase-mediated grafting of phenolic compounds. *Enz. Microb. Technol.* 43: 84–92.

El-Khouly, A.S., Kenawy, E., Safaan, A.A. et al. 2011. Synthesis, characterization and antimicrobial activity of modified cellulose-graft-polyacrylonitrile with some aromatic aldehyde derivatives. *Carbohydr. Polym.* 83(2): 346–353.

El-Sherbiny, I.M., Salama, A., Sarhan, A.A. 2009. Grafting study and antifungal activity of a carboxymethyl cellulose derivative. *Int. J. Polym. Mater.* 58(9): 453–467.

Eromosele, I.C., Bayero, S.S. 2000. Adsorption of chromium and zinc ions from aqueous solutions by cellulosic graft copolymers. *Bioresour. Technol.* 71(3): 279–281.

Esen, E., Ozbas, Z., Kasgoz, H., Gurdag, G. 2011. Thermoresponsive cellulose-g-*N,N*″-diethyl acrylamide copolymers. *Curr. Opin. Biotechnol.* 22(1): S61–S62.

Fleet, R., McLeary, J.B., Grumel, V., Weber, W.G., Matahwa, H., Sanderson, R.D. 2008. RAFT mediated polysaccharide copolymers. *Eur. Polym. J.* 44: 2899–2911.

Gao, D. 2003. Superabsorbent polymer composite (SAPC) materials and their industrial and high-tech applications. PhD dissertation, Der Technische Universität Bergakademie Freiberg, Freiberg, Germany.

Gaweł, K., Szczubiałka, K., Zapotoczny, S., Nowakowska, M. 2010. Zwitterionically modified hydroxypropylcellulose for biomedical applications. *Eur. Polym. J.* 46(7): 1475–1479.

Gcaclntov, N., Abrahamson, E.W., Stannett, V. 1960. Grafting onto cellulose and cellulose derivatives using ultraviolet irradiation. *J. Appl. Polym. Sci.* 3: 54–60.

Gorey, C., Escobar, I.C., Gruden, C., Coleman, M., Mileyeva-Biebesheimer, O. 2008. Development of smart membrane filters for microbial sensing. *Sep. Sci. Technol.* 43: 4056–4074.

Goyal, P., Kumar, V., Sharma, P. 2008. Graft copolymerization of acrylamide onto amarind kernel powder in the presence of ceric ion. *J. Appl. Polym. Sci.* 108: 3696–3701.

Gregory, A., Stenzel, M.H. 2012. Complex polymer architectures via RAFT polymerization: From fundamental process to extending the scope using click chemistry and nature's building blocks. *Prog. Polym. Sci.* 37: 38–105.

Guclu, G., Gurdag, G., Ozgumus, S. 2003. Competitive removal of heavy metal ions by cellulose graft copolymers. *J. Appl. Polym. Sci.* 90: 2034–2039.

Gullinkala, T., Escobar I.C. 2008. Desalination pretreatment using controlled-chain PEG-enhanced cellulose acetate ultrafiltration membranes, desalination and water purification research and development program report no. 138. University of Toledo, Toledo, OH.

Gupta, K.C., Khandekar, K. 2002. Graft copolymerization of acrylamide–methylacrylate comonomers onto cellulose using ceric ammonium nitrate. *J. Appl. Polym. Sci.* 86: 2631–2642.

Gupta, K.C., Khandekar, K. 2006a. Ceric(IV) ion-induced graft copolymerization of acrylamide and ethyl acrylate onto cellulose. *Polym. Int.* 55: 139–150.

Gupta, K.C., Khandekar, K. 2006b. Graft copolymerization of acrylamide onto cellulose in presence of comonomer using ceric ammonium nitrate as initiator. *J. Appl. Polym. Sci.* 101: 2546–2558.

Gupta, K.C., Sahoo, S. 2001. Co(III) acetylacetonate-complex-initiated grafting of *N*-vinyl pyrrolidone on cellulose in aqueous media. *J. Appl. Polym. Sci.* 81: 2286–2296.
Gupta, V.K., Agarwal, S., Singh, P., Pathania, D. 2013. Acrylic acid grafted cellulosic Luffa cylindrical fiber for the removal of dye and metal ions. *Carbohydr. Polym.* 98: 1214–1221.
Gurdag, G., Guçlu, G.O., Zgumus, S. 2001. Graft copolymerization of acrylic acid onto cellulose: Effects of pretreatments and crosslinking agent. *J. Appl. Polym. Sci.* 80: 2267–2272.
Gurdag, G., Yasar, M., Gurkaynak, M.A. 1997. Graft copolymerization of acrylic acid on cellulose: Reaction kinetics of copolymerization. *J. Appl. Polym. Sci.* 66: 929–934.
Hafren, J., Cordova, A. 2005. Direct organocatalytic polymerization from cellulose fibers. *Macromol. Rapid Commun.* 26(2): 82–86.
Hawker, C.J., Bosman, A.W., Harth, E. 2001. New polymer synthesis by nitroxide mediated living radical polymerizations. *Chem. Rev.* 101: 3661–3688.
Hernandez-Guerrero, M., Davis, T.P., Barner-Kowollik, C., Stenzel, M.H. 2005. Polystyrene comb polymers built on cellulose or poly(styrene-*co*-2-hydroxy ethyl methacrylate) back bones as substrates for the preparation of structured honey comb films. *Eur. Polym. J.* 41: 2264–2277.
Hsieh, M.F., Cuong, N.V., Chen, C.H., Chen, Y.T., Yeh, J.M. 2008. Nano-sized micelles of block copolymers of methoxy poly(ethylene glycol)-poly(e-caprolactone)-graft-2-hydroxyethyl cellulose for doxorubicin delivery. *J. Nanosci. Nanotechnol.* 8: 2362–2368.
Ibrahim, M.D., Mondal, H., Uraki, Y., Ubukata, M., Itoyama, K. 2008. Graft polymerization of vinyl monomers onto cotton fibres pretreated with amines. *Cellulose* 15: 581–592.
Ibrahim, M.M., Flefel, E.M., El-Zawawy, W.K. 2002. Cellulose membranes grafted with vinyl monomers in a homogeneous system. *Polym. Adv. Technol.* 13: 548–557.
Ifuku, S., Kadla, J. 2008. Preparation of a thermosensitive highly regioselective cellulose/n-isopropylacrylamide copolymer through atom transfer radical polymerization. *Biomacromolecules* 9: 3308–3313.
Isaad, J., Achari, A.E. 2011. Colorimetric sensing of cyanide anions in aqueous media based on functional surface modification of natural cellulose materials. *Tetrahedron* 67: 4939–4947.
Ishihara, K., Takayama, R., Nakabayashi, N., Fukumoto, K., Aoki, J. 1992. Improvement of blood compatibility on cellulose dialysis membrane: 2. Blood compatibility of phospholipid polymer grafted cellulose membrane. *Biomaterials* 13(4): 235–239.
Jerome, C., Lecomte, P. 2008. Recent advances in the synthesis of aliphatic polyesters by ring-opening polymerization. *Adv. Drug Deliv. Rev.* 60(9): 1056–1076.
Jun, L., Jun, L., Min, Y., Hongfei, H. 2001. Solvent effect on grafting polymerization of NIPAAm onto cotton cellulose via γ-preirradiation method. *Radiat. Phys. Chem.* 60: 625–628.
Kahovec, J., Jelinkova, M., Janout, V. 1986. Polymer-supported oligo(nacetyliminoethylenes) new phase-transfer catalysts. *Polym. Bull.* 15(6): 485–490.
Kamigaito, M., Ando, T., Sawamoto, M. 2001. Metal-catalyzed living radical polymerization. *Chem. Rev.* 101: 3689–3746.
Kang, H., Liu W., He, B., Shen, D., Ma, L., Huang, Y. 2006. Synthesis of amphiphilic ethyl cellulose grafting poly(acrylic acid) copolymers and their self-assembly morphologies in water. *Polymer* 47: 7927–7934.
Karakasyan, C., Lack, S., Brunel, F., Maingault, P., Hourdet, D. 2008. Synthesis and rheological properties of responsive thickeners based on polysaccharide architectures. *Biomacromolecules* 9: 2419–2429.
Khan, F., Ahmad, S.R. 1997. Graft copolymerization reaction of water-emulsified methyl methacrylate with pre irradiated jute fiber. *J. Appl. Polym. Sci.* 65: 459–468.
Kim, B., Kang, H., Kim, J. 2002. Thermo-sensitive microparticles of PNIPAAM-grafted ethylcellulose by spray-drying method. *J. Microencapsul.* 19: 661–669.
Kim, B.S., Mun, S.P. 2009. Effect of Ce^{4+} pretreatment on swelling properties of cellulosic superabsorbents. *Polym. Adv. Technol.* 20: 899–906.
Kubota, H., Shigehisa, Y. 1995. Introduction of amidoxime groups into cellulose and its ability to adsorb metal ions. *J. Appl. Polym. Sci.* 56: 147–151.
Kubota, H., Shiobara, N. 1998. Photografting of *N*-isopropylacrylamide on cellulose and temperature-responsive character of the resulting grafted celluloses. *React. Funct. Polym.* 37: 219–224.
Kurioz, Y., Reznikov, Y., Tereshchenko, O. et al. 2008. Highly sensitive photoaligning materials on a base of cellulose-cinnamates. *Mol. Cryst. Liq. Cryst.* 480: 81–90.
Li, P., Zhang, Y., Fa, W., Zhang, Y., Huang B. 2011. Synthesis of a grafted cellulose gel electrolyte in an ionic liquid ([Bmim]I) for dye-sensitized solar cells. *Carbohydr. Polym.* 86(3): 1216–1220.
Li, Y.X., Liu, R.G., Liu, W.Y., Kang, H.L., Wu, M., Huang, Y. 2008. Synthesis, self-assembly, and thermosensitive properties of ethyl cellulose-g-p(PEGMA) amphiphilic copolymers. *J. Polym. Sci. A: Polym. Chem.* 46: 6907–6915.

Liao, Q., Shao, Q., Qiu, G., Lu, X. 2012. Methacrylic acid-triggered phase transition behavior of thermosensitive hydroxypropylcellulose. *Carbohydr. Polym.* 89: 1301–1304.

Lin, C., Zhan, H., Liu, M., Fu, S., Zhang, J. 2009. Preparation of cellulose graft poly(methylmethacrylate) copolymers by atom transfer radical polymerization in anionic liquid. *Carbohydr. Polym.* 78: 432–438.

Lin, C., Zhan, H., Liu, M., Habibi, Y., Fu, S., Lucia, L.A. 2013. RAFT synthesis of cellulose-g-polymethyl methacrylate copolymer in anionic liquid. *J. Appl. Polym. Sci.* 127: 4840–4849.

Lin, C.X., Zhan, H.U., Liu, M.H., Fu, S.U., Huang, L.H. 2010. Rapid homogeneous preparation of cellulose graft copolymer in BMIMCL under microwave irradiation. *J. Appl. Polym. Sci.* 118: 399–404.

Liu, M., Deng, Y., Zhan, H., Zhang, X., Liu, W., Zhan, H. 2001. Removal and recovery of chromium(III) from aqueous solutions by a spheroidal cellulose adsorbent. *Water Environ. Res.* 73(3): 322–328.

Liu, M., Deng, Y., Zhan, H., Zhang, X. 2002. Adsorption and desorption of copper(II) from solutions on new spherical cellulose adsorbent. *J. Appl. Polym. Sci.* 84: 478–485.

Liu, P.S., Chen, Q. Liu, X. et al. 2009a. Grafting of zwitterion from cellulose membranes via ATRP for improving blood compatibility. *Biomacromolecules* 10(10): 2809–2816.

Liu, P.S., Chen, Q., Wu, S.S., Shen, J., Lin, S.C. 2010. Surface modification of cellulose membranes with zwitterionic polymers for resistance to protein adsorption and platelet adhesion. *J. Membr. Sci.* 350(1–2): 387–394.

Liu, S., Sun, G. 2008. Radical graft functional modification of cellulose with allyl monomers: Chemistry and structure characterization. *Carbohydr. Polym.* 71: 614–625.

Liu, W., Liu, R., Li, X. et al. 2009b. Self-assembly of ethyl cellulose-graft-polystyrene copolymers in acetone. *Polymer* 50: 211–217.

Liu, W., Liu, Y., Hao, X. et al. 2012a. Backbone-collapsed intra- and inter-molecular self assembly of cellulose-based dense graft copolymer. *Carbohydr. Polym.* 88: 290–298.

Liu, W., Liu, Y., Zeng, G., Liu, R., Huang, Y. 2012b. Coil-to-rod conformational transition and single chain structure of graft copolymer by tuning the graft density. *Polymer* 53: 1005–1014.

Ma, L., Kang, H., Liu, R., Huang, Y. 2010a. Smart assembly behaviors of hydroxypropylcellulose-graft-poly(4-vinyl pyridine) copolymers in aqueous solution by thermo and pH stimuli. *Langmuir* 26: 18519–18525.

Ma, L., Liu, R., Tan, J. et al. 2010b. Self-assembly and dual-stimuli sensitivities of hydroxypropylcellulose-graft-poly(*N,N*-dimethyl aminoethyl methacrylate) copolymers in aqueous solution. *Langmuir* 26: 8697–8703.

Majumdar, S., Adhikari, B. 2006a. Taste sensing with polyacrylamide grafted cellulose. *J. Sci. Ind. Res.* 65: 237–243.

Majumdar, S., Dey, J., Adhikari, B. 2006b. Taste sensing with polyacrylic acid grafted cellulose membrane. *Talanta* 69(1): 131–139.

Mao, C., Qiu, Y., Sang, H. et al. 2004. Various approaches to modify biomaterial surfaces for improving hemocompatibility. *Adv. Coll. Int. Sci.* 110(1–2): 5–17.

Marsano, E., Bianchi, E., Viscardi, A. 2004. Stimuli responsive gels based on interpenetrating network of hydroxypropylcellulose and poly(*N*-isopropylacrylamide). *Polymer* 45: 157–163.

Matyjaszewski, K. (ed.) 2000. ACS symposium series: Controlled/living radical polymerization: Progress in ATRP, NMP and RAFT. *Am. Chem. Soc.* 768: 2–25.

Matyjaszewski, K., Xia, J. 2001. Atom transfer radical polymerization. *Chem. Rev.* 101: 2921–2990.

Meng, T., Gao, X., Zhang, J., Yuan, J., Zhang, Y., He, J. 2009. Graft copolymers prepared by atom transfer radical polymerization ATRP from cellulose. *Polymer* 50: 447–454.

Mishra, S., Usha Rani, G., Sen, G. 2012. Microwave initiated synthesis and application of polyacrylic acid grafted carboxymethyl cellulose. *Carbohydr. Polym.* 87: 2255–2262.

Moad, G., Rizzardo, E., Thang, S.H. 2008. Radical addition–fragmentation chemistry in polymer synthesis. *Polymer* 49: 1079–1131.

Moghaddam, P.N., Avval, M.E., Fareghi, A.R. 2014. Modification of cellulose by graft polymerization for use in drug delivery systems. *Colloid Polym. Sci.* 292: 77–84.

Mondal, M.I.H., Uraki, Y., Ubukata, M., Itoyama, K. 2008. Graft polymerization of vinyl monomers onto cotton fibres pretreated with amines. *Cellulose* 15: 581–592.

Nishioka, N., Kosai, K. 1981. Homogeneous graft copolymerization of vinyl monomers onto cellulose in a dimethyl sulfoxide-paraformaldehyde solvent system I. Acrylonitrile and methyl methacrylate. *Polym. J.* 13: 1125–1133.

Nishioka, N., Matsumoto, K., Kosai, K. 1983a. Homogeneous graft copolymerization of vinyl monomers onto cellulose in a dimethyl sulfoxide-paraformaldehyde solvent system II. Characterization of graft copolymers. *Polym. J.* 15: 153–158.

Nishioka, N., Matsumoto, Y., Yumen, T., Monmae, K., Kosai, K. 1986. Homogeneous graft copolymerization of vinyl monomers onto cellulose in a dimethyl sulfoxide-paraformaldehyde solvent system IV. 2-Hydroxyethyl methacrylate. *Polym. J.* 18: 323–330.

Nishioka, N., Minami, K., Kosai, K. 1983b. Homogeneous graft copolymerization of vinyl monomers onto cellulose in a dimethyl sulfoxide-paraformaldehyde solvent system III. Methyl acrylate. *Polym. J.* 15: 591–596.

Nada, A.A.M.A., Alkady, M.Y., Fekry, H.M. 2008. Synthesis and characterization of grafted cellulose for use in water and metal ions sorption. *Bioresources* 3: 46–59.

Nagieb, Z.A., El-Gammal, A.A. 1986. Grafting of cellulose–thiocarbamate with vinyl monomers: Antimicrobial activity. *J. Appl. Polym. Sci.* 31(1): 179–187.

Navarro, R.R., Sumi, K., Matsumura, M. 1999. Improved metal affinity of chelating adsorbents through graft polymerization. *Water Res.* 33: 2037–2044.

Niu, Q., Gao, K., Lin, Z., Wu, W. 2013. Surface molecular-imprinting engineering of novel cellulose nanofibril/conjugated polymer film sensors towards highly selective recognition and responsiveness of nitroaromatic vapors. *Chem. Commun.* 49: 9137–9139.

O'Connell, D.W., Birkinshaw, C., O'Dwyer, T.F. 2006a. A chelating cellulose adsorbent for the removal of Cu(II) from aqueous solutions. *J. Appl. Polym. Sci.* 99(6): 2888–2897.

O'Connell, D.W., Birkinshaw, C., O'Dwyer, T.F. 2006b. A modified cellulose adsorbent for the removal of nickel(II) from aqueous solutions. *J. Chem. Technol. Biotechnol.* 81: 1820–1828.

O'Connell, D.W., Birkinshaw, C., O'Dwyer, T.F. 2006c. Removal of lead(II) from aqueous solutions using a modified cellulose adsorbent. *Adsorpt. Sci. Technol.* 24: 337–347.

O'Connell, D.W., Birkinshaw, C., O'Dwyer, T.F. 2008. Heavy metal adsorbents prepared from the modification of cellulose: A review. *Bioresour. Technol.* 99: 6709–6724.

Okieimen, F.E., Sogbaike, C.E., Ebhoaye, J.E. 2005. Removal of cadmium and copper ions from aqueous solution with cellulose graft copolymers. *Sep. Purif. Technol.* 44: 85–89.

Park, J.Y., Kong, B., Chi, Y.S., Kim, Y.G., Choi, I.S. 2009. Aryl azide-based photografting of β-cyclodextrin onto cellulose diacetate fibers. *Bull. Korean Chem. Soc.* 30(8): 1851–1854.

Peng, L. 2007. A novel degradable adsorbent of the hyperbranched aliphatic polyester grafted cellulose for heavy metal ions. *Turk. J. Chem.* 31: 457–462.

Peng, Z., Chen, F. 2010. Synthesis and properties of temperature-sensitive hydrogel based on hydroxyethyl cellulose. *Int. J. Polym. Mat.* 59: 450–461.

Pourjavadi, A., Zohuriaan-Mehr, M.J., Ghasempoori, S.N., Hossienzadeh, H. 2007. Modified CMC. V. Synthesis and super-swelling behavior of hydrolyzed CMC-g-PAN hydrogel. *J. Appl. Polym. Sci.* 103: 877–883.

Rani, P., Mishra, S., Sen, G. 2013. Microwave based synthesis of polymethyl methacrylate grafted sodium alginate: Its application as flocculant. *Carbohydr. Polym.* 91: 686–692.

Roy, D., Knapp, J.S., Guthrie, J.T., Perrier, S. 2008. Antibacterial cellulose fiber via RAFT surface graft polymerization. *Biomacromolecules* 9(1): 91–99.

Roy, D., Semsarilar, M., Guthrie, J.T., Perrier, S. 2009. Cellulose modification by polymer grafting: A review. *Chem. Soc. Rev.* 38: 2046–2064.

Sahoo, P.K., Samantaray, H.S., Samal, R.K.1986. Graft copolymerization with new class of acidic peroxo salts as initiators. I. Grafting of acrylamide onto cotton-cellulose using potassium monopersulfate, catalyzed by Co(II). *J. Appl. Polym. Sci.* 32: 5693–5703.

Semsarilar, M., Ladmiral, V., Perrier, S. 2010. Synthesis of a cellulose supported chain transfer agent and its application to RAFT polymerization. *J. Polym. Sci. A: Polym. Chem.* 48: 4361–4365.

Shao, D., Jiang, Z., Wang, X., Li, J., Meng, Y. 2009. Plasma induced grafting carboxymethyl cellulose on multiwalled carbon nanotubes for the removal of UO_2^{2+} from aqueous solution. *J. Phys. Chem. B* 113(4): 860–864.

Sharma, B.R., Kumar, V., Soni, P.L. 2003. Graft copolymerization of acrylonitrile onto Cassia tora gum with ceric ammonium nitrate–nitric acid as a redox initiator. *J. Appl. Polym. Sci.* 90: 129–136.

Shen, D., Yu, H., Huang, Y. 2005. Densely grafting copolymers of ethyl cellulose through atom transfer radical polymerization. *J. Polym. Sci. A: Polym. Chem.* 43: 4099–4008.

Shen, D., Yu, H., Huang, Y. 2006. Synthesis of graft copolymer of ethyl cellulose through living polymerization and its self-assembly. *Cellulose* 13: 235–244.

Shi, X., Tan, L., Xing, J. et al. 2013. Synthesis of hydroxyethylcellulose-g-methoxypoly (ethylene glycol) copolymer and its application for protein separation in CE. *J. Appl. Polym. Sci.* 128(3): 1995–2002.

Shukla, S.K. 2012. Synthesis of polyaniline grafted cellulose suitable for humidity sensing. *Ind. J. Eng. Mater. Sci.* 19: 417–420.

Shukla, S.K. 2013. Synthesis and characterization of polypyrrole grafted cellulose for humidity sensing. *Int. J. Biol. Macromol.* 62: 531–536.
Singh, R.P., Tripathy, T., Biswal, D.R. 2001. High performance flocculating agent based on carboxymethyl cellulose and polyacrylamide. Patent Appl. No. 101/Cal/2001.
Stannett, V. 1981. Grafting. *Radiat. Phys. Chem.* 18: 215–222.
Stenzel, M.H., Davis, T.P. 2002. Star polymer synthesis using trithiocarbonate functional β-cyclodextrin cores (reversible addition–fragmentation chain-transfer polymerization). *J. Polym. Sci. A: Polym. Chem.* 40: 4498–4512.
Stenzel, M.H., Davis, T.P., Fane, A.G. 2003. Honey comb structured porous films prepared from carbohydrate based polymers synthesized via the RAFT process. *J. Mater. Chem.* 13: 2090–2097.
Sui, X., Yuan, J., Zhou, M. et al. 2008. Synthesis of cellulose-graft-poly(*N*,*N*-dimethylamino-2-ethyl methacrylate) copolymers via homogeneous ATRP and their aggregates in aqueous media. *Biomacromolecules* 9: 2615–2620.
Takashi, A., Juichi, H., Saburo, N. et al. 1972. A solution of a graft copolymer of cellulose. US 3669916 A, June 13, 1972.
Tang, X., Gao, L., Fan, X., Zhou, G. 2007. Controlled grafting of ethyl cellulose with azobenzene-containing polymethacrylates via atom transfer radical polymerization. *J. Polym. Sci. A: Polym. Chem.* 45: 1653–1660.
Tankhiwale, R., Bajpai, S.K. 2009. Graft copolymerization onto cellulose-based filter paper and its further development as silver nanoparticles loaded antibacterial food-packaging material. *Colloids Surf. B Biointerfaces* 69(2): 164–168.
Tizzotti, M., Charlot, A., Fleury, E., Stenzel, M., Bernard, J. 2010. Modification of polysaccharides through controlled/living radical polymerization grafting—Towards the generation of high performance hybrids. *J. Macromol. Rapid. Commun.* 31: 1751–1772.
Wang, D., Tan, J., Kang, H. et al. 2011. Synthesis, self-assembly and drug release behaviors of PH-responsive copolymers ethyl cellulose-graft-PDEAEMA through ATRP. *Carbohydr. Polym.* 84: 195–202.
Wang, L., Yongshen, X. 2006. γ-Radiation-induced graft copolymerization of ethyl acrylate onto hydroxypropyl methylcellulose. *Macromol. Mater. Eng.* 291: 950–961.
Wen, O.H., Kuroda, S.I., Kubota, H. 2001. Temperature-responsive character of acrylic acid and *N*-isopropylacrylamide binary monomers-grafted celluloses. *Eur. Polym. J.* 37: 807–813.
Wojnárovits, L., Földváry, Cs.M., Takács, E. 2010. Radiation-induced grafting of cellulose for adsorption of hazardous water pollutants: A review. *Radiat. Phys. Chem.* 79: 848–862.
Worthley, C.H. 2012. Thesis titled: Improving the performance of cellulose acetate reverse osmosis membranes. Flinders University Adelaide, Adelaide, South Australia, Australia.
Xie, J., Hsieh, Y.L. 2003. Thermosensitive poly(n-isopropylacrylamide) hydrogels bonded on cellulose supports. *J. Appl. Polym. Sci.* 89: 999–1006.
Xin, T.T., Yuan, T., Xiao, S., He, J. 2011. Synthesis of cellulose-graft-poly(methyl methacrylate) via homogeneous ATRP. *Bioresources* 6: 2941–2953.
Yan, L., Ishihara, K. 2008b. Graft copolymerization of 2-methacryloyloxy ethyl phosphorylcholine to cellulose in homogeneous media using atom transfer radical polymerization for providing new haemo compatible coating materials. *J. Polym. Sci. A: Polym. Chem.* 46: 3306–3313.
Yan, L., Tao, W. 2008a. Graft copolymerization of *N*,*N* dimethylacrylamide to cellulose in homogeneous media using atom transfer radical polymerization for hemocompatibility. *J. Biomed. Sci. Eng.* 1: 37–43.
Yan, Q., Yuan, J., Zhang, F. et al. 2009. Cellulose-based dual graft molecular brushes as potential drug nanocarriers: Stimulus-responsive micelles, self-assembled phase transition behavior, and tunable crystalline morphologies. *Biomacromolecules* 10: 2033–2042.
Yang, R., Liu, Y., Zheng, C. 2010. Synthesis of hydroxyethyl cellulose-graft-poly(*N*,*N*-dimethyl acrylamide) copolymer by ATRP and as dynamic coating in capillary electrophoresis. *J. Appl. Polym. Sci.* 116: 3468–3472.
Yang, R., Wang, Y., Zhou, D. 2007. Novel hydroxyethyl cellulose-graft-polyacrylamide copolymer for separation of double-stranded DNA fragments by CE. *Electrophoresis* 28: 3223–3231.
Yuan, J., Zhang, J., Zang, X., Shen, J., Lin, S. 2003. Improvement of blood compatibility on cellulose membrane surface by grafting betaines. *Colloids Surf. B: Biointerfaces* 30: 147–155.
Zhang, J., Yuan, J., Yuan, Y., Shen, J., Lin, S. 2003. Chemical modification of cellulose membranes with sulfoammonium zwitterionic vinyl monomer to improve hemocompatibility. *Colloids Surf. B: Biointerfaces* 30(3): 249–257.

Zhao, Y.-H., Wee, K.-H., Bai, R. 2010. A novel electrolyte-responsive membrane with tunable permeation selectivity for protein purification. *ACS Appl. Mater. Int.* 2: 203–211.

Zoppe, J.O., Habibi, Y., Rojas, O.J. et al. 2010. Poly(*N*-isopropylacrylamide) brushes grafted from cellulose nanocrystals via surface-initiated single-electron transfer living radical polymerization. *Biomacromolecules* 11: 2683–2691.

3 Preparation of Functional Polymer-Grafted Cellulose through Azide Alkyne Cycloaddition or C–C Cross-Coupling

Jusha Ma, Qinyuan Niu, and Wenhui Wu

CONTENTS

3.1 INTRODUCTION

As an abundant natural polymer, cellulose is widely distributed in every corner of the world; it is one of the most promising raw materials with its low cost and easy availability. In the past century, scientists have paid a great deal of attention to studying its physical and chemical properties[1] (i.e., mechanical properties, thermal properties, nanostructure, etc.). But it seems that the current applications of the cellulose still could not meet the growing needs of the community. Since a lot of years, researchers have made great effort to modify the structure of cellulose and to reinforce their physical or chemical properties, like dimension stability, resistance to abrasion and wear, and oil repellency,[2,3] but it was still insufficient. The reports of extending far beyond the traditional application areas of cellulose derivatives, such as ion detectors, biosensors, or electronic devices are quite limited. It is a great chance to pay attention to value-added cellulose derivatives.[4] Let us imagine that one day we could take a piece of paper out of our pocket instead of carrying heavy equipment to detect explosives, bacteria, quality of drinking water or the air, etc.; we could browse a magazine or watch a movie on just one piece of environmentally friendly paper. Those applications will have great possibility to be realized in the near future if we keep a research eye on functional polymer-grafted cellulose. And all those applications would easily benefit from the advantages of cheaper, lighter, flexible, and green cellulose substrate.

Cellulose-based materials have the potential as raw materials if functional groups could be effectively coupled onto them. And, in fact, the most convenient method is directly grafting certain chemical groups with optoelectronic or special geometry onto cellulose substrate through chemical reactions. Utilizing these "grafting-to" or "grafting-from" tech, we could easily endow cellulose derivatives with new functions.

As we know, there are many hydroxyl groups along the backbones, which can be considered as reactive handles. Based on these chemical handles, cellulose substrates could be modified with azide-, bromophenyl-, or alkyne-based "anchor points." Furthermore, utilizing these "anchor points," various kinds of special polymer-grafted celluloses could be obtained through C–C cross-coupling reaction or click chemistry. Those synthesized cross-linked cellulose, cellulose-based dendrimer, and cellulose polymer brushes showed additional properties to the cellulose-based raw materials. In addition, a batch of practical examples of corresponding cellulose derivatives for specific applications will be introduced. It provides a wide way to design and synthesize special functional celluloses, which would offer great promise.

3.2 PREPARATION OF CELLULOSE PRECURSOR WITH REACTIVE SIDE GROUPS

Each structural unit of cellulose molecules contains three hydroxyl groups: the hydroxyl groups at position-2 and position-3 act as secondary alcohols, while the hydroxyl group in position-6 behaves as a primary alcohol. Due to the great number of hydroxyl groups, cellulose is highly hydrophilic and often poorly compatible with many solvents. However, if we considered the OH groups as chemical handles, it is also a good candidate for various chemical reactions. Usually, the reactivity of these three hydroxyl groups is not the same, which is affected by their inherent chemical reactivity or by steric effects that are produced by the reaction reagents. In general, the relative reactivity of three positions of hydroxyl groups can be expressed as position-6 $\gg$ position-2 $>$ position-3. It can be explained by the much larger free degree of rotation of primary alcoholic group at position-6. Generally, the degree of substitution (DS) is used to indicate the average number of OH groups that have been substituted by other chemical groups or graft polymeric chains on the anhydroglucose unit of the cellulose molecule.

To the best of our knowledge, it is pretty hard to attach certain functional groups onto cellulose directly. Hence, preparing cellulose precursor with special reactive side groups is of significance. So the first step of synthesizing functional polymer-grafted cellulose is to activate the hydroxyl groups in cellulose molecules and to make a special "anchor" for certain functional groups. There are several chemical groups as candidates for the further functionalizations of cellulose molecules (see Scheme 3.1). Basically, we distinguish them into three major catalogs: there are azide end for "click reaction," alkyne groups for "click reaction" or Sonogashira reaction, and aromatic bromine end for Suzuki reaction or Heck reaction. The attachment of these reactive groups could provide the essential precursors that could meet the requirement of further connecting the various functional groups or branched polymer.

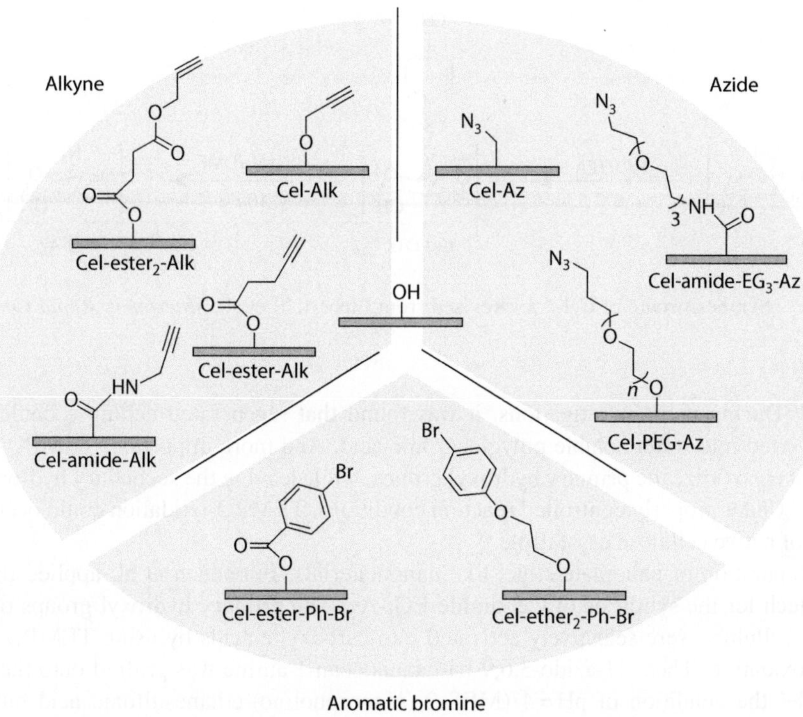

SCHEME 3.1 Cellulose precursors with different reactive groups.

3.2.1 Attachment of Azide Group

After Griess discovered organic azides in 1870, researchers showed a great interest in these energetic molecules. They designed and synthesized numerous azide derivatives. Fifty years ago, people found that except of their explosive properties, organic azides have been acted as valuable intermediates in organic syntheses. Thus, organic azides have been used in cycloadditions, in the syntheses of anilines and *N*-alkyl-substituted anilines, as well as precursors for syntheses of nitrenes. Nowadays, azide compounds are more famous for their participation in the "click reaction" and in Staudinger ligation. Because of reliability and mild condition of the reaction, the azide-group-based "click reactions" have been extended to the peptide chemistry, combinatorial chemistry, and heterocyclic syntheses.[5]

The simplest structure in this category is Cel-Az (Scheme 3.2). Liebert et al. first modified cellulose with azide moieties as the precursor for following copper-catalyzed Huisgen reaction. It was easily achieved by low-temperature tosylation of cellulose and subsequent nucleophilic displacement reaction. The IR spectrum of Cel-Az showed a significant signal at 2110 cm^{-1} typical of the azide moiety and complete disappearance of the aromatic bands of the tosyl functional groups at 1598, 1500, and 1453 cm^{-1}.[6] Elchinger group followed this synthesis route and successfully obtained the Cel-Az with a DS of 1.5 from tosyl cellulose.[7]

Another example of the introduction of azide moiety with much longer side chain is Cel-amide-EG_3-Az, synthesized by adopting TEMPO-tech and following connection of amide segment. In 1994, De Nooy et al. reported that the primary alcohol groups of carbohydrates could be selectively oxidized in aqueous media by using the 2,2,6,6-tetramethyl-1-piperidinyloxy (TEMPO) radical.[8,9] And in the following years, there were several successful samples on the modification of

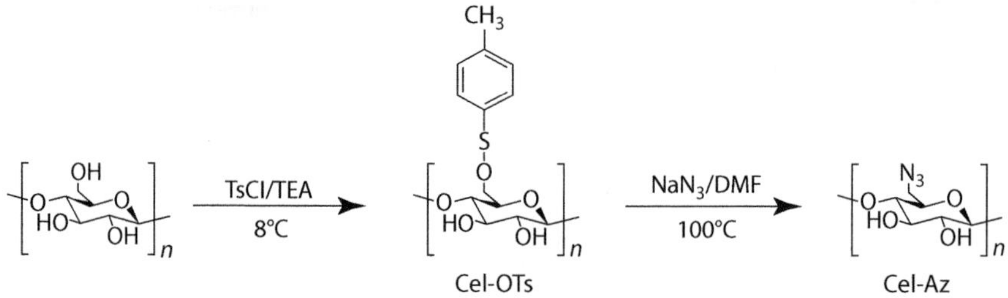

SCHEME 3.2 Synthesis route of Cel-Az. (Revised from Liebert, T. et al., *Macromol. Rapid Commun.*, 27, 208, 2006.)

cellulose.[10,11] During their investigations, it was found that regenerated cellulose could be completely converted into water-soluble polyglucuronic acid. And more important, TEMPO-oxidation could selectively oxidize the primary hydroxyl groups, while leaving the secondary hydroxyl groups unaffected.[12] Under properly controlled reaction conditions, TEMPO-oxidation could occur only on the surface of native cellulose crystalline.[13]

In the preparation of nanoplatelet-gel-like nanomaterials, Filpponen et al. applied the earlier-mentioned tech for the synthesis of Cel-amide-EG_3-Az. The primary hydroxyl groups on the surfaces of the cellulose were selectively activated into carboxylic acids by using TEMPO-mediated hypohalite oxidation. Then, 11-azido-3,6,9-tri-oxaundecan-1-amine was grafted onto the cellulose surface under the condition of pH=4 (MES 2-(*N*-morpholino)-ethanesulfonic acid buffer). The polydispersity index (PDI) of Cel-amide-EG_3-Az was 3.4 with the molecular weight of 53 kg mol^{-1} reported in the literature (Scheme 3.3).[14]

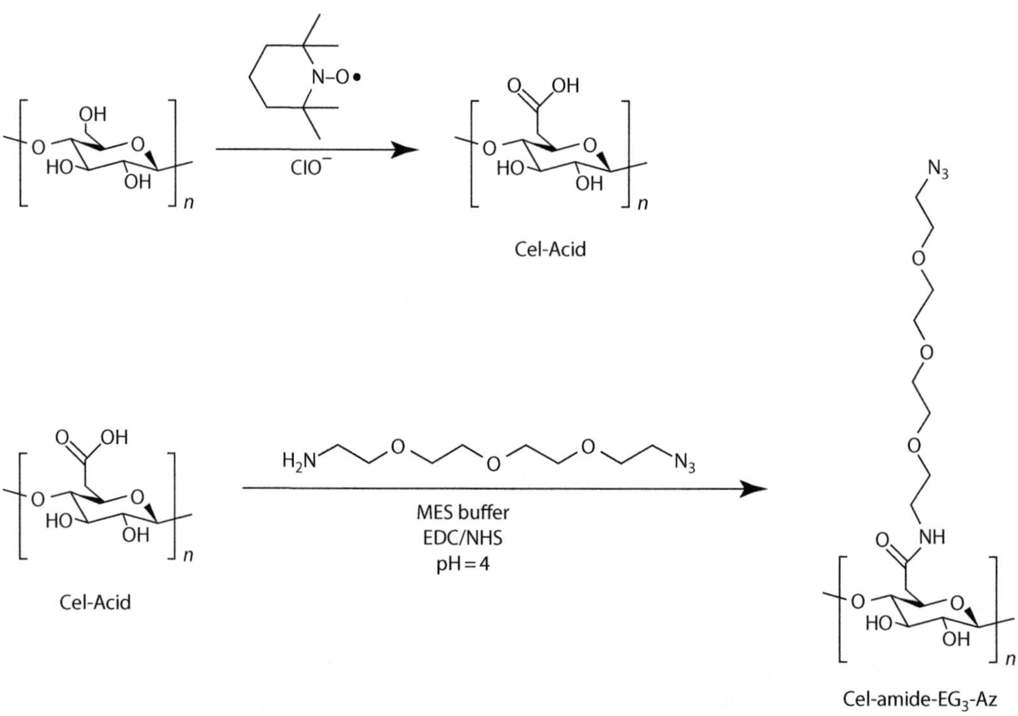

SCHEME 3.3 Synthesis route of Cel-amide-EG_3-Az. (Revised from Filpponen, I. and Argyropoulos, D.S., *Biomacromolecules*, 11, 2010, 1060.)

The third example of Cel-PEG-Az reported by Xu et al. was quite different from the last two. The azide moieties were attached to cellulose by the "grafting-to" methodology.[4] Then, pre-synthesized side chains with a controllable length were reacted onto the cellulose molecules. The reactive position of hydroxyl group at cellulose is also different from the last two examples; the azide moiety was attached on secondary hydroxyl group (position-3). From esterification studies, it has been found that the hydroxyl group at position-6 can react 10 times faster than the other two groups, and the hydroxyl group at position-2 has been observed to react twice as fast as the hydroxyl group at position-3. So after the first two occupied by (dimethylsiloxane) (DMS), the last one (position-3 of –OH group) will remain as reactive point.

The synthesis route of Cel-PEG-Az is shown in Scheme 3.4. Allyl-PEG-I was prepared from poly(ethylene-glycol) (PEG) via a three-step conversion. Accordingly, PEG was first protected by reacting allyl bromide with one of the EG hydroxyl groups to form allyloxypoly(ethylene-glycol). The second hydroxyl group was then converted to the corresponding tosylate, followed by further conversion to the iodide. Meanwhile, cellulose was modified by tridimethylsiloxane (TDMS). Because of the high reactivity, primary hydroxyl group (position-6) in cellulose will be first occupied by TDMS. A part of secondary hydroxyl group would also be reacted with TDMSCl, only leaving the hydroxyl group at position-3. The allyl-PEG-I was then reacted with regioselective TDMS-Cel to produce TDMS-Cel-PEG-Allyl. The terminal allyloxy group was subsequently oxidized to the corresponding hydroxypropoxy group and further converted to TDMS-Cel-PEG-chloride by reaction with tetrakis(triphenylphosphine)palladium (PPh_3) and tetrachloromethane (CCl_4). After reacting with NaN_3 in THF/DMA, the desirable product TDMS-Cel-PEG-Az cellulose was successfully synthesized.[15]

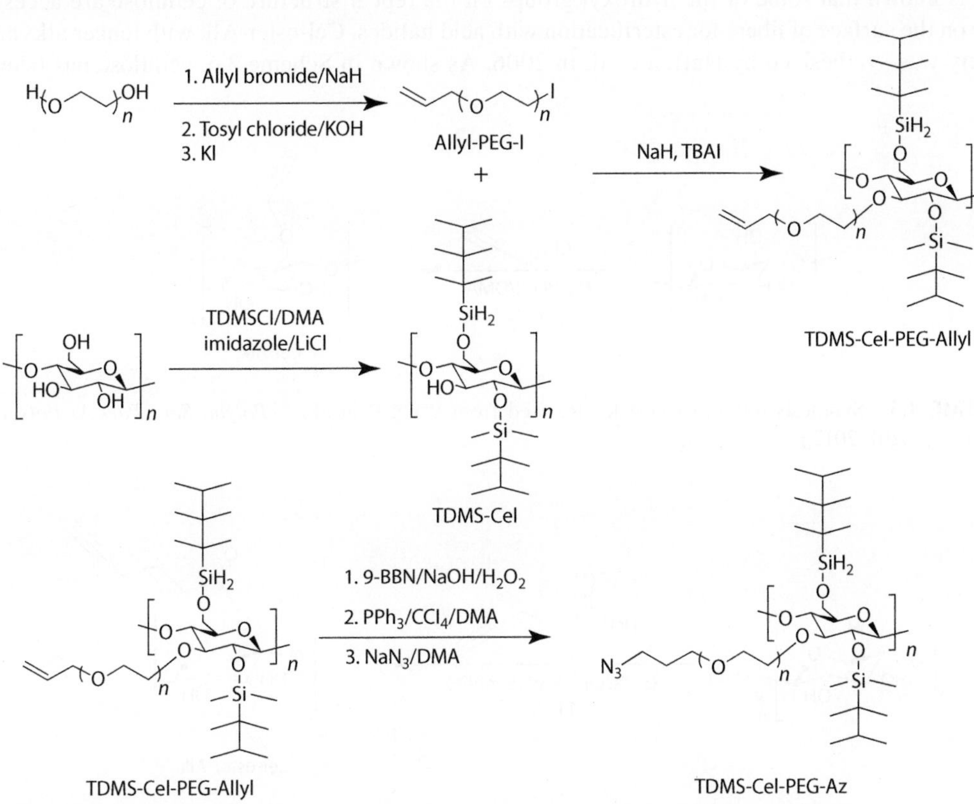

SCHEME 3.4 Synthesis route of TDMS-Cel-PEG-Az. (Revised from Xu, W.Z. et al., *Biomacromolecules*, 13, 350, 2011.)

3.2.2 Attachment of Alkyne Group

Terminal alkyne is an unsaturated hydrocarbon group with one C–C triple bond between two carbon atoms. Owing to the special structure of triple bond and the possibility of donating various numbers of electrons, chemists have been attracted to the syntheses and characterization of alkyne-derived molecules as well as studying the mechanism of the reaction. It is clear that the alkyne–ligand in molecules could offer a fascinating versatility by different coordination modes or directly participating in many organic reactions. Nowadays, the study efforts focused on more complex organic molecules such as larger conjugated molecules and the possible application to modify bioorganometallic molecules. The novel complexes were prepared involving groups such as dendrimers or pharmaceutically interesting molecules.[16] So introducing this special C–C triple bond could play an important role to provide the versatile "anchor" and further synthesize grafted cellulose copolymers.

Similar as the case of Cel-Az, the simplest structure in this category is Cel-Alk (Scheme 3.5) in which the alkyne group was directly attached onto cellulose. In the work of Peng group,[17] bamboo cellulose was propargylated with propargyl chloride (PgCl) using NaH in DMA/LiCl, as shown in Scheme 3.5. In their paper, they reported the investigation of reaction condition in detail. When adjusting the reaction parameter, the DS and yields of Pg-CE were 0.25–1.24 and 75.2%–89.8%, respectively. Clearly, an increase in the molar ratio of PgCl/anhydrous glucose unit (AGU) from 1:1 to 9:1 resulted in an increase in the DS of Cel-Alk from 0.32 to 0.87. Increasing the temperature from 20°C to 40°C would cause an increase in the DS from 0.72 to 0.97. And changing the molar ratio of NaH/AGU from 3:1 to 5:1 also promoted the etherification of cellulose, resulting in the DS value up to a maximum at 1.24.

It is known that some of the hydroxyl groups on the repeat structure of cellulose are accessible on the surface of fibers for esterification with acid halides. Cel-ester-Alk with longer alkyne moiety was synthesized by Hafrén et al. in 2006. As shown in Scheme 3.6, cellulose has been

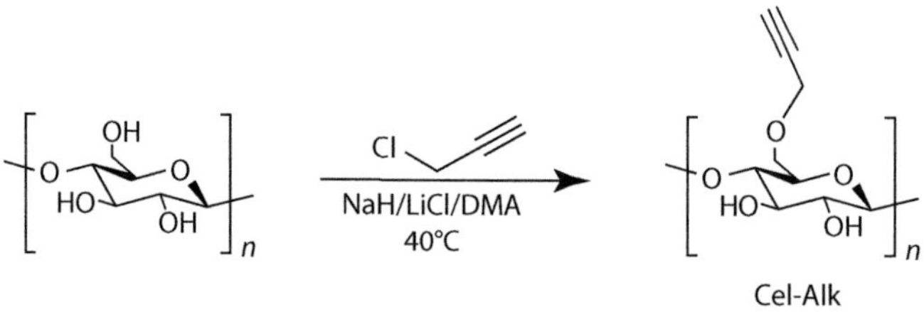

SCHEME 3.5 Synthesis route of Cel-Alk. (Revised from Peng, P. et al., *J. Polym. Sci., Part A: Polym. Chem.*, 50, 5201, 2012.)

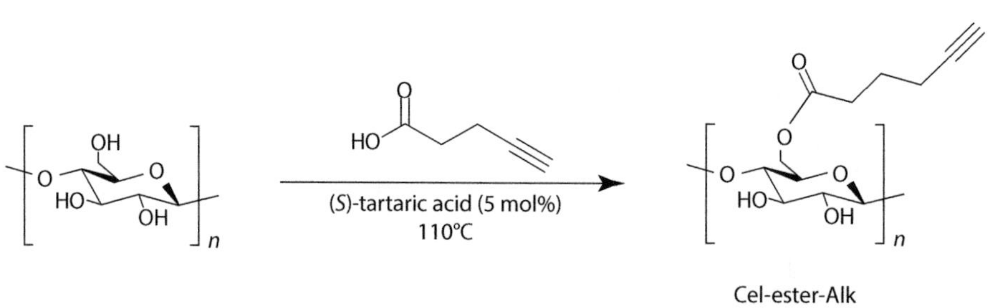

SCHEME 3.6 Synthesis route of Cel-ester-Alk. (Revised from Hafrén, J. et al., *Macromol. Rapid Commun.*, 27, 1362, 2006.)

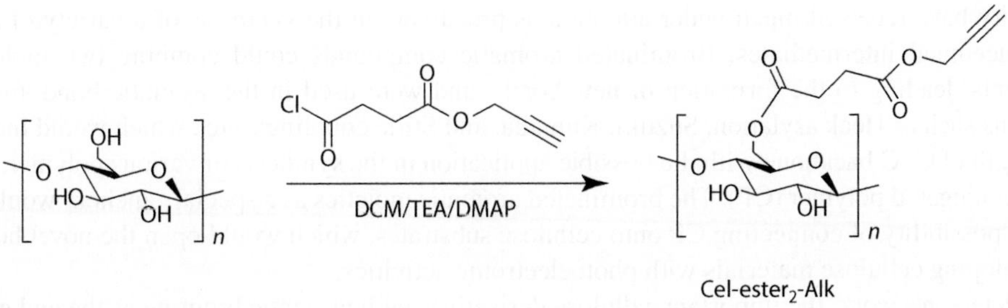

SCHEME 3.7 Synthesis route of Cel-ester$_2$-Alk. (Revised from Peterson, J.J. et al., *J. Polym. Sci., Part A: Polym. Chem.*, 49, 3004, 2011.)

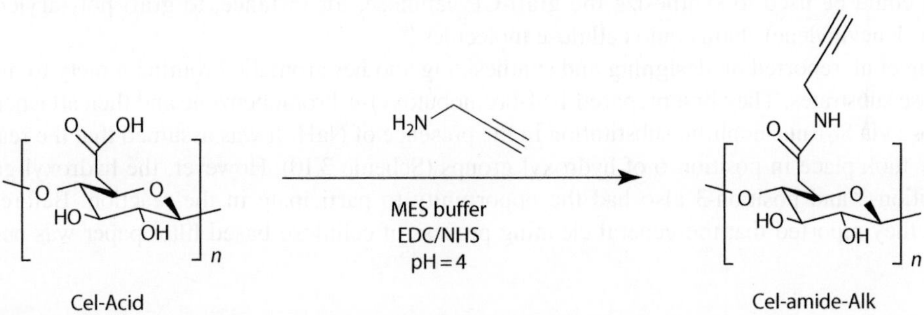

SCHEME 3.8 Synthesis route of Cel-amide-Alk. (Revised from Filpponen, I. and Argyropoulos, D.S., *Biomacromolecules*, 11, 2010, 1060.)

reacted with 5-hexynoic acid in the presence of a catalytic amount of (*S*)-tartaric acid. FT-IR analysis of the produced Cel-ester-Alk revealed a clear absorbance peak at 1730 cm^{-1} from the ester group, which indicated that the esterification successfully occurred. But no absorbance peak was observed for the sample from the blank reaction between cellulose and 5-hexynoic acid without the addition of tartaric acid catalyst.[18] So, tartaric acid catalyst is a necessary reagent for this reaction.

Peterson et al. also made a simple one-step reaction to synthesize Cel-ester$_2$-Alk with long alkyne moiety (Scheme 3.7). In their reaction, organic acid catalyst was not necessary; they chose much stronger acid (acid chloride) as reagent and used 4-(dimethylamino)pyridine (DMPA) as catalyst. After adding cellulose substrate into the solution of prop-2-ynyl-4-chloro-4-oxobutanoate with dichloromethane (DCM) and triethylamine (TEA), Cel-ester$_2$-Alk was successfully prepared.[19]

Another contribution from Filpponen et al.[14] was the preparation of Cel-amide-Alk (Scheme 3.8). They made use of TEMPO-mediated hypohalite oxidation, and the reaction routine is similar to the preparation of Cel-amide-Az. The PDI of Cel-amide-Alk was 3.5 with the molecular weight of 72 kg mol^{-1}.

3.2.3 Attachment of Aromatic Bromine Group

Halogenation of aromatic compounds is one of the significant reactions in organic synthesis. The most commonly used reagents for this purpose are bromine and chlorine in the presence of iron halide. Compared with chlorinated aromatic, brominated aromatic compounds with stronger reactivity have received much wider attention as precursors in the synthesis of a variety of active pharmaceutical intermediates. Brominated aromatic compounds could combine two molecular fragments, leading to the formation of new bonds, and were used in the aromatic bond–forming reactions such as Heck arylation, Suzuki, Kumada, and Stille couplings, etc., which would increase the length of C–C backbone with the possible application in the synthesis of various polymer, especially conjugated polymer (CP). The brominated aromatic moieties as a special "anchor" would create the possibility of connecting CP onto cellulose substrates, which would open the novel horizon of developing cellulose materials with photoelectronic activities.

In Peterson's work, the important cellulose derivatives with aromatic bromine as the end groups on the side chain were also designed and successfully synthesized (Cel-ester-Ph-Br), as shown in Scheme 3.9. The celluloses were reacted with 4-bromobenzoyl chloride in a solution of DCM/TEA, and a catalytic amount of DMPA via esterification, resulting in a chemically modified cellulose with bromo-phenyl groups. Furthermore, this work demonstrated that "grafting-from" techniques could be used to synthesize the graft-CP cellulose, for instance, to graft poly(arylene) or poly(arylenevinylene) chains onto cellulose molecules.[19]

Leng et al. reported on designing and synthesizing another aromatic bromine moiety to modify cellulose substrates. They first prepared 1-(4-bromobutoxy)-4-bromobenzene and then attached it to cellulose via S_N1 nucleophilic substitution in the presence of NaH. It was assumed that the reaction mainly took place in position-6 of hydroxyl groups (Scheme 3.10). However, the hydroxyl groups at position-2 and position-3 also had the opportunity to participate in the reaction. Before synthesis, they reported that the general cleaning process of cellulose-based filter paper was needed.

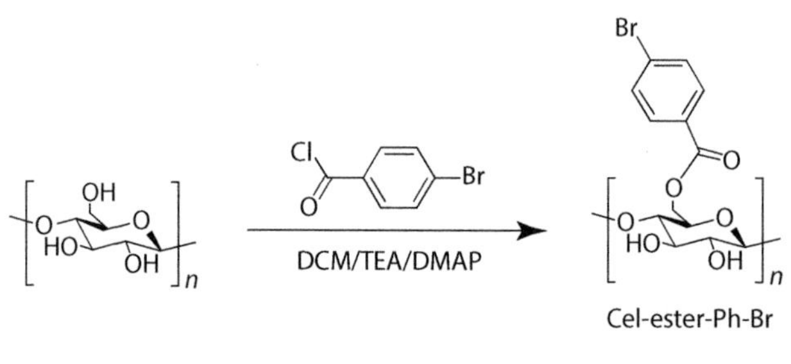

SCHEME 3.9 Synthesis route of Cel-ester-Ph-Br. (Revised from Peterson, J.J. et al., *J. Polym. Sci., Part A: Polym. Chem.*, 49, 3004, 2011.)

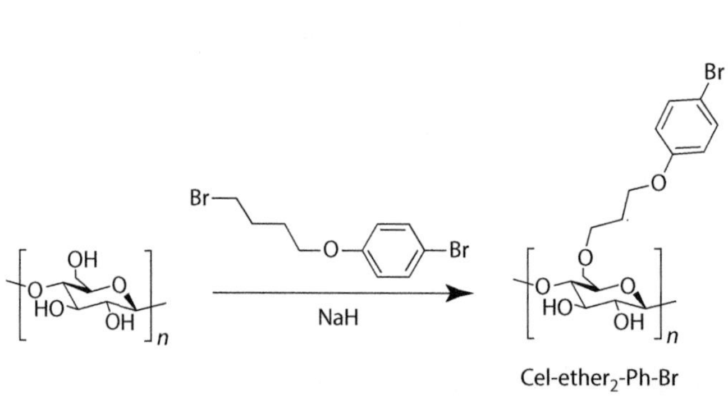

SCHEME 3.10 Synthesis route of Cel-ether$_2$-Ph-Br. (Revised from Leng, H. and Wu, W., *Imaging Sci. Photochem.*, 30, 251, 2012.)

The cellulose papers were washed by sulfuric acid solution, NaOH solution, EtOH, and distilled water, respectively, in order to remove the impurities adsorbed on the filter paper.[20]

3.3 PREPARATION OF CROSS-LINKED CELLULOSE, CELLULOSE-BASED DENDRIMER, AND CELLULOSE POLYMER BRUSHES

After cellulose precursor with reactive side groups was prepared, chemists could further synthesize the cellulose-based copolymer by azide alkyne cycloaddition or typical C–C cross-coupling reaction.

The azide alkyne cycloaddition is well known as "click chemistry," which is a powerful synthetic method with highly reliable and selective features that was developed by Sharpless et al. in 2001.[21] The 1,3-dipolar cycloaddition of an azide moiety and a triple bond (Huisgen reaction) has become the most popular "click reaction" to date.[22,23] The advantage of this reaction is experimentally simple: needing no protection from oxygen, generating almost no by-product, and requiring only stoichiometric amounts of starting materials. The nearly quantitative yields of these conversions perfectly fit the requirements of polymer-grafted cellulose.

Regarding the C–C cross-coupling reactions, there are typical organic chain growth reactions including famous Heck reaction, Suzuki coupling reaction, and Sonogashira coupling reaction. The Noble Prize of chemistry in 2010 was awarded to Heck and Suzuki, showing the significance of their research work. These famous name reactions possess many advantages for syntheses of polymer-grafted cellulose. For instance, the reaction would occur under mild reaction condition, there is the tolerance of a wide variety of function groups in the starting materials, and the unsensitivities for water or moisture. More importantly, through the coupling reaction, stereospecific features could be remained.[24]

With those significant reactions, we are able to further functionalize cellulose precursor. The functionalization of those reactive side groups will offer us various types of copolymer, typically, cross-linked polymer, dendrimer, or polymer brushes. Compared with simple physical mixture between cellulose and functional materials, grafting copolymer shows much better stability both in uniformity and in thermodynamics. Owing to random attachment of functional groups on cellulose molecules by covalent bond, functional points uniformly dispersed in nanoscale along the backbones. Cross-linked cellulose, cellulose-based dendrimer, and cellulose polymer brushes have different spatial features that would lead different physical and chemical properties, thus have the potential applications in many fields.

3.3.1 CROSS-LINKED CELLULOSE

In 2010, Filpponen et al. described the preparation of nanoplatelet gel-like nanomaterials by using cellulose nanocrystals as the starting material. They prepared grafted amine compounds that contained either terminated alkyne or terminated azide (Cel-amide-Alk or azide Cel-amide-EG_3-Az) functionalities as two sets of precursors on cellulose. Then, two parts were connected together via "click chemistry" to form Cel-click-Cel (L) (Scheme 3.11). The three-dimensional networks were created without using traditional cross-linking reactions where usually a bifunctional spacer molecule was required. Thus, the cross-linking process was well controlled without forming any intrachain. The nanoplatelet was investigated in detail by transmission electron microscopy. Interestingly, the resulting linked nanocrystals have not grown in one dimension as one would have anticipated from considering the activated position-6.[14]

In 2012, Zerrouki et al. reported a similar work, where they prepared the cross-linked cellulose from the precursor (Cel-Alk and Cel-Az) with the much shorter active side groups (Scheme 3.12). It means that we are able to adjust the inner space of cross-linked cellulose to some extent. It might

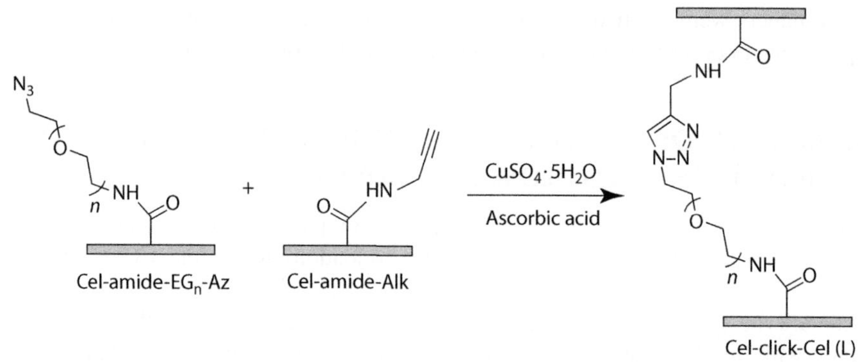

SCHEME 3.11 Synthesis route of Cel-click-Cel(L). (Revised from Filpponen, I. and Argyropoulos, D.S., *Biomacromolecules*, 11, 2010, 1060.)

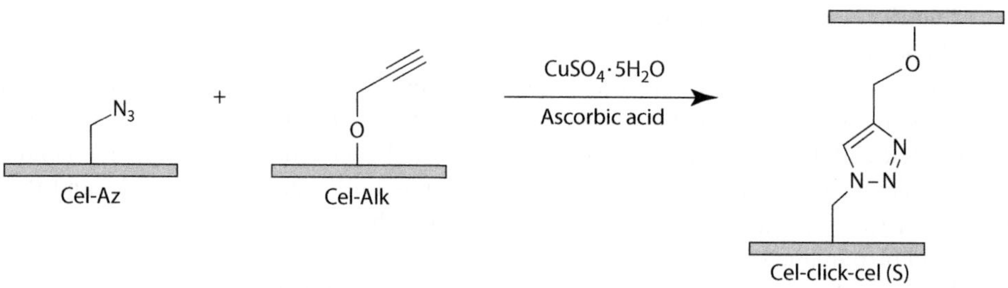

SCHEME 3.12 Synthesis route of Cel-click-Cel(S).

lead to certain effect on crystal ability or other physical properties, which have colligative properties with the pore size of polymer three-dimensional networks. To highlight the differences between functionalized celluloses and cross-linked ones, morphologies of samples were investigated by scanning electron microscopy. Both Cel-Alk and Cel-Az samples showed less uniform than the initial microcrystalline cellulose, and the resultant Cel-click-Cel (S) looked quite different from modified cellulose substrates. And the porous appearance of this materials indicated that a network with the apparent continuity of matter was created.[7,25]

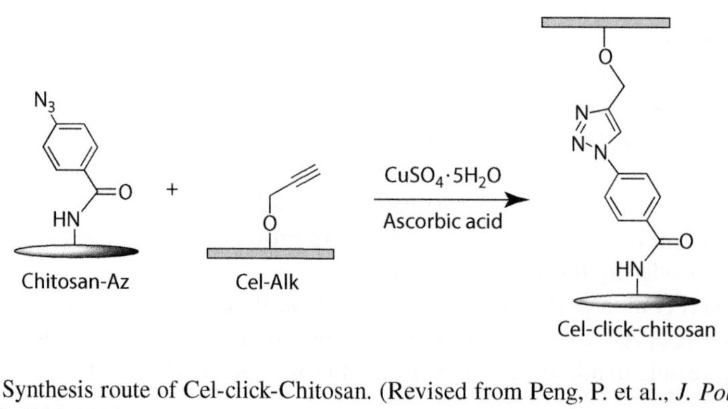

SCHEME 3.13 Synthesis route of Cel-click-Chitosan. (Revised from Peng, P. et al., *J. Polym. Sci., Part A: Polym. Chem.*, 50, 5201, 2012.)

In 2012, Peng et al. first prepared a novel cellulose-click-chitosan polymer. They chose Cel-Alk and the azido-functionalized chitosan, and obtained cellulose-click-chitosan polymer via the one-step alkyne–azide click reaction in the presence of Cu(I) (Scheme 3.13). Moreover, thermal gravimetric analysis results indicated that the cellulose-click-chitosan polymer had a higher thermal stability than that of cellulose and chitosan as well as cellulose–chitosan complex.[17] The onset degradation temperature (at the 5% weight loss) of cellulose, chitosan, mixture, and cellulose-click-chitosan were observed at 244°C, 87°C, 223°C, and 260°C, respectively. They explained the possible reason of low-onset degradation temperature of chitosan by the water present in chitosan. And the decomposition temperature occurred at 342°C, 346°C, 332°C, and 355°C (at 50% weight loss), respectively. These results indicated that chemically modified cellulose (Cel-click-Chitosan) not only showed better thermal behavior than that of its parent polymers (cellulose and chitosan) but also their complex.

3.3.2 Cellulose-Based Dendrimer

In 2008, Pohl et al. first attached dendrimer structure onto cellulose. The dendronized cellulose was synthesized by the conversion of Cel-Az cellulose (DS 0.75) with polyamidoamine (PAMAM) dendrons via the copper-catalyzed Huisgen reaction under mild conditions (homogeneously in dimethyl sulfoxide or heterogeneously in methanol) (Scheme 3.14). They successfully prepared first to third generations of cellulose derivatives Cel-PAMAM with DS values of up to 0.69. Because of the presence of large number of ester end group, this cellulose-based dendrimer could even be soluble in water. Furthermore, based on the characterization results, they claimed that there were no impurities in their products, and even no conversion occurred at the secondary positions (position-2 and position-3) of hydroxyl groups in cellulose.[26,27]

Another example worth to mention is Li group's work in 2013. They deigned and synthesized an amphiphilic peptide dendron-jacketed dextran polymer (Scheme 3.15). The alkyne-functionalized

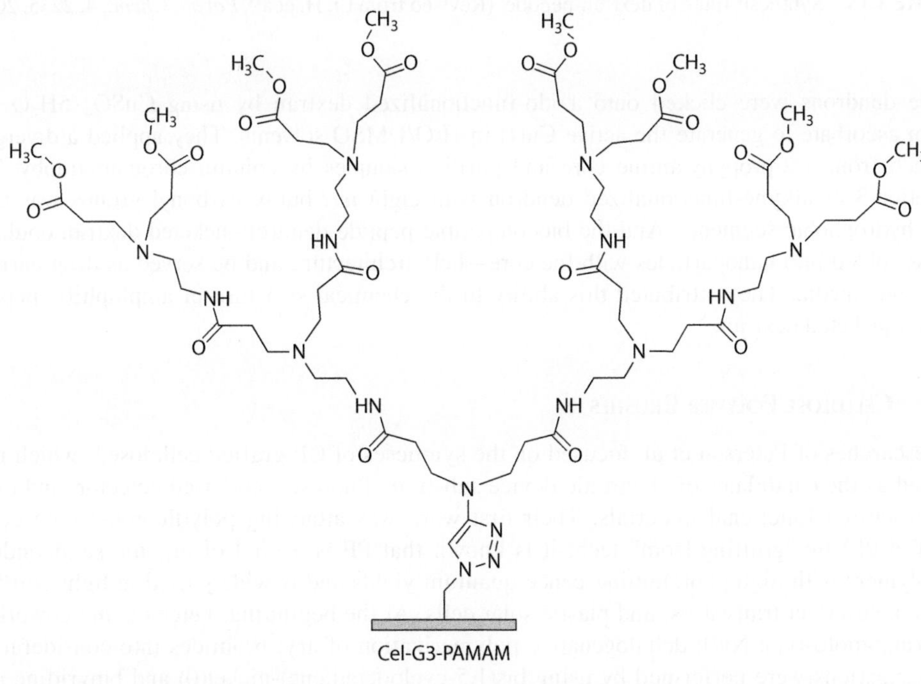

SCHEME 3.14 Synthesis route of Cel-G3-PAMAM. (Revised from Pohl, M. et al., *Macromol. Rapid Commun.*, 29, 142, 2008.)

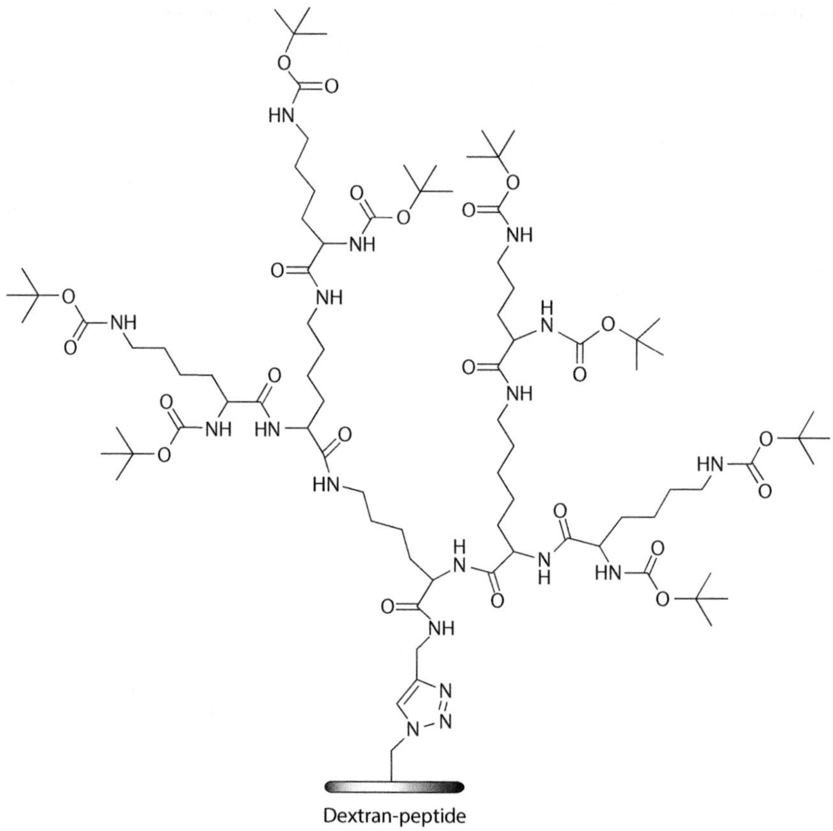

SCHEME 3.15 Synthesis route of dextran-peptide. (Revised from Li, H. et al., *Polym. Chem.*, 4, 2235, 2013.)

peptide dendrons were clicked onto azido-functionalized dextran by using $CuSO_4 \cdot 5H_2O$ and sodium ascorbate to generate the active Cu(I) in H_2O/DMSO solvents. They applied a divergent approach from a 2-propynylamine core and purified samples by column chromatography. The generation-3 of alkyne-functionalized dendron with eight *tert*-butoxycarbonyl groups was used as the hydrophobic segments. And the biocompatible peptide dendron-jacketed dextran could be self-assembled into nanoparticles with the core–shell architecture and be served as drug carriers in aqueous media. They attributed this ability to the chemical structure of amphiphilic peptide dendron-jacketed dextran.[28]

3.3.3 Cellulose Polymer Brushes

The researches of Peterson et al. focused on the syntheses of CP-grafted cellulose,[19] which may be acted as the candidates of electronic device substrate, fluorescence-based detector, and other nanostructured functional materials. Their first work was attaching poly(fluorene) onto cellulose (Cel-PF) by "grafting-from" tech; it is known that PF is a kind of organic semiconducting polymers with high photoluminescence quantum yields and is widely used in light-emitting diodes, field-effect transistors, and plastic solar cells. At the beginning, Peterson and coworkers took Yamamoto-type Ni(0) dehalogenative polymerization of aryl bromides into consideration. Polymerizations were performed by using bis(1,5-cyclooctadiene)-nickel(0) and bipyridine as a ligand to promote reductive elimination (Scheme 3.16a, upper). However, while the Ni(0) methods are generally robust and produce polymer reliably, the samples with Ni(0) appeared almost

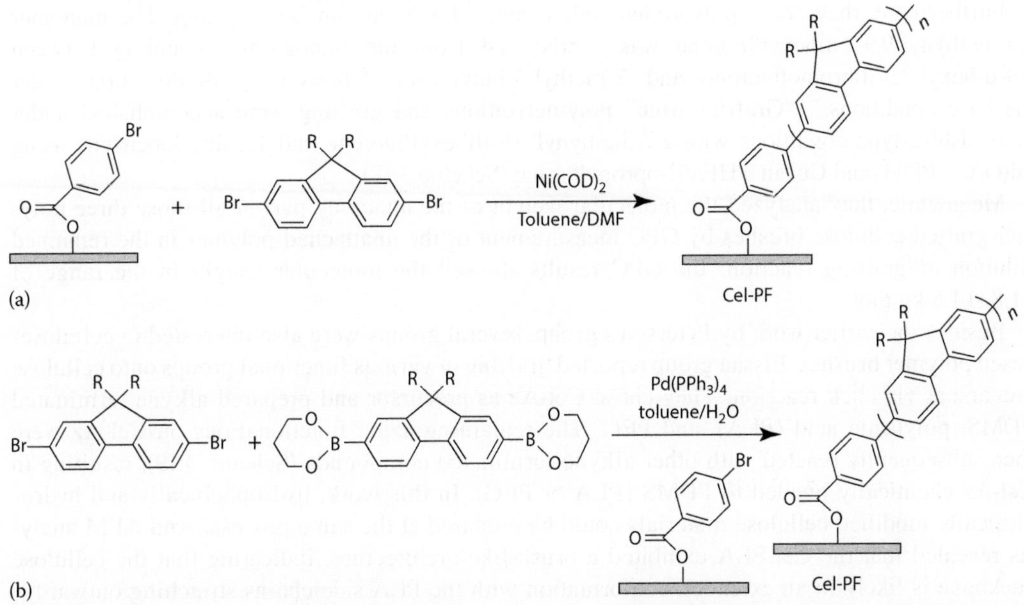

SCHEME 3.16 Two synthesis routes of Cel-PF. (a) Ni(0) dehalogenative grafting route to poly(fluorene). (b) Grafting poly(fluorene) via Suzuki polymerization. (From Peterson, J.J. et al., *J. Polym. Sci., Part A: Polym. Chem.*, 49, 3004, 2011.)

completely black after grafting polymerization and could not be easily cleaned or characterized. The impurity might affect the application of Cel-PF. Then, they changed the synthesis routine to Suzuki-coupling-based polymerization. Grafting of PF was performed via a typical Suzuki coupling polymerization of 9,9-dihexyl-2,7-dibromofluorene and 9,9-dihexylfluorene-2,7-diboronic acid bis(1,3-propanediol) ester using $Pd(PPh_3)_4$ as the catalyst (Scheme 3.16a, down). And in this reaction, by using microwave heating setup, the damage of cellulose paper was avoided. Compared with Ni(0) methods, the post-treatment of products is much easier when $Pd(PPh_3)_4$ catalyst was used.

Under typical Heck coupling conditions, they also successfully grafted poly(fluorenevinylene) onto cellulose substrate by using $Pd(OAc)_2$ and tri-*o*-tolylphosphine in dimethylformamide (DMF)/TEA (Scheme 3.17). Microwave heating was not observed to affect an exponential decrease in the time necessary to reach high microwave in this particular case.

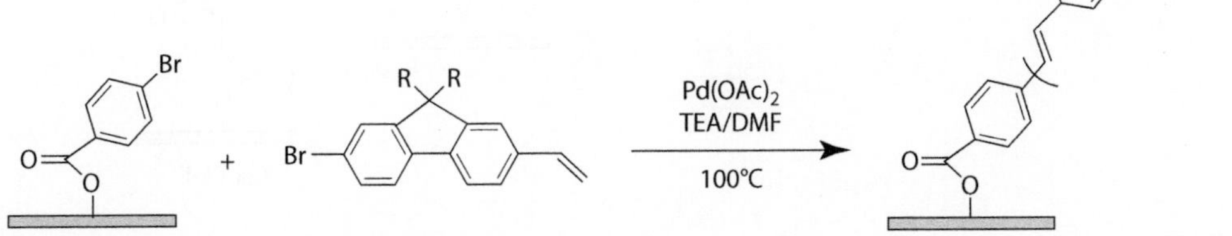

SCHEME 3.17 Synthesis route of Cel-poly(fluorenevinylene). (From Peterson, J.J. et al., *J. Polym. Sci., Part A: Polym. Chem.*, 49, 3004, 2011.)

Furthermore, they chose poly(arylene-ethynylene) (PArE) as functional group. The monomer 2,7-diethynyl-9,9- dihexylfluorene was synthesized from the Sonogashira coupling between 9,9-dihexyl-2,7-dibromofluorene and 2-methyl-3-butyn-2-ol, followed by deprotection under the base conditions.[29] "Grafting-from" polymerizations and grafting were accomplished under Sonogashira-type conditions with 2,7-diethynyl-9,9-dihexylfluorene and 1,4-diiodobenzene using Pd(OAc), PPh3, and CuI in THF/diisopropylamine (Scheme 3.18).

Meanwhile, they analyzed the molecular weight of the attaching part of all those three polymer-grafted cellulose brushes by GPC measurement of the unattached polymer in the remained solution of grafting reaction; the GPC results showed the molecular weight in the range of 11.8–14.5 kg mol^{-1}.

Besides the earlier work by Peterson's group, several groups were also interested in cellulose-based polymer brushes. Eissaa group reported grafting of various functional groups onto cellulose precursors via click reaction. They chose Cel-Az as precursor and prepared alkyne-terminated PDMS, polylactic acid (PLA), and PEG. The remaining azide functionalities on Cel-Az were then subsequently reacted with other alkyne-terminated compounds (Scheme 3.19), resulting in Cel-Az chemically bonded to PDMS (PLA or PEG). In this work, hydrophobically and hydrophilically modified cellulose materials could be prepared at the same process. And AFM analysis revealed that the Cel-PLA exhibited a brush-like architecture, indicating that the cellulose backbone is likely in an extended conformation with the PLA side chains stretching outward.[30] They expected the polymer-grafted cellulose to have some useful applications in personal care or cosmetics industries.

Koschella et al. developed novel bifunctional cellulose-based polyelectrolytes by the reactions of Cel-Az with acetylenedicarboxylic acid dimethyl ester via 1,3-dipolar cycloaddition reaction. They chose a route via the reaction of Cel-Az with acetylenedicarboxylic acid dimethyl ester and successfully obtained 6-deoxy-6-[1-triazolo-4,5-dicarboxylic acid dimethyl ester]cellulose. Then, the cellulose derivative was saponified with aqueous sodium hydroxide to get sodium Cel-dicarboxylic-acid

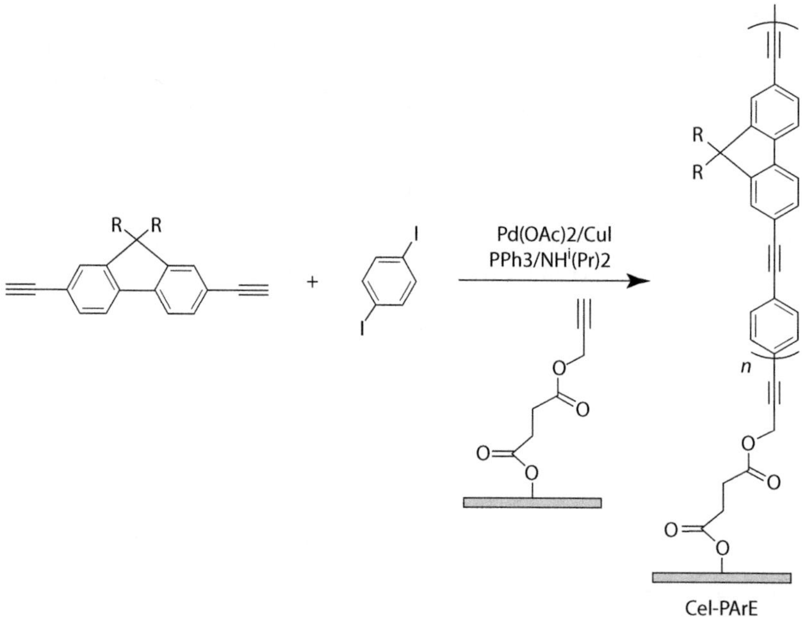

SCHEME 3.18 Synthesis route of Cel-PArE. (Revised from Peterson, J.J. et al., *J. Polym. Sci., Part A: Polym. Chem.*, 49, 3004, 2011.)

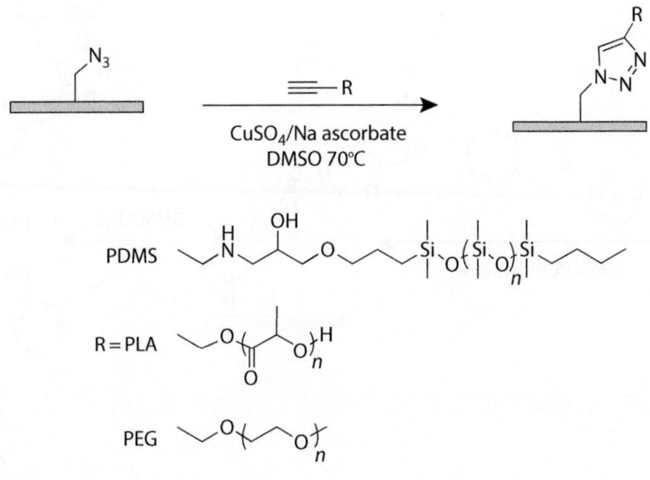

SCHEME 3.19 Synthesis route of Cel-PDMS, Cel-PLA, and Cel-PEG. (Revised from Eissa, A.M. et al., *Carbohydr. Polym.*, 90, 859, 2012.)

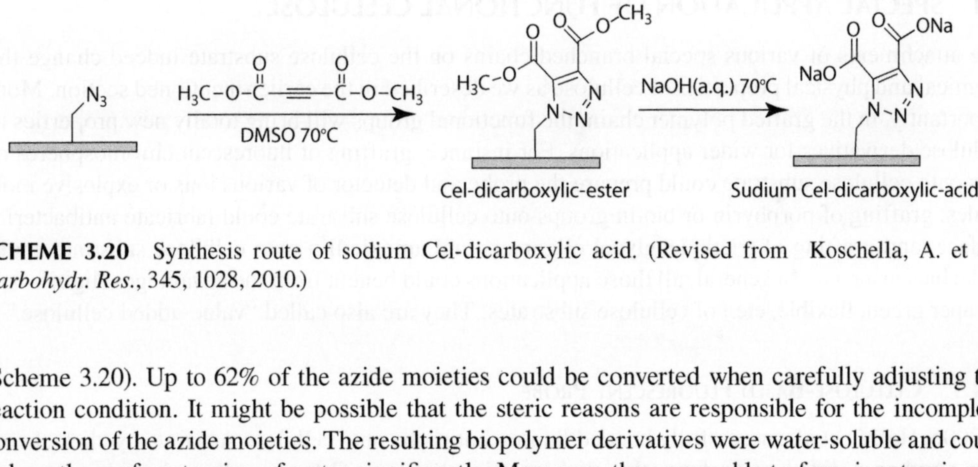

SCHEME 3.20 Synthesis route of sodium Cel-dicarboxylic acid. (Revised from Koschella, A. et al., *Carbohydr. Res.*, 345, 1028, 2010.)

(Scheme 3.20). Up to 62% of the azide moieties could be converted when carefully adjusting the reaction condition. It might be possible that the steric reasons are responsible for the incomplete conversion of the azide moieties. The resulting biopolymer derivatives were water-soluble and could reduce the surface tension of water significantly. Moreover, they were able to form ionotropic gels with multivalent metal ions. They realized the research objective to obtain polyelectrolyte-bearing bifunctional anionic moieties based on acetylenedicarboxylic acid selectively bound to position-6 of the modified anhydroglucose unit.[31]

There is a special example with the combination between cellulose-based polymer brushes and cross-linked cellulose. In 2011, Agag et al. developed side-chain-type benzoxazine-functional celluloses via a reaction of ethynyl-monofunctional benzoxazine monomer with azide-functional cellulose (Scheme 3.21). And they further cross-linked this cellulose-based polymer brushes. Interestingly, the cross-linking reaction of the benzoxazine side chain unusually took place at low temperatures in comparison to that of an ordinary benzoxazine resins. Upon cross-linking, the char yield of the modified cellulose showed a drastic increase in comparison with the unmodified cellulose. The unmodified cellulose was abruptly degraded around 320°C–360°C with the char yield of 4% at 800°C. This very narrow temperature range of degradation and nearly negligible char yield were related to the higher flammability. In contrast, the benzoxazine-modified cellulose showed broader decomposition temperature range from 270°C to 500°C with a higher char yield of 44%.[32]

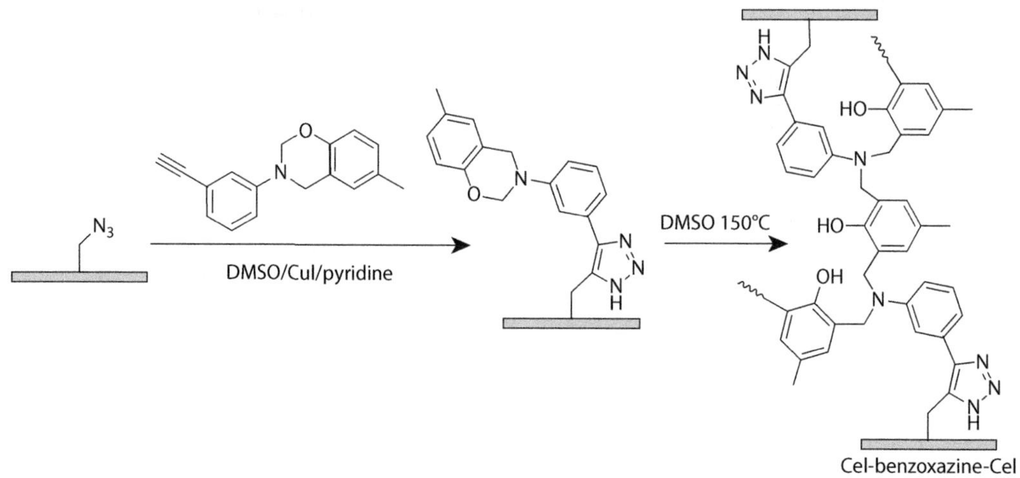

SCHEME 3.21 Synthesis route of Cel-benzoxazine-Cel. (From Agag, T. et al., *J. Appl. Polym. Sci.*, 125, 1346, 2012.)

3.4 SPECIAL APPLICATION OF FUNCTIONAL CELLULOSE

The attachments of various special branched chains on the cellulose substrate indeed change the chemical and physical properties of cellulose as we described in the earlier-mentioned section. More importantly, in the grafted polymer chain, the functional groups will bring totally new properties to cellulose derivatives for wider applications. For instance, grafting of fluorescent chromospheres or CPs onto cellulose substrate could prepare the probe and detector of various ions or explosive molecules; grafting of porphyrin or biotin groups onto cellulose substrate could fabricate antibacterial surface, and grafting of triethylenglycol oligomers and amoxicillin onto cellulose substrate could make biosensor, etc. In general, all those applications could benefit from the advantages (lighter and cheaper green, flexible, etc.) of cellulose substrates. They are also called "value-added cellulose."

3.4.1 Cellulose-Based Fluorescent Probe

In 2006, Hafrén et al. successfully bonded fluorescent probe onto cellulose substrate by click chemistry. Author decided to perform the click reaction between Cel-ester-Alk and azidocoumarin,

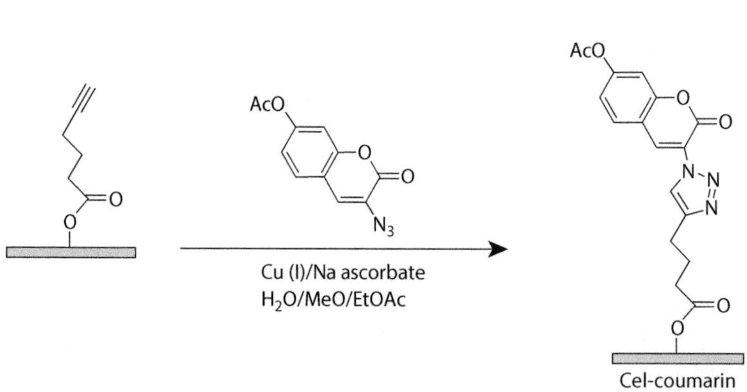

SCHEME 3.22 Synthesis route of Cel-coumarin. (Revised from Hafrén, J. et al., *Macromol. Rapid Commun.*, 27, 1362, 2006.)

expecting that the nonfluorescent azidocoumarin would form an intensely fluorescent 1,2,3-triazole product (Cel-coumarin in Scheme 3.22) upon Cu(I)-catalyzed 1,3-dipolar cycloaddition reactions with terminal alkyne cellulose. As seen in fluorescence photomicrograph, the corresponding Cel-coumarin product showed high fluorescence, and a successful derivatization was clearly demonstrated.

The reaction between Cel-ester-Alk and azidocoumarin was under mild reaction conditions in aqueous media.[18]

This environmentally friendly "organoclick" heterogeneous methodology should also be applicable to various cellulosic substrates, such as cotton and other wood fiber materials. These cellulosic materials will take an important role for the preparation of novel composite printing paper and textiles.

3.4.2 Cellulose-Based Detector

Yang et al. designed and prepared a rhodamine B–attached cellulose chemodosimeter, which could detect Hg^{2+} by sensitive reactions between Hg^{2+} and rhodamine B filter paper (Scheme 3.23). It is known that traditional method of Hg^{2+} detection needs expensive instruments like atomic absorption spectroscopy or inductively coupled plasma mass spectrometry. Furthermore, complex sample preparations and highly trained person are also necessary. Yang and coworkers took advantage of rhodamine-based fluorescent chemodosimeters for Hg^{2+} detection, which was based upon the principle of fluorescence enhancement (turn-on). The sensing property to Hg^{2+} of rhodamine B–attached cellulose paper was investigated by fluorescence spectroscopy. The color changing of the modified cellulose paper immersing in the solution containing Hg^{2+} can even be discerned by a naked eye under the irradiation of 365 nm UV light. The Hg^{2+} indicating paper displayed excellent selective detection toward Hg^{2+}, which would not be interfered by other heavy metal ions. These results suggested that the rhodamine B–grafted cellulose paper would be used as a practical fluorescent chemodosimeter for rapid and convenience detection of Hg^{2+}.[33]

The security of societies has been always an important issue for all of the world. Hongfei et al. developed a portable cellulose paper censor for detecting the explosives. They grafted conjugated functional polymer onto cellulose paper, which would generate a fluorescence response to nitroaromatic vapor. Besides the general advantage of cellulose paper, the large specific surface area and pore structure facilitate the rapid diffusion of nitroaromatic vapor inside cellulose-based sensor,

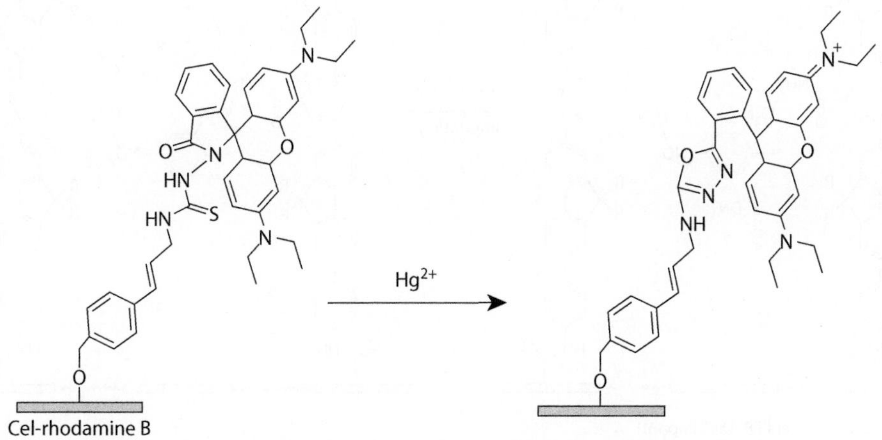

SCHEME 3.23 Structure of Cel-rhodamine B and the desulfurization of the Hg^{2+}. (From Yang, B. and Wu, W., *React. Funct. Polym.*, 73, 1553, 2013.)

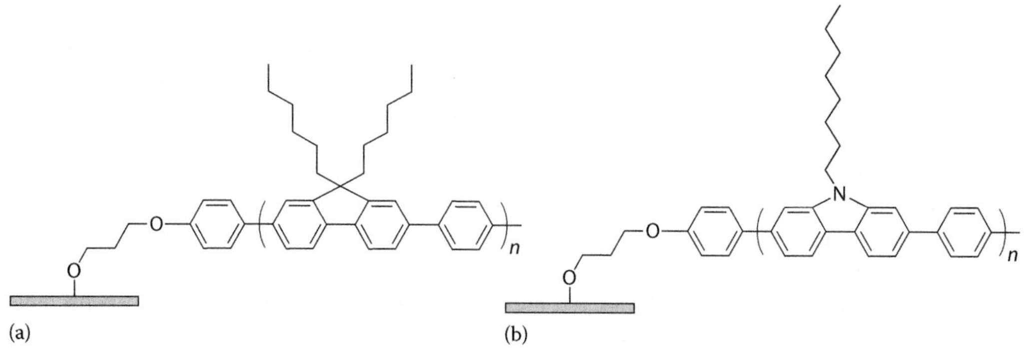

SCHEME 3.24 Structure of (a) Cel-fluorene-benzene copolymer and (b) Cel-carbazole-benzene copolymer. (Revised from Leng, H. and Wu, W., *Imaging Sci. Photochem.*, 30, 251, 2012.)

leading to the enhancement of the sensitivity and response of detection toward nitroaromatic explosive vapor. Author reported the molecular structure design and synthesis routine of Cel–fluorene–benzene copolymer and Cel–carbazole–benzene copolymer (Scheme 3.24). These two sensing cellulose products showed very good fluorescence quenching efficiency. [20]

An important contribution of cellulose-based explosives detector was reported by Niu et al. in 2013. The traditional non-imprinted CP-based sensors could produce highly sensitive but not selective fluorescent quenching toward electron-deficient nitroaromatic. So they designed and adopted a novel fluorophore-CP with a reduced possibility of π-electron delocalization as a precursor synthesized from meta-substituted phenylene monomers (Scheme 3.25). Their purpose was to diminish the nonselective fluorescence-quenching mode resulting from the amplified effect by exciton migration along the π-electron-delocalized backbones for the traditional CPs.[34]

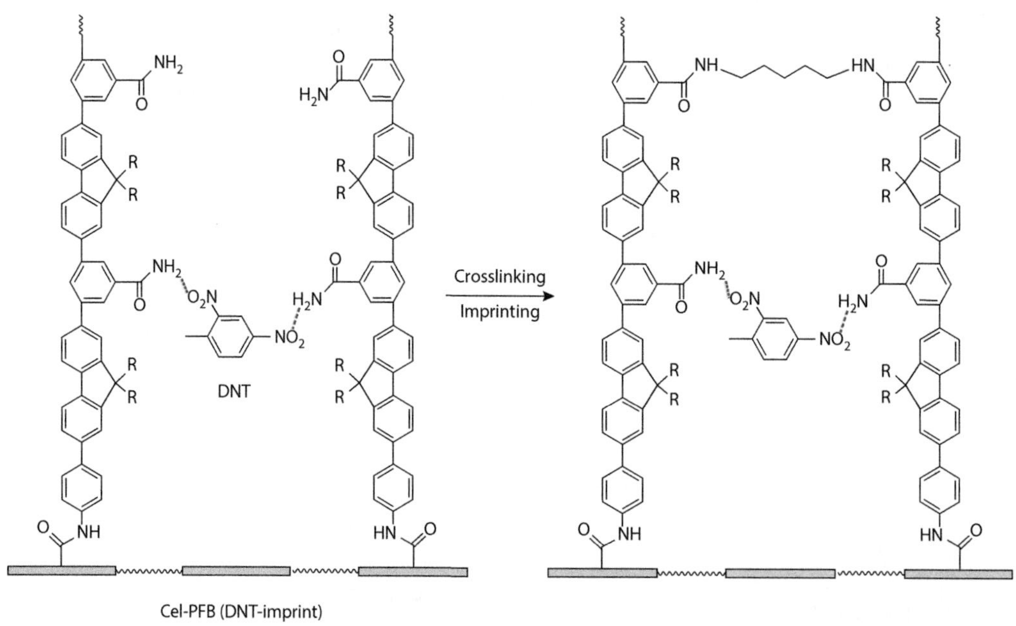

SCHEME 3.25 Schematic illustration of the preparation process of the "DNT-imprint" Cel-PFB film sensor. (Revised from Niu, Q. et al., *Chem. Commun.*, 49, 9137, 2013.)

This CP was bonded to cellulose nanofibril film via "grafting-to" tech, and a novel film sensor was fabricated. In addition, the surface molecular imprinting was formed on hydrogen bonding between amide groups of grafted polymer and nitro groups of target TNT/DNT. The vapor-phase Stern–Volmer quenching constant (KSV) of the non-imprinted Cel-PFB showed poor selectivity toward nitroaromatics. However, for the "TNT-imprinted" film, there is remarkable difference of KSV between TNT and DNT vapors. The KSV toward TNT vapor has an order of magnitude higher than that toward DNT vapor. Furthermore, the KSV of the "DNT-imprinted" Cel-PFB film toward DNT (3.7×10^{-2} s^{-1}) is up to 26 times larger than that toward TNT (1.4×10^{-3} s^{-1}). Indeed, the dramatic difference in KSV between TNT and DNT can be understood only from the standpoint of the surface molecular-imprinting intrinsic nature. Therefore, the "TNT-imprinted" Cel-PFB film exhibited highly selective recognition toward TNT, and the "DNT-imprinted" Cel-PFB film showed much more significant selectivity toward DNT. Moreover, the much enhanced responsiveness of these two sensors to target vapor may be attributed to the imprinted cavities formed by grafted and cross-linked CP chains, benefiting the diffusion-controlled target vapor penetration into the out-layer of the novel film sensor.

3.4.3 Cellulose-Based Antibacteria Surface

Adherence and survival of pathogenic bacteria on surfaces considerably increases the threat to human health, particularly by antibiotic-resistant bacteria. Consequently, more research into effective surface disinfection and alternative materials (fabrics, plastics, or coatings) with antimicrobial and other bioactive characteristics is desirable. Feese et al. described the synthesis and characterization of surface-modified cellulose nanocrystals with the cationic porphyrin (Cel-Por in Scheme 3.26). The porphyrin was appended onto the cellulose surface via the click chemistry. The reaction occurred between azide groups on the cellulosic surface and porphyrinic alkynes. The molecular structure of resulting crystalline material Cel-Por was well characteristic. And three genera of bacteria, *Staphylococcus aureus* (Gram-positive), *Escherichia coli* (Gram-negative), and *Mycobacterium smegmatis* (mycobacterium), were investigated. Five–six log units of reduction in viable cells were observed against *S. aureus*, three–four log units for *M. smegmatis*, and one–two log units for *E. coli* using Cel-Por in suspension at 20 μM solution (based on the porphyrin concentration).[35] This work developed a novel material that was capable

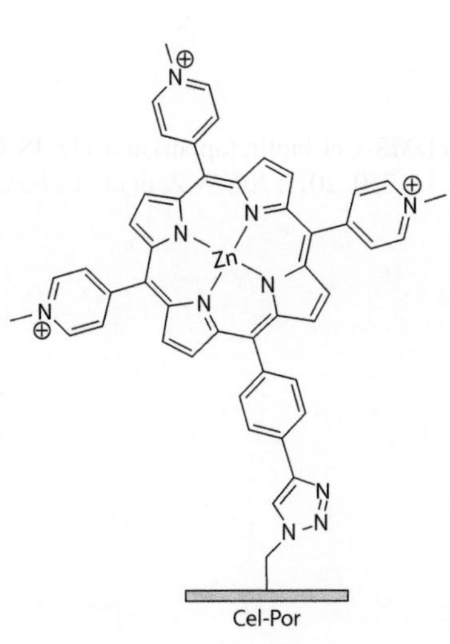

SCHEME 3.26 Structure of Cel-Por. (Revised from Feese, E. et al., *Biomacromolecules*, 12, 3528, 2011.)

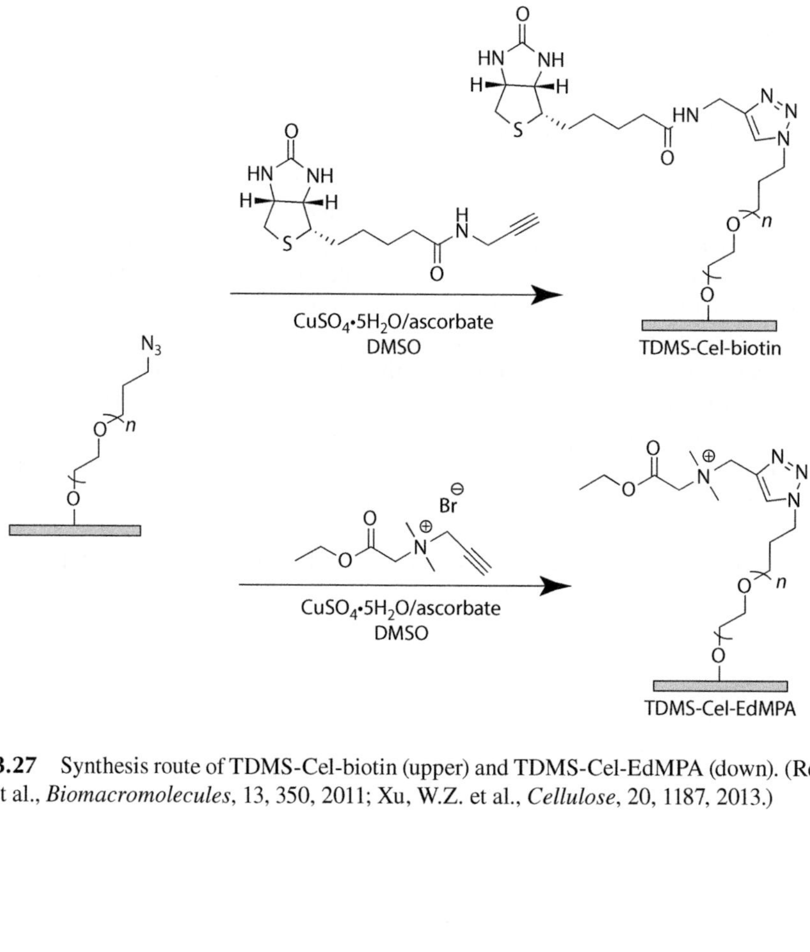

SCHEME 3.27 Synthesis route of TDMS-Cel-biotin (upper) and TDMS-Cel-EdMPA (down). (Revised from Xu, W.Z. et al., *Biomacromolecules*, 13, 350, 2011; Xu, W.Z. et al., *Cellulose*, 20, 1187, 2013.)

of sterilizing a range of bacteria with high efficacy, with potential utilization in the health care and food industries.

Kadla's group also focused on the research of bonding the antibacterial functionalities onto cellulose substrate and preparing permanent antibacterial material. They first formed open-framework structures (Cel-PEG-Az) that can be post-functionalized through click chemistry. Then, biotin was "clicked" onto the azide-functionalized cellulosic honeycomb films (Scheme 3.27, upper).[15] Note here, this grafted cellulose product had very poor solubility in commonly used solvents, owing to all the open-framework structures. And the latest work from their group described the linking of *N*-(2-ethoxy-2-oxoethyl)-*N*,*N*-dimethylprop-2yn-1-aminium bromide (EdMPABr) to the honeycomb film of TDMS-Cel-EG4-Az cellulose (Scheme 3.27, down). The cellulose derivative, TDMS-Cel-EdMPA, was also successful synthesized via site-specific modification of Cel-PEG-Az. And TDMS-Cel-EdMPA showed significant antibacterial activity against the bacteria *E. coli*.[36]

3.4.4 Cellulose-Based Biosensor

In 2011, Montañez et al. attached the other kinds of dendrimer onto cellulose substrate that acted as a biosensor[37]. They first activated cellulose surfaces with several generations of dendrons, and the terminated reactive groups were further reacted with a trifunctional orthogonal monomer. In general, the reactions were monitored by using a click dye reagent or a quartz crystal microbalance (QCM) technique. In their report, triethylenglycol oligomers and amoxicillin molecules could be easily connected to the dendritic surface (Scheme 3.28). This methodology delivers a new tool box for the design of sophisticated biosensors, with advantages of low detection limit (detection of lectin protein at concentration as low as 5 nM), versatility (i.e., triethylenglycol oligomers and amoxicillin molecules were efficiently introduced to the dendritic surface), and suppression of nonspecific interactions. The study combines defined dendrons, robust click chemistry, and dual functionality to provide highly sophisticated cellulose surfaces with unprecedented tunability. Engineered dendronized surfaces delivered multiple representations of dual functionality, which exhibited tailored hydrophilicity and in conjugation of penicillin haptens. Furthermore, mannosylated dendronized substrates were fabricated, and their subsequent specific lectin binding through QCM revealed a 10-fold stronger multivalency to Con A compared with the monomeric one (Scheme 3.28).

3.5 CONCLUSION AND PERSPECTIVE

In this chapter, we summarized the synthesis methods of pre-attaching azide, alkyne, and phenylbromo groups to cellulose substrates to make a special "anchor" for further functionalization. Based on these powerful cellulose precursors, a series of grafted cellulose copolymers including cross-linked cellulose, cellulose-based dendrimer, and cellulose polymer brushes were prepared by Heck reaction, Suzuki coupling reaction, Sonogashira reaction, as well as click chemistry. Their applications of several novel value-added cellulose products were also exemplified. Using these simple and versatile approaches to synthesize the functional polymer-grafted cellulose materials, we are able to extend much wider applications far beyond the traditional areas.

For example, bioactive polymer-grafted cellulose materials that were attached by proteins, enzymes, or antibodies could be applied as biosensors, bioreactors, or antimicrobial surface; stimuli-responsive polymer-grafted cellulose materials could be worked as smart filters; the specific optoelectronic functional cellulose, which not only remains the inherent hierarchical structure of cellulose but also keeps the special properties of functional groups could be used as a green environmentally friendly material to fabricate the batteries, super-capacitors, or organic solar cells. On the basis of the earlier-mentioned perspective, we could expect that the modified graft cellulose copolymers will have a bright future.

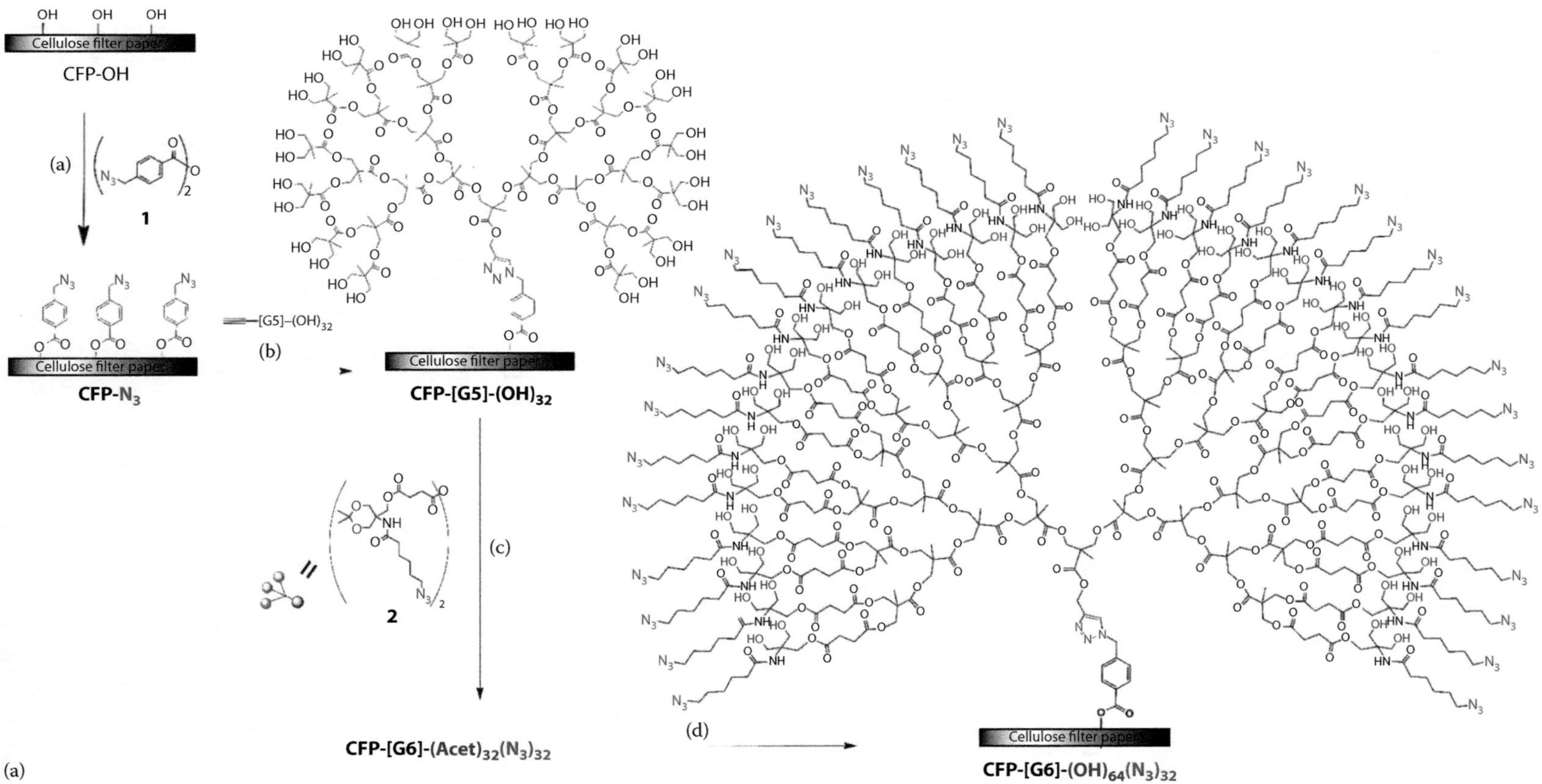

(a)

SCHEME 3.28 (a) Synthetic approach to bifunctional dendronized cellulose filter paper.

(*Continued*)

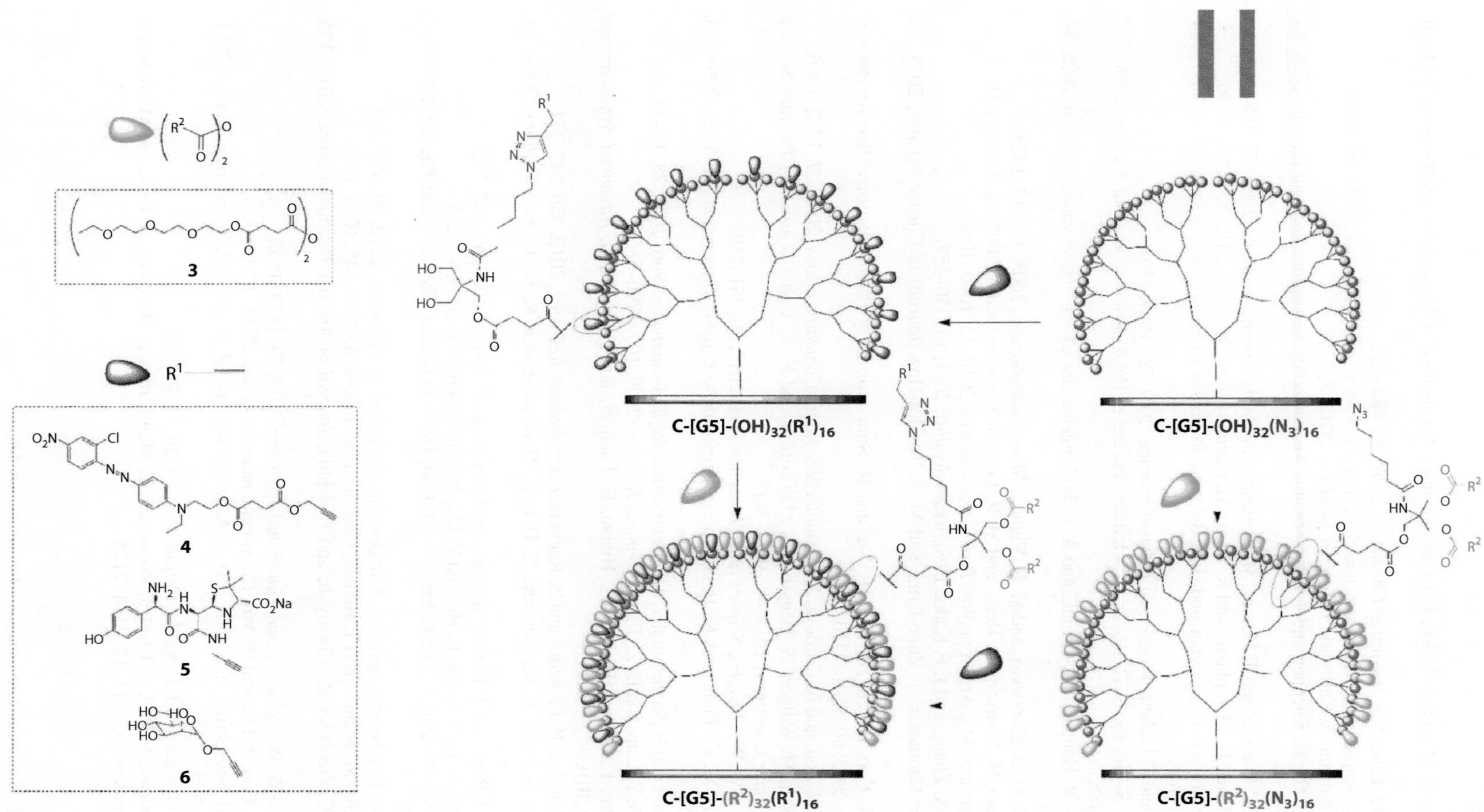

(b)

SCHEME 3.28 (Continued) (b) post-functionalization with orthogonal reactions. (Copyright 2011 American Chemical Society.)

REFERENCES

1. R. J. Moon, A. Martini, J. Nairn, J. Simonsen, and J. Youngblood, *Chemical Society Reviews*, 2011, 40, 3941.
2. A. Dufresne, *Canadian Journal of Chemistry*, 2008, 86, 484–494.
3. D. Roy, M. Semsarilar, J. T. Guthrie, and S. Perrier, *Chemical Society Reviews*, 2009, 38, 2046.
4. E. Malmström and A. Carlmark, *Polymer Chemistry*, 2012, 3, 1702.
5. S. Bräse, C. Gil, K. Knepper, and V. Zimmermann, *Angewandte Chemie International Edition*, 2005, 44, 5188–5240.
6. T. Liebert, C. Hänsch, and T. Heinze, *Macromolecular Rapid Communications*, 2006, 27, 208–213.
7. P.-H. Elchinger, D. Montplaisir, and R. Zerrouki, *Carbohydrate Polymers*, 2012, 87, 1886–1890.
8. A. E. J. De Nooy, A. C. Besemer, and H. V. Bekkum, *Recueil des Travaux Chimiques des Pays-Bas*, 1994, 113, 165–166.
9. T. Heinze and T. Liebert, *Progress in Polymer Science*, 2001, 26, 1689–1762.
10. T. Liebert, S. Hornig, S. Hesse, and T. Heinze, *Journal of the American Chemical Society*, 2005, 127, 10484–10485.
11. D. Klemm, B. Heublein, H.-P. Fink, and A. Bohn, *Angewandte Chemie International Edition*, 2005, 44, 3358–3393.
12. D. D. S. Perez, S. Montanari, and M. R. Vignon, *Biomacromolecules*, 2003, 4, 1417–1425.
13. S. Montanari, M. Roumani, L. Heux, and M. R. Vignon, *Macromolecules*, 2005, 38, 1665–1671.
14. I. Filpponen and D. S. Argyropoulos, *Biomacromolecules*, 2010, 11, 1060–1066.
15. W. Z. Xu, X. Zhang, and J. F. Kadla, *Biomacromolecules*, 2011, 13, 350–357.
16. G. Sánchez-Cabrera, F. J. Zuno-Cruz, and M. J. Rosales-Hoz, *Journal of Cluster Science*, 2013, 25, 51–82.
17. P. Peng, X. Cao, F. Peng, J. Bian, F. Xu, and R. Sun, *Journal of Polymer Science Part A: Polymer Chemistry*, 2012, 50, 5201–5210.
18. J. Hafrén, W. Zou, and A. Córdova, *Macromolecular Rapid Communications*, 2006, 27, 1362–1366.
19. J. J. Peterson, M. Willgert, S. Hansson, E. Malmström, and K. R. Carter, *Journal of Polymer Science Part A: Polymer Chemistry*, 2011, 49, 3004–3013.
20. H. Leng and W. Wu, *Imaging Science and Photochemistry*, 2012, 30, 251–259.
21. H. C. Kolb, M. G. Finn, and K. B. Sharpless, *Angewandte Chemie International Edition*, 2001, 40, 2004–2021.
22. W. H. Binder and R. Sachsenhofer, *Macromolecular Rapid Communications*, 2007, 28, 15–54.
23. J. Liu, J. W. Y. Lam, and B. Z. Tang, *Chemical Reviews*, 2009, 109, 5790–5867.
24. M. Lamblin, L. Nassar-Hardy, J.-C. Hierso, E. Fouquet, and F.-X. Felpin, *Advanced Synthesis and Catalysis*, 2010, 352, 33–79.
25. F. Pierre-Antoine, B. François, and Z. Rachida, *Carbohydrate Research*, 2012, 356, 247–251.
26. M. Pohl, J. Schaller, F. Meister, and T. Heinze, *Macromolecular Rapid Communications*, 2008, 29, 142–148.
27. D. Fenn, M. Pohl, and T. Heinze, *Reactive and Functional Polymers*, 2009, 69, 347–352.
28. H. Li, X. Xu, Y. Li, Y. Geng, B. He, and Z. Gu, *Polymer Chemistry*, 2013, 4, 2235.
29. C. Shi, Y. Wu, W. Zeng, Y. Xie, K. Yang, and Y. Cao, *Macromolecular Chemistry and Physics*, 2005, 206, 1114–1125.
30. A. M. Eissa, E. Khosravi, and A. L. Cimecioglu, *Carbohydrate Polymers*, 2012, 90, 859–869.
31. A. Koschella, M. Richter, and T. Heinze, *Carbohydrate Research*, 2010, 345, 1028–1033.
32. T. Agag, K. Vietmeier, A. Chernykh, and H. Ishida, *Journal of Applied Polymer Science*, 2012, 125, 1346–1351.
33. B. Yang and W. Wu, *Reactive and Functional Polymers*, 2013, 73, 1553–1558.
34. Q. Niu, K. Gao, Z. Lin, and W. Wu, *Chemical Communications*, 2013, 49, 9137.
35. E. Feese, H. Sadeghifar, H. S. Gracz, D. S. Argyropoulos, and R. A. Ghiladi, *Biomacromolecules*, 2011, 12, 3528–3539.
36. W. Z. Xu, G. Gao, and J. F. Kadla, *Cellulose*, 2013, 20, 1187–1199.
37. M. I. Montanez, Y. Hed, S. Utsel, J. Ropponen, E. Malmström, L. Wagberg, A. Hult, and M. Malkoch, *Biomacromolecules*, 2011, 12, 2114–2125.

4 Graft Copolymerization of Cellulose and Cellulose Derivatives

Chunmei Jian, Qiquan Ye, Meng Huo, and Jinying Yuan

CONTENTS

4.1 INTRODUCTION

With the gradual reduction of nonrenewable resources and increasing demand for structural materials, non-oil commodities, catalysts, and photoelectric devices, natural renewable resources draws the world's attention. Among them, cellulose (a linear polysaccharide of β (1 → 4) linked D-glucose) as one of the most abundant biomacromolecules in nature[1] has drawn much attention in recent years with its renewability, biocompatibility, nontoxicity, and availability.[2,3] As the major ingredient of plant cell walls, cellulose has been widely used in the traditional industries of food, medicine, transport, and architecture with is popular price. In order to fully exploit the potential functions of celluloses, much work about the multifunction of cellulose is under way. At present, the major modification methods about cellulose include derivatization, graft copolymerization, cross-linking, and alloying.[4] Among them, graft copolymers based on cellulose and cellulose derivatives have been obtained via various conventional polymerization techniques and exhibit unique properties.[5,6] Wettability, adhesion, and dyeability of the cellulose fiber could be improved by grafting hydrophilic monomer, while grafting cellulose derivatives with low wettability to oil contamination could be obtained by grafting hydrophobic monomer.[7,8]

Nowadays, researches on cellulose mainly focus on two aspects. One is finding a suitable and green solvent system for cellulose, which is insoluble in most solvents because of the hydrogen bonding between macromolecules.[1] Thereinto, *N*-methylmorpholine-*N*-oxide/water, trifluoroacetic acid/chloralkane, liquid ammonium thiocyanate, urea/sodium hydroxide,[9–11] and ionic liquid (IL)[12–14] are good solvent systems for cellulose. The other one is the functional modification of cellulose derivatives, including hydroxyethyl cellulose (HEC), hydroxypropyl cellulose (HPC), ethyl cellulose (EC), acetylcellulose (CA), and carboxymethyl cellulose (CMC).

Combining the earlier information, this chapter will introduce graft copolymerization of cellulose materials from two aspects: the graft copolymerization of cellulose and the graft copolymerization of cellulose derivatives.

4.2 GRAFT COPOLYMERIZATION OF CELLULOSE

Cellulose is one of the most abundant biopolymers in the nature. Because of its fairly good biodegradability, biocompatibility, unique mechanical property, as well as cheap price and huge output, cellulose has found a great many of applications in composite, textile, drug carrier, personal care product, and biomedical engineering.[15] Since this development, cellulose has been regarded as one of the most potential green materials that may help to alleviate the shortage of energy. However, cellulose has been suffering from some intrinsic shortages like high melt temperature, low decomposition temperature, and rather poor solubility as its basic compositional group is glucose linked with α-1,4-glucosidic bond, and this molecular structure is prone to crystallize.[16] As a result, to promote its solubility and thermal stability to obtain wider processing region is of great significance for the cellulose industry. Among the plasticization strategy, graft modification has been thought as a promising approach to solve the problems mentioned earlier. Compared with external plasticization, graft modification is enabled to effectively avoid the troublesome plasticizer bleeding as the grafts are in fact grafted chemically to the backbone of cellulose. Based on the reaction condition, graft modification of cellulose can be divided into homogeneous graft and heterogeneous graft.

4.2.1 Heterogeneous Graft Copolymerization of Cellulose

Celluloses own complex morphological structures as the coexistence of crystalline region and amorphous region. Therefore, cellulose is insoluble in most solvents because of the existence of intramolecular and intermolecular hydrogen bonds. So, most of the graft copolymerization about cellulose was conducted in heterogeneous condition. There are a large amount of reports on the heterogeneous graft copolymerization about cellulose with diverse polymerization methods. Here, two common modification methods including free radical polymerization and living polymerization will be involved.

Free radical polymerization[17–20] is a promising method for the production of synthetic polymer in industries with unique advantages including mild condition, low price, and a wider range of monomers. Anbalagan's group[19] synthesized cellulose-*g*-PAA via free radical polymerization with ceric ammonium nitrate as initiator. The brush copolymer cellulose-*g*-PAA was used as an effective low-cost adsorbent to collect metal ions such as Cu(II) and Ni(II) from the wastewater at the industrial level. Besides, 2,2-azobisisobutyronitrile (AIBN) was used to initiate the polymerization of cellulose-*g*-(PEGDMA-r-PAM).[20] The cellulose-*g*-(PEGDMA-r-PAM) was made into paper-based device to detect pesticide with excellent selectivity.

However, the traditional free radical polymerization has some weaknesses, such as the wider molecular weight distribution and the unmanageable side reactions. Living radical polymerizations have been developed to overcome these disadvantages. Among them, atom transfer radical polymerization (ATRP) and reversible addition fragmentation chain transfer (RAFT) were used to prepare graft copolymers based on cellulose.

ATRP is a promising route to obtain well-defined polymers grafted onto cellulose surface with predefined molecular weight and narrow molecular weight distribution.[21] Daneault's group[22] synthesized a cationic polymer-grafted cellulose, cellulose-*g*-poly(2-(methacryloyloxy)ethyl)-trimethylammoniumchloride (cellulose-*g*-PMeDMA), via aqueous ATRP. Then, infrared, XPS, and SEM techniques were used to analyze the cellulose-*g*-PMeDMA complex. The resulting

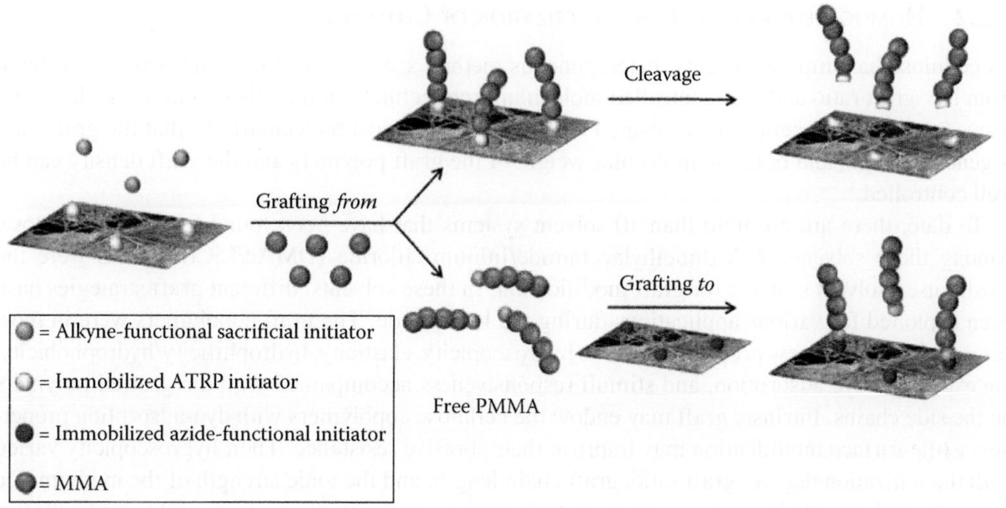

FIGURE 4.1 Schematic picture showing the "graft from" and "graft to." (From Stenzel, M.H. et al., *Macromolecules*, 40, 7140, 2007.)

cellulose-*g*-PMeDMA complex showed marked improvement in the mechanical property, which has an important potential in papermaking applications. Carlmark's group[22] has modified the cellulose through ATRP systemically. Brush copolymer cellulose-*g*-PMA[23] and brush block copolymers cellulose-*g*-(PMA-*co*-PHEMA)[24] were prepared via "graft from" of ATRP with modified cellulose as macroinitiator. Furthermore, functional cellulose materials were prepared by grafting stimulus-responsive polymer to the surface of cellulose, including cellulose-*g*-(PNIPAM-*co*-poly(acrylamidopropyltrimethylammonium chloride))[25] and cellulose-*g*-(PDMAEMA-*co*-PS).[26] Meanwhile, the "graft onto" of ATRP has also been used to synthesize cellulose grafting copolymers.[27] Comparing the two different grafting techniques shown in Figure 4.1 ("graft from" or "graft onto"), it is concluded[28] that the "graft from" was superior to the "graft to" in terms of the amount of grafted copolymers on the cellulose.

RAFT was another living radical polymerization technique that could be employed for cellulose grafting.[29,30] Perrier and coworkers[31] have grafted styrene to the cellulose substrate through RAFT in 2005. First, the cellulose fibers were converted into thiocarbonylthio chain transfer agent. Then, the modified cellulose fibers were further used to mediate the RAFT polymerization of styrene. Similarly, monomers such as MMA[31] and DMAEMA[32] were polymerized with RAFT from cellulose.

Both ATRP and RAFT require modification of the celluloses prior to the "graft from." By comparison, ring-opening polymerization (ROP) is especially advantageous as ROP reaction is initiated by hydroxyl groups with no modification of cellulose necessary prior to the grafting reaction.[33] Córdova's group[34] has developed the first direct bulk ROP of e-caprolactone (ε-CL) on solid cotton or paper cellulose with organocatalysis in 2005. The reaction provides a novel route to prepare biocompatible nanomaterials based on cellulose, which was performed without solvent—low cost, simple operation, and environmental friendly. Subsequently, related work about the grafting of cellulose using ROP was reported.[35,36] Dufresne and coworkers[37] have used a "graft from" approach to graft the ε-CL to cellulose nanocrystals by 2-ethylhexanoate($Sn(Oct)_2$)-catalyzed ROP. The obtained cellulose-*g*-PCL (poly(ε-CL)) has been characterized and demonstrated significant improvements of the mechanical property. Certainly, there was also "graft onto" method to prepare the cellulose-*g*-PCL, for example, PCL with azide group as terminal group was grafted onto cellulose backbone modified with alkynyl group via heterogeneous click reaction.[37]

4.2.2 Homogeneous Graft Copolymerization of Cellulose

As cellulose has limited solvents, heterogeneous method seemed more versatile, while it suffered from low graft ratio and less controlled molecular architecture. On the other hand, in the homogeneous graft method, cellulose is solvated into the solvent almost molecularly so that the graft ratio is generally high, and both the molecular weight of the graft polymers and the graft density can be well controlled.[3]

To date, there are no more than 10 solvent systems that have been found to solvate cellulose. Among these solvents, *N,N*-dimethylacetamide/lithium chloride (DMAc/LiCl) and IL were the mostly used solvent systems for graft modification. In these solvents, different graft strategies have been exploited for various applications during the last decade. The graft copolymers were in most cases endowed with new properties such as hygroscopicity, elasticity, hydrophilicity/hydrophobicity, ion exchange, dye adsorption, and stimuli responsiveness accompanied with the grafted polymers on the side chains. Intrinsic graft may endow the cellulose copolymers with dye-adsorption properties, while surface modification may improve their abrasive resistance. Their hygroscopicity varied with the ionization degree, graft ratio, graft chain length, and the ionic strength of the medium. On the contrary, hydrophobic polymer grafts were believed to promote their compatibility and adhesive property. As a result, these cellulose-based graft copolymers may have wide applications in body fluid adsorbents in medical application, fabrics like underwear and athletic wear, and contaminant adsorbents. In the following, we will highlight the development of homogeneous graft during the last decade.

Cellulose grafting copolymers have played a significant role in bio-separation while they usually are prone to adsorb proteins, which may hinder their separation efficiency and service life. In 2008, Yan and Tao first grafted ATRP initiator 2-bromoisobutyloyl bromide onto the cellulose backbone in DMAc/LiCl and then utilized ATRP to polymerize *N,N*-dimethylacrylamide (DMA) onto the side chains.[38] The protein-adsorption study indicated that the graft copolymers showed good protein adsorption resistance and may find applications in hemocompatibility enhancement of cellulose membranes so as to strengthen their selectively separation. Using the same macroinitiators, the same group found that graft polymerization of 2-methacryloyloxyethyl phosphorylcholine (MPC) in a homogeneous DMSO/methanol mixture solution by ATRP produced well-defined cellulose-*g*-PMPCs with similar protein adsorption resistance, which may provide an alternate approach to hemocompatibility.[39] Unfortunately, the copper ion residual after ATRP has long been the problem of ATRP in biomedical applications. Single-electron transfer living radical polymerization (SET-LRP) may help to limit the copper used in the polymerization to below ppm. Moreover, the tolerance of oxygen and the easy operation of SET-LRP have attracted more and more attention. Hiltunen's group has exploited SET-LRP for cellulose-*g*-PDMAc.[40] In their research, macroinitiators in DMSO were studied by dynamic light scattering, and the results demonstrated that they were mostly dissolved molecularly with a few aggregates. Then, they further studied the structure–property effect by light scattering and steady-shear viscosity and found that the graft chain length had little effect to the solution properties of cellulose-*g*-PDMAc, while the total molecular weight had significant effect. Moreover, the static light scattering results showed a loose and solvent-draining architecture in water.

Besides ATRP, ROP of biodegradable cyclic esters by the hydroxyl groups of cellulose was proved to be another effective method to modify the cellulose.[41] Among those polyesters, poly(L-lactic acid) (PLLA) and PCL were the most studied biodegradable polyesters. An interesting and instructive example is the cellulose-*g*-PLLA and cellulose-*g*-PCL that Mayumi et al. prepared by partial substitution of the C6-hydroxyl of cellulose with PLLA or PCL.[42] ^{13}C NMR verified that the ROP occurred regioselectively on the C6-hydroxyl of the cellulose. To achieve this, they choose to lower the degree of substitution to 0.5–0.7 and the degree of polymerization to below three. The short side chain–modified cellulose graft copolymers were easily solvated into DMSO, and some cellulose-*g*-PLLA even solvated or swelled into water, which indicated the breakage of the lateral hydrogen bonds of cellulose.

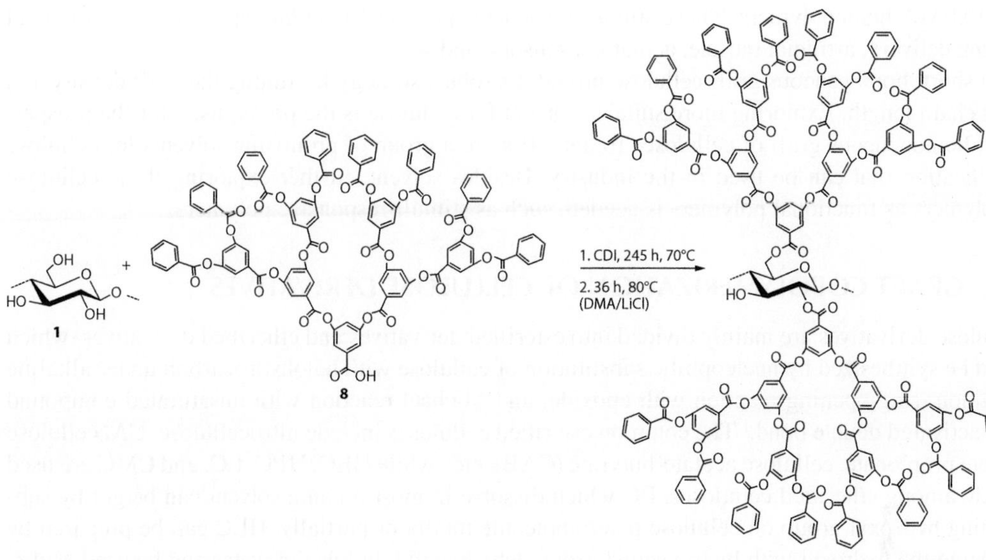

FIGURE 4.2 Preparation of the dendronized cellulose derivatives. (From Zhang, H. et al., *Macromolecules*, 38, 8272, 2005.)

Compared with "graft from" strategy, the "graft onto" method seemed less used in the homogeneous graft modification since this method has less control of the graft chains' molecular weight and graft density. In 2008, Heinze's group for the first time designed and successfully prepared the dendronized cellulose graft copolymers (Figure 4.2).[43] Since the bulky hindrance of the dendrons, the degree of substitution is 0.7 with C6- and C2-hydroxyl groups substituted with the dendrons. Taking the advantage of the low intrinsic viscosity of dendrons, these cellulose graft copolymers were soluble in aprotic solvent and could be processed to films.

To further develop the environmentally friendly solvent for cellulose modification, IL, a series of organic salts that are liquid at or near room temperature, has attracted much attention since its first use for ATRP in 2005.[44] AminCl and BminCl were two kinds of IL that have been most used in cellulose modification. Zhang's group for the first time used unmodified cellulose as the initiator for the ROP of lactide in AminCl, and they found that by controlling the ratio of lactide to cellulose, the graft density and the graft chain length can be well controlled.[45] The differential scanning calorimetry result showed only one T_g, which decreased sharply and then increased slightly upon the increment of the molecular substitution of PLLA. Specifically, the graft copolymers exhibited thermoplastic when the molecular substitution of PLLA was larger than 4.40. To further explore the application in biomedical engineering, Wang's and Liu's groups have applied these copolymers into drug delivery separately.[46,47] Both of their results showed that micelles with diameters ranging from 10 to 80 nm can be formed in solution varying the grafting density and graft chain length. Other cyclic ester analogs like ε-CL and *p*-dioxone have also been exploited to modify cellulose.[48,49] Since its use for ATRP, researches using ILs for cellulose modification by ATRP have emerged. Lin et al. have successfully prepared cellulose-*g*-poly(methyl methacrylate) in BminCl with controlled/"living" character.[50] Though there have been piles of researches dealing with the grafting modification of cellulose, few of them paid attention to utilizing the stimuli-responsive polymers to modify cellulose to construct functional polymers. We have used cellulose macroinitiators to initiate *N,N*-dimethylamino-2-ethyl methacrylate (DMAEMA) and studied their pH- and thermo-responsiveness.[14] The PDMAEMA on the side chains endowed the copolymers with not only mechanical properties, but also pH- and thermo-responsiveness similar to that of

PDMAEMA homopolymers. These stimuli-responsive polymers may find applications in the field of drug delivery, artificial muscle, actuators, sensors, and so on.

In short, homogeneous graft cellulose provides a robust strategy for tuning the graft density and graft chain length. Exploring more suitable solvent for cellulose is the prerequisite for the prosperity of homogeneous graft of cellulose. To date, ILs are a group of promising solvents for cellulose modification that can be used in the industry. Besides solvent, further exploring these cellulose copolymers as functional polymers is needed, such as stimuli-responsive polymers.

4.3 GRAFT COPOLYMERIZATION OF CELLULOSE DERIVATIVES

Cellulose derivatives are mainly divided into esterified derivatives and etherified derivatives, which could be synthesized by nucleophilic substitution of cellulose with halohydrocarbon under alkaline condition, ring-opening reaction with epoxide, and Michael reaction with unsaturated compound with activated double bond.[1] The common esterified celluloses include nitrocellulose, CA, cellulose acetate propionate, cellulose acetate-butyrate (CAB), etc., while HEC, HPC, EC, and CMC are used widely among etherified celluloses. EC which dissolve in most organic solvent can be got by substituting hydroxyl group on cellulose macromolecule totally or partially. HEC can be prepared by replacing the hydroxyl with hydroxyethyl group, which could dissolve in water and be used as dispersing agent and thickening agent. Comparing to HEC, the substituent group of HPC is hydroxypropyl, particularly, HPC possess thermo-response[1]. Ionic CMC could dissolve in water well, and it is the most utilized etherified cellulose.

Various cellulose derivatives with their unique properties are applied to military-industrial, textile industry, paint industry, and cigarette industry traditionally. And in half a century, cellulose derivatives were used as important fine chemicals all over the world. However, with the increasing demands for smart materials, biological materials, and nontoxic materials, the modification of cellulose derivatives has been invested more. So, we will introduce the development of graft modification of some important cellulose derivatives made in recent years, which include EC, HEC, HPC, CA, and CMC.

4.3.1 GRAFT COPOLYMERIZATION OF ETHYL CELLULOSE

EC shows good solubility in most organic solvents. The hydroxyl of EC could act as active site to take part in reactions for functionalization, and the degree of substitution of hydroxyl could be controlled. Different grafting reactions provide various possibilities to get multifunctional EC derivatives.

In recent years, stimuli-responsive polymers draw much attention as to the significant application potential in biomedical and environment field.[5,51,52] Yan et al.[51] designed and synthesized pH-responsive brush polymers based on EC successfully, which could be potential nanocarriers for controlled drug release. First, ECs are derived into ATRP macromolecule initiator as hydroxyl reacting with 2-bromoisobutyryl bromide partially. Then, they got ATRP macromolecule initiator initiate the polymerization of *N,N*-dimethylaminoethyl methacrylate (DMAEMA), a stimuli-responsive monomer. At last, the left hydroxyls initiate the polymerization of ε-CL through ROP, and cellulose-based dual graft molecular brushes EC-*g*-PCL-*g*-PDMAEMA with hydrophilic and hydrophobic side chains are synthesized. Dual graft molecular brushes EC-*g*-PCL-*g*-PDMAEMA exhibit different wonderful aggregation morphologies with the variation of pH value.

As showed in Figure 4.3, the cellulose-based dual graft molecular brushes exhibit responsive behaviors by forming self-assembled micelles at $pH < 4.5$ and transforming to unusual micellar aggregates at $pH > 6.2$, which may lead by the middle state of side chain PDMAEMA as pH value of the solution between 8.5 and 10. Liu et al.[52] derived EC to ATRP macromolecule initiator 2-bromoisobutyryl EC (EC-Br). EC-Br initiates the polymerization of thermosensitive polymers, poly(olig(ethylene glycol)methacrylates) (POEGMA), which possess the wide and tunable lower

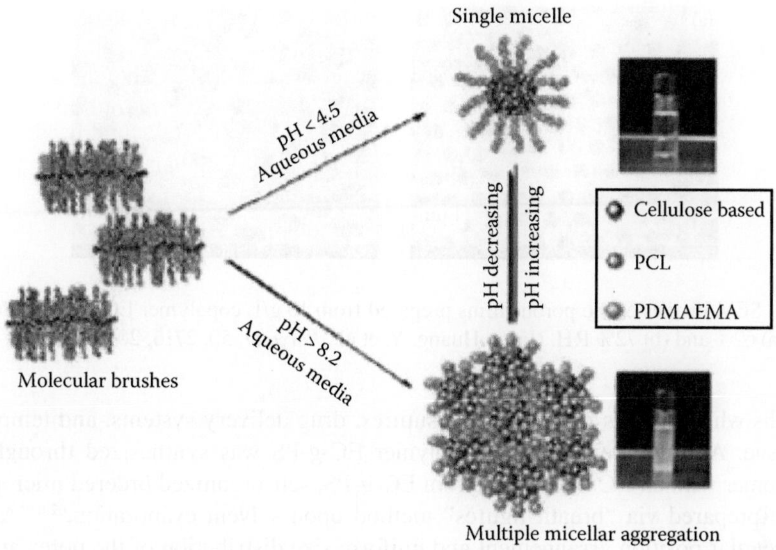

FIGURE 4.3 Schematic representation of pH-induced formation of single micelles and of the multiple micellar aggregation process. (From Yuan, J. et al., *Biomacromolecules*, 10, 2033, 2009.)

critical solution temperature (LCST), which varies in the range of 26°C–90°C with the change of ethylene oxide side chain lengths.[53,54] They got thermo-responsive brushes EC-*g*-P(POEGMA) self-assemble to nanomicelles in water with an LCST around 65°C (Figure 4.4). What's more, any LCST of the nanomicelles needed could be got by adjusting the length of PEG chain.

With the importance of environmental protection and sustainable development, the green materials are preferred with their unique advantages and of large demand.[55–61] Novel EC-*graft*-poly (ε-caprolactone)-block-poly(L-lactide) (EC-*g*-PCL-*b*-PLLA) graft-block copolymers are successfully synthesized via ROP of ε-CL and L-lactide in turn with $Sn(Oct)_2$ as catalyst.[60] EC-*g*-PCL-*b*-PLLA combined recycling of cellulose and biodegradability of both PCL and PLLA. The environment-friendly EC-*g*-PCL-*b*-PLLA with their own characteristics may make

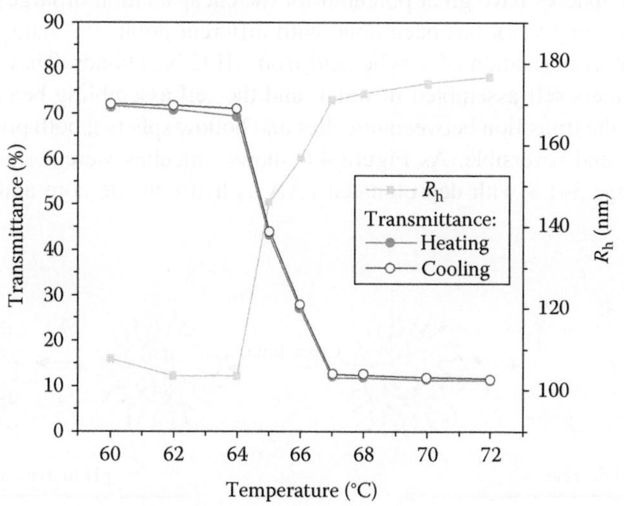

FIGURE 4.4 Hydrodynamic radius (R_h) and transmittance vary with the increase in temperature. (From Huang, Y. et al., *J. Polym. Sci. A: Polym. Chem.*, 46, 6907, 2008.)

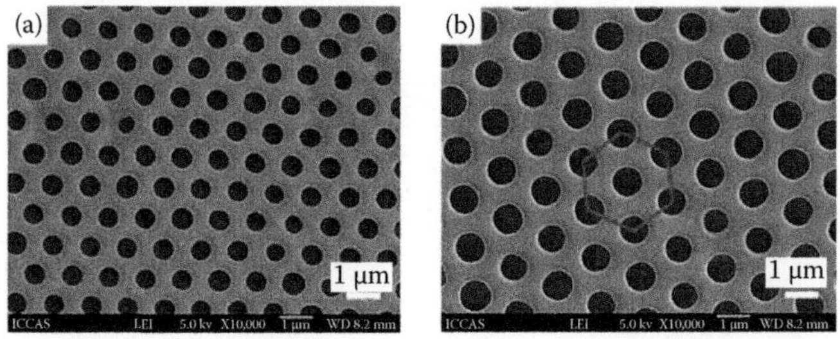

FIGURE 4.5 SEM images of the porous films prepared from 10 g/L copolymer $EC_{0.5}$-*g*-PS84/CS2 solution at the RH of (a) 62% and (b) 72% RH. (From Huang, Y. et al., *Polymer*, 50, 2716, 2009.)

breakthroughs when used as biodegradable sutures, drug delivery systems, and temporary scaffolds for tissue. Another well-defined copolymer EC-*g*-PS was synthesized through ATRP of styrene monomer with an EC initiator.[61] From EC-*g*-PS, self-organized ordered microporous thin films can be prepared via "breath figures" method upon solvent evaporation.[62,63] As shown in Figure 4.5, regular position arrangement and uniform size distribution of the pores are achieved. In addition, the average size and average depth of the pores can be controlled by adjusting copolymer concentration, length of the side chain, and relative humidity (RH). They got microporous films with regular patterned structure that have potential applications as catalyst carrier, templates, optical materials, cell culture substrates, etc.

4.3.2 Graft Copolymerization of Hydroxyethyl Cellulose

HEC is extensively studied as a nonionic and water-soluble cellulose ether. It is widely used as thickening agents, rheology modifiers, emulsifying agent, protective colloids, and a variety of other applications in the field of petroleum exploitation industry, construction industry, pharmaceutical industry, textile industry, etc.[64] Hydroxyl groups randomly distributed along the HEC backbone offer much opportunity to modify HEC by various chemical reactions. Grafting,[65,66] crosslinking,[67,68] oxidation,[69,70] glycosylation,[67] and thiolation[71–73] are the ordinary modification methods for HEC, which could improve the properties and broad range of applications of HEC.

Polymeric hollow spheres have great potential for the encapsulation of large quantities of guest molecules, and much good work has been done with different points.[74,75] Jiang's group[65] reported a free radical graft polymerization of acrylic acid from HEC backbones. They got pH-responsive HEC-*g*-PAA copolymers self-assembled in water, and the self-assembling behavior demonstrated its micellization and the transition between micelles and hollow spheres; both processes were found to be pH dependent and reversible. As Figure 4.6 shows, micelles were formed when pH value decreased to the range 3–1.8 with deprotonated PAA as hydrophobic core and hydrophilic HEC

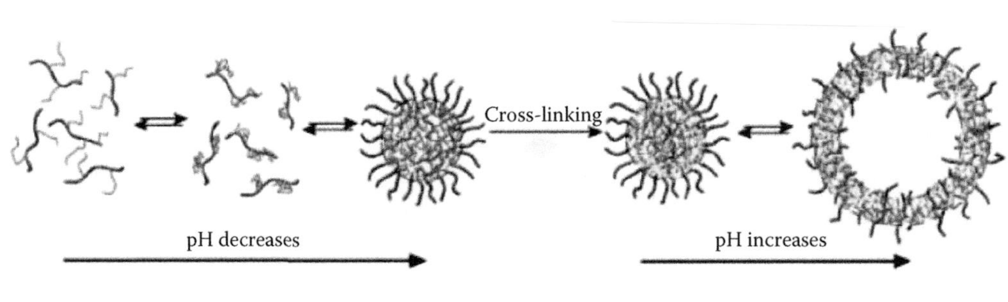

FIGURE 4.6 Scheme of the pH-dependent micellization and transition of HEC-*g*-PAA from micelle to hollow sphere. (From Jiang, M. et al., *Angew. Chem. Int. Ed.*, 42, 1516, 2003.)

backbones as shell to stable the core; then, the PAA chains of the micelles are cross-linked simply by treating them with a desired amount of cross-linkers, 2,2′-(ethylenedioxy)bis(ethylamine), and followed by increasing the pH value to 7. The hollow sphere indicated that the cross-linking has locked the integral structure and the core of the previous micelles consists of PAA dissolved in the solution with pH of 7. The pH value of the solution is the most important factor in the process of transition from micelles to hollow spheres reversibly.

Besides, hydrogel system based on HEC graft copolymer showed some particular properties and special usefulness. Chen's group[76] reported a thermo-sensitive hydrogel system that was constructed by the copolymerization of modified HEC and *N*-isopropylacrylamide. The hydrogels exhibited temperature sensitivity and could realize the controlled drug release for diverse model drugs.

HEC-*g*-PDMA brush copolymer was prepared successfully via ATRP.[69] The copolymer was applied for the separation of basic proteins in capillary electrophoresis with pH, ranging from 2.2 to 6.0, and high efficiency. Meanwhile, a brush copolymer, HEC-*g*-PCL, was synthesized by homogeneous ring-opening grafted polymerization.[77] The novel completely degradable HEC-*g*-PCL was expected to be used as a thickener and stabilizer in personal care and painting industry with strong associate ability in aqueous solution. More work about HEC graft copolymers as function materials has been reported.[78,79]

4.3.3 Graft Copolymerization of Hydroxypropyl Cellulose

HPC is regarded as nontoxic and physiologically harmless; it is applied in many industrial products in daily use such as food additives, cosmetic ingredients, and tablet. Compared with HEC, HPC shows a better dissolubility in organic solvent and possesses particular thermo-response. On this basis, grafting modification of HPC may produce some new wonderful materials.[80,81]

Similar to copolymers EC-*g*-PDEGMA mentioned earlier, the amphipathic copolymers HPC-*g*-PDEGMA with an adjustable LCST could be prepared via ARGET ATRP by altering the initial monomer feed ratio.[82] The obtained HPC-*g*-PDEGMA combines the beneficial properties of HPC with thermo-response and stealth properties of poly(ethylene glycol) methacrylates. Liu's group[83] reported a thermo-sensitive HPC-*g*-PNIPAM copolymer synthesized via SET-LRP. The successful preparation of HPC-*g*-PNIPAM with different lengths of the side chains provided an approach for the regulation of LCST to body temperature region by graft copolymerization (Figure 4.7). Liu's group[84] also synthesized the thiolated HPC (HPC-SH), which could self-associate to fabricate a dual-stimuli sensitive nanogel with thermo-response and reversible redox response.

Amphipathic brush copolymers HPC-*g*-(PLLA-*b*-PAA) are synthesized by the ROP of L-lactide and the ATRP of tertbutylacrylate (t-BA) monomer sequential.[85] The obtained HPC-*g*-(PLLA-*b*-PAA) could self-assemble into aggregations in an ethanol/water mixture (V:V = 9:1). These special properties of HPC-*g*-(PLLA-*b*-PAA) make it possible to serving as an efficient fragrance delivery system in formulations with high ethanol content. Another amphipathic brush copolymers based on HPC were also reported in some previous literatures.[86–88] A new amphiphilic grafted HPC containing polycholesteryl methacrylate side chains, HPC-*g*-(PMMA-r-PCMA), was prepared via ATRP.[88] The prepared HPC-*g*-(PMMA-r-PCMA) has potential to be used as a new platform for biodegradable and biocompatible nanocarriers.

4.3.4 Graft Copolymerization of Carboxymethylcellulose

To be different from the several cellulose derivatives provided earlier, CMC as ionic cellulose ether is a negatively charged polyelectrolyte and could dissolve in water well. Moreover, the backbone of CMC has two kinds of reactive sites carboxyl and hydroxyl, which bring more possibility for the modification of CMC.

Free radical polymerization played an important role in the grafting modification of CMC. Much work has been reported to prepare the functional brush copolymers based on CMC.[89–96]

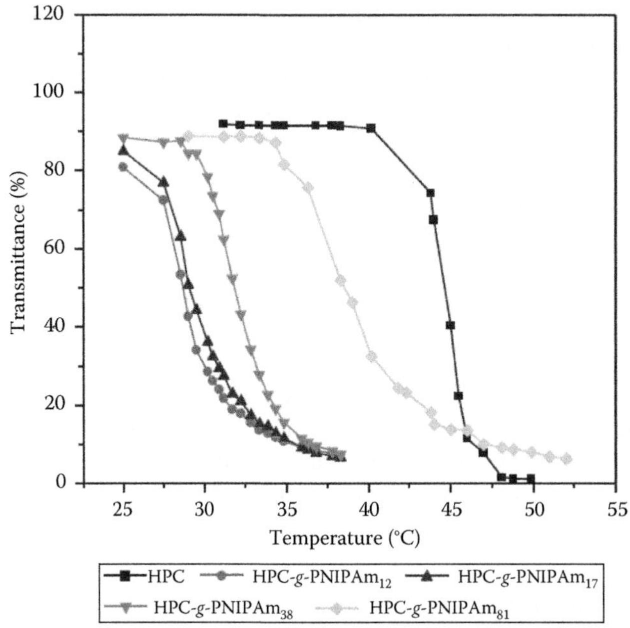

FIGURE 4.7 Transmittance of the aqueous solution of HPC and HPC-*g*-PINIPAm copolymers as a function of termperature. (From Liu, R.G. et al., *Carbohydr. Polym.*, 95, 155, 2013.)

Cheng's group[90] has synthesized a series of hydrolyzed polyacrylamide-grafted carboxymethyl cellulose (CMC-*g*-HPAM) with ammonium persulfate as the initiator. They got CMC-*g*-HPAM, which was applied as efficient flocculants to remove cationic dye in aqueous solution. Another efficient flocculants that could be used for water treatment were also prepared including CMC-*g*-PN-vinylformamide (CMC-*g*-PNVF)[92] and CMC-*g*-PAN.[94] Specifically, a CMC-*g*-PMMA[96] synthesized from knitted rags was obtained with $K_2S_2O_8$ as initiator, and the hydrophobic PMMA improved the strength properties and decreased the moisture content of CMC-*g*-PMMA films.

In addition, some special hydrogels based on CMC grafting derivatives were constructed.[97–101] Giri's group[98] introduced a highly swelling hydrogel by cross-linking the side chains of CMC-*g*-PAM. The hydrogel showed enormous swelling in aqueous medium, which could be influenced by the chemical composition of the hydrogel, pH, and ionic strength. Similar superabsorbents[99,100] were constructed by the free radical grafting solution polymerization of allyl monomer onto CMC in the presence with corresponding cross-linkers and initiators. Wang' group[101] reported a pH-, salt- and solvent-responsive superabsorbent, CMC-*g*-poly(sodium acrylate)/medical stone, which was used as reversible on–off switch for different saline solutions or different solvents (Figure 4.8).

There was also a novel thermo-responsive CMC-*g*-PNIPAM that was prepared through diverse methods.[102,103] Amino-terminated PNIPAM side chains reacted with CMC, so CMC-PNIPAM was collected via "graft onto."[103] CMC-*g*-PNIPAM exhibited thermo-thickening phenomenon because of the interconnection of PNIPAM chain, which could be useful in pharmaceutical applications.

4.3.5 Graft Copolymerization of Cellulose Acetate

CA is the product of esterification reaction of cellulose and acetic anhydride in the presence of catalyst. CA has been extensively used in synthetic fibers and plastic industry with its good thermal stability. However, the intrinsic disadvantage of high glass transition temperature (T_g), the temperature interval between its molten temperature and decomposition temperature, is too narrow to be used for processing. External plasticizations were used widely to weaken the interactions between

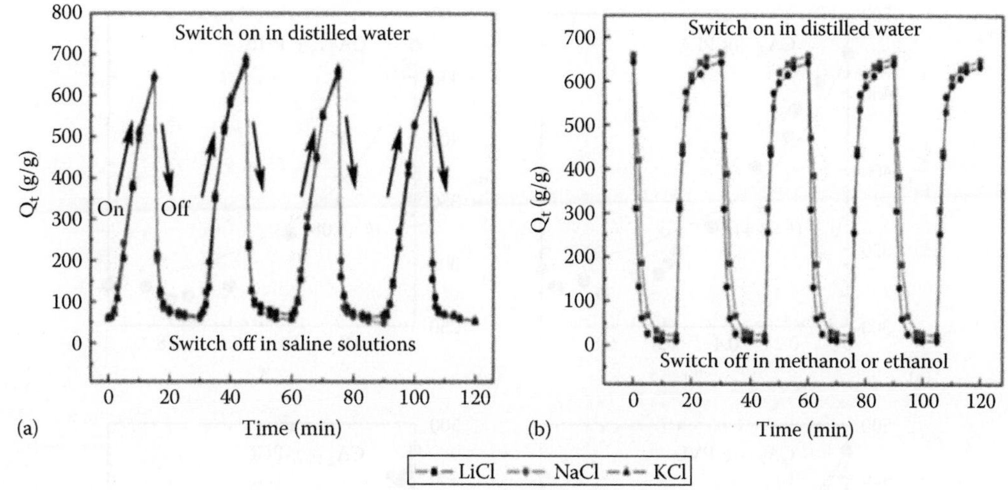

FIGURE 4.8 The reversible on–off switching swelling behaviors of the composite between (a) distilled and LiCl, NaCl, and KCl solutions, (b) distilled water and methanol or ethanol.

CA chains, which lead to a decrease in T_g. Nevertheless, the materials based on CA with external plasticization are likely to bleed during the processing and usage, leading to the changes of material properties. Moreover, the bleed plasticizer or their secondary metabolites may do harm to the environment and the users.

So, internal plasticization to plasticize the CA is urgently needed. Graft flexible polymeric chains on CA as an alternative approach realized the internal plasticization, which may impress or even overcome the plasticizer bleeding problems during the processing and usage and improve the properties of the materials. As one of the mostly used internal plasticizations for CA, ε-CL with quite long flexible alkyl chains was used to copolymerize with cellulose diacetate (CDA, DS = 2–2.7) as early as 1985 by Daicel chemistry company.[104] Grafting PCL enabled the molten temperature of CDA to decrease while the decomposition temperature increased, resulting to materials with fairly good thermal stability and wide molten temperature as well as favorable moldability and transparency for membranes and sheets. As another member of poly(hydroxyalkanoate)s (PHSs), PLLA is another internal plasticization for CDA, and its monomer L-lactic acid (LLA) is an environmentally friendly common organic acid in the nature.

There are many effective explorations[105,106] to decrease the T_g and to improve the mechanical properties and thermal stability of CDA. Teramoto's group[105] found that CDA-*g*-PLLA prepared from ROP in DMSO has the T_g decreased from 202°C to about 60°C, similar to that of PLLA homopolymers (62°C). Subsequently, Lee and coworkers[107] have studied the effect of CDA-*g*-PLLA molecular composition and thermal aging on mechanical properties by nanoindentation. They found that the hardness and elastic modulus in all CDA-*g*-PLLA were higher than those in CDA. And the hardness and elastic modulus were increased in both CDA-*g*-PLLA and PLLA, with an increase in crystallinity by thermal aging. The creep test performed, by continuous stiffness measurement, showed that the creep strain of CDA decreased by the grafting of PLLA, and the creep strain of CDA-*g*-PLLA and PLLA decreased by thermal aging. With an increase in holding time, hardness was decreased, whereas elastic modulus was kept almost constant. Then Teramoto and coworkers[107] systematically studied the approaches to CA-*g*-PHSs (lactic acid, L-lactide, (*R*, *S*)-β-butyrolactone, δ-valerolactone, and ε-CL). These polyesters could to some extent lower the T_g of CA (Figure 4.9).

In addition of ROP, some other polymerization methods have been reported to prepare the grafted CDA. Vlček's group[108] has synthesized CDA-*g*-PCL-*g*-PSt via ROP and ATRP sequentially. CDA was first partly functionalized with 2-bromoisobutyryl groups and then the unreacted hydroxyl

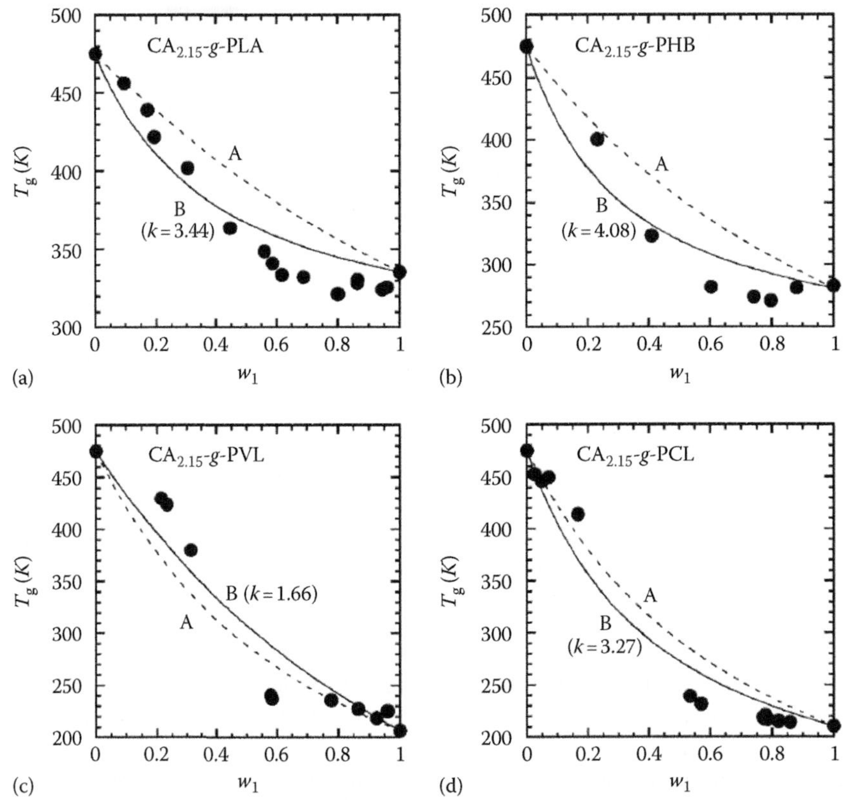

FIGURE 4.9 Glass transition temperature plotted as a function of composition (a) $CA_{2.15}$-*g*-PLA, (b) $CA_{2.15}$-*g*-PHB, (c) $CA_{2.15}$-*g*-PVL and (d) $CA_{2.15}$-*g*-PCL. The lines A (----) and B (—) are drawn according to Fox Equation and Gordon–Taylor equations, respectively. (From Rials, T.G. et al., *J. Polym. Sci. Polym. Phys.*, 45, 1114, 2007.)

initiated the ROP of ε-CL. CDA-*g*-PCL copolymers were further used as macroinitiators of ATRP for the vinyl monomer, giving densely grafted copolymers with polyester and PSt, or PBuA, or PMMA grafts.

4.4 CONCLUSION

In conclusion, this chapter introduces the graft modification of cellulose and cellulose derivatives.

The modification of cellulose can be divided into homogeneous graft and heterogeneous graft: most graft copolymerization of cellulose was conducted in heterogeneous graft resulting from the insolubility of cellulose in most solvents as the existence of intramolecular and intermolecular hydrogen bonds. During the modification process, free radical polymerization of cellulose is popular during the production of synthetic polymer in industries with its unique advantages including mild condition, low price, and a wider range of monomers. Higher graft efficiency and controlled molecular weight are needed to be investigated further. Homogeneous graft cellulose provides a robust strategy for tuning the graft density and graft chain length. Exploring more suitable solvent for cellulose is the prerequisite of the prosperity of homogeneous graft of cellulose.

Various cellulose derivatives including EC, HEC, HPC, CA, and CMC are applied to military-industrial, textile industry, paint industry, and cigarette industry traditionally. However, with the increasing demands for smart materials, biological materials, and nontoxic materials, the functional modification of cellulose derivatives is an urgent need. Compared with cellulose, cellulose derivatives have many advantages including a better solubility and higher reactivity. Therefore, more grafting methods and more suitable monomers could be utilized sufficiently to achieve multi-functional and special functional materials based on cellulose derivatives.

REFERENCES

1. B. Heublein et al., *Angew. Chem. Int. Ed.*, 2005, 44, 3358.
2. A. C. O'Sullivan, *Cellulose*, 1997, 4, 173.
3. J. Yuan et al., *Prog. Chem.*, 2010, 22, 449.
4. S. Y. Fu et al., *Trans. China Pulp Paper*, 2010, 1125, 90.
5. J. Yuan et al., *Polym. Adv. Technol.*, 2012, 23, 255.
6. J. Yuan et al., *Polym. Chem.*, 2010, 1, 423.
7. J. J. Williams et al., *J. Macromol. Sci. Chem.*, 1976, A10, 637.
8. Y. Wang et al., *Fine Spec. Chem.*, 2004, 12, 18.
9. L. Zhang et al., *Macromolecules*, 2011, 44, 1642.
10. L. Zhang et al., *Macromolecules*, 2011, 44, 4565.
11. J. Zhou et al., *Carbohydr. Polym.*, 2010, 82, 122.
12. J. Zhang et al., *Macromolecules*, 2005, 38, 8272.
13. J. Yuan et al., *Biomacromolecules*, 2008, 9, 2615.
14. J. Zhang et al., *Carbohydr. Polym.*, 2007, 69, 665.
15. S. Kalia and M. W. Sabaa (eds.), *Polysaccharide Based Graft Copolymers*, Springer-Verlag, Berlin, Germany, 2013. doi:10.1007/978-3-642-36566-9_2.
16. Y. Yang et al., *J. Cellulose Sci. Technol.*, 2009, 17, 53.
17. V. K. Thakur et al., *Int. J. Polym. Anal. Chem.*, 2013, 18, 495–503.
18. P. N. Sudha et al., *Compos. Interf.*, 2014, 21, 75.
19. J. Yu et al., *Biosens. Bioelectron.*, 2014, 50, 262.
20. S. Sahoo et al., *Cellulose*, 2001, 8, 233.
21. C. Daneault et al., *J. Colloid Interface Sci.*, 2009, 333, 145.
22. A. Carlmark et al., *Chem. Phys.*, 2013, 214, 1539.
23. A. Carlmark et al., *J. Am. Chem. Soc.*, 2002, 124, 900.
24. A. Carlmark et al., *Biomacromolecules*, 2003, 4, 1740.
25. S. Utsel et al., *Soft Matter*, 2010, 6, 342.
26. S. Utsel et al., *Eur. Polym. J.*, 2012, 48, 1195.
27. C. Barner-Kowollik et al., *Biomacromolecules*, 2013, 14, 64.
28. C. Barner-Kowollik et al., *Polym. Chem.*, 2012, 3, 307.
29. M. H. Stenzel et al., *Macromolecules*, 2007, 40, 7140.
30. S. Perrier et al., *Macromolecules*, 2005, 38, 10363.
31. Z. W. Liu et al., *Cellulose*, 2009, 16, 1133.
32. S. Perrier et al., *Aust. J. Chem.*, 2006, 59, 737.
33. E. Malmström et al., *Eur. Polym. J.*, 2012, 48, 1646.
34. A. Córdova et al., *Macromol. Rapid Commun.*, 2005, 26, 82.
35. W. Thielemans, *Cellulose*, 2011, 18, 607.
36. A. Dufresne et al., *J. Mater. Chem.*, 2008, 18, 5002.
37. N. B. Mohamed et al., *Eur. Polym. J.*, 2008, 44, 4074.
38. W. Tao et al., *J. Biomed. Sci. Eng.*, 2008, 1, 37.
39. K. Ishihara et al., *J. Polym. Sci. A: Polym. Chem.*, 2008, 46, 3306.
40. M. S. Hiltunen et al., *Polym. Int.*, 2011, 60, 1370.
41. A. Carlmark et al., *Euro. Polym. J.*, 2012, 48, 1646.
42. A. Mayumi et al., *J. Appl. Polym. Sci.*, 2006, 102, 4358.
43. M. Pohl et al., *Macromol. Symp.*, 2008, 262, 119.
44. H. Zhang et al., *Macromolecules*, 2005, 38, 8272.
45. C. H. Yan et al., *Biomacromolecules*, 2009, 10, 2013.
46. Y. Z. Guo et al., *J. Agric. Food Chem.*, 2012, 60, 3900.
47. H. Q. Dong et al., *Coll. Surf. B: Biointerfaces*, 2008, 66, 26.
48. J. Zhu et al., *Carbohydr. Polym.*, 2009, 76, 139.
49. Y. Z. Guo et al., *Carbohydr. Polym.*, 2013, 92, 77.
50. C. X. Lin et al., *Carbohydr. Polym.*, 2009, 78, 432.

51. J. Yuan et al., *Biomacromolecules*, 2009, 10, 2033.
52. Y. Huang et al., *J. Polym. Sci. A: Polym. Chem.*, 2008, 46, 6907.
53. J. F. Lutz, *J. Polym. Sci. A: Polym. Chem.*, 2008, 46, 3459.
54. A. Hoth, *Macromolecules*, 2006, 39, 893.
55. A. Boss et al., *Biomacromolecules*, 2004, 5, 1124.
56. G. H. Hsiue, *Bioconjug. Chem.*, 2005, 16, 391.
57. T. K. Bronich et al., *Bioconjug. Chem.*, 2005, 16, 397.
58. L. T. Hou et al., *Macromol. Biosci.*, 2006, 6, 90.
59. Q. Liang et al., *Macromolecules*, 2006, 39, 711.
60. J. Yuan et al., *Biomacromolecules*, 2007, 8, 1101.
61. Y. Huang et al., *Polymer*, 2009, 50, 2716.
62. M. Rawiso et al., *Nature*, 1994, 369, 387.
63. O. Pitois et al., *Adv. Mater.*, 1995, 7, 1041.
64. P. G. Wang et al., *Carbohydr. Res.*, 1999, 316, 133.
65. M. Jiang et al., *Angew. Chem. Int. Ed.*, 2003, 42, 1516.
66. C. Zheng et al., *J. Appl. Polym. Sci.*, 2010, 116, 3468.
67. M. Atoosa et al., *Biomacromolecules*, 2007, 8, 719.
68. B. Neda et al., *Polym. Bull.*, 2007, 58, 435.
69. G. Robert et al., *Carbohydr. Polym.*, 2009, 78, 938.
70. E. Ngesa et al., *Appl. Mater. Interfaces*, 2012, 4, 1043.
71. S. Alexander et al., *Eur. J. Pharm. Biopharm.*, 2010, 76, 421.
72. D. Sakloetsakun et al., *Int. J. Pharm.*, 2012, 422, 40.
73. D. Sakloetsakun et al., *Int. J. Pharm.*, 2011, 411, 10.
74. P. Liu et al., *React. Funct. Polym.*, 2012, 72, 983.
75. H. C. Chiu et al., *Langmuir*, 2012, 28, 15056.
76. F. Chen et al., *Int. J. Pharm.*, 2010, 59, 450.
77. C. Yang et al., *Int. J. Biol. Macromol.*, 2011, 48, 210.
78. P. Wang et al., *Asian J. Chem.*, 2013, 25, 4501.
79. S. Kumar et al., *J. Polym. Mater.*, 2002, 19, 403.
80. L. Zhang et al., *Carbohydr. Polym.*, 2011, 84, 40.
81. M. Geirnaer et al., *Constr. Build. Mater.*, 2011, 25, 1.
82. H. Susanne et al., *Polym. Chem.*, 2011, 2, 1114.
83. R. G. Liu et al., *Carbohydr. Polym.*, 2013, 95, 155.
84. R. G. Liu et al., *Polym. Chem.*, 2011, 2, 672.
85. H. Andreas et al., *Polym. Chem.*, 2011, 2, 2093.
86. E. E. Malmström et al., *Biomacromolecules*, 2007, 8, 1138.
87. E. Malmström et al., *Macromolecules*, 2008, 41, 4405.
88. L. Pourmirzaei et al., *Macromol. Res.*, 2013, 21, 801.
89. Y. X. Liu et al., *Pigment Resin Technol.*, 2010, 39, 156.
90. R. S. Cheng et al., *Cellulose*, 2013, 20, 2605.
91. G. X. Wang et al., *Carbohydr. Polym.*, 2009, 78, 95.
92. D. K. Mishra et al., *Carbohydr. Polym.*, 2009, 75, 604.
93. L. M. Zhang, *Macromol. Mater. Eng.*, 2000, 280, 66.
94. M. Salehi-Rad et al., *React. Funct. Polym.*, 2004, 61, 23.
95. M. Chen et al., *J. Macromol. Sci. B*, 2013, 52, 1242.
96. Md. I. H. Mondal et al., *J. Appl. Polym. Sci.*, 2013, 128, 1206.
97. T. H. Lin et al., *New Chem. Mater.*, 2013, 1, 71.
98. A. Giri et al., *Carbohydr. Polym.*, 2003, 53, 271.
99. W. G. Zhang et al., *J. Appl. Polym. Sci.*, 2007, 103, 1382.
100. H. Hosseinzadeh et al., *J. Appl. Polym. Sci.*, 2008, 108, 1142.
101. A. Q. Wang et al., *Poly. Lett.*, 2011, 5, 385.
102. G. Staikos et al., *J. Appl. Polym. Sci.*, 2003, 87, 1383.
103. G. Staikos et al., *Macromolecules*, 2001, 34, 4958.
104. O. Masaya et al., *JP* 60188401, 1985.
105. Y. Nishio et al., *Polymer*, 2003, 44, 2701.
106. Y. Nishio et al., *Macromol. Chem. Phys.*, 2004, 205, 1904.
107. T. G. Rials et al., *J. Polym. Sci. Polym. Phys.*, 2007, 45, 1114.
108. L. Toman et al., *J. Polym. Sci. Polym. Chem.*, 2008, 46, 564.

5 Cellulose Graft Copolymerization by Gamma and Electron Beam Irradiation

Dilip Kumar Kakati, Montu Moni Bora, and Chayanika Deka

CONTENTS

5.1 INTRODUCTION

Cellulose is the most abundant renewable polymer on earth. It is a linear polysaccharide with long chains, which consists of β-D-glucopyranose units joined by β-1,4-glycosidic linkages (Figure 5.1). Due to the absence of side chains or branching, cellulose chains can exist in an ordered structure. It results in the semicrystalline structure of cellulose, with both crystalline and amorphous regions. The hydrogen bonding between the cellulose chains and van der Waals forces between the glucose units give rise to crystalline regions in cellulose.[1] Cellulose is bestowed with many attractive physical and chemical properties like biocompatibility, biodegradability, hydrophilicity, stereoregularity, presence of reactive hydroxyl groups, and ability to form suprastructures.[2,3]

The main sources of cellulose are wood, cotton, and aerobic bacteria. However, the most important source of commercial cellulose is wood pulp.[3] The cellulose content of cotton fiber is 90% and that of wood is 40%–50%. Most wood pulp is utilized in making paper and cardboard. Cellulose derivatives, mainly esters and ethers, like ethyl cellulose, hydroxyethyl cellulose, hydroxyl propyl cellulose, methyl cellulose, carboxymethyl cellulose, and cyanoethyl cellulose[4–10] have been synthesized and found applications as fibers, films, coatings, laminates, optical films, and sorption media, as well as additives in building materials, pharmaceuticals, foodstuffs, and cosmetics. The scope of utility of cellulose could be further enlarged by its modification by graft copolymerization.

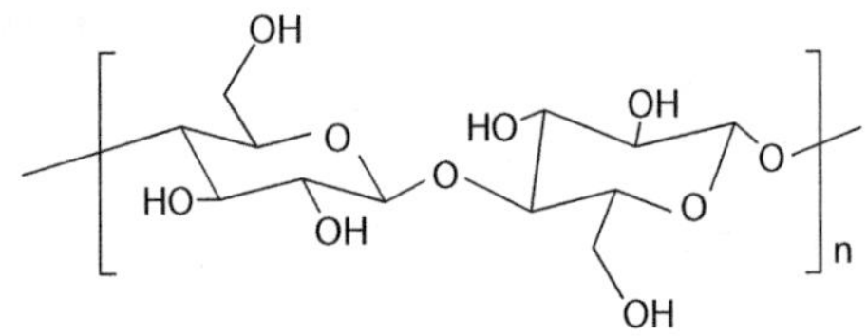

FIGURE 5.1 Structure of cellulose.

5.2 CELLULOSE GRAFT COPOLYMERS

Modification by graft copolymerization provides one of the best ways to alter physical and chemical properties of cellulose, by combining the properties of both natural cellulose and synthetic polymers. Depending on the chemical structure of the monomer grafted onto cellulose, graft copolymers[11] gain new properties such as water absorption, improved elasticity, hydrophilic or hydrophobic character, ion-exchange and dye-absorption capabilities, heat resistance, thermosensitivity, pH sensitivity, and resistance to microbiological attack. There are three approaches to prepare cellulose-based graft copolymers like grafting-from, grafting-through, and grafting-to approaches. When the propagation reaction of vinyl monomer is initiated on the active sites generated along the cellulose backbone, it is known as the "grafting-from" approach. This is the most commonly used procedure, and grafting reaction could be done with a single monomer or a binary monomer mixture. With binary monomer mixture, the reaction is carried out with either the simultaneous or sequential use of the two monomers. In the "grafting-through" approach, vinyl derivatized cellulose is polymerized with the same or different vinyl monomer. On the other hand, in the "grafting-to" method, a polymer chain with reactive functional group at the chain end reacts with the hydroxyl group of cellulose.

Various polymerization techniques have been used to prepare cellulose-based graft copolymers from cellulose and its derivatives with a great variety of monomers. These methods are generally classified into three major groups: (1) chemical grafting, (2) plasma-induced grafting, and (3) radiation-induced grafting. The area of present discourse is radiation-induced graft copolymerization of cellulose.

5.2.1 Radiation-Induced Graft Copolymerization

Radiation-induced graft copolymerization is a simple and facile method for the modification of pristine polymers and imparting new properties without affecting their inherent properties. Therefore, it has had been of particular interest for the preparation of a variety of functional membranes. Radiation-induced grafting can be achieved by using different types of radiation sources. Three types of radiations that have been commonly used are γ-radiation, electron beam, and UV-radiation. Radiation-induced graft copolymerization generally proceeds through free-radical mechanism. Under the influence of high-energy radiation, free radical sites are generated on the virgin polymer. These free radicals initiate the polymerization of vinyl monomers resulting in graft copolymers (Figure 5.2).

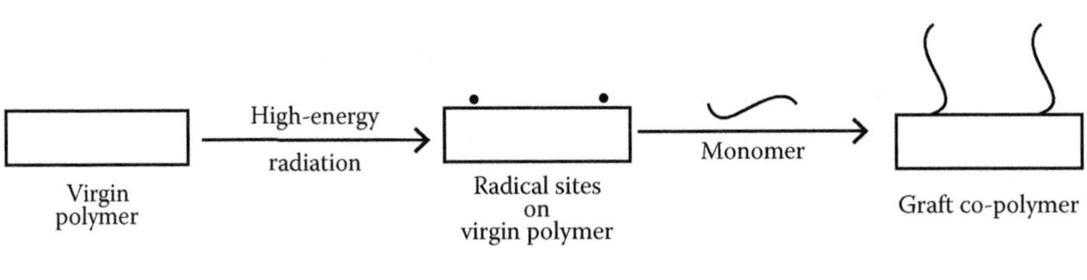

FIGURE 5.2 Graft copolymerization under high-energy radiation.

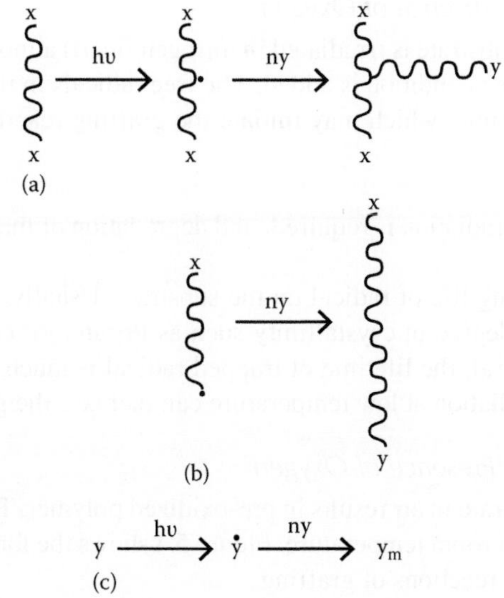

FIGURE 5.3 Schematic reaction scheme of simultaneous radiation grafting. (a) Cross-linking type, (b) degradation type, and (c) homo polymerization.

There are mainly two different methods of radiation-induced graft copolymerization: the simultaneous and pre-irradiation.

5.2.1.1 Simultaneous Radiation Grafting

In the simultaneous radiation grafting, the substrate material is irradiated in the presence of monomer or monomer solution to be grafted. While grafted chains grow from the backbone of the substrate polymer during irradiation, homopolymerization also takes place at the same time. The main reactions of simultaneous radiation grafting are illustrated in Figure 5.3.

The advantages of simultaneous radiation grafting process are as follows: easier operation, faster reaction, and lower dose of radiation. Further, the presence of a monomer can protect the polymer substrate from degradation during irradiation. Usually, homopolymerization is a serious problem during simultaneous irradiation grafting. It decreases grafting efficiency, and the homopolymers adhered to the surface of the trunk polymer are sometimes difficult to remove. The following methods are commonly used for inhibiting homopolymerization and increasing graft yields:

1. Addition of inhibitors such as Cu^{+2} and Fe^{+2}.
2. As the adsorbed dose of radiation is closely related to the density of substance, the homopolymerization is controlled by the dilution of the monomer.
3. Some solvents or mixture of solvents cannot only inhibit homopolymerization but also control the depth of grafting.

Another disadvantage associated with this process is that it is difficult to control the extent of graft copolymerization.

5.2.1.2 Pre-Irradiation Grafting

In the pre-irradiation grafting, the substrate (polymer) is irradiated first and then the grafting reaction is done by contacting the pre-irradiated substrate with monomer at a certain temperature in an oxygen-free environment. In this method, as the monomer is not irradiated, the homopolymer formation can be greatly reduced. The pre-irradiation can be performed either in the absence or the presence of oxygen.

5.2.1.2.1 Irradiation in the Absence of Oxygen

In this process, the polymer substrate is irradiated in nitrogen (inert) atmosphere or in vacuum, after which monomer in oxygen-free condition is added. The free radicals in the polymer can be trapped and retained for a period of time, which may initiate the grafting reaction. The characteristics of this method are

1. Relatively high dose of radiation is required, and degradation of the substrate is sometimes possible.
2. It requires relatively long life of radical on the substrate. Usually, the trapped radicals in polymers with a high degree of crystallinity such as PE and PP can be kept for a longer period of time. In general, the lifetime of trapped radical is much longer at low temperature. Accordingly, irradiation at low temperature can increase the grafting yield.

5.2.1.2.2 Irradiation in the Presence of Oxygen

Irradiation of a polymer substrate in air results in pre-oxidized polymer. The diperoxides and hydroperoxides are usually stable at room temperature. Figure 5.4 shows the formation of diperoxides and hydroperoxides and the main reactions of grafting.

The thermal dissociation of the hydroperoxide gives rise to an equivalent number of graft copolymer and homopolymer molecules. The homopolymer is formed from the monomer, initiated by the ·OH radicals. Usually, the homopolymerization could be controlled to a large extent by decomposing the hydroperoxide at a low temperature in a redox system such as follows:

$$\mathrm{ROOH} + \mathrm{Fe}^{+2} \longrightarrow \mathrm{RO}^{\bullet} + {}^{-}\mathrm{OH} + \mathrm{Fe}^{+3}$$

Besides the substrate itself, the other factors that influence the pre-irradiation grafting reactions are radiation dose, monomer concentration, presence of additives, reaction temperature, and reaction time.

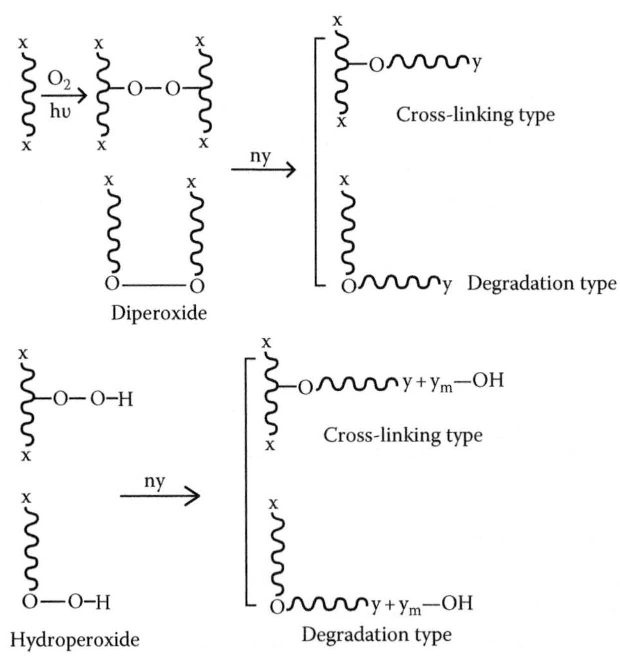

FIGURE 5.4 Schematic presentation of reactions of pre-irradiation grafting.

5.2.2 High-Energy Radiation-Induced Graft Copolymerization of Cellulose

High-energy radiation-induced grafting is advantageous over conventional chemical grafting methods. Some of the advantages are the absence of initiator, homogeneous and temperature-independent initiation, and sterilization of the product formed. This technique has been used to impart and improve flame retardancy, water impermeability, abrasion resistance, and rot resistance of cellulose.[11] It is also used to impart special properties for antibacterial and biomedical applications.[12,13] Wojnárovits et al.[14] reviewed the application of cellulose modified by radiation-induced grafting in the adsorption of pollutants from water.

The high-energy radiation-induced reactions in cellulose are initiated through rapid localization of the absorbed energy within the molecules to generate long- and short-lived free radicals. Theoretically, more than 20 different cellulose macroradicals can be formed and were distinguished.[15,16] The C(1)–H and C(4)–H bonds are the weakest carbon–hydrogen bonds in cellulose molecule. These carbons are the ones most susceptible to hydrogen abstraction,[17] and the formation of these radicals are very likely. There are also reports that carbon-centered radicals at C(2) and C(3) are also suitable for grafting.[18] The creation of radicals and their further course are strongly dependent on temperature.[19] At room temperature, they are very unstable and will immediately undergo a thermal transformation. One such possible reaction for the radical at C(4) is the formation of an allyl radical,[14] as shown in Figure 5.5. The decay of the radicals is also strongly dependent on the supramolecular structure. The decay goes very fast in the amorphous zones, while radicals formed in the crystalline regions last for a longer period of time.[20] Further, the crystalline structure of cellulose is not affected by irradiation up to several hundred kGy, and no change occurs in the ratio of crystalline to amorphous regions as a result of irradiation.[14]

In the pre-irradiation technique of grafting of the cellulose carried out in an inert atmosphere, the main active species that initiate grafting reactions are the trapped radicals at the interface of crystalline and amorphous regions.[11] However, due to the low efficiency of this technique, it is rarely used. On the other hand, pre-irradiation carried out in the presence of air or oxygen produced long-lived radicals. Under such conditions, the peroxy radicals formed on the cellulose backbone slowly convert to relatively stable hydroperoxides, ROOH- and ROOR-type peroxides. The peroxy products have a longer lifetime and could be suitably used for the initiation of grafting.[21] Grafting is initiated by immersing the irradiated cellulose in liquid monomer or monomer solution at a temperature of 40°C–70°C. The peroxy products produced alkoxy and hydroxyl radicals, which initiate the graft copolymerization:

$$\mathrm{ROOH} \longrightarrow \mathrm{RO}^{\bullet} + {}^{\bullet}\mathrm{OH}$$

$$\mathrm{ROOR} \longrightarrow 2\mathrm{RO}^{\bullet}$$

(R = Cellulose residue)

In pre-irradiation grafting of cellulose radiation, doses in the range of 10–40 kGy are applied.[21] However, in simultaneous irradiation technique of cellulose grafting, as the solvent is present in larger amount in comparison to cellulose and monomer, it is generally assumed that the energy of the ionizing radiation is absorbed by the solvent. The free radicals formed from the solvent react

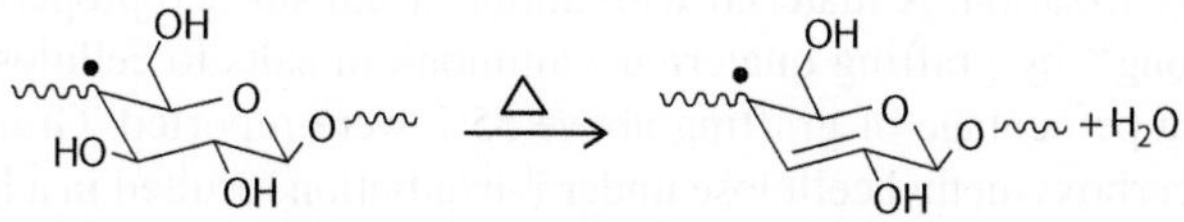

FIGURE 5.5 Dehydration of C(4) radical to an allyl radical.

both with monomer and with cellulose to form monomer radicals and cellulose macroradicals. As a result, unless suitable inhibitors are used, sufficient amount of homopolymer formation results.

5.2.2.1 Cellulose Graft Copolymerization under γ-Irradiation

γ-Radiation-induced graft copolymerization of vinylic monomers onto cellulose for the modification of cellulose properties as well as the induction of novel properties is an active area of research due to renewed interest in bio-based materials. Khan et al.[22] studied the γ-radiation-induced emulsion graft copolymerization of methyl methacrylate (MMA) onto jute fiber, composed of ~72% cellulose. The %graft wt. was significantly higher in pre-irradiation method. Further, it was observed that pre-irradiation in air produced up to 30% graft wt. compared to only 20% in nitrogen atmosphere. Sokker et al.[23] synthesized a bifunctional cellulosic material bearing $N^+ (CH_2CH_3)_3$ and COOH groups by radiation-induced graft copolymerization of glycidyl methacrylate (GMA) and methacrylic acid, followed by chemical modification with triethylamine. Grafting of GMA to cellulose under γ-irradiation and subsequent β-cyclodextrin immobilization resulted in enhanced adsorption of pesticide molecule.[24] Cellulosic fiber extracted from water hyacinth was functionalized by grafting GMA by simultaneous irradiation technique.[25] The grafting was done under nitrogen atmosphere, and GMA was used in a mixture of water and methanol. Benke et al.[26] investigated the pre-irradiation grafting of acryl amide, hydroxypropyl acrylate, propyl methacrylate, and 2-ethylhexyl methacrylate onto cellulose and slightly carboxymethylated cellulose fiber. Radiation-induced graft copolymerization of acrylonitrile (AN) and 2-acrylamido-2-methyl propane sulfonic acid (AMPS) on cellulosic fabric waste produced a material suitable for the removal of cyanide and dichromate from aqueous solution.[27] Carboxyl methyl cellulose-*graft*-polyvinyl alcohol synthesized through radiation method was used by El-Salmawi et al.[28] to investigate sorption of dye waste. Hashem et al.[29] graft-copolymerized itaconic acid onto cellulosic fabric for cationic dye removal. Pre-irradiation and mutual grafting of 2-chloro acrylonitrile on cellulose were investigated. The grafting yield was enhanced by emulsion grafting method, and a maximum of 27% grafting was reported.[30] Antibacterial properties were introduced to cellulosic materials by γ-radiation grafting of vinyl benzyl trimethyl ammonium chloride[12] and [2-(methacryloyloxy)ethyl] trimethyl ammonium chloride.[13] Takács et al.[21] modified cotton cellulose by pre-irradiation grafting of acrylamide (AAm), acrylic acid (Aac), 2-hydroxypropyl acrylate (HPA), 2-hydroxypropyl methacrylate (HPMA), and *N,N′*-methylenebisacrylamide (BAAm). They also compared the simultaneous and pre-irradiation grafting of *N*-vinylpyrrolidone to cotton cellulose.[19] γ-Radiation-induced graft copolymerization of ethyl acrylate onto hydroxypropyl methyl cellulose was reported by Wang et al.[31] Composite film of bacterial cellulose and polyvinyl alcohol was synthesized under γ-radiation from a ^{137}Cs source by Jipa and his coworkers.[32] Trimethylolpropane trimethacrylate–grafted methyl cellulose films were synthesized under γ-radiation, and films were found to be biodegradable in nature.[33] Acrylamide and cross-linking agent BAAm mixed with carboxymethyl cellulose were irradiated in nitrogen atmosphere to prepare acrylamide/carboxymethyl cellulose networks by El-Din et al.[34] MMA was grafted to biodegradable lignocellulosic fibers from jute by Khan.[35] The pre-irradiation was done in the presence of both air and nitrogen, and MMA was emulsified before polymerization. Ethyl cellulose-*g*-AN was prepared by γ-irradiation of binary mixture of ethyl cellulose and AN. Conversion of nitrile groups to amidoxime was done to investigate uranium recovery from aqueous solutions.[36] Pesticide adsorption capacity of cellulose fiber was enhanced by introducing hydrophobicity by grafting GMA under γ-radiation. The adsorption of phenol and 2,4-dichlorophenoxyacetic acid increased considerably.[37] Surface contact disinfection technique is a newly developed technique for water sterilization. A material with antibacterial surface property was developed by Xiaodong and Xiaodong[38] by grafting quaternary ammonium salts to cellulose under γ-radiation. Cellulose fibers with a percentage of grafting above 55% were reported. Grafting of cross-linked polyacrylamide onto carboxymethyl cellulose under γ-irradiation resulted in a hydrogel. The hydrogel was investigated for encapsulation and controlled release of agro-chemical potassium nitrate.[39] Cellulose isolated from pine needles was used as a substrate for graft copolymerization of styrene in a simultaneous irradiation technique. A maximum of 79.9% grafting was obtained.[40] Aly et al.[41] studied the grafting of vinyl pyrrolidone onto cellulose wood pulp in both heterogeneous and homogeneous media under γ-irradiation. They found highest grafting when cellulose was in solution in *N,N*-dimethylacetamide and lithium chloride mixture. The grafted product was investigated for wastewater treatment.

Rice straw cellulose available as waste biomass was graft-copolymerized with acrylamide under simultaneous γ-irradiation by Swantomo et al.[42] They reported that for the same dose, grafting efficiency was higher for bleached cellulose than with unbleached cellulose. An anion exchange matrix formed by radiation-induced grafting of vinyl benzyl trimethyl ammonium chloride onto cotton cellulose was investigated for protein adsorption by Kumar et al.[43] Radiation grafting of acrylic acid, 2-hydroxy ethyl methacrylate (HEMA), and polyethylene glycol methacrylate onto cellulose films improved the surface blood compatibility.[44] Jun et al.[45] investigated the grafting of *N*-isopropylacrylamide onto cotton cellulose under γ-irradiation in mixed solvents of water and alcohol or acetone. The effect of the composition of solvent mixture on the grafting was evaluated.

5.2.2.2 RAFT-Mediated Grafting from Cellulose under γ-Irradiation

γ-Radiation as initiation source at ambient temperature for reversible addition–fragmentation chain transfer (RAFT) polymerization results in polymeric materials with defined molecular weight and narrow molecular weight distribution, and a variety of monomers are reported to be polymerized by this method.[46–48] The RAFT process under γ-irradiation has also generated considerable interest in the realm of graft copolymerization. RAFT-mediated graft copolymerization results in higher graft frequencies compared to conventional methods, and it is considered as a very powerful technique for attaining tailored polymeric surfaces with well-defined properties.[49] RAFT polymerization under γ-radiation has also been investigated to produce cellulosic graft copolymers with tailored surface groups at ambient temperature. Barsbay et al.[50] applied radiation-induced RAFT polymerization to graft styrene from a pristine cellulose surface, using the chain transfer agent cumyl phenyl dithioacetate. From this experimentation, they further established an important fact that both grafted and free polystyrene have almost the same molecular weight and narrow polydispersity. The same group[51] also studied the RAFT-mediated grafting of sodium-4-styrene sulfonate from cellulose under γ-irradiation. The RAFT-mediated graft copolymerization of HEMA onto cellulose fibers, under γ-irradiation, was studied by Kodama et al.[52] The formation of the graft copolymer with a maximum of 92% (w/w) graft was reported. Barsbay et al.[53] synthesized epoxy-functionalized cellulose surface and intelligent flat cellulosic surfaces by grafting polyacrylic acid and poly-*N*-isopropyl acrylamide by the combination of radiation-induced initiation and RAFT technique.

The use of radiation as a tunable source in RAFT polymerization opens the door to designing new tunable surfaces in a controlled manner, and grafting cellulose by radiation-mediated RAFT technique offers a lot of opportunities ready to be explored by the polymer scientists.

5.2.2.3 Electron Beam–Initiated Cellulose Grafting

Electron beam irradiation has also found application as a high-energy radiation source for initiating graft copolymerization from cellulose and other polymeric substrates. As the energy used in the chemical reaction is directly injected by the electron irradiation, energy utilization efficiency is extremely high. The electron beam has directivity and high processing performance. The rate of imparted energy (the ratio of energy given to material per unit length) is extremely higher than that of other electromagnetic radiation such as UV, x-ray, or γ-ray as it is a corpuscular ray.[54] The industrial electron accelerators are usually classified according to their energy range, which are divided into low- (80–300 keV), medium- (300 keV–5 MeV), and high-energy ranges (above 5 MeV).[55] For modification of cellulose, only medium irradiation can be applied; otherwise, the chain scission will render the irradiated material mechanically weak.[56] Silver acrylate–grafted cotton fabric were tested for antibacterial activity by Mitra et al.[57] Acrylic acid was grafted using electron beam irradiation and subsequently reacted with silver nitrate.

Electron irradiation of powdered samples of cotton, flax, and viscose from textile fibers in 20–200 kGy range followed by quenching in a GMA solution resulted in epoxy-functionalized products.[58] Graft copolymerization of GMA from cellulose initiated by electron beam irradiation under different reaction conditions was also reported by others.[59,60] Kenaf fiber was de-lignified by treatment with sodium chlorite, and how the degree of de-lignification affected the extent of grafting of GMA under electron beam irradiation was investigated by Sharif et al.[61] Madrid and his coworkers[62] developed adsorbent materials from abaca, popularly known as Manila hemp. GMA was grafted onto electron beam–irradiated abaca fabric by emulsion polymerization, and the grafted product was treated with ethylenediamine to introduce amine functional groups on the grafted material.

5.3 SUMMARY

A worldwide search for environment friendly and renewable raw materials has reinvigorated research interests in cellulose and cellulose-based materials. In this context, radiation-induced graft copolymerization from cellulose to generate functionalized cellulose having multitude of applications has taken up a considerable chunk of research activities related to cellulose modification. In particular, RAFT-mediated grafting under high-energy initiation opens up a new paradigm in tailored surface modification of cellulose. Currently, radiation-induced grafting of cellulose is used for developing materials for polymeric membranes, polymeric adsorbents, and polymers for medicinal applications and applications in biotechnology.

REFERENCES

1. Bansal, P., Hall, M., Realff, M. J., Lee, J. H., Bommarius, A. S. 2010. *Bioresource Technology* 101:4461–4471.
2. Heinze, T., Liebert, T. 2001. *Progress in Polymer Science* 26:1689–1762.
3. Klemm, D., Heublein, B., Fink, H. P., Bohn, A. 2005. *Angewandte Chemie International Edition* 44:3358–3393.
4. Feng, H. Z., Zhang, L. M., Zhu, C. Y. 2013. *Colloids and Surfaces B: Biointerfaces* 103:530–537.
5. Cespi, M., Casettari, L., Bonacucina, G., Giorgioni, G., Perinelli, D. R., Palmieri, G. F. 2013. *Polymers for Advanced Technologies* 24:1018–1024.
6. Sarode, A. L., Obara, S., Tanno, F. K., Sandhu, H., Iyer, R., Shah, N. 2014. *Carbohydrate Polymers* 101:146–153.
7. Suwannateep, N., Wanichwecharungruang, S., Fluhr, J., Patzelt, A., Lademann, J., Meinke, M. C. 2013. *Skin Research and Technology* 19:1–9.
8. Hussain, P. R., Meena, R. S., Dar, M. A., Wani, A. M. 2010. *Journal of Food Science* 75:M586–M596.
9. Park, J. S., Kuang, J., Lim, Y. M., Gwon, H. J., Nho, Y. C. 2012. *Journal of Nanoscience and Nanotechnology* 12:743–747.
10. Wang, H., Shao, Z., Chen, B., Zhang, T., Wang, F., Zhong, H. 2012. *RSC Advances* 2:2675–2677.
11. Roy, D., Semsarilar, M., Guthrie, J. T., Perrier, S. 2009. *Chemical Society Reviews* 38:2046–2064.
12. Kumar, V., Bhardwaj, Y. K., Rawat, K. P., Sabharwal, S. 2005. *Radiation Physics and Chemistry* 73:175–182.
13. Goel, N. K., Rao, M. S., Kumar, V. et al. 2009. *Radiation Physics and Chemistry* 78:399–406.
14. Wojnárovits, L., Földváry, C. M., Takács, E. 2010. *Radiation Physics and Chemistry* 79:848–862.
15. Wencka, M., Wichlacz, K., Kasprzyk, H., Lijewski, S., Hofffmann, S. K. 2007. *Cellulose* 14:183–194.
16. Wach, R. A., Mitomo, H., Yoshii, F. 2004. *Journal of Radioanalytical and Nuclear Chemistry* 261:113–118.
17. Ershov, B. G., 1998. *Russian Chemical Reviews* 67:315–334.
18. Klemm, D., Philipp, B., Heinze, T., Heinze, U., Wangenknecht, W. 1998. *Comprehensive Cellulose Chemistry: Functionalization of Cellulose*. Wiley-VCH, Weinheim, Germany.
19. Takács, E., Mirzadeh, H., Wojnárovits, L., Borsa, J., Mirzataheri, M., Benke, N. 2007. *Nuclear Instruments and Methods in Physics Research Section B: Beam Interactions with Materials and Atoms* 265:217–220.

20. Vismara, E., Melone, L., Gastaldi, G., Cosentino, C., Torri, G. 2009. *Journal of Hazardous Materials* 170:798–808.
21. Takács, E., Wojnárovits, L., Borsa, J., Papp, J., Hargittai, P., Korecz, L. 2005. *Nuclear Instruments and Methods in Physics Research Section B: Beam Interactions with Materials and Atoms* 236:259–265.
22. Khan, F., Ahmad, S. R., Kronfli, E. 2002. *Advances in Polymer Technology* 21:132–140.
23. Sokker, H. H., Gad, Y. H., Ismail, S. A. 2012. *Journal of Applied Polymer Science* 126:E54–E62.
24. Desmet, G., Takács, E., Wojnárovits, L., Borsa, J. 2011. *Radiation Physics and Chemistry* 80:1358–1362.
25. Madrid, J. F., Nuesca, G. M., Abad, L. V. 2013. *Radiation Physics and Chemistry* 85:182–188.
26. Benke, N., Takács, E., Wojnárovits, L., Borsa, J. 2007. *Radiation Physics and Chemistry* 76:1355–1359.
27. El-Kelesh, N. A., Abd Elaal, S. E., Hashem, A., Sokker, H. H. 2007. *Journal of Applied Polymer Science* 105:1336–1343.
28. El-Salmawi, K. M., Zaid, M. M. A., Ibraheim, S. M., El-Naggar, A. M., Zahran, A. H. 2001. *Journal of Applied Polymer Science* 82:136–142.
29. Hashem, A., Sokker, H. H., Halim, E. S. A., Gamal, A. 2005. *Adsorption Science and Technology* 23:455–465.
30. Solpan, D., Torun, M., Güven, O. 2010. *Radiation Physics and Chemistry* 79:250–254.
31. Wang, L. L., Xu, Y. S. 2006. *Macromolecular Materials and Engineering* 291:950–961.
32. Jipa, I. M., Stroescu, M., Stoica-Guzun, A., Dobre, T., Jinga, S., Zaharescu, T. 2012. *Nuclear Instruments and Methods in Physics Research Section B: Beam Interactions with Materials and Atoms* 278:82–87.
33. Sharmin, N., Khan, R. A., Salmieri, S., Dussault, D., Bouchard, J., Lacroix, M. 2012. *Journal of Agricultural and Food Chemistry* 60:623–629.
34. El-Din, H. M. N., Abd Alla, S. G., El-Naggar, A. W. M. 2010. *Radiation Physics and Chemistry* 79:725–730.
35. Khan, F. 2005. *Macromolecular Bioscience* 5:78–89.
36. Basarir, S. S., Bayramgil, N. P. 2012. *Radiochimica Acta* 100:893–899.
37. Takács, E., Wojnárovits, L., Horvath, E. K., Fekete, T., Borsa, J. 2012. *Radiation Physics and Chemistry* 81:1389–1392.
38. Xiaodong, X., Xiaogong, W. 2009. *Huagong Jinzhan* 28:117–120.
39. Abd El-Mohdy, H. L. 2007. *Reactive and Functional Polymers* 67:1094–1102.
40. Chauhan, G. S., Dhiman, S. K., Guleria, L. K., Kaur, I. 2002. *Journal of Applied Polymer Science* 83:1490–1500.
41. Aly, A. S., Sokker, H. H., Hashem, A., Hebeish, A. 2005. *American Journal of Applied Sciences* 2:508–513.
42. Swantomo, D., Rochmadi, I., Basuki, K. T., Sudiyo, R. 2013. *Atom Indonesia* 39:57–64.
43. Kumar, V., Bhardwaj, Y. K., Jamdar, S. N., Goel, N. K., Sabharwal, S. 2006. *Journal of Applied Polymer Science* 102:5512–5521.
44. Nho, Y. C., Kwon, O. H. 2003. *Radiation Physics and Chemistry* 66:299–307.
45. Jun, L., Jun, L., Min, Y., Hongfei, H. 2001. *Radiation Physics and Chemistry* 60:625–628.
46. Barner, L., Quinn, J. F., Barner-Kowollik, C., Vana, P., Davis, T. P. 2003. *European Polymer Journal* 39:449–459.
47. Quinn, J. F., Davis, T. P., Barner, L., Barner-Kowollik, C. 2007. *Polymer* 48:6467–6480.
48. Kiani, K., Hill, D. J. T., Rasoul, F., Whittaker, M., Rintoul, L. 2007. *Journal of Polymer Science Part A: Polymer Chemistry* 45:1074–1083.
49. Barsbay, M., Güven, O. 2009. *Radiation Physics and Chemistry* 78:1054–1059.
50. Barsbay, M., Güven, O., Stenzel, M. H., Davis, T. P., Barner-Kowollik, C., Barner, L. 2007. *Macromolecules* 40:7140–7147.
51. Barsbay, M., Güven, O., Davis, T. P., Barner-Kowollik, C., Barner, L. 2009. *Polymer* 50:973–982.
52. Kodama, Y., Barsbay, M., Güven, O. 2014. *Radiation Physics and Chemistry* 94:98–104.
53. Barsbay, M., Güven, O. 2014. *Hacettepe Journal of Biology and Chemistry* 42:1–7.
54. Kashiwagi, M., Hoshi, Y. 2012. *SEI Technical Review* 75:47–54.
55. Henniges, U., Hasani, M., Potthast, A., Westman, G., Rosenau, T. 2013. *Materials* 6:1584–1598.
56. Henniges, U., Okubayashi, S., Rosenau, T., Potthast, A. 2012. *Biomacromolecules* 13:4171–4178.
57. Mitra, D., Rawat, K. P., Sabharwal, S., Majali, A. B. 2000. Antibacterial activity of cotton fabric grafted with silver acrylate by electron beam irradiation. *Proceedings of the Trombay Symposium on Radiation and Photochemistry*, Mumbai, India, January 12–17, 2000.
58. Alberti, A., Bertini, S., Gastaldi, G. et al. 2005. *European Polymer Journal* 41:1787–1797.
59. Consentino, C., Gastaldi, G., Melone, L., Torri, G., Vismara, E. 2008. *NSTI Nanotechnology* 2:110–113.

60. Parajuli, D., Hirota, K. December 2010. Electron beam initiated graft modification of cotton and preparation of high performance metal adsorbent. *International Chemical Congress of Pacific Basin Societies*, Pacifichem 2010, Honolulu, Hawaii, USA.
61. Sharif, J., Mohamad, S. F., Fatimah Othman, N. A., Bakaruddin, N. A., Osman, H. N., Güven, O. 2013. *Radiation Physics and Chemistry* 91:125–131.
62. Madrid, J. F., Ueki, Y., Seko, N. 2013. *Radiation Physics and Chemistry* 90:104–110.

6 Advances in Cellulose-Based Graft Copolymers Prepared via Controlled Radical Polymerization Methods

A Comprehensive Review

Umesh Kumar Parida, Birendra Kumar Bindhani, Susanta Kumar Biswal and Padmalochan Nayak

CONTENTS

6.1 INTRODUCTION

One trend in modern civilization is to effect gradual replacement of natural materials with either all synthetic materials or modified natural materials. In the polymeric age, it is essential to modify the properties of a polymer according to tailor-made specifications designed for target applications. There are several means to modify polymers properties, viz., blending, grafting, and curing. "Blending" is the physical mixture of two (or more) polymers to obtain the requisite properties. "Grafting" is a method wherein monomers are covalently bonded (modified) onto the polymer chain, whereas in curing, the polymerization of an oligomer mixture forms a coating that adheres to the substrate by physical forces. Curing gives a smooth finish by filling in the valleys in the surface. Grafting vinyl monomers onto natural and synthetic polymers is a challenging field of research with unlimited future prospects. During the last four decades, Nayak and coworkers have studied the graft copolymerization of several monomers onto a multitude of natural and synthetic polymers like wool, silk, cellulose, nylon and polymer (PET), and rubber to enhance their properties using various initiators like hexavalent chromium, quinquevalent vanadium, tetravalent cerium, trivalent manganese, peroxydisulfate, and peroxydiphosphate ions (Samal et al. 1975, Nayak 1976, Nayak et al. 1978a–d, 1979a–d, 1980a–c, Lenka and Nayak 1980, Panda et al. 1980, Lenka et al. 1981, Tripathy et al. 1981, Pradhan et al. 1982b).

Grafting of vinyl monomers onto natural and synthetic polymers has been suggested as a potentially effective means of altering the properties of the base polymer. In recent years, graft copolymerization of vinyl monomers onto textile fibers in particular onto silk, cellulose, nylon, and PET has gained considerable importance since it is a fascinating field of research with unlimited potential application for industrial production of various fibers.

The various properties that could be imparted to the natural macromolecules through grafting without affecting the basic properties are viscoelasticity, stereo regularity, hygroscopicity and water repellence, improved adhesion to a variety of substances, improved dye ability, stability, soil resistance, bactericidal properties, antistatic properties, and thermal stability.

The successful grafting of vinyl monomers onto the fibers involves the creation of free radicals on the backbone of the fiber. This can be achieved by various methods, that is, (1) spontaneous ignition in the presence of swelling agent, (2) radiation ignition, (3) chemical initiation, and (4) photo-initiation.

6.1.1 Definition and Potential Applications of Graft Copolymers

Graft copolymer is a special type of branched copolymer in which the side chains are structurally distinct from the main chain; one such graft copolymerization is between rick husk and methyl methacrylate (MMA; Gnanou 1996, Bhattacharya 2000, Klee 2000). An example of copolymer model is similar to that given in Figure 6.1, where respective monomer residues are coded A and B.

The nature of polymer surfaces is of great importance because it is the surface that first comes into contact with the environment and therefore determines all kinds of interactions such as wettability, adhesion, and biological response. Surface modification of polymers has recently turned in the direction of new areas involving the control of not only the surface chemistry but also the morphology in order to affect specific interactions (Xang and Silvermann 1985). Modification of properties of natural protein fibers through graft copolymerization has become an attractive means of chemical modification of these fibers, since such treatments, in general, improve some of the disadvantages associated with these fibers. Some vital changes in properties like photoyellowing, wash and wear, wrinkle recovery, water repellency, improved dyeability, soil resistance, and thermal stability can be brought about by grafting with various vinyl monomers (Samal et al. 1975).

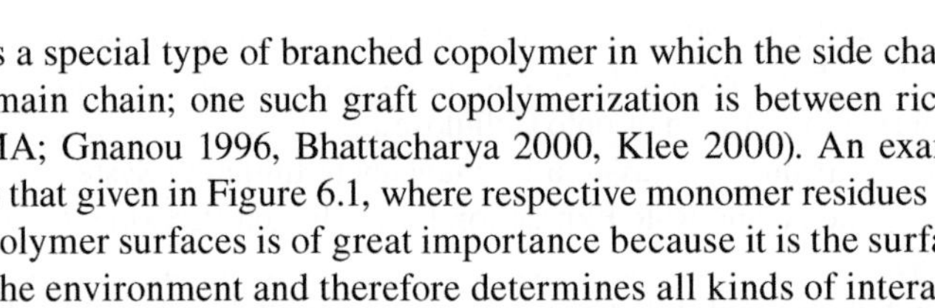

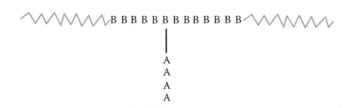

FIGURE 6.1 Structure of graft copolymer mode.

Graft copolymers are commonly used as compatibilizers in polymer blends. Their role is to stabilize the morphology of two immiscible polymers by reducing the interfacial tension and increasing the adhesion between their phases (Williams 1979). There are several types of interactions that can appear between compatibilizer and immiscible polymers. One of these interactions is the result of the same chemical structure of the graft copolymers and the polymers in an incompatible polymer blend (Williams 1976). The other possibility is that graft copolymers can make chemical bonds with the polymers in the blend whose side chains contain highly reactive functional groups (such as isocyanate). For example, by toughening of St acrylonitrile copolymer with ethylene propylene diene terpolymer (EPDM), it is difficult to achieve appropriate compatibility due to their chemically dissimilar structure. That will result in phase separation, which is larger than the optimum interfacial bonding and poor physical properties of blends (Walsh et al. 1969). Graft copolymerization enables modification of polymers and has allowed formation of various materials with unique properties. Even when a low concentration of one of the agents is added, significant changes of the structure of the graft copolymers can be observed. Such example is the addition of coagent TAC during the synthesis of EPDM-*g*-PS graft copolymers where the TAC will prevent scission of the main chain of EPDM, and then different structures of graft copolymers can be expected (Liepins et al. 1977a,b, 1978, Narayan et al. 1989, Ikeuchi et al. 1993, Peiffer and Rabeony 1994, Chung et al. 1995, Uyama et al. 1998, Xie 1998, Leger et al. 1999).

Much research has been conducted on the use of high-energy γ-radiation for the synthesis of grafted derivatives (Bhattacharya 2000). When polymeric materials are exposed to γ-radiation, radicals, cations, and free electrons can be generated, and it is the formation of free radicals on the polymer backbone that facilitates the formation of grafted chains. The radical formation upon exposure to the radiation is an extremely convenient technique from the viewpoint that no "synthetic steps" are necessary; all the reagents needed are the polymer to be grafted, the monomer, and solvent (if necessary). With this versatility, many different grafted derivatives have been synthesized for potential use in several interesting applications. Cross-linked poly (ethylene oxide), having heat shrinkable properties, can be used as a sutureless method for connecting blood vessels. Biocompatibility is an ever-present issue with biomaterials (Klee 2000); improvements in the biocompatibility of this material were observed by radiation-induced grafting of St, butadiene, and ethylene from the cross linked poly-(ethylene oxide) substrate (Xang and Silvermann 1985). For applications such as artificial heart valves, silicon rubber grafted with *N*-vinyl pyrrolidone and natural rubber grafted with 2-(*N*,*N* dimethylaminoethyl) acrylate (both synthesized with radiation techniques) appear to be useful biocompatible materials; however, the latter derivative's biocompatibility is higher than the former (Walsh 1969, Williams 1976, 1979). Graft copolymerization has several important applications for the synthesis of grafted textile industry. For instance, improved soil release and fabric comfort can be obtained from grafting fibers with hydrophilic monomers. Moisture absorbency of cellulose fibers was greatly increased (as high as 3000% water uptake) by radiation-induced grafting of acrylic acid from the fiber followed by cellulose decrystallization upon exposure to $ZnCl_2$ (Liepins et al. 1977a, 1978). Grafting a fabric's surface with the appropriate monomer can improve abrasion resistance. For example, the growth of poly (ethyl acrylate) (PEA) chains from cotton fabric by means of exposure to γ-radiation showed improved resistance to abrasion (Leger et al. 1999). Flame retardancy of fabrics is an important safety concern in many aspects of textile end uses. Due to the flame resistance of halogenated and phosphorus-based materials, radiation-induced grafting of vinyl bromide and different vinyl phosphonates from polyester and polyester/cotton-blended fabrics resulted in much improved flame retardancy (Narayan et al. 1989). Due to their influence over interfacial adhesion and friction (Nakagawa et al. 1998), graft copolymers have tremendous potential for improving the mechanical properties of composites. Since polymers of different chemical structures do not generally form intimate mixtures when blended together, the interfaces between dissimilar polymers (polyA and polyB) in a composite requires some type of adhesive for high-strength applications. Graft copolymers are ideal for this type of situation. When a hybrid branch macromolecule (polyA-*g*-polyB) is placed at the interface between polyA and polyB, the respective portions of the graft copolymer diffuse into the bulk portion of polyA and polyB. Although an overall bulk phase separation between polyA and polyB remains, the graft copolymer positioned at the interface provides a stronger bond between these two phases. Incorporating small amounts of PEA-*g*-poly (styrene) (PSt) into PEA/PSt blends increased compatibilization and results in tensile strength increases due to increased interfacial adhesion between PEA and PSt phases (Peiffer and Rabeony 1994). Commercial elastomers such as butyl rubber, poly (isobutylene-*co*-isoprene), have useful properties, such as low air permeability, but suffer however from a lack of compatibility with other polymeric materials. Grafting MMA side chains onto butyl rubber trunk polymer has been performed in an attempt to improve interfacial compatibility for possible use with other elastomers and plastics (Flory 1953, Battaerd and Tregear 1967, Chung et al. 1995). Generating composites of wood and PSt bonded with phenol formaldehyde resin still requires a compatibilizing agent in order to further bond these two dissimilar materials together. Narayan et al. observed that the placement of various cellulose-*g*-PSt derivatives at the wood/PSt interface in the presence of the phenol formaldehyde resin improved the shear strengths of layered materials (Narayan et al. 1989, Odian 1991).

An interesting medical application for graft copolymers, where reductions in frictional forces between two dissimilar surfaces are desired, is in the area of tubular devices (catheters and cytoscopes) that are, as necessary for examination, inserted into various bodily orifices (Uyama et al. 1998). For example, the surface grafting of a poly (urethane) film with dimethyl acrylamide resulted in a decrease in the coefficient of friction when the substrate was in the fully hydrated state (Ikeuchi et al. 1993). Glass-ionomer cements (GICs) have received attention for dental applications due to such properties as fluoride release, thermal compatibility, and biocompatibility. However, the current low strength and brittleness of this material make practical use difficult. Improvements in this area have been made using light-curable *N*-vinylpyrrolidone grafting of GIC, which showed improvement in both flexural and compressive strengths (Xie et al. 1998). Grafting poly (dimethyl siloxane) with st using an atom transfer radical polymerization (ATRP) mechanism, to be discussed in later sections, was performed to yield derivatives with potential applications such as supercritical CO_2 surfactants and thermoplastic elastomers (Mayo 1943, Matheson et al. 1991).

Several examples have been provided earlier to illustrate the impact graft copolymers can have on improving the properties of various end-use materials. Future applications of graft copolymers require an understanding of both intermolecular and intramolecular characteristics. These structure–property relationships are difficult to obtain without the ability to synthesize and characterize graft copolymers systematically. Besides having good control over the grafted chain molecular weight, the major problem encountered in graft copolymerization (especially with free radical–based systems) is the simultaneous formation of homopolymer. Homopolymer is essentially an unattached polymer having the same chemical structure as that of the grafted chains grown from the trunk polymer. The major sources of homopolymer result from syntheses that lack specific macro-radical formation and from the chain transfer of growing grafted chain ends. Not only is homopolymer a waste of monomer, but also the separation of it from the grafted derivative is often difficult, and it thus creates problems in characterizing the graft derivative. In fact, homopolymer formation is the major reason for the lack of a widespread industrial development of graft copolymers (Muzzarelli and Chitin 1977, Salmon and Hudson 1997, Hudson and Smith 1998).

6.1.2 Scope of This Study

In general, grafting means addition of side chains to the backbone polymer. Such side chains may be located at the surface or may be deeply penetrating. If the option is such that the grafting does not encompass the far interior of the backbone polymer, it may be envisaged that this will cause little perturbation in the molecular property of the backbone polymer. In addition, it is known that the monomer does not usually penetrate into the ordered crystalline regions of polysaccharides but enters into the disordered amorphous regions. On the other hand, if the penetration of the side chains is deeper, major changes in the properties of graft copolymer may develop. Radical chain growth mechanisms are important to polymer synthesis due to their greater versatility, relative to cationic and anionic methods, in regard to the wider range of vinyl monomers that are polymerizable by this method. The overall focus of this review is to discuss various free radical polymerization techniques that have the potential to conduct radical-based graft copolymerizations of any trunk polymer utilizing a "grafting from" mechanism in a more controlled manner with minimal homopolymerization. A substantial portion of thc chapter discusses different techniques, mostly free radical based, which have been used to graft cellulose polymers. Cellulose is underutilized renewable polysaccharides, and these grafting efforts have been performed with the intent of expanding the future applications of these biopolymers.

6.2 GRAFT COPOLYMER SYNTHESIS

A graft copolymer is a macromolecular chain with one or more species of blocks connected to the main chain as side chain(s) (Athawale and Rathi 1999). Thus, it can be described as having the general structure shown in Scheme 6.1, where the main polymer backbone poly (A), commonly referred to as the trunk polymer, has branches of polymer chain poly (B) emanating from different points along its length. The common nomenclature used to describe this structure, where poly(A) is grafted with poly(B), is poly(A)-*graft*-poly(B), which can be further abbreviated as poly(A)-*g*-poly(B). Grafting of synthetic polymer is a convenient method to add new properties to a natural polymer with minimum loss of the initial properties of the substrate. The chemistry of grafting vinyl monomers is quite different from that of grafting other monomers (or performed side chains). This section is divided into two subsections: the first dealing with grafting of vinyl monomers and the second reviewing other types of grafting methods.

6.2.1 VINYL GRAFT COPOLYMERIZATION

Grafting of polyvinylic and polyacrylic synthetic materials on the polysaccharides is mainly achieved by radical polymerization. Graft copolymers are prepared by first generating free radicals on the biopolymer backbone and then allowing these radicals to serve as macroinitiators for the vinyl (or acrylic) monomer (Scheme 6.1). Mino and Kaizerman first reported this approach in 1958 for graft copolymer preparation using a ceric ion redox initiating system (Beck et al. 1992, Mino 1958). Then, the chemistry and technology of the radical graft copolymerization technique

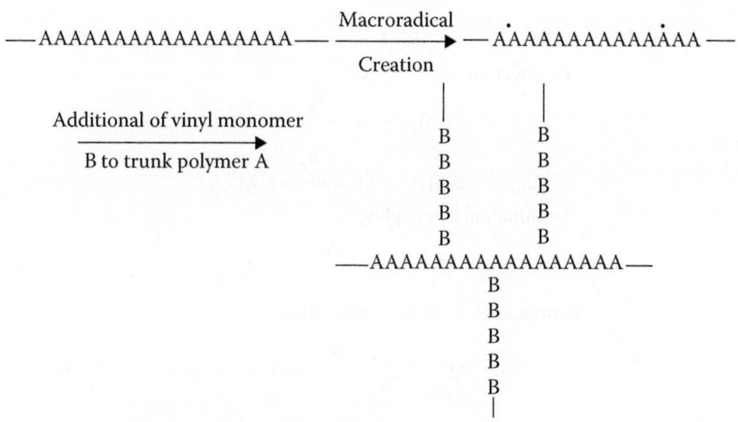

SCHEME 6.1 General mechanism of graft copolymerization of trunk polymer A with vinyl monomer B by means of a free radical mechanism.

(Berlin and Kislenko 1992) was developed especially in the case of cellulose (Hebeish and Guthrie 1981) and starch (Fanta and Doane 1986). Generally, free radical–initiated graft copolymers have medium-to-high-molecular-weight branches that are infrequently spaced along the polysaccharide backbone (Hebeish and Guthrie 1981). The copolymerizations can also be initiated anionically by allowing monomer to react with an alkali metal alkoxide derivative of polysaccharide. However, this method has not been progressed due to difficulty of the process and the low molecular weight of the grafted branches (Hebeish 1981). The properties of the resulting graft copolymers may be controlled widely by the characteristics of the side chains including molecular structures, length, number, and frequency.

6.2.2 Conventional Free Radical Polymerization

Free radical polymerization is the typical method of graft polymerization of various monomers onto existing polymer initiated by chemical initiator or by radiation (Fanta et al. 1986). During polymerization, the radical formation for initiation reactions can occur either on the backbone polymer or on the monomer to be grafted. Homopolymer will be produced if the radical formation is on monomer; therefore, initiators capable of creating radicals at various sites on the backbone are preferred (Mahdavinia et al. 2004) (Scheme 6.2).

The general mechanism for free radical vinyl polymerization utilizing an initiator that creates radicals by homolytic dissociation can be represented by Scheme 6.1. The kinetic rate laws for initiation (R_i) and termination (R_t) can be described by Equations 6.1 and 6.2, respectively (Flory 1953):

$$R_i = 2fk_d[I] \tag{6.1}$$

$$R_t = 2kt[M^\bullet]^2 \tag{6.2}$$

where

f is the initiator efficiency, k_t) $k_{tc} + k_{td}$

$M^\bullet$ is a propagating polymer chain end

Initiation

$$I \xrightarrow{K_d} 2R^\bullet$$

$$R^\bullet M \xrightarrow{K_i} M_1^\bullet$$

Propagation

$$M_1 + M \xrightarrow{K_p} M_2$$

$$Mx^\bullet + M \xrightarrow{K_p} M_{x+1}^\bullet$$

Termination by coupling

$$M_x^\bullet + M_y^\bullet \xrightarrow{K_{tc}} M_{x+y}$$

Termination by disproportionation

$$M_x^\bullet + M_y^\bullet \xrightarrow{K_d} M_x + M_y$$

SCHEME 6.2 Reaction mechanism for the classic radical polymerization of vinyl monomer, M, initiated by homolytic dissociation of species I.

Using the steady-state assumption where the radical concentration is assumed to be constant by setting R_i equal to R_t, the concentration of $M^{\bullet}$ can be removed from the rate law expression for propagation (R_p), allowing R_p to be expressed as shown in Equation 6.3.

$$R_p = k_p\left(\frac{fk_d\left[I\right]}{k_t}\right)^{1/2} \tag{6.3}$$

The kinetic chain length, *v*, is defined as the average number of monomer units that are polymerized by each initiating radical and can be quantitatively described by Equation 6.4, where the rate of polymerization is divided by either the rate of initiation or termination.

$$V = \frac{R_p}{R_i} = \frac{R_p}{R_t} \tag{6.4}$$

Qualitatively, if the only reactions that initiating and propagating radicals were allowed to undertake were the addition of monomer and termination by either disproportionation or coupling, the number-average degree of polymerization should be associated with the kinetic chain length (Flory 1953). For example, termination by disproportionation would yield average degrees of polymerization equal to *v*, whereas average degrees of polymerization equal to 2*v* would suggest termination by coupling. Experience from end group analysis indicates that the predominant mode of termination is that of coupling, with disproportionation being rather uncommon. It was observed that under certain conditions, free radical polymerizations could be conducted where termination by coupling was dominant; however, molecular weights observed were much lower than 2*v* while maintaining comparable monomer conversion as expected from the R_p. The notion of chain transfer was postulated, as follows, from these results:

$$M_y^{\bullet} + X - R' \xrightarrow{k\ tr\ X-R'} M_y - X + R'^{\bullet} \tag{6.5}$$

where

$M_y^{\bullet}$ is a propagating polymer chain with a degree of polymerization equal to *y*

X–R′ is some organic species (monomer, solvent, etc.) with X being a transferable group, typically a hydrogen or a halide

The rate of chain transfer (R_{tr}, X − R′) to X − R′ can be described as follows:

$$R_{tr,X-R'} = K_{tr,X-R'}[M_y^{\bullet}][X-R'] \tag{6.6}$$

In the chain transfer reaction, the growth of the propagating chain is stopped by capping the chain end with the X moiety. However, the polymerization as a whole has not stopped if the new radical, $R'^{\bullet}$, is capable of initiating the growth of a new polymer chain.

To quantify the occurrence of chain transfer, a relationship was developed as follows, which equates the number-average degree of polymerization ($\bar{X}_n$) to a modified form of the kinetic chain length expression (Equation 6.4), where the rate of polymerization is divided by the summation of the rate expressions for all types of chain growth breaking reactions (Odian 1991):

$$\bar{X}_n = \frac{R_p}{(R_t/2) + k_{tr,M}[M^{\bullet}][M] + k_{tr,S}[M^{\bullet}][S] + k_{tr,I}[M^{\bullet}][I]} \tag{6.7}$$

In the denominator, the terms ordered from left to right represent termination by coupling and chain transfer to monomer, solvent, and initiator. A quantity referred to as the chain transfer constant (CX – R′) for an organic substrate, (X – R′), is defined as the ratio of the rate constant for chain transfer over the rate constant for propagation. This quantity measures the likelihood of transferring the radical from the propagating polymer chain to the particular organic substrate, X – R′. Chain transfer constants for monomer, solvent, and initiator can be represented as shown in Equation 6.8, respectively.

$$C_{\mathrm{M}} = \frac{k_{\mathrm{tr,M}}}{k_{\mathrm{p}}} \qquad C_{\mathrm{S}} = \frac{k_{\mathrm{tr,S}}}{k_{\mathrm{p}}} \qquad C_{\mathrm{I}} = \frac{k_{\mathrm{tr,I}}}{k_{\mathrm{p}}} \tag{6.8}$$

Making the appropriate substitutions with Equations 6.1 through 6.3, and 6.7, 6.8 can be manipulated to provide Equation 6.9, commonly referred to as the "Mayo Equation" 6.25

Chain transfer constants have been evaluated for a wide variety of compounds based on the relationship as given, but the details of how they can be obtained are beyond the scope of this review (Mayo 1943):

$$\frac{1}{\bar{X}_{\mathrm{n}}} = \frac{k_{\mathrm{t}}R_{\mathrm{p}}}{k_{\mathrm{p}}^{2}[\mathrm{M}]^{2}} + C_{\mathrm{M}} + C_{\mathrm{S}}\frac{[\mathrm{S}]}{[\mathrm{M}]} + C_{\mathrm{I}}\frac{k_{\mathrm{t}}R_{\mathrm{p}}^{2}}{k_{\mathrm{p}}^{2} f k_{\mathrm{d}}[\mathrm{M}]^{3}} \tag{6.9}$$

6.3 CELLULOSE: STRUCTURE, SOURCES, AND USES

Cellulose is the most abundant renewable organic material produced in the biosphere, with approximately 5×10^{11} metric tons being generated yearly. Unfortunately, a mere 2% is recovered industrially (Doelker 1993, Bledzki and Gassan 1999, Mashkour et al. 2001, Belgacem and Gandini 2005, Reid et al. 2008, Kalia et al. 2009, Eichhorn et al. 2010). Cellulose is a linear syndiotactic homopolymer composed of D-anhydroglucopyranose units, which are linked by β-(1 → 4)-glycosidic bonds (Figure 6.2). Due to the high intensity of hydroxyl groups along the skeleton, the extended network of hydrogen bonds (intra- and intermolecular bonds) are formed. Consequently, two structure regions can be found: the crystalline region and the amorphous region (Klemm et al. 1998). Cellulose is a colorless, odorless, and nontoxic solid polymer, and possesses some promising properties, such as great mechanical strength, biocompatibility, hydrophilicity, relative thermostabilization, high sorption capacity, and alterable optical appearance (Klemm et al. 1998, 2005, Edgar et al. 2001, Kontturi et al. 2006, Tizzotti et al. 2010, Spence et al. 2011). These properties enable cellulose to be

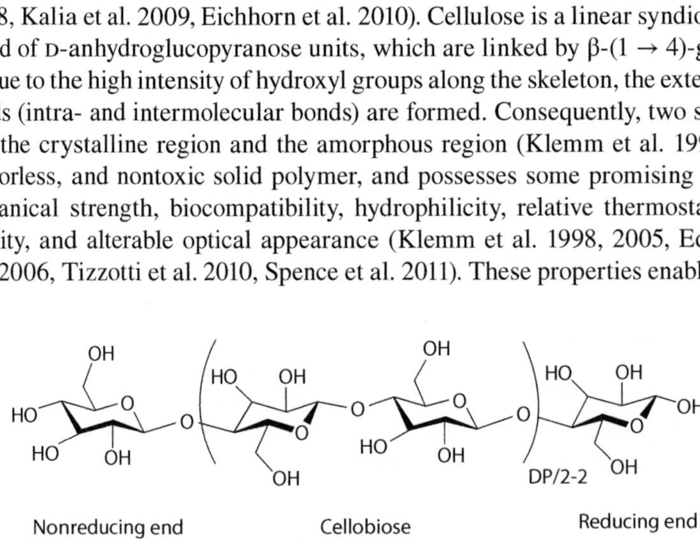

FIGURE 6.2 Molecular structure of cellulose.

TABLE 6.1
Applications of Cellulose in Different Forms Illustrated in Reviews

Material Forms	Applications	References
Fiber	Fiber, reinforcement material, biomaterial, magnetic paper, etc.	Kalia et al. (2009), Mashkour et al. (2011)
Film/membrane	Drug delivery, separation, water treatment, package, optical media, biomembrane, absorption	Huber et al. (2012), Eichhorn et al. (2011)
Nanocomposite	Biomaterials, drug delivery, reinforcement material, barrier, membrane, conductive, adhesion, etc.	Khalil et al. (2012), Gardner et al. (2008), Wojnárovits (2010)
Polymer	Drug delivery, biomaterial, water treatment, thickener, stabilizer, etc.	Zhang (2001), O'Connell et al. (2008)

applied to a vast array of fields. Some critical reviews concerning applications of materials based on cellulose in typical forms are listed in Table 6.1.

Despite those specific descriptions regarding applications of materials based on cellulose in the earlier reviews, cellulose can be used to fabricate "smart" materials, which present intelligent behaviors under environmental stimulus. "Smart" material is defined as one in which a key material property could be altered in a controlled manner in response to the introduction of a predetermined external stimulus (Czaja et al. 2007, Gardner et al. 2008, Hubbe et al. 2008, O'Connell et al. 2008, Siqueira et al. 2010, Wojnárovits 2010, Eichhorn 2011, Huber et al. 2012, Khalil et al. 2012). These stimuli-responsive materials might be utilized to undergo such changes as specimen shape, mechanical rigidity/flexibility, opacity, and porosity. Due to the intriguing property changes, "smart" materials have great potential in many applications, especially as biomaterials and drug carriers; some examples of material forms and their applications are given in Figure 6.3. Amphiphilic polymers can assemble/disassemble in water under certain stimulus changes, and drug-loaded micelles can be used as drug delivery systems. Hydrogels undergo swelling and deswelling in response to environmental changes and thus can also be applied for drug delivery and

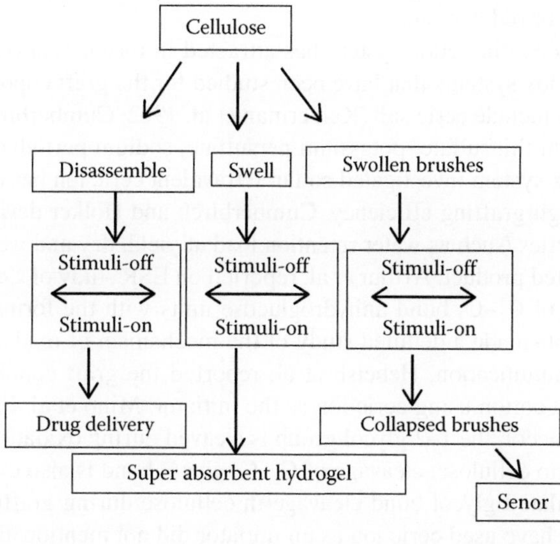

FIGURE 6.3 Examples of "smart" materials based on cellulose and their possible applications.

for super-absorbent hydrogels. And stimuli-responsive polymer-grafted membranes can regulate their pore sizes through polymer swelling and shrinking in response to stimulus. This kind of membrane can be fabricated to be separation membranes and sensors. The stimuli on/off switch can be produced by changes of pH, temperature, ionic concentration, etc. "Smart" materials based on cellulose inherit its unique properties, such as strong mechanical strength and biocompatibility; thus, studies on "smart" materials based on cellulose have bloomed during the last decade (Zhang 2001a,b, Murphy and Wudl 2010).

6.4 GRAFT COPOLYMERIZATION MONOMER ONTO CELLULOSE

Grafting is a promising field of research for modifying the properties of a number of natural and synthetic fibers (Heim et al. 2009, Marcus 2009, Moore 2010, Römer 2010, Raninen et al. 2011). During the last several years, Nayak and coworkers (Nayak et al. 1976, Nayak et al 1978a–d, 1979a–d, 1980a–c, Lenka and Nayak 1980, Panda et al. 1980, Lenka 1981, Tripathy et al. 1981, Pradhan et al. 1982, Nayak 1976) have reported the graft copolymerization of a multitude of natural and synthetic fibers using multitude of metal and nonmetal ions. The use of ultraviolet light for initiation of graft copolymerization is well known, and numerous studies have been carried out on this subject with the use of various polymers and the base material. A number of anthraquinone (Qiu et al. 2014, Testova et al. 2014), riboflavin (Hamdani et al. 2006), and other dyes have been used as photosensitizers for grafting vinyl monomers onto cellulose. The primary and secondary hydroxyl groups and β-glycosidic ether linkage present in the cellulose play an important role in defining its chemical properties and finishing treatments. Again, the formations of strong inter- and intramolecular hydrogen bonds and the natural stiffness of cellulose chain account for its high crystalline structure. The survival of cotton in competition with synthetic fiber lies in the retention of cotton as a preferred material in the eyes of the consumer, and hence it must be constantly developed and improved to retain that status. Graft copolymerization is a novel method, which has wide application in synthesizing new forms of polymeric materials and also in modifying the properties of natural polymer.

Grafting vinyl monomers to a cellulose chain could be accomplished by either ionic or free radical initiation methods. The free radicals could be created at the backbone of the cellulose by methods such as chain transfer, high-energy radiation (Arthur 1959, Brandrup 1975, Rapson 1960, Hermans1962, Demint et al. 1962) low-energy irradiation in the presence of sensitizer (Geacintov et al. 1960, Geacintov 1963, Yasuda 1963, Blousin and Arthur 1963, Kesting and Stannett 1963), mechanical degradation, or redox system.

Out of all these methods, the redox system has attracted in recent years (Nayak et al. 1978a,c, 1979a-c). Some of the redox systems that have been studied for the graft copolymerization of vinyl monomers onto cellulose include ceric salt (Kaizerman et al. 1962, Cumberbirch and Holker 1966), ferrous salt–H_2O_2, sodium thiosulfate–potassium persulfate, sodium periodate, and manganic sulfate–H_2SO_4. Of the redox system investigated so far, tetravalent ceric ion has received considerable interest because of its high grafting efficiency. Cumberbirch and Holker devoted attention mainly to the mechanical properties (such as water retention load at yield, dry and wet tenacity, and extension at break) of the grafted product. Arthur et al. reported on ESR study of Ce^{4+}-oxidized cellulose and postulated cleavage of C_2–C_3 bond anhydroglucose units with the formation of free radicals at C_2. Kulkarni and Mehta made a detailed study of the mechanism of oxidation of cellulose with Ce^{4+}. In a series of communication, Hebeish et al. reported the graft copolymerization of vinyl monomers onto modified cotton using ceric ion as the initiator. Mino et al. have shown that in the case of glycol, that is, pinacol, the 1–2 glycol group is cleaved during oxidation reaction with Ce^{4+}. Thus, during grafting onto cellulose, cleavage of C_2–C_3 glycol bond is also expected. Terasaki and Matsuki have also postulated glycol bond cleavage in cellulose during grafting initiated by Ce^{4+}. Most of the authors who have used ceric ion as an initiator did not mention about the high yield of homopolymer during the process of grafting. Since the oxidation potential of cerium is very high, it can react with vinyl monomers easily to initiate homopolymerization. Once the homopolymer is formed on the backbone of the fiber, it will be a difficult problem to remove it completely by the usual solvent extraction technique.

The main object is to find out a suitable method for grafting vinyl monomer onto cellulose eliminating completely the formation of homopolymer during the process of grafting. Nayak et al. have used a number of metal and nonmetal ions for grafting vinyl monomer onto some natural and synthetic fibers. The author has used $KMnO_4$, H_2O_2–cysteine, PP-Fe(II), PP-Mn(II), and PP-Cu(II) redox systems for monomer, oxidant, acid, temperature, nature of substrate, and solvents have been studied. The rate equations also have been derived.

Graft copolymerization reactions of cellulose are mostly carried out in aqueous and heterogeneous media. In water, the accessible, amorphous regions of cellulose swell, enabling the diffusion of monomer into these regions and the subsequent grafting reactions (Hebeish and Gutrie, 1981). By either preswelling the cellulose or performing the grafting reaction in a medium in which cellulose swells, the grafting efficiency is increased as a result of the increased ratio of monomer/cellulose. Moreover, by preswelling the cellulose, the grafting efficiency can be easily controlled. Many methods, including ozonation/oxidation, alkali, amine, and water pretreatments, have been used to improve the accessibility of cellulose toward chemical reactions.

Modification by graft copolymerization provides one of the best ways to affect the physical and chemical properties of cellulose, to combine the advantages of both natural cellulose and synthetic polymers and to use cellulose for various purposes. There are three approaches to prepare cellulose-based graft copolymers. The "grafting through" approach consists of copolymerization of premade vinyl-functionalized cellulose with a low-molecular-weight comonomer. In the "grafting to" method, a premade polymer chain with reactive end functionality reacts with a hydroxyl group of cellulose. This method usually suffers from low grafting density, due to steric hindrance. The most commonly used procedure is the "grafting from" approach, in which polymer grafts are directly grown from the initiating sites along the cellulose backbone. One of the major advantages of this approach is that a high grafting density can be achieved due to the easy access of reactive monomers to the chain ends of the growing polymers. Various polymerization techniques have been used to prepare cellulose-based graft copolymers from cellulose and its derivatives with a great variety of monomers. These methods are generally classified into three major groups: (1) conventional free radical polymerization, (2) ionic and ring-opening polymerization (ROP) and (3) controlled/living free radical polymerization (CRP). The main drawbacks of the conventional free radical polymerization are that the molecular weight and the molecular weight distribution of the grafts cannot be controlled, and the formation of homopolymer, which needs to be removed from the product, can even predominate. The ionic polymerization in preparing cellulose-based graft copolymers is challenging, since the experimental conditions needed for it are very demanding (e.g., low temperature, highly pure reagents, inert atmosphere, and anhydrous conditions). The advances in CRP techniques, such as ATRP, SET-LRP, nitroxide-mediated polymerization (NMP), and RAFT polymerization, have enabled the tailoring of macromolecules with sophisticated architectures including block, graft, comb, and star structures with predetermined molecular weights, terminal functionalities, and narrow molecular weight distributions (Hawker et al. 2001, Lindqvist and Malmstrom 2006, Gregory and Stenzel 2012). Growth of the synthetic polymer chain from a backbone has been the procedure most commonly used to prepare cellulose-based graft copolymers by CRP techniques. The "grafting from" procedure involves the preliminary conversion of hydroxyl groups of cellulose or its derivative into CRP-relevant chemical groups such as nitroxides, haloesters, or thiocarbonylthio derivatives. Control in CRP methods is based on dynamic equilibrium between dormant and active forms of the propagating chains. Under the appropriate reaction conditions, the concentration of the active propagating radicals is kept very low to reduce the irreversible termination reactions between them. Additionally, fast exchange between active and dormant species is required for good control over molecular weight, molecular weight distribution, and chain architecture in all CRP systems (Kamigaito et al. 2001). In an ideal case, propagating radicals should react with only a few monomer units within a few milliseconds before it is deactivated to a dormant state where it remains for several seconds. CRP (mainly RAFT and ATRP) methods have been successfully utilized to tune the surface properties of solid cellulose substrates in heterogeneous reaction media. However, a homogeneous reaction medium is needed to achieve a uniform structure at the molecular level. This literature survey will focus on the cellulose-based graft copolymers prepared via CRP methods, utilizing the "grafting from" approach under homogeneous reaction conditions. Most of these studies were carried out using soluble cellulose derivatives, but within recent years, a few studies in which unmodified cellulose is used have also been reported.

6.4.1 Cellulose Grafting of Potassium Permanganate Initiating System (Pradhan et al. 1982)

In a system consisting of permanganate, acid, and cellulose, Mn^{4+} might complex with cellulose, which breaks down giving rise to the cellulose macro-radicals. These cellulose macro-radicals (cell$^\bullet$) propagate giving the grafted polymer (Pradhan et al. 1982):

$$\text{Cell}-\text{H}+\text{Mn}^{4+} \xrightleftharpoons{\text{K}} \text{Complex} \xrightarrow{\text{K}_\text{d}} \text{Cell}+\text{Mn}^{3+}+\text{H}^+$$

Initiation

$$\text{Cell}^\bullet+\text{M} \xrightarrow{\text{K}_\text{i}} \text{Cell}-\text{M}^\bullet$$

Propagation

$$\text{Cell}-\text{M}^\bullet+\text{M} \quad \text{K}_\text{p} \quad \xrightarrow{\text{Cell}-\text{M}_1\cdot}$$

$$\vdots$$

$$\text{Cell}-\text{Mn}-1+\text{M} \quad \text{K}_\text{p} \quad \xrightarrow{\text{Cell}-\text{M}_\text{n}\cdot}$$

Termination

$$\text{Cell}-\text{Mn}^\bullet+\text{Mn}^{4+} \xrightarrow{\text{K}_\text{t}} \text{Grafted cellulose}$$

Oxidation

$$\text{Cell}^\bullet+\text{Mn}^{4+} \xrightarrow{\text{K}_\text{O}} \text{Oxidation products}+\text{Mn}^{3+}+\text{H}^+$$

where

Cell-H represents a reactive group in cellulose
M is isomer
Cell$^\bullet$ is cellulose macro-radical

By applying steady-state assumptions to [Cell$^\bullet$] and [Cell–M$^\bullet$], the overall rate of polymerization can be derived as follows (Scheme 6.3).

$$\frac{D[\text{cell}\bullet]}{dt} = K\,K_d[M_n{}^{4+}][\text{cell}] - K_i[\text{Cell}\bullet][M] - K_0[\text{cell}\bullet][M_n{}^{4+}] = 0$$

$$[\text{Cell}\bullet] = \frac{K\,K_d[M_n{}^{4+}][\text{Cell}]}{K_i[M] + K_0[M_n{}^{4+}]}$$

Again

$$\frac{d[\text{cell}-M\bullet]}{dt} = K_i[\text{Cell}\bullet][M] - K_t[\text{cell}-M\bullet][M_n{}^{4+}] = 0$$

(a) $$[\text{Cell}-M\bullet] = \frac{K_i[\text{Cell}\bullet][M]}{K_t[M_n{}^{4+}]}$$

$$[\text{Cell}-M^\bullet] = \frac{k\,k_d[\text{Cell}-H][M]}{K_t[M] + \frac{K_0}{K_1}[M_n{}^{4+}]}$$

Hence

$$R_p = K_p[\text{Cell}-M^\bullet][M]$$

$$= \frac{K_p}{K_t}\left\{\frac{[M]^2 K\,K_d[\text{Cell}-M]}{[M] + \frac{K_0[M_n{}^{4+}]}{K_1}}\right\}$$

(b)

SCHEME 6.3 Plot of R_p versus $[M]^2$ is linear passing through the origin that favors the above reaction scheme.

6.4.2 Reaction Scheme and Rate Expression for Hydrogen Peroxide–Cysteine Redox System

In a system consisting of hydrogen peroxide, cysteine, sulfuric acid, monomer, and cellulose, the free radical formation might take place as represented in the later text (Pradhan et al. 1982). Haber and Weiss have reported that hydrogen peroxide could be activated by the presence of reducing agents. Thus, formation of $OH^\bullet$ might be facilitated by the presence of cysteine owing to one-electron transfer with concomitant cleavage of O–O bond (Scheme 6.4).

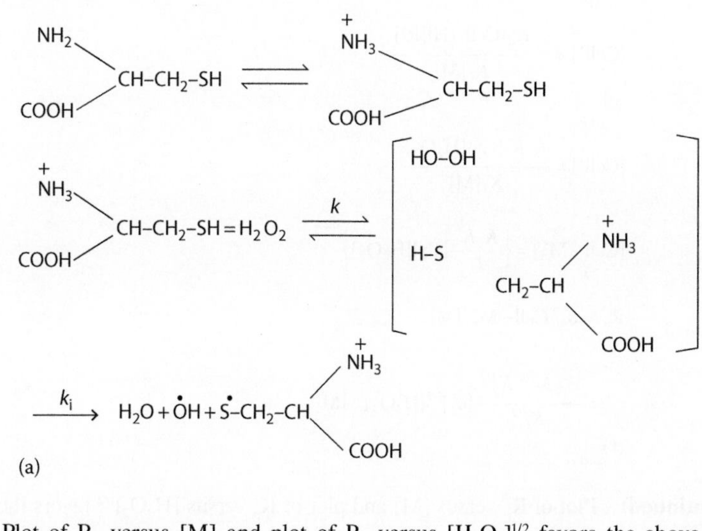

(a)

SCHEME 6.4 Plot of R_p versus [M] and plot of R_p versus $[H_2O_2]^{1/2}$ favors the above reaction scheme. (*Continued*)

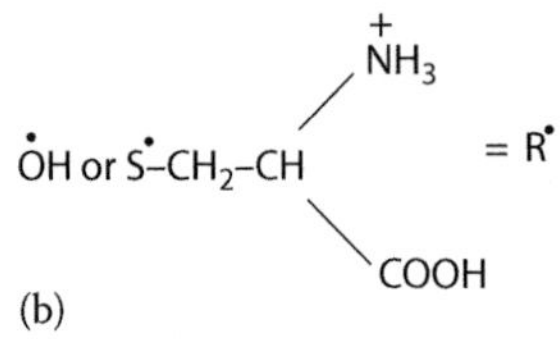

(b)

$$\text{Cell–H} + \text{R}^{\bullet} \xrightarrow{K_d} \text{Cell}^{\bullet} + \text{RH}$$

Initiation:

$$\text{Cell}^{\bullet} + \text{M} \xrightarrow{K_i} \text{Cell} - \text{M}_1^{\bullet}$$

Propagation:

$$\text{Cell} - \text{M}_1^{\bullet} + \text{M} \xrightarrow{K_p} \text{Cell} - \text{M}_2^{\bullet}$$

$$\text{Cell} - \text{M}_{n-1}^{\bullet} + \text{M} \xrightarrow{K_p} \text{Cell–M}_n$$

Termination:

$$\text{Cell–M}_{n-1}^{\bullet} + \text{Cell–M}_m^{\bullet} \xrightarrow{K_t} \text{Grafted copolymer}$$

(c)

$$\frac{d[\text{R.}]}{dt} = K_1[\text{Cy}][\text{H}_2\text{O}_2] - K_d[\text{Cell–H}][\text{R}^{\bullet}] = 0$$

$$[\text{R}^{\bullet}] = \frac{K\ K_1[\text{Cy}][\text{H}_2\text{O}_2]}{K_d[\text{Cell–H}]}$$

$$\frac{d[\text{Cell–M}_n^{\bullet}]}{dt} = K_1[\text{Cell}^{\bullet}][\text{M}] - K_t[\text{Cell} - \text{M}_n.]^2 = 0$$

$$[\text{Cell–M}_n^{\bullet}] = \left\{\frac{K_1[\text{Cell}^{\bullet}][\text{M}]}{K_t}\right\}$$

(d)

$$\frac{d[\text{Cell}^{\bullet}]}{dt} = K_d[\text{Cell–H}][\text{R}^{\bullet}] - K_1[\text{Cell}^{\bullet}][\text{M}] = 0$$

$$[\text{Cell}^{\bullet}] = \frac{K_d[\text{Cell–H}][\text{R}^{\bullet}]}{K_1[\text{M}]}$$

(e)

$$[\text{Cell}^{\bullet}] = \frac{K\ K_1[\text{Cy}][\text{H}_2\text{O}_2]}{K_1[\text{M}]}$$

$$[\text{Cell–M}_n^{\bullet}] = \left\{\frac{K\ K_1}{k_t}[\text{Cy}][\text{H}_2\text{O}_2]\right\}^{1/2}$$

$$\text{R}_p = K_p[\text{Cell–M}_n^{\bullet}][\text{M}]$$

$$= \frac{K_p K^{1/2} K_1^{1/2}}{K_t^{1/2}}[\text{cy}]^{1/2}[\text{H}_2\text{O}_2]^{1/2}[\text{M}]$$

(f)

SCHEME 6.4 (Continued) Plot of R_p versus [M] and plot of R_p versus $[H_2O_2]^{1/2}$ favors the above reaction scheme.

6.4.3 Reaction Scheme and Rate Expression for Peroxidiphosphate Me(III)) Redox System

In a system consisting of peroxydiphosphate ion, monomer, acid, and a bivalent metal ion like Fe(III) or Mn(II), the production of free radicals takes place according to the following mechanism (Scheme 6.5).

$$P_2O_8^{4-} + Me(II) \xrightarrow{K_d} HPO_4^{\bullet} - + HPO_4^{2-} + Me(III)$$

$$HPO_4^{\bullet -} + Me(III) \xrightarrow{K_a} HPO_4^{2-} + Me(III)$$

$$HPO_4^{\bullet -} + H_2O \xrightarrow{K_p} H_2PO_4^{-} + OH$$

But in case of Cu(II)

$$P_2O_8^{4-} + Cu^{2+} \xrightarrow[H+]{K_d} 2\ HPO_4^{\bullet -} + Cu^{2+}$$

$$\text{(a)}\quad HPO_4^{\bullet -} + H_2O \longrightarrow \dot{O}H + H_2PO_4^{2-}$$

Initiation:

$$Cell-OH + R^{\bullet} \xrightarrow{K_1} Cell-O^{\bullet}$$

$$\text{(b)}\quad Cell-O^{\bullet} + M \xrightarrow{K_1} Cell-OM^{\bullet}$$

Propagation:

$$Cell-OM^{\bullet} + M \xrightarrow{K_p} Cell-OM_1^{\bullet}$$

$$Cell-OM_{n-1}^{\bullet} + M \xrightarrow{K_p} Cell-OM_n^{\bullet}$$

Termination:

$$\text{(c)}\quad Cell-OM_n^{\bullet} + Cell-OM_m^{\bullet} \xrightarrow{K_t} \text{Grafted polymer}$$

$$\frac{-d[Cell-OM_n^{\bullet}]}{dt} = K_1[M][Cell-o^{\bullet}]K_t[Cell-OM_n^{\bullet}]^2 = 0$$

$$Cell-OM^{\bullet}n = \left(\frac{K_1}{K_t}\right)^{1/2}[M]^{1/2}[Cell-O^{\bullet}]^{1/2}$$

$$\frac{-d[Cell-O^{\bullet}]}{dt} = K_1[Cell-OH][R^{\bullet}]$$

$$- K_1[Cell-O^{\bullet}][M] = 0$$

$$[Cell-O] = \frac{K_1[Cell-OH][R^{\bullet}]}{K_1[M]}$$

$$\frac{K_d[P_2O_8^{4-}][Me(II)]}{K_1[M]}$$

$$R_p = K_p[Cell-OM_n^{\bullet}][M]$$

$$\text{(d)}\quad = K_p\left[\frac{K_d}{K_t}\right]^{1/2}[P_2O_8^{4-}]^{1/2}[Me(II)]^{1/2}[M]$$

SCHEME 6.5 Plot of R_p versus [M] and $[P_2O_8^{4-}]^{1/2}$ are linear indicating the validity of above reaction scheme.

6.4.4 Cellulose Grafting via NMP

NMP is one of the stable free radical polymerization processes, based on the use of a stable nitroxide radical (e.g., most commonly used nitroxide is TEMPO (2,2,6,6-tetramethyl-1-piperidinyloxy)) (Hawker et al. 2001, Kamigaito et al. 2001, Matyjaszewski and Xia 2001, Percec et al. 2006, Rosen and Percec 2009, Tizzotti et al. 2010, Malmström and Carlmark 2012). Control in NMP is achieved with dynamic equilibration between dormant alkoxyamines and actively propagating radicals (Scheme 6.6) (Hebeish and Guthire 1981, Röder et al. 2001, El Seoud and Heinze 2005, Braunecker and Matyjaszewski 2007, McCormick et al. 1985, Pinkert et al. 2009, Roy et al. 2009).

The first cellulose-based graft copolymer prepared via the CRP method was reported by Daly et al. in the early twenty-first century (Heinze and Glasser 1998, Klemm et al. 1998, 2005, Heinze and Liebert 2001, Swatloski et al. 2002, Moad et al. 2008, Pinkert et al. 2009). Authors prepared hydroxypropyl cellulose-*g*-polystyrene (HPC-*g*-PSt) using NMP. The controlled radical grafting from HPC was achieved using a TEMPO derivative formed from HPC–Barton carbonate derivative **1** (Scheme 6.7). The photolysis of **1** in the presence of styrene (St) and TEMPO yielded the TEMPO-modified HPC derivative **2**. Heating derivative **2** at 130°C with St provided the HPC-*g*-PSt copolymer **3**. An increase in the grafted polymer chain length with increasing polymerization time and the polydispersity of the grafts were observed, indicating that a certain degree of control was achieved. However, this is the only study published, so far as I know, in which cellulose-based

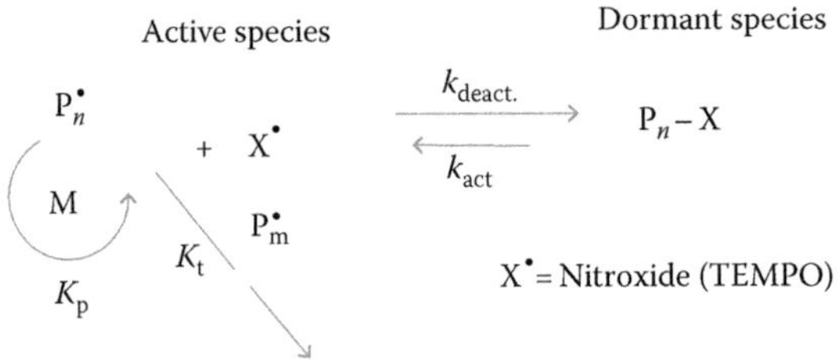

SCHEME 6.6 Accepted mechanism of NMP.

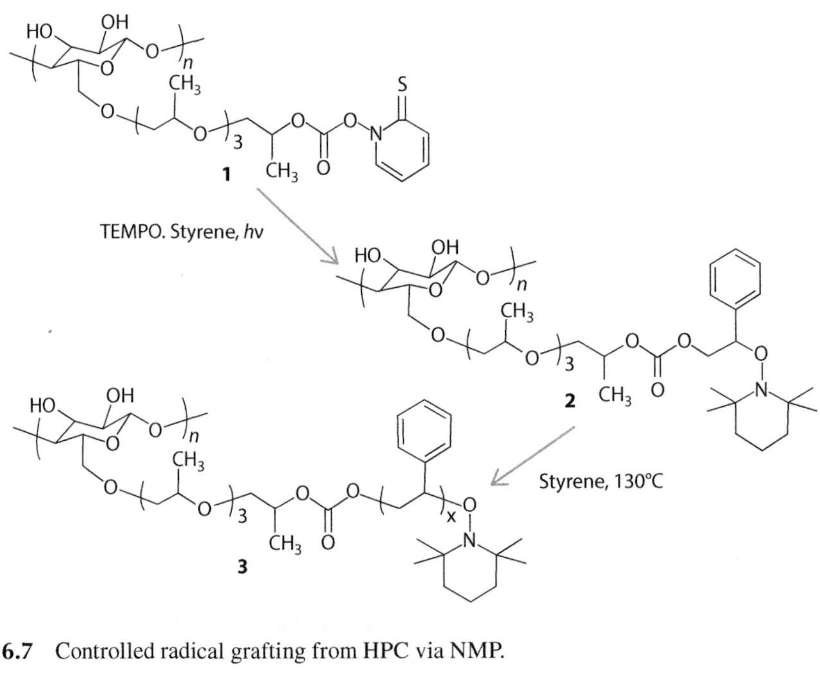

SCHEME 6.7 Controlled radical grafting from HPC via NMP.

graft copolymers were prepared using NMP. The main reason for its scarce use is probably the limited range of monomers that can be polymerized by NMP in a controlled way and the elevated temperature required for the polymerization to proceed.

6.4.5 Cellulose Grafting via RAFT Polymerization

RAFT polymerization is the most versatile and successful CRP method, due to its applicability to a wide range of radically polymerizable monomers (Carlmark and Malmstrom 2003, Roy et al. 2005, Lindqvist and Malmstrom 2006, Braunecker and Matyjaszewski 2007, Barner-Kowollik 2008, Gregory and Stenzel 2012). RAFT polymerization is based on a degenerative transfer, a thermodynamically neutral transfer process, between a minute amount of growing radicals and dormant species present at much higher concentrations via addition–fragmentation chemistry (Scheme 6.8). Rapid exchange reactions will to well-controlled systems. RAFT polymerization can be conducted under reaction conditions similar to those of conventional free radical polymerization in the presence of suitable chain transfer agents (CTAs). Various dithioesters, dithiocarbamates, trithiocarbonates, and xanthates have been effectively used as CTAs, to control molecular weights, molecular weight distributions, and even the molecular architecture of growing polymers (Heinze and Liebert 2001).

When cellulose is grafted via the RAFT polymerization method, the cellulose-based macroCTA needs to be prepared first. The CTA moiety could be attached to the cellulose backbone, either via a fragmentation bond (R-group approach) or a nonfragmenting bond (Z-group approach) (Scheme 6.9) (Matyjaszewski 2000, Daly et al. 2001, Stenzel and Davis 2002, Hernandez-Guerrero et al. 2005, Barsbay et al. 2007). The choice of synthetic method can lead to different molecular weight distributions. In both cases, after the initiation, the growing macro-radical undergoes transfer to the CTA connected to the backbone. If the CTA moiety is attached via the leaving group

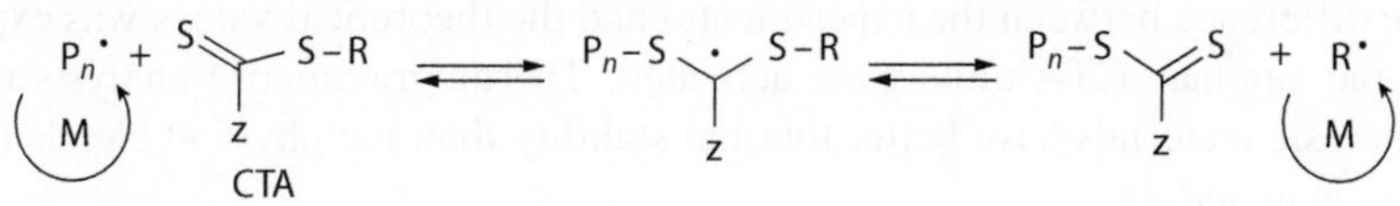

SCHEME 6.8 Mechanism of RAFT polymerization.

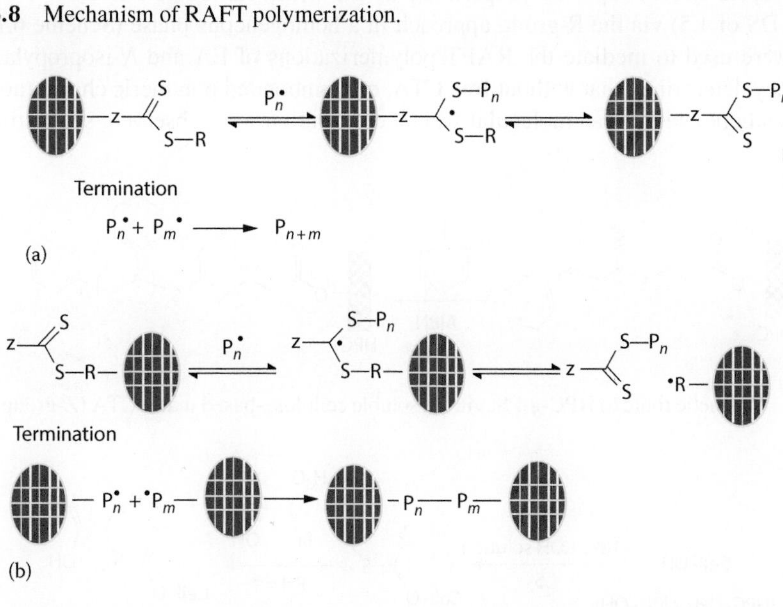

SCHEME 6.9 Graft polymerization through the (a) Z-group approach and (b) R-group approach via RAFT polymerization.

(R-group approach), the radical is located on the backbone after the first addition–fragmentation step, and the graft chains are grown directly from the backbone. This may lead to termination reactions via combination of the two growing radicals, resulting in some broadening of the molecular weight distribution especially at higher conversions. This undesirable coupling may be avoided if the Z-group approach is used. Even so, the CTA unit in this approach remains attached at the nexus of the backbone and the grafts after the transfer process, and propagation occurs extrinsic to the graft copolymer. The growing macro-radical then needs to be added again to the CTA unit on the backbone to achieve the classical RAFT equilibria. Therefore, as the side chain length increases, the steric hindrance around the CTA unit, due to the shielding effect of the grafts, may influence the control of the polymerization (Stenzel and Davis 2002, Hernandez-Guerrero 2005).

The first example of the synthesis of cellulose-based graft copolymer via RAFT polymerization in a homogeneous solution was reported by Stenzel et al. (Stenzel and Davis 2002, 2003, Hernandez-Guerrero 2005). They prepared HPC-*g*-PSt copolymer utilizing the Z-group approach. Trithiocarbonate-functionalized HPC-macroCTAs with different DS values was produced through esterification from HPC. It was then utilized in St polymerization with pseudo-first-order kinetics (Scheme 6.10). The molecular weight of the PSt grafts cleaved from the backbone showed a deviation from the theoretical molecular weight, due to reduced accessibility of the CTA unit with increasing conversion. The propagating radical was not able to reach the CTA unit and therefore terminated in preference.

Fleet et al. (2008) utilized the viscose process to introduce CTA moieties into HPC and methyl cellulose (MC) via the Z-group approach in an aqueous medium (Scheme 6.11). These thiocarbonylthio (xanthate) CTAs were used in graft copolymerizations of vinyl acetate (VAc). The cleaved PVAc grafts exhibited unexpectedly high molecular weight and molecular weight distribution. The broadness of the molecular weight distributions was attributed to the steric congestion around the CTA functionality, restricting the access of the growing macro-radical to the thiocarbonylthio functions, while the difference between the experimental and the theoretical values was explained such that not all of the xanthate CTA units were activated. Thermogravimetric analysis revealed that the grafted cellulosic materials have better thermal stability than the physical blends of PVAc and modified cellulosic materials.

Semsarilar et al. (2010) reported preparation of the trithiocarbonate-based HPC-macroCTA (with average DS of 1.5) via the R-group approach in a homogeneous phase (Scheme 6.12). These macroCTAs were used to mediate the RAFT polymerizations of EA and *N*-isopropylacrylamide (NIPAam). They determined that without free CTA, only unbonded polymeric chains (not attached to the HPC backbone) with broad molecular weight distribution were observed, suggesting that the

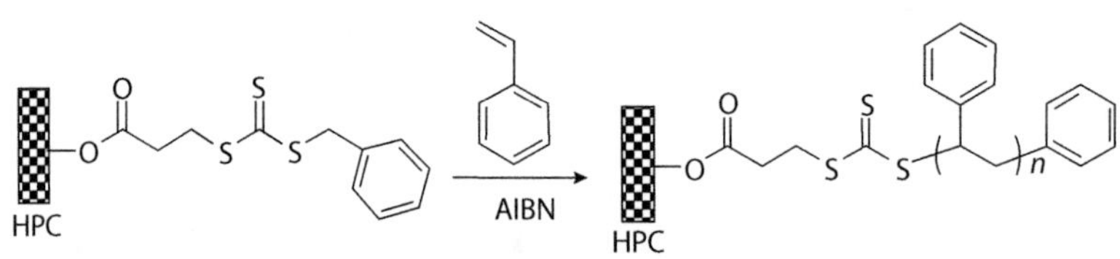

SCHEME 6.10 Synthetic route to HPC-*g*-PSt via the soluble cellulose-based macroCTA (Z-group approach).

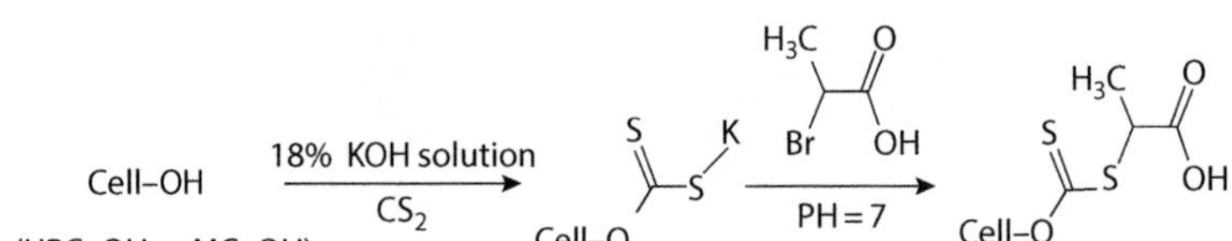

SCHEME 6.11 Synthetic route to xanthate-functionalized cellulose.

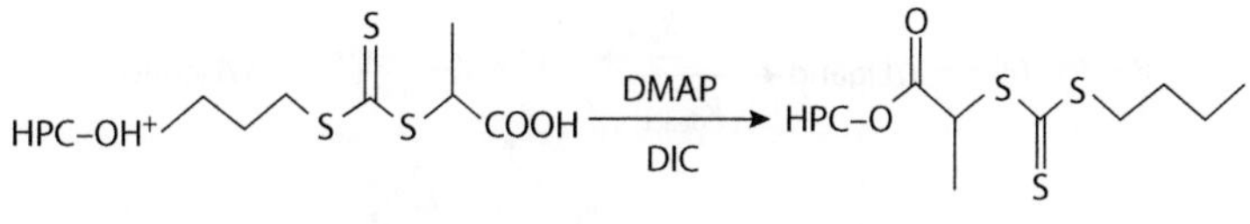

SCHEME 6.12 Synthetic route to cellulose-based macroCTA via the R-group approach.

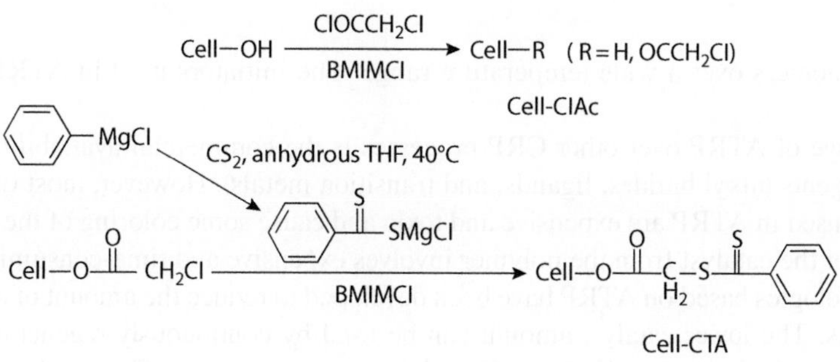

SCHEME 6.13 Synthetic route to cellulose-based macroCTA (cell-CTA) via cellulose-based ATRP initiator (Cell-ClAc).

polymer chains grow in solution via free radical polymerization. With the free CTA PNIPAam and PEA, grafts were successfully grown from the cellulosic backbone, but molecular weight distributions of the grafts and the control of the polymerizations were not analyzed. The authors pointed out that the grafted polymer chains may show relatively broad molecular weight distribution, due to the potential termination reaction between radicals' presence either in solution or in the HPC.

The first illustration for the cellulose grafting via RAFT polymerization in IL (1-*N*-butyl-3-methylimidazolium chloride, BMIMCl) solution was reported just recently by Lin et al. (2012). The authors first prepared a cellulose-based ATRP initiator (cellulose chloroacetate, cell-ClAc) from cotton linter fibers in BMIMCl, which was converted to cellulose-based macroCTA yielding a DS = 0.96 (Scheme 6.13). This macroCTA was then utilized for graft copolymerization of MMA in BMIMCl. The controlled/living polymerization character was proven by first-order kinetics of the copolymerization, linear increase in molecular weight with conversion, and quite narrow molecular weight distributions of the grafts (Mw/Mn of graft ~ 1.3) were achieved. Compared with the graft copolymerization of MMA via ATRP initiated by cell-ClAc in BMIMCl (Lin et al. 2009, 2012), polymerization via the RAFT method was more controlled, since narrower Mw/Mn grafts were produced. The static contact angle measurements revealed that cellulose-*g*-PMMA copolymers showed increase in the hydrophobicity of the modified cellulose surface.

6.4.6 Cellulose Grafting via ATRP and SET-LRP

ATRP is based on reversible cleavage of the terminal carbon–halide bond in the dormant species via a redox process catalyzed by a transition metal complex. The key step in controlling the polymerization is an atom transfer between the growing chains and a catalyst (Matyjaszewski 2000). A general mechanism of ATRP is shown in Scheme 6.14. ATRP has been successfully catalyzed by a variety of metals, including ruthenium (Ru), copper (Cu), iron (Fe), and other transition metals in combination with various types of ligands such as amines and phosphines (Matyjaszewski and Xia 2001, Kamigaito et al. 2001, Tizzotti et al. 2010). Complexes of Cu and multidentate nitrogen (N)-based ligands are the most efficient catalysts in the ATRP of a broad range of monomers in diverse media (Braunecker and Matyjaszewski 2007). ATRP can be used on a wide variety of vinyl

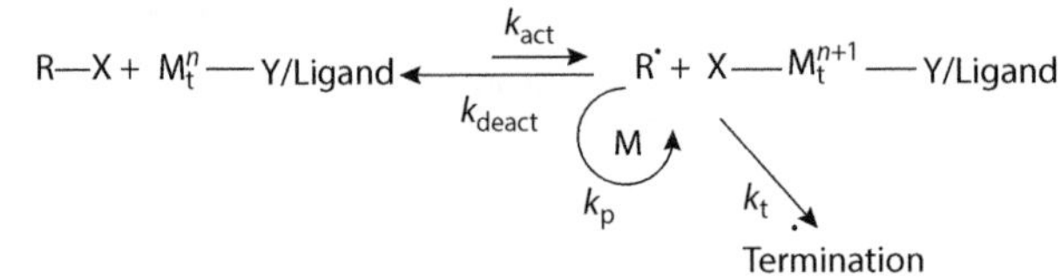

SCHEME 6.14 Mechanism of ATRP.

and acrylic monomers over a wide temperature range. The initiators used in ATRP are typically alkyl halides.

One advantage of ATRP over other CRP processes is the commercial availability of all necessary ATRP reagents (alkyl halides, ligands, and transition metals). However, most of the transition metal catalysts used in ATRP are expensive and toxic and cause some coloring of the polymer products. Removal of the catalyst from the polymer involves expensive and time-consuming techniques. Several methodologies based on ATRP have been developed to reduce the amount of catalyst needed in these systems. The lower catalyst amount can be used by continuously regenerating the Cu(I)/ligand species by reducing excess X-Cu(II)/ligand deactivator complex. This can be achieved, using a reducing agent, as in activators regenerated by electron transfer (ARGET) ATRP (Pintauer and Matyjaszewski 2008), by decomposition of free radical initiators, as in initiator for continuous activator regeneration ATRP (Pintauer and Matyjaszewski 2008), or using zero-valent transition metals or mixed transition metal catalysts, as in supplemental activator and reducing agent (SARA) ATRP (Rosen et al. 2009, Zhang et al. 2011, 2012) and SET-LRP (Percec et al. 2006, Rosen et al. 2009). During recent years, there has been lively debate between protagonists of ATRP and SET-LRP about which species [Cu(I) versus Cu(0)] is responsible for the activation of the dormant species and the role of Cu(I) disproportionation. Percec et al. proposed the SETLRP mechanism, which is based on the premise that Cu(I) X should instantaneously disproportionate into Cu(0) (activating species) and Cu(II) X2 (deactivating species) in polar aprotic solvents such as DMSO in the presence of an N-containing ligand. This facilitates LRP, in which the free radicals are generated by the nascent Cu(0) atomic species, while their deactivation is mediated by the nascent Cu(II) X2 species, and both steps proceed via an outer-sphere electron transfer mechanism (Percec et al. 2006, Rosen and Percec 2009, Rosen et al. 2009). However, Matyjaszewski et al. 2012 stated that Cu(0)-mediated CRP is a form of ARGET or SARA ATRP, in which Cu(0) acts as a supplemental and reducing agent. The mechanisms proposed for Cu-catalyzed SET-LRP and (ARGET) ATRP are shown in Scheme 6.15.

To prepare cellulose-*g*-copolymer via ATRP or SET-LRP utilizing the "grafting from" approach, cellulose-based macroinitiator needs to be synthesized first (Scheme 6.16). Haloester-based initiating sites can be straightforwardly attached to the cellulose backbone through esterification of the

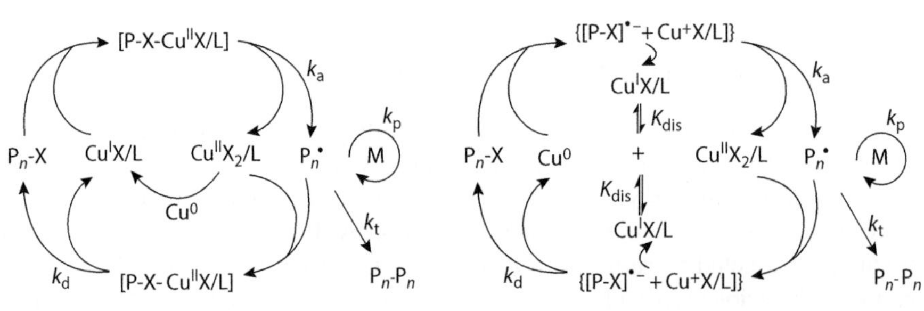

SCHEME 6.15 Proposed mechanisms of Cu-catalyzed (a) (ARGET) ATRP and (b) SET-LRP.

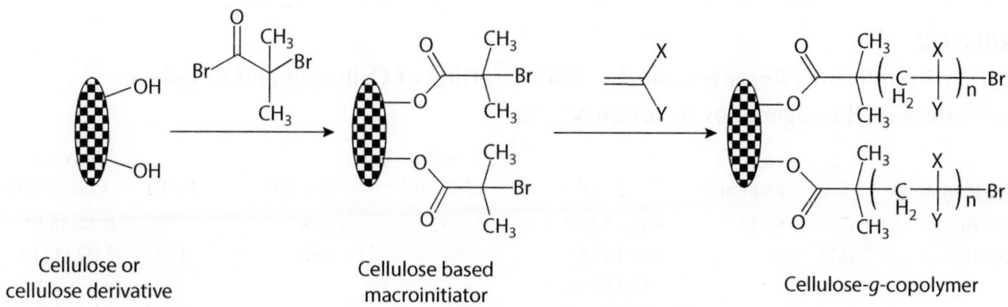

SCHEME 6.16 Synthetic route to cellulose-*g*-copolymer via ATRP or SET-LRP.

hydroxyl groups with commercially available reagents, such as 2-bromoisobutyryl bromide (BiB) or 2-chloropropionyl chloride (Tizzotti et al. 2010). ATRP has been the method most used to prepare cellulose-*g*-copolymers via CRP, since the first example reported by Carlmark and Malmström in 2002 (Matyjaszewski et al. 2007, Carlmark 2002). Most of the studies were carried out using soluble cellulose derivatives (cellulose esters and ethers) as starting material, or grafting was conducted in a heterogeneous reaction medium via surface-initiated ATRP (SI-ATRP) (Tizzotti et al. 2010). The experimental results reported for the cellulose grafting via ATRP and SET-LRP in a homogeneous reaction medium are gathered in Tables 6.2 and 6.3, respectively.

As can be seen from Tables 6.2 and 6.3, a wide variety of cellulose-based graft copolymers has been prepared via ATRP or SET-LRP. In most of the studies, kinetic analyses have confirmed living and controllable reactions that enable varying of the lengths of the grafts over a wide range when the reaction conditions are chosen properly. However, the monomer conversions need to be kept low to avoid intermolecular coupling reactions between the growing graft copolymers and loss of the control. Analysis of the real molecular weight distributions of the grafts (Mw/Mn of graft) requires cleaving off the grafts from the backbone, for example, by acid or alkaline hydrolysis. This has turned out to be challenging, since degradation of the polymer grafts and backbone in addition to hydrolysis of the ester linkage between the graft and the backbone could also occur or the graft copolymer could form an acid resistance product, due to a huge polymer graft layer wrapped around the cellulose backbone (Shen and Huang 2004, Vlček et al. 2006, 2008, Östmark et al. 2007, 2008, Billy et al. 2010, Ma et al. 2010a,b). Nevertheless, when the polymer grafts were successfully isolated from the backbone, the Mw/Mn of graft has been quite narrow (1.1–1.5) in most cases. When metallic Cu was used alone to mediate the CRP of cellulose-*g*-copolymer, the Mw/Mn of graft has been somewhat higher (Table 6.3).

6.4.7 Tailored Properties and Possible Applications of Cellulose-Based Graft Copolymers

Many of these cellulose-*g*-copolymers have self-assembling and stimuli-responsive properties that can be tuned by tailoring the length, density, and composition of the grafts. Cellulose-*g*-copolymers with tunable stimuli-responsive properties have potential applications as biomedical or smart materials. Ma et al. prepared HPC-*g*-poly (4-vinyl pyridine) (HPC-*g*-P4VP) copolymers that have reversible thermo- and pH-induced core–shell micellization properties in aqueous solutions (Shen et al. 2005, Yang et al. 2007, Ifuku and Kadla 2008, Ma et al. 2010a). For pH-induced micellization, the P_4VP side chains collapse to form the core of the micelles, and the HPC backbones remain in the shell to stabilize the micelles. In the thermo-induced micelles, the HPC backbone collapsed to form the core of the micelles upon heating, and the P4VP grafts stabilized the micelles as the shell. The cloud point (Tcp) of HPC-*g*-P4VP was tuned by changing the length of the P_4VP grafts or the pH values. The longer the P4VP grafts, the higher the Tcp, and in the case of very short P4VP grafts

TABLE 6.2
Experimental Results Reported for the ATRP Grafting of Cellulose and Cellulose Derivatives in Homogeneous Reaction Media

Macroinitiator[a]	DS	Monomer	Catalyst	Mw/Mn of Grafts[b]	Solvent	T (°C)	Maximum Conversion
CDA-Br	0.43	MMA	CuBr/PMDETA	1.12	Dioxane	70	5.4% (8 h)
CDA-Br	0.12	St	CuCl/$CuCl_2$/ HMTETA	Nr	Dioxane	110	14% (12 h)
		St	CuCl/$CuCl_2$/ HMTETA	nr	Dioxane	110	13% (9 h)
		BuA	CuCl/Cu/ PMDETA	Nr	Acetone	70	25% (5 h)
		BuA	CuCl/Cu/ PMDETA	Nr	Acetone	60	15% (8.5 h)
		MMA	CuCl/$CuCl_2$/ HMTETA	Nr	Dioxane	90	21% (2.5 h)
		MMA	CuCl/$CuCl_2$/bPy	nr	Dioxane	75	7% (18 h)
CDA-Cl	0.10	MMA	CuCl/$CuCl_2$/ HMTETA	nr	Dioxane	90	21% (2.5 h)
	0.41	MMA	CuCl/$CuCl_2$/bPy	nr	Dioxane	75	7% (18 h)
CDA-Br-*g*-PCL	0.50	St	CuCl/$CuCl_2$/ HMTETA	nr	Dioxane	110	7% (8 h)
		BuA	CuCl/PMDETA	nr	Anisole	70	10% (8 h)
		MMA	CuCl/$CuCl_2$/ HMTETA	nr	Dioxane	70	6% (8 h)
CA-Br	0.01	MDEGMA	CuCl/PMDETA	1.39	Cyclopentanone	40	18% (?)
	0.06	MDEGMA	CuCl/PMDETA	>1.5	Cyclopentanone	40	19% (?)
HPC-Br	2.26	MMA	CuBr/$CuBr_2$/ PMDETA	nr	Toluene	80	39% (19 h)
HPC-*g*-PMMA-Br		*t*-BA	CuBr/$CuBr_2$/ PMDETA	nr	Toluene	80	39% (19 h)
HPC-G1-Br	0.88	MMA	CuBr/$CuBr_2$/ PMDETA	nr	Toluene	70	3.5% (22 h)
		HDMA	CuBr/$CuBr_2$/ PMDETA	nr	Toluene	70	18% (2 h)
HPC-*g*-PCL-Br	Nr	*t*-BA	CuBr/$CuBr_2$/ PMDETA	nr	Toluene	70	32% (14 h)
HPC-Br	0.05	4VP	CuCl/Me6TREN	nr	2-Propanol	30	60% (12 h)
HPC-Br	0.10	DMAEMA	CuCl/HMTETA	nr	MeOH/H_2O	30	34.5% (12 h)
MC-Br	0.98	NIPAm	CuBr/PMDETA	nr	DMF/H_2O	RT	17.5% (12 h)
HEC-Br	Nr	Aam	CuBr/$CuBr_2$/ Me6[14]aneN4	nr	DMF/THF	30	40.5% (72 h)
EC-Br	0.50	St	CuBr/PMDETA	<1.35	Toluene	110	20% (21.5 h)
		MMA	CuBr/PMDETA	<1.35	Toluene	70	29% (48 h)
EC-Br	0.04	*t*-BA	CuBr/PMDETA	1.16	Toluene/ cyclohexanone	80	60% (5 h)
	0.25	*t*-BA	CuBr/PMDETA	1.20	Toluene/ cyclohexanone	80	45% (2.5 h)
EC-Br	0.04	St	CuBr/PMDETA	<1.20	Toluene	110	10% (10.5 h)
EC-Br	0.52	MMAzo	CuBr/PMDETA	nr	Anisole	85	18% (24 h)

(Continued)

TABLE 6.2 (*Continued*)
Experimental Results Reported for the ATRP Grafting of Cellulose and Cellulose Derivatives in Homogeneous Reaction Media

Macroinitiator[a]	DS	Monomer	Catalyst	Mw/Mn of Grafts[b]	Solvent	T (°C)	Maximum Conversion
EC-Br	0.04	HEMA	$CuCl/CuCl_2/bPy$	nr	MeOH	40	8.3% (10 h)
	0.09	HEMA	$CuCl/CuCl_2/bPy$	nr	MeOH	40	13.3% (12 h)
EC-Br	0.02	PEGMA	$CuCl/CuCl_2/$ dNbpy	nr	Toluene	60	61.7% (14 h)
	0.20	PEGMA	$CuCl/CuCl_2/$ dNbpy	nr	Toluene	60	55.6% (8 h)
EC-Br	0.10	DEAEMA	CuBr/bPy	nr	DMF	20	28% (5 h)
	0.20	DEAEMA	CuBr/bPy	nr	DMF	20	41.7% (6.5 h)
	0.06	DEAEMA	CuBr/bPy	nr	DMF	20	24.1% (4 h)
EC-Br-*g*-PCL	Nr	DMAEMA	CuBr/PMDETA	nr	THF	60	Nr
Pulp-Br	0.70	DMAEMA	CuBr/PMDETA	nr	DMF	60	34.7% (1 h)
MCC-Br	0.20	DMAam	CuBr/bPy	< 1.5	DMSO	100	55% (7 h)
Cotton-Br	0.72	MPC	CuBr/bPy	1.25	DMSO/MeOH	20	55% (3 h)
Cotton-Cl	1.11	MMA	CuBr/bPy	1.52	BMIMCl	70	15.5% (5 h)
Cell-Br	0.74	MMA	CuBr/PMDETA	1.40	DMF	60	37.8% (3 h)
MCC-Br	0.72	MMA	CuCl/bpy	1.44	Butanone	70	28.4% (3 h)
	0.93	st	CuCl/bpy	1.48	Dioxane	110	14.1% (2 h)
Cell-Cl	0.76	MMA	$CuBr_2$/TEMED/ AsAc	1.40	DMAc	50	13% (3.2 h)
MCC-Br	0.52	St	$CuCl/CuCl_2/$ PMDETA	1.24	DMSO	100	21% (nr)
	0.11	MMA	$CuCl/CuCl_2/$ HMTETA	1.35	DMSO	70	32% (nr)
	1.04	MMA	$CuCl/CuCl_2/$ HMTETA	1.28	DMAc	70	37% (1 h)

Notes: Shen and Huang (2004), Shen et al. (2005, 2006), Vlček et al. (2006, 2008), Kang et al. (2006, 2008), Tang et al. (2007), Yang et al. (2007), Östmark et al. (2007, 2008), Li et al. (2008), Sui et al. (2008), Yan and Ishira (2008), Yan and Tao (2008), Meng et al. (2009), Yan et al. (2009), Ifuku and Kadla (2010), Billy et al. (2010), Ma et al. (2010a,b), Wang et al. (2011), Xin et al. (2011), Raus et al. (2011), Zhang et al. (2012).

nr, not reported.

[a] Br and Cl refer to bromo- and chloro-functionalized initiator moieties, respectively. CDA, cellulose diacetate; CDA-Br-*g*-PCL, bromo-functionalized cellulose diacetate grafted with e-caprolactone via ring-opening polymerization; CA, cellulose acetate; HPC, hydroxypropyl cellulose; HPC-*g*-PMMA-Br, HPC-*graft*-PMMA macroinitiator prepared from HPC-Br macroinitiator; HPC-G1-Br, first-generation dendronized HPC macroinitiator; HPC-*g*-PCL-Br, end groups of PCL grafts converted into Br-containing initiating sites; MC, 2,3-di-O-methyl cellulose; HEC, hydroxyethyl cellulose; EC, ethyl cellulose; EC-Br-*g*-PCL, bromo-functionalized ethyl cellulose grafted with e-caprolactone via ring-opening polymerization; Pulp, wood pulp; MCC, microcrystalline cellulose; Cotton, cotton linter; Cell, type of cellulose unknown.

[b] The Mw/Mn of the grafts cleaved off from the backbone by hydrolysis.

(DPP4VP = 3), the Tcp is also dependent on the pH, showing higher Tcp at lower pH. Dual pH- and thermo-sensitivity of HPC-*g*-poly(*N*,*N*-dimethyl aminoethyl methacrylate) (HPC-*g*-PDMAEMA) in aqueous solution were also been detected by Ma et al. (2010). The lower critical solution temperature (LCST) of HPC0.1-*g*-PDMAEMA shifts to the lower temperature with increase in pH values, due to deprotonation of the PDMAEMA grafts at higher pH value. Sui et al. showed that cellulose-*g*-PDMAEMA also has pH- and thermoresponsive properties in H_2O similar to the expected stimuli

TABLE 6.3
Experimental Results Reported for the SET-LRP Grafting of Cellulose and Cellulose Derivatives in Homogeneous Reaction Media

Macroinitiator	DS	Monomer	Catalyst	Mw/Mn	Solvent	T (°C)	Maximum Conversion
MCC-Br	1.04	St	Cu/Me6 TREN	1.79	DMSO	25	4.8 (21 h)
CDA-Cl	0.25	MMA	Cu/Me6 TREN	1.58	DMSO	25	9% (24 h)
CDA-Cl	0.19	MMA	Cu/Me6 TREN	1.74	DMSO	25	38% (5 h)
CDA-Br	0.19	BuA	Cu/Me6 TREN	Nr	DMSO	25	86% (4.5 h)

Source: Raus, V. et al., *J. Polym. Sci. A: Polym. Chem.*, 49, 4353, 2011; Vlček, P. et al., *J. Polym. Sci. A: Polym. Chem.*, 49, 164, 2011.

responses by PDMAEMA. The copolymer formed discrete spherical particles with diameters in the range of 40–80 nm in H_2O (2 mg/mL at pH = 7), which were observed by transmission electron microscopy (TEM) and tapping mode atomic force microscopy (AFM). The dynamic light scattering (DLS) studies revealed that the aggregates had hydrodynamic radius (Rh) values ranging from 50 to 350 nm with an increase in concentration (from 0.02 to 0.2 mg/mL), indicating the interchain association of cellulose-*g*-PDMAEMA in solution (Kang et al. 2006, Shen et al. 2006, Tang 2006, Raus et al. 2011).

Ethyl cellulose-*g*-poly (2-(diethylamino) ethyl methacrylate) (EC-*g*-PDEAEMA) copolymers can self-assemble into micelles in acidic aqueous solutions. The critical micelle concentration (cmc) decreases with increase in grafting density (DSBiB of EC = 0.06, 0.1, or 0.2) at similar side chain lengths and also with increase in the side chain length at the same grafting density. The Rh of the resultant micelles increases with increasing side chain length and is independent of the grafting density at similar side chain lengths. The EC-*g*-PDEAEMA micelles showed reversible pH-sensitivity, starting to shrink at pH 6.0 and aggregating at pH > 6.9. The EC-*g*-poly(poly(ethylene glycol) methyl ether methacrylate) EC-*g*-PPEGMA copolymers formed spherical micelles in H_2O, showing thermoresponsive properties with an LCST of approximately 65°C, which was almost independent of the grafting density and the side chain length (Kang et al. 2008, Li et al. 2008, Yan et al. 2009, Wang et al. 2011). The size of the micelles (Rh) was higher (approximately 130 nm) when the grafting density was higher (EC0.2-*g*-PPEGMA), whereas the Rh of the micelles of the sparsely grafted copolymers (EC0.02-*g*-PPEGMA) was lower (approximately 60 nm). Moreover, the Rh increased slightly with increase in the side chain length. Huang et al. have studied the self-assembly of densely grafted EC-*g*-PSt (DSBiB of EC = 0.5) in acetone (Shen et al. 2005, 2006, Sui et al. 2008, Liu et al. 2009). They found that EC-*g*-PSt copolymer formed spherical core–shell micelles in acetone with the EC backbone in the shell and PSt grafts in the core of the micelles. The copolymer could self-assemble into multimolecular micelles at relatively high polymer concentration, while unimolecular micelles were formed at low concentration. The size of the micelles increased with increasing copolymer concentration and PSt side chain length. Cellulose-*g*-PMMA also tended to aggregate and self-assemble into spherical particles with a diameter range of 100–500 nm, depending on the concentration in the good solvent DMF and with a diameter range of 50–100 nm in the selective solvent acetone (Yan and Ishira 2008, Yan and Tao 2008, Meng et al. 2009, Xin et al. 2011). Huang et al. prepared amphiphilic EC-*g*-poly (acrylic acid) (EC-*g*-PAA) copolymers with two different grafting densities (DSBiB of EC = 0.5 or 0.3) by hydrolyzing the *tert*-butyl group on the poly (*tert*-butyl acrylate) side chains of the EC-*g*-PtBA copolymers (Liu et al. 2009, Raus et al. 2011, Vlček et al. 2011, Zhong 2012, Liu et al. 2012a,b). The side chain lengths also varied from short (DPPAA = 21 or 28) to long (DPPAA = 43 or 53). The influences of solvent and side chain length on the self-assembly behavior were studied by DLS and TEM. In THF/H_2O systems, the copolymers with longer side chains were intramolecularly self-assembled to form unimolecular small spherical structures that could further form larger network structures, and those with short side chains formed multimolecular large spherical aggregates by intermolecular association. The grafting density did not distinctly influence the self-assembled structures. No micelles were formed in MeOH/H_2O and DMF/H_2O systems. The chain conformation and individual chain structures of the same copolymers in MeOH were studied by static light scattering, DLS, and AFM (Liu et al. 2012b). The single-chain disk-like and rod-like structures were obtained from sparse and dense graft copolymers, respectively. It was concluded that the various conformations originated from the differing side chain density rather than the side chain length. The single-chain rods from the denser graft copolymers originated from the extended rod conformation of the backbone, whereas the unimolecular disk-like structures from the relatively sparse graft copolymers resulted from the coil conformation of the backbone.

Graft copolymerization of cellulose derivatives via combination of the ATRP and ROP approaches has also been used to modify the properties of cellulosic graft copolymers. Östmark et al. used HPC as a macroinitiator to grow poly-caprolactone (PCL) side chains (Scheme 6.17) (Mitsukami et al. 2001, Neugebauer and Matyjaszewski 2003, Östmark et al. 2008, Billy et al. 2010, Yang et al. 2010, Voepel et al. 2011, Shi et al. 2012). The PCL end groups were further functionalized with BiB and chain extended with t-BA by ATRP. Deprotection of the *tert*-butyl groups by acidic treatment yielded water-suspendable amphiphilic HPC-*g*-(PCL-b-PAA) comb block copolymers that formed unimolecular micelles with an outer PAA block. The unimolecular nanocontainers (diameter = 89–320 nm) with hydrogel-like shell were obtained after cross-linking the copolymer in dilute water solution via amidation. Somewhat different approaches were used in two other studies in which cellulose derivatives (CDA44 or EC59) were first functionalized with suitable ATRP initiator

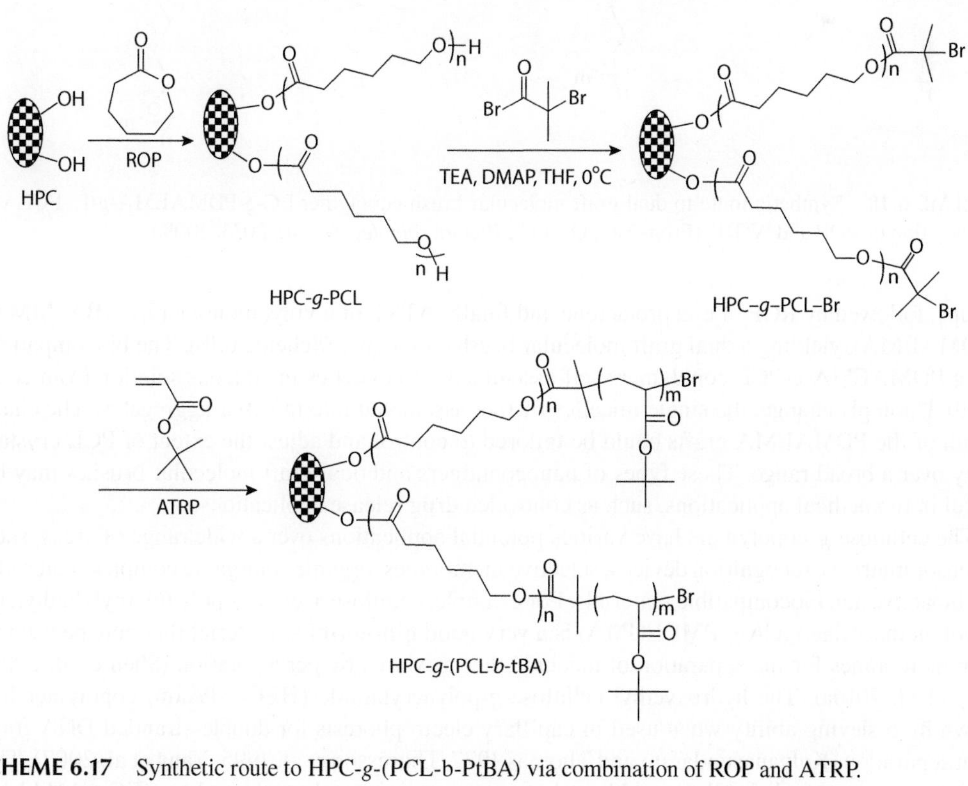

SCHEME 6.17 Synthetic route to HPC-*g*-(PCL-b-PtBA) via combination of ROP and ATRP.

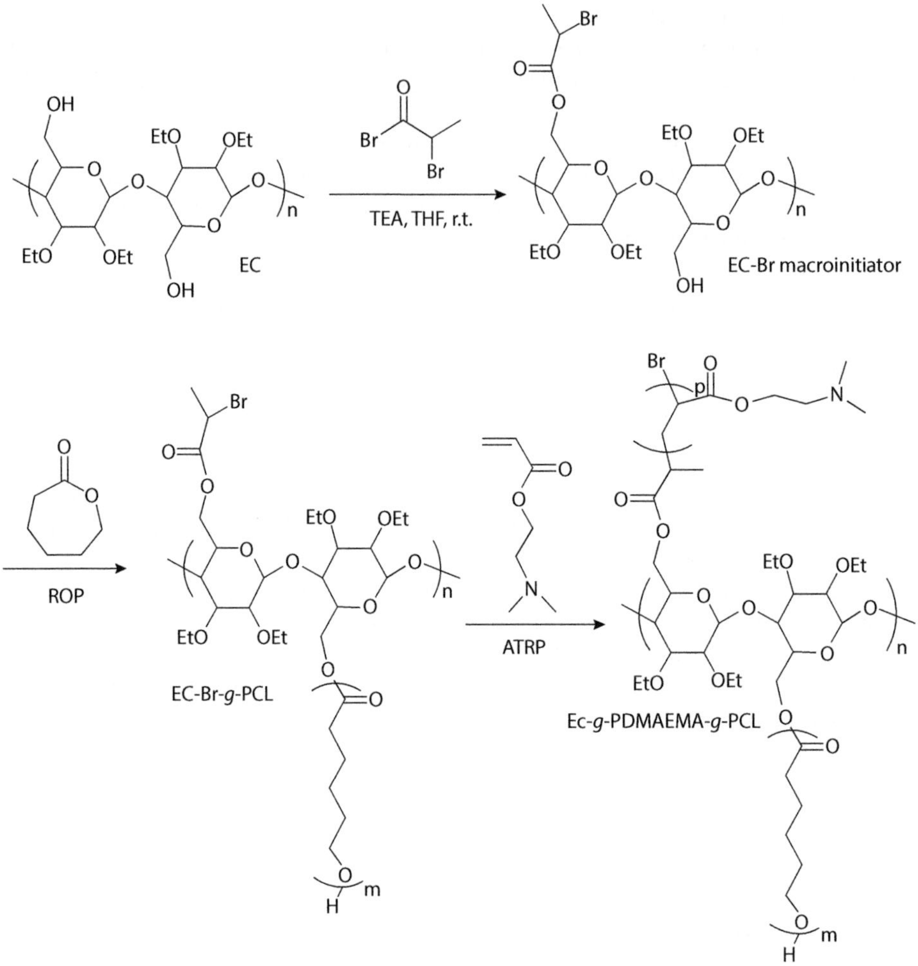

SCHEME 6.18 Synthetic route to dual graft molecular brush copolymer EC-*g*-PDMAEMA-*g*-E. PCL via combination of ROP and ATRP. (From Yan, Q. et al., *Biomacromolecules*, 10, 2033, 2009.)

groups, followed by ROP of e-caprolactone and finally ATRP of a vinyl monomer (St, tBA, MMA, or DMAEMA), yielding a dual graft molecular brush copolymer (Scheme 6.18). The biocompatible EC-*g*-PDMAEMA-*g*-PCL copolymers self-assembled into micelles in aqueous solution (Yan et al. 2009). Upon pH change, the single micelles further assembled into micellar aggregates. The chain length of the PDMAEMA grafts could be tailored to control and adjust the extent of PCL crystallinity over a broad range. These types of nanocontainers and dual graft molecular brushes may be useful in biomedical applications, such as controlled drug release applications.

The cellulose-*g*-copolymers have various potential applications over a wide range of areas, such as sensor matrices, recognition devices, selective membranes, organic–inorganic complex materials, and bioactive and biocompatible materials. For example, cellulose acetate-*g*-poly (methyl diethylene glycol methacrylate) (CA-*g*-PMDEGMA) is a very good film-forming material that may be used to form membranes for the separation of alcohol/ether mixtures by pervaporation (Shen et al. 2006, Billy et al. 2010a). The hydroxyethyl cellulose-*g*-polyacrylamide (HEC-*g*-PAam) copolymer has shown high sieving ability when used in capillary electrophoresis for double-stranded DNA fragment separation (Kalyanasundaram and Thomas 1977, Thuresson et al. 1995, Yang et al. 2007). The graft copolymers of ethyl cellulose with azobenzene-containing polymethacrylates (EC-*g*-MMAzo) have potential applications in sensors and optical materials. Silica capillaries coated with hydroxyethyl cellulose-*g*-poly(dimethyl acrylamide) (HEC-*g*-PDMAam) or with hydroxyethyl cellulose-*g*-poly(ethyl glycol) (HEC-*g*-PEG) and used in capillary electrophoresis have shown great potential for use in proteomic applications (Dong and Winnik 1984, Winnik et al. 1996, Yang et al. 2010, Shi et al. 2012). Similarly, cellulose-*g*-PDMAam and cellulose-*g*-poly (2-methacryloyloxyethyl phosphorylcholine) (cell-*g*-MPC) used as coatings for commercial cellulose membranes resulted in good hemocompatibility and protein adsorption resistance (Nishioka et al. 1993, Nishikawa et al. 1998, Evertsson and Nilsson 1999, Luda et al. 2003, Coskun and Temuz 2005, Ye et al. 2006, Yan and Ishira 2008, Yan and Tao 2008, Burchard 2009).

6.5 CONCLUSION

"Smart" materials based on cellulose show intelligent behaviors in response to stimuli in the vicinity, thus enabling them to be applied in many fields. Cellulose and/or cellulose derivatives, such as CMC, HPC, HEC, and EC, in different forms, such as CNCs and films/membranes, have been utilized to fabricate "smart" materials by chemical modifications in homogeneous or heterogeneous conditions, or by physical incorporation. Stimuli-responsive polymers have been intensively studied over the last few years, yet the research of, specifically, stimuli-responsive materials based on cellulose still needs to become the focus of more studies, because the excellent properties allow the materials to be applied in many fields, especially in bio-applications. The cellulose-*g*-copolymers have various potential applications over a wide range of areas, such as sensor matrices, recognition devices, selective membranes, organic–inorganic complex materials, coatings, adhesives, and bioactive and biocompatible materials. This will open possibilities to construct new sophisticated cellulose derivatives for a wide range of applications.

REFERENCES

Arthur, J. C. 1959. Radiation polymerization of acrylonitrile onto cotton. *Text Res. J.*, *29*, 759.

Athawale, V. D. and Rathi, S. C. 1999. Graft polymerization: Starch as a model substrate. *J. Macromol. Sci. Rev. Macromol. Chem. Phys. C*, *39*, 445–480.

Barner-Kowollik, C. (ed.) 2008. *The Handbook of RAFT Polymerization*. Wiley-VCH, Weinheim, Germany.

Barsbay, M.; Guven, O.; Stenzel, M. H.; Davis, T. P.; Barner-Kowollik, C.; and Barner, L. J. 2007. Verification of controlled grafting of styrene from cellulose via radiation-induced raft polymerization. *Macromolecules*, *40*, 7140–7147.

Battaerd, H. A. J. and Tregear, G. W. 1997. *Graft Copolymers*. Interscience Publishers, a division of John Wiley & Sons, New York, p. 238.

Beck, R. H. F.; Fitton, M. G.; and Kricheldorf, H. R. 1992. Chemical modification of polysaccharides, in *Handbook of Polymer Synthesis, Part B*, Kricheldorf, H. R. (ed.), Chapter 25. Marcel Dekker, New York.

Belgacem, M. N. and Gandini, A. 2005. The surface modification of cellulose fibers for use as reinforcing elements in composite materials. *Compos. Interfaces*, *12*, 41–75.

Berlin, A. D. A. and Kislenko, V. N. 1992. Kinetics and mechanism of radical graft polymerization of monomers onto polysaccharides. *Prog. Polym. Sci. 17*, 765–825.

Bhattacharya, A. 2000. *Prog. Polym. Sci.*, *25*, 371.

Billy, M.; Ranzani Da Costa, A.; Lochon, P.; Clement, R.; Dresch, M.; Etienne, S.; Hiver, J.M.; David, L.; and Jonquieres, A. 2010a. *Eur. Polym. J.*, *46*, 944–957.

Billy, M.; Ranzani Da Costa, A.; Lochon, P.; Clement, R.; and Dresch, M.; Jonquieres, A. 2010b. *J. Membr. Sci.*, *348*, 389–396.

Bledzki, A. K. and Gassan, J. 1999. Composites reinforced with cellulose based fibers. *Prog. Polym. Sci.*, *24*, 221–274.

Blousin, F. A. and Arthur, Jr. J. C. 1963. The effects of gamma radiation on cotton: Part V: Post-irradiation reactions. *Text. Res. J.*, *33*, 727.

Braunecker, W. A. and Matyjaszewski, K. 2007. Controlled/living radical polymerization: Features, developments, and perspectives. *Prog. Polym. Sci.*, *32*, 93–146.

Burchard, W. 1999. Solution properties of branched macromolecules. *Adv. Polym. Sci.*, *143*, 113–194.

Carlmark, A. and Malmstrom, E. 2003. ATRP grafting from cellulose fibers to create block-copolymer grafts. *Biomacromolecules*, *4*, 1740–1745.

Carlmark, A. and Malmstrom, E. 2002. Atom transfer radical polymerization from cellulose fibers at ambient temperature. *J. Am. Chem. Soc.*, *124*, 900–901.

Chung, T. C.; Janvikul, W.; Bernard, R.; Hu, R.; Li, C. L.; Liu, S. L.; and Jiang, G. 1995. Butyl rubber graft copolymers: synthesis and characterization. *J. Polym.*, *36*, 3565.

Coskun, M. and Temuz, M. M. 2005. Grafting studies onto cellulose by atom-transfer radical polymerization. *Polym. Int.*, *54*, 342–347.

Cumberbirch, R. J. E. and Holker, J. R. 1966. *J. Soc. Dyers Col.*, *82*, 59,

Czaja, W. K.; Young, D. J.; Kawecki, M.; and Brown, R. M. 2007. The future prospects of microbial cellulose in biomedical applications. *Biomacromolecules*, *8*, 1–12.

Daly, W. H.; Evenson, T. S.; Iacono, S. T.; and Jones, R. W. 2001. Recent developments in cellulose grafting chemistry utilizing Barton ester intermediates and nitroxide mediation. *Macromol. Symp.*, *174*, 155–163.

Demint, R. J.; Arthur, J. C. Jr.; Markezich, A. R.; and Mcsberry, W. F. 1962. Radiation-indoced interaction of styrene with cotton. *Text. Res. J.*, *32*, 918.

Doelker, E. 1993. Cellulose derivatives. *Adv. Polym. Sci.*, *107*, 199–265.

Dong, D. C. and Winnik, M. A. 1984. The Py scale of solvent polarities. *Can. J. Chem.*, *62*, 2560–2565.

Edgar, K. J.; Buchanan, C. M.; Debenham, J. S.; Rundquist, P. A.; Seiler, B. D.; Shelton, M. C.; and Tindall, D. 2001. Advances in cellulose ester performance and application. *Prog. Polym. Sci.*, *26*, 1605–1688.

Eichhorn, S. J. 2011. Cellulose nanowhiskers: Promising materials for advanced applications. *Soft Matter*, *7*, 303–315.

Eichhorn, S. J.; Dufresne, A.; Aranguren, M.; Marcovich, N. E.; Capadona, J. R.; Rowan, S. J.; Weder, C. et al. 2010. Review: Current international research into cellulose nanofibers and nanocomposites. *J. Mater. Sci.*, *45*, 1–33.

El Seoud, O. A. and Heinze, T. 2005. Organic esters of cellulose: new perspectives for old polymers. *Adv. Polym. Sci.*, *186*, 103–149.

Evertsson, H. and Nilsson, S. 1999. Microstructures formed in aqueous solutions of a hydrophobically modified nonionic cellulose derivative and sodium dodecyl sulfate: A fluorescence probe investigation. *Carbohydr. Polym.*, *40*, 293–298.

Fanta, G. F. and Doane, W. M. 1986. Grafted starches, in *Modified Starches: Properties and Uses*, Wurzburg, O. B. (ed.). CRC Press, Boca Raton, FL, pp. 149–178.

Fleet, R.; McLeary, J. B.; Grumel, V.; Weber, W. G.; Matahwa, H.; and Sanderson, R. D. 2008. RAFT mediated polysaccharide copolymers. *Eur. Polym. J.*, *44*, 2899–2911.

Flory, P. J. 1953. *Principles of Polymer Chemistry*. Cornell University, Ithaca, NY, Chapter 4.

Gardner, D. J.; Oporto, G. S.; Mills, R.; and Samird, M. A. S. A. 2008. Adhesion and surface issues in cellulose and nanocellulose. *J. Adhes. Sci. Technol.*, *22*, 545–567.

Geacintov, N.; Stannett, V.; Abrahamson, F. W.; and Hermans, J. J. 1960. Grafting onto cellulose and cellulose derivatives using ultraviolet irradiation. *J. Polym. Sci.*, *3*, 54.

Geacintov, N. and Stannett, V. 1963. The grafting of styrene to cellulose by mutual and preirradiation technique. *Makromol. Chem.*, *65*, 248.

Gnanou, Y. 1996. Design and synthesis of new model polymers. *J. Macromol. Sci. Rev. Macromol. Chem. Phys. C*, *36*(1), 77.

Gregory, A. and Stenzel, M. H. 2012. Complex polymer architectures via RAFT polymerization: From fundamental process to extending the scope using click chemistry and nature's building blocks. *Prog. Polym. Sci.*, *37*, 38–105.

Hamdani, J.; Goole, J.; Moës, A. J.; and Amighi, K. 2006. In vitro and in vivo evaluation of floating riboflavin pellets developed using the melt pelletization process original research article. *Int. J. Pharm.*, *323*(1–2), 86–92.

Hawker, C. J.; Bosman, A. W.; and Harth, E. 2001. New polymer synthesis by nitroxide mediated living radical polymerizations. *Chem. Rev.*, *101*, 3661–3688.

Hebeish, A. and Guthrie, J. T. 1981. *The Chemistry and Technology of Cellulosic Copolymers*. Springer, Berlin, Germany, Chapters 2–6.

Heim, M.; Keerl, D.; and Scheibel, T. 2009. Spider silk: from soluble protein to extraordinary fiber. *Angew. Chem. Int. Ed. Engl.*, *48*(20), 3584–3596.

Heinze, T. and Glasser, G. G. 1998. In *ACS Symposium Series, Cellulose Derivatives: Modification, Characterization, and Nanostructures*, Heinze, T. and Glasser, G. G. (eds.), vol. 688, pp. 2–18. American Chemical Society, Washington, DC.

Heinze, T. and Liebert, T. 2001. Unconventional methods in cellulose functionalization. *Prog. Polym. Sci.*, *26*, 1689–1762.

Hermans, J. J. 1962. Chemical mechanisms in the grafting of cellulose. *Pure Appl. Chem.*, *5*, 147.

Hernandez-Guerrero, M.; Davis, T. P.; Barner-Kowollik, C.; and Stenzel, M. H. 2005. Polystyrene comb polymers built on cellulose or poly(styrene-co-2-hydroxyethylmethacrylate) backbones as substrates for the preparation of structured honeycomb films. *Eur. Polym. J.*, *41*, 2264–2277.

Hubbe, M. A.; Rojas, O. J.; Lucia, L. A.; and Sain, M. 2008. Cellulosic nanocomposites: A review. *BioResources*, *3*, 929–980.

Huber, T.; Müssig, J.; Curnow, O.; Pang, S.; Bickerton, S.; and Staiger, M. P. 2012. A critical review of all-cellulose composites. *J. Mater. Sci.*, *47*, 1171–1186.

Hudson, S. M. and Smith, C. 1998. In *Biopolymers from Renewable Resources*, Kaplan, D. L. (ed.). Springer-Verlag, Berlin, Germany, p. 115.

Ifuku, S. and Kadla, J. F. 2008. Preparation of a thermosensitive highly regioselective cellulose/n-isopropylacrylamide copolymer through atom transfer radical polymerization. *Biomacromolecules*, *9*, 3308–3313.

Ikeuchi, K.; Takii, T.; Norikane, H.; Tomita, N.; Uyama, Y.; and Ikada, Y. 1993. Water lubrication of polyurethane grafted with dimethylacrylamide for medical use. *Wear*, *161*, 179.

Immergut, E. H. 1959. The Polymer Handbook. In *Encyclopaedia of Polymer Science and Technology*, Brandrup J., Immergut E.H. (eds.). John Wiley and Sons, New York 1975. vol. 3, 242.

Kaizerman, S.; Mino, G.; and Meinhold, F. 1962. The polymerization of vinyl monomers in cellulosic fibers. *Text. Res. J.*, *32*, 136.

Kalia, S.; Kaith, B. S.; and Kaur, I. 2009. Pretreatments of natural fibers and their application as reinforcing material in polymer composites—A review. *Polym. Eng. Sci.*, *49*, 1253–1272.

Kalyanasundaram, K. and Thomas, J. K. J. 1977. Environmental effects on vibronic band intensities in pyrene monomer fluorescence and their application in studies of micellar systems. *Am. Chem. Soc.*, 99, 2039–2044.

Kamigaito, M.; Ando, T.; and Sawamoto, M. 2001. Metal-catalyzed living radical polymerization. *Chem. Rev.*, *101*, 3689–3745.

Kang, H.; Liu, W.; He, B.; Shen, D.; Ma, L.; and Huang, Y. 2006. Synthesis of amphiphilic ethyl cellulose grafting poly(acrylic acid) copolymers and their self-assembly morphologies in water. *Polymer*, *47*, 7927–7934.

Kang, H.; Liu, W.; Liu, R.; and Huang, Y. 2008. A novel, amphiphilic ethyl cellulose grafting copolymer with poly(2-hydroxyethyl methacrylate) side chains and its micellization. *Macromol. Chem. Phys.*, *209*, 424–430.

Kesting, R. E. and Stannett, V. 1963. The grafting of styrene to cellulose by mutual and preirradiation technique. *Makromol. Chem.*, *65*, 248.

Khalil, H. P. S. A.; Bhat, A. H.; and Yusra, A. F. I. 2012. Green composites from sustainable cellulose nanofibrils: A review. *Carbohydr. Polym.*, *87*, 963–979.

Klee, D. and Hocker, H. 2000. Polymers for biomedical applications: Improvement of the interface compatibility. *Adv. Polym. Sci.*, *149*, 1.

Klemm, D.; Heublein, B.; Fink, H. P.; and Bohn, A. 2005. Cellulose: Fascinating biopolymer and sustainable raw material. *Angew. Chem. Int. Ed.*, *44*, 3358–3393.

Klemm, D.; Philipp, B.; Heinze, T.; Heinze, U.; and Wagenknecht, W. 1998. *Comprehensive Cellulose Chemistry*, 1st edn., vol. 1. Wiley-VHC, Weinheim, Germany, pp. 130–155.

Kontturi, E.; Tammelin, T.; and Österberg, M. 2006. Cellulose—Model films and the fundamental approach. *Chem. Soc. Rev.*, *35*, 1287–1304.

Leger, L.; Raphael, E.; and Hervet, H. 1999. Surface-anchored polymer chains: Their role in adhesion and friction. *Adv. Polym. Sci.*, *138*, 185.

Lenka, S. and Nayak, P. L. 1980. Grafting vinyl monomers onto cellulose. IV. Graft copolymerization of methyl methacrylate onto modified cellulose using peroxydiphosphate as the initiator. *J. Appl. Polym. Sci.*, *26*, 3135.

Lenka, S.; Nayak, P. L.; Tripathy, A. K.; and Mishra, M. K. 1981. Grafting vinyl monomers onto cellulose. V. Graft copolymerization of methyl methacrylate onto cellulose using a hexavalent chromium ion. *J. Appl. Polym. Sci.*, *26*, 2769.

Li, Y.; Liu, R.; Liu, W.; Kang, H.; Wu, M.; and Huang, Y. 2008. Synthesis, self-assembly, and thermosensitive properties of ethyl cellulose-g-P(PEGMA) amphiphilic copolymers. *J. Polym. Sci. A: Polym. Chem.*, *46*, 6907–6915.

Liepins, R.; Surles, J. R.; Morosoff, N.; and Stannett, V. T. 1977a. Localized radiation grafting of flame retardants to poly(ethylene terephthalate). I. Bromine-containing monomers. *J. Appl. Polym. Sci.*, *21*, 2529.

Liepins, R.; Surles, J. R.; Morosoff, N.; Stannett, V. T.; and Barker, R. H. 1977b. Radiation flame proofing of polyester/cotton blends. *Radiat. Phys. Chem.*, *9*, 465.

Liepins, R.; Surles, J. R.; Morosoff, N.; Stannett, V. T.; Duffy, J.; and Day, F. H. 1978. Localized radiation grafting of flame retardants to polyethylene terephthalate. II. Vinyl phosphonates. *J. Appl. Polym. Sci.*, *22*, 2403.

Lin, C.; Zhan, H.; Liu, M.; Fu, S.; and Zhang, 2009. Preparation of cellulose graft poly(methyl methacrylate) copolymers by atom transfer radical polymerization in an ionic liquid. *J. Carbohydr. Polym.*, *78*, 432–438.

Lin, C.; Zhan, H.; Liu, M.; Habibi, Y.; Fu, S.; and Lucia, L. A. 2012. RAFT synthesis of cellulose-g-polymethyl methacrylate copolymer in an ionic liquid. *J. Appl. Polym. Sci.*, *127*, 4840–4849.

Lindqvist, J. and Malmstrom, E. 2006. Surface modification of natural substrates by atom transfer radical polymerization. *J. Appl. Polym. Sci.*, *100*, 4155–4162.

Liu, W.; Liu, R.; Li, X.; Kang, H.; Shen, D.; Wu, M.; and Huang, Y. 2009. Self-assembly of ethyl cellulose-graft-polystyrene copolymers in acetone. *Polymer*, *50*, 211–217.

Liu, W.; Liu, Y.; Hao, X.; Zeng, G.; Wang, W.; Liu, R.; and Huang, Y. 2012a. Backbone-collapsed intra- and inter-molecular self-assembly of cellulose-based dense graft copolymer. *Carbohydr. Polym.*, *88*, 290–298.

Liu, W.; Liu, Y.; Zeng, G.; Liu, R.; and Huang, Y. 2012b. Coil-to-rod conformational transition and single chain structure of graft copolymer by tuning the graft density. *Polymer*, *53*, 1005–1014.

Luda, M. P.; Balabanovich, A. I.; Hornung, A.; and Camino, G. 2003. Thermal degradation of a brominated bisphenol a derivative. *Polym. Adv. Technol.*, *14*, 741–748.

Ma, L.; Kang, H.; Liu, R.; and Huang, Y. 2010a. Smart assembly behaviors of hydroxypropylcellulose-graft-poly(4-vinyl pyridine) copolymers in aqueous solution by thermo and pH stimuli. *Langmuir*, *26*, 18519–18525.

Ma, L.; Liu, R.; Tan, J.; Wang, D.; Jin, X.; Kang, H.; Wu, M.; and Huang, Y. 2010b. Self-assembly and dual-stimuli sensitivities of hydroxylpropylcellulose-graft-poly(N,N-dimethyl aminoethyl methacrylate) copolymers in aqueous solution. *Langmuir*, *26*, 8697–8703.

Mahdavinia, G. R.; Zohuriaan-Mehr, M. J.; and Pourjavadi, A. 2004. Modified chitosan. III. Superabsorbency, salt- and pH-sensitivity of smart ampholytic hydrogels from chitosang-polyacrylonitrile. *Polym. Adv. Technol.*, *15*, 173–180.

Malmstrom, E. and Carlmark, A. 2012. Surface-initiated ring-opening metathesis polymerisation from cellulose fibres. *Polym. Chem.*, *3*, 727–733.

Marcus, R. K. 2009. *J. Sci.* *32*(5–6), 695–705.

Mashkour, M.; Tajvidi, M.; Kimura, T.; Kimura, F.; and Ebrahimi, G. 2011. Fabricating unidirectional magnetic papers using permanent magnets to align magnetic nanoparticle covers natural cellulose fibers. *BioResources*, *6*, 4731–4738.

Matyjaszewski, K. 2000. In *ACS Symposium Series, Controlled/Living Radical Polymerization: Progress in ATRP, NMP and RAFT*, Matyjaszewski, K. (ed.), vol. 768, pp. 2–25. American Chemical Society, Washington, DC.

Matyjaszewski, K. 2012. Mediated CRP of methyl acrylate in the presence of metallic copper: Effect of ligand structure on reaction kinetics. *Macromolecules*, *45*, 78–86.

Matyjaszewski, K.; Trarevsky, N. V.; Braunecker, W. A.; Dong, H.; Huang, J.; Jakubowski, W.; Kwak, Y.; Nicolay, R.; Tang, W.; Yoon, J. A. 2007. Role of Cu0 in Controlled/"Living" Radical Polymerization. *Macromolecules*, *40*, 7795–7806.

Matyjaszewski, K. and Xia, 2001. Atom transfer radical polymerization. *J. Chem. Rev.*, *101*, 2921–2990.

Mayo, F. R. 1943. *J. Am. Chem. Soc.*, *65*, 2324; Mayo, F. R.; Gregg, R. A.; and Matheson, M. S. J. 1951. Chain transfer in the polymerization of styrene. VI. Chain transfer with styrene and benzoyl peroxide; the efficiency of initiation and the mechanism of chain termination 1. *Am. Chem. Soc.*, *73*, 1691.

McCormick, C. L.; Callais, P. A.; and Hutchinson, Jr., B. H. 1985. Solution studies of cellulose in lithium chloride and N,N-dimethylacetamide. *Macromolecules*, *18*, 2394–2401.

Meng, T.; Gao, X.; Zhang, J.; Yuan, J.; Zhang, Y.; and He, J. 2009. Graft copolymers prepared by atom transfer radical polymerization (ATRP) from cellulose. *Polymer*, *50*, 447–454.

Mino, G. and Kaizerman, S. 1958. A new method for the preparation of graft copolymers. Polymerization initiated by ceric ion redox systems. *J. Polym. Sci.*, *31*, 242–243.

Mitsukami, Y.; Donovan, M. S.; Lowe, A. B.; and Mc Cormick, C. L. 2001. Water-soluble polymers. 81. Direct synthesis of hydrophilic styrenic-based homopolymers and block copolymers in aqueous solution via RAFT. *Macromolecules*, *34*, 2248–2256.

Moad, G.; Rizzardo, E.; and Thang, S. H. 2008. Radical addition-fragmentation chemistry in polymer synthesis. *Polymer, 49*, 1079–1131.

Moore, H. G. 2010. Colorectal cancer: what should patients and families be told to lower the risk of colorectal cancer? *Surg. Oncol. Clin. N. Am.*, *19*(4), 693–710.

Murphy, E. B. and Wudl, F. 2010. The world of smart healable materials. *Prog. Polym. Sci.*, *35*, 223–251.

Muzzarelli, R. 1977. *Chitin*. Pergamon, New York.

Nakagawa, Y.; Miller, P. J.; and Matyjaszewski, K. 1998. Development of novel attachable initiators for atom transfer radical polymerization. Synthesis of block and graft copolymers from poly(dimethylsiloxane) macroinitiators. *Polymer*, *39*, 5163.

Narayan, R.; Biermann, C. J.; Hunt, M. O.; and Horn, D. P. 1989. In *ACS Symposium Series, Adhesives from Renewable Resources*, Hemingway, R. W.; Conner, A. H.; and Branham, S. J. (eds.), vol. 385, p. 337. American Chemical Society, Washington, DC.

Nayak, P. L. 1976. Grafting of vinyl monomers onto wool fibers. *J. Macromol, Sci.-Rev.*, *Macromol. Chem.*, *14*, 193.

Nayak P. L.; Lenka, S.; and Mishra, M. K. 1980a. Grafting vinyl monomers onto wool fibers. V. Graft copolymerization of methyl methacrylate onto wool using peroxydiphosphate as initiator. *J. Appl. Polym. Sci.*, *25*, 63.

Nayak, P. L.; Lenka, S.; and Mishra, M. K. 1980c. Grafting vinyl monomers onto wool fibers, IX. Graft copolymerization of methyl methacrylate onto wool using peroxydiphosphate-cysteine redox system. *Angew. Macromol. Chem.*, *90*, 155.

Nayak, P. L.; Lenka, S.; and Pati, N. C. 1979a. Grafting vinyl monomers onto silk fibers. II. Graft copolymerization of methyl methacrylate onto silk by hexavalent chromium ion. *J. Appl. Polym. Sci.*, *23*, 1345.

Nayak, P. L.; Lenka, S.; and Pati, N. C. 1978a. Grafting vinyl monomers onto wool fibers II. Graft copolymerization of methylmethacrylate onto wool by quinquevalent vanadium ion. *Angew Makcromol. Makromol. Chem.*, *71*, 189–199.

Nayak P. L.; Lenka, S.; and Pati, N. C. 1979b. Grafting vinyl monomers onto wool fibers. III. Graft copolymerization of methyl methacrylate onto wool using hexavalent chromium ion. *J. Polym. Sci.*, *17*, 3425.

Nayak, P. L.; Lenka, S.; and Pati, N. C. 1979c. Graft copolymerization of acrylamide onto polyethylene terephthalate (PET) with potassium permanganate as initiator. *J. Macromol. A 13*(8), 1157.

Nayak, P. L.; Lenka, S.; and Pati, N. C. 1978b. Grafting vinyl monomers onto wool fibers. I. Graft copolymerization of methyl methacrylate onto wool using V^{5+}-thiourea redox system. *J. Appl. Polym. Sci.*, *22*, 3301.

Nayak, P. L.; Lenka, S.; and Pati, N. C. 1978c. Grafting vinyl monomers onto silk fibers, I. Graft copolymerization of methyl methacrylate onto silk by quinquevalent vanadium ions. *Angew. Makromol. Chem.*, *68*, 117.

Nayak, P. L.; Lenka, S.; and Pati, N. C. 1979d. Grafting vinyl monomers onto silk fibers III. Graft copolymerization of methyl methacrylate onto silk using tetravalent cerium as initiator. *Angew. Makromol. Chem.*, *75*, 29.

Nayak, P. L.; Lenka, S.; Pati, N. C.; and Mishra, M. K. 1980b. Grafting vinyl monomers onto silk fibers, VII. Graft copolymerization of methyl methacrylate onto silk using peroxydiphosphate as initiator. *Makromol. Angew. Makromol. Chem.*, *84*, 183.

Nayak, P. L.; Lenka, S.; Pati, N. C.; and Mohanty, T. R. 1978d. Aqueous polymerization of acrylonitrile initiated by the bromate -thiourea redox system. *J. Polym. Sci.*, *16*, 343.

Nayak, P. L.; Mohanty, T. R.; and Singh, B. C. 1976. Polymerization of acrylonitrile initiated by thiourea-vanadium(V) redox system. *Eur. Polym. J.*, *12*, 371.

Nayal, P. L. 1979. Grafting of vinyl monomers onto nylon. *J. Macromol. Sci.-Rev. Macromol. Chem. C*, *17*, 267.

Neugebauer, D. and Matyjaszewski, K. 2003. Copolymerization of N,N-dimethylacrylamide with n-butyl acrylate via atom transfer radical polymerization. *Macromolecules*, *36*, 2598–2603.

Nishikawa, K.; Yekta, A.; Pham, H. H.; Winnik, M. A.; and Sau, A. C. 1998. Fluorescence studies of hydrophobically modified hydroxyethylcellulose (HMHEC) and pyrene-labeled HMHEC. *Langmuir*, *14*, 7119–7129.

Nishioka, N.; Yamaoka, M.; Haneda, H.; Kawakami, K.; and Uno, M. 1993. Thermal decomposition of cellulose/synthetic polymer blends containing grafted products. 1. Cellulose/poly(methyl methacrylate) blends. *Macromolecules*, *26*, 4694–4699.

O'Connell, D. W.; Birkinshaw, C.; and O'Dwyer, T. F. 2008. *Bioresour. Technol.*, *99*, 6709–6724.

Odian, G. 1991. *Principles of Polymerization*, John Wiley & Sons, New York, Chapter 3.

Östmark, E.; Harrison, S.; Wooley, K. L.; and Malmstrom, E. E. 2007. Comb polymers prepared by ATRP from hydroxypropyl cellulose. *Biomacromolecules*, *8*, 1138–1148.

Östmark, E.; Nystrom, D.; and Malmstrom, E. 2008. Unimolecular nanocontainers prepared by ROP and subsequent ATRP from hydroxypropylcellulose. *Macromolecules*, *41*, 4405–4415.

Panda, G.; Pradhan, A. K.; Pati, N. C.; and Nayak, P. L. 1980. Grafting vinyl monomers onto silk fibers. XII. Graft copolymerization of methyl methacrylate onto silk using hydrogen peroxidesodium thiosulfa te redox system. *J. Polym. Sci. Polym. Chem. Ed.*, *18*, 3315.

Peiffer, D. G. and Rabeony, M. 1994. Physical properties of model graft copolymers and their use as blend compatibilizers. *J. Appl. Polym. Sci.*, *51*, 1283.

Percec, V.; Guliashvili, T.; Ladislaw, J. S.; Wistrand. A.; Stjerndahl, A.; Sienkowska, M. J.; Monteiro, M. J.; and Sahoo, S. 2006. Ultrafast synthesis of ultrahigh molar mass polymers by metal-catalyzed living radical polymerization of acrylates, methacrylates, and vinyl chloride mediated by SET at 25°C *J. Am. Chem. Soc.*, *128*, 14156–14165.

Pinkert, A.; Marsh, K. N.; Pang, S.; and Staiger, M. P. 2009. Ionic liquids and their interaction with cellulose. *Chem. Rev.*, *109*, 6712–6758.

Pintauer, T. and Matyjaszewski, K. 2008. Atom transfer radical addition and polymerization reactions catalyzed by ppm amounts of copper complexes. *Chem. Soc. Rev.*, *37*, 1087–1097.

Pradhan, A. K.; Pati, N. C.; and Nayak, P. L. 1982a. Grafting vinyl monomers onto cellulose. VI. Graft copolymerization of methyl methacrylate onto cellulose using potassium permanganate as the initiator. *J. Macromol. Sci. Chem. A*, *17*(3), 501.

Pradhan, A. K.; Pati, N. C.; and Nayak, P. L. 1982b. Grafting vinyl monomers onto cellulose. VIII. Graft copolymerization of methyl methacrylate onto cellulose using H_2-O_2-cysteine redox system. *Macromol. Sci.-Chem. A* *17*(8), 1225–1236.

Pradhan, A. K., Pati, N. C.; and Nayak, P. L. 1982c. Grafting vinyl monomers onto cellulose. IX. Graft copolymerization of methyl methacrylate onto cellulose using peroxydiphosphate-Fe(ll) and Mn(ll) redox systems. *Macromol. Sci.-Chem. A*, *18*(3), 395–409.

Qiu, L.; Shao, Z.; Liu, M.; Wang, J.; Li, P.; and Zhao, M. 2014. Optimization of polysaccharides extraction from seeds of Pharbitis nil and its anti-oxidant activity. *Carbohydr. Polym.*, *102*, 986–992.

Raninen, K.; Lappi, J.; Mykkänen, H.; and Poutanen, K. 2011. Dietary fiber type reflects physiological functionality: comparison of grain fiber, inulin, and polydextrose. *Nutr. Rev.* *69*(1), 9–21.

Rapson, W. H. A. M. 1960. *Chem. Soc.138th Meeting*, New York, Sept.

Raus, V.; Panek, M.; Uchman, M.; Louf, M.; Latalova, P.; Adova, E.; Netopilik M.; Dybal, J.; and Vlček, P. 2011. Cellulose-based graft copolymers with controlled architecture prepared in a homogeneous phase. *J. Polym. Sci. A: Polym. Chem.*, *49*, 4353–4367.

Reid, M. L.; Brown, M. B.; Moss, G. P.; and Jones, S. A. 2008. *J. Pharm. Pharmacol.*, *60*, 1139–1147.

Roder, T.; Morgenstern, B.; Schelosky, N.; and Glatter, O. 2001. Solutions of cellulose in N,N-dimethylacetamide/lithium chloride studied by light scattering methods. *Polymer*, *42*, 6765–6773.

Römer, L. and Scheibel, T. 2008. *Prion*, *2*(4), 154–161.

Rosen, B. M.; Jiang, X.; Wilson, C. J; Nguyen, N. H.; Monteiro, M. J.; and Percec, V. J. 2009. The disproportionation of Cu(I)X mediated by ligand and solvent into Cu(0) and Cu(II)X2 and its implications for SET-LRP. *Polym. Sci. A: Polym. Chem.*, *47*, 5606–5628.

Rosen, B. M. and Percec, V. 2009. Single-electron transfer and single-electron transfer degenerative chain transfer living radical polymerization. *Chem. Rev.*, *109*, 5069–5119.

Roy, D.; Guthrie, J. T.; and Perrier, S. 2005. Graft Polymerization: Grafting Poly(styrene) from cellulose via reversible addition–fragmentation chain transfer (RAFT) polymerization. *Macromolecules*, *38*, 10363–10372.

Roy, D.; Semsarilar, M.; Guthrie, J. T.; and Perrier, S. 2009. Cellulose modification by polymer grafting: A review. *Chem. Soc. Rev.*, *38*, 2046–2064.

Salmon, S. and Hudson, S. M. 1997. Crystal morphology, biosynthesis, and physical assembly of cellulose, chitin, and chitosan. *J. Macromol. Sci., Rev. Macromol. Chem. Phys. C*, 37(2), 199.

Samal, R. K.; Mohanty, T. R.; and Nayak, P. L. 1975. Redox polymerization of acrylonitrile by the redox system V^{5+}-propane-1, 2-diol system in aqueous sulfuric acid. *J. Macromol. Sci. Chem. A*, *9*(7), 1149.

Semsarilar, M.; Ladmiral, V.; and Perrier, S. 2010. Synthesis of a cellulose supported chain transfer agent and its application to RAFT polymerization. *J. Polym. Sci. A: Polym. Chem.*, *48*, 4361–4365.

Shen, D. and Huang, Y. 2004. The synthesis of CDA-g-PMMA copolymers through atom transfer radical polymerization. *Polymer*, *45*, 7091–7097.

Shen, D.; Yu, H.; and Huang, Y. 2006. Synthesis of graft copolymer of ethyl cellulose through living polymerization and its self-assembly. *Cellulose*, *13*, 235–244.

Shen, D.; Yu, H.; and Huang, Y. 2005. Densely grafting copolymers of ethyl cellulose through atom transfer radical polymerization. *J. Polym. Sci. A: Polym. Chem.*, *43*, 4099–4108.

Shi, X.; Tan, L.; Xing, J.; Cao, F.; Chen, L.; Luo, Z.; and Wang, Y. 2012. Synthesis of hydroxyethylcellulose-g-methoxypoly (ethylene glycol) copolymer and its application for protein separation in CE. *J. Appl. Polym. Sci. 128*(3), 1995–2002. doi: 10.1002/app.38403.

Siqueira, G.; Bras, J.; and Dufresne, A. 2010. Cellulosic bionanocomposites: A review of preparation, properties and applications properties and applications. *Polymers*, *2*, 728–765.

Spence, K. L.; Venditti, R. A.; Rojas, O. J.; Pawlak, J. J.; and Hubbe, M. A. 2011. Water vapor barrier properties of coated and filled microfibrillated cellulose composite films. *BioResources*, *6*, 4370–4388.

Stenzel, M. H. and Davis, T. P. 2002. Star polymer synthesis using trithiocarbonate functional β-cyclodextrin cores (reversible addition–fragmentation chain-transfer polymerization). *J. Polym. Sci. A: Polym. Chem.*, *40*, 4498–4512.

Stenzel, M. H.; Davis, T. P.; and Fane, A. G. 2003. Honeycomb structured porous films prepared from carbohydrate based polymers synthesised via the RAFT process. *J. Mater. Chem.*, *13*, 2090–2097.

Sui, X.; Yuan, J.; Zhou, M.; Zhang, J.; Yang, H.; Yuan, W.; Wei, Y.; and Pan, C. 2008. Synthesis of cellulose-graft-poly(N,N-dimethylamino-2-ethyl methacrylate) copolymers via homogeneous ATRP and their aggregates in aqueous media. *Biomacromolecules*, *9*, 2615–2620.

Swatloski, R. P.; Spear, S. K.; Holbrey, J. D.; and Rogers, R. D. 2002. Dissolution of cellulose with ionic liquids. *J. Am. Chem. Soc.*, *124*, 4974–4975.

Tang, X.; Gao, L.; Fan, X.; and Zhou, G. 2007. Controlled grafting of ethyl cellulose with azobenzene-containing polymethacrylates via atom transfer radical polymerization. *J. Polym. Sci. A: Polym. Chem.*, *45*, 1653–1660.

Testova, L.; Nieminen, K.; Penttilä, P. A.; Serimaa, R.; Potthast, A.; and Sixta, H. 2014. Cellulose degradation in alkaline media upon acidic pretreatment and stabilisation. *Carbohydr. Polym.*, *100*, 185–194.

Thuresson, K.; Karlstrom, G.; and Lindman, B. 1995. Phase diagrams of mixtures of a nonionic polymer, hexanol, and water: An experimental and theoretical study of the effect of hydrophobic modification. *J. Phys. Chem.*, *99*, 3823–3831.

Tizzotti, M.; Charlot, A.; Fleury, E.; Stenzel, M.; and Bernard, J. 2010. Modification of polysaccharides through controlled/living radical polymerization grafting—Towards the generation of high performance hybrids. *Macromol. Rapid Commun.*, *31*, 1751–1772.

Tripathy, A. K.; Mishra, M. K.; and Lenka, S. 1981. Grafting vinyl monomers onto cellulose. V. Graft copolymerization of methyl methacrylate onto cellulose using a hexavalent chromium ion. *J. Appl. Polym. Sci.*, *26*, 2769.

Uyama, Y.; Kato, K.; and Ikada, Y. 1998. Surface modification of polymers by grafting. *Adv. Polym. Sci.*, *137*, 1.

Vlček, P.; Janata, M.; Latalova, P.; Dybal, J.; Pirkova, M.; and Toman, L. 2008. Bottlebrush-shaped copolymers with cellulose diacetate backbone by a combination of ring opening polymerization and ATRP. *J. Polym. Sci. A: Polym. Chem.*, *46*, 564–573.

Vlček, P.; Janata, M.; Latalova, P.; Kriz, J.; Jadova, E.; and Toman, L. 2006. Controlled grafting of cellulose diacetate. *Polymer*, *47*, 2587–2595.

Vlček, P.; Raus, V.; Janata, M.; Kriz, J.; and Sikora, A. 2011. Controlled grafting of cellulose esters using SET-LRP process. *J. Polym. Sci. A: Polym. Chem.*, *49*, 164–173.

Voepel, J.; Edlund, U.; and Albertsson, A., 2011. A versatile single-electron-transfer mediated living radical polymerization route to galactoglucomannan graft-copolymers with tunable hydrophilicity. *J. Polym. Sci. A: Polym. Chem.*, *49*, 2366–2372.

Walsh, W. K.; Siahkolah, M. A.; and Rutherford, H. A. 1969. The effect of the glass-transition temperature of conventional and radiation-deposited polymeric additives on mechanical properties of cotton fabric. *Text. Res. J.*, *39*, 1126.

Wang, D.; Tan, J.; Kang, H.; Ma, L.; Jin, X.; Liu, R.; and Huang, Y. 2011. Synthesis, self-assembly and drug release behaviors of pH-responsive copolymers ethyl cellulose-graft-PDEAEMA through ATRP. *Carbohydr. Polym.*, *84*, 195–202.

Williams, J. L. and Stannett, V. T. 1976. Polymer-monomer mixture to effect the grafting of vinyl monomers. *Text. Res. J.*, *26*, 175.

Williams, J. L. and Stannett, V. T. 1979. Highly water-absorptive cellulose by postdecrystallization. *J. Appl. Polym. Sci.*, *23*, 1265.

Winnik, F. M.; Regismode, S. T. A.; and Goddard, E. D. 1996. Interactions of cationic surfactants with a hydrophobically modified cationic cellulose polymer: A study by fluorescence spectroscopy. *Colloids Surf. A*, *106*, 243–247.

Wojnárovits, L.; Földváry, C. M.; and Takács, E. 2010. Radiation-induced grafting of cellulose for adsorption of hazardous water pollutants: A review. *Radiat. Phys. Chem. 79*, 848–862.

Xang, H. C. and Silvermann, J. 1985. Review of vinyl graft copolymerization featuring recent advances toward controlled radical-based reactions. *Radiat. Phys. Chem.*, *25*, 375.

Xie, D.; Culbertson, B. M.; and Johnston, W. M. 1998. Formulation of visible light-curable glass-ionomer cements containing N-vinylpyrrolidone. *J. Macromol. Sci., Pure Appl. Chem. A*, *35*(10), 1631.

Xin, T.; Yuan, T.; Xiao, S.; and He, J. 2011. Synthesis of cellulose-graft-poly(methyl methacrylate) via homogeneous ATR. *J. Bioresour.*, *6*, 2941–2953.

Yan, L. and Ishira, K. 2008. Graft copolymerization of 2-methacryloyloxyethyl phosphorylcholine to cellulose in homogeneous media using atom transfer radical polymerization for providing new hemocompatible coating materials. *J. Polym. Sci. A: Polym. Chem.*, *46*, 3306–3013.

Yan, L. and Tao, W. 2008. Graft copolymerization of N,N-dimethylacrylamide to cellulose in homogeneous media using atom transfer radical polymerization for hemocompatibility. *J. Biomed. Sci. Eng.*, *1*, 37–43.

Yan, Q.; Yuan, J.; Zhang, F.; Sui, X.; Xie, X.; Yin, Y.; Wang, S.; and Wei, Y. 2009. Cellulose-based dual graft molecular brushes as potential drug nanocarriers: stimulus-responsive micelles, self-assembled phase transition behavior, and tunable crystalline morphologies. *Biomacromolecules*, *10*, 2033–2042.

Yang, R.; Liu, Y.; and Zheng, C. 2010. Synthesis of hydroxyethylcellulose-graft-poly(N, N-dimethylacrylamide) copolymer by ATRP and as dynamic coating in capillary electrophoresis. *J. Appl. Poly. Sci.*, *116*, 3468–3472.

Yang. R.; Wang, Y.; and Zhou, D. 2007. Novel hydroxyethylcellulose-graft-poly acrylamide copolymer for separation of double-stranded DNA fragments by CE. *Electrophoresis*, *28*, 3223–3231.

Yasuda, H.; Wray, J. A.; and Stannett, V. 1963. Preparation and characterization of some cellulose graft. *J. Polym. Sci.*, *2*, 387.

Ye, L.; Li, Q.; and Huang, R. J. 2006. Study on the rheological behavior of the hydrophobically modified hydroxyethyl cellulose with 1,2-epoxyhexadecane. *Appl. Polym. Sci.*, *101*, 2953–2959.

Zhang, L.-M. 2001a. Cellulosic associative thickeners. *Carbohydr. Polym.*, *45*, 1–10.

Zhang, L.-M. 2001b. New water-soluble cellulosic polymers: A review. *Macromol. Mater. Eng.*, *285*, 267–275.

Zhang, Y.; Wang, Y.; and Matyjaszewski, K. 2011. ATRP of methyl acrylate with metallic zinc, magnesium, and iron as reducing agents and supplemental activators. *Macromolecules*, *44*, 683–685.

Zhang, Y.; Wang, Y.; Peng, C.; Zhong, M.; Zhu, W.; Konkolewicz, D.; Zhong, J.; Chai, X.; and Fu, S. 2012. Thermal analysis and physiological behavior of cellulose/pectin complex from Canna edulis Ker by-product. *Carbohydr. Polym.*, *87*, 1869–1873.

7 UV-Grafting
A Powerful Tool for Cellulose Surface Modification

R. Bongiovanni, A. Chiappone, and E. Zeno

CONTENTS

Cellulose is probably one of the most extensively investigated polymers: the interest for this abundant and renewable raw material spread at the beginning of the last century and renewed over the past 10 years in the frame of the conversion of the present petrol-based economy to an integrated bio-economy. In this context, cellulose has a major role to play, not only because of its availability and fascinating properties (biodegradability, biocompatibility, low density, high mechanical properties, etc.), but also because, unlike other raw materials such as starch, it is not edible so its use does not compete with human nutrition.

The large number of forms under which cellulose can be processed (polymer, derivatives, fibers, nanocellulose, etc.) makes it a potential candidate for an indefinite number of applications that take advantage of its unique features, arising from its molecular structure and its hierarchical organization. To further broaden the spectrum of cellulose products, especially in high-performance and added-value sectors (medical, electronic, energy, and transportation), its modification or functionalization is often required. The latter can also offer a window for the improvement of quite traditional products and processes, such as paper and papermaking.

However, to leave intact the potential of the cellulose as a sustainable resource, the modification routes should meet, as much as possible, the criteria of the green chemistry, and particularly the limitation to the use of non-innocuous solvents and toxic chemicals. This principle, in agreement with the ecological orientation of industrial cellulose chemistry, limits the number of strategies and reactions viable in a significant way. Among them, photografting combines the inherent benefits of photochemical initiation, namely, a fast, versatile, efficient process and the advantage of a surface grafting that does not modify the bulk properties nor degrade the cellulose structure.

Grafting has advantages over other modification methods in several points, including easy and controllable introduction of graft chains with a high density and exact localization of graft chains to the surface with the bulk properties unchanged. Furthermore, covalent attachment of graft chains onto a polymer surface avoids their delamination and assures the long-term chemical stability of introduced chains, in contrast to physically coated polymer chains [1,2]. The use of irradiation, typically UV light, appears to be an excellent method for surface grafting of polymers because of its simplicity and cleanliness. Additional reasons for the suitability of the photochemical method for surface grafting of polymers are as follows: (1) photochemically produced triplet states of carbonyl compounds can abstract hydrogen atoms from almost all polymers so that graft polymerization may be initiated; (2) high concentrations of active species can be produced locally at the interface between the substrate polymer and the monomer solution containing a sensitizer when UV irradiation is applied through the substrate polymer film; (3) in addition to the simplicity of the procedure, the cost of energy source is lower for UV radiation than for ionizing radiation [3].

In this chapter, we will first shortly explain the basics of photochemistry applied to cellulosic materials; then, we will focus on the photografting processes to modify cellulose, evidencing the advantages and the disadvantages of the approach. We will describe the different strategies of UV-induced grafting reported in the literature and the applications to which the processes are mostly oriented at present. The concluding remarks will propose future perspectives of the grafting strategy.

7.1 CELLULOSE PHOTOCHEMISTRY

Reactions of cellulosic materials induced by light are reported since the ancient times of the Egyptian and Babylonian civilizations: at the time, sunlight was used for the treatment of linen during mummification and for the preparation of papyrus boats. It is nowadays known that these early days, technologies were respectively based on a photo-induced cross-linking reaction of cellulosic fibers of linen and on a polymerization and grafting reaction of asphalt oil coated onto the papyrus leaves.

Of the sun spectrum, the most suitable radiations for triggering the formation of reactive species are in the UV range. Therefore, in modern chemistry and in industrial processes, UV light is preferred, using Hg lamps with a wide emission spectrum as reported in Figure 7.1, xenon lamps, and arc lamps. Alternatively, limiting the discussion to nonionizing radiations, chemical processes can be initiated by lasers and light-emitting diodes (LEDs) with specific wavelength usually in the UV range.

In order to make a molecule or a macromolecule to react, the UV light has to be absorbed and the absorption should result in electronic transitions to excited states. The energy acquired by the

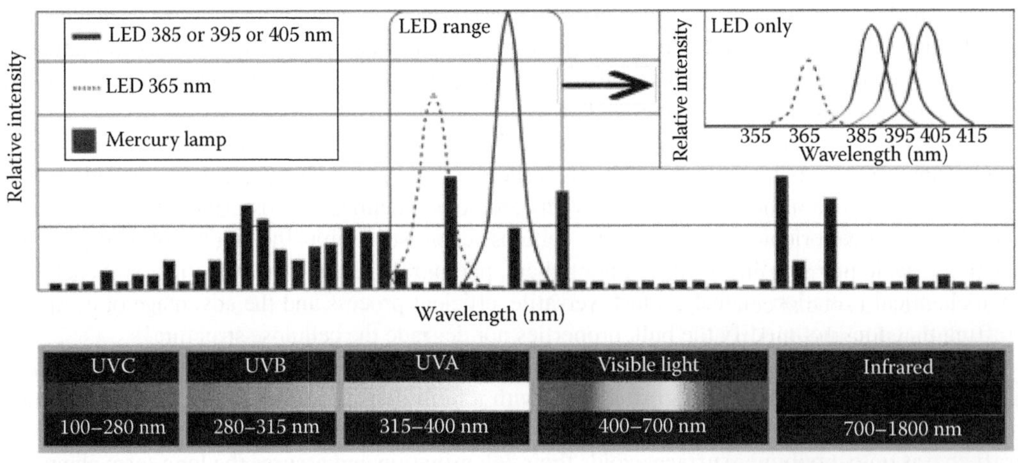

FIGURE 7.1 Hg lamp emission spectrum and comparison with LED emissions. (From Protheus Technology, http://www.phoseon.com/technology/led-uv-wavelength.htm, last accessed on January 5, 2014.)

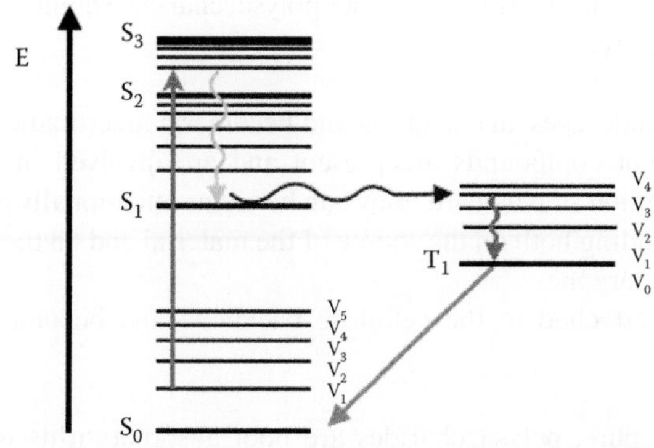

FIGURE 7.2 Jablonski diagram: a molecule at the ground electronic state S_0 absorbs light, reaching an excited state S_x. From the S_x state, by a spin change, the molecule goes to the T_x state. The weavy arrows indicate non-radiative conversions, and the $T_1 \rightarrow S_0$ transition is an example of radiative decay (phosphorescence).

molecule can be reemitted in the form of light (including fluorescence and phosphorescence emissions) or can be released through non-radiative decays. As sketched in Figure 7.2, if the excited molecule assumes a triplet state by the so-called intersystem-crossing reaction, there is a change in the spin of the electron promoted to a higher level and the molecule becomes paramagnetic. Then, reactions can take place, due to bond breaking (not always on the group involved in the light absorption). It is important to remember that the paramagnetic molecules at the triplet state can easily react with other paramagnetic species: among the many, oxygen is the most relevant co-reactant and gives triplet quenching, therefore inhibiting the reactions.

Photochemical reactions are usually classified as

- Photoscission (photocleavage, Norrish I reaction)
- Hydrogen abstraction (Norrish II reaction)
- Electron transfer

They lead to reactive chemical intermediates that are useful for further reactions. The reactions mentioned can also be induced thermally, but there are many advantages in a photochemical mechanism, already recognized at the beginning of the twentieth century by Italian chemist Ciamician in Bologna [5]:

- Radiation is the limiting agent of the reaction.
- There is a temporary control of the reaction, that is, reactions are of the type "stop and go."
- The processes are energy specific: the absorption of energy during irradiation is quantized, while thermal processes are not; the light is absorbed and converted by processes to which specified energies can be attributed (frequencies or wavelengths in spectroscopic terms) per atom, per molecule, per mole, etc.
- There is a special control of the reaction, that is, reactions take place only in the irradiated area, while the dark areas remain untreated.

Moreover, in many cases, photoreactions can be conducted in bulk. This is of main interest when cellulose is concerned. In fact, it is well known that, due to its supramolecular structure, cellulose is insoluble in water and ordinary organic solvents: therefore, it is attractive to have efficient heterogeneous phase reactions. Photo-induced reactions can be applied to the final cellulosic material, adding the photoreaction step to the production line of paper and fabrics.

The photoreactions on cellulose (as for any other polysaccharide) should be discussed taking into account that three cases apply:

- The polymer itself undergoes an excitation and becomes a macroradical/macroion.
- Low-molecular-weight compounds are present and are involved in the photoprocesses from the light absorption step onward; they can be either intentionally added or be adventitiously present depending both on the source of the material and on the processes cellulose can have already undergone.
- Chromophores are attached to the cellulose backbone and become responsible of the photoprocesses.

In fact, when chemically pure, polysaccharides are poor absorbers (this is the case of bacterial cellulose), while cellulosic pulps contain chromophores mainly due to residual lignin and to thermal-oxidative reactions happening during pulping and bleaching or any other processing step [6,7]. Chromophores are mainly aldehyde, keto, and carboxylic groups; hydroxybenzoquinone, hydroxyacetophenone, and naphthoquinone structures have been identified in many cellulosic materials: some of these structures come from keto functionalities formed during thermal treatment, in the presence of air; they are mainly independent of the natural origin of the material. In considering light absorption by cellulose, one also has to take into account that impurities such as organics and metal ions are always present in fibers. Therefore, cellulosic materials can be photosensitive to different wavelengths from deep UV (below 200 nm) to visible radiations.

Concluding remark is that photochemical processes onto cellulose (as for any chemical product) are certainly started by light absorption, but it can be very difficult or nearly impossible to establish which chromophore is involved in absorption.

The first reaction triggered by light, listed earlier, is photoscission. Photoscission is also known as Norrish type I reaction and was first studied on simple molecules such as acetone. For acetone, the chemical equation is

$$\begin{array}{l} (CH_3)_2CO(S_0) \xrightarrow{h\nu} (CH_3)_2CO(S_1) \\ \qquad\qquad\qquad\qquad \downarrow k_{ISC} \\ \qquad\qquad\qquad\qquad (CH_3)_2CO(T_1) \xrightarrow{k_{dT}} CH_3CO\bullet + CH_3\bullet \end{array} \tag{7.1}$$

where S_0, S_1 represent singlet states (ground and excited, respectively), and the intersystem crossing reaction leads to the triplet state T_1 and finally to the productions of two radicals.

As already mentioned, irradiation is often conducted in an inert atmosphere, as oxygen quenches the excited molecule. From the earlier equation, the homolytic breaking of a bond (here the light wavelength needed is 313 nm) and the formation of two radicals are evident: radicals are very reactive and will further react with species present in the reaction medium. Some typical reactions are reported in the following:

$$\begin{array}{l} H_3C{-}\overset{O}{\overset{\|}{C}}\bullet \longrightarrow H_3C\bullet + CO \\ 2H_3C\bullet \longrightarrow H_3C{-}CH_3 \\ 2H_3C{-}\overset{O}{\overset{\|}{C}}\bullet \longrightarrow H_3C{-}\overset{O}{\overset{\|}{C}}{-}\overset{O}{\overset{\|}{C}}{-}CH_3 \\ H_3C{-}\overset{O}{\overset{\|}{C}}\bullet + \bullet CH_3 \longrightarrow H_2C{=}C{=}O + CH_4 \end{array} \tag{7.2}$$

One can monitor the degradation of acetone analysing the volatiles obtained (carbon oxides, methane, etc.) and the recombination of radicals checking the formation of hydrocarbons and higher-molecular-weight species. If the radical products come in contact with oxygen (which is often the case), the formation of carboxyl, carbonyl, peroxide groups takes place through oxidative paths.

Observations on the effect of light on cellulose were reported at the end of the nineteenth century. Systematic investigations started with the development of analytical tools such as fluorescence, Fourier transform IR and UV–visible reflectance spectroscopy, electron spin resonance spectroscopy (ESR or EPR), and flash-photolysis, widely used to detect radicals [8,9]. The studies conducted using these techniques showed that when irradiation hits the cellulose (just cellulose), the photocleavage mechanism described before produces cellulose macroradicals where the unpaired electron is on a carbon and an oxygen atom of the cellulose backbone [10]. At the acetal bridge, an alkoxy radical and a carbon secondary radical form (either C1 or C4): the first consequence of this homolysis is a decrease in the molecular weight, which has been experimentally observed. Other modification effects are found, such as ring cleavage, although in negligible amount; dehydrogenation has also been proposed. One has then to take into account that the macroradicals can react with themselves and with any species present and/or added to the cellulose. Any form of cellulose (fibers, crystals, paper, whiskers, fabrics, etc.) can react in this way. In the presence of air, oxidative processes can form oxygenated groups along the chains: they can further react (as in the case of hydroperoxide groups, as will be mentioned later or); anyway, they often cause the yellowing of the material. It has also been proved that photochemical degradation gives gaseous products such as carbon oxides and hydrogen. An increase in the copper number together with an increase in solubility in alkaline solutions is also found after irradiation.

It can also be interesting to add on purpose a photosensitive species to cellulose. In this case, the products of the photodecomposition of the photosensitive molecule should be primarily considered to understand the reaction paths and control the reactions. Besides homolytic reactions leading to radical species, alternative pathways exist, causing generation of acids or bases that can intervene in many reactions, as catalysts or initiators for photodegradation, photopolymerization, photo-cross-linking, and so on.

Cellulose radical species can also form via a hydrogen abstraction mechanism, known as Norrish II reaction. It is a bimolecular reaction and can be easily represented with reference to the benzopinacolation reaction of benzophenone (BP) in the presence of an alcohol:

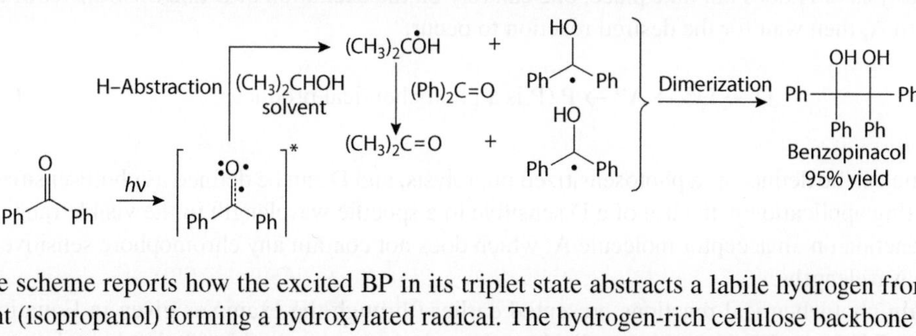

(7.3)

The scheme reports how the excited BP in its triplet state abstracts a labile hydrogen from the solvent (isopropanol) forming a hydroxylated radical. The hydrogen-rich cellulose backbone can be an ideal supplier of labile hydrogens, and the reaction can be represented as follows:

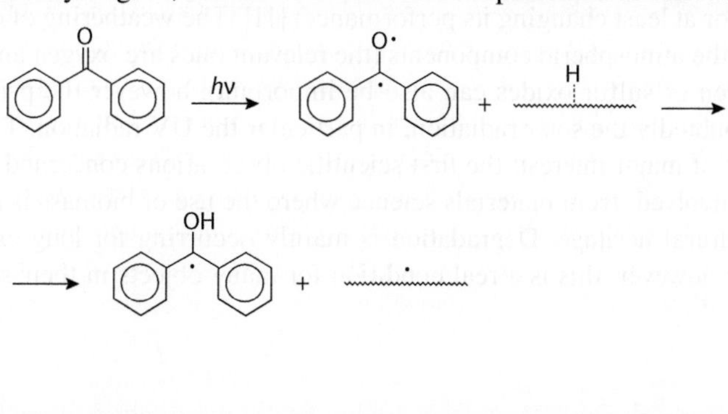

(7.4)

Upon the effect of UV, there may be possible abstraction of hydrogen from the different carbons of the glucosidic ring giving rise to radicals of different stability, therefore not involving chain scission along the backbone. Many radical transformations can eventually follow, depending on the experimental conditions, namely, wavelengths, temperature, moisture, and presence of oxygen [6].

At higher dose of UV irradiation, abstraction of CH_2OH may take place, and the radical groups may further convert to CHO or H radicals [6]. Also salts like $FeCl_3$ (besides increasing light absorption thanks to the ferric ions) can promote hydrogen abstraction via the formation of chlorine atomic radicals.

The third and last photochemical mechanisms are the electron transfer reactions. It is again a bimolecular reaction (as the H-abstraction), and a simple example is given by BP in the presence of amine, according to Equation 7.5.

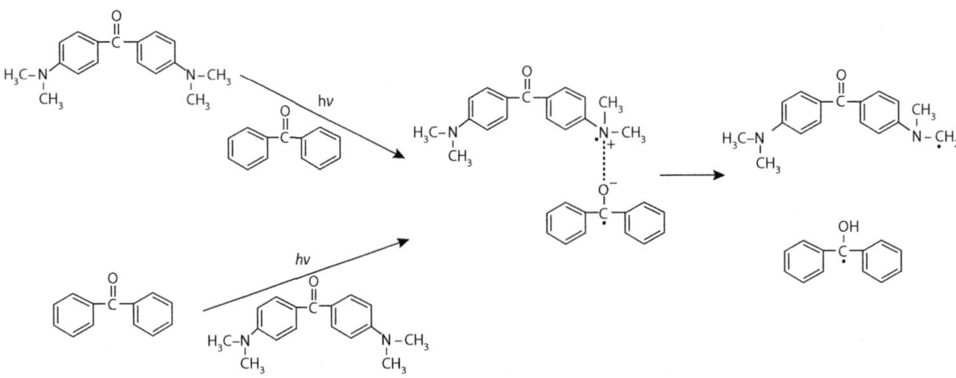

(7.5)

The excited species (in its triplet state) forms a CTC. Once the CTC is formed, there is an exchange of energy from the excited molecule, called donor D to the unexcited species, called acceptor A. A becomes excited: therefore there is a synergistic conversion to radical species. This is interesting if the formation of the excited product through a direct route is not possible, for example, if the direct photolysis of A does not take place, one can rely on the excitation of D and the transfer of the excitation to A, then wait for the desired reaction to occur:

$$D \rightarrow D^* \rightarrow A^* \rightarrow P \text{ (P is a photochemical product)} \tag{7.6}$$

The reaction can be defined as a photosensitized photolysis, and D can be defined as photosensitizer. An interesting application is the use of a D sensitive to a specific wavelength in the visible range to trigger a reaction on an acceptor molecule A, which does not contain any chromophore sensitive to the visible wavelengths.

The main photochemical reactions presented earlier (through the examples given in Equations 7.1, 7.3, and 7.5) are often generating radicals and can become responsible for the degradation of cellulose (reducing or at least changing its performance) [11]. The weathering of cellulose is caused by water, heat, and the atmospheric components (the relevant ones are oxygen and ozone; however, pollutants as nitrogen or sulfur oxides can also be important); however the primary promoter of degradation is undoubtedly the solar radiation, in particular the UV radiation. Therefore, light stability of cellulose is of major interest: the first scientific observations concerned textiles, but many other domains are involved, from materials science where the use of biomass is having an increasing attention, to cultural heritage. Degradation is mainly occurring for long exposure times and very high intensity: however, this is a real condition for many objects in their service life and for art pieces (old lines, books made of papyrus leaves, and/or modern papers after Gutenberg), if not properly stored.

Degradation can also be seen as desirable. The photolability of a material can be attractive at the time of its disposal, and photolytic processes can aid microorganism to metabolize cellulose. From a different point of view, photooxidation processes related to degradation can be advantageous as they assure functional groups that can help adhesion at the matrix–fiber interface of a composite [12].

In cellulose photochemistry, light can also promote nondegradative reactions. Modification of cellulose with chemicals properly selected is a key reaction for obtaining fully new derivatives: the preferred abstraction of OH group at C6 position due to the limited hindrance around the C6 (mentioned before) has been utilized for the synthesis of different polymers. Photochemical reactions can also be used for decorating the cellulose backbone imparting specific properties, mainly regarding the surface of fibers, paper, and fabrics [7]. This will be the topic of the next section.

Another important process is cross-linking, which can be considered as either a degradative reaction or a nondegradative reaction. It happens when cellulose macroradicals add to each other and/or by radical additions with multifunctional coreactants. In the making of materials to replace synthetic polymers, the cross-linking of cellulose is mainly exploited to form composites where a natural or a synthetic polymer forms the matrix, and cellulose fibers guarantee the reinforcement. If the polymer matrix cross-links by irradiation, the obtained product can be described as a semi-interpenetrating network (semi-IPN) with polymeric fibers entangled in the network, or as a true IPN, where a fiber physical network is combined with the light-cured one [13]. Eventually, chemical bonds between the two can be present, as a kind of grafting, as will be described further on.

7.2 UV-GRAFTING OF CELLULOSE: REACTIONS AND MECHANISMS

When grafting is considered, three basically different grafting approaches are mentioned [14]. The first approach is the "grafting-to" approach, where a monomer or an end-functional oligomer or preformed polymer with a reactive end-group is coupled with the functional group located on the polymer backbone to be modified. In the "grafting-from" approach, the growth of the polymer chain occurs from initiating sites created on the polymer backbone. The third approach is the "grafting-through" approach in which a macro monomer, for example, a vinyl derivative of cellulose, is copolymerized with a low-molecular-weight comonomer.

The grafting-to strategy is quite popular, although it gives low grafting density and yields small amounts of polymer per gram cellulose. Moreover, its use for aqueous suspensions of cellulosic substrates reduces the choice of the monomer or polymer to be grafted, which should be preferably water soluble. This is a limiting factor for conferring hydrophobicity to cellulose.

Using the grafting-from process the growing chain is attached to the cellulose, the monomer should diffuse towards its end to propagate, long brushes are formed and high grafting density can be obtained. With respect to this latter approach, a number of different polymerization methods have been proposed, including atomic transfer radical polymerization, nitroxide-mediated polymerization, or reversible addition–fragmentation polymerization [14].

Grafting can be conducted photochemically: photochemical reactions can be properly adapted to any of the previous strategies. Many kinds of polymers for as many applications have been modified by photografting, with the aid of a photoinitiator or photosensitizer. When cellulose is taken in consideration, as mentioned before, the most suitable light is in the UV range, and the term UV grafting is used.

It is necessary to underline that the grafting of various monomers or polymers using low-energy ultraviolet radiation causes negligible degradation of the backbone polymer and gives an option for better control over the grafting reaction than that can be achieved by the high-energy γ-radiation method [15,16].

As reported previously, photochemical reactions most frequently involve radical species, therefore, in the following, first the UV grafting by a radical mechanism will be described. Then, other UV grafting reactions will be described.

7.2.1 Radical Grafting of Acrylate and Vinyl Monomers

Earlier studies onto photo-induced grafting of acrylate onto cellulose showing its feasibility are reported in [17,18]. Since then, several investigations deal with the modification of natural polymers such as cellulose and cellulose derivatives with common acrylic monomers such as, for example, methyl methacrylate or 2-hydroxyethyl methacrylate monomer [19–27], mainly with the purpose of improving the tensile strength of lignocellulosic pulps. As the literature relative to the UV radical grafting of acrylates and vinyl monomers is abundant, in this part of the chapter, we will focus on the most discussed reactions carried on pure cellulose fibers.

Vinyl graft (co)polymerization and acrylic graft (co)polymerization to a cellulosic backbone are complex. Polymerization takes place via a free radical mechanism and generally involves the generation of free radical sites on the main backbone by UV radiation, which induces homolytic bond breaking as described in Section 1. The vinyl or acrylic monomer then reacts with the free radical sites to propagate a new polymer chain that is covalently anchored to the backbone. A free radical site is also formed on the newly formed branch. Many monomers may add subsequently to the free radical site of the branch. The propagation of the branch continues until termination occurs either by combination of two growing chains or by a disproportionation mechanism, where a hydrogen atom is abstracted by another growing polymeric chain. Termination may also occur by chain transfer to monomer, to initiator, to dead polymer, to additives, and to impurities. The presence of new polymeric chains gives new properties to the backbone polymer.

Such a procedure has to be carried out in an inert atmosphere in order to avoid oxygen inhibition as the rate constants for quenching of initiating and propagating radical species by oxygen is extremely fast, due to the triplet state biradical nature of oxygen [28]. The fast formation of poorly reactive peroxy radicals (RO_2^*) limits the grafting procedure.

The general mechanism of the free radical grafting of vinyl and acrylic monomers onto cellulose is illustrated in Figure 7.3: it is clearly a grafting-from approach.

Even if conducted in nitrogen atmosphere, this grafting process leads to relatively low grafting yields (<10 %wt) due to the competing homopolymerization reaction [18,29]. In fact, the monomers can grow without attaching to the cellulose. One cannot exclude that eventually the homopolymers, once formed, can graft to the cellulose, therefore the process becomes a grafting-to. Moreover, cross-linking can take place, and the chains can interpenetrate the cellulosic networks.

The problem of low grafting yield has been overcome by the use of different strategies. Garnett et al. [30] in order to enhance the MMA grafting to the cellulose substrate added styrene, enabling MMA to be grafted efficiently to the substrate with a reduction in the homopolymerization yield. Less homopolymer formation meant a less viscous solution and thus a higher MMA diffusion into the substrate backbone with a higher possibility of reaction with active sites.

Alternatively, the addition of mineral acids to the solution of monomers and solvents was proposed [31,32]. It was observed that acid enhances grafting and hinders homopolymer formation. This is mainly due to two effects. The first is a partitioning effect, that is, in the presence of the acid, the concentration of monomer available at a grafting site in the backbone polymer is increased. In addition to partitioning, an increase of radicals in the presence of acids was also found, thus influencing the kinetics of the process.

The theory developed to explain the role of acid in the grafting processes can also be extended to other additives. Photoinitiators can be favorably partitioned in the backbone polymer; they obviously enhance the grafting reactions, yielding additional radicals by exposure to UV. A wide range of photosensitive molecules have been used to produce graft copolymers of cellulose.

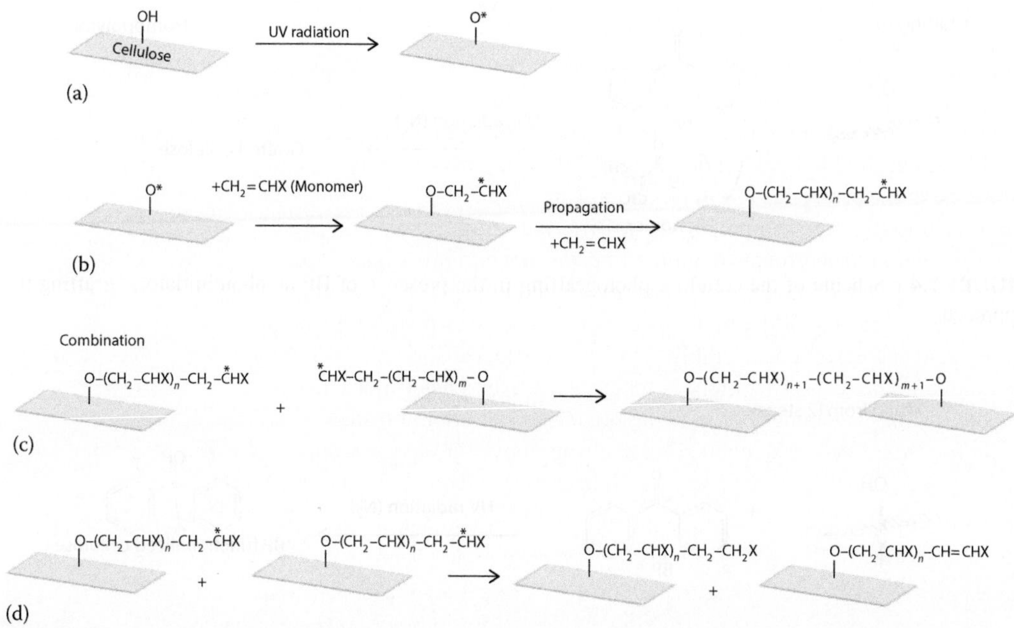

FIGURE 7.3 Scheme of the UV-induced radical grafting. (a) Initiation, (b) propagation, (c) termination, and (d) disproportionation.

Hydrogen peroxide (H_2O_2) as well as several other molecules such as ferric chloride, ferrous sulfate, ceric ammonium nitrate, sodium anthraquinone-2,7-disulfonate, and *N*-bromosuccinimide have been used as photosensitizer for MMA grafting onto cellulose in both the liquid [25,33] and vapor phases [34]. 2-Hydroxy-2-methyl-1-phenylpropan-1-one was used to promote the grafting of perfluoro-polyacrylate resins and chitosan on cotton fibers making them oil repellent [35–38]. Xanthone was used by Kubota et al. as a sensitizer for the photografting of methacrylic acid (MAA) and *N*-isopropylacrylamide (NIPAAm) on regenerated cellulose film [39].

Compared with Norrish type I photoinitiators, Norrish type II photoinitiators were more frequently used [40], predominantly because the latter results in higher grafting efficiency, while the former leads to higher polymerization yield and higher polymerization rate, but lower grafting efficiency [41]. Among the existing Norrish type II photoinitiators, probably the most widely selected have been BP and its derivatives [42–46]. It was shown that they can effectively initiate or co-initiate a number of radical-induced surface photografting polymerizations. As already described, when UV irradiated, BP or BP-based molecules are excited to a singlet state and then jump to a triplet state by intersystem crossing. Investigations have demonstrated that BP and its derivatives in a triplet state undergo hydrogen-abstracting reactions from cellulose, consequently providing surface radicals capable of initiating surface graft polymerization. The resulting benzopinacol radicals (BP–OH•) are relatively less reactive and not so prone to free radical polymerization as other photoinitiators, but tend to participate in termination by coupling reaction. When a photoinitiator like BP is used, two routes for the grafting procedure can be chosen. In the "grafting-to" approach [14,47], the photosensitive molecule is added to the monomer formulation and, during UV exposure, end-functionalized growing polymer molecules directly react with complementary functional groups located on the cellulose surface. Although this procedure is fast and reliable, it has a strong disadvantage, as seen in the cases previously discussed, since it often results in the formation of high quantities of homopolymer and even cross-linked polymer, which are in competition with the surface grafting reaction (Figure 7.4).

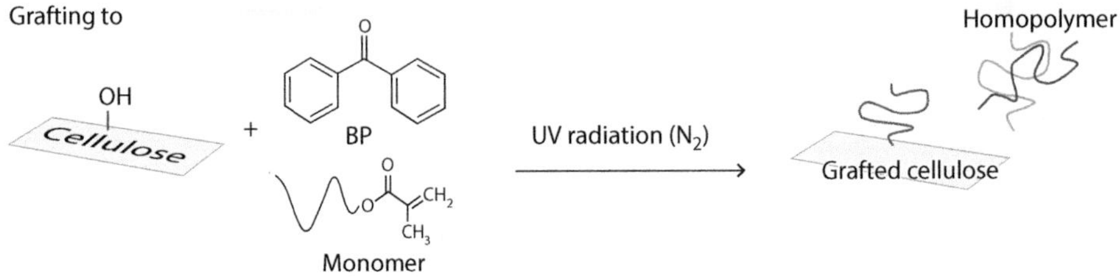

FIGURE 7.4 Scheme of the cellulose photografting in the presence of BP as photoinitiator, "grafting-to" approach.

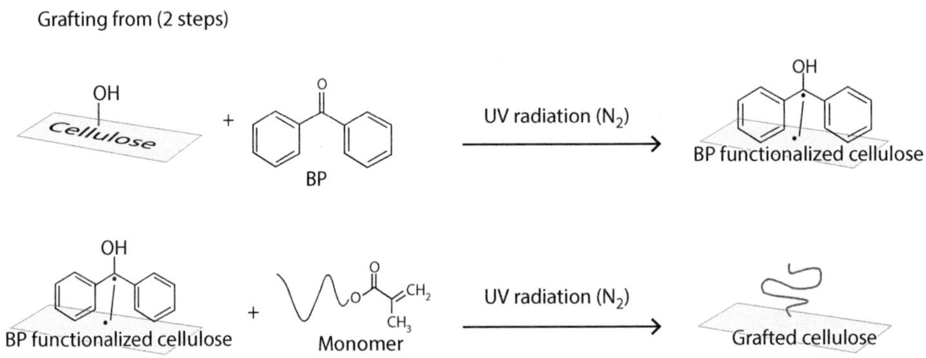

FIGURE 7.5 Scheme of the two-step cellulose photografting with BP immobilization and subsequent polymer grafting, "grafting-from" approach.

A valid alternative to the "grafting-to" is the "grafting-from" approach, which involves polymerization initiated at the substrate surface by attached initiating groups, usually covalently bonded [44,48]. The "grafting-from" method for the modification of polymeric surfaces involves the immobilization of BP on the polymer to be modified and then the growing of the grafting chains. It is a two-step process, first proposed by Ma et al. [49] for the modification of polypropylene membranes, as sketched in Figure 7.5.

According to this procedure, in the first step, BP, under UV light, abstracts hydrogen from the polymeric substrate to generate surface radicals and semipinacol radicals, which combine to form surface photoinitiators in the absence of monomers. In the second step, the monomer solution is added to the active substrate (the BP-modified cellulose), and the surface initiators initiate the graft polymerization under UV irradiation [19].

Recently, following the same chemistry described earlier, photo-reactive polymers were also used for chemical modification of paper sheets. It means that specifically designed functional polymers carrying a photo-reactive BP moiety can be transferred onto model filter papers by means of dipcoating and UV irradiation processes [50]. Interestingly, the amount of paper-attached copolymer was well controlled (from a few mg/g cellulose fibers up to several tenths of mg/g fiber) by selecting the concentration of the polymer, while physically attached chains were removed by simple solvent extraction.

Delaittre et al. [51] proposed a photo-induced macromolecular functionalization of cellulose via "nitroxide spin trapping." According to this procedure, solid cellulose is functionalized with a biocompatible Norrish type I radical photoinitiator (2-hydroxy-1-(4-(2-hydroxyethoxy)phenyl)-2-methylpropan-1-one, Irgacure® 2959). Following near-UV irradiation (λ_{max} ~311 nm), radicals are generated on the cellulose surface and trapped by a preformed nitroxide-functionalized polystyrene.

The process is efficient and elegant, and a well-controlled grafting is obtained. The limit of the technique clearly lies in the availability of nitroxide derivatives having interesting properties for cellulose modification.

An alternative type of initiator-free grafting was proposed in the late 1990s by Garnett et al. [30,32] called "cure grafting."

In practice, the technique utilizes charge transfer (CT) complex formation for the irradiation of a mixture of donor (D) and acceptor (A) monomers. The implication of this concept is that two monomers are needed for the process; however, with CT complexes, no photoinitiators are usually needed. In an alternative modification of the method, a percentage of a DA complex was used to trigger the polymerization and graft a third monomer. Other components including oligomers have also been used to tailor the grafting mixture and the surface composition of the modified cellulose. The actual grafting procedure involves coating the monomers' mixture onto the substrate, then curing the coated substrate under a UV radiation source. Cure grafting can lead to predominantly surface grafting unless the monomers swell the substrate: in this case, grafting within the bulk can be achieved [52]. Electron poor monomers such as maleimide (MI), maleic anhydride (MA), *N*-phenyl maleimide, dimethyl maleate, dimethyl fumarate have been used as acceptor components (A), while electron-rich monomers such as vinyl ethers, *N*-vinyl pyrrolidone (NVP), p-methoxy styrene (pMST), vinyl acetate (VA), and a-methyl styrene (aMST) can be preferentially chosen as donors (D).

A general overview scheme can be formulated to depict the radiation polymerization processes of the CT complexes used in this work (Figure 7.6). The scheme shows the formation of a zwitterion biradical that can participate to subsequent reactions, i.e. the direct grafting to the cellulose substrate on which radicals were formed during irradiation or the accelerated grafting of a third monomer (Figure 7.7).

One plausible mechanism for the grafting of a third monomer in the presence of a D–A complex is reported in Figure 7.7, where D is the electron-rich donor, A is the electron-poor acceptor (such as MA, MI, or NVP), M the monomer (like MMA).

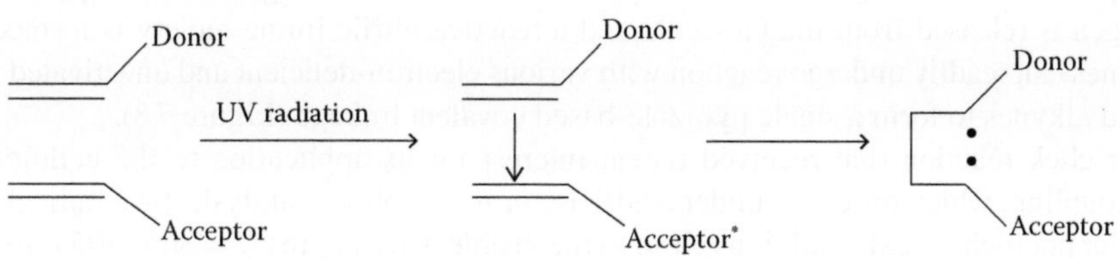

FIGURE 7.6 Scheme of the formation of biradicals after exposure to UV light of a donor and an acceptor monomer.

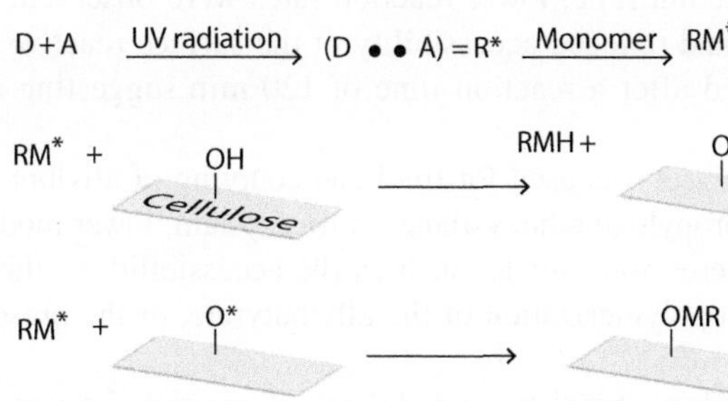

FIGURE 7.7 Scheme of the mechanism for the grafting of a third monomer in the presence of a D–A complex.

Alternatively, radical sites may be formed by abstraction reactions with the substrate involving monomer radicals, the monomer being an acrylate capable of absorbing UV. Once radicals like M* are formed, they are also capable of reacting with the D–A species, either with individual components especially D, or collectively, to give enhanced polymerization. The polymerization process involving D–A is complicated further by the fact that irradiation has been performed in air; thus, the vinyl ether D of the D–A under these conditions may readily form hydroperoxides, which will subsequently decompose in the presence of UV to give initiating radicals.

When considering the use of this grafting technique, consideration should be also given to the presence of the substrate. Thus, ease of radical formation in the backbone polymer is fundamental to the process since without the occurrence of such sites, grafting cannot be accomplished.

7.2.2 Other Grafting Processes

The grafting of cellulose based on radical reactions is definitely the most used and described in literature; however, some different procedures have also been described and will now be summarized.

7.2.2.1 Click Reactions

Numerous click reactions have already been applied to polymer chemistry and surface grafting [53,54]. Some of the proposed reactions feature a light-triggered activation process, and a few of them have been used to graft monomer onto cellulose substrates.

Dietrich and coworkers [55] exploited click methodology based on the nitrile imine-mediated 1,3-dipolar cycloaddition of tetrazole and ene (NITEC) to graft several substrates comprising cellulose. Over other more established click reactions, NITEC presents several advantages such as its simplicity of implementation since tetrazole-based molecules are rather easy to synthesize and a simple hand-held UV lamp is required, thanks to high photolysis quantum yields, the absence of metal catalyst, fast reaction times, and bioorthogonality.

In this procedure, starting from a premodified cellulose containing tetrazole, upon UV exposure, nitrogen is released from the molecule and a reactive nitrile imine moiety is formed in situ. Nitrile imines can readily undergo reaction with various electron-deficient and unactivated terminal alkenes and alkynes to form a stable pyrazole-based covalent linkage (Figure 7.8).

Another click reaction that received recent interest for its application to the cellulose is the thiol-ene coupling, which proceeds under acid/base or nucleophilic catalysis, by a radical pathway mostly under photochemical conditions close to the visible wavelengths ($\lambda = 365–405$ nm). The use of UV photoactivation allows to perform the reaction under very mild conditions. As an example, methylthioglycolate was photochemically grafted onto ene-functionalized films of microfibrillated cellulose under ambient conditions without solvent [56]. The reaction rate was very fast during the first minutes, suggesting that the reaction occurred primarily on easily accessible surface vinyl groups. By increasing the reaction time, lower reaction rates were observed, which were attributed to diffusion phenomena and reduced accessibility of the surface reactive groups. No further modification could be detected after a reaction time of 120 min suggesting a complete surface modification.

In the same work, UV catalysis was used for thiol-ene coupling of allylbutyrate with cellulose silylated with the 3-mercaptopropyltrimethoxysilane. In this system, lower modification rates were observed, and various hypotheses were made, such as the accessibility of the thiol functions on the cellulose surface, the homopolymerization of the allylbutyrate, or the presence of nonreactive sulfonic acid functions.

The combination of alkoxysilane chemistry and of the thiol-ene chemistry was recently proposed for the functionalization of cellulose nanocrystals [57].

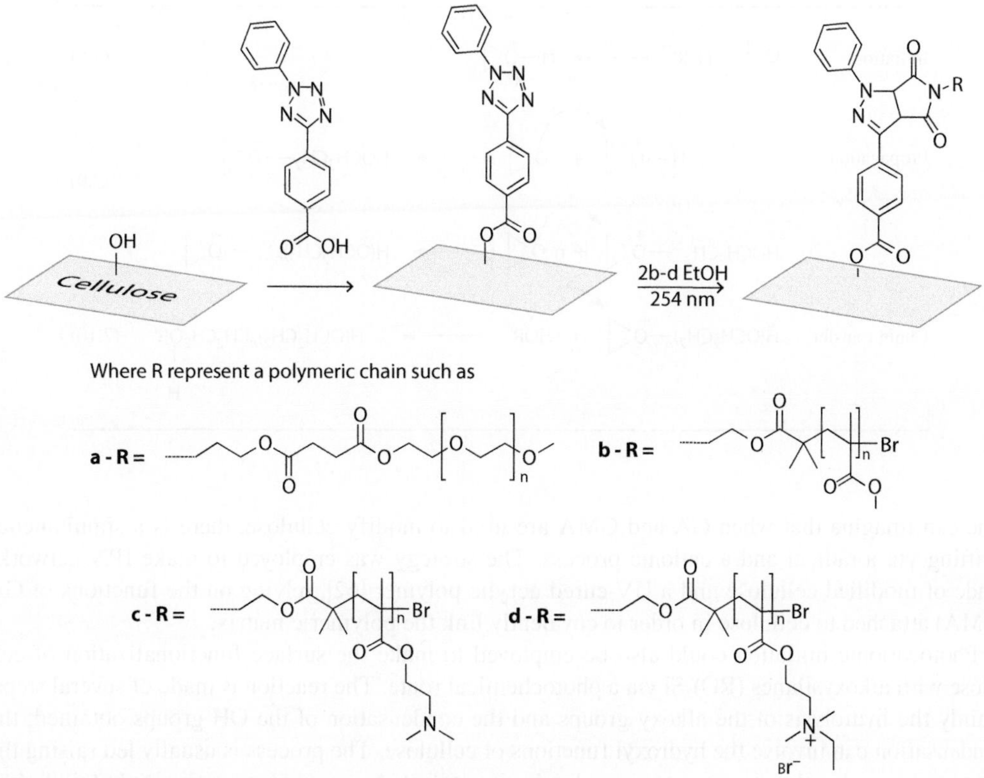

FIGURE 7.8 Scheme of the mechanism for the NITEC grafting.

7.2.2.2 Photografting via a Cationic Mechanism

Glycidyl acrylate (GA) and methacrylate (GMA) have been used to modify cellulose. These monomers presenting a (meth)acrylic group can functionalize the substrate via a radical mechanism. After grafting these monomers, the modified cellulose contains reactive epoxy groups: as described previously [58,59], the epoxide ring can open and generate new functional groups that find uses in ion exchange and chelate formation, and as pseudo-affinity ligands, acting as a "molecular anchor" for active molecular species [59]. Also the preparation of graft copolymers of cellulose with GMA and comonomers has been described [60], using radical photoinitiation. In a recent work by Chiappone et al. [61], it was shown by IR and XPS spectroscopy that in the presence of a cationic photoinitiator triarylsulfonium hexafluoro phosphate, the GA and GMA monomers can also react with cellulose via a different mechanism. The onium salt upon illumination degrades according to the following reaction:

$$Ph_3S^+X^- \xrightarrow{h\nu} \left[Ph_3S^+X^-\right]^1 \longrightarrow \left| \begin{matrix} Ph_2S^{\dot{+}}X^- + Ph^{\cdot} \\ Ph_2S + Ph^+X^- \end{matrix} \right| \rightrightarrows H^+X^- \quad (7.7)$$

The reaction provides radicals (therefore the radical grafting can take place) but mainly produces strong acids HX. As reported in Equation 7.8, by addition of the protons (initiation), the epoxy ring opens and can add either to another epoxy ring or to the OH groups of the cellulose surface. In other words, GMA and GA can propagate via a cationic mechanism (Equation 7.9) and graft to the cellulose backbone (represented by R'OH) by a chain transfer reaction (Equation 7.10):

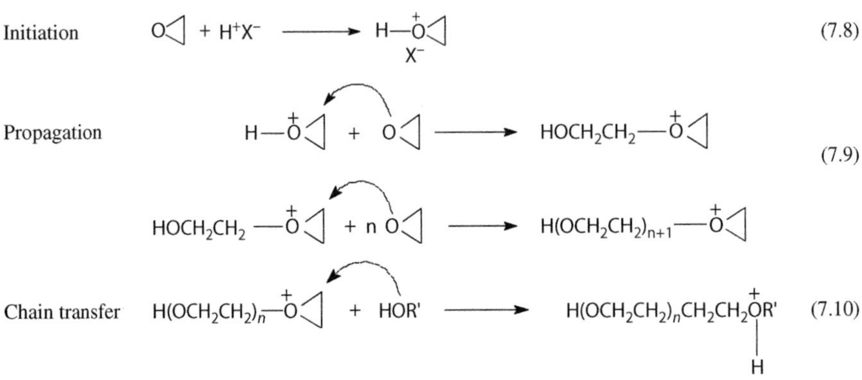

One can imagine that when GA and GMA are used to modify cellulose, there is a simultaneous grafting via a radical and a cationic process. The strategy was employed to make IPN networks made of modified cellulose and a UV-cured acrylic polymer [62], relying on the functions of GA (GMA) attached to cellulose in order to covalently link the polymeric matrix.

Photocationic initiation could also be employed to make the surface functionalization of cellulose with alkoxysilanes $(RO)_4Si$ via a photochemical route. The reaction is made of several steps, mainly the hydrolysis of the alkoxy groups and the condensation of the OH groups obtained: the condensation can involve the hydroxyl functions of cellulose. The process is usually led raising the temperature and in the presence of an acid or basic catalyst. As seen before, cationic photoinitiators can produce acidic species and therefore catalyze the hydrolysis and condensation of alkoxysilanes. There is not yet a study of this kind reported although sol–gel modification of cellulose is well known, and in the case of cellulose materials like cotton, it is based on the chemical condensation of silanol groups with the hydroxyl groups on the textile surface at above 100°C [63]. Moreover, the double role of onium salts has been employed to prepare nanocomposites based on a photocured matrix and silica nanoparticles prepared in situ by sol–gel. At the same time, the photoinitiator triggers the photopolymerization (or the photo-cross-linking of monomers if multifunctional) and at the same time causes the formation of silica [64].

7.3 UV-GRAFTED CELLULOSE APPLICATIONS

Many academic studies on the chemistry of the UV grafting reactions were carried on. Patents and publications show how photomodified cellulose can find its practical use in several fields. We will now summarize some of the proposed results and applications of UV grafting on cellulose.

Most of the data refer to acrylate and vinyl grafted cellulose. In the field of textile chemistry, many studies demonstrate the efficiency of photografting to modify fabrics: imparting new surface properties, such as hydrophobicity or hydrophilicity, grafting becomes an interesting finishing process [35–38].

Reine et al. [18] in 1975 patented the modification of cotton textiles by photo-initiated polymerization of vinylic monomers without the use of initiator. They observed that near-UV light generated a maximum number of free radical sites on the cellulose molecules of cotton with little or no detrimental effect on the physical properties of cotton; moreover in the conditions adopted the monomer exposed to near-UV light in the absence of cotton did not polymerize. This indicated that the initiating radical for polymerization of the monomer was exclusively formed on the cellulose molecule of cotton. With such a modification, the resulting textiles had improved physical and chemical properties, among which dye receptivity, moisture regain, and personal comfort.

Ferrero et al. [35] studied a semi-industrial scale-up for the antibacterial finishing of cotton fabrics by UV grafting of chitosan biopolymer on fiber surface to obtain antibacterial textiles, which could not only avoid discoloration and degradation of fabrics by microorganisms but also effectively prevent the propagation of bacteria. For this work, large textile fabric samples were impregnated by foulard with a commercial chitosan solution and then were irradiated, both dried and wet, with a high-power UV lamp, in air. Moreover, samples add-on was significantly reduced in order to hold down the finishing cost. White and dyed samples were treated and evaluated in terms of conferred antibacterial activity, yellowing, or color changes and final hand. Treatment fastness to domestic laundering was tested. A deep characterization on cotton fabrics UV-cured with chitosan confirmed the chitosan presence even after washing and revealed the great efficiency of the treatment as antibacterial agent against both *Escherichia coli* and *Staphylococcus aureus*. Obtained results showed good washing fastness by irradiation of the samples even wet and in air with a negligible affection of color or hand properties of the fabric.

By means of photografting, Kubota et al. [39] introduced stimuli-responsive polymers into regenerated cellulose film. Therefore, it demonstrated that common cellulose can become a smart material: such materials, whatever their form (copolymers, fibers, nanoparticles, gels, film/membranes), are characterized by their responsiveness to a stimulus such as pH, temperature, light, electricity, magnetic fields, and mechanical forces, and could find application in almost all the sectors of the human technology. In the work by Kubota, MAA and NIPAAm were attached on regenerated cellulose film using xanthone as photoinitiator in a water-based process. Xanthone was first coated on the film surface, and photografting was carried out in water under N_2 atmosphere. It was observed that the percentage of grafting of both monomers increased with an increase in the concentration of xanthone. The grafted chains were found to distribute homogeneously inside the film, which could shrink in acidic medium and swell in alkaline region. It clearly showed a pH-responsive character, which was not influenced by the polymerization conditions. On the other hand, NIPAAm-grafted film exhibited a temperature-responsive character: it swelled and shrank in water bringing the temperature below or above 30°C, respectively. The pH- and temperature-responsive characters of grafted films increased with increasing the percentage of grafting, making these membranes highly promising for biomedical and sensor applications.

Several works using BP are proposed in the literature for paper hydrophobicization, following a "grafting-to" approach: Bongiovanni et al. [43] introduced fluorinated monomers in order to obtain hydrophobic and oleophobic cellulose sheets. Whatman filters and softwood handsheets were UV-grafted with a highly fluorinated acrylic monomer, characterized by a long perfluoropolyether chain after soaking in a solution containing the monomer and the photoinitiator. XPS analysis showed that the outermost surface composition of the fibers was varied, surface energy was therefore dramatically reduced, and this led to interesting modifications of the paper characteristics. The wettability by different liquids was decreased, and the stain resistance improved. Moreover, anti-adhesion properties were imparted to the paper sheet. At the same time, the bulk properties of the modified fiber network, such as its tensile strength and the burst resistance, were unchanged. This kind of paper functionalization is particularly requested for packaging applications; in food packaging, where regulations are becoming very strict, grafting could avoid migration of additives from the container into food.

Nair et al. [44] developed UV-induced modification aiming to produce mechanically reinforced polymer electrolyte membranes for lithium battery applications. Cellulose handsheets were modified by using a BP-based two-step photografting procedure. In this two-step sequential photografting procedure, the cellulose handsheets were first swelled into a solution of BP in ethanol. The swelled cellulose handsheets were UV irradiated under N_2 flux and, then, dried. These pretreated handsheets were successively swelled into a solution containing a PEO-based acrylate monomer and, soon after, UV irradiated under flowing nitrogen. After thorough and prolonged washing, the obtained modified cellulose was then dried under high vacuum to assure the complete removal of water and solvent. The presence of grafted chains after washing was confirmed by an increase in weight (6%) and by FT-IR-ATR analysis. The use of a modified handsheet as a reinforcement for a polymer electrolyte containing PEO-based monomers, lithium salt, and organic solvents gave membranes with high electrochemical performances and with extremely improved mechanical properties and stability also thanks to the higher compatibility between the polymer matrix and the cellulose reinforcement given by the grafted PEO chains.

UV grafting of cellulose is interesting for the paper of the past and the paper of the future. In fact, it is interesting in the preservation of artworks from degradation such as ancient textiles and books (in this field, UV grafting has also been proposed with the aim of mechanically consolidating the fabric and/or the page [65]) and at the same time seems to be the right method for making functional paper. This novel material could interest microelectronics, actuators, and lab-on paper devices for low-cost sensing. Recently, Böhm et al. [66] exploited a previously developed [50] photochemical grafting of specifically designed functional polymers carrying a photo-reactive BP moiety to develop lab-engineered paper sheets able to control and modulate fluid transport inside microfluidic papers. The pore sizes (i.e., porosity) of the lab-sheets were adjusted by controlling the fiber density of the lab-engineered papers, and in addition, the previously mentioned photochemical attachment of barriers consisting of hydrophobic polymers, which were covalently bound to the cellulosic fibers of the preformed paper sheets, allowed the design of small millimeter-scaled channels. The analysis showed that it was possible to modulate the fluid transport process in such microfluidic papers.

BP was also used by Gashti and Almasian [67] as catalyst for the grafting of a vinylphosphonic acid monomer used to stabilize carbon nanotubes (CNTs) on a cotton surface. MWCNTs and a flame-retardant cross-linking agent were used to fabricate a flame retardant coating on the cotton through UV irradiation. The stabilization of CNTs in the composite coating was achieved by a reaction of polyvinylphosphonic acid and cellulose chains. This reaction process resulted

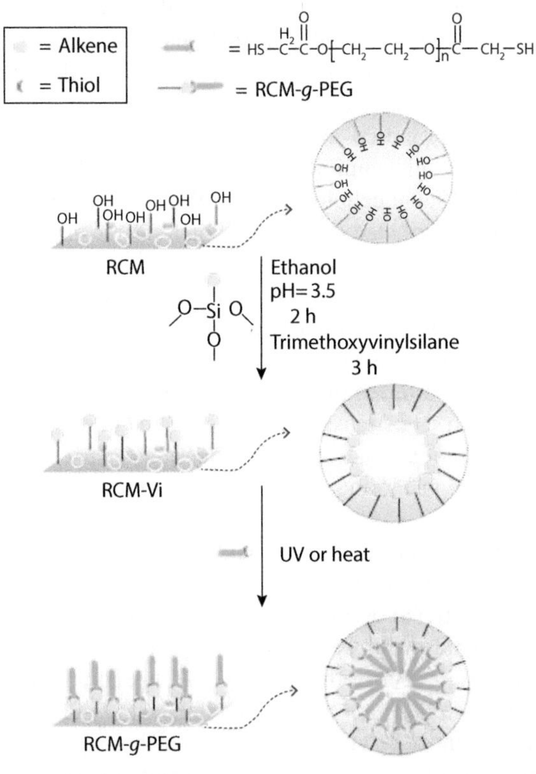

FIGURE 7.9 Scheme of the multistep thiol-ene reaction.

in the attachment of MWCNTs to the surfaces of the cellulose fibers. The successful cross-linking reaction was confirmed by FTIR spectra, which showed the bonding between the hydroxyl groups of cellulose and vinylphosphonic acid monomer to form linkages in the presence of CNTs under UV light. The results obtained from TGA and HFT tests demonstrated an improvement of the thermal properties and flammability of the coated samples. Such a textile composite coating resulted therefore very promising for civil applications as an effective lightweight flame-retardant material.

Other kinds of grafting different from the radical one were mainly presented in literature as laboratory-scale works with no proposed applications; few applications of the click chemistry reactions are reported. Thiol-ene click chemistry is described in Yuan et al. [68] to modify cellulose and change pore size of membranes made of it. The scheme of the multistep reaction is presented in Figure 7.9.

Effects of graft chain length and graft density on membrane morphology, pore size, permeation, and antifouling properties were systematically studied. The attainment of high graft density resulted to be more important than long chain length to achieve antifouling performance. We can also notice that, as proposed before, the functionalization of cellulose with trimethoxyvinylsilane in principle could also be made via a photochemically induced catalysis.

In the elegant grafting-to approach using click chemistry, called NITEC [55], the modification was mainly employed to generate fluorescence-patterned materials: as the photoreaction is dependent on light, a spatially defined polymer grafting can be achieved. The reaction, which is attractive for bio-orthogonal macromolecular conjugation, is suitable for soft matter material design, with potential applications in nanobiotechnology.

7.4 PERSPECTIVES

We have seen that photografting is a reliable strategy for an efficient surface modification as it assures the inherent benefits of photochemical reactions that are characterized by fast rates, versatility, and selectivity. Moreover, as it is a surface reaction, it does neither modify the bulk properties nor degrade the cellulose structure. In addition, in most cases, the UV-irradiation of cellulose creates some stable radicals, leading to the possibility to reduce/suppress the use of the photoinitiators. This interesting feature, combined with the use of special monomers with self-initiating abilities, allows to modify the cellulose surface, while minimizing the number of chemicals required, as green chemistry demands.

Photografting offers also the possibility, if required, to spatially confine the surface modification, allowing the formation of different patterns of functional groups (by using a photomask) and to perform the surface treatment by a continuous process, with low-energy consumption. This last point is particularly important if considering the need for upscaling the processes, which so far has been the trickiest point especially for the functionalization of cellulosic solid substrates (paper, fabrics, fibers, and nanocelluloses).

The process of upscaling is probably one of the aspects of cellulose photografting, which requires more efforts for optimizing the different parameters that affect the final efficiency of the process, such as the chemistry of the reagents and the type and concentration of the photoinitiator if needed, and the UV dose and its delivery, especially if the latter is done on a continuous roll-to-roll process.

In spite of the work that remains to do, photografting is likely to be one of the surface modification techniques closer to the industrialization for the cellulose, at least in the most traditional applications.

On the other hand, scientific research is to be done for combining this kind of grafting with the most advanced cellulose materials (nanocelluloses, defined as the "super material" of the future) and high-tech processes (i.e., additive manufacturing processes). Considering the current advances in the 3D printing, one can foresee that nanocellulose will be employed, and photografting could be an excellent way to locally modify and functionalize the scaffolds obtained in such a way.

The use of cellulose in the preparation of "smart" materials, a new challenging field, can also take advantage of the photografting. In this field, examples are not many, but certainly photografting offers a unique possibility especially for in situ modification of cellulose films/membranes and for the preparation of microdevices. In the example reported previously (photografting of MAA and NIPAm on cellulose film [39]), pH-responsive and temperature-responsive cellulose films were proposed for separation, sensor technologies, or drug delivery. Cellulose is highly suitable for this kind of applications, because of its biocompatibility and biodegradability, and photografting would be an excellent tool in the design of these materials, allowing to locally modify their surface, at a very small scale, when required.

If photografting allows envisaging a number of new advanced applications for cellulose, as the material of the future, it should not be neglected that it can also offer an irreplaceable solution for the preservation of cultural heritage items made of cellulose (paper, textile). Its use as a very innovative method of restoration for both artificially and naturally aged textiles is already known [65], but there is plenty of room for implementing it.

Thus, cellulose surface can be efficiently modified by photografting for the most advanced or traditional applications. This technique has an enormous potential for the surface functionalization, but as for the other grafting techniques, some points should be carefully evaluated. Fundamental research is necessary. First, the polymer chains covalently grafted on a substrate likely behave differently from the free polymer chains in solution or in bulk, so the performances of the grafted layers should be experimentally assessed and compared with the corresponding free polymer chains. This seems to be particularly crucial for the biomedical applications. Then, the grafted chains could reorientate in the surface region, thus resulting in a modification or even deterioration of the surface functionality; this aspect should also be investigated.

Finally, another challenging issue is the direct characterization and assessment of the grafting through a covalent link, especially considering the possible presence of branched or superbranched chains.

REFERENCES

1. A. Bhattachary, B.M. Misra, Grafting: a versatile means to modify polymers: techniques, factors and applications, *Progress in Polymer Science*, 29(2004): 767–814.
2. J.P. Fouassier, *Photoinitiation, Photopolymerization, and Photocuring Fundamentals and Applications*. Hanser Publishers, New York, 1995.
3. J. Yagci, Photografting of polymeric materials in photochemistry and photophysics of polymeric materials. N.S. Allen (ed.), *John Wiley and Sons*, Hoboken, NJ, 2010, pp. 509–540.
4. Protheus Technology. http://www.phoseon.com/technology/led-uv-wavelength.htm, (last accessed on January 5, 2014).
5. G. Ciamician, *The Photochemistry of the Future*. Rumford Press, Washington, 1913.
6. N.-S. Hon, Formation of free radicals in photoirradiated cellulose. VIII. Mechanisms, *Journal of Polymer Science: Polymer Chemistry Edition*, 14(1976): 2497–2512.
7. H. Wondraczek, A. Kotiaho, P. Fardim, T. Heinze, Photoactive polysaccharides, *Carbohydrate Polymers*, 83(2011): 1048–1061.
8. H. Tylli, I. Forsskåhl, C. Olkkonen, A spectroscopic study of photoirradiated cellulose, *Journal of Photochemistry and Photobiology A: Chemistry*, 76(1993): 143–149.
9. N. Durán, E. G6mez, H. Mansilla, Biomass photo-chemistry. A review and prospects, *Polymer Degradation and Stability*, 17(1987): 131–149.
10. G.S. Egerton, E. Attle, M.A. Rathor, Photochemistry of cellulose in the far ultra-violet, *Nature*, 194(1962): 968.
11. J. Malešič, J. Kolar, M. Strlič, D. Kočar, D. Fromageot, J. Lemaire, O. Haillant, Photo-induced degradation of cellulose, *Polymer Degradation and Stability*, 89(2005): 64–69.
12. A. Moldovan, S. Patachia, C. Vasile, R. Darie, E. Manaila, M. Tierean, Natural fibres/polyolefins composites (I) UV and electron beam irradiation, *Journal of Biobased Materials and Bioenergy*, 7(2013): 58–79.
13. M. Kamath, J. Kincaid, B.K. Mandal, Interpenetrating polymer networks of photocrosslinkable cellulose derivatives, *Journal of Applied Polymer Science*, 59(1996): 45–50.

14. D. Roy, M. Semsarilar, J.T. Guthrie, S. Perrier, Cellulose modification by polymer grafting: A review, *Chemical Society Reviews*, 38(2009): 2046–2064.
15. S.R. Shukla, G.V.G. Rao, A.R. Athalye, Mechanical and thermal behavior of cotton cellulose grafted with hydroxyethyl methacrylate using photoinitiation, *Journal of Applied Polymer Science*, 44(1992): 577–580.
16. S.R. Shukla, G.V.G. Rao, A.R. Athalye, Improving graft level during photoinduced graft-copolymerization of styrene onto cotton cellulose, *Journal of Applied Polymer Science*, 49(1993): 1423–1430.
17. A.K. Mohanty, B.C. Singh, Radiation-induced and photoinduced grafting onto cellulose and cellulosic materials, *Polymer-Plastics Technology and Engineering*, 27(1988): 435–466.
18. A.H. Reine, N.A. Portnoy, J.C. Arthur Jr., Photoinitiated Polymerization onto Cotton: Copolymerization of Acrylamide Monomers with cotton. *Textile Research Journal*, 43, 11(1973): 638–641.
19. P.L. Nayak, S. Lenka, Photoinduced graft copolymerization onto selected fibers, *Journal of Macromolecular Science, Part C*, 31(1991): 91–116.
20. M.M. Hassan, M.R. Islam, L. Drzal, M. Khan, Role of amino acids on in situ photografting of Jute Yarn with 3-(trimethoxysilyl) propylmethacrylate, *Journal of Polymers and the Environment*, 13(2005): 293–300.
21. P. Ghosh, S.K. Paul, Photograft copolymerization of methyl methacrylate (MMA) on bleached jute fiber using ferric sulfate, $Fe_2(SO_4)_3$, as initiator in limited aqueous system, *Journal of Macromolecular Science: Part A—Chemistry*, 20(1983): 169–178.
22. M. Khan, M. Hassan, *Surface Modification of Natural Fibres by Photografting and Photocuring*, in Polymer Surface Modification: Relevance to Adhesion, Volume 3 K.M. Mittal ed. CRC Press Boca Raton 2004, p. 263–283.
23. M.M. Rahman, A.K. Mallik, M.A. Khan, Influences of various surface pretreatments on the mechanical and degradable properties of photografted oil palm fibers, *Journal of Applied Polymer Science*, 105(2007): 3077–3086.
24. Y. Ogiwara, H. Kubota, Vapor phase photografting of vinyl monomers on cellulose and its derivatives, *Journal of Polymer Science: Polymer Letters Edition*, 23(1985): 15–19.
25. H. Kubota, Y. Fukushima, S. Kuwabara, Factors affecting liquid-phase photografting of acrylic acid on cellulose and its derivatives, *European Polymer Journal*, 33(1997): 67–71.
26. H. Kubota, Y. Ogiwara, S. Hinohara, Effect of water on vapor phase photografting on cellulose and its derivatives, *Journal of Applied Polymer Science*, 34(1987): 1277–1283.
27. H.L. Needles, R.P. Seiber, Photoinitiated vapor-phase grafting of acrylic-monomers onto fibrous substrates in presence of biacetyl. *Journal of Applied Polymer Science,* 19(1975): 2187–2206.
28. T.Y. Lee, C.A. Guymon, E.S. Jönsson, C.E. Hoyle, The effect of monomer structure on oxygen inhibition of (meth)acrylates photopolymerization, *Polymer*, 45(2004): 6155–6162.
29. J.A. Harris, J.C. Arthur, J.H. Carra, Photoinitiated polymerization of glycidyl methacrylate with cotton cellulose, *Journal of Applied Polymer Science*, 22(1978): 905–915.
30. V. Viengkhou, L.-T. Ng, J.L. Garnett, The effect of additives on the enhancement of methyl methacrylate grafting to cellulose in the presence of UV and ionising radiation, *Radiation Physics and Chemistry*, 49(1997): 595–602.
31. C.H. Ang, J.L. Garnett, S.V. Jankiewicz, D. Sangster, Acid effect in UV- and radiation-induced grafting of styrene to cellulose, in: *Graft Copolymerization of Lignocellulosic Fibers*. American Chemical Society, Washington, DC, 1982, pp. 141–154.
32. J.L. Garnett, L.-T. Ng, V. Viengkhou, Grafting of methyl methacrylate to cellulose and polypropylene with UV and ionising radiation in the presence of additives including CT complexes, *Radiation Physics and Chemistry*, 56(1999): 387–403.
33. S. Lenka, M. Dash, Photoinduced graft copolymerization. V. Graft copolymerization of methyl methacrylate onto cellulose in the presence of *N*-bromosuccinimide as initiator, *Journal of Macromolecular Science: Part A—Chemistry*, 18(1982): 1141–1149.
34. H. Kubota, Y. Ogiwara, S. Hinohara, Factors affecting vapor phase photografting of vinyl monomers on cellulose, *Journal of Applied Polymer Science*, 33(1987): 3045–3053.
35. F. Ferrero, M. Periolatto, S. Ferrario, Sustainable antimicrobial finishing of cotton fabrics by chitosan UV-grafting: From laboratory experiments to semi industrial scale-up, *Journal of Cleaner Production*. doi:10.1016/j.jclepro.2013.12.044 available on line.
36. F. Ferrero, M. Periolatto, C. Udrescu, Water and oil-repellent coatings of perfluoro-polyacrylate resins on cotton fibers: UV curing in comparison with thermal polymerization, *Fibers and Polymers*, 13(2012): 191–198.

37. F. Ferrero, M. Periolatto, Ultraviolet curing for surface modification of textile fabrics, *Journal of Nanoscience and Nanotechnology*, 11(2011): 8663–8669.
38. M. Periolatto, F. Ferrero, C. Vineis, Antimicrobial chitosan finish of cotton and silk fabrics by UV-curing with 2-hydroxy-2-methylphenylpropane-1-one, *Carbohydrate Polymers*, 88(2012): 201–205.
39. H. Kubota, I.G. Suka, S.-i. Kuroda, T. Kondo, Introduction of stimuli-responsive polymers into regenerated cellulose film by means of photografting, *European Polymer Journal*, 37(2001): 1367–1372.
40. J. Deng, L. Wang, L. Liu, W. Yang, Developments and new applications of UV-induced surface graft polymerizations, *Progress in Polymer Science*, 34(2009): 156–193.
41. J.-P. Deng, W.-T. Yang, B. Rĺnby, Surface photografting polymerization of vinyl acetate (VAc), maleic anhydride (MAH), and their charge transfer complex (CTC). III. VAc(3), *Journal of Applied Polymer Science*, 80(2001): 1426–1433.
42. R. Hérold, J.-P. Fouassier, Photochemical investigations into cellulosic materials III. Photografting vinyl monomers onto cotton in the presence of various photo-initiators, *Die Angewandte Makromolekulare Chemie*, 97(1981): 137–152.
43. R. Bongiovanni, E. Zeno, A. Pollicino, P.M. Serafini, C. Tonelli, UV light-induced grafting of fluorinated monomer onto cellulose sheets, *Cellulose*, 18(2011): 117–126.
44. J.R. Nair, A. Chiappone, C. Gerbaldi, V.S. Ijeri, E. Zeno, R. Bongiovanni, S. Bodoardo, N. Penazzi, Novel cellulose reinforcement for polymer electrolyte membranes with outstanding mechanical properties, *Electrochimica Acta*, 57(2011): 104–111.
45. K.H. Hong, N. Liu, G. Sun, UV-induced graft polymerization of acrylamide on cellulose by using immobilized benzophenone as a photo-initiator, *European Polymer Journal*, 45(2009): 2443–2449.
46. R. Bongiovanni, S. Marchi, E. Zeno, A. Pollicino, R.R. Thomas, Water resistance improvement of filter paper by a UV-grafting modification with a fluoromonomer, *Colloids and Surfaces A: Physicochemical and Engineering Aspects*, 418(2013): 52–59.
47. B. Zdyrko, I. Luzinov, Polymer brushes by the "Grafting to" method, *Macromolecular Rapid Communications*, 32(2011): 859–869.
48. T.B. Stachowiak, F. Svec, J.M.J. Fréchet, Patternable protein resistant surfaces for multifunctional microfluidic devices via surface hydrophilization of porous polymer monoliths using photografting, *Chemistry of Materials*, 18(2006): 5950–5957.
49. H. Ma, R.H. Davis, C.N. Bowman, A novel sequential photoinduced living graft polymerization, *Macromolecules*, 33(1999): 331–335.
50. A. Böhm, M. Gattermayer, C. Trieb, S. Schabel, D. Fiedler, F. Miletzky, M. Biesalski, Photo-attaching functional polymers to cellulose fibers for the design of chemically modified paper, *Cellulose*, 20(2013): 467–483.
51. G. Delaittre, M. Dietrich, J.P. Blinco, A. Hirschbiel, M. Bruns, L. Barner, C. Barner-Kowollik, Photoinduced macromolecular functionalization of cellulose via nitroxide spin trapping, *Biomacromolecules*, 13(2012): 1700–1705.
52. G.R. Dennis, J.L. Garnett, E. Zilic, Cure grafting—A complementary technique to preirradiation and simultaneous processes? *Radiation Physics and Chemistry*, 67(2003): 391–395.
53. J.E. Moses, A.D. Moorhouse, The growing applications of click chemistry, *Chemical Society Reviews*, 36(2007): 1249–1262.
54. B.S. Sumerlin, A.P. Vogt, Macromolecular engineering through click chemistry and other efficient transformations, *Macromolecules*, 43(2009): 1–13.
55. M. Dietrich, G. Delaittre, J.P. Blinco, A.J. Inglis, M. Bruns, C. Barner-Kowollik, Photoclickable surfaces for profluorescent covalent polymer coatings, *Advanced Functional Materials*, 22(2012): 304–312.
56. P. Tingaut, R. Hauert, T. Zimmermann, Highly efficient and straightforward functionalization of cellulose films with thiol-ene click chemistry, *Journal of Materials Chemistry*, 21(2011): 16066–16076.
57. J.-L. Huang, C.-J. Li, D.G. Gray, Functionalization of cellulose nanocrystal films via "thiol-ene" click reaction, *RSC Advances*, 4(2014): 6965–6969.
58. K. Kato, E. Uchida, E.-T. Kang, Y. Uyama, Y. Ikada, Polymer surface with graft chains, *Progress in Polymer Science*, 28(2003): 209–259.
59. K. Allmér, A. Hult, B. Rĺnby, Surface modification of polymers. II. Grafting with glycidyl acrylates and the reactions of the grafted surfaces with amines, *Journal of Polymer Science Part A: Polymer Chemistry*, 27(1989): 1641–1652.
60. G. Chauhan, L. Guleria, R. Sharma, Synthesis, characterization and metal ion sorption studies of graft copolymers of cellulose with glycidyl methacrylate and some comonomers, *Cellulose*, 12(2005): 97–110.
61. A. Chiappone, J. Nair, C. Gerbaldi, E. Zeno, R. Bongiovanni, Flexible and high performing polymer electrolytes obtained by UV-induced polymer-cellulose grafting. *RSC Advances*, 4(2014): 40873–40881.

62. A. Chiappone, Ligno cellulosic materials for energy storage, PhD thesis, Politecnico di Torino, Torino, Italy, 2012.
63. F. Ferrero, M. Periolatto, Application of fluorinated compounds to cotton fabrics via sol–gel, *Applied Surface Science*, 275(2013): 201–207.
64. A. Chemtob, D.-L. Versace, C. Belon, C. Croutxé-Barghorn, S. Rigolet, Concomitant organic—Inorganic UV-curing catalyzed by photoacids, *Macromolecules*, 41(2008): 7390–7398.
65. E. Princi, S. Vicini, E. Pedemonte, V. Arrighi, I.J. McEwen, New polymeric materials for paper and textiles conservation. II. Grafting polymerization of ethyl acrylate/methyl methacrylate copolymers onto linen and cotton, *Journal of Applied Polymer Science*, 103(2007): 90–99.
66. A. Böhm, F. Carstens, C. Trieb, S. Schabel, M. Biesalski, Engineering microfluidic papers: Effect of fiber source and paper sheet properties on capillary-driven fluid flow, *Microfluidics and Nanofluidics*, 16(2014): 789–799.
67. M. Parvinzadeh Gashti, A. Almasian, UV radiation induced flame retardant cellulose fiber by using polyvinylphosphonic acid/carbon nanotube composite coating, *Composites Part B: Engineering*, 45(2013): 282–289.
68. T. Yuan, J. Meng, X. Gong, Y. Zhang, M. Xu, Modulating pore size and surface properties of cellulose microporous membrane via thio-ene chemistry, *Desalination*, 328(2013): 58–66.

8 Graft Copolymerization of Vinyl Monomers onto Cellulosic *Cannabis indica* Fibers

Ashvinder Kumar Rana, Amar Singh Singha, Manju Kumari Thakur, and Vijay Kumar Thakur

CONTENTS

8.1 INTRODUCTION

Grafting efficiency, grafting proportion, and grafting frequency determine water absorbability [1,2], cation exchange property [3], dyeability with the basic dyes, and the degree of compatibility of lignocellulose natural fibers with a polymer matrix [4]. The products can be used as superabsorbents, ion exchange composites, or a reinforcement depending upon the type of monomers (hydrophobic/hydrophilic) graft copolymerized.

Graft copolymerization of acrylic acid (AAc) and acrylonitrile (AN) monomers onto lignocellulosic fibers has been carried out by different initiating systems [4,5]. The role of initiator is very crucial, as it determines the path of grafting process. Graft copolymerization of vinyl monomers can be initiated through the generation of free radicals on a polymeric backbone by direct oxidation of the backbone by certain transition metal ions such as Ce(IV), Cr(VI), V(V), Co(III), and Mn(III)/sulfuric acid [6–8]. Das et al. [9] have reported grafting of AN onto silk fiber by using $KMnO_4$ as an initiator. There are also other types of initiators that behave in a contrary fashion such as H_2O_2/FAS [10], FAS/KPS [11], and peroxydisulfate/ascorbic acid. These initiators initially generate free radicals, which subsequently react with polymeric backbone to produce free radical centers onto cellulosic backbone.

Graft copolymerization of vinyl monomers onto cellulosic fibers by using ceric ammonium nitrate (CAN) as an initiator has been studied by various researchers [12,13]. Ceric ion has been suggested as a very efficient redox system by Mino and Kaizerman [14] since it helps in reducing the extent of homopolymerization during graft copolymerization.

Graft copolymerization of a variety of monomers onto natural fibers has also been carried out by several other researchers [4,5,15–17]. Arifuzzaman Khan et al. [4] have reported their study on graft copolymerization of AN monomer onto bleached okra fiber under the catalytic influence of $K_2S_2O_8$ and $FeSO_4$ redox system at 70°C for different time intervals ranging from 60 to 180 min. It has been observed that grafting of bleached fiber with AN brings about a substantial increase in tensile strength. Singha and Rana [16] have carried out the graft copolymerization of methyl methacrylate (MMA) onto *Agave americana* fibers by using CAN as an initiator in aqueous nitric acid solution at 25°C, 35°C, 45°C, 55°C, and 65°C for time interval in between 30 and 180 min. Bessadok et al. [18] have studied the effect of acetylation, styrene, AAc, and maleic anhydride on water sorption characteristics of alfa fibers. They reported decrease in water uptake of alfa fibers after the surface modification. Vijay et al. [19] have modified the surface of bagasse fiber through NaOH and AAc treatment. They reported an increase in mechanical as well as in water retention properties of resulted bio-composites as compared to untreated fiber-based composites. Thakur et al. [20] have graft copolymerized MMA onto cellulosic fiber by using FAS-KPS redox initiator. They characterized grafted fibers by FTIR, XRD, SEM, and TGA techniques. Redox initiation has been successfully implemented to graft vinyl monomers onto natural fibers for the end-use application in composites [21]. Misra et al. [22] reported that methylacrylate has less accessibility to reach the active sites of the polymer backbone, thereby producing low graft yield due to less water solubility of methylacrylate as compared to AN. Monier et al. [23] have graft copolymerized natural wool with AN by using $KMnO_4$ and oxalic acid–combined redox initiator system. They have used these modified fibers for the removal of Hg(II), Cu(II), and Co(II) metal ions from aqueous solutions.

In contrast to the aforementioned results, Chaobo et al. [24] have reported an increase in water absorbance behavior after graft copolymerization of AAc onto swollen and unswollen ramie fibers. Khan [25] studied photoinduced graft copolymerization of methacrylic acid onto natural biodegradable fiber and reported a 42% increase in its hydrophilic character. Kaur et al. [26] have employed two different methods i.e. chemical and gamma radiation method for the graft copolymerization of AAc onto rayon fibers. They reported that gamma radiation induced AAc graft copolymerized rayon fibers had better hydrophilicity. Feng et al. [27] reported the synthesis of superabsorbent by a graft copolymerization reaction of cellulose from flax shive and AAc using *N,N′*-methylenebisacrylamide as a cross-linker and potassium persulfate as an initiator in aqueous solution under microwave irradiation. Grafting of AN onto the cellulosic material derived from bamboo was studied by Khullar et al. [28]. Graft copolymerization of acrylic monomers onto cotton fabric using an activated cellulose thiocarbonate-azo-*bis*-isobutyronitrile redox system has been investigated by Zahran et al. [29]. It has been found that a reaction medium of pH 2.0 and temperature of 70°C constituted the optimum conditions for grafting.

8.2 EXPERIMENTAL

8.2.1 MATERIALS

AAc/AN was purified by distillation under reduced pressure at 40°C, and the middle fraction of the distillate was used for further studies. CAN supplied by Merck chemicals was used as initiator. Weighing of the samples was done on Libror AEG-220 (Shimadzu) electronic balance. Humidity chamber of Swastika make was used to study the moisture absorbance behavior of the graft copolymers.

8.2.1.1 *Cannabis indica* Fiber

Cannabis indica is an annual plant, belonging to the *Cannabaceae* family (Figure 8.1). It is a short plant, usually less than 8 ft in height and found in India, Pakistan, Bangladesh, Afghanistan, and other surrounding areas. All of these countries have extremely variable weather conditions and fall in South Asia region.

C. indica is a bast fiber plant similar to kenaf, jute, ramie, and flax (Figure 8.2). The fibers enclose the hollow, woody core of the stalk and are extracted mostly by using water retting process.

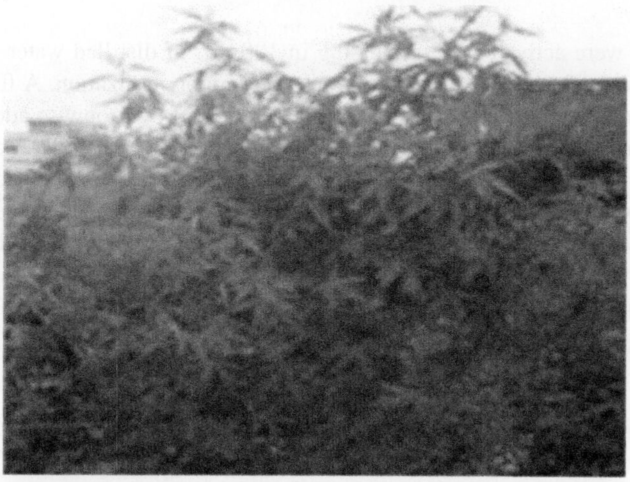

FIGURE 8.1 *Cannabis indica* plant.

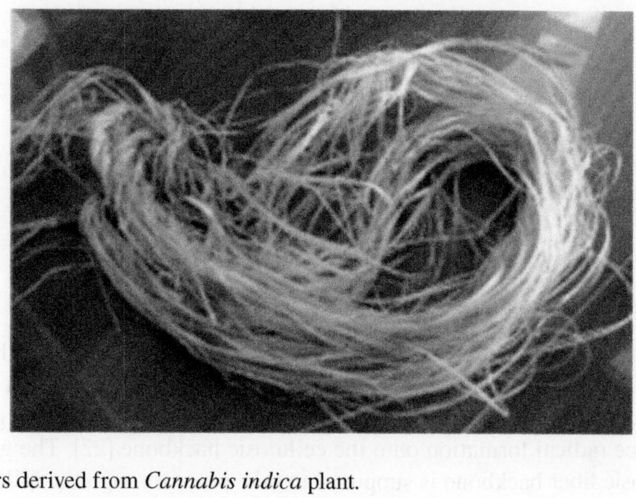

FIGURE 8.2 Fibers derived from *Cannabis indica* plant.

Water retting process involves immersing the stems in river or pond for 10–12 days, and after that, fibers are collected by gently washing gummy material. The fibers extracted from the stem of *C. indica* plant have been found to contain cellulose (65%–72%), hemicellulose (12%–20%), and lignin (5%–10%). Further, this fibrous material has been used by local people for making low-cost articles like ropes, bags, socks, boots, and mats.

8.2.1.2 Purification of Fibers

C. indica fibers were collected from higher reaches of Himalayan region in Himachal Pradesh. These fibers were initially washed thoroughly with 2% detergent solution and then dried completely in hot air oven at 70°C. Dried fibers were subjected to soxhlet extraction with acetone for 72 h followed by washing with double-distilled water and air drying to remove waxes and other water-soluble impurities prior to graft copolymerization.

8.2.2 Graft Copolymerization

Graft copolymerization on *C. indica* fiber in air has been carried out as per the procedure reported earlier [30]:

Cellulosic fibers were activated by immersing in 100 mL of distilled water in a reaction flask at room temperature for 24 h prior to carrying out graft copolymerization. A fixed amount of the CAN and nitric acid was then added to reaction flask followed by dropwise addition of monomer with continuous stirring of the reaction mixture. The reaction was carried out at definite reaction temperature and time. Optimum conditions of time, temperature, CAN, nitric acid, and monomer concentration worked out to get maximum graft yield. Homopolymer formed during the graft copolymerization was removed by extraction with hot water in case of AAc and with dimethylformamide in case of AN graft copolymerization. The grafted samples were then dried in hot air oven at 70°C to a constant weight. The percent grafting (P_g) and percent efficiency (P_e) were calculated as per the following formulas:

$$\%\ \text{Grafting}\ P_g = \frac{W_g - W}{W} \times 100$$

$$\%\ \text{Efficiency}\ P_e = \frac{W_g - W}{W_m} \times 100$$

where

W is the weight of raw fiber

W_g is the weight of grafted fiber

W_m is the weight of monomer

8.3 RESULTS AND DISCUSSION

8.3.1 Reaction Mechanism

Ce(IV) ion generate free active sites directly on the cellulosic backbone through the formation of intermediate metal–ion chelate complex. Such a complex is not restricted to a single site on the cellulose backbone; rather, it involves both primary and secondary hydroxyl groups of glucose units in inducing free radical formation onto the cellulosic backbone [22]. The grafting of AAc or AN onto the cellulosic fiber backbone is supposed to take place through the following mechanism (Scheme 8.1).

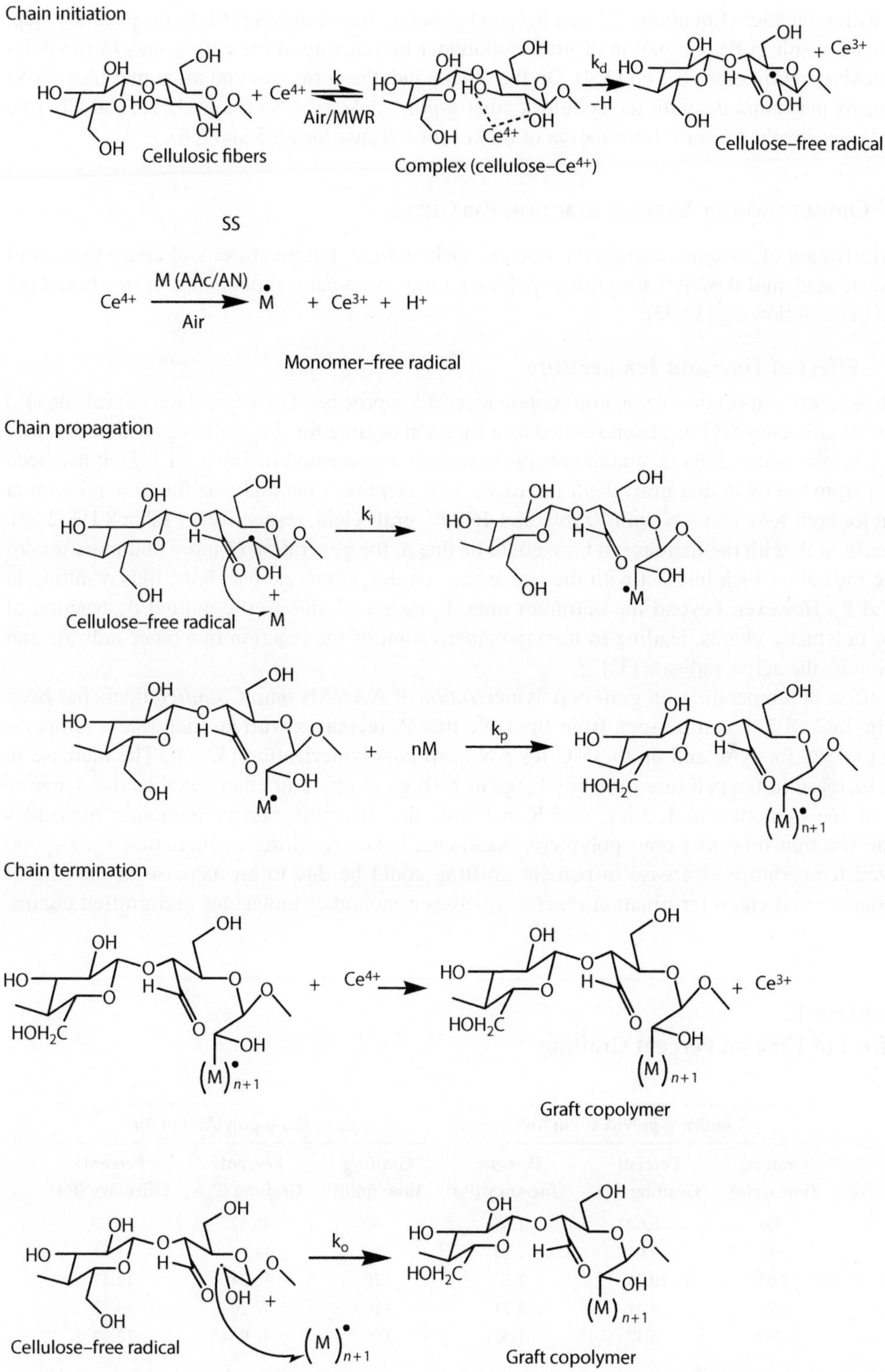

(8.1)

(8.2)

(8.3)

(8.4)

(8.5)

(8.6)

SCHEME 8.1 A proposed mechanism for graft copolymerization of acrylonitrile/acrylic acid onto *cellulosic* fiber. (From Singha, A.S. and Rana, A.K., *Iran. Polym. J.*, 20, 913, 2011.)

In chain initiation step, ceric ions form complexes with the carbon chain of polymer backbone as well as with monomer (Equations 8.1 and 8.2) and generate free radicals [26]. In propagation step, free radicals result in the formation of graft copolymer by reacting at the active sites of the polymeric backbone (Equations 8.3 and 8.4). On the other hand, the ceric ions and monomer (AAc/AN) free radicals may combine with the cellulosic fiber-g-poly (AAc or AN) free radicals and CH-free radicals, respectively, to cause termination of the reaction (Equations 8.5 and 8.6).

8.3.2 Optimization of Various Reaction Parameters

The optimization of various reaction parameters such as time, temperature, and concentration of CAN, nitric acid, and AAc/AN for graft copolymerization onto natural fibers has been worked out as given in the following [32,33].

8.3.2.1 Effect of Time and Temperature

Time plays a very important role on graft copolymerization process. The percentage of grafting (P_g) and percent efficiency (P_e) has been studied as a function of time for the graft copolymerization of AN or AAc onto natural fibers, and the results have been represented in Table 8.1 [32]. It has been observed from the table that graft yield increases with increase time and was found maximum at 120 min for both AAc and AN with 10.76% and 46.24% graft yield, respectively (Table 8.1) [32,33].

Increase in P_g with the increase in time could be due to the generation of more and more monomer free radicals, which interact with the active sites on the polymeric backbone thus resulting in increased P_g. However, beyond the optimum time, P_g decreases due to the mutual destruction of growing polymeric chains, leading to homopolymerization of the reaction monomer radicals and backbiting by the active radicals [32].

The effect of temperature on graft copolymerization of AAc/AN onto *C. indica* fibers has been shown in Table 8.2. It can be seen from the table that P_g increases with an increase in temperature up to 45°C for AAc and up to 35°C for AN graft copolymerization [32,33]. The increase in P_g with increase in temperature probably happens as high temperature can enhance the dynamic energy of the monomer molecules, which increases the diffusion rate of monomer molecules from the reaction mixtures onto polymeric backbone, hence resulting in increased P_g. Beyond optimized temperature, decrease in percent grafting could be due to an increase in the rate of chain transfer and chain termination reactions between monomer molecules and grafted chains.

TABLE 8.1
Effect of Time on Percent Grafting

	A			B		
	C. indica-g-poly(AAc) in Air[a]			*C. indica*-g-poly(AN) in Air[b]		
Sr. No	Grafting Time (min)	Percent Grafting (P_g)	Percent Efficiency (P_e)	Grafting Time (min)	Percent Grafting (P_g)	Percent Efficiency (P_e)
1.	60	5.69	1.35	60	36.32	11.20
2.	90	9.64	2.29	90	44.10	13.61
3.	**120**	**10.76**	**2.55**	**120**	**46.24**	**14.27**
4.	150	9.31	2.21	150	43.16	13.32
5.	180	6.40	1.52	180	41.90	12.93

Note: Bold numbers indicate optimize values.

[a] [CAN]: 0.91×10^{-2} mol L^{-1}; [HNO_3]: 2.88×10^{-1} mol L^{-1}; [AAc]: 2.91×10^{-1} mol L^{-1}; temp: 45°C.

[b] [CAN]: 1.82×10^{-2} mol L^{-1}; [AN]: 3.05×10^{-1} mol L^{-1}; [HNO_3]: 2.88×10^{-2} mol L^{-1}; temp: 45°C.

TABLE 8.2
Effect of Temperature on Percent Grafting

	A			B		
	C. indica-g-poly(AAc) in Air[a]			*C. indica*-g-poly(AN) in Air[b]		
Sr. No	**Grafting Temp (°C)**	**Percent Grafting (P_g)**	**Percent Efficiency (P_e)**	**Grafting Temp (°C)**	**Percent Grafting (P_g)**	**Percent Efficiency (P_e)**
1.	25	7.30	1.73	15	28.02	12.22
2.	35	7.96	1.89	25	40.12	13.00
3.	**45**	**10.76**	**2.55**	**35**	**47.36**	**14.61**
4.	55	8.62	2.04	45	46.24	14.27
5.	65	8.11	1.92	55	38.24	11.80

[a] [CAN]: 0.91×10^{-2} mol L^{-1}; [HNO_3]: 2.88×10^{-1} mol L^{-1}; [AAc]: 2.91×10^{-1} mol L^{-1}; Time: 120 min.
[b] [CAN]: 1.82×10^{-2} mol L^{-1}; [AN]: 3.05×10^{-1} mol L^{-1}; [HNO_3]: 2.88×10^{-2} mol L^{-1}; Time: 120 min.

Coupling of monomer free radicals at higher temperature may also be responsible for decreased graft yield beyond optimum value.

8.3.2.2 Effect of CAN

Both P_g and P_e have been studied as a function of CAN concentration, and results are shown in Table 8.3. It has been observed from the table that P_g increases with increase in initiator concentration and was found maximum at CAN = 1.82×10^{-2} mol L^{-1} for both AAc and AN graft copolymerization with 16.68% and 47.36% graft yield, respectively (Table 8.3) [32,33].

Increase in P_g with increase in CAN may be due to the generation of free radical active sites on the polymeric backbone, where grafting takes place. However, a further increase in CAN concentration beyond the optimum value accelerates the dissociation rate of Ce(IV), which reduces the concentration of CAN participating in the graft copolymerization. Additionally, a higher concentration of CAN makes it easier for Ce(IV) to be involved in a termination reaction, thereby causing a decrease in P_g (Scheme 8.1, Equation 8.5).

TABLE 8.3
Effect of CAN on Percent Grafting

	A			B		
	C. indica-g-poly(AAc) in Air[a]			*C. indica*-g-poly(AN) in Air[b]		
Sr. No	**[CAN] × 10^{-2} mol L^{-1}**	**Percent Grafting (P_g)**	**Percent Efficiency (P_e)**	**[CAN] × 10^{-2} mol L^{-1}**	**Percent Grafting (P_g)**	**Percent Efficiency (P_e)**
1.	0.91	10.76	2.55	0.91	26.74	8.25
2.	1.36	14.56	3.46	1.36	33.2	10.24
3.	**1.82**	**16.68**	**3.96**	**1.82**	**47.36**	**14.61**
4.	2.27	15.94	3.79	2.27	45.18	13.94
5.	2.73	12.90	3.06	2.73	44.4	13.70

[a] [HNO_3]: 2.88×10^{-1} mol L^{-1}; [AAc]: 2.91×10^{-1} mol L^{-1}; Time: 120 min; temp: 45°C.
[b] [AN]: 3.05×10^{-1} mol L^{-1}; [HNO_3]: 2.88×10^{-2} mol L^{-1}; Time: 120 min; temp: 35°C.

TABLE 8.4
Effect of Nitric Acid on Percent Grafting

	A			B		
	C. indica-g-poly(AAc) in Air[a]			*C. indica*-g-poly(AN) in Air[b]		
Sr. No	$[HNO_3] \times 10^{-1}$ mol L^{-1}	Percent Grafting (P_g)	Percent Efficiency (P_e)	$[HNO_3] \times 10^{-1}$ mol L^{-1}	Percent Grafting (P_g)	Percent Efficiency (P_e)
1.	2.16	12.42	2.95	1.44	36.74	11.33
2.	2.88	16.68	3.96	2.16	42.42	13.09
3.	**3.60**	**17.24**	**4.10**	**2.88**	**47.36**	**14.61**
4.	4.32	16.36	3.89	3.60	43.8	13.51
5.	5.04	14.78	3.51	4.32	43.64	13.46

[a] [CAN]: 1.82×10^{-2} mol L^{-1}; [AAc]: 2.91×10^{-1} mol L^{-1}; time: 120 min; temp: 45°C.
[b] [CAN]: 1.82×10^{-2} mol L^{-1}; [AN]: 3.05×10^{-1} mol L^{-1}; time: 120 min; temp: 35°C.

8.3.2.3 Effect of Nitric Acid

Effect of nitric acid concentration on graft copolymerization of vinyl monomers (AAc or AN) onto *C. indica* fibers has been represented in Table 8.4. The maximum P_g (17.24%) was found at 3.60×10^{-1} mol L^{-1} for AAc, whereas with AN, the maximum grafting was observed at 2.88×10^{-1} mol L^{-1} nitric acid concentration (Table 8.4) [32,33].

The initial increase in P_g with increase in nitric acid concentration was due to the increase in the concentration of Ce^{4+}, which forms a complex with natural fiber, thus increasing the number of reaction sites and hence P_g. In aqueous medium, CAN exists as Ce^{4+}, $[Ce(OH)]^{3+}$, and $[Ce–O–Ce]^{6+}$ ions (Equations 8.7 and 8.8). Due to the large size, these ions are not able to form complexes with polymer backbone. However, in the presence of HNO_3, equilibrium shifts more and more toward Ce^{4+} ions; therefore, graft copolymerization increases with increase in nitric acid concentration:

$$Ce^{4+} + H_2O \rightleftharpoons [Ce(OH)^{3+}] + H^+ \quad (8.7)$$

$$2[Ce(OH)^{3+}] \rightleftharpoons [Ce-O-Ce)^{6+} + H_2O \quad (8.8)$$

However, decrease in P_g with further increase in the nitric acid concentration beyond optimum value occurred probably due to the termination of growing grafted chains. Also the increased concentration of nitric acid may result in the hydrolysis (Scheme 8.2) of the fiber thereby resulting in decreased percent grafting [31].

8.3.2.4 Effect of Monomer

P_g and P_e for graft copolymerization of monomers (AAc or AN) onto cellulosic fibers has also been studied as a function of monomer concentration, and the results are shown in Table 8.5. It has been observed from the table that percent graft yield for graft copolymerization of monomers increases with an increase in monomer concentration, giving a maximum P_g (21.08%) at 2.91×10^{-1} mol L^{-1} concentration of AAc, whereas maximum grafting (47.36%) with AN was obtained at 3.05×10^{-1} mol L^{-1} molar concentration [32,33].

This increase in P_g with an increase in monomer concentration may be due to the generation of more and more free radicals, which reach onto the polymeric backbone and thus resulting in an increased P_g. However, a decrease in P_g beyond the optimum value was probably due to the predominance of homopolymerization over graft copolymerization.

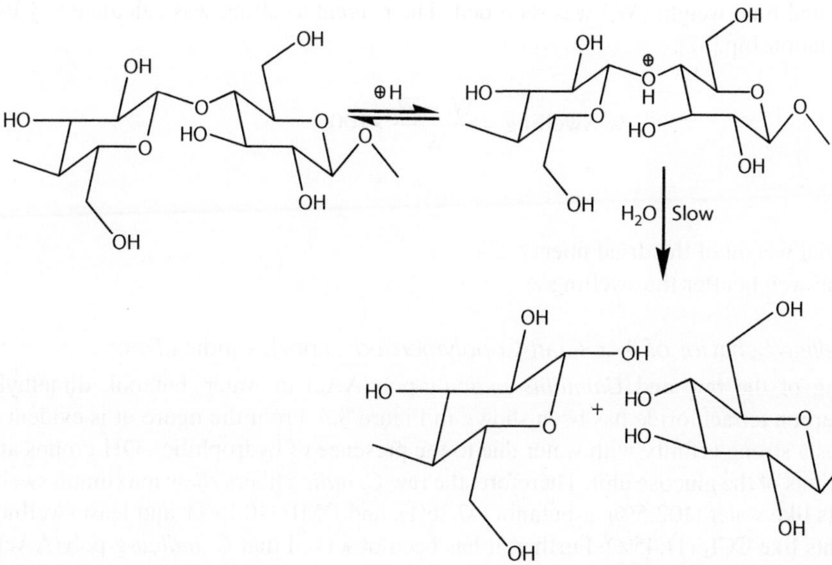

SCHEME 8.2 Hydrolysis of the cellulosic fiber due to increased HNO_3 concentration. (From Nevell, T.P., Cellulose—its structure and properties, in: *The Dyeing of Cellulosic Fibers*, C. Preston (ed.), Dyers' Company Publication Trust, London, U.K., 1986, pp. 1–4.)

TABLE 8.5
Effect of Monomer Concentration on Percent Grafting

	A			B		
	C. indica-g-poly(AAc) in Air[a]			*C. indica*-g-poly(AN) in Air[b]		
Sr. No	[AAc] × 10^{-1} mol L^{-1}	Percent Grafting (P_g)	Percent Efficiency (P_e)	[AN] × 10^{-1} mol L^{-1}	Percent Grafting (P_g)	Percent Efficiency (P_e)
1.	1.75	11.2	2.66	1.83	31.12	16.08
2.	2.33	14.66	3.48	2.44	40.92	15.78
3.	**2.91**	**21.08**	**5.01**	**3.05**	**47.36**	**14.61**
4.	3.50	20.18	4.80	3.66	43.90	11.29
5.	4.08	12.88	3.06	4.27	41.80	9.21

[a] [CAN]: 1.82×10^{-2} mol L^{-1}; [HNO_3]: 3.60×10^{-2} mol L^{-1}; time: 120 min; temp: 45°C.
[b] [CAN]: 1.82×10^{-2} mol L^{-1}; [HNO_3]: 2.88×10^{-2} mol L^{-1}; time: 120 min; temp: 35°C.

8.3.3 Physical and Chemical Properties

8.3.3.1 Swelling Behavior

Swelling behavior of raw and graft copolymerized fibers was studied for 24 h as per standard method reported earlier. The swelling behavior of samples was studied in water, butanol, dimethyl formamide, and carbon tetra chloride. Dried samples of raw and grafted copolymerized fibers of known weight (W_i) were immersed in known amounts of different solvents for 24 h. The samples were then taken out, and excess of the solvent was removed by pressing them between the folds of the filter paper, and final weight (W_f) was recorded. The percent swelling was calculated by using the following relationship [32]:

$$\% \text{ Swelling} = \frac{W_f - W_i}{W_i} \times 100$$

where

W_i is the initial weight of the dried fiber
W_f is the final weight after the swelling

8.3.3.1.1 Swelling Behavior of AAc Graft Copolymerized Cannabis indica *Fibers*

Percent swelling of the raw and *Cannabis indica*-g-poly(AAc) in water, butanol, dimethylformamide, and carbon tetrachloride has been shown in Figure 8.3. From the figure, it is evident that the raw fiber has a strong affinity with water due to the presence of hydrophilic –OH groups at C_2, C_3, and C_6 positions of the glucose unit. Therefore, the raw *C. indica* fibers show maximum swelling in polar solvents like water (102.5%), n-butanol (47.26%), and DMF (40.16%), and least swelling in nonpolar solvents like CCl_4 (11.45%). Further, it has been observed that *C. indica*-g-poly(AAc)-IA (P_g: 21.24%) exhibit 132%, 71.15%, 60.23%, and 6.98% swelling in water, n-butanol, DMF, and CCl_4, respectively [32].

The percent swelling in water, butanol, and DMF for *C. indica*-g-poly(AAc) fibers has been found to increase with increase in P_g, while the percent swelling for AAc-grafted fiber in CCl_4 has been found to be less than that of the raw fiber. This increase in percent swelling for *C. indica*-g-poly(AAc) fibers in water, DMF, and n-butanol may be due to interaction between carboxyl groups of poly(AAc) chains and polar groups of solvent. The lower percent swelling of *C. indica*-g-poly(AAc) fibers in carbon tetrachloride may be due to less interaction of nonpolar CCl_4 with polar carboxyl groups in comparison to the hydroxyl groups of the raw fiber. Further, it has also been observed that the percent swelling of *C. indica*-g-poly(AAc) fibers in water, butanol, and DMF decreases beyond P_g of 14.66%. This may be due to the formation of inter- and intramolecular hydrogen-bonded structures between the pendant carboxyl groups (Figure 8.4).

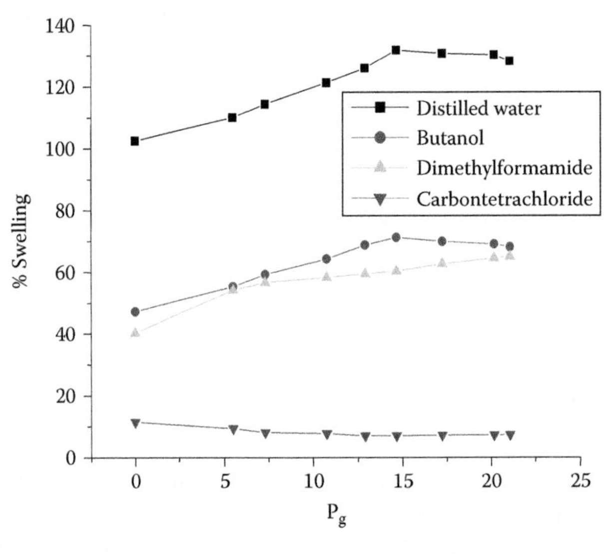

FIGURE 8.3 Effect of percent grafting of AAc on the swelling behavior of *Cannabis indica*-g-poly(AAc)-fibers in different solvents.

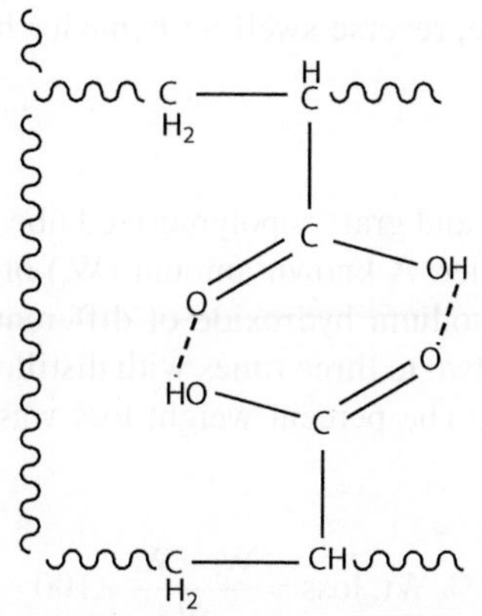

FIGURE 8.4 Formation of inter- and intramolecular hydrogen bonding between carboxyl groups. (From Kaur, I. et al., *Carbohydr. Res.*, 345, 2164, 2010.)

8.3.3.1.2 Swelling Behavior of Cannabis indica*-g-poly(AN) Fibers*

The percent swelling of AN-grafted fibers in different solvents varies as a function of percent grafting and follows the trend: DMF > H_2O > CCl_4 > C_2H_5OH (Figure 8.5). It has been observed that *C. indica*-g-poly(AN) fibers (47.3%) showed reverse swelling trend when compared with that of raw fiber. *C. indica*-g-poly(AN) fibers show 43.47%, 20.46%, 130.56%, and 60.48% swelling in the earlier-mentioned solvents, respectively (Figure 8.5) [33]. This happens due to the increase in hydrophobicity of fiber on account of the blockage of the hydroxyl groups (active sites) on polymer backbone by poly(AN) chains. Higher percent swelling in DMF occurs due to solvolysis of grafted fiber in DMF as it is dipolar aprotic in nature. Further swelling of grafted fibers in carbon tetrachloride increases as a function of P_g due to the development of the hydrophobic character on the polymeric backbone. Also unlike AAc-grafted fiber, there are not any polar groups

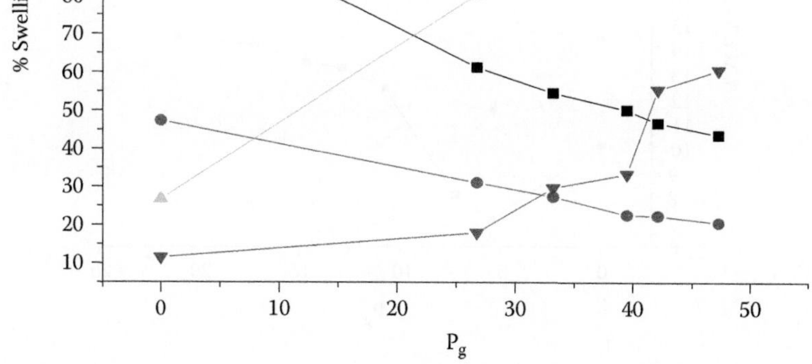

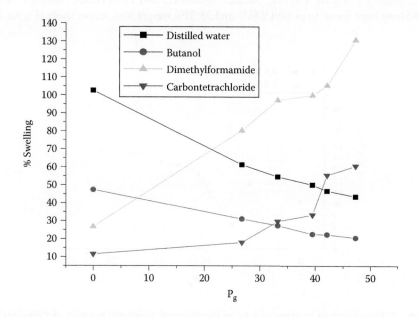

FIGURE 8.5 Effect of percent grafting of AN on swelling behavior of *Cannabis indica*-g-poly(AN) fibers in different solvents.

present on poly(AN) chains; hence, reverse swelling behavior has been observed in case of AN graft copolymerized fibers.

8.3.3.2 Chemical Resistance

The chemical resistance of the raw and graft copolymerized fibers was studied in accordance with the standard method reported earlier. A known amount (W_i) of sample was treated with a fixed volume of hydrochloric acid and sodium hydroxide of different strengths for a time interval of 24 h. The fibers were then washed two to three times with distilled water, dried, and were weighed again to get the final weight (W_f). The percent weight loss was determined using the following formula [32]:

$$\% \text{ Wt. loss} = \frac{W_i - W_f}{W_i} \times 100$$

where

W_i is the initial weight of the dried fiber
W_f is the final weight after the swelling

8.3.3.2.1 *Chemical Resistance Behavior of AAc Graft Copolymerized* Cannabis indica *Fibers*

The chemical resistance behavior of raw *C. indica* fibers was studied in terms of weight loss in NaOH and HCl solutions of different strengths for 24 h. The weight loss has been found to increase with an increase in the normality of solution as well as with P_g. Raw *C. indica* fibers have been found to show 10.08% and 14.25% weight loss against 0.5 and 1.0 N NaOH solution, while against 0.5 and 1.0 N HCl solutions, the weight loss was found to be 8.89% and 13.02%, respectively (Figures 8.6 and 8.7).

From Figures 8.6 and 8.7, it has been observed that chemical resistance of AAc-grafted fibers decreases with increase in percent grafting both with acid and with base. *C. indica*-g-poly(AAc)-IA (P_g: 14.66%) have been found to exhibit 14.4% and 18.19% weight loss against 0.5 and 1.0 N NaOH solutions, respectively (Figure 8.6) [32]. Further, against 0.5 and 1.0 N HCl, *C. indica*-g-poly(AAc)-IA (14.66%) have been found to exhibit 9.81% and 23.32% weight loss, respectively (Figure 8.7) [32].

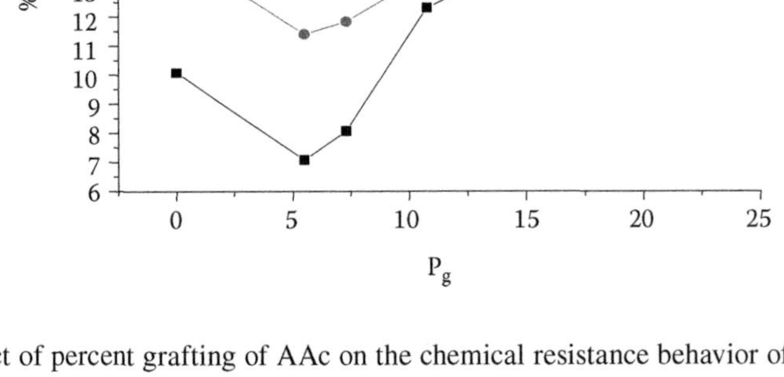

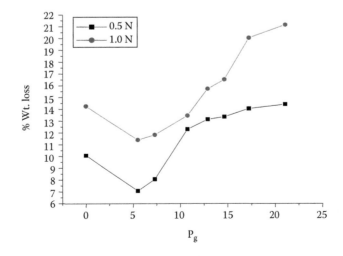

FIGURE 8.6 Effect of percent grafting of AAc on the chemical resistance behavior of *Cannabis indica*-g-poly(AAc)-IA against 0.5 and 1.0 N NaOH solutions. (From Singha, A.S. and Rana, A.K., *Iran. Polym. J.*, 20, 913, 2011.)

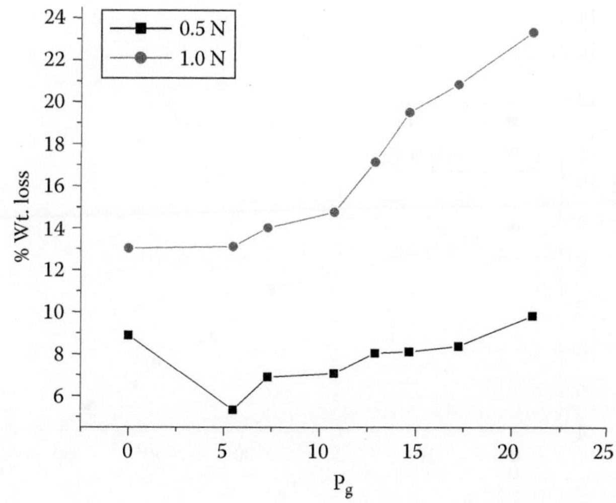

FIGURE 8.7 Effect of percent grafting of AAc on the chemical resistance behavior of *Cannabis indica*-g-poly(AAc)-IA against 0.5 and 1.0 N HCl solutions. (From Singha, A.S. and Rana, A.K., *Iran. Polym. J.*, 20, 913, 2011.)

This decrease in chemical resistance behavior with increase in P_g could be due to the formation of the corresponding sodium salts and, to some extent, due to the solubility of the poly(AAc) chain.

8.3.3.2.2 Chemical Resistance Behavior of AN Graft Copolymerized Cannabis indica *Fibers*

It has been observed that *C. indica*-g-poly(AN)-IA (47.3%) showed 5.47% and 6.83% weight loss against 0.5 and 1.0 N NaOH solutions, respectively (Figure 8.8) [33]. The chemical resistance in case of *C. indica*-g-poly(AN)-IA (47.3%) graft copolymers against 0.5 and 1.0 N HCl has been found to be 4.57% and 6.65%, respectively (Figure 8.9) [33]. Further, the chemical resistance of AN

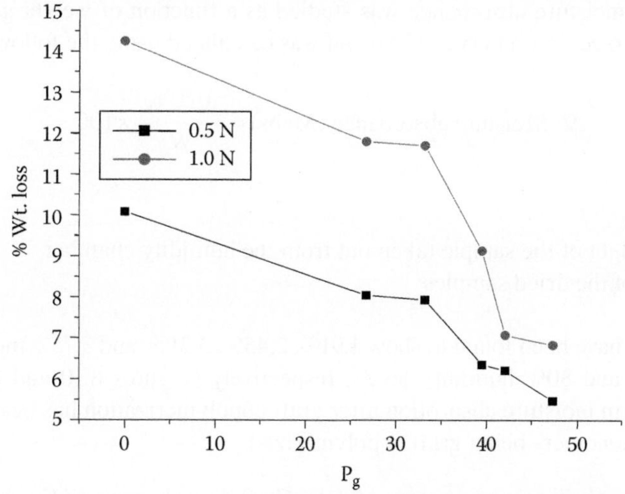

FIGURE 8.8 Effect of percent grafting of AN on the chemical resistance behavior of *Cannabis indica*-g-poly(AN)-IA against 0.5 and 1.0 N NaOH solutions. (From Singha, A.S. and Rana, A.K., *J. Reinf. Plast. Compos.*, 31, 1538, 2012.)

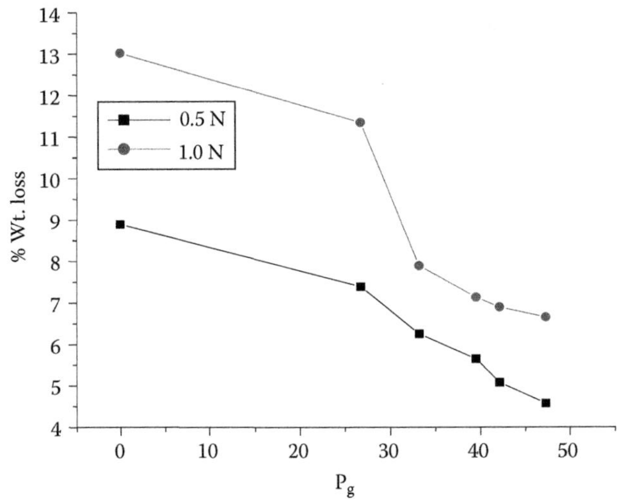

FIGURE 8.9 Effect of percent grafting of AN on the chemical resistance behavior of *Cannabis indica*-g-poly(AN)-IA against 0.5 and 1.0 N HCl solutions. (From Singha, A.S. and Rana, A.K., *J. Reinf. Plast. Compos.*, 31, 1538, 2012.)

graft copolymers has been found to be higher than that of raw fibers. It has also been observed that chemical resistance of graft copolymers increases with increase in P_g. It could be due to the blockage of the active sites by poly(AN) chains, which are prone to attack on the fiber backbone.

Further, it has also been observed that chemical resistance of fibers was more toward HCl as compared to NaOH solutions. This behavior may be due to high reactivity of lignin and hemicellulose toward NaOH solution.

8.3.3.3 Moisture Absorbance

The moisture absorbance study of the raw and graft copolymerized fibers was performed at different humidity levels ranging from 20% to 80% in humidity chamber as per the method reported earlier. The percent moisture absorbance was studied as a function of weight gain at a particular humidity level for a fixed time interval of 2 h and was calculated using the following formula [23]:

$$\% \text{ Moisture absorbance (Mabs)} = \frac{W_f - W_i}{W_i} \times 100$$

where

W_f is the final weight of the sample taken out from the humidity chamber
W_i is the weight of the dried samples

Raw *C. indica* fibers have been found to show 1.91%, 2.45%, 3.21%, and 3.75% moisture absorbance at 20%, 40%, 60%, and 80% humidity levels, respectively (Figures 8.10 and 8.11). The percent increase or decrease in moisture absorption after graft copolymerization has been found to depend upon the nature of monomers being graft copolymerized.

8.3.3.3.1 Moisture Absorption Behavior of AAc Graft Copolymerized Cannabis indica *Fibers*

The moisture absorbance for AAc graft copolymerized fibers has been found to increase with the increase in P_g. *C. indica*-g-poly(AAc)-IA (P_g: 14.66%) showed 2.15%, 2.67%, 3.45%, and 3.96% moisture absorbance at 20%, 40%, 60%, and 80% humidity levels, respectively

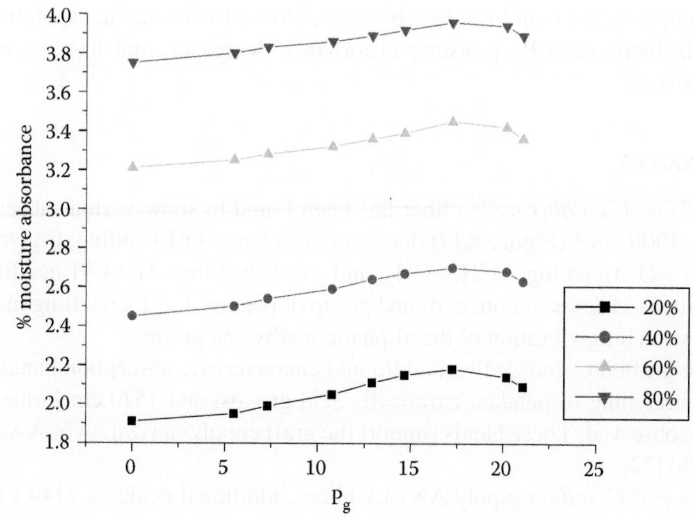

FIGURE 8.10 Effect of percent grafting of AAc on the moisture absorption behavior of *Cannabis indica*-g-poly(AAc)-IA at different humidity levels. (From Singha, A.S. and Rana, A.K., *Iran. Polym. J.*, 20, 913, 2011.)

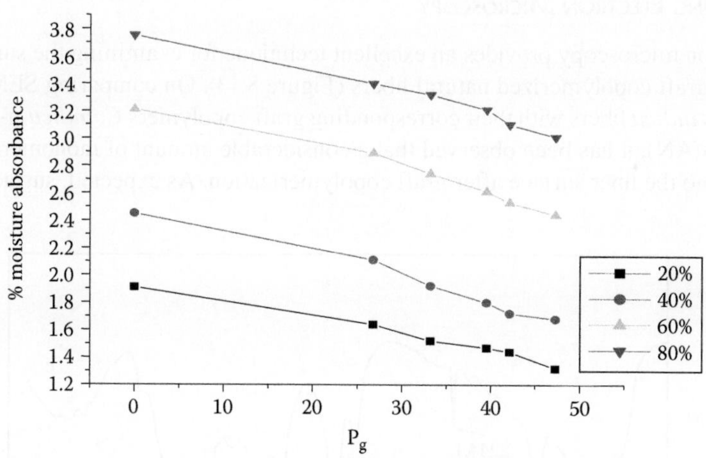

FIGURE 8.11 Effect of percent grafting of AN on moisture absorption behavior of *Cannabis indica*-g-poly (AN)-IA at different humidity levels. (From Singha, A.S. and Rana, A.K., *J. Reinf. Plast. Compos.*, 31, 1538, 2012.)

(Figure 8.10) [32]. This increase in moisture absorbance with the increase in graft yield could be due to availability of more carboxyl groups for the formation of the hydrogen bond with the water molecules.

8.3.3.3.2 Moisture Absorption Behavior of AN Graft Copolymerized Cannabis indica *Fibers*

In case of AN graft copolymers, it has been observed that *C. indica*-g-poly(AN)-IA (47.3%) showed 1.32%, 1.68%, 2.44%, and 3.01% moisture absorbance at 20%, 40%, 60%, and 80% humidity levels, respectively (Figure 8.11) [33]. It is evident from the earlier results that moisture absorbance behavior decreases with increase in P_g. Raw fibers contain active –OH groups and thus have high affinity toward moisture absorbance. However, upon graft copolymerization, these –OH groups (active groups) on the cellulosic backbone got blocked with the incorporation of poly(AN) chains. Thus, with increase in P_g, moisture absorbance decreases, and fiber becomes more and more moisture resistant.

8.3.4 FTIR Analysis

The IR spectra of raw *Cannabis indica* fiber has been found to show various absorption peaks in the range of 400–4000 cm^{-1} (Figure 8.12) due to out of plane –OH bending, β-glycosidic linkage, –C–O–C– and –C=O stretching, –CH, $-CH_2$, and $-CH_3$ bending, H–O–H bending of absorbed water and for lignin C–H deformation, carbonyl group of pectins, C–H stretching in polysaccharide chains, and C–H stretching vibration of the aliphatic methylene group.

In case of AAc-grafted *C. indica* fiber, additional characteristic absorption bands at 1729.9 cm^{-1} (due to carbonyl stretching of pendant carboxylic acid groups) and 1570 cm^{-1} (due to unsaturated groups) have been observed. These bands support the graft copolymerization of AAc onto *C. indica* fiber (Figure 8.12b) [32].

However, in case of *C. indica*-g-poly(AN)-IA fibers, additional peaks at 2244.1 cm^{-1} have been observed due to the presence of the nitrile group in the grafted structure (Figure 8.12c). Also increase in the intensity of peak around 2922 cm^{-1} after graft copolymerization of AN, which is a characteristic of $-CH_2$ group, has been observed [33].

8.3.5 Scanning Electron Microscopy

Scanning electron microscopy provides an excellent technique for examining the surface morphology of raw and graft copolymerized natural fibers (Figure 8.13). On comparing SEM micrographs of raw *Cannabis indica* fibers with their corresponding graft copolymers *C. indica*-g-poly(AAc) and *C. indica*-g-poly(AN), it has been observed that a considerable amount of monomers (AN or AAc) got deposited onto the fiber surface after graft copolymerization. As expected, surface morphology

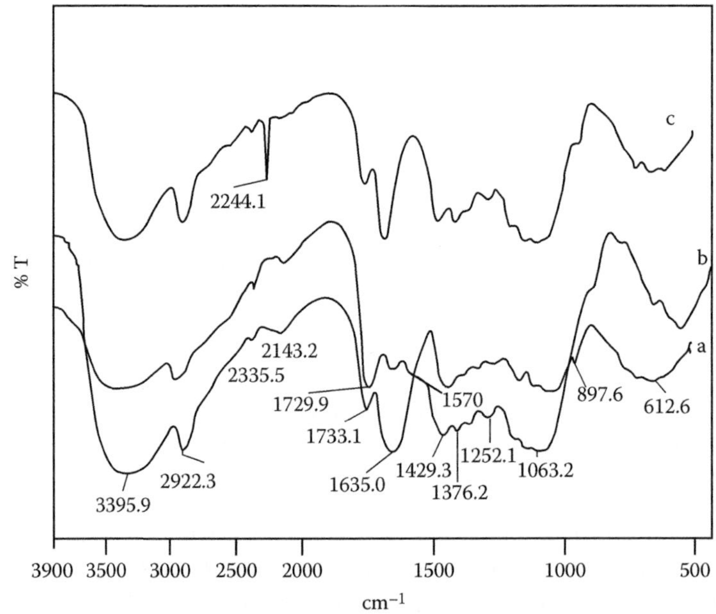

FIGURE 8.12 FTIR spectra of (a) raw, (b) *Cannabis indica*-g-poly(AAc), and (c) *Cannabis indica*-g-poly(AN).

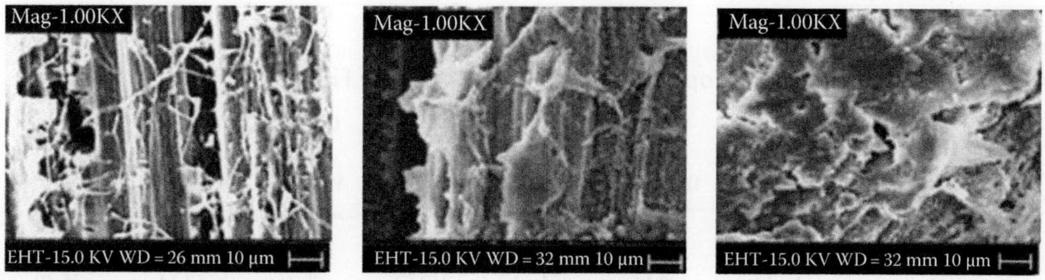

FIGURE 8.13 Scanning electron micrographs of (a) raw, (b) *Cannabis indica*-g-poly(AAc), and (c) *Cannabis indica*-g-poly(AN).

of raw *C. indica* fibers has been found to be different from their corresponding graft copolymerized samples in terms of roughness and smoothness.

8.3.6 Thermal Stability

Thermogravimetric analysis (TGA) of the raw and graft copolymerized *Cannabis indica* fibers was conducted on a TGA with autosampler (Mettler Toledo) analyzer at a heating rate of 15°C min^{-1}. Thermograms were recorded over a temperature range of 25°C–800°C in the presence of nitrogen atmosphere with the flow rate of 20 mL min^{-1}. Thermal behavior of raw, AAc, and AN graft copolymerized *C. indica* fibers was studied as a function of percent weight loss with the increase in temperature (Figure 8.14). Table 8.6 shows the initial decomposition temperature (IDT), final decomposition temperature (FDT), and decomposition temperature (DT) at 20%, 40%, and 60% weight loss for *C. indica* fibers.

For raw *C. indica* fiber, IDT and FDT have been found to be 250.33°C (6.91% weight loss) and 383.25°C (61.12% weight loss), respectively, whereas for *C. indica*-g-poly(AAc) and

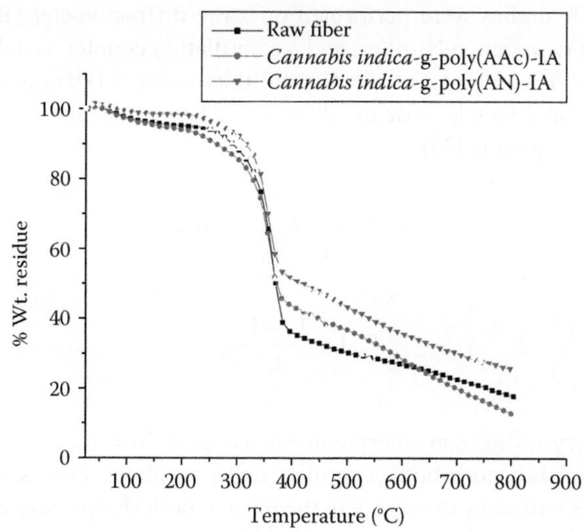

FIGURE 8.14 TGA thermograms of raw *Cannabis indica* and its graft copolymers with AN and AAc. (From Singha, A.S. and Rana, A.K., *Iran. Polym. J.*, 20, 913, 2011; Singha, A.S. and Rana, A.K., *J. Reinf. Plast. Compos.*, 31, 1538, 2012.)

TABLE 8.6
TGA Data of Raw and Graft Copolymerized *Cannabis indica* Fibers

Sr. No	Sample Designation	IDT (°C)	FDT (°C)	DT (°C) at 20% Wt. Loss	DT (°C) at 40% Wt. Loss	DT (°C) at 60% Wt. Loss	Residual Weight (%) at 600°C
1.	Raw *C. indica* fiber	250.33	383.25	329.61	362.56	383.25	27.04
2.	*C. indica*-g-poly(AAc)-IA	236.9	388.68	329.18	364.23	447	27.84
3.	*C. indica*-g-poly(AN)-IA	290.11	395.43	342.64	539.18	552.14	35.40

Sources: Singha, A.S. and Rana, A.K., *Iran. Polym. J.*, 20, 913, 2011; Singha, A.S. and Rana, A.K., *J. Reinf. Plast. Compos.*, 31, 1538, 2012.

C. indica-g-poly(AN), IDT and FDT were found to be 236.9°C (7.88% weight loss) and 388.68°C (54.85% weight loss), and 290.11°C (6.31% weight loss) and 395.43°C (48.25% weight loss), respectively [32,33]. It has also been observed that upon graft copolymerization of AAc onto *C. indica* fiber, a decrease in the IDT and an increase in FDT have been observed for the resulted *Grewia optiva*-g-poly(AAc) fibers. Also if we compare DT at 20% and 60% weight loss (Table 8.6), AAc-grafted fibers have been found to possess less thermal stability at lower temperature. Poor thermal stability of grafted fibers at a lower temperature (IDT) may be because of the decomposition of anhydride (formed due to dehydration of carboxylic acid groups) of grafted poly(AAc) chains to carbon dioxide at lower temperature, accompanied by an overall decrease in the AAc content [34].

Also on comparing DT of AN graft copolymerized fibers at 20% and 60% weight loss, then it has been observed that *C. indica*-g-poly (AN) fibers are thermally more stable than the raw fibers, which could be due to the decomposition of grafted poly(AN) chains at high temperature [33].

8.3.7 Crystallinity Study

X-ray diffraction (XRD) studies were performed on x-ray diffractometer (Bruker D8 Advance), using Cu Kα (1.5418 Å) radiation, a Ni-filter, and a scintillation counter as a detector at 40 kV and 40 mA on rotation from 10° to 50° at 2θ scale. Crystallinity index (CI) was determined by using the wide-angle XRD counts at 2θ angle close to 22° and 15°. Percent crystallinity and CI were calculated using the following equation [35]:

$$\%\ C_r = \frac{I_C}{I_C + I_A} \times 100$$

$$C \cdot I = \frac{I_C - I_A}{I_C}$$

where I_C and I_A are the crystalline and amorphous intensities at 2θ scale close to 22° and 15° angles.

Since cellulosic materials contain both crystalline and amorphous regions, it is evident that XRD pattern of such materials will show the region in the form of both sharp peaks and diffused patterns. Graft copolymerization has been known to decrease the percent crystallinity.

It has been observed from Table 8.7 that on graft copolymerization of *C. indica* fibers with vinyl monomer, there is a decrease in percent crystallinity. This change in diffraction pattern occurs due to the creation of disorder in the crystalline pattern of the main polymeric backbone by the grafted units of poly(AN) and poly(AAc) chains.

TABLE 8.7
X-RD Data of Raw and Graft Copolymerized *Cannabis indica* Fibers

		At 2θ Scale			
Sr. No	Sample Designation	I_{22}	I_{15}	% Crystallinity	CI
1.	Raw *C. indica* fiber	709	348	67.07	0.5091
2.	*C. indica*-g-poly(AAc)-IA	603	314	65.71	0.4792
3.	*C. indica*-g-poly(AN)-IA	535	302	63.91	0.4355

Sources: Singha, A.S. and Rana, A.K., *Iran. Polym. J.*, 20, 913, 2011; Singha, A.S. and Rana, A.K., *J. Reinf. Plast. Compos.*, 31, 1538, 2012.

8.4 CONCLUSION

From the earlier studies, it has been observed that percent graft yield was higher with AN as compared to AAc monomers. Higher graft yield in case of AN monomer may be due to the generation of more number of active sites/free radical sites on the polymeric backbone as compared to AAc monomer. AN also shows lower affinity to solvent than AAc, which is soluble in water and undergoes homopolymerization more readily in comparison to graft copolymerization, which ultimately results in poor graft yield.

Further, AN graft copolymerized fibers have been found to be more stable than the AAc-grafted one. It has been also found that percent crystallinity of *C. indica*-g-poly(AN) fibers was lower than that of *C. indica*-g-poly(AAc). This indicates that incorporation of poly(AN) chains into the fiber causes more disturbance in the crystalline structure of cellulosic fibers as compared to incorporation of poly(AAc) chains.

REFERENCES

1. Vitta SB, Stahel EP, and Stannett VT, The preparation and properties of acrylic acid and methacrylic acid grafted cellulose prepared by ceric ion initiation. II. Water retention properties, *J Appl Polym Sci*, **32**, 5799–5810, 1986.
2. Yoshinoba M, Morita M, and Higuchi M, Morphological study of hydrogels of cellulosic water absorbents by CRY-SEM observation, *J Appl Polym Sci*, **53**, 1203–1209, 1994.
3. Ibrahim NA and Abo Shosha MH, Polymerizations of ethylene and propylene initiated by milled metallic oxides characterizations of the mechanochemically produced polymers, *J Appl Poly Sci*, **49**, 291–298, 1993.
4. Arifuzzaman Khan GM, Shaheruzzaman MD, Rahman MH, Abdur Razzaque SM, Islam MS, and Alam MS, Surface modification of Okra bast fiber and its physico-chemical characteristics, *Fibers Polym*, **10**, 65, 2009.
5. Kalia S, Kaushik VK, and Sharma RK, Effect of benzoylation and graft copolymerization on morphology, thermal stability and crystallinity of sisal fibers, *J Nat Fibers*, **8**, 27, 2011.
6. Taghizadeh MT and Mehrdad A, Kinetic study of graft polymerization of acrylic acid and ethyl methacrylate onto starch by ceric ammonium nitrate, *Iran J Chem Chem Eng*, **25**, 1, 2006.
7. Giri G, Nanda CN, and Samal RK, Graft copolymerization onto wool fibers: Graft copolymerization of acrylic acid onto wool fibers initiated by quinquivalent vanadium, *Poymers* **21**, 883, 1989.
8. Samal RK, Nanda CN, Satrusallya SC, Nayak BL, and Suryanarayan GV, Grafting of vinyl monomers onto silk fibers: Trivalent-manganese—Initiated graft copolymerization of acrylamide onto silk fibers, *J Appl Polym Sci*, **28**, 1311, 1983.
9. Das AM, Chowdhury PK, Saikia CN, and Rao PG, Silk fibre modification through graft copolymerization using vinyl monomer, *Indian J Fibre Text Res*, **35**, 107, 2009.
10. Fanta GF, Rober CB, Russell RC, and Rist CE, Copolymers of starch and polyacrylonitrile: Influence of granule swelling on copolymer composition under various reaction conditions, *J Macromol Sci Chem*, **4**, 331, 1970.

11. Kalia S, Sharma S, Bhardwaj B, Kaith BS, and Singha AS, Potential use of graft copolymers of mercerized flax as filler in polystyrene composite materials, *BioResources*, **3**, 1010, 2008.
12. Taghizadeh MT and Darvishi MA, Kinetics and mechanism of heterogeneous graft copolymerization of acrylonitrile onto polyvinyl alcohol initiated with ceric ammonium nitrate, *Iran Polym J*, **10**, 283, 2001.
13. Huang RYM and Chandramouli P, Structure and properties of cellulose graft copolymers. III. Cellulose–methyl methacrylate graft copolymers synthesized by ceric ion method, *Polym Chem*, **7**, 1393, 2003.
14. Mino G and Kaizerman S, A new method for the preparation of graft copolymers. Polymerization initiated by ceric ion redox systems, *J Polym Sci*, **31**, 242, 1958.
15. Guan J and Chen G, Flame resistant modification of silk fabric with vinyl phosphate, fibers and polymers, *Fibers Polym*, **9**, 438, 2008.
16. Singha AS and Rana RK, Graft copolymerization of methylmethacrylate (MMA) onto Agave Americana fibers and evaluation of their physicochemical properties, *Int J Polym Anal Charact*, **14**, 1, 2009.
17. Kaith BS, Jindal R, and Maiti M, Graft copolymerization of methylmethacrylate onto acetylated *Saccharum spontaneum* L, using FAS-KPS as a redox initiator and evaluation of physical, chemical and thermal properties, *Int J Polym Anal Charact*, **14**, 210, 2009.
18. Bessadok A, Marais S, Gouanve F, Colasse L, Zimmerlin I, Roudesli S, and Metayer M, Effect of chemical treatments of alfa (*Stipa tenacissima*) fibers on water absorption properties, *Compos Sci Technol*, **67**, 685, 2007.
19. Vijay V, Mariatti M, Taib RM, and Mitsugu T, Effect of fiber treatment and fiber loading on the properties of bagasse fiber-reinforced unsaturated polyester composites, *Compos Sci Technol*, **68**, 631, 2008.
20. Thakur VK, Singha AS, and Misra BN, Graft copolymerization of methyl methacrylate onto cellulosic biofibers, *J Appl Polym Sci*, **122**, 532, 2011.
21. Mohanty AK, Khan MA, Sahoo S, and Hinrichsen G, Effect of chemical modification on the performance of biodegradable jute yarn, *J Mater Sci*, **35**, 2589, 2000.
22. Misra BN, Kaur I, Gupta A, John V, and Singha AS, Graft copolymerization of methyl acrylate and methyl methacrylate onto polyamide film by the mutual method, *Polym Polym Compos*, **4**, 411, 1996.
23. Monier M, Nawar N, and Abdel-Latif DA, Preparation and characterization of chelating fibers based on natural wool for removal of Hg(II), Cu(II) and Co(II) metal ions from aqueous solutions, *J Hazard Mater*, **184**, 118, 2010.
24. Chaobo X, Lili W, and Shaozhi R, Studies on graft copolymerization of acrylic acid onto ramie fibers with chromic acid initiation system, *Wuhan Univ J Nat Sci*, **3**, 359, 1998.
25. Khan F, Photoinduced graft-copolymer synthesis and characterization of methacrylic acid onto natural biodegradable lignocelluloses fiber, *Biomacromolecules,* **5**, 1078, 2004.
26. Kaur I, Kumar R, and Sharma N, A comparative study on the graft copolymerization of acrylic acid onto rayon fiber by a ceric ion redox system and a γ-radiation method, *Carbohydr Res*, **345**, 2164, 2010.
27. Feng H, Li J, and Wang L, Preparation of biodegradable flax shive cellulose-based superabsorbent polymer under microwave irradiation, *BioResources*, **5**, 1484, 2011.
28. Khullar R, Varshney VK, Naithani S, and Soni PL, Grafting of acrylonitrile onto cellulosic material derived from bamboo (*Dendrocalamus strictus*), *Expr Polym Lett*, **2**, 12, 2008.
29. Zahran MK, Morsy M, and Mahmoud RI, Grafting of acrylic monomers onto cotton fabric using an activated cellulose thiocarbonate-azobisisobutyronitrile redox system, *J Appl Polym Sci*, **91**, 1261, 2004.
30. Singha AS and Rana AK, A study on benzoylation and graft copolymerization of lignocellulosic *Cannabis indica* fiber, *Polym Environ*, **20**, 361, 2012.
31. Nevell TP, Cellulose—its structure and properties, in: *The Dyeing of Cellulosic Fibers*, C. Preston (Ed.), Dyers' Company Publication Trust, London, U.K., pp. 1–4, 1986.
32. Singha AS and Rana AK, Kinetic study on acrylic acid (AAc) graft copolymerized *Cannabis indica* fiber, *Iran Polym J*, **20**, 913–919, 2011.
33. Singha AS and Rana AK, Preparation and characterization of graft copolymerized *Cannabis indica L.* fiber reinforced unsaturated polyester matrix based bio-composites, *J Reinf Plast Compos*, **31**, 1538–1553, 2012.
34. McGaugh MC and Kottle S, The thermal degradation of poly(acrylic acid), *J Polym Sci Part B: Polym Lett*, **5**, 817, 1967.
35. Mwaikambo LY and Ansell MP, Chemical and surface modification of hemp, sisal, jute and kapook fibers alkalization, *J Appl Polym Sci*, **84**, 2222, 2002.

9 Advances, Development, and Characterization of Cellulose Graft Copolymers

Vicente de Oliveira Sousa Neto, Diego de Quadros Melo, Paulo de Tarso C. Freire, Marcos Antônio Araujo-Silva, and Ronaldo Ferreira do Nascimento

CONTENTS

9.1 INTRODUCTION

In recent years, many researchers and scientists have paid attention to develop a variety of advanced and hybrid polymeric materials for their industrial applications (Liu et al., 2009) due to their unlimited availability, much higher specific strength, lower cost, and their potential applications such as biomaterials, drug delivery (Dong et al., 2008; Liu et al., 2011; Das and Pal, 2013), coatings, films, membranes, drilling techniques, pharmaceuticals and foodstuffs (Klemm et al., 2005; Hiltunen et al., 2012), packaging, bioenergy, bioplastics, and aerospace industry (Alila et al., 2009; Akar et al., 2012; Bao et al., 2012; Thakur et al., 2013). Of these materials, one of the most important is graft copolymer (Liu et al., 2011; Thakur et al., 2013). Graft copolymers by definition consist of a long sequence of one polymer (often referred to as the backbone polymer) with one or more branches (grafts) of another (chemically different) polymer (Gowariker et al., 1986; Odian, 2002). Graft copolymers can associate to form micelles in selective solvents, which are thermodynamically good solvents for one of the components and comparatively poor solvents for the other (Tang et al., 2007; Gao et al., 2008).

Natural cellulosic polymers such as lignocellulosic natural fibers offer well-known advantages as compared to the traditional synthetic materials, which include toxicologically harmless, eco-friendliness, biodegradability, easy availability, noncorrosive nature, enhanced energy recovery, and usually lower cost (Singha and Thakur, 2010; Thakur et al., 2013). Various modification techniques have been reported to improve the physicochemical properties of natural polymers (Eissa et al., 2012; Zhong et al., 2012), and among these, graft copolymerization has received much more attention during the last few decades (Sand et al., 2010; Abdel-Halim, 2012). It is one of the most facile methods to incorporate desired functional groups onto natural polymers depending upon the targeted application (Oza et al., 2012; Thakur et al., 2013). This chapter describes the advances, development, and characterization of the cellulose graft copolymers. The chapter discusses grafting to cellulose. The various methods of grafting, including both chemical and radiation initiation, are discussed in some detail.

9.2 GRAFT COPOLYMERS

A graft copolymer consists of a polymeric backbone with covalently linked polymeric side chains. In principle, both backbone and side chains could be homopolymers or copolymers. Grafting can be carried out in such a way that the properties of the side chains can be added to those of the substrate polymer without changing the latter. The process of graft copolymer synthesis starts with a preformed polymer (polysaccharide in case of grafted polysaccharides). An external agent is used to create free radical sites on this preformed polymer. The agent should be effective enough to create the required free radical sites and, at the same time, should not be too drastic to rupture the structural integrity of the preformed polymer chain (Mishra et al., 2012). Thus, cellulose fibers can be grafted with sodium polyacrylate, polyacrylonitrile, polyacrylamide, etc., while still maintaining their fibrous nature and most of their mechanical properties.

9.2.1 Techniques of Grafting

The synthesis of a polymer-grafted cellulose is an effective way to modify cellulose's properties and combine the advantages of natural cellulose and synthetic polymers. Graft copolymerization of cellulose and its derivatives can be generally classified into three major groups: (1) free radical polymerization, (2) ionic and ring-opening polymerization (ROP), and (3) controlled/living radical polymerization (CRP) (Roy et al., 2009).

9.2.2 Grafting Initiated by Chemical Means

By chemical means, the grafting can proceed along two major paths, viz., free radical and ionic. In the chemical process, the role of initiator is very important as it determines the path of the grafting process. Apart from the general free radical mechanism, grafting in the melt and atom transfer radical polymerization (ATRP) are also interesting techniques to carry out grafting.

9.2.2.1 Free Radical Grafting

Radical polymerization has received the greatest amount of attention among all of the polymerization methods. Five years ago, about 60% of all available polymers were still obtained by this method. This position is due to its many attractive characteristics, including

1. Ability to provide an unlimited number of copolymers; it is simple to implement and inexpensive compared with competitive technologies
2. Tolerance to water or other impurities in contrast to the great sensitivities of ionic polymerization and coordination polymerization
3. Applicability to the polymerization of a wide range of monomers such as (meth)acrylates, (meth)acrylamides, styrene (Sty), butadiene, vinyl acetate (VAc), and the water-soluble monomers such as acrylic acid, the hydroxyacrylates, and *N*-vinyl pyrrolidone
4. Tolerance to a wide range of functional groups (e.g., OH, NR_2, COOH, $CONR_2$) and reaction conditions (bulk, solution, emulsion, mini-emulsion, suspension), the convenient, mild reaction conditions and wide temperature range under which it can be conducted

In the chemical process, free radicals are produced from the initiators and transferred to the substrate to react with monomer to form the graft copolymers. In general, one can consider the generation of free radicals by indirect or direct methods. An example of free radicals produced by an indirect method is the production through redox reaction, viz., M^{n+}/H_2O_2, persulfates.

9.2.2.1.1 Indirect Method

Aqueous solutions of peroxides, persulfates, and redox systems (e.g., Ce^{4+} or Fe^{2+}/H_2O_2) can be used in the initiation step: however, depending on the olefin chemical nature, other suitable solvents, such as acetic acid, dimethylsulfoxide, sulfuric acid, or mixed polar solvents, may replace water. The final product, after separation from the reaction medium, is always a mixture of graft copolymer, unreacted cellulose, and olefin homopolymer, the proportion among the three components depending on the processing conditions. Schemes 9.1 and 9.2 show the formation of the active species in the indirect method:

$$Fe^{2+} + H_2O_2 \rightarrow Fe^{3+} + OH^- + OH^{\bullet} \quad (9.1)$$

$$Fe^{2+} + {}^-O_3S-OO-SO_3^- \rightarrow Fe^{3+} + SO_4^{2-} + SO_4^{-\bullet} \quad (9.2)$$

It may be observed that the active species in the decomposition of H_2O_2 (1) and potassium persulfate (2) induced by Fe^{2+} are $OH^{\bullet}$ and $SO_4^{-\bullet}$, respectively. There are different views regarding the activity of $SO_4^{-\bullet}$. Some authors reported that initially formed $SO_4^{-\bullet}$ reacts with water to form $OH^{\bullet}$, subsequently producing free radicals on the polymeric backbone (Scheme 9.3):

$$SO_4^{-\bullet} + H_2O \rightarrow HSO_4^- + OH^{\bullet} \quad (9.3)$$

According to Bhattacharya and Misra (2004), an alternate view is that $SO_4^{-\bullet}$ reacts directly with the polymeric backbone (e.g., cellulose) to produce the requisite radicals (Scheme 9.4):

$$SO_4^{-\bullet} + R_{polymer} - OH \rightarrow HSO_4 + R_{polymer} - O^{\bullet} \quad (9.4)$$

However, Mishra et al. (1984) established that during grafting of vinyl monomers onto wool/cellulose, $OH^{\bullet}$ is more reactive than $SO_4^{-\bullet}$.

Mishra et al. (2003) applied a free radical copolymerization initiated (indirect methods) by ammonium cerium (IV) nitrate $(NH_4)_2Ce(NO_3)_6$ to get nanofibrillated cellulose with acrylic monomers. This mechanism is illustrated in Figure 9.1. In this process, the initiation occurs via a redox reaction as the cerium ion chelates with two adjacent hydroxyl groups in a cellulose chain, resulting in radical formation on an opened glucose ring.

9.2.2.1.2 Direct Method

Free radical sites may be generated on a polymeric backbone by direct oxidation of the backbone by certain transition metal ions (e.g., Ce^{4+}, Cr^{6+}, V^{5+}, and Co^{3+}). The redox potential of the metal ions is the important parameter in determining the grafting efficiency. In general, metal ions with low oxidation potential are preferred for better grafting efficiency. The proposed mechanism for such a process has been ascribed to the intermediate formation of a metal ion–polymer chelate complex, viz., ceric ion is known to form a complex with hydroxyl groups on a polymeric backbone, which can dissociate via one-electron transfer to give free radicals (Zhang et al., 2003).

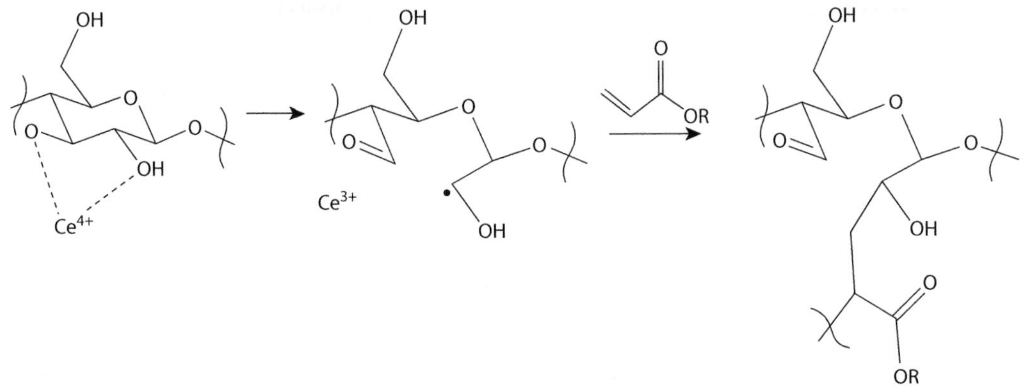

FIGURE 9.1 Mechanism of cerium-initiated copolymerization. (Reprinted from Mishra, A. et al., *J. Polym. Sci. Part A: Polym. Chem.*, 22, 2767, 1984. With permission; Mishra, A. et al., *Colloid Polym. Sci.*, 281(2), 187, 2003.)

9.2.2.1.2.1 Direct Oxidation via Ce(IV) Ions Among the various chemical initiation methods, the formation of free radicals on the cellulose molecules by direct oxidation with Ce(IV) ions has gained considerable importance, due to its ease of application and its high grafting efficiency compared with other known redox systems such as the Fe(II)–hydrogen peroxide system (Mino and Kaizerman, 1958). Gupta and Khandekar (2006) call attention to the importance of using the acidic medium. According to these authors quoting from Okieimen and Idehen (1989), the use of ceric(IV) ion as initiator has shown a substantial decrease in ungrafted polymer due to the participation of a single-electron process in the formation of active sites on cellulose. The ceric(IV) ions produce free radicals on the cellulose backbone in the presence of acid, but their efficiency is low in aqueous media due to hydrolysis of the ceric(IV) ions (Gupta and Khandekar, 2006). In principle, no homopolymer should be formed, as the radicals are almost exclusively formed on the cellulose backbone (Hebeish and Guthrie, 1981). However, small amounts of homopolymer are always observed due to direct reactions of the Ce(IV) ions with the monomers (McDowall et al., 1984). The proposed mechanism for such a process has been ascribed to the intermediate formation of a metal ion–polymer chelate complex, viz., ceric ion is known to form a complex with hydroxyl groups on a polymeric backbone, which can dissociate via one-electron transfer to give free radicals. The process is shown in Schemes 9.5 and 9.6:

$$Ce^{4+} + R_{polym}OH \rightarrow \text{complex} \rightarrow R_{poly}O^{\bullet} + Ce^{3+} + H^{+} \tag{9.5}$$

$$R_{poly}O^{\bullet} + M \rightarrow R_{cell}OM^{\bullet} \rightarrow R_{poly}OMM^{\bullet} \tag{9.6}$$

where

R_{poly} is the polymer
R_{cell} is cellulose
M is the monomer

Imai et al. (1970) proposed that the oxidation of cellulose by ceric ions occurred primarily at the hemiacetal unit, as illustrated in Figure 9.2.

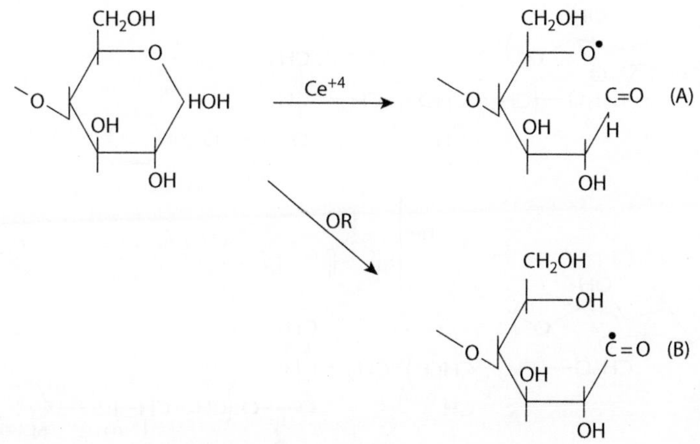

FIGURE 9.2 Oxidation of cellulose by Ce(IV). (Reprinted from Imai, Y. et al., *J. Polym. Sci.: Part B*: Polymer Letters, 8, 75, 1970. With permission.)

$$\text{Cellulose–OOH} \longrightarrow \text{Cellulose–O}^{\bullet} + \text{HO}^{\bullet}$$

$$\text{HO}^{\bullet} + \text{M} \longrightarrow \text{Homopolymer}$$

$$\text{Cellulose–O}^{\bullet} + \text{M} \longrightarrow \text{Graft copolymer}$$

Homopolymer reduction via reducing agent:

$$\text{Cellulose–OOH} + \text{Fe}^{2+} \longrightarrow \text{Cellulose–O}^{\bullet} + \text{Fe}^{3+} + \text{OH}^{-}$$

FIGURE 9.3 General mechanism of graft polymerization via decomposition of a cellulosic hydroperoxide initiator. (Reprinted from Roy, D. et al., *Chem. Soc. Rev.*, 38, 2046, 2009. With permission.)

9.2.2.1.2.2 Cellulosic Initiators If the cellulose material can be chemically converted into an initiator such as a peroxide (cellulose hydroperoxide), it can then decompose into radicals and initiate either graft copolymerization, or homopolymerization as shown in Figure 9.3.

Esters or carbonates of *N*-hydroxypyridine-2-thione (Barton esters) have been immobilized onto carboxymethyl cellulose or onto hydroxypropyl cellulose (HPC). Irradiation of the cellulose-immobilized Barton esters in the presence of a monomer initiated the free radical graft copolymerization of Sty, acrylamide, and *N*-isopropyl acrylamide (NIPAAm) (Daily et al., 2001). The graft copolymerization of Sty with the HPC–Barton ester derivative is shown in Figure 9.4.

Other method involves the introduction of an aromatic amine onto the cellulose backbone, followed by its conversion to its corresponding diazonium salt. Upon heating, the diazonium salt decomposes to produce free radicals, leading to graft copolymerization, when a suitable monomer is present. The reactions involved in this method are illustrated in Figure 9.5.

9.2.2.2 Ionic and Ring-Opening Polymerization

9.2.2.2.1 Ionic Polymerization

This method requires a strict control of experimental conditions. The stringent reaction conditions required by the method certainly explain why relatively few studies based on this approach to grafting have been undertaken.

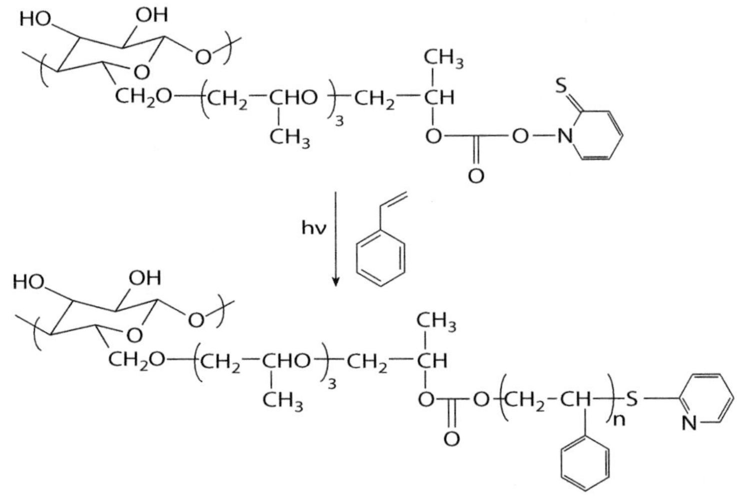

FIGURE 9.4 Grafting of styrene to a hydroxypropyl cellulose–Barton ester derivative. (Reprinted from Daily, H. et al., *Macromol. Symp.*, 174, 155, 2001. With permission.)

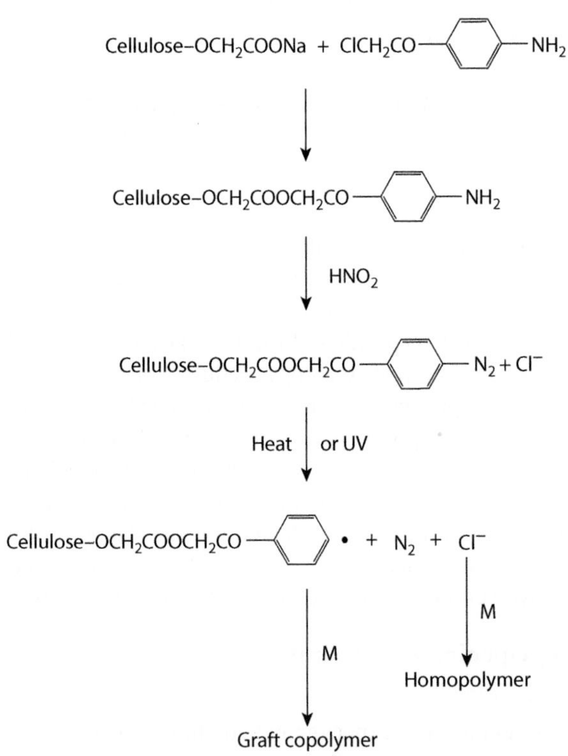

FIGURE 9.5 Introducing a diazonium group onto cellulose to make a cellulosic initiator. (Reprinted from Roy, D. et al., *Chem. Soc. Rev.*, 38, 2046, 2009. With permission.)

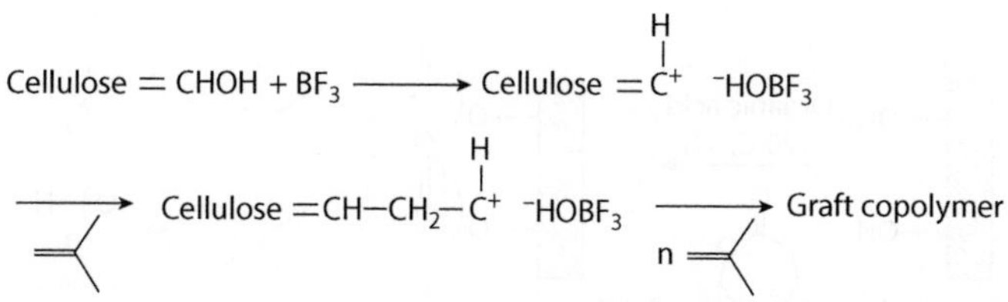

FIGURE 9.6 General mechanism of cationic graft copolymerization of cellulose with isobutylene. (Reprinted from Roy, D. et al., *Chem. Soc. Rev.*, 38, 2046, 2009. With permission.)

Descriptions of ionic polymerization often employ the terminology used for radical polymerization (initiation, chain growth, chain termination, and chain transfer) although the mechanisms of the two types of polymerization are entirely different.

Lewis acids, such as $AlCl_3$ or BF_3, can also initiate polymerization. In this case, a trace amount of a proton donor (cocatalyst), such as water or methanol, is normally required. For example, water combined with BF_3 forms a complex that provides the protons for the polymerization reaction. An important difference between free radical and ionic polymerization is that a counterion appears only in the latter case. For example, the intermediate formed from the initiation of propene with BF_3–H_2O could be represented as Scheme 9.7:

$$H^+[BF_3OH]^- + CH_2{=}CH-CH_3 \rightarrow (CH_3)_2CH^+[BF_3OH]^- \quad (9.7)$$

The cationic-initiated grafting of isobutylene and of α-methyl Sty onto a cellulosic substrate was studied by (Rausing and Sunner 1962; Roy et al., 2009). In this experimental process, the initiator was formed through the chemical reaction of a Lewis acid (boron trifluoride) with a Lewis base (cellulose hydroxyl groups). Boron trifluoride was adsorbed on the cellulose surface. The resulting complex catalyst systems initiated the graft copolymerization by reacting the cellulose reactive sites with isobutylene and α-methyl Sty. The resulting cellulosic substrate exhibited excellent water resistance properties. Figure 9.6 summarizes the cationic graft polymerization of cellulose with isobutylene (Hebeish and Guthrie, 1981).

9.2.2.2.2 Ring-Opening Polymerization

ROP produces a small number of synthetic commercial polymers. Although no small molecule gets eliminated, the reaction can be considered a condensation polymerization. Monomers suitable for polymerization by ring-opening condensation normally possess two different functional groups within the ring. Examples of suitable monomers are lactams (such as caprolactam), which produce polyamides, and lactons, which produce polyesters. In this technique, an alcohol (or hydroxyl group) is generally used as the initiator for ROP, which makes it especially interesting to utilize ROP of cyclic monomers for the polymer modification of cellulose or cellulose derivatives (Jerome and Lecomte, 2008).

Hafrén and Cordova (2005) reported the direct organic acid-catalyzed, ROP of cyclic monomers such as ε-caprolactone (ε-CL) with solid cotton and paper cellulose as initiators (Figure 9.7). Tartaric acid was used as the most efficient catalyst for the production of PCL-grafted cellulose. PCL is poly(ε-CL).

Yuan et al. (2007) grafted a block copolymer of ε-CL and L-lactide (L-LA) from ethyl cellulose (EC) using ROP (Figure 9.8).

Grafts were produced with varying lengths of the PCL and PLLA (poly-L-LA) blocks to investigate whether varying the sizes and proportions of the blocks could give control over the thermal properties and the biodegradation time. The results showed that grafted EC containing longer blocks of PCL had higher melting temperatures than those with shorter PCL blocks.

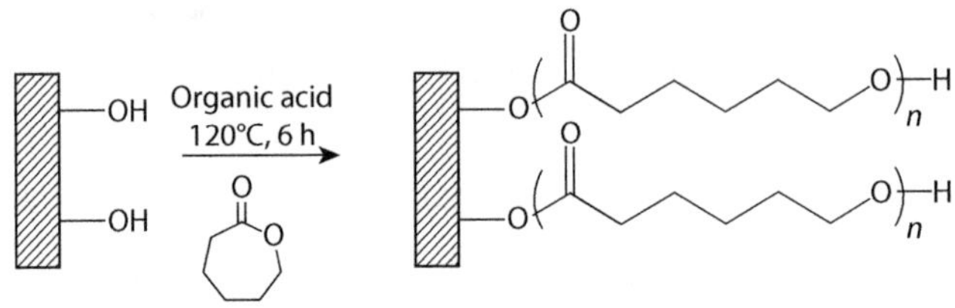

FIGURE 9.7 Organic acid–catalyzed ROP from cellulose fiber. (Reprinted from Hafrén, J. and Cordova, A., *Macromol. Rapid Commun.*, 26, 82, 2005. With permission.)

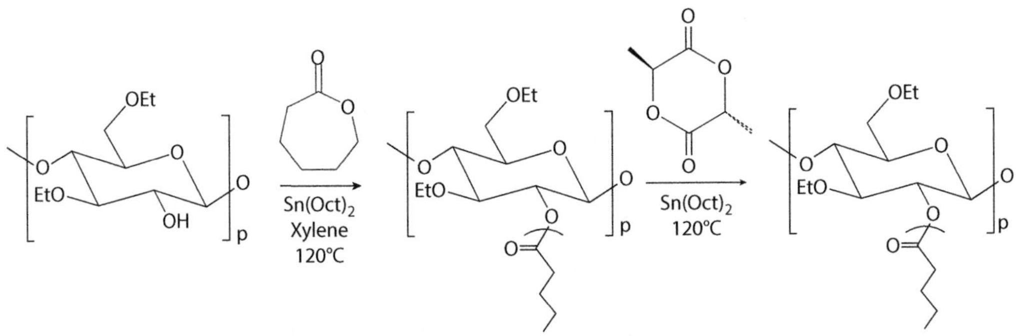

FIGURE 9.8 ROP of ε-CL from HEC (hydroxyethyl cellulose) and subsequently ROP of L-LA from HEC-graft-PCL. (Reprinted with permission from Yuan, W., Yuan, J., Zhang, F., and Xie, X., Syntheses, characterization, and in vitro degradation of ethyl cellulose-graft-poly (e-caprolactone)-block-poly (L-lactide) copolymers by sequential ring-opening polymerization, *Biomacromolecules*, 8(4), 1101–1108. Copyright 2007 American Chemical Society.)

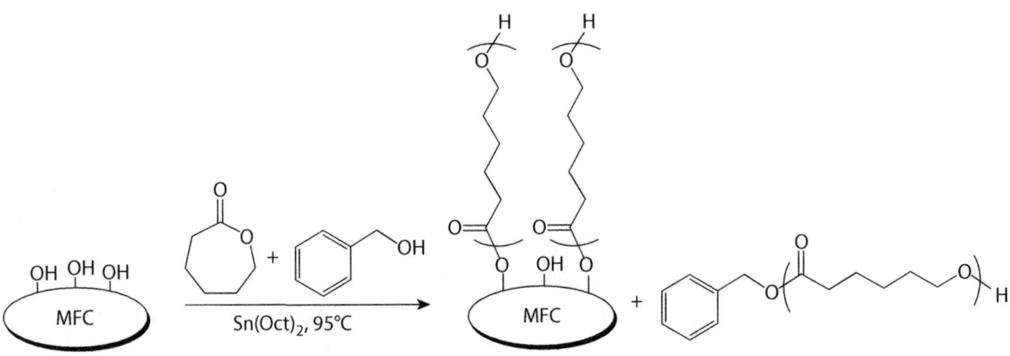

FIGURE 9.9 ROP of ε-caprolactone from microfibrillated cellulose. (Reprinted from Lönnberg, H. et al., *Eur. Polym. J.*, 44, 2991, 2008. With permission.)

The results also showed that the introduction of a PLLA block increased the degradation time of the material.

Lönnberg et al. (2008) were the first to report ROP from microfibrillated cellulose (MFC) (Lönnberg et al., 2008; Carlmark et al., 2012). The grafting was performed by SI-ROP (where SI indicates surface-initiated) of ε-CL in the presence of benzyl alcohol as a free initiator (Figure 9.9), which created grafts on the MFC as well as an unbound free polymer.

Goffin et al. (2012) employed ROP catalyzed by $Sn(Oct)_2$ to graft successively PCL and then PLLA from the surface of CNCs—cellulose nanocrystals (Figure 9.10). Despite the prolonged

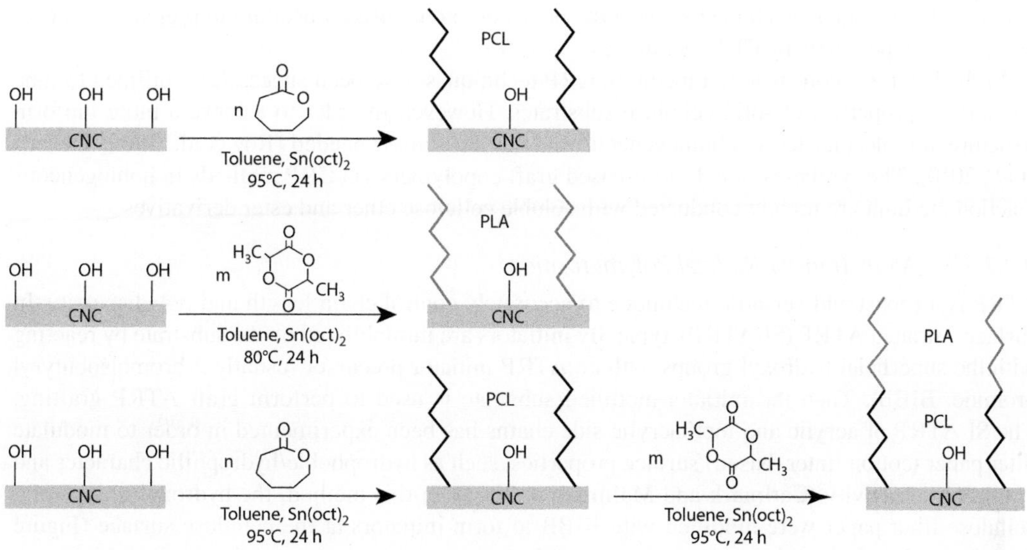

FIGURE 9.10 Illustration of the ROP of PCL, PLA, and PCL-b-PLA initiated from the surface of CNCs. (Reprinted from Goffin, A.-L., *Appl. Mat.*, 4, 3364, 2012. With permission.)

reaction time under metal-catalyzed ROP conditions, the morphology and crystalline structure of the CNCs were preserved. These CNCs grafted with PCL-b-PLA copolymer showed distinct crystallization behavior and dispersion ability when blended with a mixture of immiscible blend of PCL and PLA.

ROP operates through different mechanisms depending on which monomer, initiator, and catalytic system are utilized. Tin(II) 2-ethylhexanoate ($Sn(Oct)_2$) is a commonly used catalyst for the polymerization for monomers such as ε-CL, LA, and *p*-dioxanone. Several different mechanisms have been hypothesized for this system, but the most commonly accepted mechanism for the initiation is that $Sn(Oct)_2$ is converted into tin alkoxide, the actual initiator, by reaction with alcohols or other protic compounds.

9.2.2.3 Controlled/Living Radical Polymerization

The term "living polymerization" was first defined by Szwarc (1956) as a chain growth process, without chain-breaking reactions such as chain transfer or irreversible termination. Living polymerization mechanisms provide polymers of controlled composition, architecture, and molecular weight distribution. Thus, end-functional polymers with narrow polydispersity can be achieved easily. Further, high-purity block copolymers, graft, stars, and other polymers with complex architectures can be obtained. The combination of a living mechanism with the versatile radical process gives more freedom in choosing a wide range of monomers and reaction conditions (Moad and Solomon, 2006).

The CRP techniques, such as ATRP (Matyjaszewski and Xia, 2001), single-electron-transfer living radical polymerization (SET-LRP) (Rosen and Percec, 2009; Nguyen and Percec, 2010), nitroxide-mediated polymerization (NMP) (Hawker et al., 2001), and reversible addition–fragmentation chain transfer (RAFT) polymerization (Barner et al., 2007; Barner-Kowollik, 2008), have been applied to cellulose grafting. These approaches allow the tailoring of the properties of cellulose-based graft copolymers by tuning the synthetic graft length, the architecture, and also the chemical composition of the product (Tizzotti et al., 2010). The "grafting from" procedure involves the preliminary conversion of cellulose hydroxyl groups into CRP-relevant chemical groups such as nitroxides, haloesters, or thiocarbonyl-thio derivatives. Moreover, the growth of the synthetic polymer chain from a backbone has been the most commonly used procedure to prepare cellulose-based graft copolymers by CRP techniques.

In the heterogeneous reaction medium, CRP techniques have been successfully utilized to tune the surface properties of solid cellulose substrates. However, in order to achieve a more uniform structure at molecular level, a homogeneous reaction medium is needed (Roy et al., 2009; Tizzotti et al., 2010). The syntheses of cellulose-based graft copolymers via CRP methods in homogeneous reaction medium are mainly conducted with soluble cellulose ether and ester derivatives.

9.2.2.3.1 Atom Transfer Radical Polymerization

ATRP is a robust and versatile technique to accurately control chain length and polydispersity. In surface-initiated ATRP (SI-ATRP), typically initiators are immobilized on the substrate by reacting with the superficial hydroxyl groups with an ATRP initiator precursor (usually 2-bromoisobutyryl bromide, BIBB). Then the initiator-modified substrate is used to perform graft ATRP grafting. The SI-ATRP of acrylic and methacrylic side chains has been experimented in order to modulate filter paper (cotton linter–based) surface properties, such as hydrophobic/hydrophilic character and antibacterial activity (Carlmark and Malmstrom, 2003). In this method, the hydroxyl groups of a cellulose filter paper were modified with BIBB to form initiators at the cellulose surface (Figure 9.11). Methyl acrylate (MA) was grafted from the surface in the presence of a sacrificial initiator. The resulting PMA-grafted paper showed excellent hydrophobicity.

ATRP has also been used to modify a variety of cellulosic substrates, cellulose powder (Coskun et al., 2005), EC (Shen and Huang, 2006), HPC (Ostmark et al., 2007), and hydroxyethyl cellulose (HEC; Yang et al., 2007).

Coskun et al. (2005) modified a cellulose powder. In this study, Sty, methyl methacrylate (MMA), methacrylamide (MAm), and acrylomorpholine were grafted onto powder cellulose by ATRP. It is known that the chloroacetyl group in any ester is an effective initiator for ATRP (Kamigaito et al., 2001). According to this study, cellulose chloroacetate (Cell-ClAc), as a macro-initiator, was first prepared by the reaction of chloroacetyl chloride with primary alcoholic OH groups on powder cellulose. CuBr and 1,2-dipiperidinoethane were used as a transition metal compound and as a ligand, respectively. Cellulose chloroacetate was first obtained, and then a series of grafting studies onto cellulose were carried out using a 1,2-dipiperidinoethane–Cu(I) complex as a catalyst of atom-transfer radical graft copolymerization. The 1,2-dipiperidinoethane-Cu(I) complex has also successfully catalyzed the grafting of poly[styrene-co-(*p*-chlorostyrene)] with ethyl methacrylate by ATRP, and the growth from chloromethyl groups provided the graft copolymers with relatively low dispersities (Mw/Mn = 1.60 – 2.05) in the case of poly[styrene-co-(*p*-chlorostyrene)] (62:38 by mole) macro-initiator. All reactions of grafting on cellulose are indicated in Figure 9.12. Chloroacetate groups here act as initiator sites.

Although most of the studies have concentrated on the modification of cellulose in its solid state, recent work has shown that ATRP polymerization can also be applied to soluble polysaccharides, in homogeneous reaction conditions.

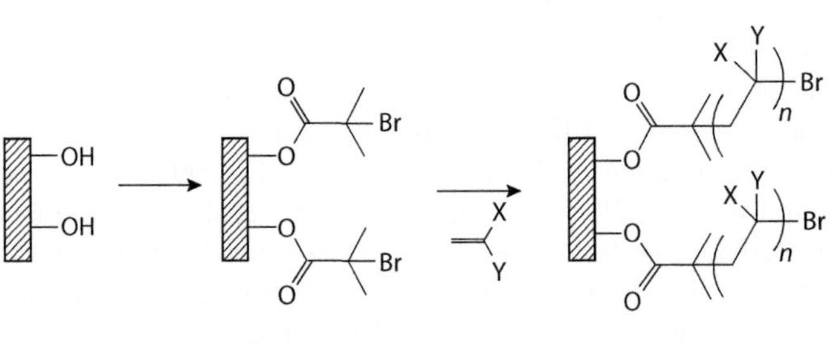

FIGURE 9.11 Formation of graft copolymers on cellulose fibers using ATRP. (Reprinted from Roy, D. et al., *Chem. Soc. Rev.*, 38, 2046, 2009. With permission.)

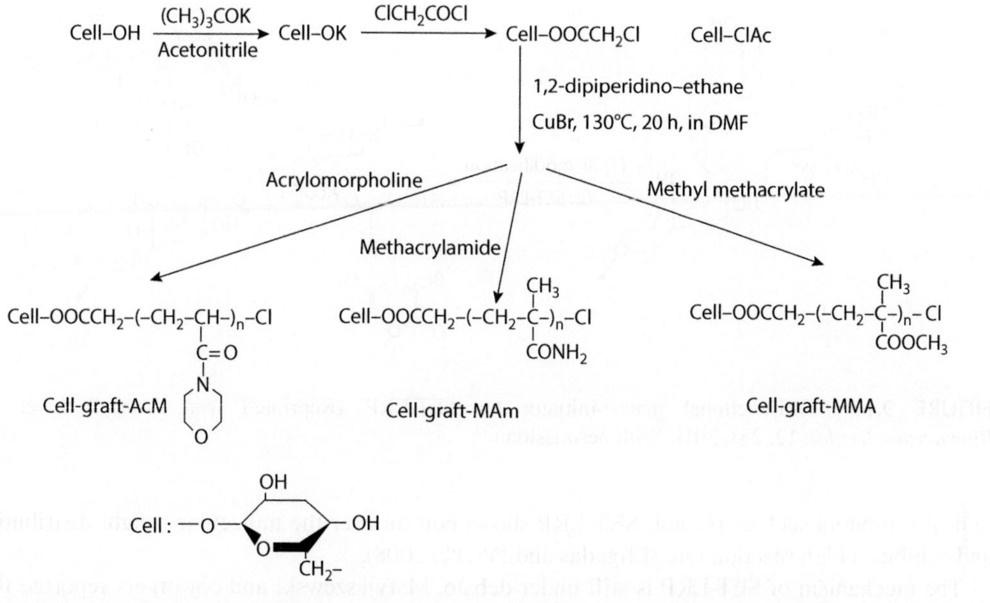

FIGURE 9.12 Reactions of grafting on cellulose by ATRP. (Reprinted from Coskun, M. et al., *Polym. Int.*, 54, 342, 2005. With permission.)

Rannard et al. (2007) reported the atom transfer radical graft copolymerization at ambient temperature in water from a soluble polysaccharide such as locust bean gum. The hydroxyl groups of the polysaccharide were modified with an acid imidazolide to form ATRP initiators for the polymerization of a series of water-soluble methacrylates and styrenic monomers. High-molecular-weight graft copolymers with targeted graft lengths were achieved.

9.2.2.3.2 *Single-Electron-Transfer Living Radical Polymerization*

SET-LRP was introduced by Percec et al. (2006). The authors claim that SET-LRP is catalyzed by extremely reactive Cu (0), which is formed by low-activation-energy outer-sphere SET. The reaction is controlled or deactivated by Cu (II) species that are formed via the same process (see Figure 9.13). It has been reported that SET-LRP is very effective at room temperature and that extremely high molecular weights can be obtained in conjunction with a low PDI. Even in the presence of typical

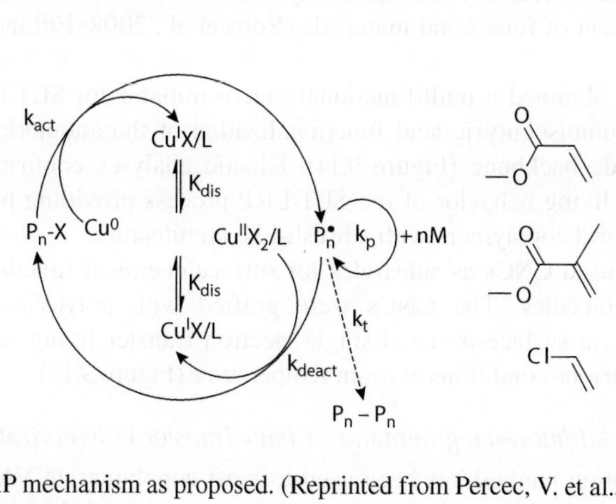

FIGURE 9.13 SET-LRP mechanism as proposed. (Reprinted from Percec, V. et al., *J. Am. Chem. Soc.*, 128, 14156, 2006. With permission.)

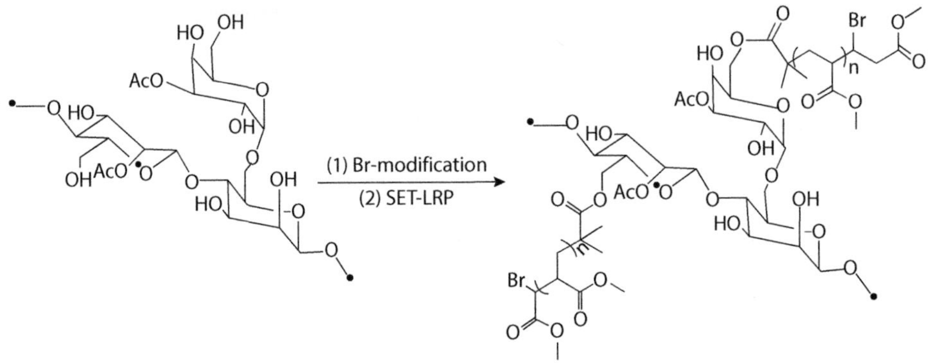

FIGURE 9.14 Multifunctional macro-initiator for SET-LRP. (Reprinted from Voepel, J. et al., *Biomacromolecules*, 12, 253, 2011. With permission.)

radical inhibitors such as phenol, SET-LRP shows control over the molecular weight distribution and exhibits a high reaction rate (Lligadas and Percec, 2008).

The mechanism of SET-LRP is still under debate. Matyjaszewski and coworkers reported that according to their results the reaction follows the same mechanism as activators regenerated by electron transfer ATRP, and the role of Cu (0) is limited to that of the reducing agent.

According to Percec et al.'s (2006) work, SET-LRP occurs under very mild reaction conditions, at room temperature and below, uses a catalytic rather than a stoichiometric amount of catalyst, and, although proceeds ultrafast, generates polymers with unprecedentedly high molecular weight. SET-LRP is general and applies to both nonactivated and activated monomers containing electron-withdrawing functional groups, such as vinyl chloride and other halogenated monomers, acrylates, and methacrylates. It also applies to organic reactions and tolerates a diversity of functional groups.

The versatility and controllability of the SET-LRP strategy open up a range of possibilities to use this method for the site-specific controlled grafting from functionalized sites on macromolecules thereby producing graft copolymers and brush-like structure. As such, the method is appealing for the design of hybrid materials from macromolecules that do not otherwise lend themselves to vinyl copolymerization, such as polymers based on sugar moieties, known as polysaccharides. An abundant, inexpensive, renewable, and green candidate from this family is acetylated galactoglucomannan (AcGGM), a softwood hemicellulose. Hartman et al. (2006) have previously demonstrated its viability and versatility as a candidate for various chemical modifications and the development of functional materials (Roos et al., 2008; Edlund et al., 2010; Voepel et al., 2011).

Voepel et al. (2011) obtained a multifunctional macro-initiator for SET-LRP. It was designed from AcGGM by α-bromoisobutyric acid functionalization of the anomeric hydroxyl groups on the heteropolysaccharide backbone (Figure 9.14). Kinetic analyses confirmed high conversions of up to 99.98% and a living behavior of the SET-LRP process providing high-molecular-weight hemicelluloses/MA hybrid copolymers with a brush-like architecture.

Zoppe et al. (2010) used CNCs as substrates for surface chemical functionalization with thermoresponsive macromolecules. The CNCs were grafted with poly(*N*-isopropylacrylamide)—PolyNiPAAm brushes via surface-initiated single-electron transfer living radical polymerization (SI-SET-LRP) under various conditions at room temperature (Figure 9.15).

9.2.2.3.3 Reversible Addition–Fragmentation Chain Transfer Polymerization

The RAFT polymerization method has been used to graft-copolymerize VAc, Sty, acrylates, and acrylamides from soluble cellulose ethers such as hydroxypropyl, ethyl hydroxyethyl, and methyl

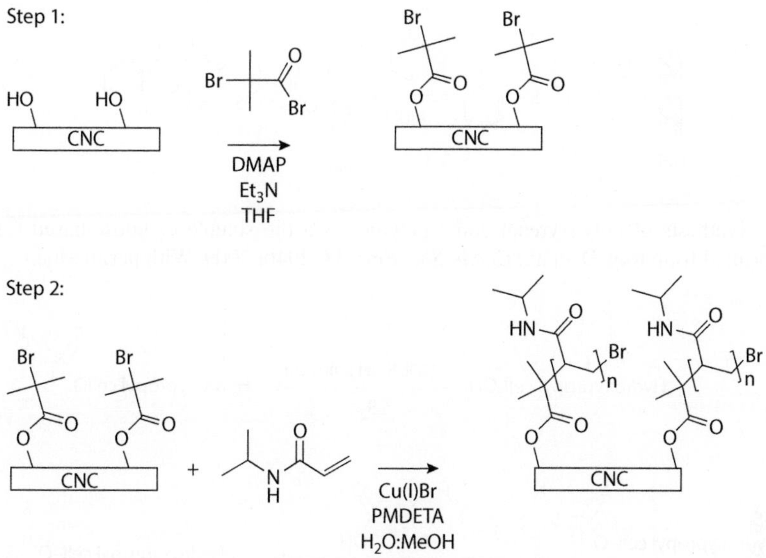

FIGURE 9.15 Synthesis route for the grafting of poly(NiPAAm) from the surface of cellulose nanocrystals where PMDETA—*N,N,N′,N″,N″*-pentamethyldiethylenetriamine (PMDETA), DMAP—2-dimethylaminopyridine (DMAP). (Reprinted from Zoppe, J. et al., *Biomacromolecules,* 11, 2683, 2010. With permission.)

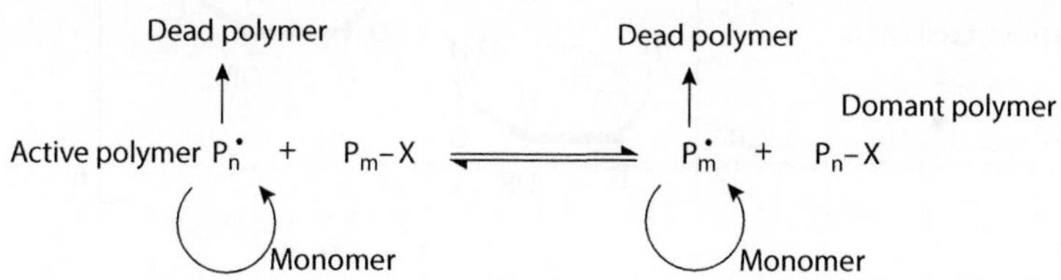

FIGURE 9.16 Polymerization with reversible deactivation by degenerate chain transfer. (From Moad, G. et al., 2008.)

cellulose. It is an effective method for providing living characteristics to radical polymerization (Barner-Kowollik, 2008; Moad et al., 2008, 2009). RAFT provides reversible deactivation of propagating radicals by degenerate chain transfer for which a general mechanism is shown in Figure 9.16 (Moad et al., 2008). The chain transfer step has been termed degenerate because the process involves an exchange of functionality, and the only distinction between the species on the two sides of the equilibrium is molar mass.

Stenzel et al. (2003) and Hernandez-Guerrero et al. (2005) were the first to report the preparation of a trithiocarbonate chain transfer agent based on the soluble cellulose derivative, hydroxysopropyl cellulose (HPC), by attaching the RAFT agent to cellulose through its stabilizing "Z"-group (Z-group approach), to obtain poly(Sty) comb polymers. Since the chain transfer agent was attached via its Z-group, the molecular weight of the poly(Sty) branch showed a pronounced deviation from the theoretical molecular weight due to reduced accessibility of the RAFT group at high polymerization conversions (Figure 9.17).

Fleet et al. (2008) studied the synthesis and characterization of hybrid cellulose-based materials using existing cellulose modification technology together with advanced LRP techniques. According to the authors, it was the first time VAc has been grafted onto cellulosic materials via the RAFT process, where xanthate was used as RAFT agent.

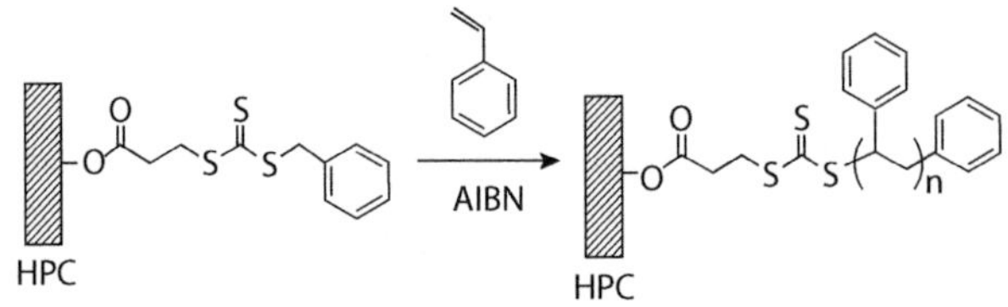

FIGURE 9.17 Synthesis of poly(styrene) comb polymers via the soluble cellulose-based CTA (Z-group approach). (Reprinted from Roy, D. et al., *Chem. Soc. Rev.*, 38, 2046, 2009. With permission.)

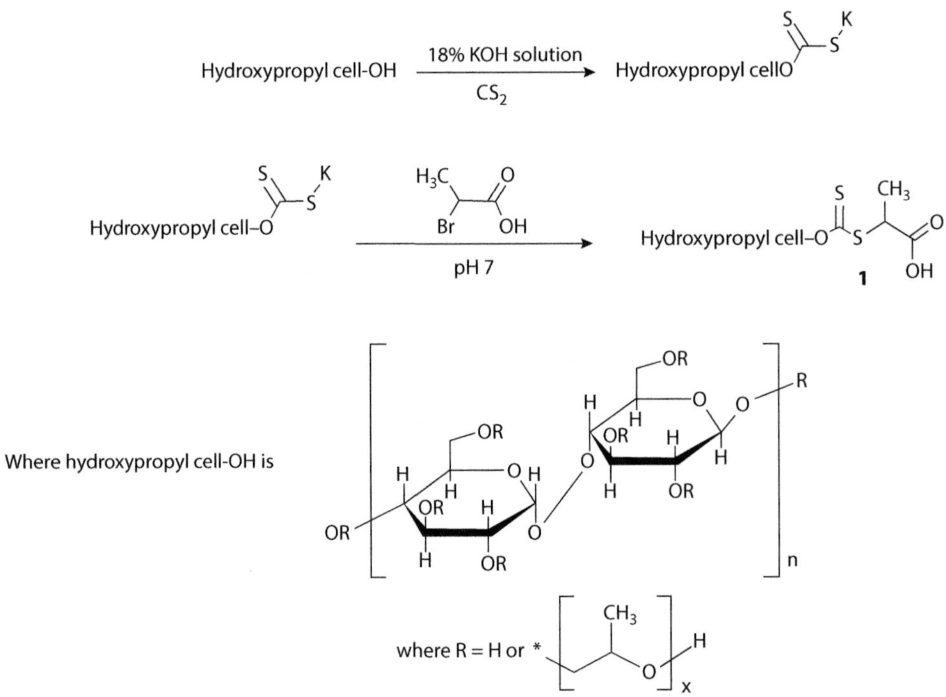

FIGURE 9.18 Preparation of S-sec propionic acid hydroxypropyl cellulose xanthate RAFT agent (**1**). (Reprinted from Fleet, R. et al., *Eur. Polym. J.*, 44, 2899, 2008. With permission.)

Xanthate RAFT agents were synthesized through the formation of xanthate salts directly on a cellulosic substrate and subsequent alkylation to the cellulosic materials (Figure 9.18).

The cellulosic materials are combined with a nonpolar vinyl polymer (polyvinyl acetate) via Z-group approach to yield an amphiphilic graft copolymer. The resulting graft copolymers are complex multicomponent hybrid materials with a molar mass distribution as well as a chemical composition distribution.

Perrier and coworkers performed grafting of Sty from cellulose substrate via RAFT polymerization. The hydroxyl groups of cellulose fiber were converted into thiocarbonyl-thio chain transfer agent and were further used to mediate the RAFT polymerization of Sty. Figure 9.19 illustrates the outline of the synthesis of the cellulose-based RAFT agent and of cellulose-g-poly(Sty) copolymer, mediated by the RAFT process.

9.2.2.3.4 Commercial Availability of RAFT Agents

A range of RAFT agents (Figure 9.20) including the carboxylic acid functional RAFT agents **a, b,** and **c** are now commercially available in research quantities (Moad et al., 2010, 2011).

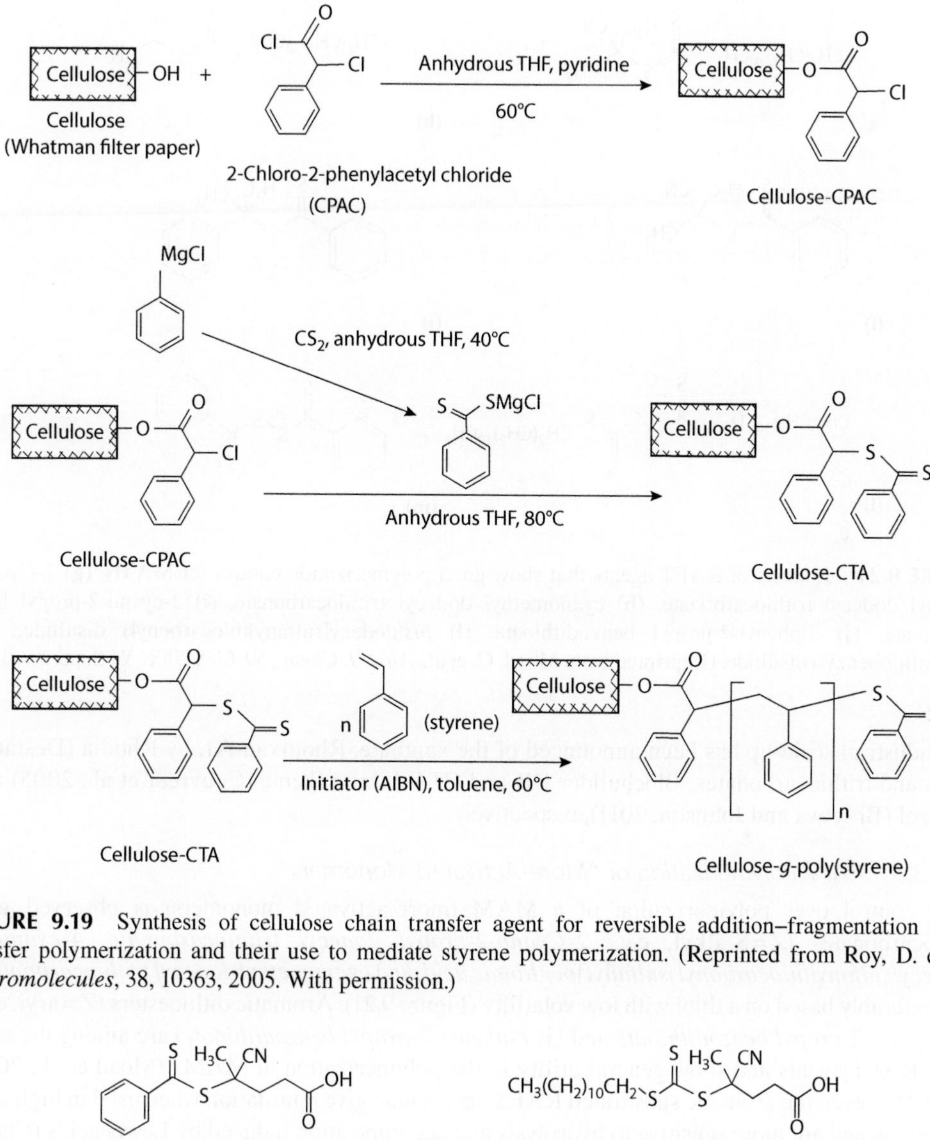

FIGURE 9.19 Synthesis of cellulose chain transfer agent for reversible addition–fragmentation chain transfer polymerization and their use to mediate styrene polymerization. (Reprinted from Roy, D. et al., *Macromolecules*, 38, 10363, 2005. With permission.)

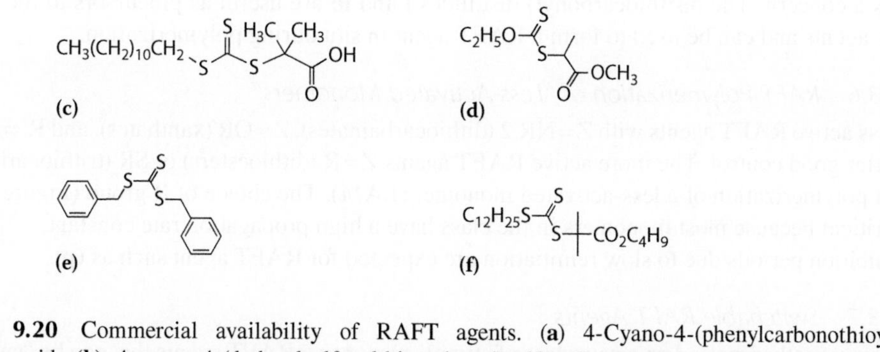

FIGURE 9.20 Commercial availability of RAFT agents. (**a**) 4-Cyano-4-(phenylcarbonothioylthio) pentanoic acid, (**b**) 4-cyano-4-(dodecylsulfanylthiocarbonyl)sulfanyl] pentanoic acid, (**c**) 2-(dodecylthio carbonothioylthio)-2-methylpropionic acid, (**d**) Rhodixan A1, (**e**) Blocbuilder DB, and (**f**) Lubrizol CTA-1. (Reprinted from Moad, G. et al., *Mater. Matters*, 5, 2, 2010. With permission.)

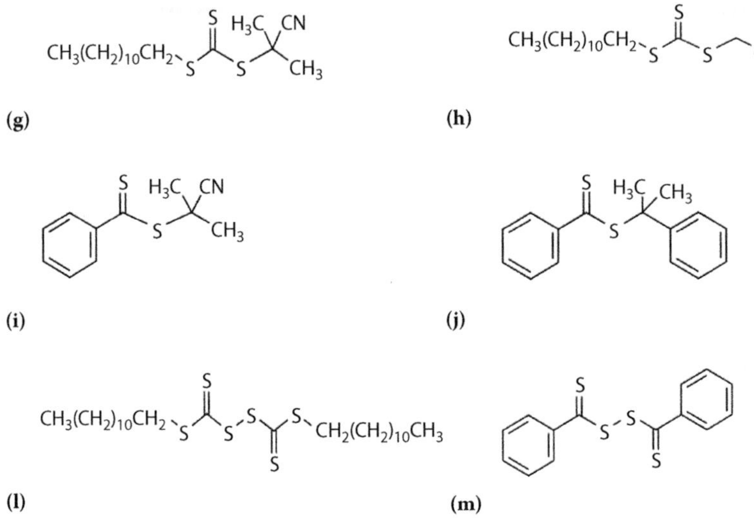

FIGURE 9.21 A series of RAFT agents that show good polymerization control for MAMs. (**g**) 2-Cyano-2-propyl dodecyl trithiocarbonate, (**h**) cyanomethyl dodecyl trithiocarbonate, (**i**) 2-cyano-2-propyl benzodithioate, (**j**) 2-phenyl-2-propyl benzodithioate, (**l**) *bis*(dodecylsulfanylthiocarbonyl) disulfide, and (**m**) *bis*(thiobenzyl) disulfide. (Reprinted from Moad, G. et al., *Aust. J. Chem.*, 59, 669, 2006. With permission.)

The industrial scale-up has been announced of the xanthate, Rhodixan-A1, by Rhodia (Destarac, 2010), and trithiocarbonates, Blocbuilder DB and CTA-1, by Arkema (Couvreur et al., 2005) and Lubrizol (Brzytwa and Johnson, 2011), respectively.

9.2.2.3.5 RAFT Polymerization of "More-Activated Monomers"

Good control over polymerization of a MAM (more-activated monomers) is observed with trithiocarbonates (Z=S-alkyl, e.g., 2-*Cyano-2-propyl dodecyl trithiocarbonate,* 4-*cyano*-4-*[(dodecylsulfanylthiocarbonyl)sulfanyl]pentanoic acid*, and *cyanomethyl dodecyl trithiocarbonate*). Z is preferably based on a thiol with low volatility (Figure 9.21). Aromatic dithioesters (Z=aryl, e.g., [**i**] 2-*cyano-2-propyl benzodithioate* and [**j**] 2-*phenyl-2-propyl benzodithioate*) are among the most active RAFT agents and show general utility in the polymerization of MAMs (Moad et al., 2005, 2006). However, the aromatic substituted RAFT agents may give retardation when used in high concentrations and are more sensitive to hydrolysis and decomposition induced by Lewis acids (Chong et al., 2007; Rizzardo et al., 2007). Alkyl-substituted RAFT agents (**b**, **g**, **h**) can be tried if hydrolysis is a concern. The bis(thiocarbonyl) disulfides **l** and **m** are useful as precursors to the tertiary RAFT agents and can be used to form a RAFT agent in situ during polymerization.

9.2.2.3.6 RAFT Polymerization of "Less-Activated Monomers"

The less active RAFT agents with Z=NR′2 (dithiocarbamates), Z=OR′(xanthates), and R′=alkyl or aryl offer good control. The more active RAFT agents Z=R (dithioesters) or SR (trithiocarbonates) inhibit polymerization of a less-activated monomer (LAM). The choice of R group (Figure 9.22) is also critical because most monomers in the class have a high propagation rate constant.

Inhibition periods due to slow reinitiation are expected for RAFT agent such as (**p**).

9.2.2.3.7 Switchable RAFT Agents

We have recently reported on a new class of stimuli-responsive RAFT agents that can be "switched" to offer good control over polymerization of both MAMs and LAMs and thus a more convenient route to polyMAM-block-polyLAM polymers with narrowed molecular weight distributions.

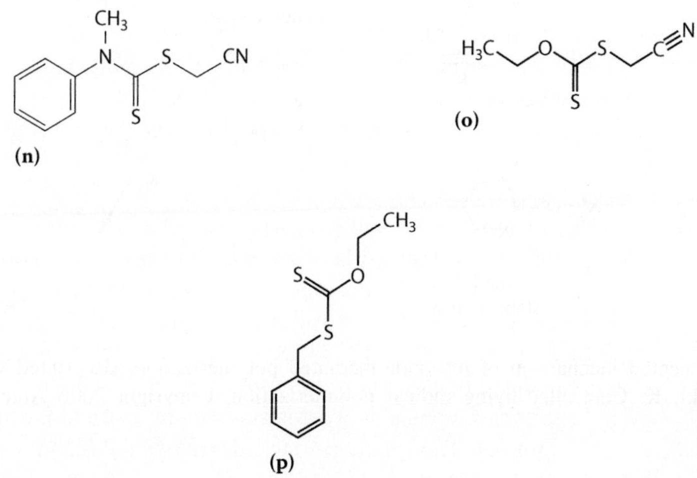

FIGURE 9.22 A series of RAFT agents that show good polymerization control for LAMs. (**n**) Cyanomethyl methyl(phenyl)carbamodithioate, (**o**) S-(cyanomethyl) O-ethyl carbonodithioate, and (**p**) S-benzyl O-ethyl carbonodithioate. (Reprinted from Moad, G. et al., *Aust. J. Chem.*, 59, 669, 2006. With permission.)

This approach was demonstrated with the use of 4-pyridinyl-*N*-methyldi-thiocarbamate derivatives to prepare PMMA-block-PVAc and PMA-block-PNVC. The *N*-4-pyridinyl-*N*-methyldithiocarbamates provide effective control over polymerization of LAMs (Scheme 9.2) and when protonated also provide excellent control over the polymerization of MAMs.9

9.2.2.3.8 Nitroxide-Mediated Polymerization

NMP belongs to a large family of stable free radical polymerization processes and is based on the use of a stable nitroxide radical. It is a very attractive CRP system (Hawker et al., 1996) because it is metal free and effective in the polymerization of a broad range of monomers with various functionalities. This system provides colorless and odorless polymers with no demanding purification. This control of the NMP process relies on the reversible capture of the propagating species by nitroxides with formation of dormant chains (alkoxyamines) (Figure 9.23). Whenever this equilibrium is shifted toward the dormant form, the stationary concentration of the active species is low, and the irreversible chain termination is limited (Sciannamea et al., 2008).

Either bimolecular or unimolecular initiators can be used in NMP (Hawker et al., 2001). The bimolecular initiation requires combining a traditional free radical initiator (e.g., benzoyl peroxide [BPO] and 2,2′-azobis(isobutyronitrile) [AIBN]) with a nitroxide (e.g., 2,2,6,6-tetrame thylpiperidinyloxy—TEMPO) (Georges et al., 1993).

TEMPO (2,2,6,6-tetramethyl-1-piperidinyloxy) is one the more commonly used nitroxide radicals in this respect. In this method, the propagating species ($P_n^{\bullet}$) reacts with a stable radical ($X^{\bullet}$) to form

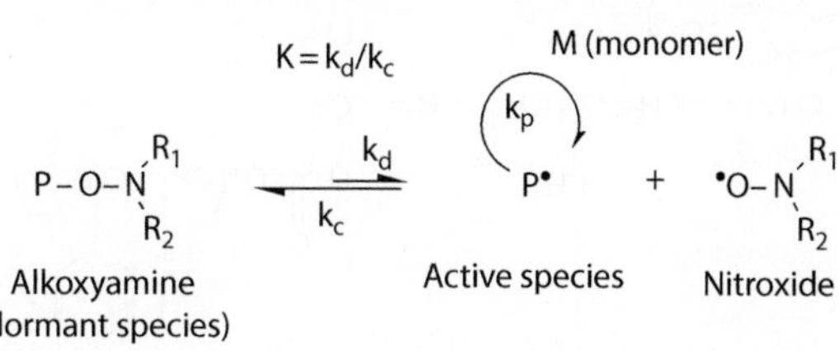

FIGURE 9.23 Reversible capture of the propagating species by nitroxides with the formation of dormant chains (alkoxyamines).

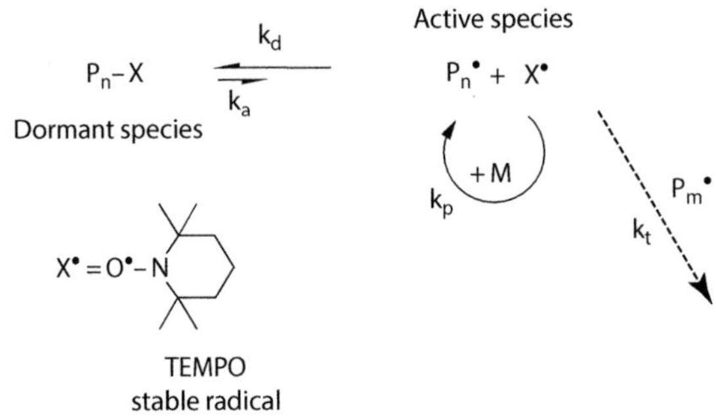

FIGURE 9.24 Accepted mechanism of nitroxide-mediated polymerization. (Reprinted with permission from Matyjaszewski, K. Controlled/living radical polymerization. Copyright 2006 American Chemical Society, 2000.)

dormant species (P_n–X). Thus, deactivation of propagating radicals occurs. The resulting dormant species can then reversibly cleave to reform the free radicals. Once $P_n^\bullet$ forms, it can propagate by reacting with a monomer (M), or it can terminate with other growing radicals. NMP requires only the addition of an appropriate alkoxyamine to the polymerization system. Polymerization is usually undertaken at high temperatures (>120°C) (Matyjaszewski, 2000). This method is widely applicable

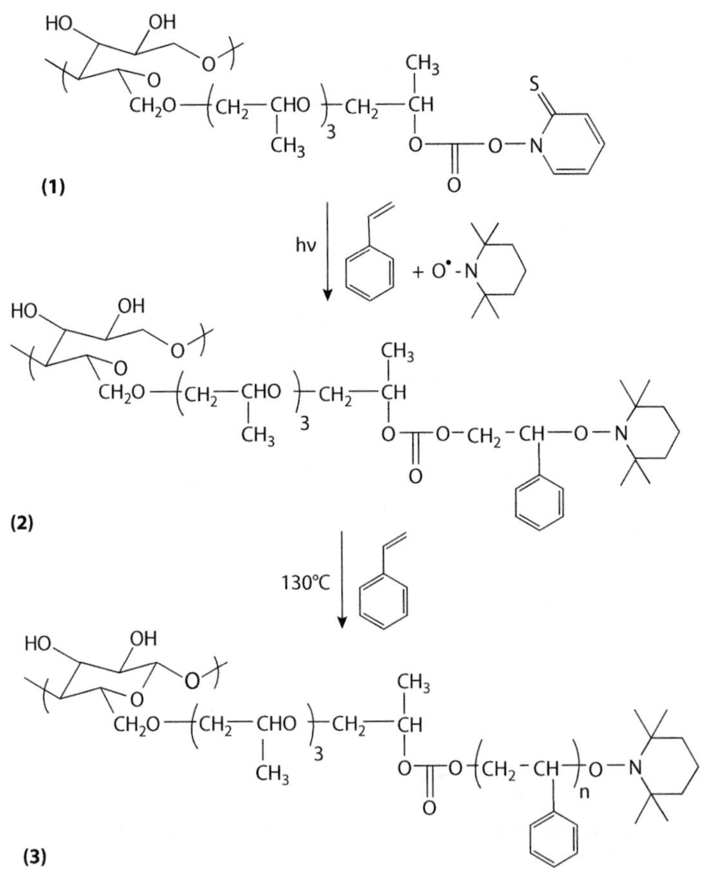

FIGURE 9.25 NMP-mediated controlled radical grafting from hydroxypropyl cellulose. (Reprinted from Roy, D. et al., *Chem. Soc. Rev.*, 38, 2046, 2009. With permission.)

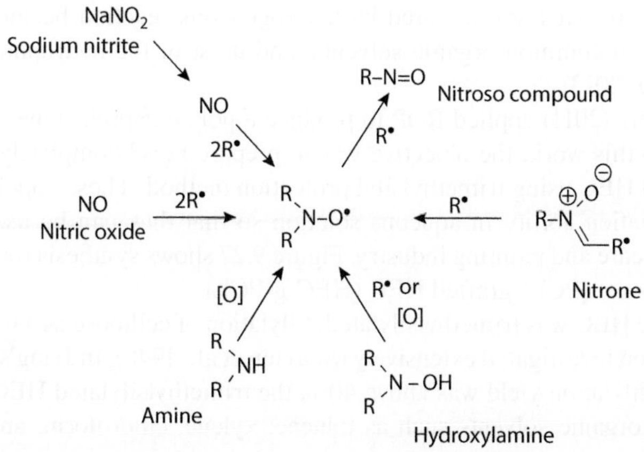

FIGURE 9.26 Nitroxide precursors: most of these precursors are known as inhibitors of radical polymerization. (Reprinted with permission from Chauvin, C. et al., Controlled/living radical polymerization. Copyright 2006 American Chemical Society; Sciannamea, V. et al., *Chemical Reviews*, 108, 1104, 2008.)

to Sty and acrylate monomers. Its use for the polymerization of methacrylates and MAms requires the presence of specially designed nitroxides (Chauvin, 2006). A simplified mechanism of NMP is shown in Figure 9.24.

Daly et al. (1992) reported the first use of nitroxide-mediated, controlled radical grafting from cellulose and cellulose derivatives. The controlled radical grafting from HPC was performed using TEMPO monoadducts, formed from the HPC–Barton carbonate derivative (carbonates of *N*-hydroxypyridine-2-thione) **1** (Figure 9.25). The photolysis of **1** in the presence of Sty and TEMPO provided adduct **2**. Heating the macro-initiator at 130°C provided Sty–HPC graft copolymers **3**. An increase in grafted polymeric chain length with increasing polymerization time was observed. The polydispersity of the poly(Sty) grafts ranged from 1.3 to 1.5. However, the grafting was limited to Sty monomer only and required the use of high temperatures.

Although NMP is now extremely efficient for the preparation of a variety of well-defined (co) polymers, availability and cost of nitroxides and/or alkoxyamines remain a concern. Indeed, alkoxyamines are commonly synthesized by the coupling of an alkyl radical to a nitroxide that must be synthesized (usually by a multistep reaction) and purified (Sciannamea et al., 2008).

As an alternative strategy, several researchers have contemplated the direct formation of nitroxides and alkoxyamines in the polymerization medium from readily and/or commercially available and inexpensive precursors. Both the initiating radicals and the mediators would be produced in a one-pot technique, designated as in situ nitroxide-mediated polymerization (in situ NMP). A large variety of nitroxide precursors have been considered, which includes nitrones, nitroso compounds, hydroxylamines, amines, sodium nitrite, and nitric oxide (Figure 9.26). Most of these precursors are known as inhibitors of radical polymerization (Tanczos et al., 1982).

9.3 GRAFT COPOLYMERS FROM CELLULOSE: APPLICATIONS AND CHARACTERIZATION METHODS

Hydrophobically modified cellulose derivates have been investigated extensively. Though the substitution degree of hydrophobic groups is low, these hydrophobically modified cellulose derivates exhibit interesting rheological behaviors such as a much stronger viscosity enhancement with increasing concentration as compared with the corresponding unmodified parent polymer. With the addition of the surfactant, the strength of hydrophobic interaction of the hydrophobically modified cellulose derivates can be modulated easily. However, so far, most of the hydrophobically modified cellulose derivatives are prepared by heterogeneous reaction because cellulose derivatives cannot dissolve in common organic solvents, and most of the hydrophobic parts are undegradable (Qiu and Hu, 2013).

Jiang and coworkers (2011) applied ROP to produce a poly(ε-caprolactone)-grafted HEC copolymers. According to this work, the objective was to prepare novel completely degradable poly(ε-caprolactone)-grafted HEC using trimethylsilyl protection method. These copolymers are expected to have strong association ability in aqueous solution so that they can be used as thickener and stabilizer in personal care and painting industry. Figure 9.27 shows synthesis routes for HEC-g-PCL (poly(ε-polycaprolactone) (PCL)-grafted HEC (HEC-g-PCL).

In the first step, the HEC was trimethylsilylated. Silylation of cellulose as a route to reactive soluble derivatives has been investigated extensively (Shuyten et al., 1948). In Jiang's experiments, it was found that when the silylation yield was above 40%, the trimethylsilylated HEC (TMSHEC) could dissolve in common organic solvents such as toluene, xylene, chloroform, and acetone. Because

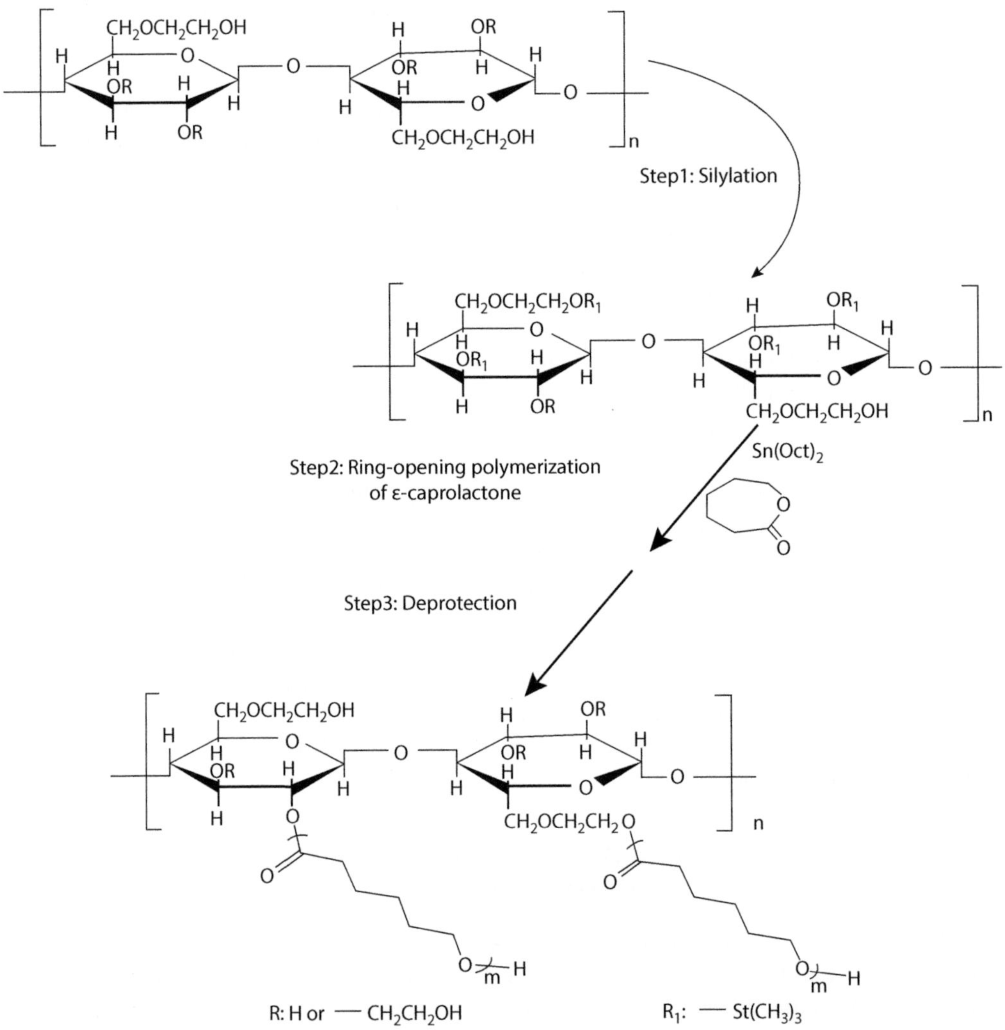

FIGURE 9.27 Synthesis of HEC-g-PCL copolymers. (Reprinted from Jiang, C. et al., *Int. J. Biol. Macromol.*, 48, 210, 2011. With permission.)

the goal was to prepare amphiphilic HEC-g-PCL copolymers, TMSHEC with high silylation yield of 83.2% was used to synthesize TMSHEC-g-PCL so that a limited amount of PCL grafts can grow away from the remaining free alcohol functions (Ydens et al., 2000). In the second step, the PCL was grafted on the HEC through the ROP of CL (ε-polycaprolactone) and the condensation between the PCL and rest –OH of HEC in the homogeneous solution. In the third step, HEC-g-PCL copolymers were obtained by deprotecting trimethylsilylation. Both gravimetry methods and ^{1}H NMR were used to determine the PCL weight fraction in the copolymers (FPCL). According to Ydens et al. (2000), ^{1}H NMR usually leads to higher FPCL value than gravimetry ones due to the ^{1}H NMR instrument reason, gravimetry is better suited than ^{1}H NMR to determine the FPCL, especially when initial CL weight fraction is higher than 0.3. Table 9.1 shows the polymerization conditions of HEC-g-PCL copolymers. Three HEC-g-PCL copolymers, namely, G1–G3, were prepared. Therefore, gravimetric analysis was used to determine the FPCL values of G1, G2, and G3, and their values were 16.3%, 25.7%, and 32.2%, respectively.

Figure 9.28 is the FTIR spectra of HEC, TMSHEC, TMSHEC-g-PCL, and HEC-g-PCL. Compared with the spectrum of HEC, the spectrum of TMSHEC shows additional absorption peaks at 1251, 877, 840, and 750 cm^{-1}. All these peaks originated from the Si–Me group. After the TMSHEC-g-PCL was deprotected, these peaks disappeared as is shown in Figure 9.28, spectra D. FTIR spectra of TMSHEC-g-PCL and HEC-g-PCL show the C double bond; length as m-dash O absorption peak at 1730 cm^{-1}, this indicates that the PCL has been grafted on the HEC.

The ^{1}H NMR spectra of the HEC, TMSHEC-g-PCL , and HEC-g-PCL can confirm the above information. The methyl proton of the TMS groups could be observed at δ_f=0.1 ppm. Peaks at

TABLE 9.1
Polymerization Conditions of Grafted Copolymer

Samples	TMSHEC (g)	CL (mL)	[CL]/[OH]	Sn(Oct)$_2$/OH	T (°C)	t (h)	F_{PCL} (%)
G1	1	0.3	3.5	0.05	100	24	16.3
G2	1	0.5	5.8	0.05	100	24	25.7
G3	1	0.7	8.2	0.05	100	24	32.2

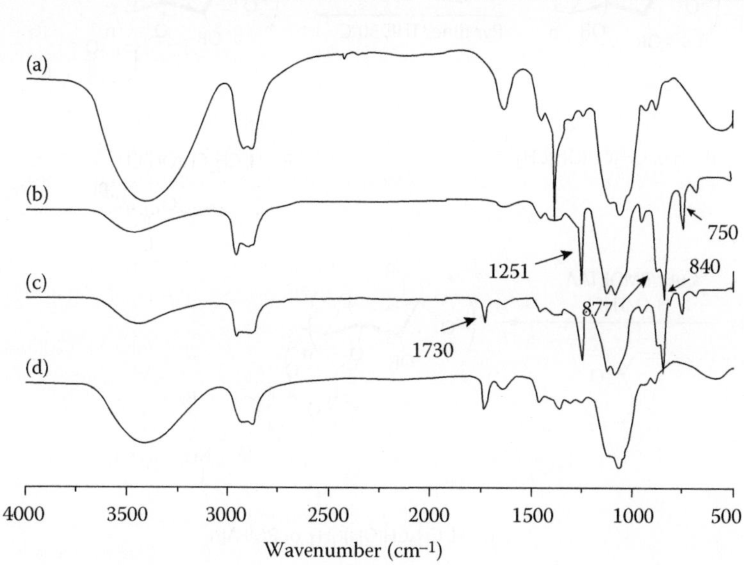

FIGURE 9.28 FTIR spectra of (a) HEC, (b) TMSHEC, (c) TMSHEC-g-PCL, and (d) HEC-g-PCL. (Reprinted from Jiang, C. et al., *Int. J. Biol. Macromol.*, 48, 210, 2011. With permission.)

$\delta_a = 2.27$ ppm, $\delta_b = 1.38$ ppm, $\delta_c = 1.27$ ppm, $\delta_d = 1.51$ ppm, and $\delta_e = 4.1$ ppm were contributed from the methylene proton of PCL. This confirms that the grafting of PCL on the HEC is successful. After the TMSHEC-g-PCL was deprotected, the methyl proton of the TMS groups ($\delta_f = 0.1$ ppm) disappeared. This is in agreement with the results of the FTIR spectrum.

For the other work, Jin et al. (2013) applied SET-LRP method to get copolymer hydroxypropyl cellulose graft poly(*N*-isopropylacryamide) (HPC-g-PNIPAm). According to these authors, the thermal sensitivity of HPC is attractive as biomaterial. However, the lower critical solution temperature (LCST) of HPC is around 42°C in aqueous solution, and there is a gap to the physiological temperature (25°C–38°C) (Crespy and Rossi, 2007), which limits the applications of HPC as a promising biomaterial. Efforts have been tried to regulate the LCST of HPC to the physiological temperature region or even to body temperature (Xu et al., 2010), among which graft modification of HPC seems more effective (Ma et al., 2010a,b). Aiming to improve this property of HPC, Jin et al. (2013) have obtained copolymer HPC-g-PNIPAm. According to this work, the LCST of the HPC-g-PNIPAm copolymers can be regulated to an LCST close to body temperature by controlling the PNIPAm side chains to a proper length. The synthesis route of HPC-g-PNIPAm copolymers is shown in Figure 9.29. The macro-initiator HPC-Br for SET-LRP graft copolymerization was synthesized according to previous works (Ma et al., 2010a,b). Briefly, HPC (5.0 g) was dissolved in 100 mL anhydrous tetrahydrofuran (THF) with continuous stirring overnight. The solution was then cooled down to 0°C in an ice bath, and then 0.5 mL BIBB in 5 mL anhydrous THF was added dropwise into the flask over a period of 30 min. The flask was then sealed and allowed to react at room temperature for another 3 h. The final reaction mixture was condensed by rotary evaporation and then dialyzed against water. The resultant solution was lyophilized to result purified macro-initiator HPC-Br. The degree of substitution of the bromide groups can be tailored via varying the feeding molar ratio of BIBB and hydroxyl groups of HPC. In present work, HPC-Br with a relatively low degree of substitution of bromide groups (DS–Br = 0.1, about 1 bromide group per 10 glucose units of HPC) was selected as the initiator for the purpose to preserve the properties of HPC.

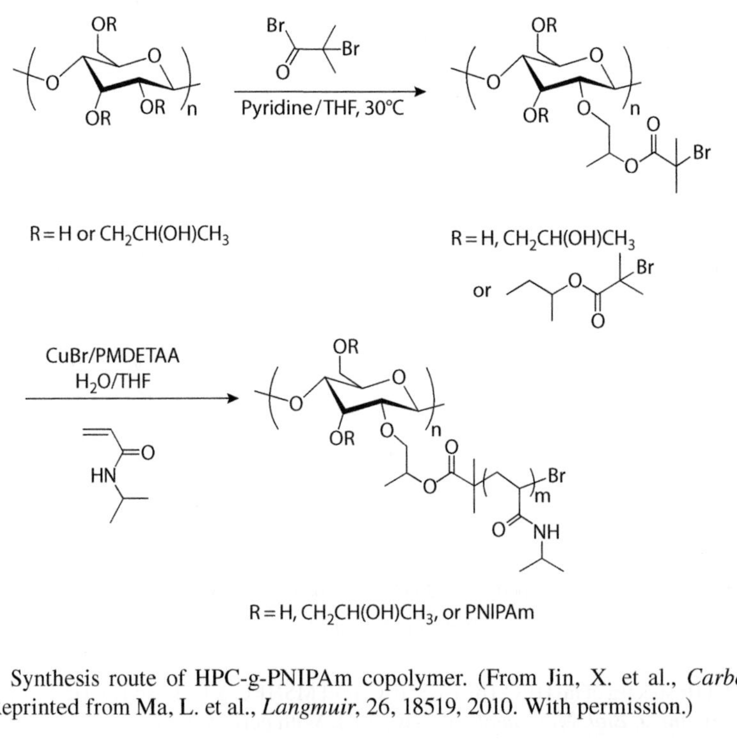

FIGURE 9.29 Synthesis route of HPC-g-PNIPAm copolymer. (From Jin, X. et al., *Carbohydr. Polym.*, 95, 155, 2013; Reprinted from Ma, L. et al., *Langmuir*, 26, 18519, 2010. With permission.)

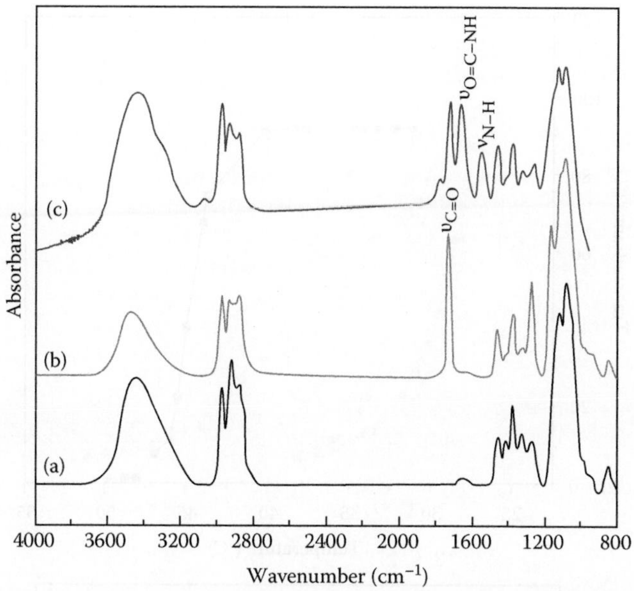

FIGURE 9.30 FTIR spectra of (a) HPC, (b) HPC-Br, and (c) HPC-g-PNIPAm (band 1730 cm^{-1}, $\upsilon_{O=C-O}$; band 1650 cm^{-1}, $\upsilon_{O=C-NH}$; band 1540 cm^{-1}, υ_{N-H}). (Reprinted from Jin, X. et al., *Carbohydr. Polym.*, 95, 155, 2013. With permission.)

The synthesis route of HPC-g-PNIPAm copolymers is shown in Figure 9.29. The first step is to synthesize the macro-initiator HPC-Br via the esterification between hydroxyl groups on HPC backbone and BIBB. The resultant HPC-Br macro-initiators were characterized by FTIR and ^{1}H NMR spectroscopies (Figure 9.30). On the FTIR spectrum of HPC-Br, the absorbance peak at 1735 cm^{-1} comes from the C=O stretching vibration of the ester (Figure 9.30b), which is unavailable on the spectrum of HPC (Figure 9.30a). On the ^{1}H NMR spectra, a new single peak at $\delta_d = 1.90$ ppm appears on the ^{1}H NMR spectrum of HPC-Br, which comes from the methyl protons in the ester group. Both FTIR and ^{1}H NMR results confirm the success of the esterification. The substitution degree of the 2-bromoisobutyryl groups (DS–Br, defined as the number of bromide groups per glucose ring) on the HPC backbone was estimated by comparing the integral area of the signal for the methyl group of HPC around $\delta_d = 1.10$ ppm to that of the methyl proton of the 2-bromoisobutyryl group around $\delta_d = 1.90$ ppm. In present work, macro-initiator with DS–Br = 0.1 was used for the initiation of graft copolymerization. At low DS–Br, the properties of the HPC are less influenced by the substitution of hydroxyl groups.

The LCST of the HPC-g-PNIPAm samples was determined by transmittance and differential scanning calorimetry (DSC). Plotting the transmittance of HPC and HPC-g-PNIPAm copolymers as a function of temperature (shown in Figure 9.31), Jin and coworkers showed that the temperature at which the transmittance changed for 50% was taken as the LCST or cloud point of the graft copolymers. The results indicated that the LCST of HPC-g-PNIPAm copolymers decreases with the decrease in the length of PNIPAm side chains.

DSC measurements resulted in a similar phenomenon (Figure 9.32). The HPC used in them work as an LCST around 44°C, which is similar to that in literature (Gao et al., 2001). For HPC itself, the good solubility in water at room temperature is due to the abundant hydrophilic hydroxyl groups on HPC chains, which can form hydrogen bond with water at room temperature. When the HPC solutions are heated to a higher temperature, hydrogen bonds between water and HPC molecular chains will be broken, and the HPC molecules become more hydrophobic simultaneously. The loss

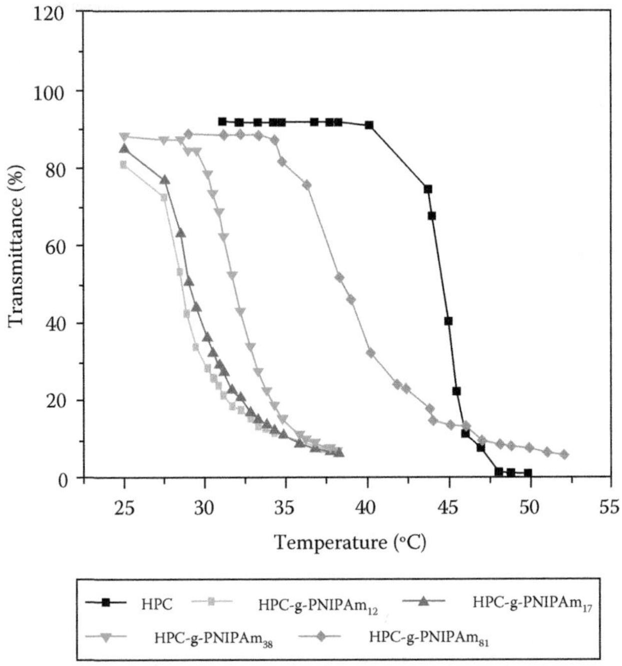

FIGURE 9.31 Transmittance of the aqueous solution of HPC and HPC-g-PNIPAm copolymers as a function of temperature. (Reprinted from Jin, X. et al., *Carbohydr. Polym.*, 95, 155, 2013. With permission.)

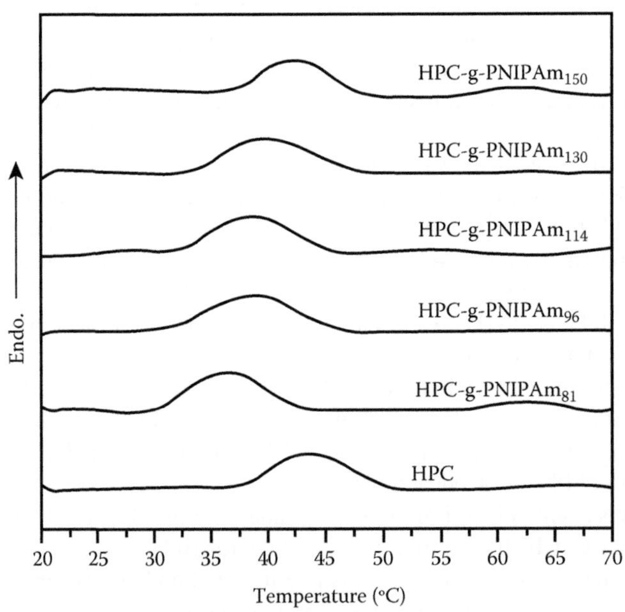

FIGURE 9.32 DSC traces of HPC and HPC-g-PNIPAm at a heating rate of 2°C/min in the temperature range from 20°C to 70°C. (Reprinted from Jin, X. et al., *Carbohydr. Polym.*, 95, 155, 2013. With permission.)

of hydrogen bonds between HPC chains and the water molecules leads to a collapse and hereafter the aggregation of HPC chains, which results in an LCST at around 44°C (Gao et al., 2001).

According to Jin and coworkers, the SET-LRP has a relatively lower polymerization rate in the mixture solvents with low water content. Through the thermal sensitivity of the HPC-g-PNIPAm copolymers, it was found that the shorter side PNIPAm chains correlate to a relatively lower LCST of the copolymers in aqueous solution. The LCST of the HPC-g-PNIPAm copolymers can be regulated to an LCST close to body temperature by controlling the PNIPAm side chains to a proper length.

9.4 CONCLUSION

The properties of the cellulose graft copolymers can be tailored by varying the structure of the cellulosic backbone, the chemical structure and length of the side chains, and the graft density. The cellulose graft copolymers can self-assemble into spherical micelles in selective solvents or can self-assemble with the trigger of temperature, pH, and ionic strength. The grafting can be performed in heterogeneous or homogeneous medium. In the grafting performed in heterogeneous medium, the reaction is carried out in aqueous medium using a suitable initiator. In this chapter, the latest advances, development, and characterization of the cellulose graft copolymers are shown.

REFERENCES

Abdel-Halim, E.S. 2012. An effective redox system for bleaching cotton cellulose. *Carbohydrate Polymers* 90: 316–321.

Akar, E., Altinisik, A., and Seki, Y. 2012. Preparation of pH- and ionic-strength responsive biodegradable fumaric acid crosslinked carboxymethyl cellulose. *Carbohydrate Polymers* 90: 1634–1641.

Alila, S., Ferraria, A.M., do Rego, A.M.B., and Boufi, S. 2009. Controlled surface modification of cellulose fibers by amino derivatives using *N,N′*-carbonyldiimidazole as activator. *Carbohydrate Polymers* 77: 553–562.

Bao, Y., Ma, J., and Sun, Y. 2012. Swelling behaviors of organic/inorganic composites based on various cellulose derivatives and inorganic particles. *Carbohydrate Polymers* 88(2): 589–595.

Barner, L., Davis, T.P., Stenzel, M.H., and Barner-Kowollik, C. 2007. Complex macromolecular architectures by reversible addition fragmentation chain transfer chemistry: Theory and practice. *Macromolecular Rapid Communications* 28(5): 539–559.

Barner-Kowollik, C., ed. 2008. *The Handbook of RAFT Polymerization*. Weinheim, Germany: Wiley-VCH.

Bhattacharya, A. and Misra, B.N. 2004. Grafting: A versatile means to modify polymers: Techniques, factors and applications. *Progress in Polymer Science* 29(8): 767–814. ISSN 0079-6700, http://dx.doi.org/10.1016/j.progpolymsci.2004.05.002.

Brzytwa, A.J. and Johnson, J. 2011. Scaled production of RAFT CTA—A star performer. *Polymer Preprints* 52(2): 533–534.

Carlmark, A. and Malmström, E. 2003. ATRP grafting from cellulose fibers to create block-copolymer grafts. *Biomacromolecules* 4(6): 1740–1745.

Carlmark, A., Larsson, E., and Malmström, E. 2012. Grafting of cellulose by ring-opening polymerization—A review. *European Polymer Journal* 48(10): 1646–1659.

Chauvin, F., Couturier, J.-L., Dufils, P.-E., Gerard, P., Gigmes, D., Guerret, O., Guillaneuf, Y., Marque, S.R.A., Bertin, D., and Tordo, P. 2006. In: Matyjaszewski, K. (ed.) ACS Symposium Series, *Controlled/Living Radical Polymerisation-From Synthesis to Materials*. Washington, DC: American Chemical Society, Vol. 944, pp. 326–341.

Chong, Y.K., Moad, G., Rizzardo, E., and Thang, S. 2007. Thiocarbonylthio end group removal from RAFT-synthesized polymers by radical-induced reduction. *Macromolecules* 40: 4446–4455.

Coskun, M. et al. 2005. Grafting studies onto cellulose by atom-transfer radical polymerization. *Polymer International* 54: 342–347.

Crespy, D. and Rossi, R.M. 2007. Temperature responsive polymer with LCST in the physiological range and their applications in textiles. *Polymer International* 56: 1461–1468.

Daily, H., Evenson, T.S., Iacono, S.T., and Jones, R.W. 2001. Recent developments in cellulose grafting chemistry utilizing Barton ester intermediates and nitroxide mediation. *Macromolecular Symposia* 174: 155–163.

Das, R. and Pal, S. 2013. Hydroxypropyl methyl cellulose grafted with polyacrylamide: Application in controlled release of 5-amino salicylic acid. *Colloids and Surfaces B: Biointerfaces* 110: 236–241. ISSN 0927–7765, http://dx.doi.org/10.1016/j.colsurfb.2013.04.033.

Destarac, M., Guinaudeau, A., Geagea, R., Mazieres, S., Van Gramberen, E., Boutin, C., Chadel, S., and Wilson, J. 2010. Aqueous MADIX/RAFT polymerization of diallyldimethylammonium chloride: Extension to the synthesis of poly(DADMAC)-based double hydrophilic block copolymers. *Journal of Polymer Science Part A: Polymer Chemistry* 48: 5163–5171.

Dong, H., Xu, Q., Li, Y., Mo, S., Cai, S., and Liu, L. 2008. The synthesis of biodegradable graft copolymer cellulose-graft-poly(l-lactide) and the study of its controlled drug release. *Colloids and Surfaces B: Biointerfaces* 66(1): 26–33. ISSN 0927-7765, http://dx.doi.org/10.1016/j.colsurfb.2008.05.007.

Edlund, U., Ryberg, Y.Z., and Albertsson, A.C. 2010. Barrier films from renewable forestry waste. *Biomacromolecules* 11: 2532–2538.

Eissa, A.M., Khosravi, E., and Cimecioglu, A.L. 2012. A versatile method for functionalization and grafting of 2-hydroxyethyl cellulose (HEC) via click chemistry. *Carbohydrate Polymers* 90: 859–869.

Fleet, R., McLeary, J.B., Grumel, V., Weber, W.G., Matahwa, H., and Sanderson, R.D. 2008. RAFT mediated polysaccharide copolymers. *European Polymer Journal* 44: 2899–2911.

Gao, J.P., Wei, Y.H., Li, B.Y., and Han, Y.C. 2008. Fabrication of fibril like aggregates by self-assembly of block copolymer mixtures via interpolymer hydrogen bonding. *Polymer* 49: 2354–2361.

Gao, J., Haidar, G., Lu, X., and Hu, Z. 2001. Self-association of hydroxypropylcellulose in water. *Macromolecules* 34: 2242–2247.

Georges, M.K., Veregin, R.P.N., Kazmaier, P.M., and Hamer, G.K. 1993. Free radical polymerizations for narrow polydispersity resins: Electron spin resonance studies of the kinetics and mechanism. *Macromolecules* 26: 2987.

Goffin, A.-L., Habibi, Y., Raquez, J.-M., and Dubois, P. 2012. Polyester-grafted cellulose nanowhiskers: A new approach for tuning the microstructure of immiscible polyester blends. *ACS Appllied Materials and Interfaces* 4(7): 3364–3371. doi: 10.1021/am3008196. Epub July 16, 2012.

Gowariker, V.R., Viswanathan, N.V., and Sreedhar, J. 1986. *Polymer Science*. New Delhi, India: Wiley Eastern Ltd.

Gupta, K.C. and Khandekar, K. 2006. Ceric(IV) ion-induced graft copolymerization of acrylamide and ethyl acrylate onto cellulose. *Polymer International* 55(2): 139–150.

Hafrén, J. and Cordova, A. 2005. Direct organocatalytic polymerization from cellulose fibers. *Macromolecular Rapid Communications* 26: 82–86.

Hartman, J., Albertsson, A.-C., Lindblad, M.S., and Sjöberg, J. 2006. Oxygen barrier materials from renewable sources: Material properties of softwood hemicellulose-based films. *Journal Applied Polymer Science* 100(4): 2985–2991.

Hawker, C.J., Barclay, G.G., Orellana, A., Dao, J., and Devonport, W. 1996. Initiating systems for nitroxide-mediated "Living" free radical polymerizations: Synthesis and evaluation. *Macromolecules* 16: 5245–5254.

Hawker, C.J., Bosman, A.W., and Harth, E. 2001. New polymer synthesis by nitroxide mediated living radical polymerizations. *Chemical Reviews* 101(12): 3661–3688.

Hebeish, A. and Guthrie, J.T. 1981. *The Chemistry and Technology of Cellulose Copolymers*, No. 4 of the series "Polymers—Properties and Applications" (Chemie und Technologie der Cellulose-Copolymere, Nr. 4 der Serie Polymere—Eigenschaften und Anwendung). Berlin, Germany: Springer-Verlag, p. 351.

Hernandez-Guerrero, M., Davis, T.P., Barner-Kowollik, C., and Stenzel, M.H. 2005. Polystyrene comb polymers built on cellulose or poly(styrene-co-2-hydroxyethylmethacrylate) backbones as substrates for the preparation of structured honeycomb films. *European Polymer Journal* 41(10): 2264–2277.

Hiltunen, M., Siirilä, J., Aseyev, V., and Maunu, S.L. 2012. Cellulose-g-PDMAam copolymers by controlled radical polymerization in homogeneous medium and their aqueous solution properties. *European Polymer Journal* 48(1): 136–145, ISSN 0014-3057, http://dx.doi.org/10.1016/j.eurpolymj.2011.10.010.

Imai, Y., Masuhara, E., and Iwakura, Y. 1970. Initiation mechanism of cerium-initiated grafting onto cellulosic materials. *Journal of Polymer Science, Part B: Polymer Letters* 8: 75–79.

Jerome, C. and Lecomte, P. 2008. Recent advances in the synthesis of aliphatic polyesters by ring-opening polymerization. *Advanced Drug Delivery Reviews* 60(9): 1056–1076.

Jiang, C. et al. 2011. Synthesis and solution behavior of poly(ε-caprolactone) grafted hydroxyethyl cellulose copolymers. *International Journal of Biological Macromolecules* 48: 210–214.

Jin, X. et al. 2013. Regulation of the thermal sensitivity of hydroxypropyl cellulose by poly(*N*-isopropylacryamide) side chains. *Carbohydrate Polymers* 95: 155–160.

Kamigaito, M., Ando, T., and Sawamoto, M. 2001. Metal-catalyzed living radical polymerization. *Chemical Review* 101: 3689–3745.

Klemm, D., Heublein, B., Fink, H.P., and Bohn, A. 2005. Cellulose: Fascinating biopolymer and sustainable raw material. *Angewandte Chemie International Edition* 44(22): 3358–3393.

Liu, G., Jin, Q., Liu, X., Lv, L., Chen, C., and Ji, J. 2011. Biocompatible vesicles based on PEO-b-PMPC/[small alpha]-cyclodextrin inclusion complexes for drug delivery. *Soft Matter* 7: 662–669.

Liu, H., Wu, Q., and Zhang, Q. 2009. Preparation and properties of banana fiber-reinforced composites based on high density polyethylene (HDPE)/Nylon-6 blends. *Bioresource Technology* 100: 6088–6097.

Lligadas, G. and Percec, V.A. 2008. Comparative analysis of SET-LRP of MA in solvents mediating different degrees of disproportionation of Cu(I)Br. *Journal of Polymer Science Part A: Polymer Chemistry* 46: 6880–6895.

Lönnberg, H., Fogelström, L., Berglund, L., Malmström, E., and Hult, A. 2008. Surface grafting of microfibrillated cellulose with poly (Î-caprolactone)—Synthesis and characterization. *European Polymer Journal* 44(9): 2991–2997.

Ma, L. et al. 2010. Self-assembly and dual-stimuli sensitivities of hydroxypropylcellulose-graftpoly(*N*,*N*-dimethyl aminoethyl methacrylate) copolymers in aqueous solution. *Langmuir* 26: 18519–18525.

Ma, L., Kang, H.L., Liu, R.G., and Huang, Y. 2010a. Smart assembly behaviors of hydroxypropylcellulose-graft-poly(4-vinyl pyridine) copolymers in aqueous solution by thermo and pH stimuli. *Langmuir* 26: 18519–18525.

Ma, L., Liu, R.G., Tan, J.J., Wang, D.Q., Jin, X., Kang, H.L. et al. 2010b. Self-assembly and dual-stimuli sensitivities of hydroxypropylcellulose-graftpoly(N,N-dimethyl aminoethyl methacrylate) copolymers in aqueous solution. *Langmuir* 26: 8697–8703.

Matyjaszewski, K. (ed.) 2000. *Controlled/Living Radical Polymerization: Progress in ATRP, NMP and RAFT*, In ACS Symposium Series. Washington, DC: *American Chemical Society*, Vol. 768, pp. 2–25.

Matyjaszewski, K. and Xia, J. 2001. Atom transfer radical polymerization. *Chemical Reviews* 101(9): 2921–2990.

McDowall, D.J., Gupta, B.S., and Stannett, V.T. 1984. Grafting of vinyl monomers to cellulose by ceric ion initiation. *Progress in Polymer Science* 10(1): 1–50. ISSN 0079-6700, http://dx.doi.org/10.1016/0079-6700(84)90005-4.

Mino, G. and Kaizerman, S. 1958. A new method for the preparation of graft copolymers. Polymerization initiated by ceric ion redox systems. *Journal of Polymer Science* 31: 242–243.

Mishra, A., Srinivasan, R., and Gupta, R. 2003. *P. psyllium*-g-polyacrylonitrile: Synthesis and characterization. *Colloid and Polymer Science* 281(2): 187–189.

Mishra, B.N., Mehta, I.K., and Khetrapal, R.C. 1984. Grafting onto cellulose. VIII. Graft copolymerization of poly(ethylacrylate) onto cellulose by use of redox initiators. Comparison of initiator reactivities. *Journal of Polymer Science Part A: Polymer Chemistry* 22: 2767–2775.

Mishra, S., Rani, G.U., and Sen, G. 2012. Microwave initiated synthesis and application of polyacrylic acid grafted carboxymethyl cellulose. *Carbohydrate Polymers* 87(3): 2255–2262. ISSN 0144-8617, http://dx.doi.org/10.1016/j.carbpol.2011.10.057.

Moad, G., Chong, Y.K., Postma, A., Rizzardo, E., and Thang S.H. 2005. Advances in RAFT polymerization: The synthesis of polymers with defined end-groups. *Polymer* 46: 8458–8468.

Moad, G., Rizzardo, E., and Thang. S.H. 2006. Living radical polymerization by the RAFT process—A first update. *Australian Journal of Chemistry* 59: 669–692.

Moad, G. and Solomon, D.H. 2006. *The Chemistry of Radical Polymerization*, 2nd edn. Oxford, U.K.: Elsevier Ltd.

Moad, G. et al. 2010. Reversible addition fragmentation chain transfer (RAFT) polymerization. *Material Matters* 5: 2–5.

Moad, G., Rizzardo, E., and Thang, S.H. 2008. Radical addition–fragmentation chemistry in polymer synthesis. *Polymer* 49: 1079–1131.

Moad, G., Rizzardo, E., and Thang, S.E. 2009. Living radical polymerization by the RAFT process—A second update. *Australian Journal of Chemistry* 62: 1402–1472.

Moad, G., Rizzardo, E., and Thang, S.H. 2011. End-functional polymers, thiocarbonylthio group removal/transformation and reversible addition–fragmentation–chain transfer (RAFT) polymerization. *Polymer International* 60: 9–25.

Nguyen, N.H. and Percec, V. 2010. Dramatic acceleration of SET-LRP of methyl acrylate during catalysis with activated Cu(0) wire. *Journal of Polymer Science Part A: Polymer Chemistry* 48(22): 5109–5119.

Odian, G. 2002. *Principles of Polymerization,* 3rd edn. John Wiley & Sons, New York.

Okieimen, F.E. and Idehen, K.I. 1989. Studies in the graft copolymerization of vinyl monomers on cellulosic materials. *Journal of Applied Polymer Science* 37(5): 1253–1258.

Östmark, E., Harrisson, S., Wooley, K.L., and Malmström, E.E. 2007. Comb polymers prepared by ATRP from hydroxypropyl cellulose. *Biomacromolecules* 8(4): 1138–1148.

Oza, M.D., Meena, R., and Siddhanta, A.K. 2012. Facile synthesis of fluorescent polysaccharides: Cytosine grafted agarose and kappa-carrageenan. *Carbohydrate Polymers* 87: 1971–1979.

Percec, V. et al. 2006. Ultrafast synthesis of ultrahigh molar mass polymers by metal-catalyzed living radical polymerization of acrylates, methacrylates, and vinyl chloride mediated by set at 25°C. *Journal of the American Chemical Society* 128: 14156–14165.

Qiu, X. and Hu, S. 2013. "Smart" materials based on cellulose: A review of the preparations, properties, and Aapplications. *Materials* 6: 738–781.

Rannard, S.P., Rogers, S.H., and Hunter, R. 2007. Synthesis of well-defined Locust Bean Gum-graft-copolymers using ambient aqueous atom transfer radical polymerisation. *Chemical Communications* 4: 362–364.

Rizzardo, E., Moad, G., and Thang, S.H. 2007. RAFT polymerization in bulk monomer or in (organic) solution. In: Barner-Kowollik, C. (ed.) *Handbook of RAFT polymerization*. Weinheim, Germany: Wiley-VCH.

Roos, A.A., Edlund, U., Sjöberg, J., Albertsson, A.-C., and Stålbrand, H. 2008. Protein release from galactoglucomannan hydrogels: Influence of substitutions and enzymatic hydrolysis by β-mannanase. *Biomacromolecules* 9: 2104–2110.

Rosen, B.M. and Percec, V. 2009. Single-electron transfer and single-electron transfer degenerative chain transfer living radical polymerization. *Chemical Reviews* 109(11): 5069–5119.

Roy, D. et al. 2005. Graft polymerization: Grafting poly(styrene) from cellulose via reversible addition–fragmentation chain transfer (RAFT) polymerization. *Macromolecules* 38: 10363–10372.

Roy, D., Semsarilar, M., Guthrie, J.T., and Perrier, S. 2009. Cellulose modification by polymer grafting: A review. *Chemical Society Reviews* 38(7): 2046–2064.

Sand, A., Yadav, M., and Behari, K. 2010. Preparation and characterization of modified sodium carboxymethyl cellulose via free radical graft copolymerization of vinyl sulfonic acid in aqueous media *Carbohydrate Polymers* 81: 97–103.

Schuyten, H.A., Reid, D.J., Weaver, J.W., and Frick, J.G. 1948. Imparting water-repellsmcy to textiles by chemical methods: A review of the literature. *Textile Research Journal* 18(7): 396–415.

Sciannamea, V., Jerome, R., and Detrembleur, C. 2008. In-situ nitroxide-mediated radical polymerization (NMP) processes: Their understanding and optimization. *Chemical Reviews* 108: 1104–1126.

Shen, D., Yu, H., and Huang, Y. 2006. Synthesis of graft copolymer of ethyl cellulose through living polymerization and its self-assembly. *Cellulose* 13: 235–244.

Singha, A.S. and Thakur, V.K. 2010. Synthesis and characterization of short Grewia optiva fiber based polymer composites. *Polymer Composites* 31: 459–470.

Stannett, V.T. and Hopfenberg, H.B. 1971. In *Cellulose and Cellulose Derivatives*, eds. N.M. Bikales and L. Segal, John Wiley & Sons, Vol. 5, pp. 907–936.

Stenzel, M.H., Davis, T.P., and Fane, A.G. 2003. Honeycomb structured porous films prepared from carbohydrate based polymers synthesized via the RAFT process. *Journal of Materials Chemistry* 13: 2090–2097.

Szwarc, M. 1956. Living' polymers. *Nature* 178: 1168–1169.

Tanczos, E. et al. 1982. Kinetics of radical polymerization. *European Polymer Journal* 18(6): 487–491.

Tang, X.Z., Hu, Y.H., and Pan, C.Y. 2007. Multiple morphologies of self-assembled star aggregates of amphiphilic PEO-b-PNPMA diblock copolymers in solution, synthesis and micellization. *Polymer* 48: 6354–6365.

Thakur, V.K., Thakur, M.K., and Gupta, R.K. 2013. Graft copolymers from cellulose: Synthesis, characterization and evaluation. *Carbohydrate Polymers* 97(1): 18–25. ISSN 0144-8617, http://dx.doi.org/10.1016/j.carbpol.2013.04.069.

Tizzotti, M.,Charlot, A., Fleury, E., Stenzel, M., and Bernard, J. 2010. Modification of polysaccharides through controlled/living radical polymerization grafting—Towards the generation of high performance hybrids. *Macromolecular Rapid Communications* 31(20): 1751–1772.

Voepel, J. et al. 2011. Hemicellulose-based multifunctional macroinitiator for single-electron-transfer mediated living radical polymerization. *Biomacromolecules*12: 253–259.

Xu, F.J., Zhu, Y., Liu, F.S., Nie, J., Ma, J., and Yang, W.T. 2010. Comb-shaped conjugates comprising hydroxypropyl cellulose backbones and low-molecular-weight poly(N-isopropylacryamide) side chains for smart hydrogels: Synthesis, characterization, and biomedical applications. *Bioconjugate Chemistry* 21: 456–464.

Yang, R., Wang, Y., and Zhou, D. 2007. Novel hydroxyethylcellulose-graft-polyacrylamide copolymer for separation of double-stranded DNA fragments by CE. *Electrophoresis* 28: 3223–3231.

Ydens, I., Rutot, D., Degee, P., Six, J.L., Dellacherie, E., and Dubois, P. 2000. Controlled synthesis of poly(epsilon-caprolactone)-grafted dextran copolymers as potential environmentally friendly surfactants. *Macromolecules* 33: 6713–6721.

Yuan, W., Yuan, J., Zhang, F., and Xie, X. 2007. Syntheses, characterization, and in vitro degradation of ethyl cellulose-graft-poly (e-caprolactone)-block-poly (L-lactide) copolymers by sequential ring-opening polymerization. *Biomacromolecules* 8(4): 1101–1108.

Zhang, J., Youling, Y., Shen, J., and Lin, S. 2003. Synthesis and characterization of chitosan grafted poly(*N*, *N*-dimethyl-*N*-methacryloxyethyl-*N*-3-sulfopropyl ammonium) initiated by Ce(IV) ion. *European Polymer Journal* 39(4): 847–850.

Zhong, F., Chai, X.-S., and Fu, S.-Y. 2012. Homogeneous grafting poly(methyl methacrylate) on cellulose by atom transfer radical polymerization. *Carbohydrate Polymers* 87: 1869–1873.

Zoppe, J. et al. 2010. Poly(*N*-isopropylacrylamide) brushes grafted from cellulose nanocrystals via surface-initiated single-electron transfer living radical polymerization. *Biomacromolecules* 11: 2683–2691.

10 Modification of Cellulose-Based Fibers by the Graft Copolymerization Method

Mehlika Pulat

CONTENTS

10.1 INTRODUCTION

Natural fibers originate from animal, vegetable, or mineral sources. Vegetable fibers are derived from plants. The basic chemical component in plants is cellulose, and therefore they are also named as cellulosic fibers. Cellulose, a fibrous carbohydrate found in all plants, is the structural component of plant cell walls. It is a polysaccharide made up of repeating 1,4-8-anhydro glucose units connected to each other by eight ether linkages. The fibers are usually bound by a natural phenolic polymer, lignin, which also is frequently present in the cell wall of the fiber; thus, vegetable fibers are also often referred to as lignocellulosic fibers, except for cotton, which does not contain lignin.

Natural cellulosic fibers are classified as bast, leaf, and seed-hair fibers. The bast fibers form the fibrous bundles in the inner bark of the plant stems. The leaf fibers run lengthwise through the leaves of monocotyledonous plants, and the seed-hair fibers, the source of cotton, are the most important vegetable fiber.

Cellulose, which has been known to have good physical properties, has been widely used as construction material, paper, and clothes. However, chemical modification of cellulose fibers by introducing new functional groups or compounds is still needed in order to improve its performance characteristics, for example, swelling, dye fixation, water and soil repellence, crease resistance, flame retardance, etc. Numerous chemical compounds are currently used for specific needs and applications of the fibers.

Synthesis of cellulose graft copolymers is one of the important means of modifying physical and chemical properties of cellulose. This is usually achieved by modifying the cellulose molecules through the creation of branches (grafts) of synthetic polymers that impart specific properties onto the cellulose substrate, without destroying its intrinsic properties. Free radical polymerization, ionic and ring-opening polymerization, and living radical polymerization methods could be used to graft different monomers onto cellulose fibers.

The main objective of this chapter is to study the graft copolymerization of various monomers onto cellulose fibers and evaluate their modified properties.

10.2 FIBERS

Fiber is a rope or string used as a component of composite materials, or matted into sheets to make products such as paper or felt [1]. Fibers are often used in the manufacture of other materials. Fibers are broadly classified into natural fibers and man-made fibers, as shown in Figure 10.1.

Natural fibers include those produced by plants, animals, and geological processes. They are biodegradable over time. They can be classified according to their origin:

- Vegetable fibers are generally based on arrangements of cellulose, often with lignin: examples include cotton, hemp, jute, flax, ramie, sisal, and bagasse. Plant fibers are employed in the manufacture of paper and textile, and dietary fiber is an important component of human nutrition.
- Wood fiber, distinguished from vegetable fiber, is from tree sources. Forms include ground wood, thermo-mechanical pulp, and bleached or unbleached kraft or sulfite pulps.
- Animal fibers consist largely of particular proteins. Instances are silkworm silk, spider silk, sinew, catgut, wool, and sea silk; hair such as cashmere wool, mohair, and angora; fur such as sheepskin, rabbit, mink, fox, and beaver.
- Mineral fibers include the asbestos group. Asbestos is the only naturally occurring long mineral fiber. Six minerals have been classified as "asbestos" including chrysotile of the serpentine class and those belonging to the amphibole class: amosite, crocidolite, tremolite, anthophyllite, and actinolite. Short, fiber-like minerals include wollastonite and palygorskite.

Vegetable fibers are usually bound by a natural phenolic polymer, lignin, which also is frequently present in the cell wall of the fiber; thus, vegetable fibers are also often referred to as lignocellulosic fibers, except for cotton, which does not contain lignin [2]. Vegetable fibers are classified according to their source in plants as follows:

1. The bast or stem fibers, which form the fibrous bundles in the inner bark (phloem or bast) of the plant stems, are often referred to as soft fibers for textile use.

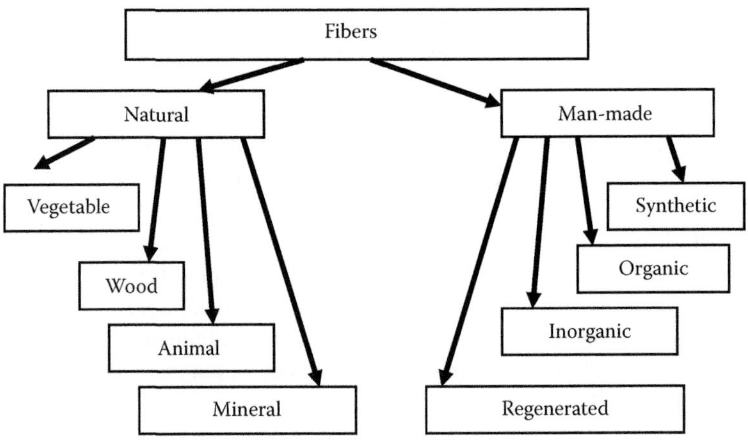

FIGURE 10.1 Classification of fibers.

TABLE 10.1
Chemical Component (%) of Vegetable Fibers

Vegetable Fiber	Cellulose	Hemicelluloses	Pectin	Lignin	Extractives
Bast fibers					
Flax	71.2	18.6	2.0	2.2	6.0
Hemp	74.9	17.9	0.9	3.7	3.1
Jute	71.5	13.4	0.2	13.1	1.8
Kenaf	63.0	18.0	—	17.0	2.0
Ramie	76.2	14.6	2.1	0.7	6.4
Leaf fibers					
Abaca	70.1	21.8	0.6	5.7	1.8
Phormium	71.3	—	—	—	—
Sisal	73.1	13.3	0.9	11.0	1.6
Seed-hair fibers					
Coir	43.0	0.1	—	45.0	—
Cotton	92.9	2.6	2.6	—	1.9
Kapok	64.0	23.0	23.0	13.0	—

2. The leaf fibers, which run lengthwise through the leaves of monocotyledonous plants, are also referred to as hard fibers.
3. The seed-hair fibers, the source of cotton, are the most important vegetable fiber.

The principal chemical component in plants is cellulose; therefore, vegetable fibers are also referred to as cellulosic fibers. Because the earth is covered with vegetation, cellulose is the most abundant of all carbohydrates, accounting for over 50% of all the carbon found in the vegetable kingdom. Chemically, all vegetable fibers consist mainly of cellulose, although they also contain varying amounts of such substances as hemicellulose, lignin, pectins, and waxes that must be removed or reduced by processing [3]. The chemical components of some vegetable fibers are presented in Table 10.1.

Chemically, cotton is the purest vegetable fiber, containing >90% cellulose with little or no lignin. The other fibers contain 40%–75% cellulose, depending on processing. Boiled and bleached flax and degummed ramie may contain >95% cellulose. Kenaf and jute contain higher contents of lignin, which contributes to their stiffness. Although the cellulose contents are fairly uniform, the other components, for example, hemicelluloses, pectins, extractives, and lignin vary widely without obvious pattern. These differences may characterize specific fibers. Except for the seed-hair fibers, the vegetable fibers of bast or leaf origins are multicelled and are used as strands.

In contrast to the bast fibers, leaf fibers are not readily broken down into their ultimate cells. The ultimate cells are composites of micro-fibrils, which, in turn, comprised groups of parallel cellulose chains. Bast and leaf fibers are stronger (higher tensile strength and modulus of elasticity) but lower in elongation (extensibility) than cotton. Vegetable fibers are stiffer but less tough than synthetic fibers. Kapok and coir are relatively low in strength; kapok is known for its buoyancy.

10.3 CELLULOSE

Cellulose is the most abundant organic raw material and finds applications in areas as diverse as composite materials, textiles, drug delivery systems, and personal care products [4]. It was isolated in 1838 from plant matter and determined its chemical formula. Cellulose was used to produce

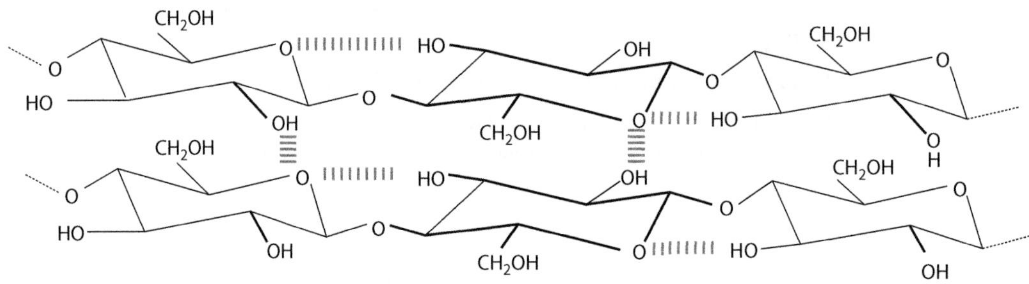

FIGURE 10.2 Hydrogen bonds in cellulose structure.

the first successful thermoplastic polymer, celluloid, by Hyatt Manufacturing Company, Newark, New Jersey, in 1870. Production of rayon (artificial silk) from cellulose began in the 1890s, and cellophane was invented in 1912. Hermann Staudinger determined the polymer structure of cellulose in 1920. The compound was first chemically synthesized (without the use of any biologically derived enzymes) in 1992 by Kobayashi and Shoda [5–8].

Cellulose has no taste, is odorless, is hydrophilic with the contact angle of 20°–30°, is insoluble in water and most organic solvents, is chiral, and is biodegradable. It can be broken down chemically into its glucose units by treating it with concentrated acids at high temperature. Cellulose requires a temperature of 320°C and pressure of 25 MPa to become amorphous in water [9].

Since cellulose was first characterized in 1838, this inexpensive, biodegradable, and renewable resource has received a great deal of attention for its physical properties and chemical reactivity [4,5,10]. The chemical and physical properties of the cellulose biopolymer are largely dependent on its specific structure. Cellulose is derived from D-glucose units, which condense through β(1→4)-glycosidic bonds. This linkage motif contrasts with that for α(1→4)-glycosidic bonds present in starch, glycogen, and other carbohydrates. Cellulose is a straight-chain polymer: unlike starch, no coiling or branching occurs, and the molecule adopts an extended and rather stiff rod-like conformation, aided by the equatorial conformation of the glucose residues. The multiple hydroxyl groups on the glucose from one chain form hydrogen bonds with oxygen atoms on the same or on a neighbor chain, holding the chains firmly together side by side and forming microfibrils with high tensile strength (Figure 10.2). This confers tensile strength in cell walls, where cellulose microfibrils are meshed into a polysaccharide matrix.

Many properties of cellulose depend on its chain length or degree of polymerization, the number of glucose units that make up one polymer molecule. Cellulose from wood pulp has typical chain lengths between 300 and 1,700 units; cotton and other plant fibers as well as bacterial cellulose have chain lengths ranging from 800 to 10,000 units. Molecules with very small chain length resulting from the breakdown of cellulose are known as cellodextrins; in contrast to long-chain cellulose, cellodextrins are typically soluble in water and organic solvents [11].

10.4 MODIFICATION OF CELLULOSE FIBERS BY GRAFT POLYMERIZATION METHOD

Cellulose is itself a unique polymeric product and possesses several attributes such as a fine cross section, the ability to absorb moisture, high strength and durability, high thermal stability, good biocompatibility, relatively low cost, and low density yet good mechanical properties. However, cellulose has some inherent drawbacks. These include poor solubility in common solvents, poor crease resistance, poor dimensional stability, lack of thermoplasticity, high hydrophilicity (not desirable for several composite applications), and lack of antimicrobial properties. To overcome such drawbacks, the controlled physical and/or chemical modification of the cellulose structure is necessary [12].

Chemical modification of cellulose fibers by introducing new functional groups or compounds is needed in order to improve their performance characteristics, for example, dye fixation, water and soil repellence, crease resistance, handle, flame retardance, and others. For this purpose, a large number of chemical compounds are used depending on the specific application of the fibers [13].

The industrial history of the chemical modification of cellulose to impart new properties can be traced back to 1870 with the production of the first thermoplastic polymeric material "celluloid," which was manufactured by the Hyatt Manufacturing Company. The formation of cellulose nitrate involves the esterification of cellulose with nitric acid in the presence of sulfuric acid, phosphoric acid, or acetic acid. Currently, other commercially important cellulose esters are cellulose acetate, cellulose acetate propionate, and cellulose acetate butyrate [4].

The synthesis of cellulose graft copolymers marked the first departure from the traditional means of modifying cellulose, until then undertaken via the chemical reactions. In 1943, Ushakov attempted to copolymerize some ally esters and vinyl esters of cellulose with the esters of maleic acid. He obtained some insoluble products that were probably the first graft copolymers ever reported [4]. Since this invention, extensive studies have been carried out on the synthesis, properties, and applications of cellulose graft copolymers. Research studies on the cellulose graft copolymers through to 1986 have been reviewed by Hebeish and Guthrie and by Samal et al. [12,14–17].

The main purpose of preparing monomer-grafted cellulose is to gain new properties such as water absorption, improved elasticity, hydrophilic or hydrophobic character, ion-exchange and dye adsorption capabilities, heat resistance, thermosensitivity, pH sensitivity, antibacterial effect, and resistance to microbiological attack. While the internal grafting changes the dyeing behavior of cellulose fibers, surface grafting improves the abrasion resistance [18–30].

In order to obtain a cellulose graft copolymer with high water or moisture absorbency, hydrophilic monomers such as acrylic acid (AA), acrylamide (AAm), and 2-acrylamidomethylpropane sulfonic acid ($AASO_3H$) should be grafted onto cellulose. In order to improve the compatibility and adhesion of hydrophilic cellulose fibers to the components of hydrophobic composites, hydrophobic monomers such as methyl methacrylate (MMA), styrene, acrylonitrile (AN), butadiene, isobutyl vinyl ether, and vinyl acetate should be grafted onto the surface of cellulose [31–33].

The graft copolymerization of many monomers onto cellulose and cellulose derivatives has been carried out by different methods that can be generally classified into three major groups: (1) free radical polymerization, (2) ionic and ring opening polymerization, and (3) living radical polymerization [18].

Graft copolymerization is a well-established and commonly used technique for the modification of polymer surface [34]. Grafting can be performed in a homogeneous or in a heterogeneous medium [18]. A general schematic representation for grafted cellulose is shown in Figure 10.3.

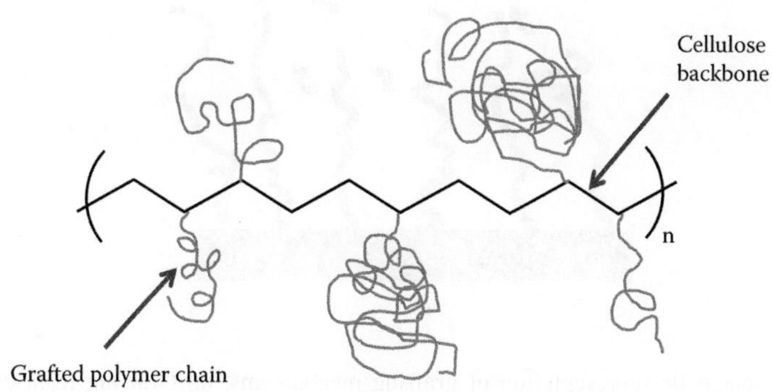

FIGURE 10.3 A schematic representation of the grafting of cellulose backbone.

As represented in Figure 10.4, grafting mechanisms can be investigated in three groups [4,35,36]:

1. In the "grafting from" approach, the growth of polymer chain occurs from initiating sites on the polymer backbone. The polymerization of a vinyl monomer in the presence of a polymer in which the propagation reaction is initiated on the polymer backbone by a chain transfer and the growth of graft chains begin from the active sites on the polymer backbone. In that approach, the grafting is performed either with a single monomer or with a binary monomer mixture. With single monomer, the grafting usually occurs in a single step. But in the grafting with binary monomer mixture, the reaction is carried out with either the simultaneous or sequential use of the two monomers. In the mosaic grafting, two kinds of monomer are grafted side by side to obtain the required property. This is the origin of bipolar membranes [37].
2. In the "grafting through" approach, a macro monomer, for example, a vinyl derivative of cellulose, is copolymerized with the same or another vinyl monomer. The polymerization of a vinyl monomer in the presence of a polymer is initiated with reactive functional end

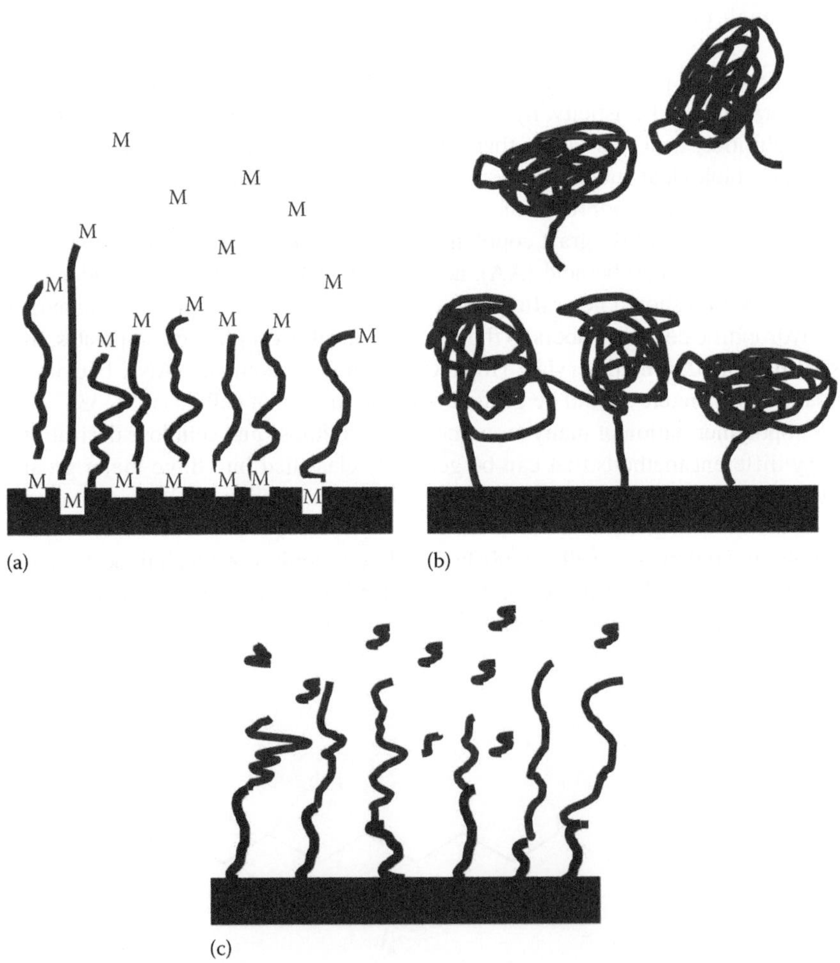

FIGURE 10.4 A schematic representation of grafting mechanisms. (a) Grafting from cellulosic surface, (b) grafting onto cellulosic surface, and (c) grafting through cellulosic surface.

groups. These functional end groups can be activated by means of heat, light, or other ways [4].

3. In the "grafting onto" approach, an end-functional preformed polymer with a reactive end group is coupled with the functional group located on the polymer backbone. The grafting of a monomer onto a polymer backbone is initiated by high-energy irradiation. The radiation grafting can be performed by direct/mutual method in which the monomer and the polymer (graft substrate) are irradiated simultaneously to create the radicals that are starting the polymerization or by preirradiation/indirect grafting in which the monomer is contacted with the polymer backbone irradiated alone before. Grafting onto allows a preformed polymer, generally in a "mushroom regime," to adhere to the surface of either a droplet or bead in solution. Due to the larger volume of the coiled polymer and the steric hindrance this causes, the grafting density is lower for "onto" in comparison to "grafting from." The surface of the bead is wetted by the polymer, and the interaction in the solution causes the polymer to become more flexible. The "extended conformation" of the polymer grafted, or polymerized, from the surface of the bead means that the monomer must be in the solution and therefore lyophilic. This results with a polymer that has favorable interactions with the solution, allowing the polymer to form more linearly.

10.5 OVERVIEW TO THE LITERATURE

In 1999, mercuric ions' absorption from aqueous solutions by PAAm-grafted cellulose was studied by Biçak et al. The mercury-uptake capacity of the graft polymer is as high as 3.55 mmol/g, and sorption is also reasonably fast. The Hg(II) sorption is selective, and no interferences have been observed in the presence of Ni(II), Co(II), Cd(II), Fe(III), Zn(II) ions in 0.1 M concentrations at pH 6 [21].

In 1999, the properties of cellulose fiber and PMMA- or PBA-grafted cellulose fibers are investigated as a function of the initiator (ceric ammonium nitrate) concentration and the amount of grafted polymer onto cellulose fiber by Canché-Escamilla. The grafting of PMMA or PBA on the fiber results in lower mechanical properties than those of the ungrafted cellulose fiber [38].

In 2005, several approaches to the modification of cellulose fibers are studied, namely, (1) physical treatments such as corona or plasma treatments under different atmospheres; (2) grafting with hydrophobic molecules using well-known sizing compounds; (3) grafting with bifunctional molecules, leaving one of the functions available for further exploitation; and (4) grafting with organometallic compounds by Belgacem and Gandini. These different tools provided clear-cut evidence of the occurrence of chemical reactions between the grafting agent used and the hydroxy functions of the cellulose surface, as well as of the existence of covalent bonding in the ensuing composite materials between the matrix and the fibers through the use of doubly reactive coupling agents [39].

In 2006, Lönnberg graft epsilon-caprolactone (epsilon-CL) and L-lactide (L-LA) onto the surface of cellulose fibers by ring-opening polymerization method. Results showed an improved grafting efficiency after activation of the cellulose surface with *bis*-methylpropanamide and showed that the amount of grafted polymer could be controlled by the ratio of added free initiator to monomer [40].

In 2006, Pulat and Isakoca investigated the chemically induced graft copolymerizations of AA, AAm, crotonic acid, and itaconic acid (IA) onto cotton fibers. Benzoyl peroxide (BPO) was used as an initiator. The effects of grafting temperature, grafting time, and monomer and initiator concentrations on the grafting yields were studied, and optimum grafting conditions were determined for the sample material. The maximum grafting yield value obtained was 23.8% for AA [41].

The swelling percentage value of the ungrafted cotton fibers was 155%. The swelling values of the grafted fibers increased according to the grafting percentage. IA-grafted fibers were measured

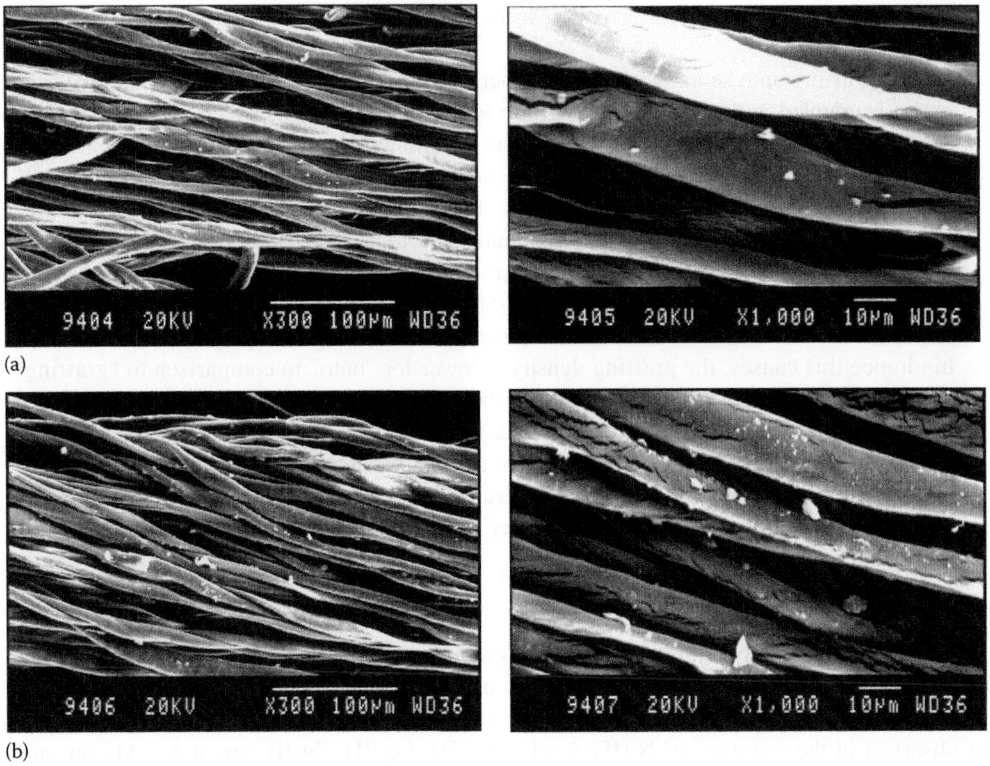

FIGURE 10.5 SEM micrographs of (a) AA-grafted cotton fibers at 300X and 1000X and (b) AAm-grafted fibers at 300X and 1000X.

as the most swollen fibers, with a swelling value of 510%. The AAm-grafted fibers were the least swollen fibers. A comparison of swelling percentage values shows that the swelling capacities of the grafted fibers were nearly three times higher than the capacity of the ungrafted cotton fibers.

Scanning electron micrographs of the grafted fibers are presented in Figure 10.5. As clearly shown in the micrographs, the rough and scaly tissue of the grafted fibers and bonded fibrils indicated the grafted copolymers.

In 2007, a novel degradable adsorbent for the removal of heavy metal ions from wastewater, a hyperbranched aliphatic polyester-grafted cellulose (HAPE-Cell), was successfully prepared by the simple one-pot method for the first time by Liu. The hyperbranched aliphatic polyester was grafted from the surface hydroxyl groups of natural cotton fibers via the solution polycondensation. The adsorption properties of the HAPE-Cell toward the heavy metal ions [Cu(II), Hg(II), Zn(II), and Cd(II)] were also preliminarily investigated [42].

In 2008, the chemical modification of cellulose by grafting reaction with AA considering different reaction factors was investigated by Neira et al. Maximum grafting yield was obtained as 90% at pH 7.0 [43].

In 2008, optimization of grafting of AN onto cellulosic material, isolated from bamboo (*Dendrocalamus strictus*), was performed by varying the process parameters such as duration of soaking of cellulosic material in ceric ammonium nitrate solution, ceric ammonium nitrate concentration, and polymerization time, temperature of reaction, and AN concentration by Khullar et al. The optimum reaction conditions obtained for the grafting of AN onto cellulosic material were duration of dipping cellulosic material in ceric ammonium nitrate solution 1 h, ceric ammonium nitrate concentration 0.02 M, AN concentration 24.6 mol/anhydroglucose units, temperature of reaction 40°C, and polymerization time 4 h. The percent grafting for optimized samples is 210.3%, and grafting efficiency is 97% [44].

In 2009, a facile method to graft biodegradable starch on fiber surface through the hydrogen bond formation among cellulose, starch, and ammonium zirconium (IV) carbonate was developed by Song et al. The effects of grafting conditions, including pH, temperature, fiber consistency, cross-linker, starch dosage, and mechanical agitation on the grafting yield, were systematically investigated. Optical and electron microscopes clearly revealed that, after grafting, the fiber surface was covered by hydrogel of starch. The significant improvements of water retention value of fibers with starch grafting were also demonstrated in this study [45].

In 2010, two cellulosic substrates (microcrystalline cellulose, MCC, and bleached kraft softwood pulps, BSK) were grafted by polycaprolactone (PCL) chains with different molecular weights, following a three-step procedure using nonswelling conditions in order to limit the reaction to their surface by Paquet et al. First, one of the two OH PCL ends was blocked by phenyl isocyanate, and the reaction product was subsequently reacted with 2,4-toluene diisocyanate to provide it with an NCO function, capable of reacting with cellulose. The polar component of the surface energy of cellulosic substrates before treatment was found to be about 32 and 10 mJ/m^2, for MCC and BSK, respectively [46].

In 2011, hyperbranched poly(3-methyl-3-oxetanemethanol) (HBPO) was directly grafted from the surface of cellulose fibers through a surface hydroxyl group–initiated ring-opening polymerization of 3-methyl-3-oxetanemethanol by Yang et al. Consuming only one surface hydroxyl, the grafting introduced a great number of new terminal hydroxyl groups. Because of three-dimensional architecture of the grafted HBPO, it can act as an effective macro-spacer from the cellulose surface, which makes the introduced hydroxyl groups highly reactive for further chemical modifications [47].

In 2011, ceric-induced grafting of AN onto alpha cellulose isolated from stems of *Lantana camara* was carried out with AN as monomer and ceric ammonium nitrate as initiator by Bhatt et al. The water retention value of grafted alpha cellulose pulp was obtained as 5.10 g/g, which is much lower than that obtained with ungrafted alpha cellulose pulp. *L. camara*, therefore, seems to be a potential feedstock for the production of alpha cellulose, which can be subsequently converted into grafted cellulose for several applications [48].

In 2011, the alkali-scoured cotton fabric was grafted with 2-(dimethylamino) ethyl acrylate (DMAEA) monomer using ceric ammonium nitrate as an effective initiator by free radical polymerization by Kathirvelan et al. The optimum reaction conditions for the grafting of DMAEA onto cellulosic material were studied. The percentages of graft yield and graft efficiency for the optimized sample were found to be 101.8 and 88.3, respectively. Thermal stability of grafted sample was increased [49].

In 2012, the heterogeneous grafting of cellulose fibers through controlled radical polymerization methods was highlighted by Malmström and Carlmark. Techniques such as atom transfer radical polymerization (ATRP) and reversible addition–fragmentation chain-transfer (RAFT) allow for fibers with tailorable properties and built-in functionality to be produced [50].

In 2012, Zhong et al. grafted MMA on a cellulose-based macro-initiator, cellulose chloroacetyl chloride, by the ATRP at a mild reaction temperature. The molecular weights and their distributions of the PMMA grafted onto the cellulose backbone were determined by gel permeation chromatography. The results confirmed that the generation of the cellulose-grafted PMMA at 50°C in the given solvent system was a controlled/living ATRP process [51].

In 2012, BPO-initiated grafting of MMA, 2-hydroxyethyl methacrylate (HEMA), and glycidyl methacrylate (GMA) onto cellulose extracted from pine needles along with their binary monomer mixtures with AAm, AA, and AN has been reported earlier by Sharma. Graft copolymers improved thermal stability as compared to cellulose as has been observed from initial decomposition temperature of the graft copolymers. Higher initial decomposition temperature of graft copolymers along with appreciable amount of residue left reflects on retardation in flammability and enhanced thermal stability of the graft copolymers. The binary monomer graft copolymers show different degradation pattern, and it has been observed that grafting of other monomer with MMA increases initial decomposition temperature, indicative of improved thermal stability than other graft copolymers. The highest initial decomposition temperature is recorded at 283.2°C for cell-*g*-poly(GMA-*co*-AN) [52].

In 2012, cellulose was used for the preparation of adsorbent of organic impurities in wastewater treatment. Hydrophobic surface of cellulose substrate was developed by grafting GMA in simultaneous grafting using gamma irradiation initiation by Takacs et al. Water uptake of cellulose significantly decreased, while adsorption of phenol and a pesticide molecule (2,4-dichlorophenoxyacetic acid: 2,4-D) increased upon grafting [53].

In 2014, RAFT-mediated free-radical graft copolymerization of HEMA onto cellulose fibers in a "grafting-from" approach under γ-irradiation was investigated by Kodama et al. The effects of absorbed dose and monomer concentration on the graft ratios were investigated at different monomer-to–RAFT agent (cumyldithio benzoate) ratios. Cellulose-g-PHEMA copolymers with various graft ratios up to 92% (w/w) have been synthesized [54].

In 2014, cellulose cotton fibers were first modified through graft copolymerization of polyacrylonitrile (PAN) and then by insertion of phenyl thio-semicarbazide (C-PTS) moieties to finally produce chelating fibers by Monier et al. The obtained C-PTS were employed in the removal and extraction of Au^{3+}, Pd^{2+}, and Ag^{+} precious metal ions from their aqueous solutions using batch experiments [55].

In our last research in 2014, graft copolymerization of HEMA monomers onto cotton fibers was performed, by using BPO, which is an original initiator for the HEMA/cotton system. The polymerization conditions were investigated, and the optimum grafting conditions were found as 0.25 M of HEMA concentration, 50°C, 2 h of grafting time, and 0.08 M of BPO concentration. The maximum grafting yield and grafting efficiency values were obtained as 47.6% and 51.2%, respectively. Swelling percentage values showed that the swelling capacities of grafted fibers were nearly three times higher than the capacity of ungrafted cotton fiber [56].

Scanning electron micrographs of ungrafted and PHEMA-grafted fibers are presented in Figure 10.6. A change in the morphology of fiber surface before and after grafting can be evidently observed. Both grafted and ungrafted cotton samples present fiber bundles (ribbon-like structure). No polymer chain or mound is detected on the ungrafted cotton fiber surfaces. Some apparent aggregates of PHEMA fibrils on the surface of grafted fibers are a good evidence for the successive

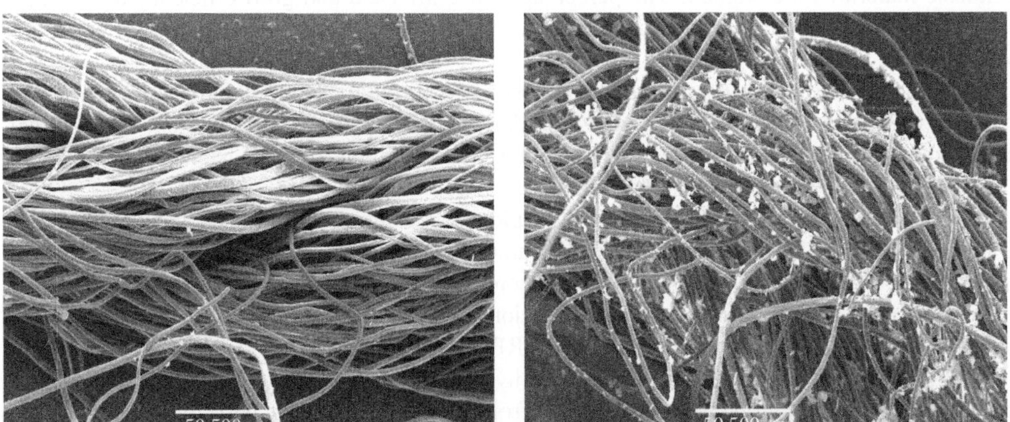

(a) (b)

FIGURE 10.6 SEM micrographs of (a) ungrafted cotton fibers and (b) HEMA-grafted cotton fibers.

TABLE 10.2
Comparative Fastness Rates of Grafted and Ungrafted Cotton Fibers

Sample	Weather Fastness	Washing Fastness	Wet Rubbing Fastness	Dry Rubbing Fastness
Ungrafted cotton fibers	5	4	3	5
HEMA-grafted cotton	5	5	5	5

grafting process. The bonded PHEMA fibrils on the cotton fibers indicate that the grafting was successfully performed.

Fastness tests were performed, and satisfactory results were obtained, in comparison with those reported in the literature. Although the grafted and ungrafted cotton fibers present similar weather and dry rubbing fastness ratings, the grafted cotton fibers had higher ratings of wet rubbing and washing fastness than the ungrafted cotton fibers. The ratings of rubbing, washing, and weather fastness of the cotton fibers are presented in Table 10.2. The results obtained from dry rubbing fastness, washing fastness, and weather fastness tests showed that the grafted and ungrafted cotton fibers appeared to have similar fastness values, with the exception of wet rubbing and washing fastness. The wet rubbing fastness value for HEMA-grafted cotton fiber was 5, while the wet rubbing fastness value for ungrafted cotton fiber was 3. The washing fastness rating of the grafted sample presents better rating than that of the ungrafted sample. The results given in the table indicate that the color of HEMA-grafted cotton fiber is more stable to wet rubbing and washing. Consequently, fastness results show that the ratings obtained from the fastness tests are satisfactory if compared with the values given in the literature.

REFERENCES

1. H. F. Mark, *Encyclopedia of Polymer Science and Technology, Concise*, John Wiley & Sons, Hoboken, NJ, 2007.
2. A. K. Mohanty, M. Misra, and L. T. Drzal, *Natural Fibers, Biopolymers, and Biocomposites*, April 8, CRC Press, Boca Raton, FL, 2005.
3. D. W. Ball, J. W. Hill, and R. J. Scott, *The Basics of General, Organic, and Biological Chemistry*, Chapter 16, Section 7, Flat World Knowledge, Washington, DC, 2011.
4. D. Roy, M. Semsarilar, J. T. Guthriea, and S. Perrie, Cellulose modification by polymer grafting: A review, *Chem. Soc. Rev.*, 38, 2046–2064, 2009.
5. D. Klemm, B. Heublein, H. P. Fink, and A. Bohn, *Angew. Chem., Int. Ed.*, Cellulose: Fascinating Biopolymer and Sustainable Raw Material, 44(22), 3358–3393, 2005.
6. R. L. Crawford, *Lignin Biodegradation and Transformation*, John Wiley & Sons, New York, 1981.
7. R. Young, *Cellulose Structure Modification and Hydrolysis*, Wiley, New York, 1986.
8. S. Kobayashi, K. Kashiwa, J. Shimada, T. Kawasaki, and S.-i. Shoda, Enzymatic polymerization: The first in vitro synthesis of cellulose via nonbiosynthetic path catalyzed by cellulase, *Makromolekulare Chemie. Macromolecular Symposia*, 54–55(1), 509–518, 1992.
9. S. Deguchi, K. Tsujii, and K. Horikoshi, Cooking cellulose in hot and compressed water, *Chem. Commun.*, 21(31), 3293, 2006.
10. H. A. Krassig, *Cellulose—Structure, Accessibility and Reactivity*, Gordon & Breach Science Publisher, Yverdon, Switzerland, 1993.
11. D. Klemm, B. Heublein, H.-P. Fink, and A. Bohn, Cellulose: Fascinating biopolymer and sustainable raw material, *Chem. Inform.*, 36(36), September 6, 2005.
12. A. Hebeish and J. T. Guthrie, *The Chemistry and Technology of Cellulosic Copolymers*, Springer-Verlag, Berlin, Germany, 1981.
13. T. Tzanov and A. Cavaco-Paulo, Surface modification of cellulose fibers with hydrolases and kinases, in: J. V. Edwards et al. (eds.), *Modified Fibers with Medical and Specialty Applications*, Chapter 10, pp. 159–180. Springer, Dordrecht, the Netherlands, 2006.

14. K. Ward Jr., *Chemical Modification of Papermaking Fibers*, Marcel Dekker Inc., New York, 1973.
15. R. K. Samal, P. K. Sahoo, and H. S. Samantaray, Graft copolymerization of cellulose, cellulose derivatives and lignocelluloses; *J. Macromol. Sci. R. M. C.*, 26, 81–141, 1986.
16. V. T. Stannett and H. B. Hopfenberg, in: N. M. Bikales and L. Segal (eds.), *Cellulose and Cellulose Derivatives*, Part. 5, pp. 907–936. John Wiley & Sons, New York, 1971.
17. E. H. Immergut, H. F. Mark, N. G. Gaylord, and N. M. Bikales, (ed.), *Encyclopedia of Polymer Science and Technology*, vol. 3: Casting to Cohesive Energy Density, pp. 242–284. Interscience, New York, 1965.
18. G. Gürdağ and S. Sarmad, Polysaccharide based graft copolymers, in: S. Kalia and M. W. Sabaa (eds.), *Cellulose Graft Copolymers: Synthesis, Properties, and Applications*, Chapter 2. Springer-Verlag, Berlin, Germany, 2013.
19. G. N. Richards and E. F. White, Graft polymerization on cellulosic materials. Part I. Cation exchange membranes from paper and acrylic acid, *J. Polym. Sci.*, 4, 1251–1260, 1964.
20. A. Waly, F. A. Abdel-Mohdy, A. S. Aly, and A. Hebeish, Synthesis and characterization of cellulose ion exchanger. II. Pilot scale and utilization in dye–heavy metal removal, *J. Appl. Polym. Sci.*, 68, 2151–2157, 1998.
21. N. Biçak, D. C. Sherrington, and B. F. Senkal, Graft copolymer of acrylamide onto cellulose as mercury selective sorbent, *React. Funct. Polym.*, 41, 69–76, 1999.
22. E. F. Okieimen, Studies on the graft copolymerization of cellulosic materials, *Eur. Polym. J.*, 23, 319–322, 1987.
23. B. B. Samal, S. Sahu, B. B. Chinara, S. Nanda, P. K. Otta, L. M. Mohapatro, T. R. Mohanty, A. R. Ray, and K. C. Singh, Grafting of vinyl monomers onto sisal fiber in aqueous solution, *J. Polym. Sci. Part A: Polym. Chem.*, 26, 3159–3166, 1988.
24. M. Misra, A. K. Mohanty, and B. C. Singh, A study on grafting of methyl methacrylate onto jute fiber ($S_2O_8^{2-}$-thiourea redox system), *J. Appl. Polym. Sci.*, 33, 2809–2819, 1987.
25. J. Xie and Y. L. Hsieh, Thermosensitive poly(*n*-isopropylacrylamide) hydrogels bonded on cellulose supports, *J. Appl. Polym. Sci.*, 89, 999–1006, 2003.
26. S. Ifuku and J. Kadla, Preparation of a thermosensitive highly regioselective cellulose/nisopropylacrylamide copolymer through atom transfer radical polymerization, *Biomacromolecules*, 9, 3308–3313, 2008.
27. D. Wang, J. Tan, H. Kang, L. Ma, X. Jin, R. Liu, and Y. Huang, Synthesis, self-assembly and drug release behaviors of pH-responsive copolymers ethyl cellulose-graft-PDEAEMA through ATRP, *Carbohydr. Polym.*, 84, 195–202, 2011.
28. D. W. Ball, J. W. Hill, and R. J. Scott, *The Basics of General, Organic, and Biological Chemistry*, v.1.0, Chapter 16: Carbohydrates, Section 7, Flat World Knowledge, Irvington, NY, 2011.
29. D. J. Mcdowall, B. S. Gupta, and V. T. Stannett, Grafting of vinyl monomers to cellulose by ceric ion inhibition, *Prog. Polym. Sci.*, 10, 1–50, 1984.
30. C. N. Saikia and F. Ali, Graft copolymerization of methyl methacrylate onto high α-cellulose pulp extracted from *Hibiscus sabdariffa* and *Gmelina arborea*, *Bioresour. Technol.*, 68, 165–171, 1999.
31. D. Roy, J. T. Guthrie, and S. Perrier, Graft polymerization: Grafting poly(styrene) from cellulose via reversible addition-fragmentation chain transfer (RAFT) polymerization, *Macromolecules*, 38, 10363–10372, 2005.
32. L. M. Zhang and L. Q. Chen, Water-soluble grafted polysaccharides containing sulfobetaine groups: Synthesis and characterization of graft copolymers of hydroxyethyl cellulose with 3-dimethyl(methacryloyloxyethyl)ammonium propane sulfonate, *J. Appl. Polym. Sci.*, 83, 2755–2761, 2002.
33. N. Tsubokawa, T. Iida, and T. Takayama, Modification of cellulose powder surface by grafting of polymers with controlled molecular weight and narrow molecular weight distribution, *J. Appl. Polym. Sci.*, 75, 515–522, 2000.
34. F. Khan, Photoinduced graft-copolymer synthesis and characterization of methacrylic acid onto natural biodegradable lignocellulose fiber, *Biomacromolecules*, 5, 1078–1088, 2004.
35. L. Wojnarovits, Cs. M. Földvary, and E. Takacs, Radiation-induced grafting of cellulose for adsorption of hazardous water pollutants: A review, *Radiat. Phys. Chem.*, 79, 848–862, 2010.
36. F. Khan, S. R. Ahmad, and E. Kronfli, UV-radiation-induced preirradiation grafting of methyl methacrylate onto lignocellulose fiber in an aqueous medium and characterization, *J. Appl. Polym. Sci.*, 91, 1667–1675, 2004.
37. A. Bhattacharya and B. N. Misra, Grafting: A versatile means to modify polymers techniques, factors and applications, *Prog. Polym. Sci.*, 29, 767–814, 2004.

38. G. Canché-Escamilla, J. I. Cauich-Cupul, E. Mendizábal, J. E. Puig, H. Vázquez-Torres, and P. J. Herrera-Franco, Mechanical properties of acrylate-grafted henequen cellulose fibers and their application in composites, *Compos. A: Appl. Sci. Manuf.*, 30(3), 349–359, 1999.
39. M. N. Belgacem and A. Gandini, Surface modification of cellulose fibers, *Polímeros*, 15(2), 114–121, 2005.
40. H. Lönnberg, Q. Zhou, H. Brumer, T. T. Teeri, E. Malmström, and A. Hult, Grafting of cellulose fibers with poly(epsilon-caprolactone) and poly(L-lactic acid) via ring-opening polymerization, *Biomacromolecules*, 7(7), 2178–2185, 2006.
41. M. Pulat and C. Isakoca, Chemically induced graft copolymerization of vinyl monomers onto cotton fibers, *J. Appl. Polym. Sci.*, 100, 2343–2347, 2006.
42. L. I. U. Peng, A novel degradable adsorbent of the hyperbranched aliphatic polyester grafted cellulose for heavy metal ions, *Turk. J. Chem.*, 31, 457–462, 2007.
43. A. Neira, M. Tarraga, and R. Catalan, Degradation of acrylic acid-grafted cellulose in aqueous medium with radical initiators, *J. Chil. Chem. Soc.*, 53, 1, 2008.
44. R. Khullar, V. K. Varshney, and S. Naithani, Grafting of acrylonitrile onto cellulosic material derived from bamboo (*Dendrocalamus strictus*), *eXPRESS Polym. Lett.*, 2(1), 12–18, 2008.
45. D. Song, Y. Zhao, C. Dong, and Y. Deng, Surface modification of cellulose fibers by starch grafting with crosslinkers, *J. Appl. Polym. Sci.*, 113(5), 3019–3026, 2009.
46. O. Paquet, M. Krouit, J. Bras, W. Thielemans, and M. N. Belgacem, Surface modification of cellulose by PCL grafts, *Acta Mater.*, 58(3), 792–801, 2010.
47. Q. Yang, X. Pan, F. Huang, and K. Li, Synthesis and characterization of cellulose fibers grafted with hyperbranched poly(3-methyl-3-oxetanemethanol), *Cellulose*, 18, 1611–1621, 2011.
48. N. Bhatt, P. K. Gupta, and S. Naithani, Ceric-induced grafting of acrylonitrile onto alpha cellulose isolated from *Lantana camara*, *Cellulose Chem. Technol.*, 45(5–6), 321–327, 2011.
49. D. Kathirvelan, S. Senthivel, and B. S. R. Reddy, Graft copolymerization of 2-(dimethylamino) ethyl acrylate onto cellulose (alkali scoured cotton) material, *Int. J. Fiber Textile Res.*, 1(2), 31–38, 2011.
50. E. Malmström and A. Carlmark, Controlled grafting of cellulose fibres—An outlook beyond paper and cardboard, *Polym. Chem.*, 3, 1702, 2012.
51. J.-F. Zhong, X.-S. Chai, and S.-Y. Fu, Homogeneous grafting poly(methylmethacrylate) on cellulose by atom transfer radical polymerization, *Carbohydr. Polym.*, 87(2), 1869–1873, January 15, 2012.
52. R. K. Sharma, A study in thermal properties of graft copolymers of cellulose and methacrylates, *Adv. Appl. Sci. Res.*, 3(6), 3961–3969, 2012.
53. E. Takacs, L. Wojnarovits, E. K. Horvath, T. Fekete, and J. Borsa, Improvement of pesticide adsorption capacity of cellulose fiber by high-energy irradiation-initiated grafting of glycidylmethacrylate, *Radiat. Phys. Chem.*, 81(9), 1389–1392, September 2012.
54. Y. Kodama, M. Barsbay, and O. Güven, Radiation-induced and RAFT-mediated grafting of poly(hydroxyethylmethacrylate) (PHEMA) from cellulose surfaces, *Radiat. Phys. Chem.*, 94, 98–104, 2014.
55. M. Monier, M. A. Akl, and W. M. Ali, Modification and characterization of cellulose cotton fibers for fast extraction of some precious metal ions, *Int. J. Biol. Macromol.*, 66, 125–134, 2014.
56. M. Pulat and F. Nuralin, Synthesis of 2-hydroxy ethyl methacrylate grafted cotton fibers and their fastness properties, *Cellulose Chem. Technol.*, 48(1–2), 137–143, 2014.

11 Modification of Jute Fibers by Radiation-Induced Graft Copolymerization and Their Applications

Mubarak A. Khan, Md. Saifur Rahaman, Abdullah-Al-Jubayer, and Jahid M.M. Islam

CONTENTS

11.1 INTRODUCTION

Jute belongs to the genus *Corchorus*, family Tiliaceae. *Corchorus capsularis* L. and *C. olitorius* L.—these two species of *Corchorus* are grown commercially. The chemical compositions of *olitorius* and *capsularis* jute are very similar (Kundu et al., 1959; Majumder et al., 1980; Ghose and Ganguly, 1996). Generally, jute plants grow to about 2.5–3.5 m in height. Jute fiber runs in the form of a lacework sheath along the length of the stem. In South Asia, the major jute-producing countries are Bangladesh, India, China, and Thailand. Over 90% of the world's raw jute and allied fiber is exported by Bangladesh. In terms of usage, global consumption, production, and availability, it is the second most important vegetable fiber after cotton. It is one of the cheapest and the strongest of all natural fibers (Kundu et al., 1959). Jute fiber has traditionally been used for the manufacturing of sacks, Hessian cloth, carpet and twines, ropes, and cords. Automotive, construction, and packaging industries are also using this fiber as a reinforcing material.

Jute fiber is renewable, cheap, biodegradable, and eco-friendly. Jute products compare well with other fibers in terms of energy use, greenhouse gas (GHG) emissions, eutrophication, and acidification. One hectare of jute plants absorb tons of CO_2 from the atmosphere and add 11 tons of O_2 during their lifespan of 120 days. Additionally, decomposed leaves and roots of jute plants enhance the fertility of the soil and reduce fertilizer costs. The manufacture of 1 kg of fabric of jute shopping bags saves 80 MJ of energy in comparison to 1 kg of polyhydroxy alkanoid (Chavez et al., 2012). Jute Hessian cloth consumes lesser amounts of energy and emits negligible amounts of GHG compared with thermoplastic polypropylene (PP) resin (Saha and Sagorika, 2013).

Jute fiber is chemically composed of cellulose (61%–71%), hemicelluloses (13.6%–20.4%), lignin (12%–13%), ash (0.5%–2%), pectin (~0.2%), wax (~0.5%), and moisture (~12.6%) (Rowell et al., 2000). The properties of the fiber are rolled by its different structural components. This fiber has two desirable properties—high cellulose content and low microfibril angle (~8.0°). This is important to be used as reinforcement in a polymer matrix (Rowell et al., 2000). The crystalline portion of cellulose shows resistance to strong alkali (17.5 wt%) but is hydrolyzed by acid easily (Heitner, 1993; Hon, 2000; Rowell and Stout, 2007). On the other hand, cellulose is relatively resistant to oxidizing agents. The cellulose fibrils facilitate rigidity and high tensile and flexural strength (FS). These fibrils are composed of microfibrils. Microfibrils form a microfibrillar angle with respect to the fiber axis. The stiffness of the fibers is determined by microfibrillar angle, which in turn governs the mechanical properties of the composite (Figure 11.1).

Low microfibril angle ensures the fiber to be more rigid, inflexible, and mechanically more strong. The value of the microfibrillar angle varies from fiber to fiber (Nevell and Zeronian, 1985; Rowell et al., 2000; Goda et al., 2009). Cellulose has a large number of hydroxyl groups that gives a hydrophilic character to jute fiber, which is responsible for its poor compatibility with hydrophobic polymer matrices and also for its dimensional instability. These hydroxyl groups make the fiber more reactive toward the different surface modifiers. The nature of cellulose and its crystallinity determine the reinforcing efficiency of jute fiber.

Being an amorphous, highly complex substance, lignin consists mainly of aromatic phenyl propane units, is very sensitive to oxidation, and readily undergoes condensation reactions (Joseph et al., 2000). Jute lignin contains predominantly sinapyl alcohol. A small portion of jute lignin can be dissolved in dilute alkali at room temperature (Ghose and Ganguly, 1996). Lignin is responsible for the ultraviolet (UV) degradation and is also considered to resist microbial degradation (Heitner, 1993; Hon, 2000).

Properties of jute fiber depend mainly on the nature of the plant, the locality in which it is grown, the age, and the extraction methods used. Additionally, the fiber aspect ratio, the volume fraction of fibers, and the orientation of fibers must be considered in the design of a fiber-reinforced composite (Netraveli and Chabba, 2003; Gupta and Gupta, 2005; Jacob et al., 2009). In comparison to glass, carbon, and aramid fibers, jute fiber has low density and is light with high specific

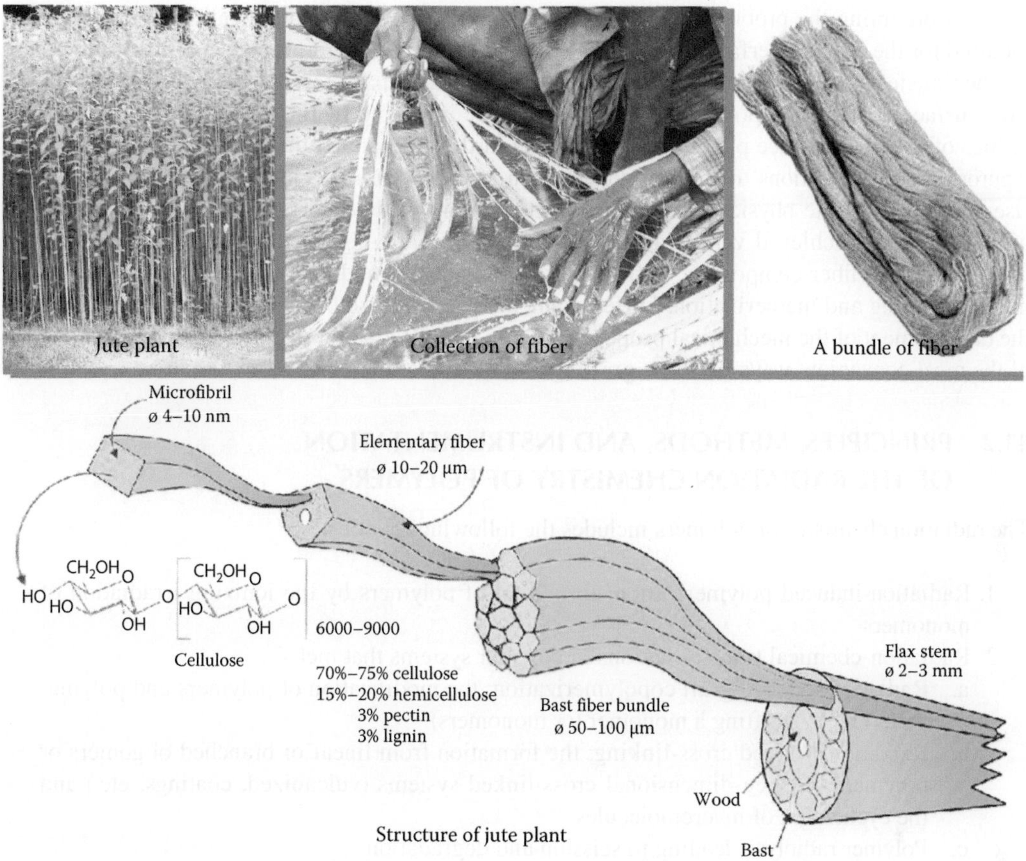

FIGURE 11.1 Structure of a jute plant and jute fiber.

strength and stiffness. Some important mechanical parameters of jute fiber are as follows: density 1.3–1.46 g cm^{-3}, elongation 1.5%–1.8%, tensile strength (TS) 393–800 MPa, Young's V modulus 10–30 GPa, specific TS 302–547 MPa/g cm^{-3}, and specific Young's modulus 8–20.5 GPa/g cm^{-3} (Paul et al., 1997; Bledzki and Gassan, 1999; Frederick and Norman, 2004).

Jute fiber can be degraded biologically by organisms. This results into weakening the fiber cell wall of the high-molecular-weight cellulose. Strength is lost through oxidation, hydrolysis, and dehydration reactions. Jute fiber also undergoes photochemical degradation by UV light when exposed outdoors. Exposure to UV can cause changes in the surface chemistry of the composite, which may result into discoloration, making the products aesthetically unappealing. Mechanical integrity may be lost due to prolonged UV exposure (Matuana et al., 2001; Matuana and Kamdem, 2002; Stark and Matuana, 2003).

Several disadvantages are associated with jute fibers as a reinforcement in polymer matrices. The presence of hydroxyl and other oxygen-containing groups in the fiber makes it polar and hydrophilic. But polymer matrices are mostly nonpolar thermoplastics. This results in poor dispersion and interfacial adhesion between the fiber and matrix phases. This is a major disadvantage of jute fiber–reinforced composites. High moisture absorption is another drawback of jute fibers. It results in poor mechanical properties and reduces dimensional stability of the composites. Higher processing temperature (above 250°C) results in the degradation of jute fiber, which restricts the choice of matrices. The variations in properties within the same fiber also work as a barrier in producing composites with uniform properties.

For overcoming the problems associated with jute fibers, surface modification of jute fibers is required for the strong interfacial adhesion between the matrix and reinforcement phases, essential for the transfer of load from the former to the latter. Surface characteristics such as wetting, adhesion, surface tension, and porosity of the fibers can be improved by the modification. The irregularities of the fiber surface play an important role in the mechanical interlocking at the interface. Appropriate modifications to the components can improve the interfacial properties, which give rise to changes in the physical and chemical interactions at the interface. Surface modifications of jute fiber have achieved various levels of success in improving fiber strength and fiber/matrix adhesion in jute fiber composites. Different types of surface modification have been carried out, mainly grafting and mercerization. Different chemicals have also been successfully employed for the development of the mechanical properties of jute fiber. Radiation processing technology is one of the most convenient ways for these grafting and modifications.

11.2 PRINCIPLES, METHODS, AND INSTRUMENTATION OF THE RADIATION CHEMISTRY OF POLYMERS

The radiation chemistry of polymers includes the following sections:

1. Radiation-induced polymerization: formation of polymers by the ionizing irradiation of monomers
2. Radiation-chemical transformations in polymer systems that include
   a. Radiation-induced graft copolymerization: the modification of polymers and polymer materials by grafting a monomer (or monomers)
   b. Radiation-induced cross-linking: the formation from linear or branched oligomers or polymers of three-dimensional cross-linked systems (vulcanized, coatings, etc.) and the cyclization of macromolecules
   c. Polymer radiolysis leading to scission and degradation
   d. Polymer-analogous transformations proceeding (or intensified) by ionizing radiation
3. Protection of polymers against radiation and their radiation resistance

Each of these sections, apart from its theoretical content, is mainly considered as specific manifestations of the main problem of chemistry: the dependence of the properties on the structure of the substance also has some practical aspects. They show the possibility of useful application of atomic energy to the synthesis or modification of polymers and polymer materials. Thus, it is possible to synthesize, modify, cross-link, or degrade polymers by using ionizing radiation.

Radiation processing is a promising technology that can be used to produce new composite materials using other better means and in an environmentally friendly way. This technology has been used in multilayer tables and is under investigation in numerous other areas, such as structural ports for use as automotive panels and for the electro-optical devices, health-care products, and many other areas.

The basic advantages of using radiation for industrial processing depend on actual application. There are some general facts such as it offers significant energy savings and reliability, gives products of superior quality, and can be used to obtain new products.

The basic requirements for successful radiation application depend on actual industrial process. Some conditions are common for all applications such as radiation treatment should produce no induced radioactivity, should be safe for operating personnel, and should be cheaper and more reliable than that of alternative technique.

Additionally, radiation sources and material handling equipment have to match capacity and reliability of standard industrial production.

In this chapter, mainly two types of radiation sources for the production of radiation-induced graft copolymers are going to be discussed:

1. Gamma radiation source: the energy of Co-60 rays is below the threshold level of other nuclear photon-induced reactions. Inducing radioactivity in irradiated materials is not possible theoretically or practically.
2. UV light source: here energy carried out by UV photon (between 200 and 450 nm) is used to form one or many radicals that are reactive enough to initiate polymerization reaction.

This technology relies on the use of radiation energy to initiate chemical reactions that induce biological or chemical or physical changes of materials. Extremely high efficiency of energy conversion results from the transfer of high quanta, comparable to electron bonding energies in atoms and molecules. Elementary processes of interactions induce molecular and atomic excitations and ionizations that result in the production of a multitude of reactive species such as free radicals, radical ions, and excited species at different levels of excitations. Depending on the system and irradiation conditions, these species initiate favorable or unfavorable chemical reactions.

11.2.1 Physicochemical Properties of Composites: Definition and Impacts

11.2.1.1 Tensile Strength

The TS of a material is the maximum amount of tensile stress that it can bear before failure, for example, breaking. It is an important property for polymers. For example, fibers must have good TS. In comparison to other composites, jute composites have a higher TS. Sometimes TS is also expressed by tensile factor (Tf), which is the ratio of the TS of samples and control.

11.2.1.2 Elongation at Break

Elongation at break (Eb) is the ratio between changed length and initial length after breakage of the test specimen. It is also known as fracture strain or ultimate elongation. It expresses the capability of a material to resist changes of shape without forming crack. This usually is expressed as a percentage. Fibers generally have a low Eb, for example, jute composites have an Eb of 1-2%.

11.2.1.3 Water Retention/Capture

The water retention value (WRV) test provides an indication of fibers' ability to absorb water and swell. The WRV is also highly correlated to the bonding ability of fibers. Jute composites show good water retention capacity, which is up to 70%. The WRV or water absorption capacity is determined by the following equation:

$$\text{Water absorption capacity} = \left[\left(\text{Final weight} - \text{Initial weight}\right) / \text{Initial weight}\right] \times 100\%$$

11.2.1.4 Grafting

When two or more chemically different polymeric parts form a polymer, it is called graft copolymer. These are segmented copolymers with a linear backbone of one composite and randomly distributed branches of other composites. The percentage of grafting is defined as follows:

$$\%\ \text{Grafting} = \frac{\text{Final cellulose weight} - \text{Initial cellulose weight}}{\text{Initial cellulose weight}} \times 100$$

11.2.1.5 Polymer Loading

The loading capacity of a composite polymer is a measure of the number of anchoring sites per gram of polymer. It is expressed in units of millimole per gram ($mmolg^{-1}$). High polymeric loading is advantageous to reduce the total expenditure of polymer supports and to allow manageable amounts of material in medium- or large-scale application. It also reduces the solubilizing capacity. Jute fiber has a high polymer-loading capacity than many other fibers.

11.2.1.6 Charpy Impact

The Charpy impact test determines the amount of energy absorbed by a material during fracture. This test is used to study temperature-dependent ductile–brittle transition and can be used to measure the toughness of the material. It cannot be expressed by a standard formula. The apparatus consists of a pendulum of known mass and length that is dropped from a known height to impact a notched specimen of material. The energy transferred to the material can be inferred by comparing the difference in the height of the hammer before and after the fracture (energy absorbed by the fracture event).

11.2.1.7 Impact Strength

The impact strength (IS) describes the ability of a material to absorb shock and impact energy without breaking; simply saying, it is a measure of the impact resistance of materials. The IS is calculated as the ratio of impact absorption to test specimen cross section. The test is similar to the Charpy impact test but uses a different arrangement of the specimen under test. The impact test differs from the Charpy impact test in that the sample is held in a cantilevered beam configuration as opposed to a three-point bending configuration.

11.2.2 Composite Manufacturing Processes

Process of manufacturing composites can be of different kinds. Among them, the followings are very common:

1. *Hand layup*: The most commonly used method for the manufacture of both small and large reinforced products is the hand layup technique. A flat surface, a cavity, or a positive-shaped mold made from wood, metal, plastic, or a combination of these materials are used for the method (Al-Kafi et al., 2006).
2. *Pultrusion*: This is used for manufacturing composite materials into continuous, constant cross-sectional profiles as it is an automated process. The product is pulled from the dice rather than forced out by pressure. A large number of profiles such as rods, tubes, and various structural shapes can be produced using appropriate dice.
3. *Injection molding*: Both thermoplastic and thermosetting plastic materials can be prepared by this method and is the best for producing high volumes of the same object (Heitner, 1993). Composites are fed into a heated barrel, mixed and forced into a mold cavity where it cools and hardens to the configuration of the mold cavity.
4. *Spray-up*: The spray-up method allows rapid formation of uniform composite coating. However, the mechanical properties of the material are moderate as the method is unable to use continuous reinforcing fibers. Liquid resin matrix and chopped reinforcing fibers are sprayed by separate sprays onto the mold surface in this process. The fibers are chopped into 1–2″ (25–50 mm) length and then sprayed by an air jet simultaneously with a resin spray at a predetermined ratio between the reinforcing and matrix phases (Khan et al., 2006; Doan et al., 2007).
5. *Compression molding*: This is also known as "heat-pressed" molding and is a conventional and simple method for the manufacture of jute fiber–reinforced composites. Use of molds allows for the production of composites with simple shapes and curved surfaces. In this method, the sandwich is prepared by placing jute fabric (JF) or yarn between the polymer sheets. This is then laid inside the mold and heat-pressed at pressure.

11.2.3 Methods of Cellulose Grafting

Cellulose and cellulose derivatives have been grafted by various initiator systems. The grafting methods of cellulose and cellulosic materials basically fall into three major types: (1) initiation by chemical method, (2) initiation by irradiation, and (3) initiation by thermal method. Initiation of grafting by chemical means is preferred owing to its simple nature and less requirement of special equipment. Chemical initiation methods yield free radicals that are necessarily a part of the monomer or the polymer. They are classified as (1) free radical-producing initiator systems and (2) redox systems.

Free radical initiation is a primary method of forming cellulose graft copolymers. In some cases, macrocellulosic radicals are formed directly and initiate polymerization of vinyl monomers onto cellulose. In other cases, free radicals are formed, which may abstract hydrogen atoms from cellulose to form macrocellulosic radical sites. Ionic-initiated grafting of vinyl monomers onto cellulose by formation of active sites on cellulosic molecule has been reported. Two important factors in free radical initiation of grafting reactions of vinyl monomers with fibrous cellulose are (1) the lifetimes of macrocellulosic radicals are formed and (2) the soaking time of fibrous cellulose in solutions of monomers. The short-lived radicals, usually more accessible, are probably scavenged by the solvent, and the long-lived radicals predominate in initiating polymerization. The long-lived radicals are present in the more molecularly oriented regions of the fiber.

Graft copolymerization using conventional chemical methods of initiation has been an accepted technology for many years, whereas physical activation processes are the modern and graduating technology. Physical activation processes include

1. Use of low-energy irradiation methods (like UV light in the presence of photosensitizer)
2. Use of high-energy irradiation methods (like gamma rays and electron beam)
3. Mechanical treatment methods (like mastication and ultrasonic wave–induced degradation)

11.2.4 UV-Curing Mechanism

Techniques involving UV are particularly attractive since the UV sources are relatively cheap, flexible, and easy to install. Photo-initiation is also unique in that it allows a precise control of the duration and the rate at which initiating species are produced. This explains that photo-induced polymerization has attracted so much interest during the last decade and has found a growing numbers of industrial applications. An advantage of using UV radiation is the fact that rather inexpensive radiation sources such as mercury lamps or germicidal lamps can be used to initiate grafting. Owing to the low energy of this type of radiation, the degradation of cellulose substrate is almost negligible. On the other hand, this method is applicable only for surface grafting because of the low penetrating power of the UV radiation. It is therefore most useful for modifying the surface properties of films and fibers but cannot be used where a change in bulk properties is desired.

Grafting of different monomers onto cellulose is a typical free radical mechanism. Irradiation grafting is the most convenient method. The initial effects of radical formation on cellulose are to depolymerize the molecule and increase the concentration of carbonyl and carboxyl groups. The grafting reaction starts with the photolysis of carbonyl group. The degree of grafting and the apparent number of grafting chains vary with the species and position of carboxyl groups. Free radical mechanism involves three distinct aspects—initiation, propagation, and termination.

11.2.4.1 Initiation

UV radiation can be used to initiate grafting since the type of radiation is not sufficiently of high energy to break C–C or C–H bonds. A photosensitizer must be added in the system. Initiation consists of the production of free radicals on the cellulose backbone. The initiator in the photo-activated system gives excited initiator (having high energy) that transfers energies to cellulose samples thereby causing free radical formation by hydrogen abstraction and glucosidic bond scission. These cellulose macroradicals can then diffuse to points on the trunk polymer and abstract hydrogen atoms leaving radical sites for grafting.

$$\text{Cell-OH} \rightarrow \text{Cell-OH}^{*} \rightarrow \text{CellO}^{\bullet} + \text{OH}^{\bullet}$$

$$\text{M (Monomer)} \rightarrow \text{M}^{*} \rightarrow \text{M}^{\bullet} + \text{H}^{\bullet}$$

$$\text{Photo initiator} \xrightarrow{\text{hv}} \text{P}^{*} \rightarrow \text{P}^{\bullet} + \text{H}^{\bullet}$$

$$\text{Cell-OH} + \text{P}^{\bullet} \rightarrow \text{Cell O}^{\bullet} + \text{PH}$$

$$\text{M} + \text{P}^{\bullet} \rightarrow \text{M}^{\bullet} + \text{P}^{\bullet}$$

where CellO• and M• represent the cellulose and monomer redeemer radicals, respectively.

11.2.4.2 Propagation

The cellulose macroradical thus formed reacts with an unexcited monomer molecule and adds to it, forming a new radical capable of further interaction with the initial monomers.

$$\text{CellO}^{\bullet} + \text{M}^{\bullet} \rightarrow \text{CellOM}^{\bullet}$$

$$\text{Cell-OH} + \text{M} \rightarrow \text{CellOM}$$

$$\text{CellOM}^{\bullet} + \text{nM} \rightarrow \text{CellOM}^{\bullet}_{\text{n+1}}$$

$$\text{M}^{\bullet} + \text{nM} \rightarrow \text{M}^{\bullet}_{\text{n+1}}$$

11.2.4.3 Termination

Termination occurs by combination, where the radicals of two growing polymer chains are coupled:

$$\text{CellOM} \cdot \text{x} + \text{CellOM} \cdot \text{y} \rightarrow \text{CelloMx} - \text{MyOCell (Grafted structure)}$$

$$\text{M}^{\bullet}_{\text{n+1}} + \text{H}^{\bullet} \rightarrow \text{M}_{\text{n+1}}\text{H}$$

Chain transfer of disproportionate:

$$\text{M}^{\bullet} + \text{H}^{\bullet} \rightarrow \text{MH}$$

$$\text{M}^{\bullet} + \text{M}^{\bullet} \rightarrow \text{MM (Homopolymer)}$$

11.2.5 Mechanism of Grafting by Gamma Radiation

The influence of ionizing radiation on polymers, particularly γ-radiation, has been studied quite extensively over the past few decades. Ionizing radiation such as γ-radiation is known to deposit energy in solid cellulose by Compton scattering, and the rapid localization of energy within molecules produced trapped macrocellulosic radicals. The radicals thus generated are responsible for changing the physical, chemical, and biological properties of cellulose fibers.

Mechanism of gamma-irradiated grafting of jute fibers is similar to that of UV curing, except that the gamma radiation treatment does not need any photoinitiator to induce the grafting as it is a high-energy radiation. The modification of jute surface by gamma radiation thus can be summarized as follows, which is based upon the principle of free radical polymerization:

Initiator	$RH \xrightarrow{\gamma\text{-radiation}} R^\bullet$
Propagation	$R^\bullet + O_2 \rightarrow ROO^\bullet$
	$RH + ROO^\bullet \rightarrow ROOH + R^\bullet$
	$ROOH \rightarrow RO^\bullet + {}^\bullet OH$
	$2ROOH \rightarrow ROO^\bullet + RO^\bullet + H_2O$
	$RO^\bullet + RH \rightarrow ROH + R^\bullet$
	${}^\bullet OH + RH \rightarrow R^\bullet + H_2O$
Termination	$R^\bullet + R^\bullet \rightarrow R_2$
	$R^\bullet + ROO^\bullet \rightarrow ROOR$
	$ROO^\bullet + ROO^\bullet \rightarrow ROOR + O_2$

Here RH = jute cellulose and $R^\bullet$ is the possible free radical formed by the abstraction of $H^\bullet$ and OH from jute cellulose cleavage of C2–C3 bonds and chain scission of cellulose backbone.

11.2.6 Mechanism of Grafting by Thermal Method

Peroxidases are used in thermal process for initiating free radicals. In this work, benzoyl peroxide (catalyst) was used as a source of free radicals to initiate the polymerization of the monomer ethylene glycol (EG). Dissociation energies of C–H, C–C, and O–O are 100, 83, and 35 kcal per mole, respectively. Therefore, the weakest and most heat-sensitive bond of benzoyl peroxide is O–O. Thus, a benzoyl peroxide molecule can produce two phenyl free radicals on heat treatment:

$$Ph-CO-O-O-CO-Ph \rightarrow 2Ph-CO-O^\bullet \rightarrow 2Ph^\bullet + 2CO_2 \quad (11.1)$$

Each phenyl radical ($R^\bullet$) can then initiate polymerization reaction:

$$R^\bullet + M \rightarrow R-M^\bullet \quad (11.2)$$

where M is a monomer.

Propagation step can be represented by the following addition of monomer to the aforementioned growing chain:

$$R-(M)_n-M^\bullet + M \rightarrow R-(M)_{n+1}-M^\bullet \quad (11.3)$$

Chain termination may take place in three ways:

1. Recombination of radicals:

$$R-(M)_n-M^\bullet + R-(M)_n-M^\bullet \rightarrow R-(M)_n-M-M-(M)_n-R \quad (11.4)$$

2. By chain transfer (or radical transfer) to the cellulose molecule:

$$R-(M)_n-M + H{:}Cellulose \rightarrow R-(M)_n-M-H + Cellulose \quad (11.5)$$

One H can be extracted from the jute yarn cellulose, and in this case, there would be a polymer branch growing on the jute yarn.

$$R-M+\text{Cellulose}\rightarrow R-M-\text{Cellulose grafted} \quad (11.6)$$

3. Termination by disproportion:

$$-CH_2-CH_2^{\bullet}+{}^{\bullet}CH_2-CH_2\rightarrow -CH=CH_2+CH_3-CH_2 \quad (11.7)$$

11.3 RADIATION-INDUCED GRAFTING OF JUTE FIBER

11.3.1 Modification by UV Radiation

11.3.1.1 Monomer and Oligomer Grafting

UV radiation–induced monomer and oligomer grafting to improve surface characteristics such as wetting, adhesion, surface tension, and porosity of jute fibers is the most common technique for surface modification. The irregularities of the fiber surface play an important role in the mechanical interlocking at the interface. Appropriate modifications to the components can improve the interfacial properties, which give rise to changes in the physical and chemical interactions at the interface.

Several studies have been conducted to improve the quality of jute fiber by UV radiation technique. Especially modification by monomers like acrylamide (AA), 2-hydroxyethylmethacrylate (HEMA), methylmethacrylate (MMA), 2-hydroxyethylacrylate (HEA), 1,6-hexanedioldiacrylate (HDDA), 3-(trimethoxysilyl)propylmethacrylate (TMSPM), and urethane acrylate (UA) has been well characterized and documented.

By modification with vinyl monomers like HEMA (Khan et al., 2003a; Khan and Drzal, 2004) using UV radiation, monomer solutions of different concentrations in methanol along with photoinitiator (Irgacure-184) were prepared and optimized. Degree of grafting of the Hessian cloth was found to increase with increase in radiation time as well as monomer concentration. For HEMA, the maximum grafting occurs at five UV passes at 3% concentration (Figure 11.2).

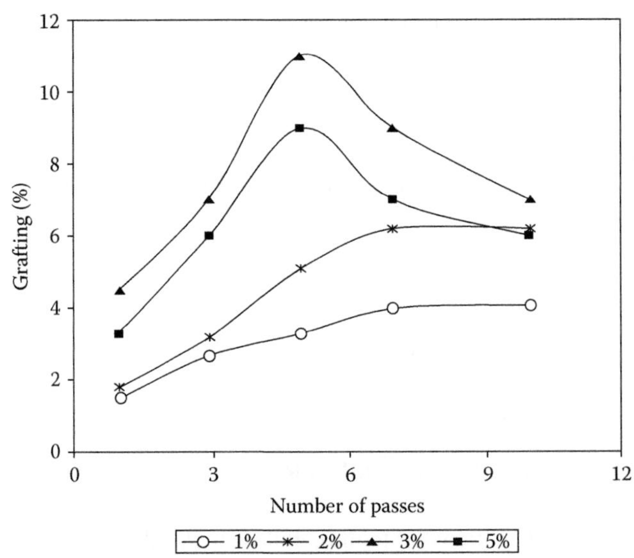

FIGURE 11.2 Grafting versus radiation dose (number of passes) with respect to HEMA concentration.

The radiation-induced graft copolymerization reaction on vinyl monomer onto cellulose backbone is affected by the diffusion of monomer into the fiber. The swelling of trunk polymer cellulose and the Trommsdorff effect of solvent on grafting also affect grafting of monomer onto cellulose. Soaking increases the cross-sectional area of the fiber at the same time the fiber surface becomes lustrous. As a result, the monomer can easily diffuse in the fiber and react with cellulose in a lower soaking time. In higher soaking time, the fiber becomes twisted, shrinks, and changes its outer fibrillar layer.

After achieving the highest polymer loading (PL) value, PL value decreases with increasing monomer concentration. The vinyl monomer promotes rapid free radical propagation reaction with the help of photoinitiator, leading to a network of (cross-linking) polymer structures through grafting via their double bonds. When concentration of vinyl monomer is increased, the amount of residual unsaturation also increases as a consequence of the faster rate of formation of the three-dimensional network causing restricted mobility in the early stage. The cross-linking rate especially during the early stages of radiation is proportional to monomer concentration. Increase in the concentration of monomer increases the radical–radical reaction termination and hence decreases the extent of secession reaction and oxidation. Solvent also plays a pivotal role in the decreasing trend of polymer load with monomer concentration increase. The swelling of the cellulose backbone with MeOH is insufficient due to low MeOH concentration. As a result, monomer molecules are incapable of penetrating the cellulose molecules in the presence of low solvent concentrations. This may cause a smaller number of reacting sites at the cellulose backbone and thus continue to reduce the active sites as MeOH concentration decreases with higher monomer concentration.

TS of the monomer-treated Hessian cloth decreases in higher monomer concentration, which can be rationalized by the homo-polymerization reaction between the monomer and monomer radicals that is dominated over the monomer–cellulose reaction at higher monomer concentration. The highest mechanical properties of grafted fiber (80% increase of TS and 93% increase of Eb) were found for 3% HEMA in methanol at the fifth pass of UV radiation.

In simulated weathering test of the samples, tensile properties, particularly TS and Eb, were periodically monitored. The losses of TS and Eb resulting from the weathering treatment are plotted in Figure 11.3. During the initial period of the weathering test, the strength increases with the treated samples (but not with the untreated one). This means that some unreacted radicals and

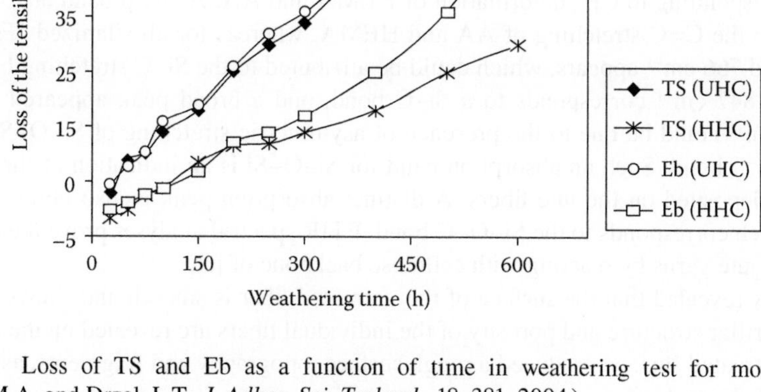

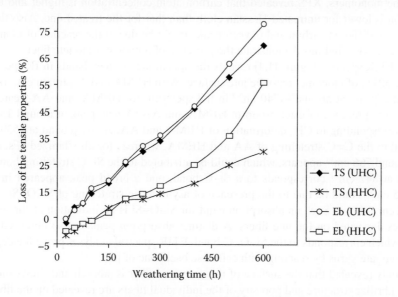

FIGURE 11.3 Loss of TS and Eb as a function of time in weathering test for monomer HEMA. (From Khan, M.A. and Drzal, L.T., *J. Adhes. Sci. Technol.*, 18, 381, 2004.)

other entities produced during grafting reaction under UV radiation were present in the treated samples, and these radicals/entities were reactivated further under the UV lamp used during the weathering test. Thus, there were some increases in the tensile properties at the initial stage, and then these started to decrease, due to weathering effect. The maximum losses of TS and Eb for virgin fiber were found to be 70% and 78%, respectively, and those for treated samples were found to be 30% and 56%.

The variations of dielectric properties with temperature were also measured at 10 kHz frequency. It was observed that dielectric constant and loss tangent (tan) increased with increasing temperature up to the transition temperature and then decreased, and at the end became almost constant. Both the dielectric constant and loss tangent depend on the number of radiation pass. For both dielectric constant and loss tangent, there is a transition at the same temperature. This transition is very likely associated with ferroelectric to paraelectric phase transition. Jute is composed of cellulose whose skeletal backbone is linked by intramolecular hydrogen-bonded material. As temperature increases, these bonds break up to split the chain into smaller units of dipoles. The dipoles so formed trend to align them with the applied electric field and thus increase the dielectric constant and loss tangent. At the transition temperature, the formation of dipoles and alignment toward the field are maximum, giving rise to maximum dielectric constant and loss tangent values. Above the transition temperature, the dipoles trend to be oriented random. As the randomness increases with increasing temperature, the dielectric constant and loss tangent decrease and eventually become constant. The maximum dielectric constant and loss tangent were found at a lower transition temperature because UV radiation of the composites might be due to the photo-cross-linking between the neighboring cellulose molecules and polymer matrix that occurs under UV exposure.

The water uptake value of untreated jute sample was higher than that of treated sample because monomer reacts with the OH groups of cellulose of the jute through graft copolymerization and reduces the hydrophilic nature of jute resulting in a decrease in the water uptake.

To further establish the relationship between the mechanical properties with modification, modified and virgin jute fiber surfaces are characterized by x-ray photoelectron spectroscopy (XPS), Fourier transform infrared spectroscopy (FTIR), and environmental scanning electron microscopy (ESEM).

For all the monomers, XPS revealed that carbon atom concentration is higher and the oxygen concentration is lower for untreated Hessian cloth than that for the treated one. Also the changes in total areas of different carbon and oxygen peaks might be due to the reaction of monomer with cellulose. These XPS findings demonstrate the presence of monomer onto jute fiber.

Study of FTIR spectra (Figure 11.4) reveals the appearance of new bands in IR spectra, which proves the grafting of monomer onto the jute surface. With HEMA and AA treatment, the carbonyl (C=O) band appears at around ~1740 cm^{-1} in the spectrum for HEMA- and AA-treated Hessian cloth, due to the presence of ester group in HEMA and AA. A new peak at around 1396 cm^{-1} is observed, corresponding to CH_3 deformation of HEMA and AA. A sharp band at 1539 cm^{-1} may be attributed to the C=C stretching of AA and HEMA, whereas for all silanized JFs, absorption peaks at around 766 cm^{-1} appears, which could be attributed to the Si–C stretching bond. A weak peak found at 847 cm^{-1} corresponds to a Si–C bond, and a broad peak appeared in the range of 925–1105 cm^{-1} could be due to the presence of asymmetric stretching of Si–O–Si or Si–O–C (1014–1090 cm^{-1}) bond. Such an absorption band for Si–O–Si is an indication of the existence of polysiloxanes deposited on the jute fibers. A distinct absorption peak is also observed at around 1200 cm^{-1}, which corresponds to the Si–O–C bond. FTIR spectral analyses prove the deposition of monomer onto jute yarns by reacting with cellulose backbone of jute.

ESEM study revealed that the surface of the untreated fiber is smooth and shows multicellular nature. The fibrillar structure and porosity of the individual fibers are revealed on the fiber surface. The monomer-treated surface produced a rough surface topography and fragments, as well as shallow and cut-off channels.

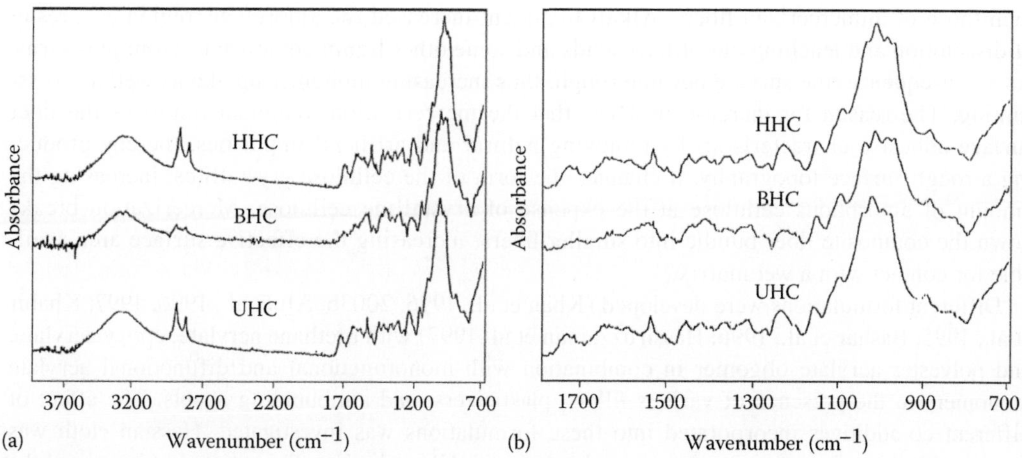

FIGURE 11.4 (a) FTIR spectra of unbleached (UHC), bleached (BHC), and HEMA-treated (HHC) Hessian cloth from 4000 to 700 cm^{-1} and (b) FTIR spectra of unbleached (UHC), bleached (BHC), and HEMA-treated (HHC) Hessian cloth from 1800 to 700 cm^{-1}.

Studies with some other different monomers like HEA (Khan et al., 2010), (MMA, butyl acrylate (BA), and styrene [ST]) (Khan et al., 2002) showed that similar trends in mechanical and electrical properties due to grafting of jute (Hessian cloth) under UV radiation at different intensities were observed and rationalized likewise. The concentrations of the monomers and oligomer, radiation dose, and soaking time were optimized with respect to mechanical property such as TS of the treated and untreated Hessian cloth. The 73% HEA, 25% oligomer urethane acrylate (M-1200), and 2% photoinitiator (Darocur-1116) in 1 min soaking time showed the highest TS at 50th UV pass, which was found to be about 190% of the untreated sample. The highest PL values for MMA, BA, and ST (2.9%, 5.0%, and 4.75%) were obtained with the monomer concentrations 50%, 10%, and 20% for MMA, BA, and ST, respectively. Maximum TS enhancement was observed for the sample treated by 70% MMA followed by 10% BA. Five types of additives (1%) of different chemical nature, such as 2-hydroxyethyl methacrylate (HEA), ethylhexyl acrylate, AA, *N*-vinyl pyrrolidine, and urea (U), were added into the bulk monomer (MMA, BA, and ST) solutions, and their effects on grafting and mechanical properties of jute yarn were also investigated by Khan et al. (2002). Among all additives, only U showed better properties in MMA + MeOH system. This enhancement could be caused by the augmentation preprocess rendered by the carbamide group (=N–CO–) present in U. Water uptake of the treated and untreated samples was also measured, and BA-grafted samples showed lower water uptake to that of virgin as well as other treated samples. The sample with 70% MMA showed the maximum (42%) water uptake. The acrylated monomer reacts with OH groups of cellulose through graft copolymerization reaction and hence reduces the hydrophilic nature of the cellulose of jute yarn.

Effect of alkali on the grafting of jute yarn with 1,6-hexanediol diacrylate (HDDA) in methanol in the presence of a small quantity of photoinitiator (Darocur-1664) by UV radiation pretreatment was investigated by Khan et al. (2004). Jute yarns were pretreated with alkali solution, and after that, they were treated under UV radiation of various intensities to investigate the change in mechanical properties of jute yarn. The pretreated samples were grafted with optimized monomer concentration. Increase in properties of alkali and UV-pretreated and grafted samples such as PL (12%), TS (103%), Eb (46%), and tensile modulus (TS; 114%) were achieved over those of virgin jute yarn. During alkali–UV monomer treatment, PL values increased because more monomer may be introduced into the cellulose backbone as a result of mercerization and application of a UV radiation—induced modified surface. Mercerized fibers yielded higher PL values than those of unmercerized fibers. Alkali treatment increased the amorphous region as a result of dissolution and leaching out of fatty acids and some other lignin components from jute yarns. As a consequence, the surface became rough, thus increasing monomer uptake as well as cross-linking. The reason for increase in TS is that the mercerization treatment improves the fiber surface-adhesive characteristics by removing natural and artificial impurities, thereby producing a rough surface topography. It changes the form of the cellulose crystallites, increasing the amount of amorphous cellulose at the expense of crystalline cellulose. Mercerization breaks down the composite fiber bundle into smaller fibers, increasing the effective surface area available for contact with a wet matrix.

Different formulations were developed (Khan et al., 1996, 2003b; Ali et al., 1996, 1997; Khabir et al., 1995; Bashar et al., 1996; Hassiruzzaman et al. 1997) with urethane acrylate, epoxy acrylate, and polyester acrylate oligomer in combination with monofunctional and difunctional acrylate monomers in the presence of various fillers, plasticizers, and antibubbling agents. The effect of different co-additives incorporated into these formulations was investigated. Hessian cloth was coated with these formulated solutions and cured with UV radiation. This treatment improved the rheological properties of the Hessian cloth. Incorporation of certain amide additives and inorganic salts further improved the tensile properties of the Hessian cloth with enhanced water absorption resistivity.

A new and interesting study was done by Hassan et al. (2003c, 2005). They reported the UV-irradiated grafting of TMSPM and AA monomers on lignocellulosic jute yarn in the presence of various amino acids (1%) as additives. The PL and tensile properties like TS and Eb of treated samples were enhanced by incorporation of amino acids, and the highest properties (TS = 300% and Eb = 386%) were achieved by the sample treated with L-arginine (Arg) with 32.5% PL value (Figure 11.5).

It is believed that an equilibrium concentration of the impregnation solution is attained in the copolymerizing region of the backbone polymer (cellulose) of the substrate. The condition of the region may continually change depending on various factors prevailing during the time of the copolymerization. The partitioning/diffusion of the monomer and/or components of

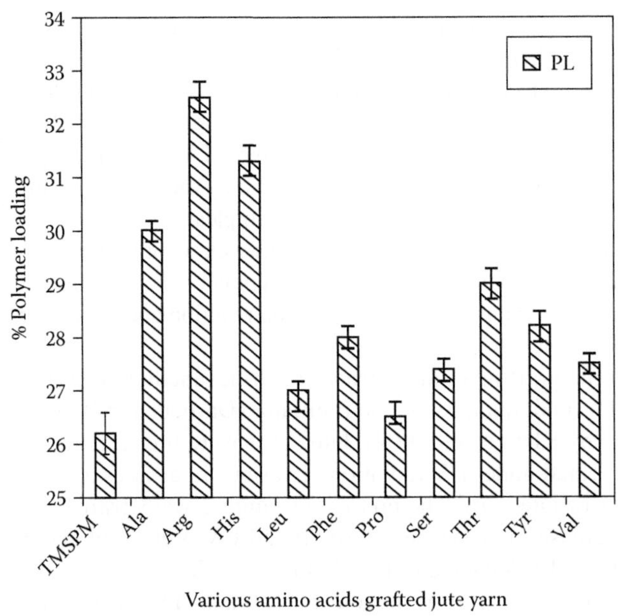

FIGURE 11.5 Effect of additives (amino acids) on polymer loading.

the impregnating solution are one of the factors in such a copolymerization process. Thus, the structural shape, ionic mobility, and possible affinity for interactions among the components of the impregnating solution are some of the factors to be considered. Additives like Arg, His, and Thr have possibly the most favorable partitioning/diffusion ability among the 10 amino acids due to their inherent natural and structural advantages. The improvement in Tf values of amino acid (additives)–treated jute yarn can be represented by the series Arg > His > Thr > Tyr > Leu > Ala > Phe > Pro > Ser > Val > TMSPM, and thc improvement in elongation factor values of amino acid (additives)–treated jute yarn can be represented by the series Arg > His > Thr > Tyr > Ala, Leu > Phe, Pro > Ser > Val > TMSPM. It may be noted that the lone pair electrons in nitrogen atom are activated to form a bridge between the monomer and the cellulose through additives like Arg, His, and Thr and may create some favorable conditions for the augmentation of the bulk monomers (TMSPM and AA) and additive units with the cellulose backbone polymer of the jute yarn. It is registered that the high TS of skin and bone is due to the presence of fibrous protein. The >C=O group of each amino acid is hydrogen bonded to the NH group of the amino acid that is situated four residues ahead in the linear sequence (Scheme 11.1). The carbonyl carbon atom and the nitrogen atom of the peptide link have partial double bond character (Scheme 11.2). Hence, during the grafting process, molecular structure of TMSPM and AA and additive amino acid has played a significant role, and a peptide chain may be formed, which can penetrate cellulose backbone. Thus, it could be concluded that not only the nitrogen atom alone makes this favorable condition for achieving high TS, but the carbamide group also. More elaborate investigation is also needed for ascertaining the proper function of jute cellulose at the equilibrium condition of the impregnating solution of bulk monomer TMSPM containing different amino acids.

Weak acid like 3% acetic acid and inorganic acid like 1% sulfuric acid were also incorporated in the optimized system of TMSPM grafting and compared their effect on the tensile properties with amino acid–treated samples. It was observed that enhanced PL values of 31% were achieved by 1% sulfuric acid but suppressed the tensile properties, even lower than the TS and Eb values of the virgin jute yarn. The enhanced PL value is due to the formation of more homopolymers in the presence of acid, thereby making the system unable to graft the monomer on the jute yarn. Sulfuric acid as a strong acid readily breaks the cellulose backbone and some polymer chains having condensed inter-unit linkages. It was also noticed that, generally, strong acids like sulfuric acid and nitric acid reduce the TS of the composites based on cellulose substrates. Addition of acetic acid as additives in TMSPM has also enhanced the PL values with increased mechanical properties of jute yarn. It is an important point of view that in any grafting system at any one time, there is an equilibrium concentration of monomer absorbed within the grafting region of the polymer backbone. This grafting region may be continually changing as grafting proceeds. The degree of monomer

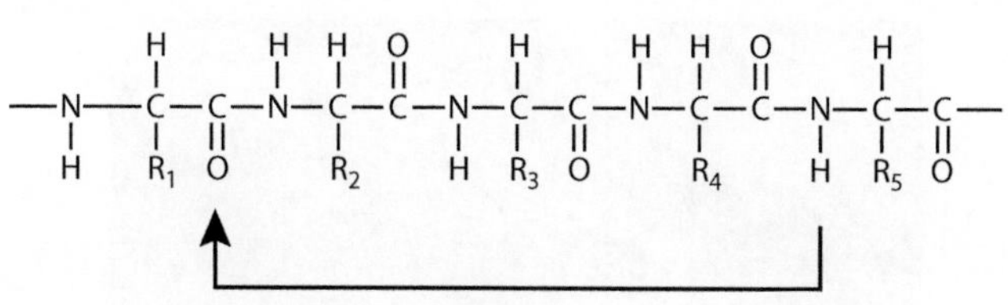

SCHEME 11.1 Linear structure of protein.

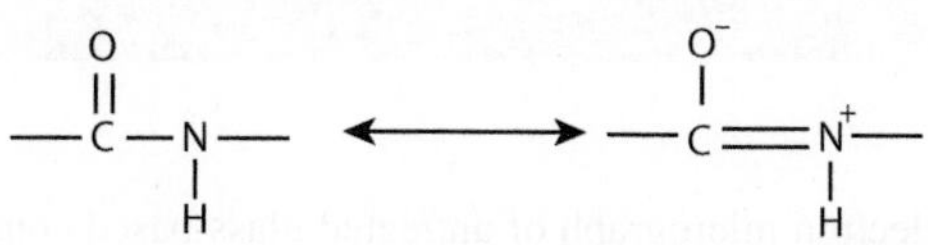

SCHEME 11.2 Partial double bond character of peptide link.

depends on the polarity of the monomer, substrate, solvent, and the concentration of the acid. In the presence of nitrogen-containing monomer such as TMSPM, acetic acid will protonate the nitrogen to give different reactivity. Acid can also attack the polymer backbone under certain conditions. Hence, the effect of acids used in the current work can be interpreted, at least partially, in terms of partitioning phenomena.

Water absorption and weathering resistance of treated and untreated samples were also determined, and treated sample showed lesser water uptake as well as less weight loss and mechanical properties as compared to untreated samples. Lower water absorption by amino acid–treated samples indicated that amino acid might have entered into the process of the polymer chain of jute cellulose in grafting system.

11.3.1.2 Polymer Grafting

Effects of UV radiation on jute fiber (Hessian cloth) reinforced with unsaturated polyester (USP) resin along with additives and initiator composites prepared by the hand layup technique were reported by Al-Kafi et al. (2006). Jute fiber content in the composites was optimized with the extent of mechanical properties, and composites with 25% jute showed higher mechanical properties. The mechanical properties were found to increase with the incorporation of dissimilar portions of glass fiber into the jute fiber–reinforced composite. Among all the resulting hybrid composites, the composite with jute to glass ratio of 1:3 demonstrated improved mechanical properties, such as TS 125%, TM 49%, bending strength (BS) 162%, and bending modulus (BM) 235% over untreated jute composite. To further improve the properties, the surface of jute and glass fiber was irradiated under UV radiation of different intensities. UV-pretreated jute and glass fibers (1:3) at optimum intensities showed the highest mechanical properties, such as TS 70%, TM 33%, BS 40%, and BM 43%

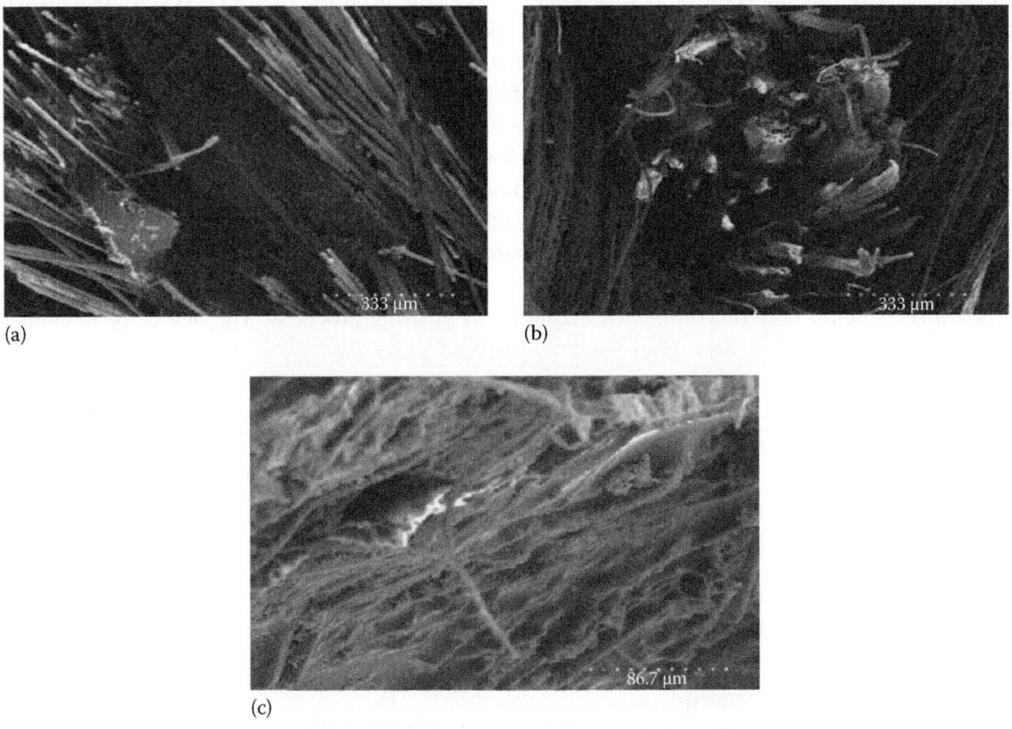

FIGURE 11.6 (a) Scanning electron micrograph of untreated glass-based composite, (b) scanning electron micrograph of untreated jute-based composite, and (c) scanning electron micrograph of UV-pretreated jute/glass-based hybrid composite.

compared to untreated jute- and glass-based hybrid composites. UV-modified jute/glass-reinforced hybrid composites also showed the best of Charpy IS (40 kJ/m^2). The interfacial adhesion between jute/glass and USP is monitored by a scanning electron microscope (SEM). Interfacial properties, such as fiber–matrix interaction, fracture behavior, and fiber pullout of different samples, are observed in the case of jute/glass-reinforced hybrid composites. Figure 11.6a and b show the tensile fracture surfaces of untreated jute and glass composites. Owing to the substantial difference in chemical and physical characters and the formation of hydrogen bonds between untreated jute and glass fiber, the fibers agglomerate into the bundles and become unevenly distributed through the matrix. So the untreated composite (UC) shows a higher extent of pullout. Figure 11.6c shows the tensile fracture surfaces of optimum UV-treated jute/glass-based hybrid composites. A better dispersion and pullout of the fibers in the matrix is observed when both jute and glass are UV-treated at optimum intensities and hybridized at an optimum ratio (1:3). Physical modification, such as nonionizing UV radiation of the fibers, usually prevents hydrogen bond formation and increases the number of free radical active sites by which better dispersion and interfacial bonding are significantly observed as in Figure 11.6c.

11.3.2 Modification by Gamma Radiation

11.3.2.1 Monomer and Oligomer Grafting

Gamma-radiation-cured graft copolymerization of UV-pretreated jute (Hessian cloth) with a mixture of HEMA (monomer) and aliphatic urethane diacrylate oligomer (EB-204) was reported by Khan et al. (2006). The concentrations of the monomer and oligomer along with the radiation doses were optimized on the basis of their mechanical properties. Among all resulting composites prepared from the combination of different ratios of monomer and oligomer, the composite with 38% jute content at monomer:oligomer = 50:50 (w/w) ratios showed better mechanical properties, such as 108% increase in TS, 58% increase in BS, 138% increase in TM, and 211% increase in BM relative to pure polymer film. The increase in both the TS and BS of pure polymer and composite with the increase in radiation dose may have occurred by the formation of a number of free radicals, which subsequently increases the degree of cross-linking. The decrease in both the TS and BS after attaining the maximum value may be associated with the degradation of the backbone of the cellulose structure. The loss of strength during degradation is due to the breakage of the primary bonds of the cellulose constituents. Both TM and BM showed continuous increasing trends but no decrease in properties after 500 krad of total gamma radiation. This different case of moduli can be explained by the Eb of composites. Eb for both tensile and bending decreases with the increase in radiation dose. These decreasing values of elongation usually decrease the strain or deformation of the resulting composites, which was likely to be responsible for its increasing modulus.

The gel content values were also found to increase with the increase in jute content in the composite. But the Eb for both tensile and bending was found to decrease with increasing jute content. Best mechanical properties were obtained when UV-pretreated 38% of jute (Hessian cloth) was reinforced using formulation (oligomer:monomer = 50:50) and cured under 500 krad of total gamma radiation dose at 600 krad/h dose rate. In this case, 150% increase in TS, 90% increase in BS relative to polymer film, 19% increase in TS, and 15% increase in BS relative to untreated jute-based composites were observed. The effects of UV radiation as a method of surface treatment on the TS and BS of the composites were investigated by comparing UV-pretreated and untreated jute composites as shown in Figure 11.7. Surface modification of jute by UV treatment usually increased the polarities of fiber surface, which increased the fiber wettability as well as composite strength. The higher the number of active sites generated on the polymeric substrate, the greater was the grafting efficiency. An intense UV radiation resulted in loss of TS and a reduced degree of polymerization was observed, and two opposing phenomena such as photo-cross-linking and photo-degradation took place simultaneously when UV radiation was used as a method of surface pretreatment.

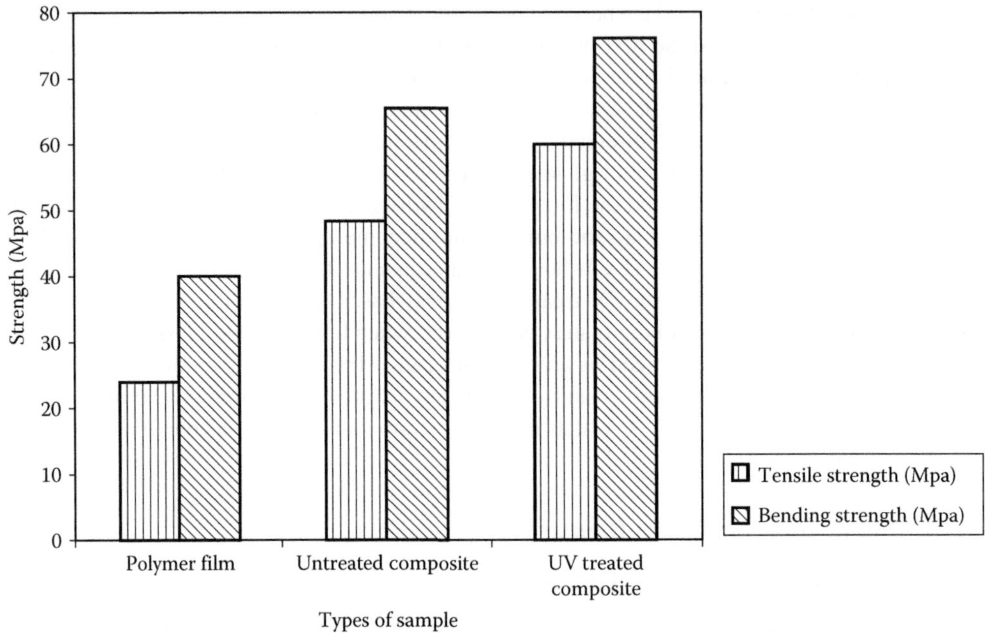

FIGURE 11.7 Effect of pretreatment of jute by UV radiation on the tensile and bending strength of composites prepared by gamma radiation.

Sheherzade and Khan (2003) studied the effect of ionizing gamma radiation to improve the physico-mechanical properties of jute yarns. Procedure same as earlier was maintained to optimize the grafting conditions and were cured under UV lamp at different UV radiation intensities. It was observed that only gamma-pretreated samples exhibit higher TS. But when gamma-pretreated samples were grafted with HDDA and cured with UV, then the tensile properties decreased but PL increased considerably. It was obtained that the PL increased with total doses and that the highest PL (21%) was exhibited by the sample pretreated under 1 Mrad gamma radiation. Under higher doses of gamma radiation, the polymer may undergo scission, and the polymer molecules may be broken into smaller fragments. As a result, reaction sites are opened, and more monomer can be introduced into the reaction, which increases PL. And as polymer breaks into smaller fragments, the ultimate loss of TS occurs.

Effect of alkali (5% NaOH)-pretreated jute yarn grafting by gamma radiation with two types of monomer such as TMSPM (silane) and AA under UV radiation has also been studied (Hassan et al., 2003a,b). The surface of jute yarns was pretreated by alkali along with UV and gamma radiation with different intensities and grafted with silane and AA to improve the tensile properties of the jute yarn. The jute yarns were pretreated with alkali and UV radiation and grafted with silane showed the best properties such as TS (360%), EB (380%), and PL (31%). Simulated weathering test and water uptake of untreated and treated jute yarns were studied. The alkali + UV-pretreated silanized jute yarn showed lesser water uptake as well as less weight loss and mechanical properties as compared with treated samples. The weathering test demonstrated that untreated jute yarn samples lost both weight and tensile properties (TS and Eb), whereas the grafted samples retained tensile properties even though these were subjected to severe weathering for 600 h.

11.3.3 Polymer Grafting

Gamma radiation induces a faster and efficient grafting having higher degree of grafting. Effects of gamma radiation on JF-reinforced poly(caprolactone) (PCL) biocomposites (30%–70% jute) fabricated by compression molding were investigated by Islam et al. (2009). The irradiated composites containing 50% jute showed improved physico-mechanical properties. TS, TM, BS, BM, and IS of the nonirradiated composites were found to be 65 MPa, 0.75 GPa, 75 MPa, 4.2 GPa, and 6.8 kJ/m^2, respectively. An increase in TS and BS of both the pre-irradiated and post-irradiated composites was observed in the radiation dose ranging from 50 to 500 krad. The maximum values of TS and BS for the pre-irradiated composite were 78 and 86 MPa, respectively, at the dose of 500 krad, and at the same dose, maximum TS and BS of the post-irradiated composite were 82 and 92 MPa, respectively, although after 500 krad, both TS and BS decreased. A similar thing happens for the TM, BM, and IS of the composites. Both the TM and BM of both pre- and post-irradiated samples were maximum at 500 krad, but after 500 krad, both TM and BM decreased. IS value of pre- and post-irradiated composites also increased with increasing radiation intensity from 50 to 500 krad. Then, IS value showed a decreasing trend with increasing radiation dose. Maximum IS value was found to be 7.25 and 7.35 kJ/m^2 for pre- and post-irradiated composites, respectively, at 500 krad. TS, BS, TM, BM, and IS of the composite are influenced by the interfacial bond strength of the PCL matrix and jute fiber. Gamma treatment improved interfacial bond strength by producing active sites. Consequently, the mechanical properties of the irradiated composites were improved up to 500 krad dose due to cross-linking. Crack propagation in the impact test is very sensitive to adhesion between the matrix and the reinforcing fiber. It can be assumed that stress transfer between matrix and fiber was good at 500 krad, leading to cracks stopping at the fiber. But above 500 krad dose, the mechanical properties of both the pre- and post-irradiated composites decreased on exposure to high-energy gamma radiation, which causes degradation of PCL by breaking the polymer chains. In the case of pre-irradiated composites, gamma radiation removes the moisture of jute fiber, which in turn contributed to the fiber matrix adhesion. Gamma irradiation affects the polymeric structure of the cellulose fiber and produces active sites that increase the intra-chain bond in the fiber that causes the polymeric chain to group together in highly ordered (crystal-like) structure. The intra-chain bonds are strong and give the fiber strength.

Another way of explaining the variation of mechanical properties induced by gamma irradiation is active site formation in the PCL matrix that may contribute to jute fiber—PCL bonding at fabrication temperature. For these reasons, the mechanical properties of the pre-irradiated composite increased up to 500 krad dose. In the case of post-irradiated composite, gamma radiation alters the mechanical properties through main-chain scission and cross-linking in the amorphous region or recombination in the crystalline region. Both the process chain scission and cross-linking take place simultaneously. The degree of crystallization is affected by the amount of main chain scission induced by different radiations doses, and the rate of crystallization is related to the radiation dose and degree of cross-linking.

Water absorption of nonirradiated composites was found higher than that of irradiated composites. The irradiated composites showed better stability to deterioration of mechanical properties than nonirradiated composites after 6 weeks of degradation in water. As PCL is hydrophobic in nature, the percentage of water uptake of the composites mainly depends on the water uptake properties of jute fiber and the degree of fiber matrix adhesion. The intermolecular spaces in the jute fiber are too small that the water molecule cannot penetrate in this region. So the water molecule can penetrate only the amorphous region and get linked with the available hydroxyl (–OH) groups. Decreased water absorption by pre- and post-irradiated composites attributed to the fact that gamma radiation reduced the –OH group as well as increased crystalline regions in jute fiber through cross-linking, which in turn decreased amorphous regions. The weight loss of the nonirradiated samples was found to be about 25% after 5 months, whereas about 19% and 16% weight loss were found for pre- and post-irradiated composites, respectively, after 5 months.

The morphology was evaluated by SEM, as shown in Figure 11.8a and b. The figure reveals large-scale variations in the aspect ratio, diameter, and the morphology among jute samples. It is observed that the diameters of the fibers are ranging from 5 to 50 mm, and the surface of the fibers is rough with the adhesion of some smaller jute fibers and jute particles. These variations are probably on

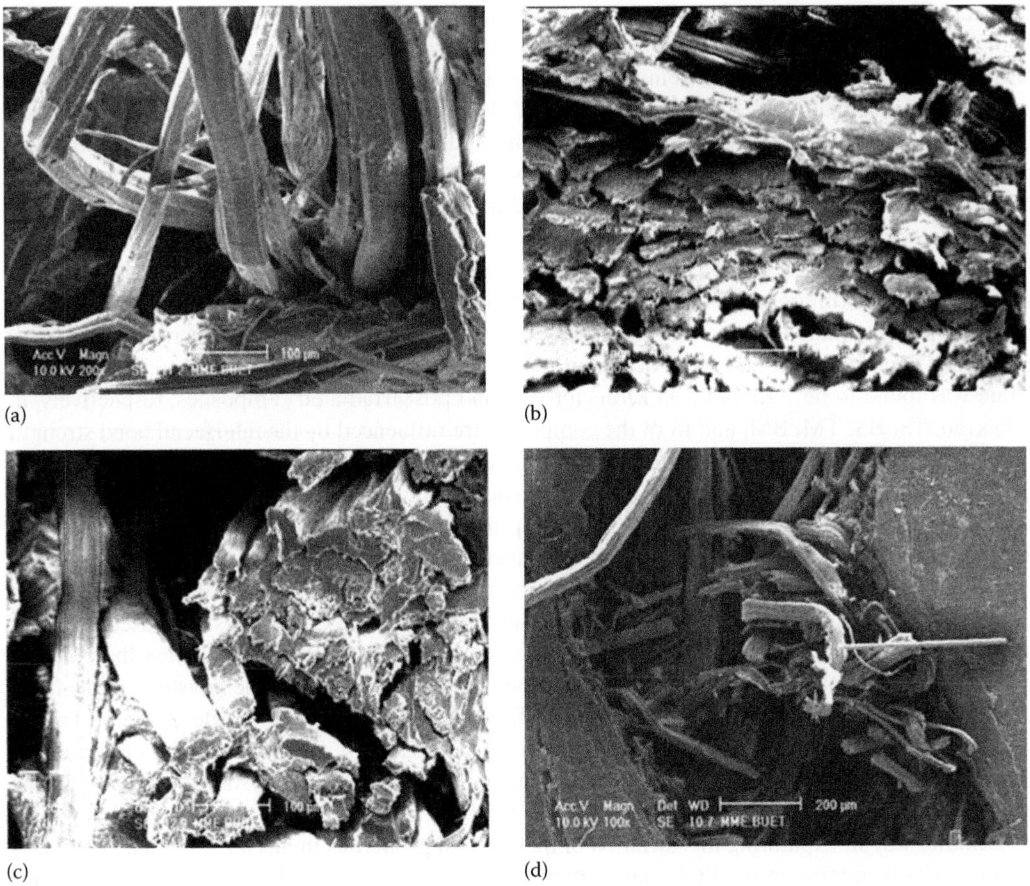

FIGURE 11.8 SEM micrographs of jute fiber (a), pure PCL (b), freshly fractured surface of nonirradiated PCL=jute composite (c), and irradiated PCL=jute (d).

account of the different sources and the processing history of the fibers. Furthermore, the morphology and fracture mechanism of the materials were evaluated by SEM. The SEM micrographs of the tensile fractured surfaces of the neat PCL and PCL:jute (50:50) composite are presented in Figure 11.8. As shown in Figure 11.8c, the fracture surface of pure PCL is regular. Besides, the craze and fibril are observed in the surface, signifying that the fracture of PCL is in the "ductile" manner, the surface of jute is smooth in the composite, and the fibrils linking the fiber surface to the matrix can be observed in Figure 11.8c and d. Furthermore, it can be seen from Figure 11.8d that the fiber is obviously covered by a thin layer of PCL matrix. These all suggest that the fiber and polymer matrix are in good adhesion, which leads to better stress transfer between the matrix and reinforcing fibers. On the other hand, as seen in Figure 11.8d, the fracture surface is irregular and the fiber pullout is prevailed over fiber fracture. In addition, as shown in Figure 11.8d, the de-bonding of the PCL matrix and fiber is observed. These signify that the interface interaction between the fibers and the polymer matrix can be further improved. The mechanical properties of composite greatly depend on the state of the filler dispersion and the strength of the interfacial interaction. The interfacial interaction between bulk polymer and nucleating agent has a significant influence on the crystallization rate. Therefore, it is considered that the mechanical properties as well as the crystallization behavior can be further optimized through the use of compatibilizers or coupling agents.

Another investigation was conducted by Khan and Khan (2009a), which showed the effect of gamma radiation on Hessian cloth (jute fiber)—reinforced PP composites. The fiber content in the composites was about 50%. The resulting composites and also PP sheets were irradiated under gamma radiation of various total doses (250–1000 krad) at the rate of 600 krad/h. It was found that by using gamma radiation, the mechanical properties of the PP sheets and composites were improved. Gamma radiation dose of 500 krad showed better mechanical properties than that of other doses. TS and TM of the PP sheets improved 28% and 26%, respectively, and for composites 16% and 45%, respectively. On the other hand, BS and BM of the PP sheet improved 16% and 125%. For composites, BS, BM, and IS improved 12%, 38%, and 62%, respectively. Water uptake of the composites at 25°C was measured, and it was found that treated samples had lower water uptake properties. The dielectric constant was higher for the treated composite compared to that of the untreated one. The transition temperatures were found to be 80°C for untreated and 75°C for irradiated composites, respectively. This phase transition is likely to be ferroelectric to para-electric transitions. It is likely that free charges remain bound up to the transition temperature, but with further increase in temperature, trapped charges become released and contribute to the conductivity, and hence conductivity increases. As a result of gamma irradiation on composites, more cross-linking happened inside the polymer matrix and jute fibers, so resistivity increased and hence conductivity decreased. Explanation of conductivity can be rationalized as we know that jute is composed of cellulose whose skeletal backbone is linked by intramolecular hydrogen bonding. When temperature increased, dipoles formed and tended to align themselves with the applied electric field and thus increase the dielectric constant. At the transition temperature, the formation of dipoles and alignment toward the field are maximum, giving rise to maximum dielectric values, whereas above the transition temperature, the dipoles tend to be oriented randomly and hence lower the dielectric values. At an optimum temperature, the dielectric values then become constant. It was observed that the conductivity rapidly decreased with increasing temperature up to transition temperature, and above the transition temperature, it increased with some fluctuations and remained almost constant.

Again, Mina et al. (2013) illustrated the incorporation of untreated JF and triple-super-phosphate (TSP)-treated JF in isotactic PP to prepare sandwich composites. Illustrative mechanisms for the effect of γ-radiation on the basis of spectroscopic analyses were proposed (Schemes 11.3 and 11.4). Both, TSP-treated composite (TC) and UC were irradiated by γ-rays at various doses to produce γTC and γUC. The highest TS, FS, and Young's modulus (E) were observed at a radiation dose of 5.0 kGy. The maximum increases in TS, FS, and E of γTC from UC are 17%, 18%, and 69%, while those of TC from UC are 12%, 13%, and 12%, respectively. Thermal degradation temperature of γTC and TC was found to increase significantly from that of UC, suggesting an improved thermal stability of the treated composites. All these findings are explained on the basis of fiber–matrix interactions developed by the formation of physical and chemical bonds among JF and PP, as demonstrated by means of the FTIR. The most notable changes in the spectra are found in the wavenumber ranges of 3200–3600 and 1000–1200 cm^{-1}. A reduction in the intensity of C–O vibrations from crystalline part in the region of 1113 and 910 cm^{-1} as compared to the UC and TC proves a breaking of crystalline cellulose by γ-ray irradiation. An increase in the intensity of 1162 cm^{-1} band, which can be related to the antisymmetric stretching of C–O–C glycoside bonds, may indicate the formation of this bond with PP molecules. Besides, changes in the intensity of C–O stretching (at 910 cm^{-1}) of amorphous cellulose and that of hydrogen-bonded O–H stretching are also noticeable. C–H stretching of cellulose at 1375 cm^{-1} is found to be changed after γ-ray irradiation. To explain these results, we invoke the cross-linking mechanism between JF and PP molecules by ionizing radiation process. According to this mechanism, free radicals (as marked by small black circles) are formed after C–H, C–O, and C–C bond cleavages of the monomeric units of β-D-glucopyranose of jute through hydrogen and hydroxyl abstraction (a), cycle opening (b), and chain scission (c) by c-radiation (Scheme 11.3). Thereafter, JF and PP molecules join together through the C–C and C–O–C bonds (Scheme 11.4). The observed increase in C–O–C bond intensity confirms the formation of this bond, whereas the intensity increase at the downward solid arrow (1050 cm^{-1}) may indicate the C–C stretching mode of the JF–PP link. Thus, the observed findings of FTIR spectra corroborate the proposed cross-linking mechanism between cellulose and PP.

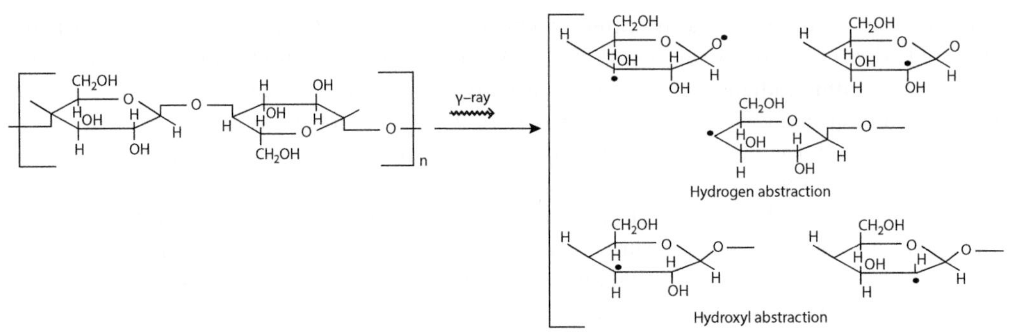

(a)

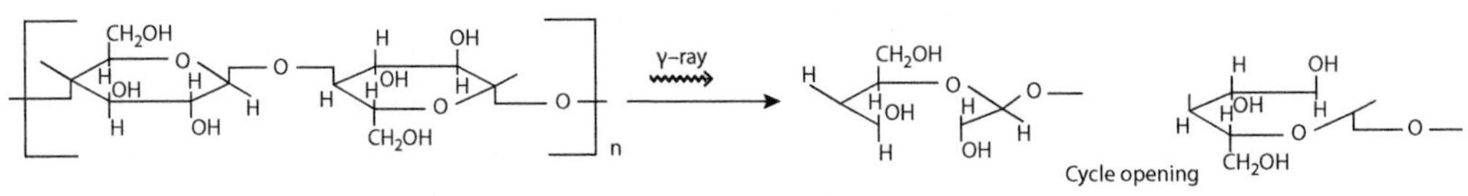

(b)

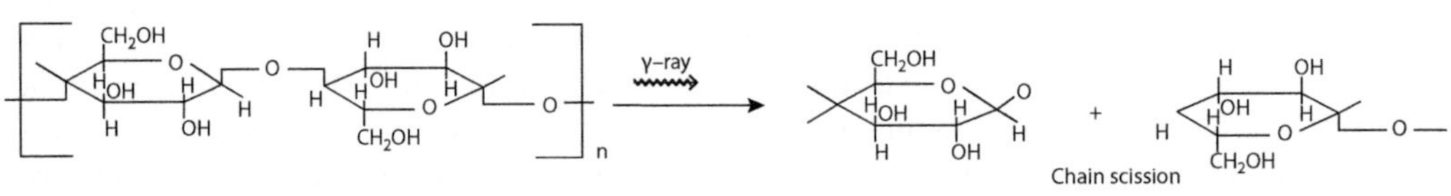

(c)

SCHEME 11.3 (a) Hydrogen and hydroxyl abstraction, (b) cycle opening, and (c) chain scission mechanisms of cellulose molecules in JF after γ-ray irradiation.

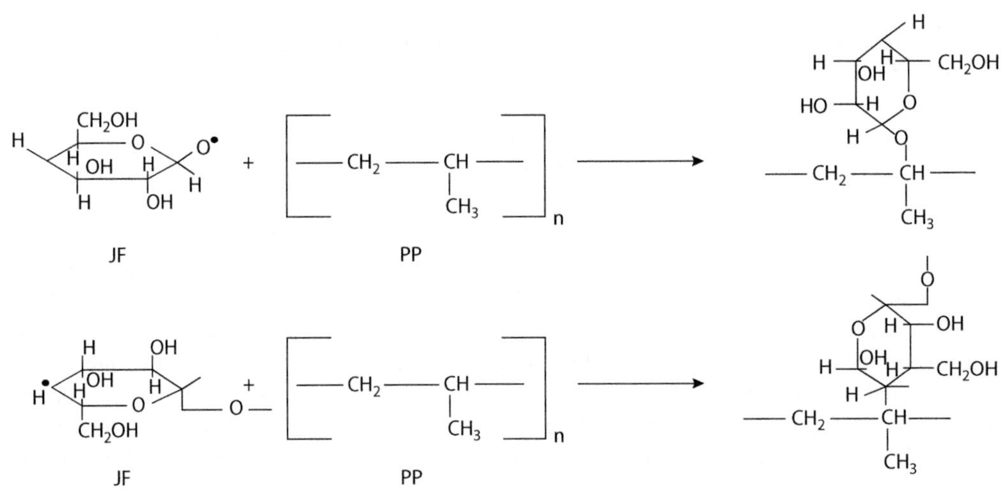

SCHEME 11.4 The cross-linking mechanism between the cellulose and PP molecules.

The differential thermal analysis thermograms of PP and others contained several peaks that correspond to melting temperature of the solid sample and degradation temperature of the molecules of this solid. The most striking observations found here are the disappearance of the water release peak at 85°C and a slight shift of all peaks. The melting temperature of composites was found to be lower than that of PP. This result might be associated with the disordered crystalline structures possibly developed in the lamellae of PP and the cellulose of JF during fabrication. The melting temperature of γTC slightly increased with increasing γ-ray doses. This increase was possibly related to the breaking of chemical and adhesive bonds, whose formation by γ-rays has been suggested and discussed earlier.

Further thermogravimetric analyses exhibited the weight loss with increasing temperature for PP, untreated JF, UC, TC, and γTC, respectively. Untreated natural fibers suffered thermal degradation in a two-stage process of which the first part occurred in the temperature range 200°C–310°C and the second part in the range 310°C–400°C. In contrast to the untreated ones, JF-based PP composites exhibited a three-step degradation process, which is a commonly practiced indication to characterize the structural degradation or destabilization. Analysis showed that the thermal degradation increased for TC and γTC from UC are 17°C and 21°C, respectively. This increase demonstrated the formation of physical and chemical bonds among JF and PP molecules by surface treatment and γ-ray irradiation, respectively. More interestingly, the weight loss pattern for the γ-ray-treated composites was unlike that of other samples, immediately after the rapid weight loss. The mechanism of this disintegration also gives us a sign of the bond formation in the composites due to γ-ray irradiation. The low-temperature degradation process is associated with the degradation of hemicellulose, whereas the high-temperature process corresponds to the degradation of cellulose and is also associated with the pyrolysis of lignin involving fragmentation of interunit linkages (releasing monomeric phenols into the vapor phase), decomposition, and condensation of the aromatic rings. The formation of char residues may involve initial physical desorption of water, intramolecular dehydration, formation of carboxyl and carbon–carbon double bonds, cleavage of glycosidic linkage and rupture of C=O and C=C bonds, and condensation and aromatization of carbon atoms from each original pyranose ring to form discrete graphite layers.

Khan et al. (2009b) experimented the effect of gamma radiation on starch solution—treated jute yarn—reinforced PP composites. To prepare the composites, jute yarns were treated with 1%–5% aqueous starch solution (w/w) varying different soaking time (1–5 min). The yarn content in the composite was about 50% by weight. Starch-treated jute composites showed higher mechanical properties than that of the untreated jute composites. Composites prepared with 3% starch-treated yarns (for 3 min soaking time) demonstrated the highest mechanical properties (optimized), that was, TS 52 MPa, TM 700 MPa, BS 50 MPa, and BM 1406 MPa. Optimized composite was then treated with gamma radiation (Co-60) at a dose of 500 krad and found further improvement of the mechanical properties. Water uptake of the composites at room temperature was measured and found that starch-treated samples showed higher water uptake properties than the control sample. After 500 h of simulating weathering testing, optimized composites retained its 75% TS and 93% TM.

Use of natural rubber (NR) for the preparation of JF-reinforced composites and effects of gamma radiation on the composites were investigated by Rahman et al. (2012). TS, TM, Eb BS, BM, and softness of the composite were 30 MPa, 395 MPa, 65%, 10 MPa, 2130 MPa, and 79 Shore-A, respectively. Degradation nature of the composite was investigated in soil and aqueous medium. Composites showed the same trend of water uptake as the jute fibers. Since only a fraction of the surface of jute fiber of the composite came in contact with aqueous medium, water uptake of composite was significantly lower than that of jute fiber. NR is biodegradable, which consists of more than 90% of cis-1,4-isoprene and less than 10% of nonrubber constituents, like proteins, lipids, carbohydrate, resins, and inorganic salts. Since soaking was done for a long time in aqueous medium, leaching out of nonrubber constituents took place. These are causes for the significant loss of TS and TM of the composite due to degradation in aqueous medium. The rate of loss of both TS and TM in soil burial test was much lower than that in aqueous medium, which indicated that other incidents like enzymatic attack might not have taken place during soil burial test. To improve the compatibility between fiber and matrix, the composites were irradiated with gamma rays. Total radiation dose varied from 50 to 1000 krad. Tensile properties of the irradiated (250 krad) composites improved significantly (TS and TM increased 47% and 147%). The reason behind this variation of TS and TM after gamma radiation is deposition of energy in solid cellulose by Compton scattering and rapid localization of energy within molecules producing trapped macrocellulosic radicals, which has been already discussed in section under the name mechanism of grafting by gamma radiation.

11.4 APPLICATIONS OF JUTE COMPOSITES

Jute has been in use mainly as a packaging material, and for roping and household purposes. Jute fiber composites have also been used for producing door panels, roofing, and sanitary products. Jute-reinforced thermoplastic laminates and composites represent a promising substitution for thermoplastic and synthetic fiber-reinforced composites with good physical properties and excellent performance at low weight. Potential future applications of jute fiber composites include the automobile industry, the footwear industry, construction, home/garden furniture, and the toy sectors. Bangladesh Atomic Energy Commission has successfully made a wide range of products from jute-reinforced polymer composite.

The products include the following:

- Jute/polymer corrugated sheet (Jutin) (Khan and Khan, 2010)
- False ceilings, roof tiles, kitchen sinks
- Durable chairs, tables, etc.
- Sanitary latrine accessories such as the slab, ring, etc.
- Decorative materials
- Helmets, chest guards, leg guards, etc.
- Bullet-proof materials, etc.

"Jutin" can also be used extensively for hut making in coastal areas because of their saline-resistant properties and in earthquake regions for their lightweight.

11.5 CONCLUSION

Jute has been widely regarded as a versatile, useful, and valuable agro-fiber. It is difficult to suggest another natural fiber possessing such diverse properties and basic utilities as jute in solicitous use in carpets, ropes, sacks, Hessian clothes, etc. With the invention of different types of new synthetic materials, their vast use has adversely affected jute products in the world market. The use of jute and jute products are declining by 5% annually due to the availability of the new synthetic substances that are cheap and attractive. Marketing of traditional jute products like bags and Hessian clothes is facing serious challenge, causing shrinkage of jute market due to the disadvantages like low mechanical properties. However, in this chapter, we have reviewed some works on jute fiber reinforcement by environmental friendly radiation-induced graft copolymerization and found that the radiation technology is very promising in improving the quality of jute products and thus making it viable against synthetic product available in the market, which are threats to our very existence.

REFERENCES

Ali, K. M. I., Khan M. A., and Ali, M. A. (1997). Study on jute material with urethane acrylate by UV curing, *Radiation Physics and Chemistry*, 49(3): 383–388.

Ali K. M. I., Khan M. A., and Islam M. N. (1996). Improvement of Physicomechanical Properties of Hessian Cloth (Jute) by Graft Copolymerization of Urethane Acrylate With Ultraviolet Radiation, *Polymer-Plastics Technology and Engineering*, 35(1): 53–65.

Al-Kafi, A., Abedin, M. Z., Beg, M. D. H., Pickering, K. L., and Khan, M. A. (2006). Study on the mechanical properties of jute/glass fiber-reinforced unsaturated polyester hybrid composites: Effect of surface modification by ultraviolet radiation, *Journal of Reinforced Plastics and Composites*, 25(6): 575–588.

Bashar, A. S., Khan, M. A., and Ali, K. M. I. (1996). UV-cured films of epoxy, polyester and urethane oligomers and their applications on hessian cloth (jute), *Radiation. Physics and Chemistry*, 48(3): 349–354.

Bledzki, A. K. and Gassan, J. (1999). Composites reinforced with cellulose based fibres, *Progress in Polymer Science*, 24: 221–274.

Chavez, C. R. A., Edwards, S., Eraso, R. M., and Geiser, K. (2012). Sustainability of bio-based plastics: General comparative analysis and recommendations for improvement, *Journal of Cleaner Production*, 23: 47–56.

Doan, T. T. L., Brodowsky, H., and Mäder, E. (2007). Jute fiber/polypropylene composites II. Thermal, hydrothermal and dynamic mechanical behaviour, *Composites Science and Technology*, 67: 2707–2714.

Frederick, T. W. and Norman W. (2004). *Natural Fibers Plastics and Composites*, Kluwer Academic Publishers, New York.

Ghose, P. and Ganguly, P. K. (1996). Jute, in: *Polymeric Materials Encyclopedia*, J. C. Salamone (ed.), vol. 5, CRC Press, Boca Raton, FL, pp. 3504–3513.

Goda, K., Takagi, H., and Netravali, A. N. (2009). Fully biodegradable green composites reinforced with natural fibers, in: *Natural Fiber Reinforced Polymer Composites*, S. Thomas and L. A. Pothan (eds.), Old City Publishing, Philadelphia, PA, pp. 329–360.

Gupta, C. and Gupta, A. P. (2005). *Polymer Composite*, New Age International (P) Ltd., New Delhi, India.

Hassan, M. M., Islam, M. R., Drzal, L. T., and Khan, M. A. (2005). Role of amino acids on in situ photografting of jute yarn with 3-(trimethoxysilyl) propylmethacrylate, *Journal of Polymers and the Environment*, 13(3): 293–300.

Hassan, M. M., Islam, M. R., Sawpan, M. A., and Khan, M. A. (2003a). Effect of silane monomer on the improvement of mechanical and degradable properties of photografted jute yarn with acrylamide, *Journal of Applied Polymer Science*, 89: 3530–3538.

Hassan, M. M., Islam, M. R., Shehrzade, S., and Khan, M. A. (2003b). Influence of mercerization along with ultraviolet (UV) and gamma radiation on physical and mechanical properties of jute yarn by grafting with 3-(trimethoxysilyl) propylmethacrylate (silane) and acrylamide under UV radiation, *Polymer-Plastics Technology and Engineering*, 42(4), 515–531.

Hassan, M. M., Islam, R., and Khan, M. A. (2003c). Role of amino acids on in situ photografting of jute yarn with acrylamide using ultraviolet radiation, *Polymer-Plastics Technology and Engineering*, 42(5): 779–793.

Hassiruzzaman, M., Khan, M. A., and Ali, K. M. I. (1997). Effect of benzohydroxamato-ethylenediamine-titanium complex on modification of jute and cotton yarns by UV-radiation-induced urethane acrylate, *Journal of Applied Polymer Science*, 65: 1571–1580.

Heitner, C. (1993). Light induced yellowing of wood containing papers, in *Photochemistry of Lignocellulosic Materials, ACS Symposium Series 531, Journal of the American Chemical Society*, Ch-15: 192–204.

Hon, D. N. S. (2001). Weathering and photochemistry of wood, in: *Wood and cellulosic chemistry*, Hon, D. N. S., Shiraishi, N. (eds.), 2nd edition. Marcel Dekker, New York, pp. 512–546.

Islam, T., Khan, R. A., Khan, M. A., Rahman, M. A., Fernandez-Lahore, M., Huque Q. M. I., and Islam, R. (2009). Physico-mechanical and degradation properties of gamma-irradiated biocomposites of jute fabric-reinforced poly (caprolactone), *Polymer-Plastics Technology and Engineering*, 48(11): 1198–1205.

Jacob, M., Anandjiwala, R. D., and Thomas, S. (2009). Lignocellulosic fiber reinforced rubber composites, in: *Natural Fiber Reinforced Polymer Composites*, S. Thomas and L. A. Pothan (eds.), Old City Publishing, Philadelphia, PA, pp. 256–257.

Joseph, K., Mattoso, L. H. C., Toledo, R. D., Thomas, S., de Carvalho, L. H., Pothan, L., Kala, S., and James, B. (2000). Natural fiber reinforced thermoplastic composites, in: *Natural Polymers and Agrofibers Based Composites*, E. Frollini, A. L. Leão, and L. H. C. Mattoso (eds.), EAI, São Carlos, Brazil, pp. 159–201.

Khabir, M. U., Khan, M. A., and Ali, K. M. I. (1995). Modification of jute yarn by graft-copolymerization with ultraviolet radiation, *Radiation Physics and Chemistry*, 48(4): 511–517.

Khan, M. A., Das, L. R., Khan, A. H., Ahmed, F., and Rahman, S. M. B. (2003a). Study on the mechanical and dielectric properties of photocured jute fabrics with 2-hydroxyethyl methacrylate, *Journal of Applied Polymer Science*, 89: 655–661.

Khan, M. A. and Drzal, L. T. (2004). Characterization of 2-hydroxyethyl methacrylate (HEMA)-treated jute surface cured by UV radiation, *Journal of Adhesion Science and Technology*, 18(3): 381–393.

Khan, M. A., Haque, N., Al-Kafi, A., Alam, M. N., and Abedin, M. Z. (2006). Jute reinforced composite by gamma radiation: Effect of surface treatment with UV radiation, *Polymer-Plastics Technology and Engineering*, 45(5): 607–613.

Khan, M. A., Islam, N. A., Hossain, A., and Ali, K. M. I. (1996). Effect of additives in the improvement of hessian cloth by UV-induced copolymerization, *Radiation Physics and Chemistry*, 48(3): 337–342.

Khan M. A., Islam M. N., and Ali K. M. I. (1996). Graft Copolymerization of Urethane Acrylate on Hessian Cloth (Jute) by UV Radiation, *Polymer-Plastics Technology and Engineering*, 35(2): 299–315.

Khan, M. A. and Khan, J. A. (2010). Jute reinforced polymer corrugated sheet (JUTIN) and its opportunities, in: *Eighth Global WPC and Natural Fiber Composites Congress and Exhibition*, June 22–23, Stuttgart, Germany.

Khan, M. A. and Khan, R. A. (2009a). Effect of gamma radiation on the physico-mechanical and electrical properties of jute fiber-reinforced polypropylene composites, *Journal of Reinforced Plastics and Composites*, 28(13): 1651–1660.

Khan, M. A., Khan, R. A., Zaman, H. U., Ghoshal, S., Siddiky, M. N. A., and Saha M. (2009b). Study on the physico-mechanical properties of starch-treated jute yarn-reinforced polypropylene composites: Effect of gamma radiation, *Polymer-Plastics Technology and Engineering*, 48(5): 542–548.

Khan, M. A., Majumder, S. C., Rahman, M. A., Noor, F. G., Zaman, H. U., Mollah, M. Z. I., Khan, R. A., and Das, L. R. (2010). Mechanical and electrical properties of photocured jute fabric with 2-hydroxy ethylacrylate, *Fibers and Polymers*, 11(3): 391–397.

Khan, M. A., Rahman, M. M., and Akhunzada, K. S. (2002). Grafting of different monomers onto jute yarn by in situ UV-radiation method: Effect of additives, *Polymer-Plastics Technology and Engineering*, 41(4): 677–689.

Khan, M. A., Rahman, M. S., and Islam, M. N. (2003b). Influence of coadditives on physical and mechanical properties of jute fabrics improved by UV-cured coating with urethane acrylate, *Polymer-Plastics Technology and Engineering*, 42(3): 399–413.

Khan, M. A., Shehrzade, S., and Hassan, M. M. (2004). Effect of alkali and ultraviolet (UV) radiation pretreatment on physical and mechanical properties of 1,6-hexanediol diacrylate—Grafted jute yarn by UV radiation, *Journal of Applied Polymer Science*, 92: 18–24.

Kundu, B. C., Basak, K. C., and Sarkar, P. B. (1959). *Jute in India*, Indian Central Jute Committee, Calcutta, India.

Majumder, A., Samajpati, S., Ganguly, P. K., Sardar, D., and Gupta, P. C. D. (1980). Swelling of jute: Heterogeneity of crimp formation, *Textile Research Journal*, 50: 575–578.

Matuana, L. M., Kamdem, D. P., and Zhang, J. (2001). Photoaging and stabilization of rigid PVC/wood–fibre composites, *Journal of Applied Polymer Science*, 80(11): 1943–1950.

Mina, M. F., Shohrawardy, M. H. S., Khan, M. A., Alam, A. K. M. M., and Beg, M. D. H. (2013). Improved mechanical performances of triple super phosphate treated jute-fabric reinforced polypropylene composites irradiated by gamma rays, *Journal of Applied Polymer Science*, 130: 470–478.

Netraveli, A. N. and Chabba, S. (2003). Composites get greener, *Materials Today*, 6: 22–29.

Nevell, T. P. and Zeronian, S. H. (1985). *Cellulose Chemistry and Its Application*, Wiley, New York.

Paul, A., Joseph, K., and Thomas, S. (1997). Effect of surface treatments on the electrical properties of low-density polyethylene composites reinforced with shorts is Al fibers, *Composites Science and Technology*, 57(1): 67–79.

Rahman, M. M., Sharmin, N., Khan, R. A., Dey, K., and Haque, M. E. (2012). Studies on the mechanical and degradation properties of jute fabric-reinforced natural rubber composite: Effect of gamma radiation, *Journal of Thermoplastic Composite Materials*, 25: 249–264.

Rowell, R. M., Han, J. S., and Rowell, J. S. (2000). Characterization and factors affecting fiber properties, in: *Natural Polymers and Agrofibers Based Composites*, E. Frollini, A. L. Leão, and L. H. C. Mattoso (eds.), EAI, São Carlos, Brazil, pp. 115–134.

Rowell, R. M. and Stout, H. P. (2007). Jute and Kenaf, in: *Handbook of Fiber Chemistry*, M. Lewin (ed.), Taylor & Francis, Boca Raton, FL.

Saha, C. K. and Sagorika, S. (2013). Carbon credit of jute and sustainable environment, *Jute Matters*, 1: 1–4.

Shehrzade, S. and Khan, M. A. (2003). Effect of pretreatment with gamma radiation on the performance of photocured jute yarn with 1,6-hexanediol diacrylate (HDDA), *Polymer-Plastics Technology and Engineering*, 42(5): 795–810.

Stark, N. M. and Matuana, L. M. (2003). Ultraviolet weathering of photostabilized wood-flour filled high-density polyethylene, *Journal of Applied Polymer Science*, 90(10): 2609–2617.

12 Chemically Modified Cotton Fibers for Antimicrobial Applications

Surinder Pal Singh, Bhawna Soni, and S.K. Bajpai

CONTENTS

12.1 INTRODUCTION

Cotton fiber–based gauze has been used to dress wounds for hundreds of years because it is naturally soft, pliable, and absorbent. Cotton fiber consists mainly of cellulose, which is a linear chain of several hundreds to over 9000 β (1→4)-linked D-glucose units. The hydroxyl groups of glucose in cellulose molecular can be partially or fully reacted with various reagents to afford derivatives with useful properties. Unfortunately, cotton fiber is also an ideal place for settling and growing pathogenic bacteria because of its porous and hydrophilic structure. Therefore, antibacterial finishing is also of importance, especially in some specific applications like medical usage. There are many antibacterial agents used in this field, including metal nanoparticles like silver and copper (Chen and Chiang 2008, Grace et al. 2009, Perelshtein et al. 2009, Chattopadhyay and Patel 2010, El-Rafie et al. 2010, Ravindra et al. 2010, Hebeish et al. 2011, Xu et al. 2011). The antimicrobial activity of silver and copper nanoparticles is widely reported and is linked with ions that leach out from these nanoparticles. The activity is further enhanced due to their small size and high surface area-to-volume ratio, which allows them to interact closely with microbial membranes. In fact, copper has been the most familiar antibacterial agent used for centuries. Bioactive copper nanomaterials are an emerging class of nano-antimicrobials providing complimentary effects and characteristics, as compared to other nano-sized metals, such as silver or zinc oxide nanoparticles (Daniela et al. 2012). Since the eighteenth century, copper had come into wide clinical use in the Western world, being for the treatment of mental disorders and afflictions of the lungs. Early American pioneers moving West across the continent put silver and copper coins in large wooden water casks to provide them with safe drinking water for their long voyage. In the Second World War, Japanese soldiers put pieces of copper in their water bottles to help prevent dysentery. Copper sulfate is highly prized by some inhabitants of Africa and Asia for healing sores and skin diseases. NASA first designed an ionization copper–silver sterilizing system for its *Apollo* flights. Today copper is used as a water purifier, algaecide, fungicide, nematocide, and molluscicide, and as an antibacterial and antifouling agent (Cooney 1995, Stout et al. 1998, Cooney and Tang 1999, Fraser et al. 2001, Weber and Rutala 2001). Copper is considered safe to humans, as demonstrated by the widespread and prolonged use of copper intrauterine devices by women (Hubacher et al. 2001, Bilian 2002). In contrast to the low sensitivity of human tissue (skin or other) to copper (Hostynek and Maibach 2003), microorganisms are extremely susceptible to copper.

Recent past has witnessed several studies involving different types of strategies to load metal nanoparticles into the cotton cellulose fiber networks for antibacterial applications. Danijela et al. (2012) have proposed a novel two-step procedure utilizing the pad-dry-cure method to apply an inorganic–organic hybrid sol–gel precursor (reactive binder, RB) followed by the in situ synthesis of AgCl particles on the RB-treated fibers. The antimicrobial activity against the bacteria *Escherichia coli* and *Staphylococcus aureus* was estimated according to the ISO 20645:2004 (E) and AATCC 100-1999 methods. The results showed that this application process yields the following important benefits: (1) the presence of the RB silica matrix increased the fiber capacity for adsorbing AgCl particles compared with the same fibers without RB; (2) the in situ synthesis enabled a simple and environmentally friendly preparation of AgCl particles from $AgNO_3$ and their embedment into the fibers; (3) the AgCl particles were bound to the RB silica matrix by physical forces, which allowed for their controlled release from the fibers; (4) the capacity of the RB-modified cotton samples to hold embedded AgCl particles was sufficient to provide a 100% bacterial reduction even after 10 repeated washing cycles; and (5) the chemical modification of the cotton fibers did not significantly change their whiteness, wet ability, or softness. Similarly, polyvinyl alcohol/regenerated silk fibroin/$AgNO_3$ composite nanofibers were prepared by electrospinning (Wenli et al. 2012). A large number of nanoparticles containing silver were generated in situ, and well-dispersed nanoparticles were confirmed by transmission electron microscopy (TEM) intuitively. Ultraviolet (UV)–visible spectroscopy and x-ray diffraction (XRD) patterns indicated that nanoparticles containing Ag were present both in blend solution and in composite nanofibers after heat treatment and after subsequent UV irradiation. By annealing the nanofibers, Ag^+ therein was reduced so as to produce nanoparticles containing silver. By combining heat treatment with UV irradiation, Ag^+ was transformed into Ag clusters and further oxidized into Ag_3O_4 and Ag_2O_2. Especially size of the nanoparticles increased with heat treatment and subsequent UV irradiation. This indicated that the nanoparticles containing silver could be regulated by heat treatment and UV irradiation. The antimicrobial activity of heat-treated composite nanofibers was evaluated by halo test method, and the resultant nanofibers showed very strong antimicrobial activity. Most recently, in a report from Bajpai et al. (2012), calcium alginate—impregnated cotton fabric has been loaded with copper nanoparticles to impart antimicrobial properties. The fabric, so prepared, has been characterized by TEM and FTIR analyses. There has been no adverse effect found on the mechanical properties of fabric due to alginate impregnation. The release of Cu(II) ions has been studied in the physiological fluid at 37°C under different experimental conditions, such as varying concentrations of sodium alginate and the cross-linker calcium chloride. The fabrics showed an appreciable release of Cu(II) ions, extended over a period of 50 h. The amount of Cu(II) ions released showed a negative dependence on the amount of alginate present within the fabric network and the concentration of cross-linker calcium chloride used. The release data were fitted on the Higuchi diffusion-controlled release model successfully. Finally, the antibacterial activity of fabric was tested by zone inhibition method against *E. coli* as model bacteria.

Thus, in order to use cotton fibers as an effective material for wound healing applications, we hereby propose a strategy, which involves attachment of a monomer, acrylic acid (AAc), to the cellulosic backbone via graft copolymerization followed by entrapment of Cu(II) ions into the synthesized polymer network and their subsequent reduction to copper nanoparticles. Not only the poly(AAc) graft chains act as templates for incoming Cu(II) ions but the three-dimensional cross-linked grafted network also provides them enough space for accommodation.

Recently, there has been growing interest to develop antibacterial fibers that could be used in a number of biomedical applications such as personal care products, military and biodefense protective suits and coatings, and burn and wound dressings (Lee et al. 2007, Rujitanaroj et al. 2008, Tao et al. 2008, Wiegand et al. 2009). The antimicrobial fibers are usually made from natural and biodegradable polymers such as gelatin (Yin et al. 2009), sodium alginate (Bajpai et al. 2009, Grace et al. 2009, Fen et al. 2010), cellulose (Hou et al. 2009, Xing et al. 2009), and chitosan (Qin 2008), as well as synthetic polymers such as polylactide (Elsner and Zilberman 2009, Hong et al. 2009). Of these, cellulose has been the most frequently used biopolymer used in antibacterial dressing materials, due to its biocompatibility, nontoxicity, easy availability, and above all low cost (Bajpai et al. 2010). In addition, the fair susceptibility of cellulose toward chemical modification to attach or incorporate any desired functionality is an extraordinary plus point that makes it most acceptable to be used in biomedical applications, particularly in wound and burn dressings (Borbely 2005). Finally, fair mechanical strength, sweat absorption, feeling like human skin, and comfort are also additional features that cannot be overlooked.

In the recent past, the cationic antibiotic drug gentamicin sulfate (GS) has been frequently used in wound dressing materials. For example, Campos et al. (2009) have prepared chitosan cross-linked film and investigated it for the controlled release of gentamicin while covering and protecting the wound. In vitro gentamicin release from the cross-linked films, at physiological conditions of pH and temperature, was studied for 2 weeks. The effect of initial drug concentration and cross-linking ratio on the kinetics of drug release was also studied. Similarly, Simovic et al. (2010) developed a mathematical model to estimate the release of GS from chitosan hydrogel, using Franz diffusion technique. The diffusive transport of drug through three connected compartments, that is, chitosan hydrogel, membrane, and solution, was considered by using Fick's second law. The value of diffusion coefficient of drug was considered for every initial drug concentration. In a study by Zilberman et al. (2009), gentamicin-eluting bioresorbable core/shell fiber structures were developed using a technique involving freeze-drying of inverted emulsions. These structures were composed of a polyglyconate core and a porous poly(DL-lactic-co-glycolic acid) shell loaded with the antibiotic agent GS. The investigation was focused on the effect of the emulsion's composition (formulation) on the fibers and on bacterial inhibition. The release profiles exhibited an initial burst effect accompanied by a decrease in release rate.

In the present work, a cationic antibacterial drug GS has been loaded into poly(AAc)-grafted cotton cellulose fibers to develop a wound dressing material that could release the active ingredient and target it at the contain wound. As these fibers contain exchangeable or free H^+ ions in their grafted network, the cationic antibiotic drug GS can conveniently be loaded into these fibers. In addition, the amount of poly(AAc) grafted onto cotton cellulose fibers can also act as one of the rate-controlling parameters. The drug has been frequently used as an effective antibacterial agent in wound dressings. Gentamicin is a broad-spectrum antibiotic that is active against both gram-positive and gram-negative bacteria. It functions by inhibiting DNA gyrase, a type II topoisomerase, and topoisomerase IV enzyme necessary to separate bacterial DNA, thereby inhibiting cell division drug-load.

In the recent past, there have been serious efforts made to develop efficient, nontoxic, durable, and cost-effective antibacterial fibers with increased applications in medical, health care, and hygienic products as well as protective textile materials (Czajka 2005, Pim-on Rujitanaroj et al. 2008). These fibers are usually made from manmade and natural polymers, which mainly include proteins (Fan et al. 2010) and polysaccharides (Teo et al. 2011), and some other polymers with biodegradable nature (Mary et al. 2010). Of these, cellulose has been the most frequently used biopolymer as antibacterial dressing materials due to its low cost, easy availability, biodegradability, and nontoxicity (Elsner and Zilberman, 2009). These fibers are usually loaded with some suitable antibacterial agent that is released over a long time period on coming into contact with wound fluid (Kraitzera et al. 2008, He et al. 2009, Elsner et al. 2010).

Most recently, we reported the release of antibiotic drug GS from poly(AAc)-grafted cotton fiber (PAc-GCF) for wound dressing applications (Bajpai and Das 2011). In spite of obtaining satisfactory results, there was a major drawback in the work. The poly(AAc)-grafted fibers suffered from an appreciable loss in their mechanical strength due to Ce(IV)-induced grafting onto cellulosic backbone. However, a fair mechanical strength is an essential requirement for using fibers as dressing materials. Therefore, in the present study, we hereby report a unique approach to prepare cotton cellulose/poly(AAc) CC/PAAc fibers loaded with antibiotic drug GS. The strategy, followed, involves soaking of cotton fibers into the aqueous solution that contains monomer, initiator, cross-linking agent, and drug. The soaked fibers are then exposed to microwave (MW) radiation for a definite time period to induce in situ polymerization of AAc within the cotton fiber's network. This strategy is based on the logical presumption that when the soaked polymerization solution, containing initiator, monomer, and cross-linker in dissolved state, is exposed to MWs, there starts formation of cross-linked network within the ultrafine pores of cotton fibers. To the best of our information, this is the first study of its own kind where polymer network has been produced within cotton fibers without involving cleavage of any bond in cellulosic backbone, thus restoring full mechanical strength.

12.2 PHYSICAL PROPERTIES OF COTTON FIBERS

Cotton today is the most used textile fiber in the world. Its current market share is 56% for all fibers used for apparel and home furnishings. Another contribution is attributed to nonwoven textiles and personal care items. Some important properties are the following.

TABLE 12.1
Staple Length of Cotton

Sea Island	5.0 cm and More (cm)
Egyptian	3.8–4.4
Brazilian	2.5–3.8
American	2.5–3.0
Indian	2.0–2.5
Chinese	1.5–2.0

12.2.1 Staple Length

Staple length is one of the important primary properties of any textile fiber. The staple length of cotton varies from 1 to 8 cm for different classes, which is shown in Table 12.1.

12.2.2 Fiber Uniformity

Cotton cannot be considered a uniform material even though sufficiently large number of fibers may have a characteristic average behavior. Each fiber must be regarded as an individual with its own characteristic length, strength, fineness, and other properties. For this reason, sampling methods are extremely important, and test data must be handled by statistical method. It has been observed that longer cotton tends to become uniform in length than the shorter ones. The varying percentage of immature fiber also indicates nonuniformity of wall thickness for the same variety of fibers. Also there are considerable differences between cotton grown from the same seed in the same location from time to time.

12.2.3 Porosity

Cotton fibers are porous and exhibits capillary effects to a higher degree. The fibrils themselves are dense as a result of the higher packing density of the molecules and so nonporous. This part of the structure constitutes approximately 70% or more of the fiber. The arrangement of denser fibrils in the fiber may be visualized as analogous to the packing of fibers in well-made yarn. So the porosity of the unoccupied space in the fiber ranges from 20% to 40% of the fiber volume. The fine cottons are more compacted than the coarse variety. Also, the lumen is generally small, about one-third of the unoccupied space. The pore space is largely between the fibrils as capillaries of small diameter. The pore arises from imperfections in the lateral packing of the microstructural elements. Pores of cotton fiber influence properties and reactivity of the fiber in the presence of water. Pores are generally expressed in terms of average surface area. The surface area of dry cotton is 0.6–0.7 m^2/g. The internal surface area can be developed and can be made larger by immersing cotton fiber in water, acetic acid, or ethanol. The surface of cotton fiber in water is around 137 m^2/g.

12.2.4 Density

Cotton fiber has a density of 1.54 g/cc, which corresponds to a specific volume of 0.64 cc/g.

12.2.5 Strength

The load required to break, that is, tensile strength of single cotton fiber varies widely. It depends upon the thickness of wall, prior damage to the fiber, and cellulose degradation. Matured fibers with coarse and heavy wall are the strongest fibers. Their strength ranges from 9 to 13 g/fiber.

The strength of the mature fibers of intermediate and fine types is between 4 g and 9 g/fiber. On the other hand, immature fiber strength can be as low as 0.5–1.0 g/fiber.

The strength of the fiber increases at higher humidity or at higher moisture. In general, the tensile strength increases up to a relative humidity of 60%, and then it remains mostly constant. At higher humidity or moisture pickup, moisture or water penetrates inside amorphous region, breaks the intermolecular forces and also internal stresses, and improves its strength as well as deformability because of more uniform load transfer action.

With the same cotton, yarn strengths can be augmented by changes in friction at fiber surface, by increasing the yarn density and by the selection of uniform staple length of the fibers. Long staple cottons with their fineness and higher fiber bundle strength can be expected to make the yarn stronger.

12.2.6 Maturity and Fineness

The term fiber maturity is generally understood to refer to the degree of development or thickening of the fiber secondary wall (Pierce and Lord 1939, Lord and Heap 1988). Fiber maturity is a function of the growing conditions that can control the rate of wall development and of catastrophic occurrences such as premature termination of growth due to such factors as insect infestation, disease, or frost. As we have seen, the fiber develops as a cylindrical cell with a thickened wall. As the diameter of the fiber cylinder is largely genetic or species dependent, a simple absolute measure of the thickness of the fiber secondary wall is not sufficient to define maturity. Probably the best definition of cotton fiber maturity has been proposed by Raes and Verschraege (1981), who state "the maturity of cotton fibers consists in defining it as the average relative wall thickness." What is implied in this statement is that maturity is the thickness of the cell wall relative to the diameter or perimeter of the fiber.

A term that has more recently gained popularity is the degree of thickening, *U*, defined as the ratio of the area of the cell wall to the area of a circle having the same perimeter as the fiber cross section or $\Theta = 4\pi A/P^2$, where *A* is the wall area (μm²) and *P* is the fiber perimeter (μm). In selecting cotton to be used in the manufacturing process, it is important to have knowledge of the maturity of cotton, which will determine the ultimate quality of the product as related to dye ability and ease of processing. Immature cottons tend to not dye uniformly and result in large processing wastes in large numbers of spinning and weaving breaks and faults. Fiber maturity can be measured directly or indirectly. In general, the direct methods are more accurate and precise, but are much slower and more tedious than the indirect methods. In practice, direct methods are used to calibrate or standardize the indirect methods.

Three of the most significant direct methods include the following:

1. The caustic swelling Smith et al. (1956) test, in which whole fibers are swollen in 18% caustic soda (NaOH) and examined under the light microscope with a specific assessment of the relative width of the fiber versus its wall thickness used to identify a fiber as mature, immature, or dead.
2. The polarized light test (Calkins 1946), in which beards of parallel fiber are placed on microscope slides on a polarized light microscope using crossed polar and a selenite retardation plate. The interference color of the secondary wall will be a direct measure of its thickness and thus maturity. Generally, mature fibers appear orange to greenish yellow, whereas immature fibers appear as blue-green to deep blue to purple.
3. The absolute reference method of image analysis of fiber bundle cross sections (Thibodeaux and Evans 1986, Thibodeaux and Price 1989, Boylston et al. 1993), wherein an image analysis computer system is used to automatically measure the area and perimeter of several hundred fiber sections and statistically analyzed to measure the average *U* and perimeter. The indirect methods are characterized by the need to be rapid as well as accurate and be reliable enough to be used in the cotton marketing system. These methods may be divided

into the double compression airflow approach and near-infrared reflectance spectroscopy (NIRS). Examples of the former (airflow) method are the Shirley Developments Fineness and Maturity Tester Lunenschloss et al. (1980), and the Spinlab Arealometer (Hertel and Craven 1951). The NIRS approaches have been developed and discussed by (Ghosh 1985, Montalvo et al. 1987).

The term fiber fineness has had many interpretations and understanding in fiber science. Some of the most important parameters used to define fineness include

1. Perimeter
2. Diameter
3. Cross-sectional area
4. Mass per unit length
5. Specific fiber surface

Of all of these five parameters, the perimeter has proven to be the least variable with growing conditions and is essentially an invariant property with respect to genetic variety. For this reason, perimeter has become recognized by many as inherent or intrinsic fiber fineness. Because of the irregularity of cotton fiber cross sections, it is very difficult to measure a real diameter (this would presuppose that the fiber was circular in cross section). Similarly, cross-sectional area, mass per unit length, and specific fiber surface are dependent on maturity and thus are not real independent variables that we desire. However, from the standpoint of the spinner, the most important of the possible fineness parameters listed earlier is mass per unit length. Knowledge of this parameter allows the selection of fibers based on the minimum numbers of fibers required to spin a certain size yarn, that is, the finer the yarn, the finer the fiber required.

Fiber fineness or mass per unit length can be measured both directly and indirectly. The direct method consists of selecting five separate bundles from the sample. In each bundle or tuft, the fibers are combed straight, and each is cut at the top and bottom to leave 1 cm long bundles. The fibers from each bundle are laid out on a watch glass beneath a low-magnification lens, and 100 fibers are counted out from each of the bundles, compacted together, and weighed separately on a sensitive microbalance. For each bundle, we obtain the fiber fineness in 10^{-8} g/cm. The closest thing to an indirect method for measuring fineness is the micron ire test (Lord 1956). However, as we will show, the micron ire test actually measures the product of fineness and maturity. It is based upon the measurement of airflow through a porous plug of cotton fibers. In the standard micron ire test, 50 g (3.24 g) of fiber is loosely packed into a cylindrical holder. The cylinder and the walls enclosing it are both perforated to allow the flow of air under pressure that compresses the fiber into a 1 in. diameter by 1 in.–long porous plug that will offer resistance to the flow of air under 6 lb/in.^{2} Research has shown that the flow through the cotton is given by $Q=aMH$, where a is a constant, M is the maturity, and H is the fineness. These results imply that for a constant maturity, a micron ire instrument will be nearly linearly dependent on fineness. However, for samples of various finenesses and maturity, it has been demonstrated that there is a quadratic relationship between the product of fineness and maturity (MH) and micron ire. This relationship is best expressed by the quadratic $MH=aX^2+bX+c$, where X is micron ire and a, b, and c are constants (Lord and Heap 1988). Thus, given that any two of the parameters (fineness, maturity, or micron ire) are known, the third can be determined, and the processor will have a much more complete picture of the quality of the cotton being processed.

12.2.7 Tensile Strength

An accurate knowledge of the tensile behavior of textile fibers (their reaction to axial forces) is essential to select the proper fiber for specified textile end-use applications. However, to have meaningful comparisons between fibers, experience has shown that it is necessary to conduct measurements under known, controlled, and reproducible experimental conditions (Morton and Hearle 1976). These include mechanical history, relative humidity and temperature of the surrounding air, test or breaking gauge length, rate of loading, and degree of impurities. Mechanical history is important because fiber could be annealed, extended beyond its elastic limit, or otherwise affected by mechanical manipulation. Cotton is the only significant textile fiber whose strength increases with humidity, while most others are weakened by increased moisture. Textile fibers universally lose strength with increasing temperature. It seems logical that the longer the breaking or gauge length, there is more chance for an imperfection to occur that will cause a failure. Likewise, the presence of impurities in a material will tend to lead to disorder and weakness.

One definition of strength is the power to resist force. In the case of an engineering material such as textile fibers, this can be translated as a breaking strength or the force or load necessary to break a fiber under certain conditions of strength. Although textiles will be forced to endure a wide variety of forces and stresses, experience is that tensile breaking load is an excellent benchmark of fiber strength. The general approach to relative ranking of the strength of materials is with breaking stress, that is, the tensile load necessary to break a material normalized for its cross-sectional area. This is expressed by the equation, $\sigma = T_b/A$, where T_b is the breaking tension and A is the cross-sectional area. The crystallinity index (CI) units for s are N/m^2 (or Pa). However, when dealing with textiles, it is often more convenient to think of strength in terms of force per mass rather than per area. When dealing with fibers, this translates into force per mass (m) per fiber length (l), which defines specific stress (tenacity) as given by $\sigma_{sp} = T_b/(m/l)$ (N m/kg or Pa m^3/kg). Because of the magnitude of quantities dealing with textiles, it has been found to be more convenient to go to the tex system for linear density (1 tex = 1 mg/m) and for single fibers to measure load in millinewtons with the resultant stress units of mN/tex or gf/tex. Here gf refers to grams force or grams weight, which is the force necessary to give 1 g mass an acceleration of 980 cm/s^2.

The values for the tensile strength of single fibers range from about 13 gf/tex (127.5 mN/tex) to approximately 32 gf/tex (313.7 mN/tex) (Meredith 1945). Calculations based purely upon bond strengths of the cellulose molecule would predict much higher strengths for cotton, but other factors also contribute significantly to determine ultimate fiber tenacity. These include crystallite orientation, degree of crystallinity, fiber maturity, fibrillar orientation, and other features of the fiber structure. Although single-fiber testing is quite tedious and time-consuming, considerable studies in the past show rather consistent findings including

1. Fiber breaking load increases with fiber coarseness, though not in direct proportion to fiber cross section
2. Breaking tenacity correlates well with fiber length and fineness
3. There is a correlation between fiber breaking load and fiber weight within any single variety (Hearle 1991)

Although, as mentioned earlier, the procedures for measuring single fiber breaks have made this type of investigation nearly prohibitive, especially in the case of quality control testing, a new instrument has been designed that shows potential for making single-fiber testing more feasible. The most significant advance in the technology of fiber strength measurements has been the development of the Mantis, a single-fiber tensile tester (Hebert et al. 1995). Mantis's unique design allows for rapid loading of single fibers between the breaker jaws without the use of glue and has computer system to control single-fiber breaks and record both stress–strain curves and other pertinent data. The single fiber test used by the Mantis consists of two measurement modes: mechanical and optical. Fiber mounting is semiautomatic, that is, the operator places a fiber across the jaw faces, and the fiber is straightened by a transverse airflow caused by two lateral vacuum pipes. Small jaws clamp the fiber ends, and a slight stress (<0.2 g) is applied to remove crimp.

Optical measurements are accomplished by the detection of the attenuation of infrared radiation by the presence of the fiber. The degree of attenuation is proportional to the fiber's projected profile (ribbon width). A uniform stress is applied, causing the elongation of the fiber until it breaks. A plot of grams force versus elongation is provided until the fiber breaks. In addition to the stress–strain curve, Mantis supplies the force to break, T_b (g), the fiber ribbon width, *RW* (μm), and the work of rupture (J).

The main purpose of testing raw cotton's strength is to predict the strength of yarn spun from the fiber. As yarn strength is determined by not only fiber strength but also by fiber-to-fiber interactions as induced by length, friction, and degree of twist, it has been found that breaking bundles of parallel fibers gives a better predictor of yarn strength by simulating the combination of fiber tenacity and interaction. The two most commonly used bundle testers are the Pressley and the Stelometer testers (Lord 1961). The Pressley operates with a flat bundle of parallel fibers clamped between a set of jaws that may be operated such that there is essentially no gap (zero gauge) between the clamps holding the fibers or that there is a 0.125 in. spacing (one-eighth-inch gauge) between the clamps. The loading on the jaws is initiated by a weight rolling down an inclined plane. When the breaking load is reached, the bundle breaks, the jaws separate, and the breaking force is read from an attached scale.

The force is determined by the length of travel of the carriage weight and is thus applied to the bundle specimen at a nearly constant rate of loading. The mass of the broken bundle is also measured, and the breaking tenacity is calculated. There are, however, some mechanical problems with the Pressley, and as a result, an alternative bundle tester has been developed that is almost universally accepted as the method of choice. The Stelometer operates on the principle of a pendulum and by proper adjustment can be set to operate at a constant rate of loading of 1 kg/s. The fiber bundle to be tested is mounted between Pressley clamps set to 1/8 inches. The clamps are mounted between a pendulum and beam that are set to allow the pendulum to rotate about a fulcrum. When the beam is released, it rotates about a point, causing the pendulum to rotate in such a fashion as to produce a constantly increasing rate of loading of the bundle under test.

Cotton bundle strengths range from a low of about 18 gf/tex (176.5 mN/tex) for short coarse Asian cottons to a high of approximately 44 gf/tex (431.5 mN/tex) for long fine Egyptian cottons. The degree of crystallite orientation, the fine structural parameter obtained by XRD, is directly related to the bundle strength (Meredith 1946). This parameter is a measure of the angle of the fibrils spiraling around the fiber axis. The angle varies from about 25° for Egyptian cottons to about 45° for the coarser and weaker species. The degree of crystallite orientation increases with decreasing spiral angle. In general, the more highly oriented fibers are stronger and more rigid. In general, cotton strength increases with moisture content and decreases with temperature.

The reaction of a material to a tensile stress is to stretch or elongate. This is measured as tensile strain, defined as the elongation or increased length per initial length. Strain is a dimensionless unit that is usually expressed as a percentage (percent elongation).

12.2.8 Elongation, Elasticity, Stiffness, Resilience, Toughness, and Rigidity

In the previous section, we discussed the evaluation of the strength of cotton under conditions of static or steady loading. In practice, textile fibers are exposed to a variety of dynamic forces, and their response to "stress in motion" will better characterize their performance during processing or in end use. To quantify a material's dynamic response, it is necessary to record the elongation corresponding to increasing load. A typical load–elongation or stress–strain curve Figure 12.1. This represents the response of cotton loaded to the point of breaking. It begins with a curvilinear region (AB) in which fiber crimp or kinkiness is removed as load is applied. The crimp of a cotton fiber is a minor parameter compared with the other factors in the stress–strain properties of cotton, and consequently little quantitative consideration has been given to it (Alexander et al. 1956). However, it has long been recognized that the crimp of a fiber plays a major role, leading to the phenomenon

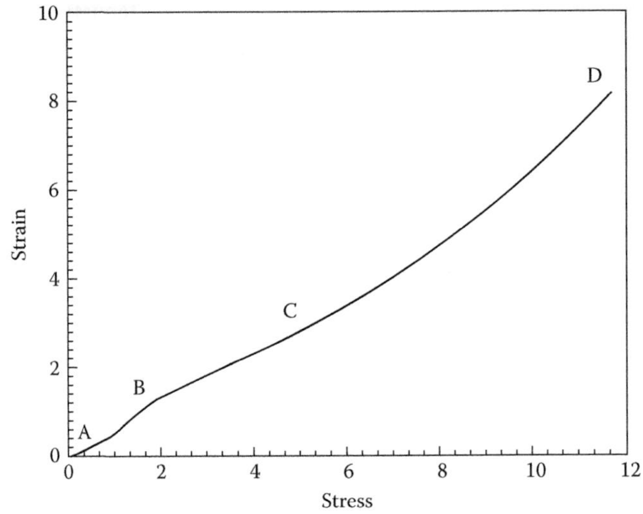

FIGURE 12.1 A typical load–elongation or stress–strain curve.

of fiber cohesion, a property that causes materials to cling together. Without cohesion, it would literally be impossible to spin yarn from staple fibers. In the case of the synthetic fibers, crimp must be artificially induced by elaborate texturing schemes. With further loading of the fiber, the curve (BC) becomes linear. In this region, stress is proportional to strain with the ratio referred to as the Hookean slope (i.e., follows Hooke's law). The point C at which the curve becomes nonlinear is referred to as the yield point where the loaded elements begin to deform in a nonelastic or irreversible fashion and redistribute the stresses. From here to the breaking point (D), the curve becomes essentially linear. The stress–strain curve is strongly influenced by any of several conditions as the rate of loading, sample moisture content, specimen length (where structural imperfections in the fiber come into effect), and extent of mechanical preconditioning.

12.2.9 Typical Load–Elongation or Stress–Strain Curve

The elongation of cotton is expressed as percent elongation taken at the point of breaking, hence the term elongation at break (Morton and Hearle 1976). For most cotton, elongation at break, or just elongation, is in the range 6%–9%. The effect of moisture is most pronounced on elongation. An elongation of about 5% at low relative humidity will increase to about 10% when the relative humidity is almost at the saturation point. The adsorption of water in the pores and amorphous regions of the fiber serves to reduce interfibrillar cohesion and to relieve internal fiber stresses. A more uniform distribution of applied stresses is thereby realized. The internal fibrillar orientation can be seen with XRD. Swelling treatments, such as mercerization, ethylamine, and liquid ammonia treatments, affect the fiber elongation in a far greater fashion than water does. Whereas the parameter elongation is the ability of the fiber to undergo deformation, elasticity is fiber's ability to return to its original shape when the loading is released. This property is highly time dependent. Young's modulus, the ratio of stretching stress per unit cross-sectional area to elongation per unit length, may be calculated from data taken at either the beginning of elongation (initial modulus) or at the breaking point. Initial Young's moduli for cotton range from about 80 g/den for Sea Island down to 40 g/den for Asian cottons. The elasticity of cotton is imperfect because it does not return to its original length after stretching. When a fiber is stressed and allowed to recover, Young's modulus is found to be approximately one-third of the initial value, indicating that some permanent deformation is now present in the fiber.

Elastic recovery of the fiber can be estimated by two methods. In one method, fibers are preconditioned mechanically by cyclic loading to specific levels. The recoveries after stretching and releasing to zero stress give elastic recovery, the ratio of recoverable elongation after a specified cycle to total elongation at the end of the cycle. In this method, elastic recovery is a function of percent elongation; elastic recovery drops curvilinearly from 0.9 at about 1% elongation to about 0.4 at the elongation at break (approximately 6%). In the second method, elastic recovery is resolved into three components: immediate elastic recovery, delayed elastic recovery (5 min after removal of load), and permanent set (or stretch). There is no mechanical preconditioning; a new sample is tested at each successive cycle to higher loadings. Percent elongation at each load is plotted against percent of total elongation to give a plot resembling a phase diagram.

The resilience of a fiber is the ratio of the energy absorbed to the energy recovered when the fiber is stretched and then released. To obtain this index, the areas under the stress–strain curves for the extension phase as well as the recovery phase are measured. The ratio of extension to recovery areas is the index of resilience. As would be expected, cotton is not a very resilient fiber. Another parameter from the stress–strain curve is toughness or the energy to rupture. Toughness is determined from the area under the stress–strain curve measured up to the point of break. It may be closely approximated by the product of the breaking stress and the strain at break divided by 2. The units of toughness are therefore also gf/tex or mN/tex (CI). Values for cotton's toughness range from about 5 to 15 mN/tex. Compared to unswollen fibers, toughness is increased considerably by swelling treatments that end in drying without tension.

However, swelling of fibers followed by drying under tension decreases toughness. Rigidity of the fiber is another elastic parameter that is of great significance in describing a fiber's resistance to twisting. Thus, rigidity will obviously have applications to the spinning of textile fibers. Sometimes referred to as "tensional rigidity," it is defined as torque necessary to impart unit twist or unit angular deflection between the ends of a specimen of unit length (Morton and Hearle 1976). In analogy to Young's modulus, the shear modulus or modulus of rigidity is defined as the ratio of shear stress to shear strain or as the ratio of torsion force per unit area to the angle of twist (displacement) produced by the torque. The finer varieties show less rigidity than coarser fiber: fine Egyptian cottons are in the range 1.0–3.0 mN/m^2; American cottons, 4.0–6.0 mN/m^2; and coarse Indian cottons, 7.0–11.0 mN/m^2. It may be convenient to introduce a specific torsion rigidity of unit linear density (tex) that is independent of fiber fineness. This may be defined as $R_t = \varepsilon n/\rho$, where R_t is the specific torsion rigidity (mN/mm^2/tex^2), ε is the shape factor that equals approximately 0.7 for cotton, n is the shear modulus, and ρ is the density. Rigidity will vary with growth conditions and fiber maturity. Fiber rigidity increases with temperature and decreases with moisture content. Difficulties in fiber rigidity during spinning are thus eased by maintaining a reasonably warm and humid atmosphere.

The elastic properties discussed so far relate to stresses applied at relatively low rates. When forces are applied at rapid rates, then dynamic modules are obtained. The energy relationships and the orders of magnitude of the data are much different (Smith et al. 1956). Because of the experimental difficulties, only little work at rapid rates has been carried out with cotton fiber compared to that done with testing at low rates of application of stress. In contrast, cotton also responds to zero rate of loading, that is, the application of a constant stress. Under this condition, the fiber exhibits creep that is measured by determining fiber elongation at various intervals of time after the load has been applied. Creep is time dependent and may be reversible upon removal of the load. However, even a low load applied to a fiber for a long period of time will cause the fiber to break.

12.2.10 Electrical Properties

Electrical properties of fibers were first considered important because of the effects associated with the buildup of static charges that could hinder mechanical processing and with certain discomfort and hazards associated with electrical charges in clothing, carpets, upholstery, etc. The degree to which a material is susceptible to electrical charging is referred to as its electrical permittivity or dielectric constant. Another factor, closely related to dielectric constant, is the electrical resistivity, which describes the degree to which electrical charges can be conducted through a material to which an electrical potential or voltage differential is applied (Morton and Hearle 1976). In practice, the dielectric constant, «*r*, is determined from the measurements of electrical capacitance as the ratio C_p/C_o, where C_p is the capacitance with the material between the plates of the condenser and C_o is the capacitance of the empty space. The capacitance and thus dielectric constant of cotton are dependent on three parameters including electrical frequency, moisture content, and temperature. The dielectric constant of all materials decreases within creasing frequency. As the moisture content increases, dielectric increases. Thus, in the case of cotton at 0% RH, the dielectric constant ranges from 3.2 at 1 kHz to 3.0 at 100 kHz. At 65% RH, cotton's dielectric constant decreases from 18 at 1 kHz to 6.0 at 100 kHz (Hearle 1954).

The electric resistance of a material is defined as the ratio of the voltage applied across a material to the current (measured in amperes) that flows as a result. The unit of resistance is $V(V=A)$. It is more convenient to use specific resistance *r*, defined as the resistance between opposite faces of a 1 m cube. However, as was the case for fibers, it is more convenient to base the measurement on the linear density rather than cross-sectional area. This leads to the mass specific resistance, R_S 1/4 rd, where *d* is the mass density. R_S is usually expressed in Ω g/cm^2. Under standard conditions, R_S for raw cotton is approximately 0.5×10^6 Ω g/cm^2. As raw cotton is washed and otherwise purified, its resistance increases at least 50-fold (Walker and Quell 1933). Moisture content has even a greater role in resistance with $R_S = 10^{11}$ Ω g/cm^2 at 10% RH decreasing a million-fold to $R_S = 10^5$ Ω g/cm^2 at 90% RH (Hearle 1953).

12.3 CHEMICAL PROPERTIES OF COTTON

The cotton fiber is predominantly cellulose, and its chemical reactivity is the same as that of the cellulose polymer, a β-(1–4)-linked glucan Figure 12.2. The chemical structure shows that the 2–OH, 3–OH, and 6–OH sites are potentially available for the same chemical reactions that occur with alcohols. If the glucan were water soluble, the primary 6–OH, for steric reasons, would be the most available hydroxyl for the reaction. However, as discussed earlier, the chains of cellulose molecules associate with each other by forming intermolecular hydrogen bonds and hydrophobic bonds. These coalesce to form microfibrils that are organized into macrofibrils. The macrofibrils are organized into fibers.

12.3.1 Chemical Structure of Cotton Fiber

The cotton fiber is subjected to many treatments that affect swelling and change its crystal structure. The agents employed must be able to interact with and disrupt the native crystalline structure in order to change it to different polymorphs. The chemical reactions of commerce generally involve the water-swollen fiber, which retains a highly crystalline structure. Reactions with this highly

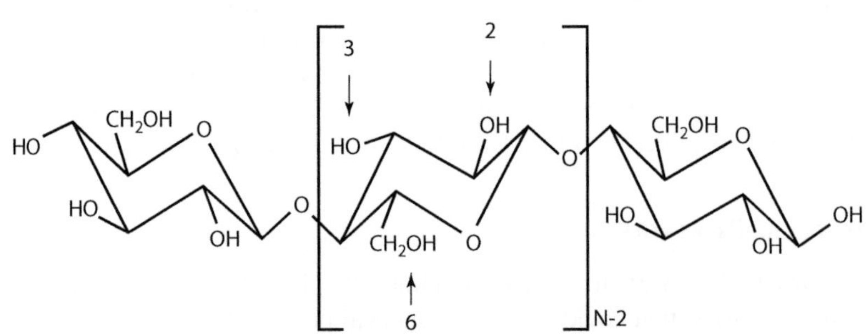

FIGURE 12.2 Chemical structure of cotton fiber.

crystalline, water-insoluble polymer are therefore heterogeneous. Chemical agents that have access to the internal pores of the fiber find many potential reactive sites unavailable for reaction because of involvement in hydrogen bonding. Considerable light has been shed on this subject in research conducted using the chemical microstructural analysis (CMA) technique discussed earlier. Here chemical measurements based on reaction with DEAE chloride under mild conditions showed that decreasing availability of the hydroxyl groups in cotton is 2–OH > 6–OH > 3–OH. The total reactivity of the hydroxyls of cellulose and the relative reactivity of the 2–OH, 3–OH, and 6–OH differ depending on the swelling pretreatment, the reagent, and the reaction conditions. These have not been delineated for all systems.

12.3.2 Swelling

12.3.2.1 Water

Cellulose is hydrophilic and swells in the presence of water. Normally cellulose–water interactions are considered to occur either in intercrystalline regions or on the surfaces of the crystallites and the gross structures. Water vapor adsorption isotherms have been obtained on cotton from room temperature up to 150°C (Jeffries 1960, Zeronian 1985). Theoretical models for explaining the water vapor sorption isotherms of cellulose have been reviewed (Zeronian 1985). Only adsorption theories will be discussed here at ambient temperatures. The shape of the isotherm indicates that multilayer adsorption occurs and thus the Brunauer, Emmett, and Teller (BET) or the Guggenheim, Anderson, and de Boer (GAB) theory can be applied. In fact, the BET equation can be applied only at relative vapors pressures (RVPs) below 0.5 and after modification up to an RVP of 0.8 (Babbett 1943). The GAB equation, which was not discussed in the chapter in the book *Cellulose Chemistry and Its Applications* (Zeronian 1985), can be applied up to RVPs above 0.9 (Zeronian and Kim 1987). Initially, as the RVP increases, a monomolecular layer of water forms in the cellulose. By an RVP of 0.19–0.22, the monomolecular layer is complete, and the moisture regain, when a monomolecular layer has just formed, for cotton and mercerized cotton is 3.27% and 4.56%, respectively. By an RVP of 0.83–0.86, about three layers of water molecules are formed, and at higher RVPs, it is thought that condensation occurs in the permanent capillary structure of the sample (Weatherwax 1974).

It is well known that at low moisture uptakes, the water associated with the cellulose exhibits properties that differ from those of liquid water, and it has been called by such terms as bound water, non-solvent water, hydrate water, and nonfreezing water. From a review of the literature, which included determinations by such techniques as NMR and calorimetric, Zeronian (1985) concluded that between 0.10 and 0.20 g/g of the water present in the fiber cell wall appeared to be bound. Such regains are obtained at RVPs between 0.85 and 0.98. The fiber saturation point (FSP) of cotton is the total amount of water present within the cell wall expressed as a ratio of water to solid content. It is equivalent to the water of imbibitions of the fiber, also called its water retention value. The FSP has been measured using solute exclusion, centrifugation, porous plate, and hydrostatic tension techniques. It occurs at RVP greater than 0.997, and from the review of the papers, it has been concluded that the studies have yielded a value for FSP in the range of 0.43–0.52 g/g (Zeronian 1985).

At equilibrium and at a particular RVP, the amount of adsorbed water held by a cellulose generally will be greater if it has been obtained following desorption from a higher RVP and not by adsorption from a lower RVP. The cause of this hysteresis is not fully established (Zeronian 1985). One explanation is based on the internal forces generated when dry cellulose swells, limiting the amount of moisture adsorbed, whereas when swollen cellulose shrinks, stress relaxation occurs since the cellulose is plastic and permits a higher uptake of moisture.

12.3.2.2 Sodium Hydroxide

The swelling of cotton with an aqueous solution of sodium hydroxide is an important commercial treatment. It is called mercerization after its discoverer, John Mercer, who took a patent on the process in 1850 (Mercer 1850). Other alkali metal hydroxides, notably lithium hydroxide and potassium hydroxide, will also mercerize cotton, but normally sodium hydroxide is used. Mercerization is utilized to improve such properties as dye affinity, chemical reactivity, dimensional stability, tensile strength, luster, and smoothness of the cotton fabrics (Abrahams 1994). The treatment is normally applied either to yarn or to the fabric itself either in the slack state to obtain, for example, stretch products, or under tension to improve such properties as strength and luster. The interaction of alkali metal hydroxides and cellulose has been extensively reviewed. Earlier reviews can be traced from relatively recent ones (Freytag and Donzé 1983, Zeronian 1985).

The term mercerization has to be used with care. One of the changes that occur to the treated cotton is that its crystal structure can be converted from cellulose I to II. To the searcher, the term implies that the caustic treatment has induced close to complete, or full, conversion of the crystal structure to cellulose II. On the other hand, the industrial requirement is improvement in the properties described earlier, and these changes can be produced without full conversion of the crystal structure. For a given temperature and concentration of sodium hydroxide, the amount of swelling that occurs depends on the form of the sample. Swelling deceases in the order fiber > yarn > fabric. In addition, properties are affected by whether the material is treated in slack condition or under tension. Finally, depending on the processing time, the material, and other conditions (e.g., caustic concentration, temperature, slack, or tension treatment), mercerization, as defined by researchers, might not extend beyond peripheral regions. In mercerizing fabrics industrially, the following variables need to be considered: caustic strength, temperature, time of contact, squeeze, framing and washing, and the use of penetrate. Abrahams (1994) has provided the following guidelines. The caustic concentration should preferably be in the range of 48°–54° T_w (approximately 6.8–7.6 M), although if improved dye affinity is the objective, 30°–35° T_w (roughly 4.0–4.7 M) can be used. Temperature may vary in the range of 70°F–100°F (21.1°C–37.8°C) at higher concentrations but has to be monitored more closely when the concentration is 30° T_w. A contact time of 30 s can be used normally. A penetrate is essential if the fabric is in the grease state to permit wetting. Washing on the frame is enhanced by using a mercerizing penetrate that is an active detergent over a wide caustic range.

Hot mercerization allows better penetration of the alkali into the fibers than the ambient temperatures used normally (Vigo 1994). However, to obtain optimum improvement in properties, the caustic has to be washed out after the fabric is cooled. During mercerization, the swelling induced by the caustic is inhibited from outward expansion by the presence of the primary wall of the cotton fiber. The changes observed in fiber morphology by mercerization include deconvolution, decrease in the size of the lumen, and a more circular cross section. Changes in the fine structure that occur when cotton is mercerized include a conversion of the crystal lattice from cellulose I to II, a marked reduction in crystallite length, a marked increase in moisture regain, and a reduction in the degree of crystallinity (Zeronian 1985). A higher concentration is required to induce the optimum changes as the temperature is increased from subambient to room temperature. The conversion from cellulose I to II is substantially complete in cotton yarn treated at 0°C for 1 h, with 5 M LiOH, NaOH, or KOH (Zeronian and Cabradilla 1973). In the case of the sample treated with 5 M NaOH, the following changes were noted: the extent of swelling, measured by the 2-propanol technique, roughly tripled; the moisture regain increased by about 50%; and the crystallite length decreased by approximately 40% (Zeronian and Cabradilla 1973). An estimate of the loss in crystallinity on mercerization determined by moisture regains measurements.

The effect of mercerization on tensile properties depends on the type of cotton tested. In one study, six *Gossypium barbadense* samples were slack mercerized, and the breaking forces and tenacities of the fibers relative to their non-mercerized counterparts ranged from 88% to 122% and from 80% to 114%, respectively (Aboul-Fadl et al. 1985). A larger change was found in the case of a *Gossypium hirsutum* Deltapine Smooth Leaf sample. In this case, the relative breaking force and tenacity were 186% and 134%, respectively. Relative breaking strains ranged from 160% to 189% for the *G. barbadense* samples and 150% for the *G. hirsutum*. The increased strength and extensibility of slack mercerized cotton have been attributed partly to the deconvolution that has occurred and partly to the relief of internal stresses (Sarko et al. 1986). The reduction in crystallinity and crystallite length that results from mercerization contributes to the relief of stresses in the fiber as well as in giving a product of higher extensibility.

There is some evidence that the degree of hydration of alkali hydroxide ions affects their ability to enter and swell cellulose fibers (Freytag and Donzé 1983). At low concentrations of sodium hydroxide, the diameters of the hydrated ions are too large for easy penetration into the fibers. As the concentration increases, the number of water molecules available for the formation of hydrates decreases, and therefore their size decreases. Small hydrates can diffuse into the high-order or crystalline regions, as well as into the pores and low-order regions. The hydrates can form hydrogen bonds with the cellulose molecules.

Ternary complexes called soda celluloses can form between cellulose, sodium hydroxide, and water. In these complexes, some of the water molecules of the sodium hydroxide hydrates are replaced by the hydroxyl groups of the cellulose (Freytag and Donzé 1983). The XRD diagrams have been obtained for five soda celluloses as intermediates in the formation of cellulose II from cellulose I (Freytag and Donzé 1983, Sarko et al. 1986).

12.3.2.3 Liquid Ammonia

Another swelling reagent for cotton cellulose, which is also used industrially, is liquid ammonia. This treatment has been extensively reviewed and discussed (Schuerch 1964, Lewin and Roldan 1971, Lewin et al. 1974, Stevens and Roldán-González 1983, Zeronian 1985, Bredereck 1991, Vigo 1994). Anhydrous ammonia penetrates the cellulose relatively easily and reacts with the hydroxyl groups after breaking the hydrogen bonds. The reaction occurs first in the less-ordered regions (LORs), and gradually later in the crystalline regions of the fibers. An intermediate ammonia–cellulose (A–C) complex, held together by strong hydrogen bonds, is formed. This complex can decompose in several ways and yield different products, depending on the condition of the removal of the ammonia. Lewin and Roldan developed a phase diagram of the four major phases represented in the four corners of a tetrahedron.

The directions of the transitions between the various phases are indicated by the arrows, that is, a transition from D to III is possible on application of dry heat. A transition from III to D is impossible unless a strong swelling agent like ammonia is used. A transition from III to I is possible by the application of water and heat or by a prolonged application of water at ambient conditions. The reverse transition is impossible without an intermediate swelling step. The transitions are usually not complete, especially in industries, and a wide range of products can be obtained as indicated by the phase diagram. The ammonia–cellulose complex and cellulose III can also be obtained from cellulose II. There is, however, no reversion to cellulose I.

The CI decreases upon liquid ammonia treatment and rinsing with water with or without heating, from 79 to 30–40 Å, and the crystallite size decreases from 54 to 37–34 Å. The circularity and homogeneity are also increased. The tensile strength is greatly increased, and the elongation is decreased upon stretching the ammonia-treated fibers. The accessibility and consequently the dye ability of the fibers are also greatly increased as shown in Figure 12.3.

12.3.3 Action of Heat

Cotton fiber ignites easily and burns with an odor similar to that of burning paper. It burns with bright flame, which continues even after the fiber is removed from fire. After the flame has been extinguished, the fiber continues to smolder and smoke. This is a typical test of cellulose. Cotton can be heated in dry state to 150°C without any decomposition. But if heating continues, a brown color on cotton develops gradually. A slight brown discoloration can occur at temperatures lower than 150°C, which does not deteriorate the fiber. However, it is sufficient to spoil the effects of bleaching. So care should be taken to control the temperature of drying. The temperature should

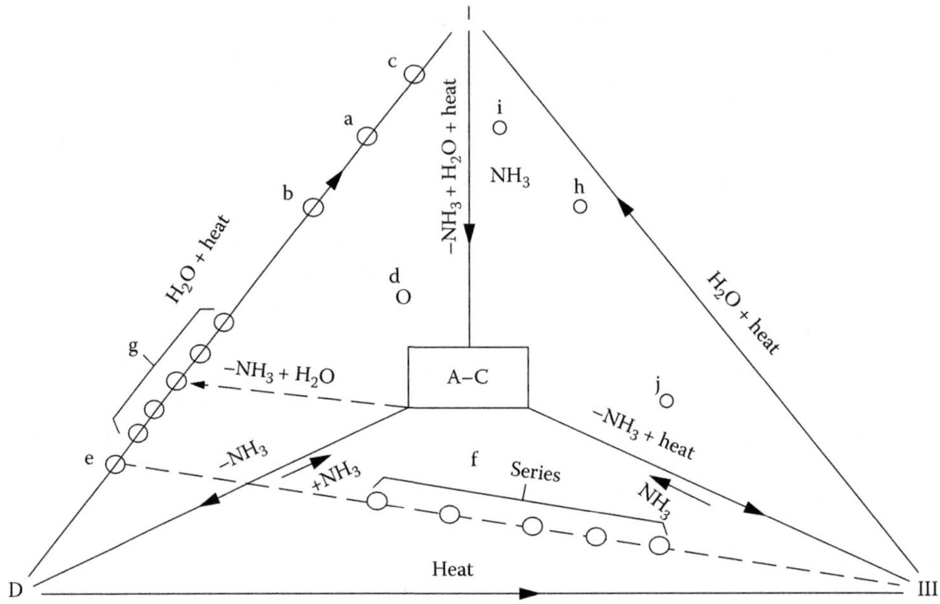

FIGURE 12.3 Phase diagram of ammonia–cellulose (A–C), disordered cellulose (D), cellulose I (I), and cellulose III (III). A–C is the vertex of a tetrahedron and is placed above the plane of the paper. The various samples studied are placed in the basal plane. Arrows show the transition directions.

not exceed more than 93°C. Prolonged exposure at high temperature to an atmosphere containing oxygen causes tendering due to the formation of oxycellulose.

At about 170°C, cotton begins to scorch even in a short time. If cotton is heated out of contact with air, the cotton cellulose molecules break down to form gaseous hydrocarbons, methyl alcohol, acetic acid, and carbon dioxide. The mechanism of thermal degradation of cellulose may be assumed to include two main reactions. One reaction consists of dehydration, and the other scissions of C–O bond in the chain, that is, either in the rings or between the rings. The C–O bond is weaker than the C–C bond and so are more likely to be ruptured. Scission of C–O bond in the ring results in the disintegration of the ring as per the scheme given in Figure 12.3. Scissoring of the external C–O bond degrades the chain molecule with the formation of laevoglucose unit and another glucose unit with hydroxyl end.

12.3.4 Action of Light

Exposure to air in the presence of sunlight for a long period has an effect on cotton like that of heat. Oxycellulose is gradually formed accompanied by tendering because of atmospheric oxygen. The tendering effect by light and air is accelerated by traces of metals like copper.

12.3.5 Action of Water

Raw cotton is very hard to wet because the wax present on the surface of the fiber, that is, cuticle is difficult to wet. Wax can be removed by scouring. So unsecured cotton will not absorb water as easily as scoured cotton. Cold water swells cotton without any chemical damage. The swelling is accompanied by the disappearance of the natural twist, that is, deconvolution (Figure 12.3). The irregular cross section becomes more circular, which reappears on drying. Structurally, swelling is due to the intercrystalline areas, which means only amorphous regions are affected by swelling. Seawater can sometimes degrade cellulose and form hydrocellulose.

12.3.6 Action of Acids

Cold dilute solutions of mineral acids at boil have no effect on cotton cellulose, provided the acids are neutralized or washed out completely before drying. However, if traces of mineral acid like 0.01% be allowed to dry in, tendering soon becomes apparent due to the formation of hydrocellulose. Boiling with dilute acids will ultimately hydrolyze cellulose to glucose. At low temperature, the action by acid is mild and hydrocellulose forms. Cold concentrated sulfuric acid dissolves cellulose and forms cellulose hydrate. If this solution is poured in cold water, the cellulose hydrate is precipitated in a gelatinous form. This principle is used for parchmentising paper to give a transparency effect with higher strength. Hydrochloric acid affects cotton much more severely than sulfuric acid. Degradation is more rapid and severe in the presence of hydrochloric acid than sulfuric acid. Nitric acid, on account of its oxidizing action, differs from other acids in its behavior toward cellulose. Immersion for a short time in concentrated nitric acid results in partial shrinkage with higher tensile strength and affinity for dyestuffs. Prolonged action oxidizes cellulose to oxycellulose and finally breaks it down to oxalic acid. The reaction rate is higher at higher temperature. If nitric acid is allowed to dry in cotton, the material will tender on storage in a similar manner like that of other mineral acids.

12.3.7 Action of Alkali

One of the main advantages of cotton is its resistance to alkali solutions. Mild alkalis like sodium carbonate have no action on cotton in the absence of air either at low temperature or at high temperature. However, in the presence of oxygen or air, oxycellulose is formed with gradual tendering of cotton. On the other hand, the action of string alkalis on cotton fiber is very interesting. Dilute solution of strong alkalis like sodium hydroxide with concentration of 2%–7% can be boiled without least tendering in the absence of air. Generally, dilute solution of sodium hydroxide is used for scouring, that is, removal of waxy and other impurities from cotton fiber. The scouring process purifies cellulose and imparts hydrophilic character and permeability to cotton fiber. In this range, the fiber will have moderate swelling depending upon the concentration of alkali used. Strong alkalis with higher concentration induce structural and physical changes in cotton fiber. Sodium hydroxide as well as potassium hydroxide form different hydrated forms in association with water. The diameter of these hydrated forms depends on the concentration of the alkali used. For small concentration of alkali, that is, less than 5%, the diameter of hydrated ions is too large. So it cannot penetrate into the structure of cotton. As the concentration of alkali increases, the number of water molecules per molecule of alkali decreases for the formation of smaller hydrates. Thus, the diameter of the hydrated form of alkali decreases. The penetration of the hydrated molecule inside the structure, that is, amorphous and or crystalline phase depends on the diameter of the hydrates. Because of the penetration, the fiber swells. When cotton fiber is treated with 7%–15% sodium hydroxide solution, the selling increases to a maximum value with deconvolution. For alkalis with a concentration of 15%–23%, swelling remains constant. The maximum swelling occurs at 13% sodium hydroxide and is related to the penetration of the hydrate to the amorphous region only, which is generally referred to as "intercrystalline swelling."

Cotton is attacked and degraded by strong hot alkalis. The rate of degradation varies depending upon the presence or absence of air. The degradation is slow and in a stepwise manner in the absence of air. However, the degradation is very serious in the presence of air. The oxidative degradation of cotton results in chain scission and weight loss, lowers the molecular length of cotton, and forms oxycellulose. The extent of degradation is higher at higher temperature. Mercerization cotton can be mercerized by treating with or without tension in a strong solution of alkali like sodium hydroxide. The properties can be improved like shrinkage in yarn or cloth due to swelling, improvement in luster with a silky look, improvement in tensile strength, improvement in dye ability and uniformity in dyeing, improvement in dimensional stability, and improvement in elasticity and stretch ability. Mercerization is generally defined as subject of cotton, linen, and other vegetable fiber, either in fiber form or any other stage of its manufacture to the action of caustic soda, caustic potash, dilute sulfuric acid, or zinc chloride of a temperature and strength sufficient to produce a new effect.

The changes that take place during mercerization are a physical one, though there is some chemical change. Solvated dipole hydrates form in this alkali concentration. The hydrates penetrate inside cotton fiber. Two to three hydrated molecules combine with the hydroxyl groups of cotton cellulose. In this manner, cellulose, sodium hydroxide, and water form a ternary complex, generally referred to as soda cellulose. During washing, soda cellulose decomposes with the formation of cellulose II. Washing is also an equally important process for the decomposition of soda cellulose.

12.3.8 Action of Microorganism

Much microorganisms attack cotton. Numerous fungi cause mildew. The mildew discolors rots and weakens the fiber. Most fungi reproduce by means of spores, largely present in air, and are attracted to cotton, wherever found. Certain bacteria also cause microbiological rotting and appear to be its main cause in waterlogged conditions.

12.3.8.1 Modification of Cotton

Cotton fibers have the following inherent drawbacks:

1. Poor solubility in common solvents, which restricts the improvement in fiber and yarns.
2. Poor crease resistance, which makes garments made from cellulosic fibers crumple easily during wear.
3. Lack of thermoplasticity, which is a requirement for heat setting and shaping of garments.
4. Poor dimensional stability, resulting in distortion of the garments during laundering and ironing.

These drawbacks have directed attention toward improving the properties of cotton by modification of its physical and chemical structures.

The physical structure of the fiber can be changed either by swelling or by regeneration. Cotton or cellulose can be swollen in a suitable swelling agent and then partially deswollen by removal of the swelling agent. Change in physical structure enhances strength, luster, and reactivity. The chemical structure of cotton can be modified in several ways like substitution, cross-linking, and grafting reactions.

12.3.9 Substitution

The cellulose hydroxyls in cotton can be substituted. In this process, hydroxyl groups in cellulose molecules are altered through introduction of side groups by an etherification or by an etherification reaction. Some of the drawbacks of cellulose or cotton such as flammability, susceptibility to rot and mildew, and swell ability can be eliminated or reduced. Chemical reaction rate of cellulose hydroxyls is generally low and nonuniform. So conditions for chemical modification must prevent the decrease in molecular mass or chain length. Acetylating involves treatment of cellulose with a mixture of acetic anhydride, acetic acid, and a catalyst such as sulfuric acid or perchloric acid. The reaction of cellulose with acetic anhydride may be written as

$$\text{Cell-OH} + \left(CH_3CO_2\right)O \rightarrow \text{Cell-O} - CO - CH_3 + CH_3COOH$$

Acetylated cellulose possesses several useful properties such as heat resistance, mildew resistance, and rot resistance. Modification of cellulose by cyano-ethylation results in cyano-ethylated cotton.

In this procedure, cotton is first impregnated with dilute sodium hydroxide solution and then treated with acrylonitrile at 55°C, followed by rinsing with dilute acetic acid and further washing with water. The reaction between cellulose hydroxyl and acrylonitrile is as follows:

$$\text{Cell-OH} + (CH_2 = CHCN) \rightarrow \text{Cell-O} - CH_2 - CH_2 - CN$$

Cyano-ethylated cotton possesses improved resistance to rot, heat, and damage by acids and abrasion. Also, these fibers are better dyeable. Carboxyl methylation is one of the common methods of chemical modification. Partially carboxymethylated cotton may be prepared by padding the material with monochloro acetic acid or its sodium salt, followed by padding it with sodium hydroxide. The reaction is as follows:

$$\text{Cell-OH} + NaOH \rightarrow \text{Cell-O} - Na + H_2O$$

$$\text{Cell-O} - Na + Cl - CH_2 - COO - Na \rightarrow \text{Cell-O} - CH_2 - COO - Na + NaCl$$

Carboxymethylated cotton shows improvement in properties like moisture regain, water absorbency, water permeability, dyeing, soil resistance, and soil removal. Cellulose reacts with acrylamide in an alkaline medium to give carboxyethylated cellulose:

$$\text{Cell-OH} + CH_2 = CH - CO - NH_2 \rightarrow \text{Cell-O} - CH_2 - CH_2 - CO - NH_2$$

The carboxyethylated cellulose possesses better rot resistance and heat resistance properties. Cellulose phosphate can be prepared by reacting with suitable phosphorylating agents like phosphoric acid and ammonium phosphate. Phosphorylated cotton shows better fire resistance and soil resistance qualities. Cross-linking cotton can be reacted bi- or polyfunctional compounds. This results in the production of cross-linked or resinification products and stabilizes its structure. The interaction of cellulose and formaldehyde at higher temperature leads to the formation of methylene ether cross-links with secondary hydroxyl groups of cellulose. The cross-linking reaction takes place in highly disordered regions. In the presence of swelling agents, the cross-linkages appear to be located in the ordered regions, that is, crystalline regions. Also, formaldehyde condensate with urea, phenol, or melamine gives rise to urea-formaldehyde, phenol-formaldehyde, and melamine-formaldehyde resins. These resins are generally applied and cross-linked with cotton as well as other cellulose material to obtain crease resistance and low shrinkable fabrics. In a similar manner, epoxy resins are cross-linked with cotton and other cellulosic materials to retain fabric feel in addition to the crease resistance and anti-shrink properties.

12.4 CHEMICAL MODIFICATION OF COTTON FIBERS

In this chapter, we discuss cellulose-based fibers (e.g., cotton fibers) as an alternative material to be developed and used in wound dressing. We developed four methods for composites.

a. Grafting of acrylamide (AAm) and *N*-vinyl-2-pyrrolidone (VP) onto cotton fibers
b. Poly(AAc)-GCFs
c. Preparation of chitosan-attached cotton fibers
d. Preparation of alginate-attached cotton fibers

a. Grafting of (AAm) and (VP) on to cotton fibers: All procedures, from solution preparation to the graft copolymerization, were performed at room temperature. In this procedure, pre-weighed cotton fibers were put in monomer solution. After graft copolymerization reaction, grafted fibers are ready to further reactions (shown in Figures 12.4 and 12.5).

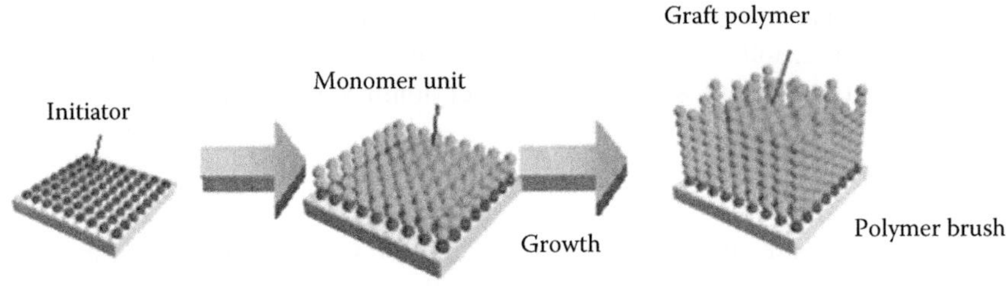

FIGURE 12.4 Grafting mechanism of cotton fibers.

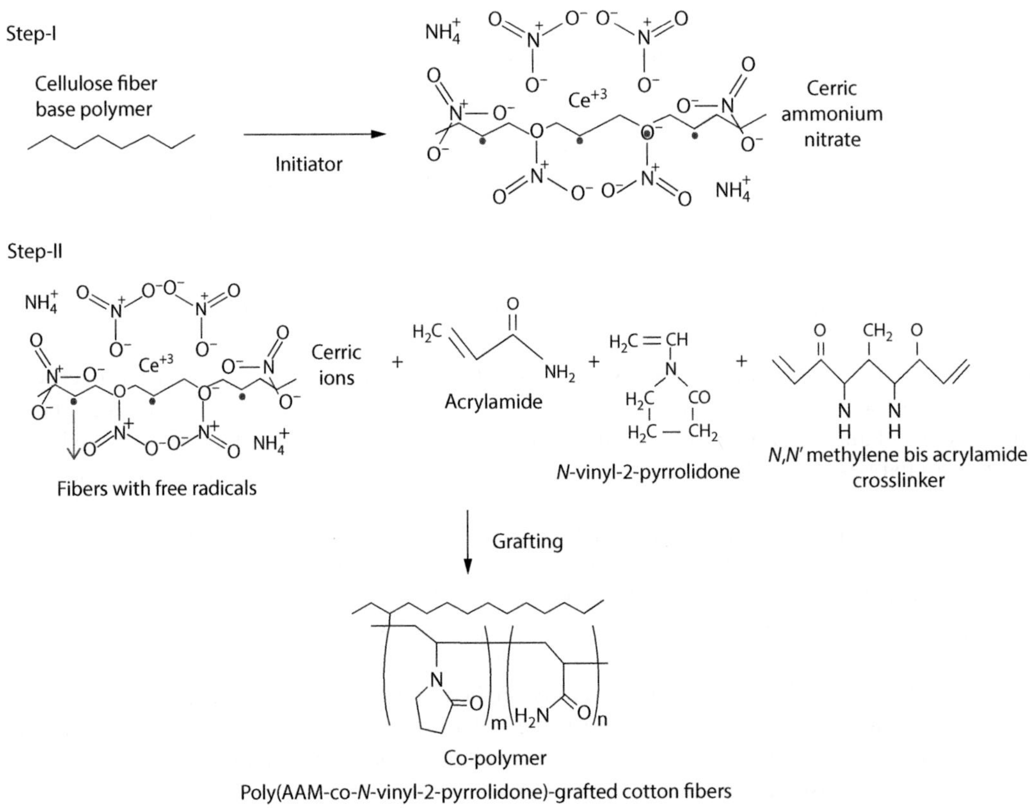

FIGURE 12.5 Grafting procedure of cotton fibers.

b. Poly(AAc)-GCFs: Pre-weighed cotton fibers were placed in 10 mL of 20 mM CAN for 30 min, blotted with tissue paper to remove extra CAN, and then immersed in 25 mL of a solution containing pre-weighed quantities of monomer AAc and cross-linker MB. After the grafting reaction was over, each substrate was equilibrated in distilled water to remove unreacted salts. Finally, the grafted fibers were put in 50% methanol solution to remove any homopolymer formed (Taghizadeh and Darvish 2001) and placed at 40°C in a dust-free chamber until the fibers were completely dry (shown in Figure 12.6). The percent grafting was calculated using the following expression:

$$\text{P.G.} = (W_g - W_0) / W_0 \times 100$$

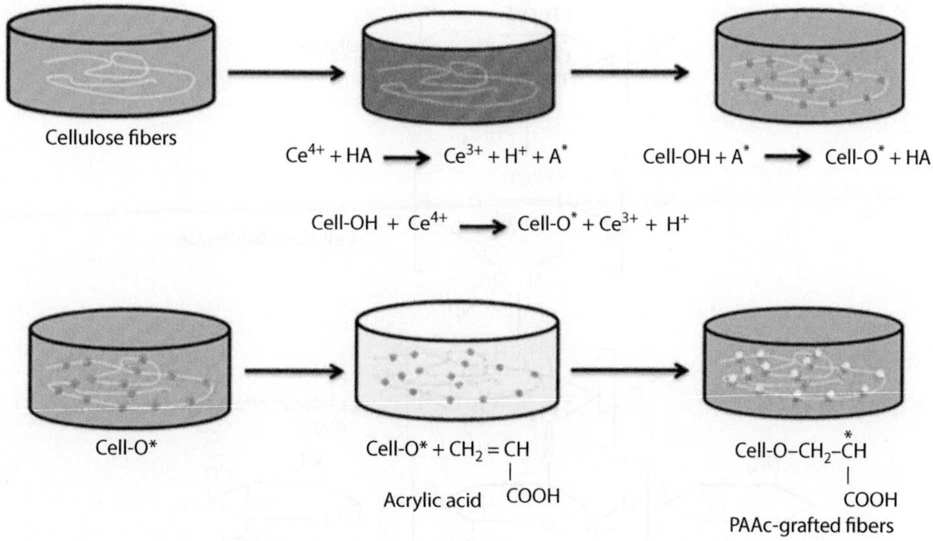

FIGURE 12.6 Poly(acrylic acid)-grafted cotton fibers.

c. *Preparation of chitosan-attached cotton fibers*: In this procedure, the covalent attachment of chitosan to the cellulose has been carried out by periodic acid–induced oxidation of cellulose to dialdehyde group of chitosan and aldehyde group of oxidized cellulose as shown in Figures 12.7 and 12.8.

d. *Alginate-attached cotton cellulose fibers*: Alginate is an anionic linear polysaccharide with 1,4-linked D-mannuronic acid and L-guluronic acid. In this procedure, cotton cellulose fibers are placed in dilute solution of sodium alginate and macromolecular chains of alginate get absorbed onto the surface of the ultrafine cellulose fibers as shown in Figures 12.9 and 12.10.

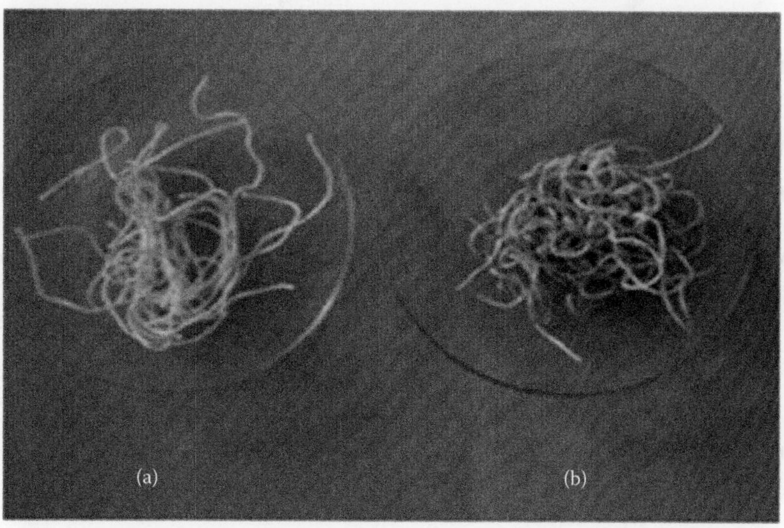

FIGURE 12.7 (a) Plain cotton fibers and (b) Cu(II) ion-bound chitosan-attached fibers.

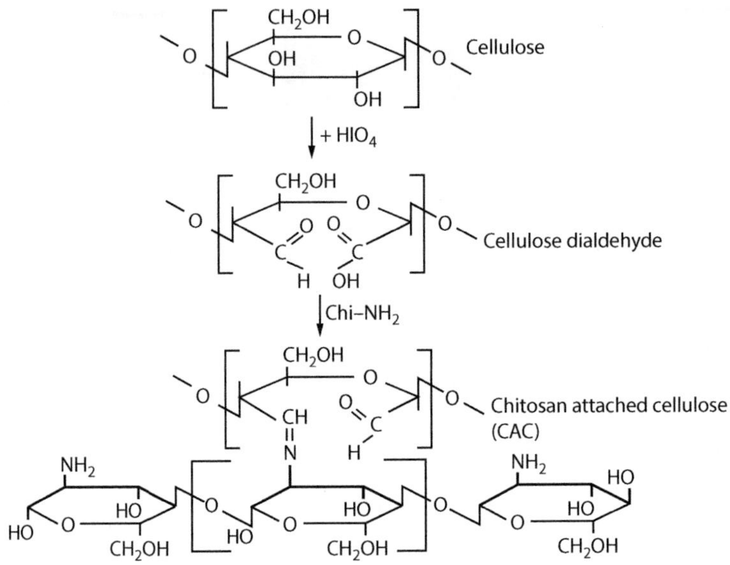

FIGURE 12.8 Chitosan-attached cotton cellulose fibers.

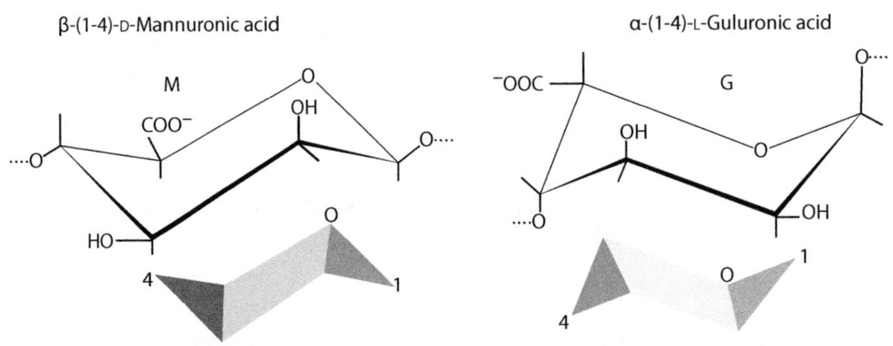

FIGURE 12.9 Structure of alginate.

12.4.1 Graft Copolymerization

Cotton can be grafted to prepare a branched cellulose chain in combination with synthetic polymers. This process is known as grafting, usually done by modifying the cellulose molecules through creation of branches of synthetic polymers. Grafting confer certain desirable properties on the fiber without destroying its intrinsic properties.

Grafting on cellulose is heterogeneous reaction because of the structure of cellulose or cotton. Grafting can be done by

1. Chain transfer
2. Activation of the macromolecule
3. Introduction of functional groups

Chain transfer reaction involves the interaction of reactive centers in the middle of cellulose macromolecule with the grafting agent. Activation of cellulose consists of introduction of active

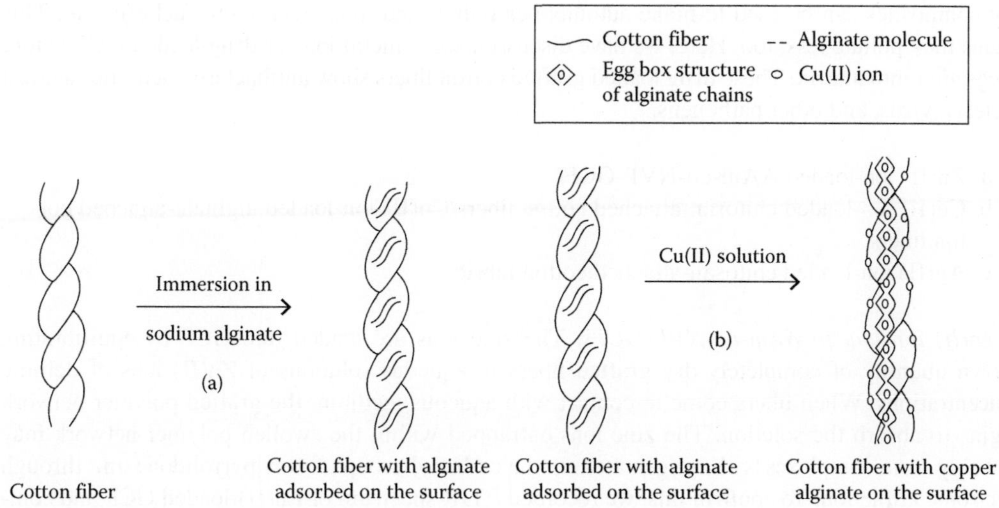

FIGURE 12.10 (a) Sorption of alginate chains into cotton cellulose fibers and (b) cross-linking of alginate chains by Cu(II) ions thus forming "egg-box" cavities.

centers in the macromolecules by thermal, mechanical, chemical, photochemical, or radiation energy like gamma or UV rays. The third method consists of introducing groups into the macromolecule, which will decompose to form free radicals. These free radicals induce grafting. The mechanisms proposed for graft are graft initiation, propagation, that is, chain growth, and termination. Mostly, vinyl and acrylic monomers are used for grafting. Initiation consists of formation of free radical on the cellulose free radical. This results in the formation of a covalent bond between cellulose and monomer unit with a free radical on the newly formed branch. This is followed by subsequent additions of monomer molecule to the initiated chain, thereby propagating the chain. Termination occurs by reaction with impurities, initiator or activated monomer, or by a chain transfer process.

There are different types of polymers used for grafting cotton or cellulose for different applications. Some of the examples are

Flammability—poly(methyl vinyl pyridine), phosphorous containing vinyl polymers like poly(vinylpyrrolidone) and phosphorous-containing monomer like vinyl phosphate monomers, phosphate acrylamide.

Water-proofing—Fluorine-containing polymers, poly(isoprene), and polyolefins.

Moth and mildew—Silver or copper salts of poly(AAc) or poly(methyl methacrylate), poly(acrylonitrile).

12.5 INCORPORATION OF ANTIMICROBIAL AGENT INTO MODIFIED FIBERS

12.5.1 Metal Ions

Modern composites are usually made of two components, a fiber and a matrix. The fiber is most often glass, but sometimes Kevlar, carbon fiber, or polyethylene. The matrix is usually a thermoset like an epoxy resin, polydicyclopentadiene, or a polyimide. The fiber is embedded in the matrix in order to make the matrix stronger. Fiber-reinforced composites have two things going for them. They are strong and light. They are often stronger than steel, but weigh much less. This means that composites can be used to make automobiles lighter and thus much more fuel efficient. This means they pollute less, too. Here, we have discussed some metal ions or drug-loaded GCF before integration into matrix. These drug loaded grafted cotton fibers show antibacterial activities against bacteria, virus, and other pathogens.

a. Zn(II) ion-loaded AAm-co-NVP-GCFs
b. Cu(II) ion-loaded chitosan-attached cotton fibers/Cu(II) ion-loaded alginate-attached cotton fibers
c. Ag(II) ion-loaded chitosan-attached cotton fabric

a. Zn(II) ion-loaded AAm-co-NVP-GCFs: The zinc ions are loaded into GCF by equilibrating known quantity of completely dry grafted fibers in aqueous solutions of Zn(II) ions of definite concentrations. When fibers come in contact with aqueous medium, the grafted polymer network begins to absorb the solution. The zinc ions entrapped within the swollen polymer network may probably form complexes with oxygen atom in the carbonyl group of vinylpyrrolidone unit through electronic attraction. To confirm this, we recorded FTIR spectrum of Zn(II)-loaded GCF and compared it with that of grafted fibers. It was observed that the peak, appearing at 1705 cm^{-1} for CO group of *N*-vinyl-2-pyrrolidone in grafted GCF, was shifted to 1633 cm^{-1} in Zn(II)-loaded grafted GCF (as shown Figure 12.11). The binding of Zn(II) with oxygen of CO group of NVP in Zn(II)-loaded grafted fibers is shown in Figure 12.12. Recently, silver ions have also been reported to form complex with *N*-vinyl-2-pyrrolidone (Borbely 2005).

b. Cu(II) ion-loaded chitosan/alginate cotton fibers: Copper ions, either alone or in copper complex, have been used for centuries to disinfect liquid, solids, and human tissues. Copper has been frequently exploited to impart antimicrobial properties to various polymeric substances. Apart from showing strong antibacterial properties, Cu(II) is also playing a key role in collagen cross-linking thus aiding in the normal formation of bone matrix. Among the various fibrous products, alginate- and chitosan-based products are currently the most popular ones used in developing antibacterial agent-releasing system or dressing materials (shown in Figures 12.13 through 12.15).

Thomas et al. have done an excellent work on silver nanoparticle-loaded chitosan-attached cotton fabric for antibacterial property. This work will be beneficial for medical area in near future (shown Figure 12.16).

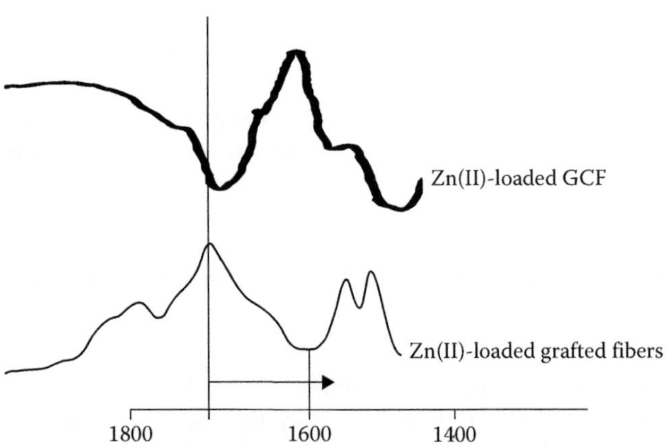

FIGURE 12.11 FTIR spectrum of Zn(II)-loaded GCF and grafted fibers.

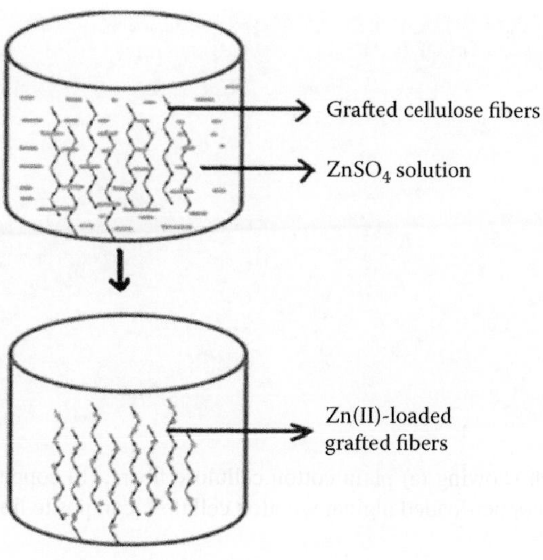

FIGURE 12.12 Entrapment of Zn(II) ions in grafted cotton fibers.

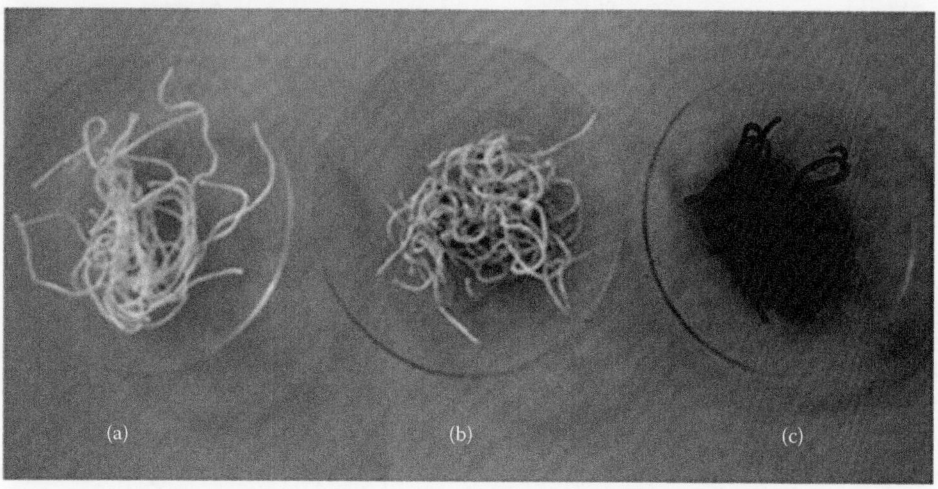

FIGURE 12.13 Photograph showing (a) plain cotton cellulose fibers, (b) copper-bound chitosan-attached cellulose (CBCAC) fibers, and (c) nanocopper-loaded chitosan-attached cellulose (NCLCAC) fibers.

12.5.2 Antibiotic Drug

12.5.2.1 Gentamicin-Loaded AAc-GCFs

GS is a water-soluble drug with a fair solubility of nearly 50 mg/mL H_2O (28). In aqueous medium, it is present in the form of cation.

$$G.SO_4 \rightleftharpoons G^{++} + SO_4^{--}$$

The poly(AAc)-grafted-fibers have carboxylic groups attached along the poly(AAc)-grafted chains with free or counter H^+ ions.

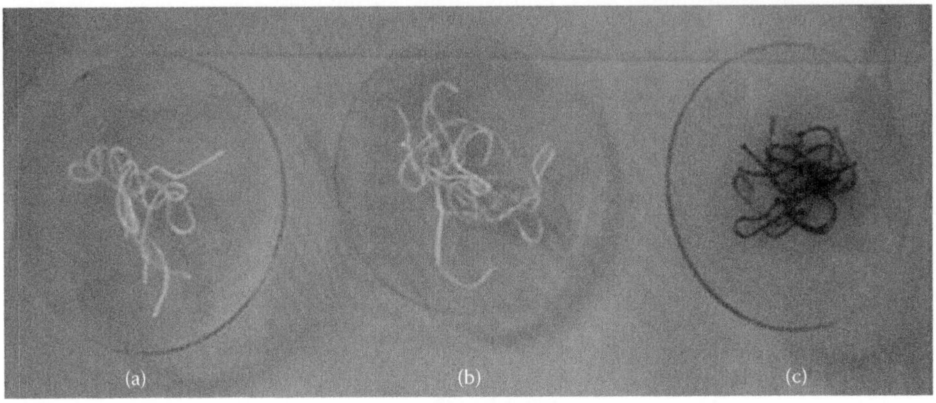

FIGURE 12.14 Photograph showing (a) plain cotton cellulose fibers, (b) copper alginate–cotton cellulose (CACC) fibers, and (c) nanocopper-loaded alginate–cotton cellulose composite fibers.

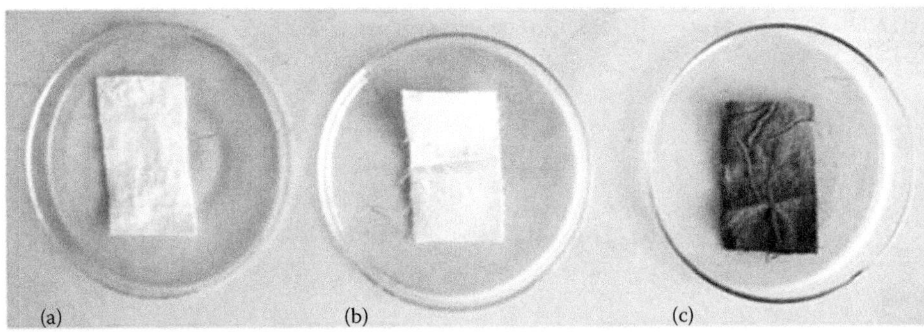

FIGURE 12.15 (a) Plain fabric, (b) chitosan-attached fabric, and (c) nanosilver-loaded fabric.

$$\text{fibers} - \text{COOH} \rightleftharpoons \text{fibers} - \text{COO}^- + \text{H}^+$$

When grafted fibers are placed in aqueous solution of drug GS, there occurs ion-exchange process between counter H^+ ions attached along the fibers and G^{++} ions present in the aqueous solution, as shown in the following:

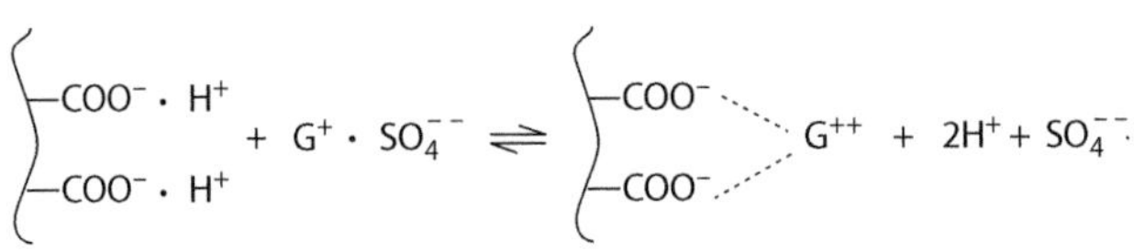

Therefore, the drug is loaded into grafted fibers via ion-exchange mechanism (Figure 12.17).

12.5.3 Halamines

N-halamines are heterocyclic organic compounds containing one or two covalent bonds formed between nitrogen and a halogen (N–X), in which the latter is usually chlorine (Sun et al. 1995). N–Cl bonds of different stabilities can be formed by the chlorination of amine, amide, or imide groups in dilute sodium hypochlorite. *N*-halamines are biocides that are active for a broad spectrum of bacteria, fungi, and viruses. Their antimicrobial properties are based on the electrophilic

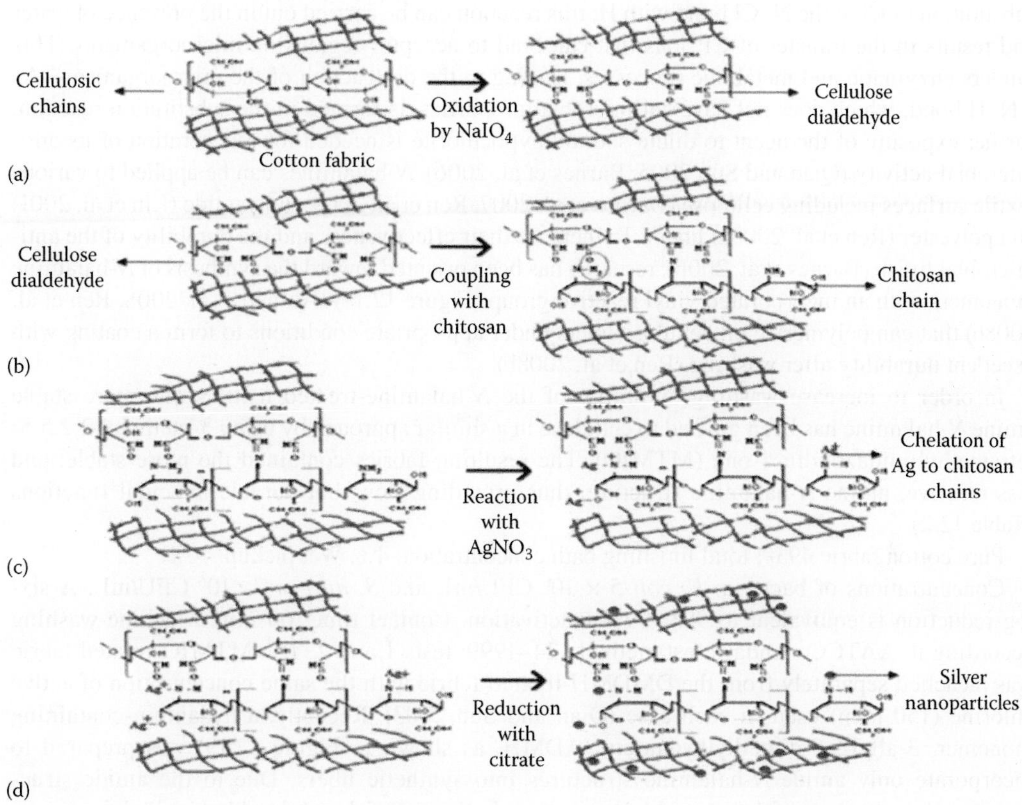

FIGURE 12.16 Matrix form of nanosilver-loaded fabric (a) cellulosic chain oxidation by $NaIO_4$, (b) cellulose dialdehyde coupling with chitosan, (c) reaction with $AgNO_3$, and (d) reduction with citrate.

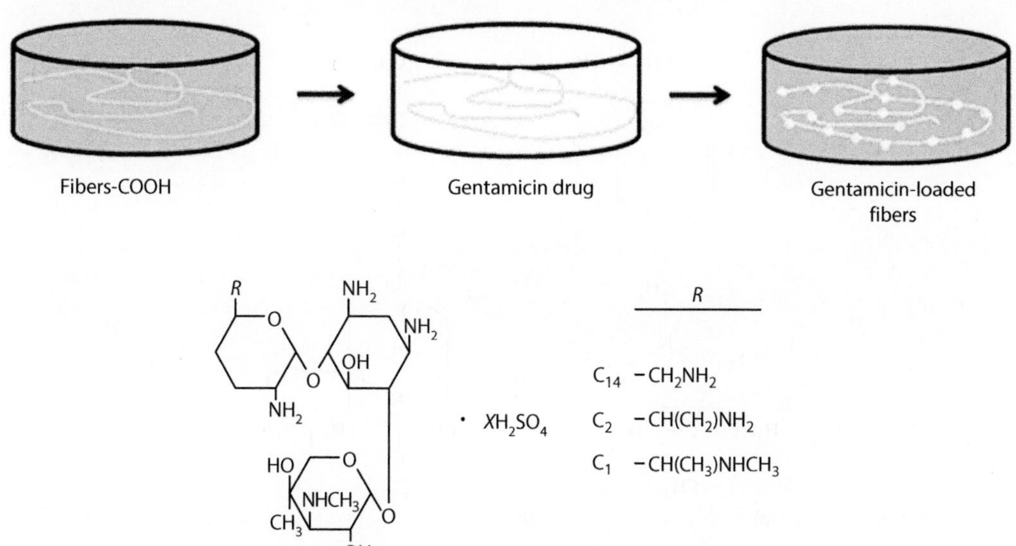

FIGURE 12.17 Gentamicin drug-loaded grafted cotton fibers.

substitution of Cl in the N–Cl bond with H; this reaction can be carried out in the presence of water and results in the transfer of Cl^+ ions that can bind to acceptor regions on microorganisms. This hinders enzymatic and metabolic processes, leading to the destruction of the microorganisms. As a N–H bond, which does not have antimicrobial properties, is formed in the substitution reaction, further exposure of the agent to dilute sodium hypochlorite is needed for regeneration of its antimicrobial activity (Qian and Sun 2005, Barnes et al. 2006). *N*-halamines can be applied to various textile surfaces including cellulose (Barnes et al. 2007, Ren et al. 2009), polyamide (Lin et al. 2001) and polyester (Ren et al. 2008a) fibers. To increase their effectiveness and the durability of the antimicrobial finish (Barnes et al. 2006), research has been oriented toward the synthesis of *N*-halamine monomers with an incorporated vinyl reactive group (Figure 12.18) (Ahmed et al. 2008, Ren et al. 2008b) that can polymerize on cellulose fibers under appropriate conditions to form a coating with excellent durability after washing (Ren et al. 2008b).

In order to increase washing durability of the *N*-halamine-treated textiles, the more stable amine *N*-halamine has been grafted to cellulose in a similar approach by using 3-methylol-2,2,5,5-tetramethylimidazolidin-4-one (MTMIO). The resulting fabrics contained the more stable, and less reactive, amine *N*-halamine structure, thus providing slow, but durable, biocidal functions (Table 12.2).

Pure cotton fabric 493#; total finishing bath concentration: 4%. Wet pickup: 70%.

Concentrations of bacteria: *E. coli* 5×10^6 CFU/mL and *S. aureus* 7×10^6 CFU/mL. A six-log reduction is equivalent to 99.9999% inactivation. Contact time: 60 min. Machine-washing according to AATCC standard test method 124–1999; tests 1 and 2. The MTMIO-treated fabric was bleached separately from the DMDMH-treated fabric with the same concentration of active chlorine (150 ppm) used in each case (Qian and Sun 2003). Recently, a hydantoin-containing monomer, 3-allyl-5,5-dimethylhydantoin (ADMH, as shown in Figure 12.19) was prepared to incorporate only amide *N*-halamine structures into synthetic fibers. Due to the amide structure, the thus-produced fabrics could demonstrate both powerful and durable biocidal functions. Synthetic fabrics such nylon-66, polyester (PET), polypropylene (PP), acrylics, and amide fibers, as well as pure cotton fabrics, were used in the chemical modification. The ADMH can be incorporated in the surfaces of fibers by a controlled radical grafting reaction, which can ensure short-chain grafts instead of long-chain self-polymerization of the monomers (Figure 12.19) (Sun and Sun 2002, 2003).

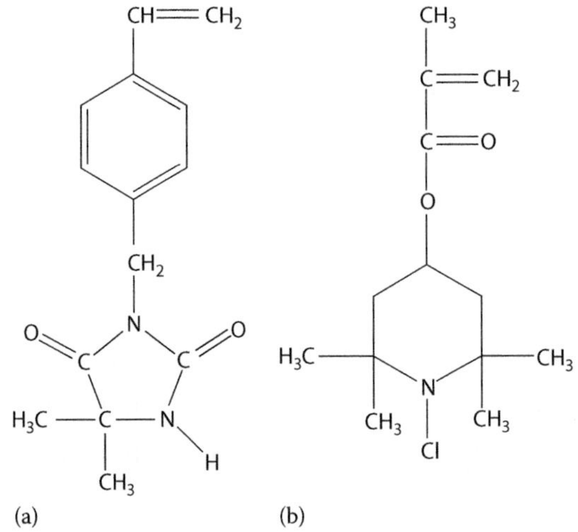

FIGURE 12.18 Chemical structures of (a) 3-(4′-vinylbenzyl)-5,5-dimethylhydantoin and (b) *N*-chloro-2,2,6,6-tetramethyl-4-piperidinyl methacrylate.

TABLE 12.2
Chlorine Loss and Antimicrobial Effects of MTMIO- and DMDMH-Modified Cotton Samples

		Against *Escherichia coli*			Against *Staphylococcus aureus*		
Chemical	**Washing Cycles**	**Cl ppm**	**Cl loss %**	**Log reduction**	**Cl ppm**	**Cl loss %**	**Log reduction**
MTMIO	0	565	—	6	654	—	6
	2	507	10.2	5	616	6.1	6
	5	498	11.9	4	601	8.4	4
	0	863	—	6	934	—	6
DMDMH	2	218	74.7	1.5	380	59.3	3
	5	157	81	0.9	274	70.7	2

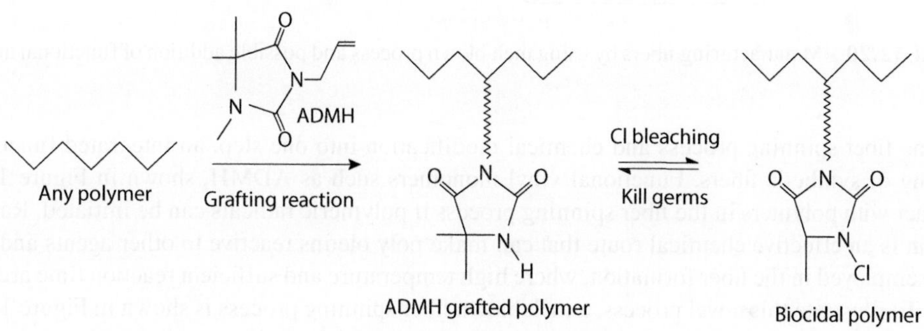

FIGURE 12.19 Structure of ADMH and its grafting reactions on synthetic polymers.

Biocidal properties of the modified fibers could be demonstrated after a chlorination reaction by exposing the grafted fibers to a diluted chlorine solution, with which the grafted hydantoin rings were converted to *N*-halamine structures. The polymeric *N*-halamines could provide powerful and rapid antibacterial activities against *E. coli* and *S. aureus*. Most of the fibers could completely inactivate a large number of bacteria (1 × 10^6 CFU) in a 10–30 min contact time. In addition, the antibacterial activities of these polymeric *N*-halamines could be easily recovered after usage by simply exposing to chlorine solution again.

Currently used chemical and biological protective clothing is mostly made of nonwoven fabrics (Rigby et al. 1993, Leonas 1998). The nonwoven fabrics could resist liquid and aerosol microorganisms and toxic chemicals penetrating through the fabrics due to the dense fiber entanglements and hydrophobic structures. These nonwoven fabrics are widely employed in most personal protective gear such as disposable protective clothing, filters, and respirators with different performance against different toxicants and biological agents. Novel technologies have been developed to incorporate self-decontamination functions to many woven fabric materials, but failed to treat nonwoven fabrics. In addition, most nonwoven fabrics are made of poly olefins, which are the polymers that are hardly modified in regular textile chemical finishing processes. The only possible approach is to introduce the functions of the nonwovens during fiber formation processes, where thermoplastic polymers are molten and extruded through spinnerets to form fine fibers.

In order to incorporate the self-decontaminating functions to the currently used biological and chemical protective clothing, we propose to develop an innovative manufacturing process that can

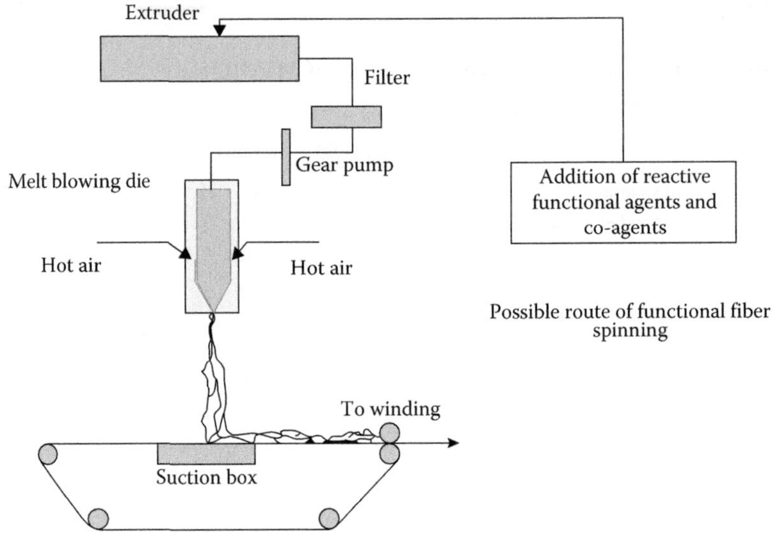

FIGURE 12.20 Manufacturing fibers by using melt blown process and possible addition of functional agents.

combine fiber spinning process and chemical modification into one step, an integrated functional spinning of synthetic fibers. Functional vinyl monomers such as ADMH, shown in Figure 12.19, can react with polymers in the fiber spinning process if polymeric radicals can be initiated. Radical reaction is an effective chemical route that can make poly olefins reactive to other agents and thus can be employed in the fiber formation, where high temperature and sufficient reaction time are provided. To illustrate this novel process, a melt blown fiber spinning process is shown in Figure 12.20. The functional agents are added into and mixed with the polymers in extruders and co-spun into chemically modified fibers.

12.6 ASSESSING THE PERFORMANCE OF THE COMPOSITE

Cotton fiber composites can perform fair antibacterial activity against bacteria, virus, fungus, etc. We are using these cotton fibers as burn and wound dressing materials. Zinc-based enzymes and protein that direct the process of skin generation are especially evident during wound healing and inflammation reduction. In a study by the authors, gentamicin drugs have been employed for preparing Zn(II) and gentamicin loaded cotton fibers as dressing materials (shown in Figures 12.21 and 12.22, respectively) (Grace et al. 2008). Moreover, we have also used cotton, chitosan, and alginate fibers, loaded with copper ions and nanosilver for antibacterial, antiviral, antifungal properties (Bajpai et al. 2012 and Grace et al. 2009) (see Figures 12.23 through 12.25).

12.7 APPLICATIONS

Cotton is one of the oldest known natural fibers. According to Cotton Council International, cotton is a natural, renewable, biodegradable, and sustainable fiber. Some major applications of cotton fibers are shown in Figures 12.26 and 12.27. Cotton fabrics with specialty applications include, for example, fire-proof (flame-resistant) apparel, which is suitable for professional uses and provides effective protection against potential risks associated with high temperature and particularly flashover. Flame-resistant cotton fabrics are treated with chemicals.

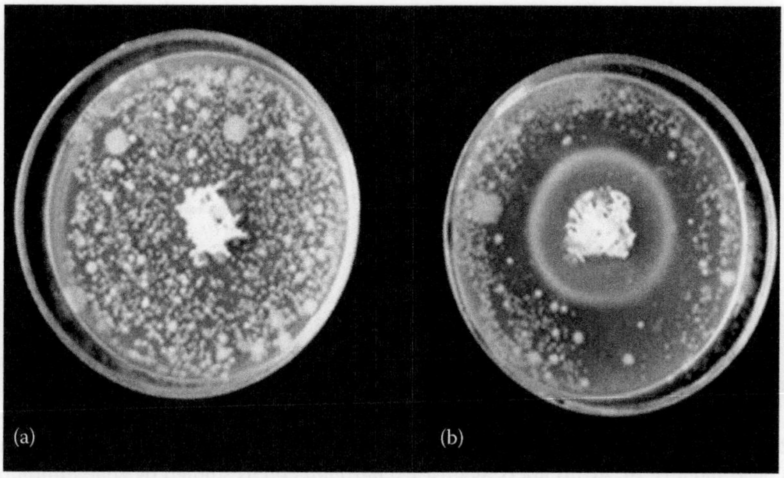

FIGURE 12.21 Photograph showing bacterial growth in the plates (a) containing plain fibers and (b) containing Zn(II)-loaded fibers. A clear zone of inhibition appears around the Zn(II)-loaded fibers in the plate shown in (b).

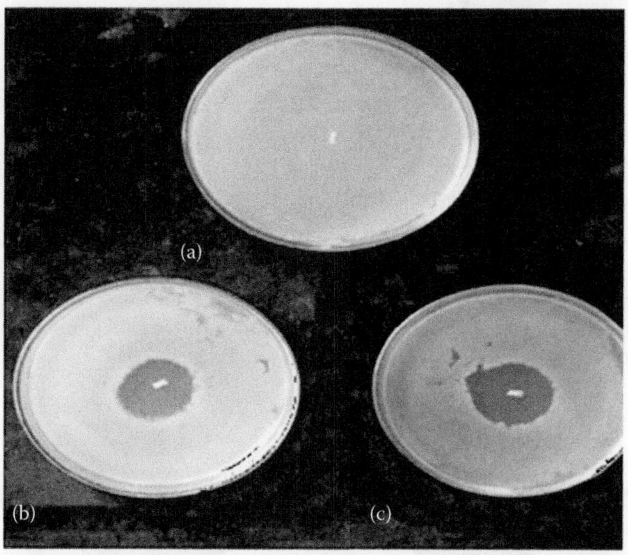

FIGURE 12.22 Antibacterial activity of drug-loaded grafted fibers: (a) plain fiber, (b) 2% drug-loaded fiber, and (c) 4% drug-loaded fiber.

Without chemical treatment, cotton would burn up releasing very strong heat, just like the major part of synthetic fibers, which melt when they are exposed to high temperatures. Cotton also finds specialty applications in medical and hygienic uses. Most notably, the fiber is used to manufacture hydrophilic cotton (cotton wool), compress, gauze bandages, tampons or sanitary towels, and cotton swabs. In this field, the most suitable cotton variety is the species *G. herbaceum* with short-staple thick fibers.

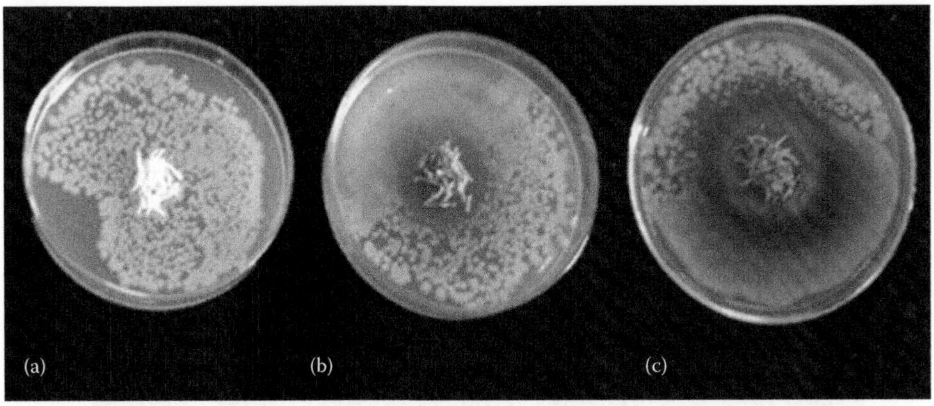

FIGURE 12.23 Biocidal action of (a) plain cellulose fibers, (b) chitosan-bounded copper-attached cotton fibers (CBCAC)(2), and (c) CBCAC(4) fibers against *Escherichia coli* as studied by zone inhibition method.

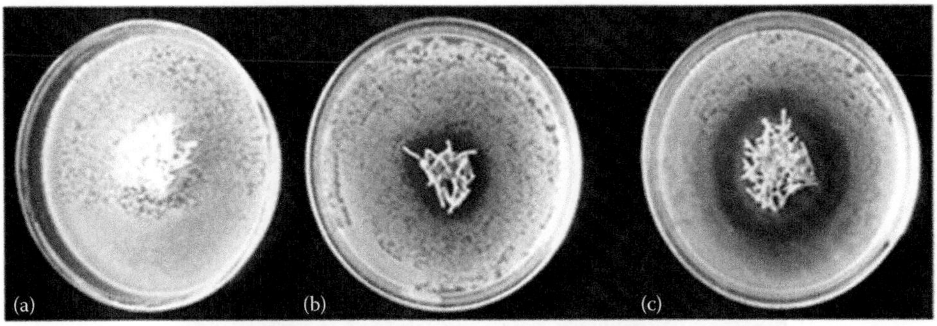

FIGURE 12.24 Biocidal action of (a) plain cotton fibers, (b) copper alginate-coated cotton CACC(2), and (c) CACC(4) fibers against *Escherichia coli* as studied by zone inhibition method (number in parenthesis denotes % copper solution used for loading onto alginate coated cotton fibers).

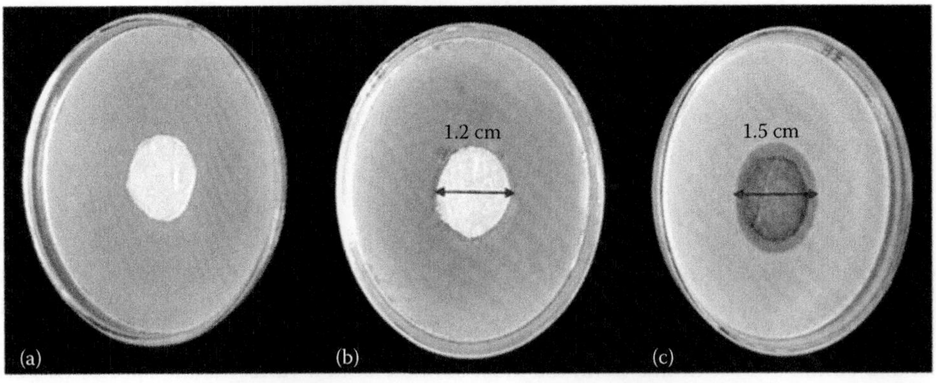

FIGURE 12.25 Photograph showing the inhibition zone of (a) plain cotton fabric disk, (b) chitosan attached cotton fabric disk, (c) nanosilver-loaded 1% chitosan-attached fabric disk.

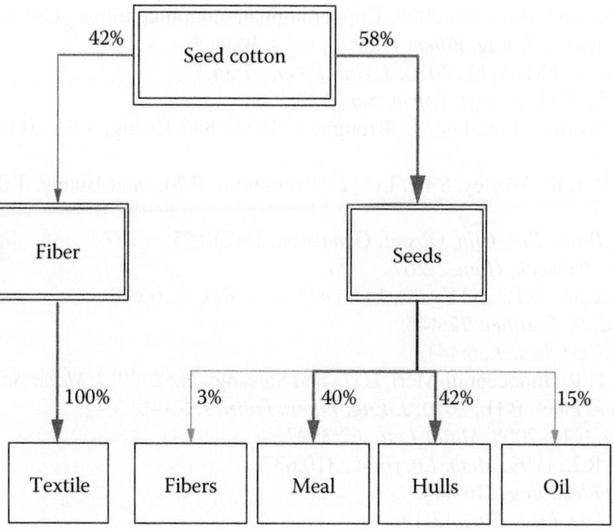

FIGURE 12.26 Products derived from cotton fiber.

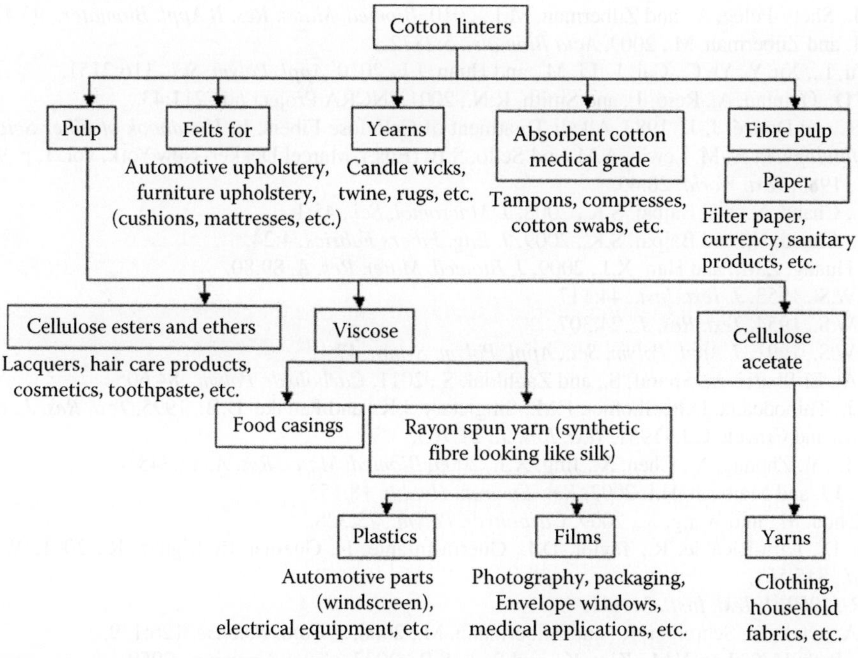

FIGURE 12.27 Application of cotton.

REFERENCES

Aboul-Fadl, S.M., Zeronian, S.H., Kamal, M.M., Kim, M.S., and Ellison, M.S., 1985, *Text. Res. J.*, 55:461–485.
Abrahams, D.H., 1994, *Am. Dyestuff Reptr.*, 83:78.
Ahmed, A.E.I., Hay, J.N., Bushell, M.E., Wardell, J.N., and Cavalli, G., 2008, *React. Funct. Polym.*, 68:248.
Alexander, E., Lewin, M., Musham, H.V., and Shiloh, M., 1956, *Text. Res. J.*, 26:606.
Babbett, J.D., 1943, *Can. J. Res.*, 20:143.
Bajpai, S.K., Bajpai, M., and Sharma, L., 2012, *J. Appl. Polym. Sci.*, 126:319.

Bajpai, S.K., Chand, N., and Mary, G., 2009, Copper alginate-cotton cellulose (CACC) fibers with excellent antibacterial properties. *J. Eng. Fibers Fabrics*, vol.4, Issue 3.
Bajpai, S.K., Chand, N., and Mary, G., 2010, *J. Nat. Fibers*, 7:34.
Bajpai, S.K. and Das, P., 2011, *J. Appl. Polym. Sci.*, 122:366.
Barnes, K., Liang, J., Worley, S.D., Lee, J., Broughton, R.M., and Huang, T.S., 2007, *J. Appl. Polym. Sci.*, 105:2306.
Barnes, G., Liang, J., Wu, R., Worley, S.D., Lee, J., Broughton, R.M., and Huang, T.S., 2006, *Biomaterials*, 27:4825.
Bilian, X., 2002, *Best. Pract. Res. Clin. Obstet. Gynaecol.*, 16(2):155.
Borbely, E., 2005, *Acta Polytech. Hung.*, 2:67.
Boylston, E.K., Thibodeaux, D.P., and Evans, J.P., 1993, *Text. Res. J.*, 60:80.
Bredereck, K., 1991, *Mell. Textilber.* 72:446.
Calkins, E.W.S., 1946, *Text. Res. J.*, 6:441.
Campos, G.N., Rawls, H.R., Innocentini-Meri, L.H., and Satsangi, N., 2009, *J. Mater Sci. Mater. Med.*, 20:537.
Chattopadhyay, D.P. and Patel, B.H., 2010, *J. Eng. Fibers Fabrics*, 5:1–6.
Chen, C.Y. and Chiang, C.L., 2008, *Mater Lett.*, 62:3607.
Cooney, J.J. and Tang, R.J., 1999, *Meth. Enzymol.*, 310:637.
Cooney, T.E., 1995, *Epidemiology*, 16:444.
Czajka, R., 2005, *Fib. Text. East. Eur.*, 13:13.
Daniela, L., Nicoletta, D., Luigia, S., Luisa, T., and Nicola, C., 2012, *Synthesis and antimicrobial activity of copper nano materials*, Springer, p. 85.
Danijela, K., Barbara, S., Brigita, T., and Franci, K., 2012, *Cellulose*, 19:1715.
El-Rafie, M.H., Mohamed, A.A., Shaheen, Th.I., and Hebeish, A., 2010, *Carbohydr. Polym.*, 80:779.
Elsner, J.J., Shefy-Peleg, A., and Zilberman, M.J., 2010, *Biomed. Mater. Res. B Appl. Biomater.*, 93:425.
Elsner, J.J. and Zilberman, M., 2009, *Acta Biomatr.*, 5:2872.
Fen, L., Yu, L., Xu, Y., Yi, C., Cai, J., Li, M., and Huan, J.J., 2010, *Appl. Polym. Sci.*, 116:2151.
Fraser, W.D., Quinlan, A., Reid, J., and Smith, R.N., 2001, INCRA Project no., 211:43.
Freytag, R. and Donzé, J.-J., 1983, Alkali Treatment of Cellulose Fibers. In *Handbook of Fiber Science and Technology*, Pt A, M. Lewin, A.M. and Sello, S.B. (Eds.), Marcel Dekker, New York, vol. 1, p. 93–165.
Ghosh, S., 1985, *Text. World*, 28:45.
Grace, M., Chand, N., and Bajpai, S.K., 2008, *J. Macromol. Sci.*, 45:1.
Grace, M., Chand, N., and Bajpai, S.K., 2009, *J. Eng. Fibers Fabrics*, 4:24.
He, C.L., Huang, Z.M., and Han, X.J., 2009, *J. Biomed. Mater. Res. A*, 89:80.
Hearle, J.W.S., 1953, *J. Text. Inst.*, 44:117.
Hearle, J.W.S., 1954, *Text. Res. J.*, 24:307.
Hearle, J.W.S., 1991, *J. Appl. Polym. Sci., Appl. Polym. Symp.*, 47:1.
Hebeish, A., El-Shafei, A., Sharaf, S., and Zaghloul, S., 2011, *Carbohydr. Polym.*, 84:605.
Hebert, J.J., Thibodeaux, D.P., Shofner, F.M., Singletary, J.K., and Patelke, D.B., 1995, *Text. Res. J.*, 65:440.
Hertel, K.L. and Craven, C.J., 1951, *Text. Res. J.*, 21:765.
Hong, Y., Li, Y., Zhuang, X., Chen, X., Jing, X.J., 2009, *Biomed. Mater. Res. A*, 89:345.
Hostynek, J.J. and Maibach, H.I. 2003, *Rev. Environ. Health*, 18:153.
Hou, A., Zhou, M., and Wang, X., 2009, *Carbohydr. Polym.*, 75;328.
Hubacher, D., Lara-Ricalde, R., Taylor, D.J., Guerra-Infante, F., Guzman-Rodriguez, R., 2001, *N. Engl. J. Med.*, 345:561.
Jeffries, R., 1960, *J. Text. Inst.*, 51:441.
Kraitzer, A., Ofek, L., Schreiber, R., and Zilbermann, M., 2008, *J. Cont. Release*, 126:139.
Lee, H.Y., Park, H.K., Lee, Y.M., Kim, K., and Park, S.B., 2007, *Chem. Commun.*, 2959.
Leonas, K.K., 1998, *Am. J. Infect. Cont.*, 26:495.
Lewin, M., Rau, R.O., and Sello, S.B., 1974, *Text. Res. J.*, 44:680.
Lewin, M. and Roldan, L.G., 1971, *J. Polym. Sci., Part C*, 36:213.
Lin, J., Cammarata, V., and Worley, S.D., 2001, *Polymer*, 42:7903.
Lord, E., 1956, *J. Text. Inst.*, 47:16.
Lord, E., 1961, *Manual of Cotton Spining, vol. II part - I - The Characteristics of Raw Cotton,* Textile Book Publishers, Inc., New York, vol. 1, p. 214.
Lord, E. and Heap, S.A., 1988, *Manchester*, England, U.K.
Lunenschloss, J., Gilhaus, K., and Hoffman, K., 1980, *Melli Textilber.*, 61:5.
Mercer, J., 1850, *British Patent*, 132:96.

Meredith, R., 1945, *J. Text. Inst.*, 36:107.
Meredith, R., 1946, *J. Text. Inst.*, 37:205.
Montalvo, J.G., Faught, S.E., Buco, S.M., and Saxton, A.M., 1987, *Appl. Spectrosc.*, 41:645.
Morton, W.E. and Hearle, J.W.S., 1976, *Physical Properties of Textile Fibres,* John Wiley & Sons, New York.
Perelshtein, I., Applerot, G., Perkas, N. et al. 2009, *Surf. Coat. Tech.*, 204:54–57.
Pierce, F.T. and Lord, E., 1939, *J. Text. Inst.*, 30:173.
Pim-on Rujitanaroj, Pimpha, N., and Supaphol, P., 2008, *Polymer*, 49:4723.
Qian, L. and Sun, G., 2003, *J. Appl. Polym. Sci.*, 89:2418.
Qian, L. and Sun, G., 2005, *Ind. Eng. Chem. Res.*, 44:852.
Qin, Y., 2008, *J. Appl. Polym. Sci.*, 107:993.
Raes, G.T.J. and Verschraege, L., 1981, *J. Text. Inst.*, 72:191.
Ravindra, S.Y., Murali, M., Narayana, R.N., Mohana Raju, K., 2010, *Colloids Surf. A Phys. Eng. Aspec.*, 367:31.
Ren, X., Kocer, H.B., Kou, L., Worley, S.D., Broughton, R., Tzou, Y.M., and Huang, T.S., 2008a, *J. Appl. Polym. Sci.*, 109:2756.
Ren, X., Kocer, H.B., Worley, S.D., Broughton, R.M., and Huang, T.S., 2009, *Carbohydr. Polym.*, 75:683.
Ren, X., Kou, L., Kocer, H.B., Zhu, C., Worley, S.D., Broughton, R.M., and Huang, T.S., 2008b, *Colloids Surf.*, 317:711.
Rigby, A.J., Anand, S.C., and Miraftab, M., 1993, *Textile Horizons*, 42.
Rujitanaroj, P., Pimpha, N., and Supaphol, P., 2008, *Polymer*, 49:4723.
Sarko, A., Young, R.A., and Rowell, R.M., eds., 1986, Cellulose: Structure and Distribution. In *Encyclopedia of Life Science,* John Wiley & Sons, New York, p. 29.
Schuerch, C., 1964, *For. Prod. J.*, 14:377.
Simovic, L., Skundric, P., Pajic-Lijakovic, I., Ristic, K., Medovic, A., Tasi, G., 2010, *J. Appl. Polym. Sci.*, 117:1424.
Smith, J.C., McCracken, F.L., Schiefer, H.F., and Stone, W.K., 1956, *Text. Res. J.*, 26:281.
Stevens, C.V. and Roldán-González, L.G., 1983, Liquid ammonia treatment of textiles. *Handbook of Fiber Science and Technology*, vol. 1, Pt Lewin, A.M. and Sello, S.B. (Eds.), Marcel Dekker, New York, pp. 167–203.
Stout, J.E., Lin, Y.S., Goetz, A.M., and Muder, R.R., 1998, *Infect. Cont. Hosp. Epidemiol.*, 19:911.
Sun, G., Chen, T.Y., Wheatley, W.B., and Worley, S.D., 1995, *J. Bioact. Compat. Polym.*, 10:135.
Sun, Y.Y. and Sun, G., 2002, *J. Appl. Polym. Sci.*, 84:1592.
Sun, Y.Y. and Sun, G., 2003, *J. Appl. Polym. Sci.*, 88:1032.
Taghizadeh, M.T. and Darvish, M.A., 2001, *Iranian Polym. J.*, 10:283.
Tao, T.X, Xin, H.Q, Zhang, Y.D, Chen, P.G, Wang, E.L, Wu, Z.C., 2008, *J. Funct. Mater.*, 39:148.
Teo, E.Y, Ong, S.Y., Chong, M.S, Zhang, Z.J, Lu, S., Moochala, B., Hoanal, S., and Teoh, H., 2011, *Biomaterials*, 32:279.
Thibodeaux, D.P. and Evans, J.P., 1986, *Text. Res. J.*, 56:130.
Thibodeaux, D.P. and Price, J.B., 1989, *Melli Textilber.*, 70:243.
Thomas, V., Bajpai, S.K., Mohan, Y.M., and Sreedhar, B., 2007, *J. Colloids. Interf. Sci.*, 315:389.
Vigo, T.L., 1994, *Textile Processing and Properties*, Elsevier, Amsterdam.
Walker, A.C. and Quell, M.H., 1933, *J. Text. Inst.*, 24:123.
Weatherwax, R.C., 1974, *J. Colloids Interf. Sci.*, 49:40.
Weber, D.J. and Rutala, W.H., 2001, *Disinfection, Sterilization, and Preservation*, 5:415.
Wenli, L. Jianjun, W., Hengxuan, C. et al. 2012, *J. Appl. Polym. Sci.*, 123:20.
Wiegand, C., Heinze, T., and Hipler, U.C. 2009, *Wound Repair Regen.*, 17:511.
Xing, X., Lu, D., Wang, X., and Liu, Z., 2009, *J. Macromol. Sci. Part A*, 46:560.
Xu, H., Shi, X., Ma, H.L., Zhang, Y., and Mao, L., 2011, *Appl. Surf. Sci.*, 257:6799.
Yin, R., Huang, Y., Huang, C., Tong, Y., and Tian, N., 2009, *Mater. Lett.*, 63:1335.
Zeronian, S.H., 1985, Ellis Horwood Ltd., Chichester, England and Halsted Press, New York, vol. 5, p. 138.
Zeronian, S.H. and Cabradilla, K.E., 1973, *J. Appl. Polym. Sci.*, 17:539.
Zeronian, S.H. and Kim, M.S., 1987, *International Dissolving and Specialty Pulps Conference,* TAPPI Press, Atlanta, GA, p. 125.
Zilberman, M., Golerkansky, E., Elsner, J.J, and Berdicevsky, I.J, 2009, *Biomed. Mater. Res. Part A*, 89:645.

13 Cellulose-Based Graft Copolymer for Toxic Ion and Organic Persistent Pollutants Removal

Iñaki Urruzola, Eduardo Robles, Luis Serrano, and Jalel Labidi

CONTENTS

13.1 INTRODUCTION

Chemical contamination of water by the presence of aromatic molecules from industrial wastes nowadays represents a topic of concern. Different processes are currently being used for the removal of pollutants from wastewater, such as biological treatments, membrane processes, or adsorption. Among all proposed treatments, adsorption using sorbents is one of the most commonly applied methods since it is an effective, efficient, and economical method for water decontamination. In the last few years, adsorption using activated carbon as adsorbent has been widely employed due to its large surface area. Nowadays, numerous studies have been performed to develop a cheaper and biodegradable adsorbent containing natural polymers (Alila and Boufi 2009a; Aloulou et al. 2004a; Boufi and Belgacem 2006; Jonker 2007).

The use of cellulose as adsorption support is not recent. Cellulose is one of the most important biopolymers that can be found in nature due to its natural character, biocompatibility, biodegradability, and low price. It is a polysaccharide composed exclusively of glucose molecules, is rigid, insoluble in water, and contains from several hundred to several thousand units of β-glucose. It is the most abundant organic biomolecules as it forms the bulk of terrestrial biomass (Bidlack et al. 1992; Fratzl 2003; Vincent 1999). In recent years, the study of cellulose has been increased due to its high availability; annual produce is about 100 million tons of cellulose in plants around the world (Delmer and Amor 1995), and this number is in constant rise as every year more countries tend to invest in annual plants as source of materials.

Cellulose has different applications in industry. One important aspect is the conversion of cellulose into ethanol for the productions of alternative biofuels, which have little environmental impacts (Annergren 1996). It is also used in the manufacture of explosives—the most famous is nitrocellulose—artificial silk, and varnish, and as thermal and acoustic insulators. The principal application of cellulose is the production of pulp and paper, using different bleached wood pulps obtained from different raw materials. Industrially, bleached cellulose pulp is obtained through two process stages, the pulping and bleaching. The objective of pulping is the removal of lignin to release cellulose fibers, and so separating cellulose from other components of wood by using mechanical or chemical processes. The most widely used pulping method in the world is the Kraft process. Moreover, the main reason for bleaching pulp is to remove the residual lignin content because lignin produces a brown coloration in the final paper. The bleaching is a chemical treatment performed usually in different stages and under different operating conditions. The main chemical reagents used are chlorine (Cl_2), chlorine dioxide (ClO_2), and hydrogen peroxide (H_2O_2).

The individualization of cellulose nanofibers from renewable sources has gained more attention in recent years because of their exceptional mechanical properties (high specific strength and modulus), large specific surface area, low coefficient of thermal expansion, high aspect ratio, environmental benefits, and low cost (Nishino et al. 2004). Suitable applications of cellulose nanofibers, such as reinforcement components in flexible display panels (Iwamoto et al. 2007) and oxygen-barrier layers (Fukuzumi et al. 2009) have been proposed as well. Cellulose nanofibers have shown considerable potential in several applications, including biomedical, bioimaging, nanocomposites, gas barrier films, and optically transparent functional materials. Chemical and mechanical treatments or combinations are used for the collection of cellulose nanofiber (Joonobi et al. 2009). Different series of chemical treatments using either acids or bases promote hydrolysis and improve the yield of glucose from hemicellulose or lignin during pretreatment (Serrano et al. 2011).

Mechanical treatments such as high-pressure homogenization and ultrasound techniques are used to reduce the size of the cellulose fibers to the nano size scale where the properties of the cells vary considerably (Chen et al. 2011; Lee et al. 2009).

The adsorption capacity of cellulose is an aspect that has attracted considerable interest in recent years (Alila et al. 2005; Bel-Hassen et al. 2008; Brochier et al. 2005). This is because of the possibility of removal of organic matter by adsorption onto waste materials at low cost (Aloulou et al. 2004a–c; Bras et al. 1999; Xu et al. 2007). Also, it has demonstrated the ability of cellulose to fix metal ions by adsorption (Al-Ghouti et al. 2010; Chakravarty et al. 2008; Gerente et al. 2000; Marshall and Campagne 1995). However, the characteristics of adsorption of native cellulose are not constant and vary depending on the origin of the cellulose and the preliminary treatments. Native cellulose has a relatively low adsorption capacity that can be increased by chemical functionalization of the fibers, where the adsorption capacity of modified cellulose fibers increases even 10 times than those without any treatment. This can be achieved by introducing chemical groups that exhibit a high affinity for chemical species in aqueous solution such as acrylamide and acrylic acid to adsorb water, chitin to adsorb heavy metals, or sorption of Cu^{2+} ions by cellulose graft copolymer (Chauhan and Lal 2003; Chauhan et al. 2000; Zhou et al. 2004). These modifications are made possible by the special structure of cellulose. The numerous studies on this subject (Aloulou et al. 2006; Alila et al. 2011; Boufi and Belgacem 2006) have shown that the retention capacity can reach 300–600 μmol/g substrate. However, to reach this relatively high level, it is necessary to increase the surface area beyond 300–500 m^2/g. To achieve this surface, used nanoparticles or microporous (50–100 nm) are relatively expensive. Different studies have shown that there are different factors that influence the adsorption capacity of cellulose. Two important factors are the hydrophobicity and their water solubility of organic solute, but they are not the only factors to take into account, but the hydrodynamic volume, the shape of the molecule, and the interaction potential between the adsorbent and adsorbate are also likely to play an important role (Alila and Boufi 2009a).

13.2 CELLULOSE SOURCES

In the present day, cellulose is extracted from different lignocellulosic biomass (Kennedy et al. 2000), wood has been the most common source for industrial cellulosic fibers, but recently the use of fiber crops has increased as the growing time is drastically reduced and the impact on deforestation is considerably lower compared to traditional silviculture. There are two main groups of wood in forestry that include nearly all the species: hardwood and softwood.

13.2.1 Woody Materials

For many years, fiber length has been a factor of critical importance in order to determine the quality of paper pulps; hardwoods provide shorter fibers, with a length between 0.75 and 1.5 mm. This is the reason why hardwood has been traditionally relegated from pulp and paper industry. However, in recent years, there has been an increasing tendency to use short fiber pulps because of the availability of forest resources, high derivative costs, and world demand for paper supplies (García Hortal 2007). Hardwoods are composed by fibers divided in two main categories: libriform and fiber tracheids (vascular and vasicentric). Libriform fibers are found in every species and are the main component. Unlike softwood fibers, hardwoods have a high content of nonfibrous components (vessels, vessel elements, and cell wall remains) that affect either paper manufacturing or final paper properties. Vessels are an important component of hardwoods as they represent the longitudinal conduction system of plants and are composed by individual cells connected vertically to form a continuous tubular vessel whose main function is the ascending water and nutrient conduction. Their length is between 0.4 and 0.8 mm reaching a maximum of 1.3 mm, and diameter is between 20 and 500 μm. Unlike fibers, vessels do not generate bonds; therefore, they do not contribute to the resistance of the paper, and this can be an inconvenience in elaborating printing paper. Even though hardwood has shorter fibers and for that reason has been relegated by softwoods for pulping, their low lignin content has attracted attention in recent years; also it has been proved that short fibers improve the printing properties of paper, which is the reason why this pulp is widely used for printing (Krzysik and Gonet 1954).

Probably, the most used hardwoods in the world are those of eucalyptus family; this includes blue gum (*Eucalyptus globulus*), river red gum (*Eucalyptus camaldulensis*), and Sydney blue gum (*Eucalyptus saligna*). Eucalyptus species pulps are hardwoods commonly called deciduous or broadleaf (García Hortal 2007). There are almost 700 species in the *Eucalyptus* species distributed all over the world and are used widely because of their fast growth in the pulp and paper industry, wood industry, or for chemical purposes. Other hardwoods used in pulping include birches (*Betula papyrifera*), aspen (*Populus tremula*), and acacia (*Acacia mangium*), which are also widely used (Doran and Turnbull 1997). The availability of the raw material and the climatic conditions in the case of arboriculture are important factors that determine the species used for pulping.

Softwood has longer fibers that provide better tensile strength (Horn 1974); it also improves the performance of paper during its manufacturing. In northern countries like Norway and Canada, which have tough climatic conditions, the use of softwood as raw materials for pulping is mainly focused in softwoods as there are great extensions of slash pine (*Pinus elliottii*) forests and spruces such as black spruce (*Picea mariana*), and Norwegian spruce (*Picea abies*) (Li et al. 2011).

13.2.2 Nonwood

Concerns on sustainability have let to the industrial use of crop fibers or agricultural residues as a complement or even as a substitute for conventional pulping wood. Traditionally, the use of non-wood fibers has been a practice in countries with limited access to wood supply and was used as the last resource as the quality of the obtained fibers was not as good as that of wood (Sabharwal and Young 1996). However, the environmental concerns have increased in developed countries, and disposal of agricultural by-products has become an issue of greater interest among producers; recent researches have focused in enhancing properties of crop fibers to make them more competitive with wood pulp (Finell et al. 2000). Advantages from nonwood pulp and paper industry include little strain in ecological balance as they are based on fast-growing renewable raw materials that are abundant; this also ensures the availability of the fiber, either crop fibers or agricultural residues. The sales of agricultural residues also provide to the farmers additional income that increases the value of the crop, and at last, the localization of mills near the agricultural exploitations can reduce the cost of raw material transport thus making the pulp economically competitive (Judt 1991).

Fiber-dedicated crops are grown mostly for fabrics or paper manufacturing: plant fibers may include hairs such as cotton (*Gossypium hirsutum*), fiber-sheafs or dicotylic plants or vessel sheafs, or monocotylic plants such as bast fibers, that is, kenaf (*Hibiscus cannabinus*), flax (*Linum usitatissimum*), hemp (*Cannabis sativa*), and ramie (*Boehmeria nivea*), and there are also hard fibers as sisal (*Agave sisalana*) and henequen (*Agave fourcroydes*) among others (Bledzki and Gassan 1999). Kenaf is one of the most promising fiber crops; for many years, it has been used as fiber source for ropes and sacks, but recently, it has been considered as a reinforcing agent for composites. Therefore, it has reached the target of many governments from Southeast Asian countries, as Malaysia, to develop new applications. Also, hemp and sisal have proved their performance as pulping raw materials; sisal is a leaf plant native to Mexico, although the main producers are Brazil and Tanzania. Sisal as henequen or blue agave is a slow-growing plant, and usually 4–6 years are needed before the first harvesting (Gutierrez et al. 2008).

On the other hand, agricultural residues, also called harvesting residues or agricultural by-products (Hunter 2007), are either materials left in an agricultural exploitation after the crop has been harvested as the case of sugarcane (*Saccharum officinarum*) and blue agave (*Agave tequilana*) bagasse, or waste left after agricultural products have been processed into a usable product as coconut (*Cocos nucifera*) husk or almond (*Prunus dulcis*) shell. This kind of products are characterized by their low price as the growing cost is already absorbed by the main purpose industry, the relatively cheap harvesting costs, especially in the case of industrial residues, as they already are in factories and the medium-high quality of the obtained pulp (Wong and Chiu 1995). Besides, the use of harvesting residues in the elaboration of pulp and paper products averts the need of disposal from these products in the large European and American exploitations, which currently represent an

TABLE 13.1
Composition of the Different Raw Materials

Type of Fiber	Cellulose (%)	Lignin (%)	Hemicellulose (%)	Ash (%)
Aspen	52.1	21.4	20.6	0.4
Acacia	46.5	27.1	24.4	0.22
Birch	45	18	33	0.3
Slash pine	46	27	18	0.2
Spruce (heartwood)	45.5	28.3	25.7	—
Kenaf	58	17.5	22	2.4
Flax	64.1	2.0	16.7	—
Sisal	65.8	9.9	12	—
Hemp	60.09	12.36	23.83	3.16
Ramie	68.6	0.6	13.1	—
Cotton	82.7	—	5.7	—
Sugarcane bagasse	54.3	24.3	16.8	1.1
Blue agave bagasse	64.8	15.9	5.1	2
Coconut husk	44.2	32.8	12.1	2.2

environmental issue as pollution and fires are a constant risk when disposing of this kind of materials (Alcaide et al. 1991). Sugarcane bagasse is one of the most promising agricultural fibers used for pulping as it is easily accessible and available in several locations, especially in regions where lack of wood represents a challenge for pulping industry; after the cane processing through roller mills to extract sugar juice, bagasse is usually burned in sugar-mill boilers (Siqueira et al. 2010). Coir or coconut husk is characterized for its toughness and durability due to high lignin content; huge quantities of coconut palm residues are burned, but recent works have focused in finding a further use for its less used components, such as coir or other fibrous parts (Maheswari et al. 2012).

Table 13.1 shows some of the most used raw materials for cellulose obtention with their respective composition (Bertaud and Holmbom 2004; Bledzki and Gassan 1999; Iñiguez-Covarrubias et al. 2001; Jonoobi et al. 2011; Kopania et al. 2012; Livca et al. 2012; Maheswari et al. 2012; Pettersen 1984; Pinto et al. 2005; Siqueira et al. 2010; Malinen et al. 2006).

13.2.3 Pulping

Cellulose fibers are often cemented inside the middle layer—composed mainly by lignin—so for its isolation, there are two main processes for pulping, consisting of chemical and mechanical pulping (Casey 1980), but usually for papermaking, both types of pulp are used, and even a considerable percent of recycled fiber can be added to the pulp. The type of pulp is always selected depending on the further use of paper.

Mechanical processes include wood logs being processed with a millstone or chopped up to splinters with a disk mill; in these processes, the original structural components of wood remain in the pulp, thus giving an efficiency of 95% (García Hortal 2007). Mechanical pulp produces papers with high lignin content, thus being very rigid, which limits the bond capacity of the pulp. On the other hand, they are sensitive to optical aging (high tendency to yellow pigmentation because of exposure to light as a consequence of residual lignin, and other pulp components, being oxidized). However mechanical pulp has long fibers with good aspect ratio, and is easy to print in, that is why it is widely used in the newspaper industry as the main resource for papermaking. It can also be used as a blend with chemical pulping, that can be obtained from a very wide varieties of treatments (Ragauskas 1994). During chemical pulping, lignin modification occurs by the action of chemical agents under alkali or acid conditions. Nowadays the most used method is Kraft pulping (sodium hydroxide and sodium sulphur) that allows the removal of a high amount of lignin, the residual quantities and chromophores remaining can be eliminated with bleaching processes, thus giving very white pulps with high mechanical resistance. Legal environmental pressure has forced pulp and paper industry to find delignification methods that are less aggressive to the environment than those using high-impact pollutants (Kordsachia et al. 1992). Therefore, many studies have been made to minimize pollutant impacts of the pulp and paper industry on the environment and to improve the efficiency of its processes by recovering the highest percent of the original lignocellulosic components for their further employment. These methods are called organosolv or solvent cooking, where solvents are used along with biomass in high-temperature cooking operations (Sundquist et al. 1998). Most used solvents are methanol, ethanol, acetic acid, and formic acid, along with phenols, amines, glycols, nitrobenzene, dioxane, dimethylsulfoxide, sulfolene, and carbon dioxide, or different blend combinations of the previous solvents of them with water (Hergert 1992). Among these methods, the most used are ethanol and methanol as they are easy to obtain and have a considerably low price (Akgul and Kirci 2009). While large-scale commercial viability had been demonstrated decades ago from a technical and operational perspective, organosolv extraction has not, to date, been widely adopted.

Another types of methods less harmful for the environment based on biotechnology can contribute to plant biomass deconstruction by providing biocatalysts being able to degrade or modify lignin using enzymatic mechanisms have been studied in recent years (Ruiz-Dueñas and Martinez 2009). A large number of microbials have been studied in order to determine their potential use in enzymatic bio-refinery processes: *P. chrysosporium* is a fungus of growing interest. It is a basidiomycete that is involved in lignin biodegradation, and it provides a low redox-potential peroxidase (Kersten and Cullen 2007). Other enzymes used are *Pleurotus ostreatus* and *Ceriporiopsis subvermispora*, two white-rot fungi secreting ligninolytic enzymes (Martinez et al. 2005). Until now, laccases and peroxidases stemming from nature are not well suited for industrial use as substrate specifications and application conditions are required to ensure repeatability (Ayala et al. 2008). Lignin-degrading oxidoreductases, including laccases and oxidases, are enzymes of industrial interest in bio-refineries for cell wall delignification in cellulose and ethanol production, functionalization of fibers, and modification of lignins and other aromatic compounds (Jonsson 2007; Palonen and Viikari 2004; Widsten and Kandelbauer 2008).

13.2.4 Bleaching

To obtain paper for writing quality, residual lignin elimination is essential from the chemical pulps via a bleaching process; the main objective of this stage is to increase the whiteness of the pulp either with elimination or modification of residual lignin and its degradation products (Fengel and Wegener 1984). Diatomic chlorine (Cl_2) is the main oxidizing agent used for bleaching, but the liberation of chlorophenol and other organochlorides in the process effluents and the recent environmental legislation have restricted its use. For these reasons diatomic chlorine was substituted by chlorine dioxide in denominated elemental chlorine free (ECF) (Valchev et al. 1999). Continuous technological advances in this area have contributed to the elimination of chlorine and its derivatives in the bleaching stages known as totally chlorine free (TCF), process that reduces the organochlorinated compounds to acceptable levels according to environmental legislation (Ragnar et al. 2004; Roncero and Vidal 2007; Yadav et al. 2006). Bleaching sequences include the use of oxygen (O), ozone (Z) (Torres et al. 2004), and hydrogen peroxide (P), and the introduction of biotechnological enzymes (treatments) such as xylanase (Kuligowski et al. 2006; Roncero et al. 2003; Valls 2008) and oxidoreductase (Ibarra et al. 2006; Sigoillot et al. 2005; You et al. 2008), have great advantages in bleaching as they reduce toxicity of the effluents and diminish the consumption of chemical agents. Enzymatic treatments are potentially more selective for lignin elimination (Fillat 2008; Moldes and Vidal 2008).

In chemical pulping processes—pulping and bleaching operations—it is of main interest to preserve the resistance of the fibers in order to avoid the formation of weaknesses in paper. The best conditions for further paper production are obtained when lignin is eliminated, but high amounts of hemicelluloses are retained. To impulse the capacity of interfibrillar bonding and optimizing their contribution to physical and mechanical properties of the paper, a "refining" stage is included as the final resistance of the paper not only depends on the individual resistance of the fibers but also on the linking between them.

13.2.5 Cellulose Nanofibers

Cellulose nanofibers are obtained from cellulosic materials with the use of mechanical treatments in order to increase the surface area of the fibers. Their diameter range is between 2 and 10 nm and a length of several micrometers. Various mechanical treatments have been used to extract nanofibers from cellulose fibers, depending on the properties desired for the obtained nanofibers. These treatments can be classified in three main families, depending of the device used for their obtaining: homogenization systems which may also include the microfluidization, ultrasonic systems and grinding devices (Alemdar and Sain 2008). Grinder devices involve the breakdown of the cell wall structure because of the shearing forces generated by two grinding stones in counter-rotation. The pulp is passed between a static grinding stone and a rotating grinding stone at about 1500 rpm. Other grinding devices may include the ZETA RS agitator bed mill by Netzsch GmbH. The mill is equipped with a grinding media separator, which ensures separation of grinding media from the suspension by centrifugal forces (Mende 2011). Missoum et al. (2013) sum up also the different pre–post treatments applied to different cellulosic fibers to obtain nanofibrillar cellulose (NFC) using a grinder device. To submit cellulose fibers to homogenization, strong mechanical shearing combined with high pressure is used to enhance the fibrillation of fibers. In most of the current homogenizing equipments, fibers enter a small-diameter orifice at high pressure and low velocity. The pressure is then increased by a pneumatic valve shaft, closing the adjustable gap between the impact head and the passage head. Homogenizing effect is produced when the product entering the valve inlet at a high pressure passes through the minute gap causing a velocity increases while the pressure rapidly decreases to atmospheric pressure. Homogenized product impinges on the impact ring and exits at a sufficient pressure for moving to the next processing stage. The ensuing fibrillated fibers are cooled at room temperature. Several passes are needed before obtaining a stable gel (Lavoine et al. 2012). For ultrasonic mechanical treatment, ultrasonic energy is transferred to cellulose chains through a process called cavitation; this refers to the forming, growing, and violent collapse of cavitations in water. Energy provided by cavitation is approximately 10–100 kJ/mol, which is within the energy scale of hydrogen bonds. Therefore, ultrasound impacts can disintegrate cellulose fibers, reducing their size up to nanoscale.

13.2.6 Cellulose Nanowhiskers

Whiskers are fibers that have been grown under controlled conditions that lead to the formation of high-purity single crystals. The resultant highly ordered structure produces, among other properties, unusual high strengths (Milewski et al. 1994). The isolation of these crystals that are surrounded by paracrystalline or amorphous regions containing both cellulose and other polysaccharides can be achieved with a controlled chemical pretreatment to destroy the molecular bonds whereby microcrystals are hinged together in a network structure followed by mechanical treatments to disperse the crystal in a water colloidal solution (Battista and Smith 1962; Lynd et al. 2002). Aqueous suspensions of cellulose crystallites can be prepared by acid hydrolysis of cellulose, a treatment consisting of the disruption of amorphous regions surrounding and embedded within cellulose microfibrils while leaving the microcrystalline segments intact (Schroeder et al. 1985). The characteristics of the raw material, along with the treatment conditions such as time, temperature, and purity, determine the morphology and properties of the final whisker (Dong et al. 1998). For this purpose, different solutions are used to break the amorphous part of the cellulose; most common are sulfuric acid and hydrochloric acid. However, as $H_2SO_4^-$ prepared whiskers present negative charged surface due to the presence of sulfuric ester groups in the surface of microcrystals that leads to a more stable whisker aqueous suspension than the whiskers prepared with HCl that are not charged (Araki et al. 1998). Therefore, whiskers prepared with HCl need further treatments to achieve a stable suspension, as can be oxidation of the surface or sulfation (Araki et al. 1999; Saito et al. 2007).

13.3 NANOCELLULOSE SURFACE MODIFICATIONS

The interest in obtaining cellulose nanofibers has increased in the last few decades due to the unique characteristics they endow as can be: high surface-area-to-volume ratio, high surface area, high Young's modulus, high tensile strength, and low coefficient of thermal expansion (Nishino et al. 2004). Recent researches have shown the great potential of cellulose nanofibers in several applications, including biomedical, bioimaging, nanocomposite reinforcement, gas barrier films, and optically transparent functional materials. Cellulose nanofibers cannot be dispersed uniformly in most nonpolar solvents due to their hydrophilic nature. When dispersed in very low concentrations, a structure similar to a gel is obtained, and when it is dried, aggregates or films can be obtained. Consequently, the modification of nanofibers prior to their further use is of high interest in order to limit this phenomenon and open new applications. Despite the existence of many proposed methods for cellulose surface modification, including a recent review on the functionalization of cellulose nanocrystals (Lin et al. 2012), reports on the surface modification of nanocellulose fibers are very limited in number. The adsorption capacity of nanocellulose is an aspect that has attracted considerable interest in recent years (Alila et al. 2005; Bel-Hassen et al. 2008; Brochier et al. 2005). Native cellulose has a relatively low adsorption capacity, but this can be increased by chemical functionalization of the fibers. The potential of the adsorption capacity of modified nanocellulose fibers suggests an increment of even 10 times than that of the same fibers without any treatments. These modifications are possible because of the particular structure of nanocellulose. The surface of cellulose nanoparticles can be modified by various methods: on the one hand by the use of chemical methods to produce covalent bonds between cellulosic substrates and the grafting agent, and on the other hand by physical interaction or adsorption on the surface of molecules or macromolecules.

Since the chemical composition of the surface of the nanofibers depends, in first place, on the process used for their production, several approaches to decrease the energy consumption in the fibrillation have been proposed. For example, TEMPO oxidation of cellulose introduces carboxylic acid groups on the surface of the fibrillated cellulose. Moreover, carboxymethylation has also been used as a pretreatment prior to mechanical defibrillation (Wagberg et al. 2008) and also to induce chemical modification of the surface. All this is related to nanoscale dimensions of the nanocellulose as it exhibits high surface area, usually of about 50–70 m^2/g, which greatly increases the amount of hydroxyl groups available in the surface for its modification and change in the classical grafting conditions. The esterification is a reaction that introduces an ester functionality (O–C=O) on the surface of cellulose by condensation of the cellulose with a reactive alcohol group. This esterification process has a positive effect on the surface hydrophobicity of cellulose by using carboxylic acid, acid anhydrides, or acid chlorides as reactants. The main objective of this strategy is to maintain the nanofibrillar structure of nanocellulose, while the grafting of functional groups is performed only on the surface of the nanofibers. On the other hand, there are different studies that have shown the presence of many factors that influence the adsorption capacity of cellulose. Two main factors are the hydrophobicity and the water solubility of organic solutes; therefore, the esterification as it increases hydrophobicity provides higher retention capacity, allowing the organic compounds to be absorbed within cellulose fibers. Still, they are not the only factors to take into account as the hydrodynamic volume, the shape of the molecule, and the interaction potential between the adsorbent and adsorbate, are likely to play an important role (Alila et al. 2009b).

In order to maintain the structure and properties, esterification reaction mechanism needs a non-swelling medium due to the heterogeneousness of this kind of reactions. In this case, as the reaction occurs only on the cellulose chains located on the surface of the nanoparticles, the limitation on the extent of grafting resides in the susceptibility and accessibility of the surface, which can produce several grades of modified materials with different degrees of substitution (DSs). For example, in a research published by Boufi (Boufi and Belgacem 2006), commercial microcrystalline cellulose was grafted with aliphatic anhydrides having C6, C8, C12, and C16 chain length using a heterogeneous solvent exchange acylation procedure. In this case, the evolution of the acylation degree is presented as a function of the catalyst and the amount of triethylamine percent, which is related to the degree of substitution; therefore, a greater DS implies a higher acylation degree. This considerably influences the adsorption capacity of the fibers, with the adsorption capacity of the fibers increasing with the same anhydride when the DS is higher. The same conclusion was also reported in other works, where in addition to the solvent, it also influences the reaction time (Freire et al. 2006; Tome et al. 2010). When adsorption capacity of the modified cellulose fibers used in the work of Boufi with different aliphatic anhydrides is analyzed, it can be observed that the adsorption equilibrium is amplified with increased acyl chain length, namely, about 2, 3, 4, and 6 h for Cell-C6, Cell-C12, Cell-C16, and Cell-C18, respectively. The relatively long adsorption time indicates that the mechanism is based on the slow diffusion of the organic solute molecule inside the microporous structure of the fibers. This assumption is corroborated by the high expansion capacity of the modified fibers when they are immersed into water. The driving force of the adsorption process is expected to be largely by the van der Waals interactions between the grafted chains and the organic solute. Therefore, any magnification of these interactions contributes to an improvement in the adsorption capacity. In particular, the planar structure of the aromatic organic solutes studied tends to favor the intercalation of molecules within the domain formed by the grafted chains. This may account for the significant improvement in adsorption capacity after grafting of linear alkyl chains on the surface of the fibers.

In other works, this modification method for cellulose fibers by using anhydrides has been modified with the purpose of saving time and enhancing the treatment performance by eliminating the synthesis of the acid anhydride stage. In the recent work of Urruzola, it has been observed that after the fiber and solvent dehydration by azeotropic distillation with a Dean–Stark distiller, the corresponding fatty acid with catalyst and a desiccant agent can be introduced in the same stage, where similar results can be obtained by saving a stage in the esterification process (Urruzola et al. 2013a,b). The adsorption capacity of the fibers studied by Fadhel Aloulou (Aloulou et al. 2006) obtained by the modification of commercial microcrystalline cellulose with previously prepared octanoic anhydrid, were compared with fibers prepared by Urruzola (Urruzola et al. 2013a), where octanoic acid was used in a one-stage modification of commercial microcrystalline cellulose. It can be observed that in both cases, the retention capacity is comparable. Fibers modified with a two-stage process can adsorb a maximum of 250 μmol/g of benzene, while fibers modified with a one-stage process can retain up to 400 μmol/g of benzene.

Another aspect to consider when performing a modification is the size of the cellulose fibers. Previous works (Urruzola et al. 2013b) show how the most complete esterification can be obtained when cellulose nanofibers are used. This is caused because nanocellulose exhibits high surface area, usually of about 50–70 m^2/g, which widely increases the amount of surface hydroxyl groups available for modification of the surface and change of the classical grafting conditions. This is well demonstrated by the contact angle technique, which allows seeing how hydrophobicity of modified nanocellulose is increased reaching values near 100°. This is the reason why modified cellulose nanofibers have considerable adsorption capacity. Focusing on the elimination of herbicides from water, another kind of esterification has been performed, like those studied by Sabrine Alila (Alila and Boufi 2009a, Alila et al. 2009b). In this work, different modified cellulose fibers were prepared, and their efficiency as adsorbent for the removal of several aromatic organic compounds and three herbicides, that is, Alachlor (ACH), Linuron (LNR), and Atrazine (ATR), was investigated. For this purpose, the modification was carried out under heterogeneous conditions using *N,N′*-carbonyldiimidazole (CDI) as an activator and different amino derivatives as grafting agent. The particularity of CDI is its ability to react with alcohol, carboxylic acid, and amine groups giving rise to reactive carbonyl imidazole intermediates that are more easily handled and may be isolated, if necessary. The ensuing carbonyl imidazole could subsequently undergo selective reactions with primary amines or primary alcohols to form amide, carbonate, or ester derivative (Rannard and Davis 1999, 2000). The advantages of this method include mild reaction conditions that minimize secondary reaction, the lack of formation of amine hydrochloride when using acid chlorides, and the avoidance of lengthy purification stages. Moreover, imidazole, the by-product obtained both when CDI reacts with hydroxyl and carboxylic acid and after the reaction of carbonyl imidazole with alcohol or amine, is easily removed from the reaction mixture by an acidic wash. These advantages, coupled with the relatively low cost of CDI, render this method an attractive alternative to the carbodiimide-based reagents such as *N,N*-dicyclohexylcarbodiimide (Samaranayake and Glasser 1993) or acid chloride. By varying the structure of the amino derivative and the reaction sequence, different organic structures bearing diverse functional groups were generated on the surface. In this case, longer chains up to 24 carbons can be obtained. These chains positively influence the adsorption capacity, where adsorption values of up to 730 μmol/g of fiber for Linuron (LNR) herbicide or 456 μmol/g of fiber fort the Alachlor (ACH) herbicide could be achieved.

TABLE 13.2
Adsorption Capacities of Modified Nanofibers

Fiber	Modification	Contaminant	Maximum Adsorption (μmol/g)	Reference
Technocel-150DM	Esterification with aliphatic anhydrides having C6, C8, C12, and C16 chain length	Organic solutes	Trichlorobenzene (470)	Boufi and Belgacem (2006)
Jute/Avicel	Esterification with palmitic acid	Organic solutes	Toluene (580)	Urruzola et al. (2013a)
Bleached eucalyptus pulp	Esterification with palmitic acid	Organic solutes	Trichlorobenzene (610)	Urruzola et al. (2013b)
Technocel-150DM	Esterification with octanoic anhydride	Organic solute	Quinoline (313)	Aloulou et al. (2006)
Bleached soda pulp	Esterification with differing-length hydrocarbon chains bearing amino terminal functionalities	Organic solutes and herbicides	Linuron (LNR) (730)	Alila and Boufi (2009a)
Microfibrillated cellulose	Modification with succinic anhydride under pyridine reflux	Heavy metals	Cd (720)	Hokkanen et al. (2013)
Commercial cellulose	Precipitation of cellulose in the presence of Fe(II)/Fe(III) mixture	Heavy metals	Hg (2000)	Donia et al. (2008)

Table 13.2 summarizes the most relevant modification method and obtained adsorption capacities.

In recent years, the investigation of water polluted with heavy metals has become an essential focus of environmental scientists. The heavy metals in water could be derived not only from natural sources like volcanoes, weathering, and erosion of bedrocks and ore deposits but also from numerous anthropogenic activities, such as mining, industries, wastewater irrigation, and agriculture activities (Huang et al. 2008, 2009; Muhammad et al. 2011). Adsorption has demonstrated to be one of the most efficient and technically feasible methods for the metal removal from aqueous solutions. In this perspective, Hokkanen et al. (2013) describe the preparation and evaluation of mercerized and succinic anhydride–modified micro/nano cellulose to adsorb Zn(II), Ni(II), Cu(II), Co(II), and Cd(II) ions in aqueous solutions. For this purpose, mercerized cellulose was reacted with succinic anhydride under pyridine reflux. The modified cellulose was centrifuged and washed. In order to liberate carboxylate functions for a better chelating function than the carboxylic group, succinylated cellulose was treated with a saturated sodium bicarbonate solution. The removal of metal ions from aqueous solutions by adsorption depends on the pH of the solution since acidity of the solution affects the ionization of the metal ions and concentration of the counter H^+ ions of the surface groups. To maximize the removal of heavy metals by the adsorbents, knowledge of an optimum pH is important. The adsorption capacities of metals on modified nanocellulose increased while increasing the pH. When the pH values were lower to 3, the concentration of protons competing with metal ions for the active sites was higher (Iqbal et al. 2009). The adsorbent surface was positively charged, and metal ions with positive charge had difficulties to approach the functional groups due to electrostatic repulsion. Thus, adsorption capacities were found to be lower at lower pH values. With increasing pH above 3, the concentration of protons decreased, and the adsorbent surface charge became negative when electrostatic attraction increased between the metal ions and the adsorbent. The maximum adsorption of metals occurred at a pH range from 3 to 7. Analyzing the adsorption capacity of these modified fibers, it can be observed that the maximum metal retention capacity ranged from 0.72 to 1.95 mmol/g, which followed the order of Cd > Cu > Zn > Co > Ni. Another totally different method, but with the same focus on eliminating heavy metals from water, is the one performed by Donia et al. (2008), where a nanomagnetic cellulose hybrid was obtained from the precipitation of cellulose in the presence of Fe(II)/Fe(III) mixture. The hybrid material obtained was then functionalized with amino group through successive treatments by glycidyl methacrylate and tetraethylenepentamine.

For this purpose, dissolution of cellulose was carried out dispersing 4 g of cellulose into a pre-cooled solution of distilled water, NaOH, and urea (Cai et al. 2008). Next, preparation of regenerated magnetic cellulose was carried out dissolving in aqueous solution of ferrous sulfate and ferric chloride. Then, magnetic cellulose was grafted by GMA-polymer as reported by Dahou; magnetic cellulose was dispersed in distilled water, and GMA was added, stirred, and followed by the addition of CAN solution (Dahou et al. 2010). Finally, the immobilization of grafted magnetic cellulose was elaborated with tetraethylenepentamine. The modified magnetic cellulose obtained in the earlier step was loaded by tetraethylenepentamine as follows: grafted magnetic cellulose was suspended in amine and dissolved in DMF; the product obtained was referred as MCGT. In this case, the maximum uptake was observed at pH 5.4 and 6.3 for Cu(II) and Ag(I), respectively (Donia et al. 2008). The conclusion of this study shows that the retention capacity was found to be 2, 1.5, and 1.2 mmol/g for Hg(II), Cu(II), and Ag(I), respectively. On the other hand, the adsorption reaction has fast kinetics and follows the pseudo-second-order model. The equilibrium of adsorption as a function of time was achieved within 3–5 min. Thermodynamic parameters obtained indicates that the adsorption process is spontaneous with exothermic nature. The MCGT obtained has excellent durability and can be easily separated and regenerated from adsorption medium by an external magnetic field. The MCGT was also applied for a real sample of industrial wastewater and displayed high removal efficiency. These characteristics make the prepared nanomagnetic cellulose promising in the field of wastewater treatment.

13.4 CONCLUSIONS

For many years, chemical modification of substrates has emerged as a new technique to produce adsorbents with high chemical pollutant adsorption capacity in aqueous solution. The use of cellulose as adsorption support is not new as it is one of the most important biopolymers that can be found in nature. In recent years, many works have been developed in different levels from the ranked structure of cellulose. One of its most promising derivates is, without any doubt, cellulose nanofibers. Cellulose nanofibers due to of their exceptional mechanical properties are being used in numerous applications such as paper reinforcement and nanocomposite elaboration, and in adsorption processes. Adsorption properties of the cellulose can be highly increased by chemical modification of the surface of the fiber by the introduction of chemical groups that exhibit strong affinity toward certain chemical compounds in aqueous solution. Due to the abundance of cellulose, its excellent adsorption properties, low regenerating costs, and possibility of reuse can be considered as a future alternative for the elimination of pollutants present in aqueous media.

REFERENCES

Akgul, M. and Kirci, H. 2009. An environmentally friendly organosolv (ethanol-water) pulping of poplar wood. *Journal of Environmental Biology* 30:735–740.

Alcaide, L.J., Baldovin, F.L., and Parra, I.S. 1991. Characterization of cellulose pulp from agricultural residues. *TAPPI* 74:217–221.

Alemdar, A. and Sain, M. 2008. Isolation and characterization of nanofibers from agricultural residues—Wheat straw and soy hulls. *Bioresource Technology* 99(6):1664–1671.

Al-Ghouti, M.A., Li, J., Salamh, Y., Al-Laqtah, N., Walker, G., and Ahmad, N.M. 2010. Adsorption mechanisms of removing heavy metals and dyes from aqueous solution using date pits solid adsorbent. *Journal of Hazardous Materials* 176:510–520.

Alila, S., Aloulou, F., Thielemans, W., and Boufi, S. 2011. Sorption potential of modified nanocrystals for the removal of aromatic organic pollutant from aqueous solution. *Industrial Crops and Products* 33:350–357.

Alila, S. and Boufi, S. 2009a. Removal of organic pollutants from water by modified cellulose fibres. *Industrial Crops and Products* 30:93–104.

Alila, S., Boufi, S., Belgacem, M.N., and Beneventi, D. 2005. Adsorption of a cationic surfactant onto cellulosic fibers I. Surface charge effects. *Langmuir* 21:8106–8113.

Alila, S., Ferraria, A.M., Botelho do Rego, A.M., and Boufi, S. 2009b. Controlled surface modification of cellulose fibers by amino derivatives using N,N′-carbonyldiimidazole as activator. *Carbohydrate Polymers* 77:553–562.

Aloulou, F., Boufi, S., Belgacem, N., and Gandini, A. 2004a. Adsorption of cationic surfactants and subsequent adsolubilization of organic compounds onto cellulosic fibers. *Colloid and Polymer Science* 283:344–350.

Aloulou, F., Boufi, S., and Beneventi, D. 2004b. Adsorption of organic compound onto polyelectrolyte immobilized-surfactant aggregates onto cellulosic fibres. *Journal of Colloid and Interface Science* 280:350–358.

Aloulou, F., Boufi, S., and Chachouk, M. 2004c. Adsorption of octadecyltrimethylammonium chloride and adsolubilization onto cellulosic fibres. *Colloid and Polymer Science* 282:699–707.

Aloulou, F., Boufi, S., and Labidi, J. 2006. Modified cellulose fibres for adsorption of organic compound in aqueous solution. *Separation and Purification Technology* 52:332–342.

Annergren, G.E. 1996. Strength properties and characteristics of bleached chemical and (chemi)mechanical pulps. In: *Pulp Bleaching—Principles and Practice*, Section VII: The Properties of Bleached Pulp. Atlanta, GA: Tappi Press, pp. 717–748.

Araki, J., Wada, M., Kuga, S., and Okano, T. 1998. Flow properties of microcrystalline cellulose suspension prepared by acid treatment of native cellulose. *Colloids and Surfaces* 142:75–82.

Araki, J., Wada, M., Kuga, S., and Okano, T. 1999. Influence of surface charge on viscosity behavior of cellulose microcrystal suspension. *Journal of Wood Science* 45:258–261.

Ayala, M., Pickard, M.A., and Vazquez-Duhalt, R. 2008. Fungal enzymes for environmental purposes, a molecular biology challenge. *Journal of Molecular Microbiology and Biotechnology*15:172–180.

Battista, O.A. and Smith, P.A. 1962. Microcrystalline cellulose. *Industrial and Engineering Chemistry* 54:20–29.

Bel-Hassen, R., Boufi, S., Brochier, M.C., Abdelmouleh, M., and Belgacem, M.N. 2008. Adsorption of silane onto cellulose fibers. II. The effect of pH on silane hydrolysis, condensation and adsorption behaviour. *Journal of Applied Polymer Science* 108:1958–1968.

Bertaud, F. and Holmbom, B. 2004. Chemical composition of earlywood and latewood in Norway spruce heartwood, sapwood and transition zone wood. *Wood Science and Technology* 38:245–256.

Bidlack, J., Malone, M., and Benson, R. 1992. Molecular structure and component integration of secondary cell walls in plants. *Proceedings of the Oklahoma Academy of Science* 72:51–56.

Bledzki, A.K. and Gassan, J. 1999. Composites reinforced with cellulose based fibres. *Progress in Polymer Science* 24:221–274.

Boufi, S. and Belgacem, M.N. 2006. Modified cellulose fibres for adsorption of dissolved organic solutes. *Cellulose* 13:81–94.

Bras, I.P., Santos, L., and Alves, A. 1999. Organochlorine pesticides removal by pinus bark sorption. *Environmental Science and Technology* 33:631.

Brochier, M.C., Abdelmouleh, M., Boufi, S., Belgacem, M.N., and Gandini, A. 2005. Silane adsorption onto cellulose fibers: Hydrolysis and condensation reactions. *Journal of Colloid and Interface Science* 289:249–261.

Cai, J., Zhang, L., Liu, S., Liu, Y., Xu, X., Chen, X., Chu, B. et al. 2008. Dynamic self-assembly induced rapid dissolution of cellulose at low temperatures. *Macromolecules* 41:9345–9351.

Casey, J.P. 1980. *Pulp and Paper: Chemistry and Chemical Technology*, Vol. 2. New York: John Wiley & Sons, 1446pp.

Chakravarty, S., Pimple, S., Chaturvedi, H.T., Singh, S., and Gupta, K.K. 2008. Removal of copper from aqueous solution using newspaper pulp as an adsorbent. *Journal of Hazardous Materials* 159:396–403.

Chauhan, G.S. and Lal, H. 2003. Novel grafted cellulose-based hydrogel for water technologies. *Desalination* 159:131–138.

Chauhan, G.S., Mahajan, S., and Guleria, L.K. 2000. Polymer from renewable resources: Sorption of Cu^{2+} ions by cellulose graft copolymers. *Desalination* 16:331–334.

Chen, W., Yu, H., Liu, Y., Chen, P., Zhang, M., and Hai, Y. 2011. Individualization of cellulose nanofibers from wood using high-intensity ultrasonication combined with chemical pretreatments. *Carbohydrate Polymer* 83:1804–1811.

Dahou, W., Ghemati, D., Oudia, A., and Aliouche, D. 2010. Preparation and biological characterization of cellulose graft copolymers. *Biochemical Engineering Journal* 48:187–194.

Delmer, C. and Amor, Y. 1995. Cellulose biosynthesis. *The Plant Cell* 7:987–1000.

Dong, X.M., Revol, J.F., and Gray, D.G. 1998. Effect of microcrystallite preparation conditions on the formation of colloid crystals of cellulose. *Cellulose* 5:19–32.

Donia, A.M., Atia, A.A., and Heniesh, A.M. 2008. Efficient removal of Hg(II) using magnetic chelating resin derived from copolymerization of bisthiourea/thiourea/glutaraldehyde. *Separation and Purification Technology* 60:46–53.

Doran, J.C. and Turnbull, J.W. 1997. Australian trees and shrubs: Species for land rehabilitation and farm planting in the tropics. ACIAR Monograph No. 24.

Fengel, D. and Wegener, G. 1984. *Wood: Chemistry, Ultrastructure, Reactions*. New York: Walter de Gruyter Inc., 613pp.

Fillat, U. 2008. Aplicación de biotecnología para la obtención de pastas de alta calidad. Estudio de sistemas enzimáticos en secuencias de blanqueo respetuosas con el medio ambiente. Tesis doctoral. Departamento de Ingeniería Textil y Papelera. Universidad Politécnica de Cataluña. Terrassa, España.

Finell, M., Hedman, B., and Nilsson, C. 2000. Effect of dry fractionation on pulping conditions and fibre properties of reed canary grass. In: Kennedy, J.F. et al. (eds.), *Cellulosic pulps, fibres and materials. Proceedings of the 10th international cellucon conference*, December 14–17, 1998. Turku, Finland. Wood-head Publishing Ltd. 261–266.

Fratzl, P. 2003. Cellulose and collagen: From fibres to tissues. *Current Opinion in Colloid and Interface Science* 8:32–39.

Freire, C.S.R., Silvestre, A.J.D., Pascoal Neto, C., Belgacem, M.N., and Gandini, A. 2006. Controlled heterogeneous modification of cellulose fibers with fatty acids: Effect of reaction conditions on the extent of esterification and fiber properties. *Journal of Applied Polymer Science* 100:1093–1102.

Fukuzumi, H., Saito, T., Iwata, T., Kumamoto, Y., and Isogai, A. 2009. Transparent and high gas barrier films of cellulose nanofibers prepared by TEMPO-mediated oxidation. *Biomacromolecules* 10:162–165.

García Hortal, J.A. 2007. *Fibras Papeleras*. Barcelona, Spain: Edicions UPC, 243pp.

Gerente, C., Mesnil, P.C., Andres, Y., Thibault, J.F., and Le Cloirec, P. 2000. Removal of metal ions from aqueous solution on low cost natural polysaccharides sorption mechanism approach. *Reactive and Functional Polymers* 46:135.

Gutierrez, A., Rodriguez, J., and Rio, J. 2008. Chemical composition of lipophilic extractives from sisal (*Agave sisalana*) fibers. *Industrial Crops and Products* 28:81–87.

Hergert, H.L. 1992. *Solvent Pulping Symposium Notes*. Atlanta, GA: Tappy Press, p. 1.

Hokkanen, S., Repo, E., and Sillanpää, M. 2013. Removal of heavy metals from aqueous solutions by succinic anhydride modified mercerized nanocellulose, *Chemical Engineering Journal* 223:40–47.

Horn, R.A. 1974. Morphology of wood pulp fiber from softwoods and influence on paper strength. USDA Forest Service Research Paper FPL 242. Madison, WI: Forest Products Lab.

Huang, X., Sillanpää, M., Duo, B., and Gjessing, E.T. 2008. Water quality in the Tibetan Plateau: Metal contents of four selected rivers. *Environmental Pollution* 156:270–277.

Huang, X., Sillanpää, M., Gjessing, E.T., and Vog, R.D. 2009. Water quality in the Tibetan Plateau: Major ions and trace elements in the headwaters of four major Asian rivers. *Science of the Total Environment* 407:6242–6254.

Hunter, N. 2007. 'Fuels Plus' from the forest. *Journal of the Technical Association of the Australian and New Zealand Pulp and Paper Industry* 60:10–12.

Ibarra, D., Romero, J., Martinez, M.J., Martinez, A.T., and Camarero, S. 2006. Exploring the enzymatic parameters for optimal delignification of eucalypt pulp by laccase-mediator. *Enzyme and Microbial Technology* 39:1319–1327.

Iniguez-Covarrubias, G., Diaz-Teres, R., Sanjuan-Dueñas, R., Anzaldo-Hernandez, J., and Rowell Roger, M. 2001. Utilization of by-products from the tequila industry. Part 2: Potential value of *Agave tequilana* Weber azul leaves. *Bioresource Technology* 77:101–108.

Iqbal, M., Saeed, A., and Kalim, I. 2009. Characterization of adsorptive capacity and investigation of mechanism of Cu^{2+}, Ni^{2+} and Zn^{2+} adsorption on mango peel waste from constituted metal solution and genuine electroplating effluent. *Separation Science and Technology* 44:3770–379.

Iwamoto, S., Nakagaito, A.N., and Yano, H. 2007. Nano-fibrillation of pulp fibers for the processing of transparent nanocomposites. *Applied Physics A: Materials Science and Processing* 89:461–466.

Jonker, M.T.O. 2007. Absorption of polycyclic aromatic hydrocarbons to cellulose. *Chemosphere* 70:778–782.

Jonsson, U. 2007. Functional studies of a membrane anchored cellulase from poplar. Royal Institute of Technology, School of Biotechnology, Department of Wood Biotechnology, Stockholm, Sweden.

Joonobi, M., Harun, J., Paridah, M.T., Shakeri, A., Sayfulazry, S., and Makinejad, M.D. 2011. Physicochemical characterization of pulp and nanofibers from kenaf stem. *Materials Letters* 65:1098–1100.

Joonobi, M., Harun, J., Shakeri, A., Misra, M., and Oksman, K. 2009. Chemical composition, crystallinity, and thermal degradation of bleached and unbleached kenaf bast pulp and nanofibers. *Bioresources* 4:626–639.

Judt, M. 1991. Raising paper output without wood. *Pulp and Paper International* 33:75–77.

Kennedy, J.F., Phillips, G.O., Williams, P.A., and Lönnberg, B. 2000. *Cellulosic Pulps, Fibres and Materials*. Cambridge, U.K.: Woodhead Publishing Ltd., pp. 261–266.

Kersten, P. and Cullen, D. 2007. Extracellular oxidative systems of the lignin-degrading Basidiomycete Phanerochaete chrysosporium. *Fungal Genetics and Biology* 44:77–87.

Kopania, E., Wietecha, J., and Ciechańska, D. 2012. Studies on Isolation of Cellulose Fibres from Waste Plant Biomass. Fibres and Textiles in Eastern Europe 20, 6B (96):167–172.

Kordsachia, O., Wandinger, B., and Patt, R. 1992. Some investigations an ASAM pulping and chlorine free bleaching of Eucalyptus from Spain. *Holz als Roh und Werkstof* 50:85–92.

Krzysik, F. and Gonet, B. 1954. Poplar as a raw material for pulp and paper. *Przeglad Papierniczy Lodz* 10:161–168.

Kuligowski, C., Brochier, B., Petit-Conil, M., and Housen, I. 2006. Development and optimization of biotechnology use in the manufacture of bleached chemical pulps. *TAPPI Engineering, Pulping and Environmental Conferences, Proceedings*, Tappi Press, Philadelphia, PA, pp. 16–20.

Lavoine, N., Desloges, I., Dufresne, A., and Bras, J. 2012. Microfibrillated cellulose—Its barrier properties and applications in cellulosic materials: A review. *Carbohydrate Polymers* 90:735–764.

Lee, S.Y., Chun, S.J., Kang, I.A., and Park, J.Y. 2009. Preparation of cellulose nanofibrils by high-pressure homogenizer and cellulose-based composite films. *Journal of Industrial and Engineering Chemistry* 15:50–55.

Li, B., Bandekar, R., Zha, Q., Alsaggaf, A., and Ni, Y. 2011. Fiber quality analysis: OpTest fiber quality analyzer versus L&W fiber tester. *Industrial and Engineering Chemistry Research* 50:12572–12578.

Lin, N., Huang, J., and Dufresne, A. 2012. Preparation, properties and applications of polysaccharide nanocrystals in advanced functional nanomaterials: A review. *Nanoscale* 4:3274–3294.

Livča, S., Verovkins, A., Shulga, G., Neiberte, B., and Vitolina, S. 2012. Characteristics and properties of soda lignin obtained from aspen wood by products. *Latvian Journal of Chemistry* 4:421–427.

Lynd, L.R., Weimer, P.J., Willem, H.Z., and Pretorius, I.S. 2002. Microbial cellulose utilization: Fundamentals and biotechnology. *Microbiology and Molecular Biology Reviews* 63:506–577.

Maheswari, C., Obi Reddy, K., Muzenda, E., Guduri, B.R., and Rajulu, A. 2012. Extraction and characterization of cellulose microfibrils from agricultural residue e *Cocos nucifera* L. *Biomass and Bio Energy* 46:555–563.

Malinen, R.O., Pisuttipiched, S., Kolehmainen, H., and Kusuma, F.N. 2006. Potential of acacia species as pulpwood in Thailand. *Journal of the Technical Association of the Australian and New Zealand Pulp and Paper Industry* 59:190–196.

Marshall, W.E. and Campagne, E.T. 1995. Agricultural byproducts as adsorbent for metal ions in laboratory prepared solution and in manufacturing waste water. *Journal of Environmental Science and Health A* 30:241.

Martínez, A.T., Speranza, M., Ruiz-Dueñas, F.J., Ferreira, P., Camarero, S., Guillén, F., Martínez, M.J., Gutiérrez, A., and del Río, J.C. 2005. Biodegradation of lignocellulosics: Microbial, chemical, and enzymatic aspects of the fungal attack of lignin. *International Microbiology* 8:195–204.

Mende, S. 2011. New generation of grinding media separation in agitator bead mills. *Deutsche Keramische Geselschaft* 10:E1–E4

Milewski, J.V., Meyer, J.A., Schniewind, A.P., and Chou, W. 1994. Whiskers. In *Concise Encyclopedia of Composite*, A. Kelly (ed.). Oxford: Pergamon, pp. 311–326.

Missoum, K., Belgacem, M.N., and Bras, J. 2013. Nanofibrillated cellulose surface modification: A review Materials, 6 (5):1745–1766.

Moldes, D. and Vidal, T. 2008. Laccase-HBT bleaching of eucalyptus kraft pulp: Influence of the operating conditions. *Bioresource Technology* 99:8565–8570.

Muhammad, S., Shah, M.T., and Khan, S. 2011. Health risk assessment of heavy metals and their source apportionment in drinking water of Kohistan region, northern Pakistan. *Microchemical Journal* 98: 334–343.

Nishino, T., Matsuda, I., and Hirao, K. 2004. All-cellulose composite. *Macromolecules* 37:7683–7687.

Palonen, H. and Viikari, L. 2004. Role of oxidative enzymatic treatments on enzymatic hydrolysis of softwood. *Biotechnology and Bioengineering* 86:550–557.

Pettersen, R.C. 1984. *The Chemical Composition of Wood*. Madison, WI: U.S. Department of Agriculture, Forest Service, Forest Products Laboratory.

Pinto, P.C., Evtuguin, D.V., and Pascoal, C. 2005. Chemical composition and structural features of the macromolecular components of plantation *Acacia mangium* wood. *Journal of Agricultural and Food Chemistry* 53:7856–7862.

Ragauskas, A.J. 1994. Brightness reversion of mechanical pulps. Part 2: Thermal aging of ascorbic acid-impregnated lignin-retaining pulps. *Cellulose Chemistry and Technology* 28:265–272.

Ragnar, M., Dahllof, H., and Lundgren, S. 2004. Towards an environmentally sustainable bleaching of kraft pulp exploring alternative ECF and TCF bleaching sequences. *58th Appita Annual Conference*, Vol. 2, Canberra, Australian Capital Territory, Australia, pp. 477–485.

Rannard, S.P. and Davis, N.J. 1999. Controlled synthesis of asymmetric dialkyl and cyclic carbonates using the highly selective reactions of imidazole carboxylic esters. *Organic Letters* 1:933–936.

Rannard, S.P. and Davis, N.J. 2000. The selective reaction of primary amines with carbonyl imidazole containing compounds: Selective amide and carbamate synthesis. *Organic Letters* 2:2117–2120.

Roncero, M.B., Torres, A.L., Colom, J.F., and Vidal, T. 2003. TCF bleaching of wheat straw pulp using ozone and xylanase. Part A: Paper quality assessment. *Bioresource Technology* 87:305–314.

Roncero, M.B. and Vidal, T. 2007. Optimizaciόn del tratamiento con ozono en el blanqueo TCF de pastas para papel. *Afinidad* 64:420–428.

Ruiz-Dueñas, F.J. and Martínez, A.T. 2009. Microbial degradation of lignin: How a bulky recalcitrant polymer is efficiently recycled in nature and how we can take advantage of this. *Microbial Biotechnology* 2:164–177.

Sabharwal, H.S. and Young, R.A. 1996. International agro-fiber research initiative. *TAPPI* 79:66–67.

Saito, T., Kimura, S., Nishiyama, S., and Isogai, A. 2007. Cellulose nanofibers prepared by TEMPO-mediated oxidation of native cellulose. *Biomacromolecules* 8:2485–2491.

Samaranayake, G. and Glasser, W.G. 1993. Cellulose derivatives with low DSI. A novel acylation system. *Carbohydrate Polymers* 22:1–7.

Schroeder, H.A., Chum, H.L., Douglas, L.J., and Feinberg, D.A. 1985. *Evaluation of Pretreatments of Biomass for Enzymatic Hydrolysis of Cellulose*. Golden, CO: Solar Energy Research Institute, US. Department of Energy.

Serrano, L., Urruzola, I., Nemeth, D., Belafi-Bako, K., and Labidi, J. 2011. Modified cellulose microfibrils as benzene adsorbent. *Desalination* 270:143–150.

Sigoillot, C., Camarero, S., Vidal, T., Record, E., Asther, M., Perez-Boada, M., Martinez, M.J. et al. 2005. Comparison of different fungal enzymes for bleaching high-quality paper pulps. *Journal of Biotechnology* 115:333–343.

Siqueira, G., Bras, J., and Dufresne, A. 2010. Cellulosic bionanocomposites: A review of preparation, properties and applications. *Polymers* 2:728–765.

Sundquist, J., Laamanen, L., and Poppius, K. 1998. Problem of non-conventional pulping processes in the peroxyformic acid cooking experiments. *Paperi Ja Puu* 70:143–148.

Tomé, L., Brandao, L., Mendes, A., Silvestre, A., Pascoal Neto, C., Gandini, A., Freire, C., and Marrucho, I. 2010. Preparation and characterization of bacterial cellulose membranes with tailored surface and barrier properties. *Cellulose* 17:1203–1211.

Torres, A.L., Roncero, M.B., Colom, J.F., Martinez, J.A., and Vidal, T. 2004. Application of an experimental design to modeling of ozone bleaching stage in TCF processes. *Ozone: Science and Engineering* 26:443–451.

Urruzola, I., de Andres, M.A., Nemeth, D., Belafi-Bako, K., and Labidi, J. 2013a. Multicomponents adsorption of modified cellulose microfibrils. *Desalination and Water Treatment* 51:10–12.

Urruzola, I., Serrano, L., Llano-Ponte, R., Andrés, M.A., and Labidi, J. 2013b. Obtaining of eucalyptus microfibrils for adsorption of aromatic compounds in aqueous solution. *Chemical Engineering Journal* 229:42–49.

Valchev, I., Valchev, V., and Ganev, I. 1999. Improved elemental chlorine-free bleaching of hardwood kraft pulp. *Cellulose Chemistry and Technology* 33:61–66.

Valls, C. 2008. Aplicaciό de nous sistemas enzimàtics pel blanqueig de pasta kraft d'eucaliptus. Tesis doctoral. Departamento de Ingeniería Textil y Papelera. Universidad Politécnica de Cataluña. Terrassa, España.

Vincent, J.F. 1999. From cellulose to cell. *The Journal of Experimental Biology* 202:3263–3268.

Wagberg, L., Decher, G., Norgren, M., Lindstrom, T., Ankerfors, M., and Axnas, K. 2008. The build-up of polyelectrolyte multilayers of microfibrillated cellulose and cationic polyelectrolytes. *Langmuir* 2008:784–795.

Widsten, P. and Kandelbauer, A. 2008. Laccase applications in the forest products industry: A review. *Enzyme and Microbial Technology* 42:293–307.

Wong, A. and Chiu, C. 1995. Pulping and bleaching of hemp, TAPPI Nonwood Plant Fiber Progress Report No. 22, pp. 165–176.

Yadav, S.K., Singh, N., Prasad, K.D., and Arora, S.S. 2006. Chlorine dioxide substitution during bleaching of pulp—An attempt towards AOX reduction in effluent. *IPPTA: Quarterly Journal of Indian Pulp and Paper Technical Association* 18:111–117.

You, J., Meng, J., Chen, X., and Ye, H. 2008. Study on direct delignification with laccase/xylanase system. *Journal of Wood Chemistry and Technology* 28:227–239.

Xu, M., Wang, Q., and Hao, Y. 2007. Removal of organic carbon from wastepaper pulp effluent by lab-scale solar photo Fenton process. *Journal of Hazardous Materials* 148:103–109.

Zhou, D., Zhang, L., Zhou, J., and Guo, S. 2004. Cellulose/chitin beads for adsorption of heavy metals in aqueous solution. *Water Research* 38:2643–2650.

14 Use of Oxidized Regenerated Cellulose in Controlling Bleeding during Neurosurgical Procedures

Roberto Gazzeri, Marcelo Galarza, Marika Morabito, and Alex Alfieri

CONTENTS

14.1 INTRODUCTION

Adequate hemostasis is of utmost importance in neurosurgery to prevent major postoperative bleedings and their consequences. The use of hemostatic agents during surgery has a lot of advantages as they minimize blood loss, improve visualization of the surgical area, save operation time, reduce or avoid blood transfusions, handle anticoagulated patients (i.e., hemophiliacs), decrease postoperation drainage, and decrease length of hospital stay. Controlling bleeding during neurosurgical procedures is a matter of life, because hematoma in the central nervous system in the postoperative course can cause neurological damages, while more copious bleeding can raise intracranial pressure, leading to coma and death.[1] During most of intraspinal (intramedullary and extradural) procedures, bleeding from venous vessels into the spinal canal may produce devastating neurological damages. Furthermore, continuous bleeding can hide visualization and identification of target structures, such as nerve roots during removal of a herniated disk.[2]

The conventional mechanical methods of hemostasis, such as direct pressure and ligature, are mostly impractical in cranial and spinal surgery because of the depth at which the surgery is performed and the critical neurological structures involved. For most of this century, the mainstay of control of intraspinal and brain bleeding has been bipolar cautery, allowing precise coagulation of small vessels and, compared to monopolar cautery, minimizing the dangerous spread of heat to adjacent nervous tissue. Though bipolar cautery is most effectively used to occlude identifiable vessels, it has minimal efficacy in controlling diffuse capillary bleeding that characterizes most intraspinal pathologies.[2] Bipolar electric coagulation allows subcutaneous bleeding control. Muscular dissection is often performed by monopolar electric coagulation. Hemostasis of the muscular layers is performed by bipolar coagulation and maintained by mechanical compression of spreaders. Each procedure on the bone (laminectomy, screw placement, etc.) carries the risk of conspicuous bleeding, mostly from cancellous bone. Its control is achieved by means of bone wax. The epidural phase of spinal procedures probably carries the longest and highest risk of bleeding due to the deep surgical field and difficulty to find bleeders. Iatrogenic damage of the epidural venous plexus increases the risk of managing against low pressure. However, continuous venous bleeding is difficult to control and time consuming. From the beginning of the neurosurgical practice, local hemostatic agents have proved to be very useful completing the more classical use of the electrocoagulation whatever its type, mono or bipolar. During this step, oxidized regenerated cellulose (ORC) and fibrillar collagen are very useful.[3] ORC is a flexible hemostatic agent that adheres readily to bleeding surfaces: it has a long history of safe use in surgical procedures. The mechanism by which the ORC accomplishes hemostasis is due to activation of the intrinsic coagulation pathway, the formation of a gel-like layer that holds the clot in place, and the vasoconstriction triggered by the low pH of the hemostatic agent. One major concern about the use of hemostatic agents in spine surgery is that there is danger of aggravating compression of the neural structures. The present study evaluates the efficacy, safety, and handling of ORC in a wide range of cranial and spinal procedures such as surgery of traumatic intracranial hematomas, brain tumors, and degenerative and traumatic spinal diseases.

14.2 HISTORICAL BACKGROUND

Hemostasis is achieved by different mechanisms: vasoconstriction, platelet plug formation, blood clot composition, and fibrinous tissue growth into the blood clot to definitively close injury of the damaged side. More than 50 substances have been identified in the blood, which influence active (procoagulant) or inhibit (anticoagulant) coagulation progress. In the blood stream, in an intact vessel, anticoagulants prevail; when a vessel is damaged, areas that have suffered damage get activated, and procoagulants prevail.[4] Hemostasis is a complex process: it can be divided into two distinct processes, primary and secondary hemostases. Primary hemostasis results in the formation of soft platelet plugs, which in turn are stabilized and cross-linked during secondary hemostasis. Of central importance in both primary and secondary hemostases is the activation of the clotting cascade, which can be broken down into two basic pathways, the intrinsic pathway and the extrinsic pathway.[5] The intrinsic pathway is activated by collagen, which is exposed when a blood vessel is damaged. The extrinsic pathway is similarly activated by tissue damage and the resultant release of tissue factor. The intrinsic and extrinsic pathways converge into the common pathway, which begins with the conversion of Factor X to Xa and ultimately results in the conversion of prothrombin to thrombin, which is integral in clot stabilization via fibrin.[6] The common pathway is facilitated by Factor V, which surgeons often think of due to the relatively common heritable coagulation disorder, Factor V Leiden.[7]

It is very important to know hemostatic cascade agents and moments because hemostatic agents stand by mechanism and time of action.

The hemostatic cascade is characterized by

1. Vessel injury
2. Vasoconstriction
3. Platelet plug formation
4. Fibrin clot formation
5. Fibrinolysis

The hemostatic agents work on the hemostatic cascade in different ways of action:

- ORC acts at second and third steps: provides a matrix for platelet adhesion and aggregation.
- Flowable gelatin acts at third and fourth steps: provides a matrix for platelet adhesion and aggregation; aids in fibrin clot formation when used with thrombin.
- Thrombin acts in the fourth step: aids in fibrin clot formation.
- Fibrin sealant acts in the fourth step: provides all the component necessary for fibrin clot formation.

Historically, the introduction of those and other topical absorbable hemostatic (TAH) agents has provided an innovative means for controlling intraoperative hemostasis and an advantage in managing bleeding during surgery when compared to gauze pads, ligature, or digital pressure. TAH agents provide a physical barrier to blood loss, which helps to stimulate platelet aggregation and clotting. The mechanism of action appears to be a physical effect rather than an alteration of the normal physiologic clotting mechanism. Inherently, TAH will swell after being saturated with blood and become a gelatinous mass that aids in the formation of a clot. In addition, the acidic properties of TAH products lower blood pH, leading to vasoconstriction. The pH of oxidized cellulose varies between 2 and 4. When exposed to blood, oxidized cellulose turns a dark brown or black color. This results from degradation of red blood cells and the subsequent formation of acid hematin.[8] The regenerated cellulose is obtained through the viscose process, which affords very pure cellulosic fibers as the end products. Compared with cotton cellulose, regenerated cellulose is of lower molecular weight and lower crystallinity. Also, regenerated cellulose fibers are continuous and have uniform diameters throughout the fiber length, while cotton cellulosic fibers have tapered shapes and different diameters. These properties of regenerated cellulose fibers achieve uniform and consistent oxidation. Twisted into yarns, regenerated cellulose can be knitted with different basis weights. ORC, which could be obtained by partial oxidation of the primary hydroxyl groups on the anhydroglucose rings to produce the monocarboxyl cellulose, is a kind of natural topical biomaterial. Within the range of 16%–24% carboxylic acid content, all the ORC materials represent an important class of biocompatible and bioabsorbable polymers, and they have been available in a sterilized knitted fabric or powder form for use to stop bleeding[9], which have been proved to hold an excellent bio-security. ORC was prepared and studied for the first time in the late 1930s. Research into the mechanism of blood coagulation led to the development of oxidized cellulose in 1942,[10] whereas ORC was developed in 1960 and is manufactured from wood pulp, which contains about 50% cellulose by mass. Johnson & Johnson has pioneered an industrial-scale oxidation process using nitrogen dioxide to manufacture ORC absorbable hemostat.[11]

The greatest use of this material has been for the control of oozing from broad surfaces, but it can also be pressed under osteoplastic flaps to supplement bone waxing or used to stop oozing from dural surfaces. It can also be applied directly on brain surfaces, to control bleeding from small vessels.[12] ORC in the fibrillar form is not markedly different from the other Surgicel cellulose-based products currently available.[13] Additional advantages are related to the physical properties of the loosely knit regenerated cellulose. This allows placement in certain areas where the product will rapidly conform to the recipient surface, giving a favorable three-dimensional structure for the clot organization. ORC also seems to confer hemostasis by decreasing the pH and acting as a caustic, thus generating an artificial clot. The clot is brownish because of the production of acid hematin.[14] ORC presents multiple mechanisms of action, including physical and mechanical actions in tamponade, food absorption, swelling and gel formation, and then surface interactions with proteins, platelets, and intrinsic and extrinsic pathway activation. One major advantage of oxidized cellulose is its definite and potent action against a wide variety of pathogenic organisms, both in vivo and in vitro.[15]

14.3 TYPE OF CELLULOSE

Since 1960, when Surgicel Absorbable Hemostat (Johnson & Johnson Wound Management, a Division of Ethicon, Inc, Somerville, NJ) has been approved for use in the United States, the company has developed three other similar products (Fibrillar in 1986, Nu-Knit in 1996, and SNoW in 2010). However, at the same time, other companies have raised analogous hemostatic agents to control hemorrhage in surgical procedure.

The present chapter is going to focus the attention on the three Surgicel types actually in commerce: Original, Fibrillar, and Nu-Knit.

14.3.1 Product Characteristics

Surgicel Original has a flexible texture. Thanks to its simplicity to being cut, without fraying or discard, it can be used easily in any surgical procedure for bleeding control. The sheer wave allows visualization of the bleeding site. Also, it is well suited for electrocautery, and if passed through a trocar, it does not slit.

Mixing is not required. Applied dry, Surgicel Original has no adherence to gloves or instruments (Figure 14.1). Once hemostasis has been achieved, Surgicel Original excess can be easily removed, while the surplus in the wound will completely reassimilate by 2 weeks. The extreme manageability attributed by the homogeneous structure of the fibers allows Surgicel Original to adhere also to irregular surfaces (Figure 14.2).[1] Surgicel Fibrillar is a kind of fibrous oxidized regenerated

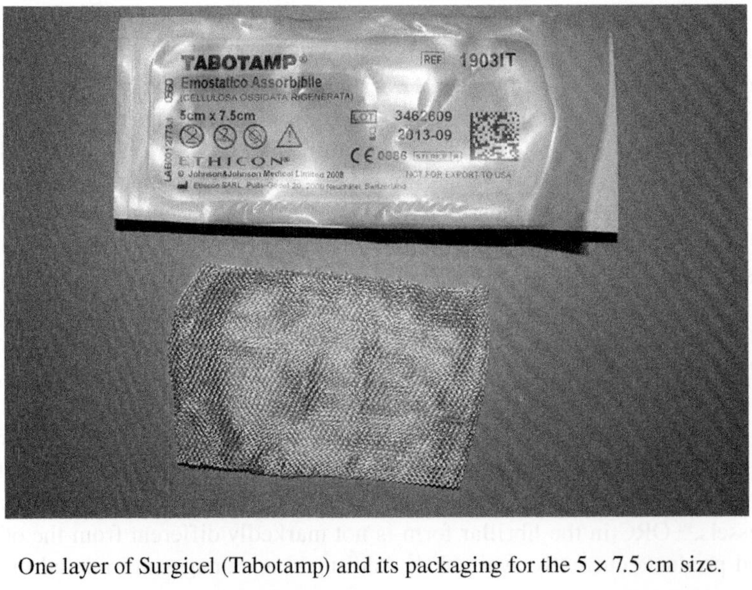

FIGURE 14.1 One layer of Surgicel (Tabotamp) and its packaging for the 5 × 7.5 cm size.

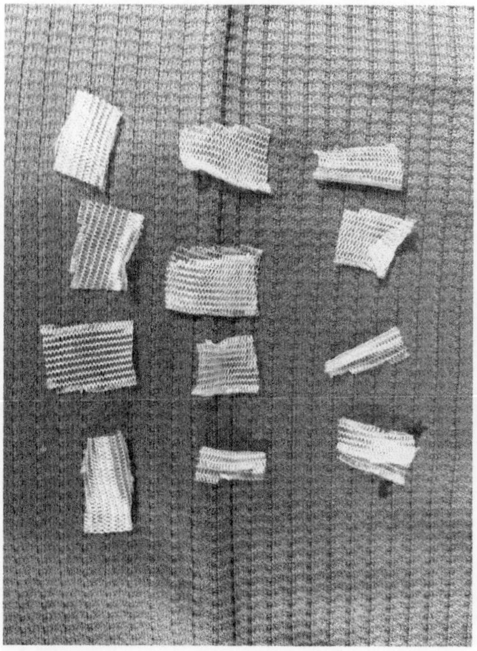

FIGURE 14.2 Oxidized regenerated cellulose is cut in different sizes and ready to use in the operating room.

cellulose that makes it comfortable and provides broad surface area coverage. It can obtain hemostasis with 39% faster than Surgicel Original. It is the seven-layer microfibrillar structure that makes Surgicel Fibrillar the most versatile product of Surgicel family (Figure 14.3). The seven lightweight layers can be separated to obtain any shape (strips, ball, or wad) or thickness, to satisfy different needs in wound management: in fact, Surgicel Fibrillar perfectly adheres to any surface as in difficult to access point. "Melts in" to bleeding tissue, but it can be easily removed if necessary. Moreover, it is suitable for use with electrocautery. This is especially helpful in cases of venous or cortical oozing, or when used to help identify a bleeding point where coagulation can be achieved

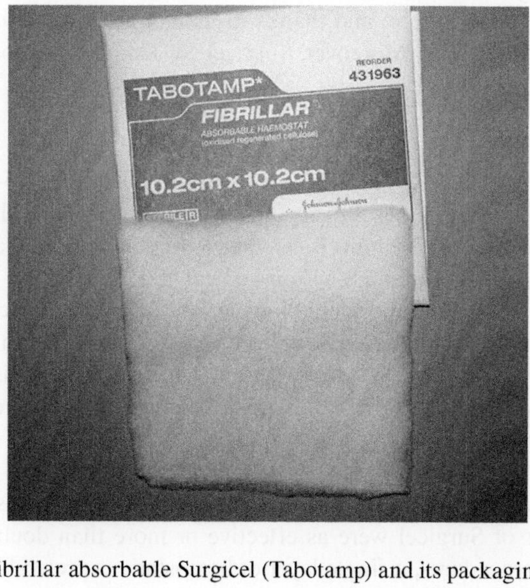

FIGURE 14.3 Squared fibrillar absorbable Surgicel (Tabotamp) and its packaging.

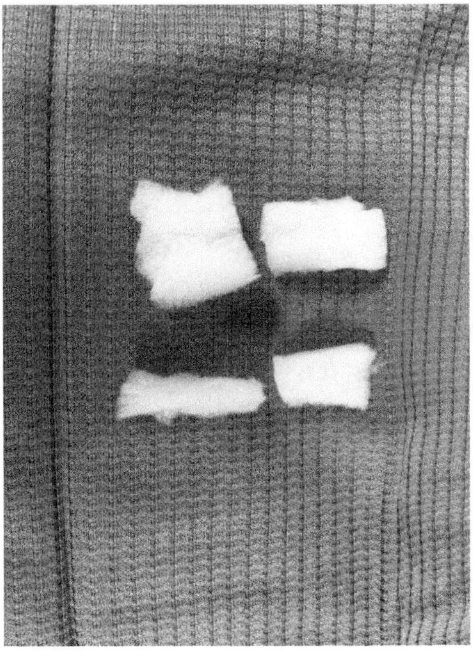

FIGURE 14.4 Oxidized regenerated cellulose fibrillar is prepared by the scrub nurse in different shapes and sizes.

with Surgicel Fibrillar held in place with a Fukushima-type sucker. Surgicel Fibrillar is ideal for controlling venous bleeding and oozing from cortical surfaces after lobectomies or tumor resection (Figure 14.4).[13]

Surgicel Nu-Knit has a denser and stronger stitch if compared to Surgicel Original: this awards hemostatic ability 29% faster than Surgicel Original. Three times thicker than Surgicel Original, Surgicel Nu-Knit guarantees greater endurance and coverage in case of profuse bleeding; also, it can be saturated in situ to offer another suture carrier.

Surgicel Nu-Knit is a good choice in case of trauma; also, it can be rolled and put in tiny injury of perforation. It can support a suture, and thanks to its increased density, it preserves structural integrity during surgery operation.[16] Moreover, Surgicel Nu-Knit can be slot with a trocar.

14.3.2 Hemostatic Activity

To compare time to hemostasis (TTH) of Surgicel® family (Original, Nu-Knit®, Fibrillar™, and SNoW™) and others, competitive TAH agents—GELITACEL and Curacel® (Gelita Medical B.V.), Traumastem and Emoxicel TAF Reticulum (Bioster, a.s.), Arista® AH (Medafor, Inc.), BloodSTOP® iX (LifeScience Plus, Inc.), Equitamp® (Equimedical B.V.), OKCEL H-T (Synthesia, a.s.), BLOODCARE (Lifeline Plus s.r.o.), Oxycel (Woundcare Ltd.), and Reoxcel (Skyteks TeksilL)—were evaluated by a linear incision on a swine spleen model study: in 10 animals, each received 17 incisions (15 tests and 2 control sites). Surgicel products achieved hemostasis in an average of 7 min for all the engraved areas. Except for 1 of 10 Arista AH-treated sites and 2 out of 10 sites receiving Equitamp, all competitors achieved hemostasis in less than 10 min.

Surgicel Nu-Knit, Fibrillar, and SNoW were applied in single layer, while for all the other mesh-like products, a double layer was applied: equivalent TTH were observed in both, demonstrating than single layer of Surgicel were as effective or more than double layer of competitors tested. In neurosurgical procedures, a single layer of hemostatic is preferable to avoid compression of the healthy neural structures. No different liability was observed during intraoperative period. In this test, Arista AH was applied in powered form with manufacturer's aspiration tools, while BloodSTOP was applied with a wet gauze, dry and covered.

14.3.3 Safety

ORC is generally safe and well-tolerated, save few reports of adverse reactions in neurosurgical use. Rare granulomatous foreign body reactions have been reported in patients undergoing surgical brain tumor resection. However, all were removed with positive results, and most of them were histologically formed by cellulose remnants, multinuclear giant cells, and monocytes.[17,18]

Furthermore, it is generally nonantigenic because it is a plant-derived agent and does not contain human components.[19] Risks of viral disease transmission have not been reported yet.

14.3.4 Enlargement

TAH agents may be left in situ although when hemostasis is achieved, it is better to remove any excess product, mostly if used near spinal cord or optic nerve and chiasm because swelling can increase pressure that can fall into paralysis or nerve damage. Surgicel, Curacel, and Gelitacel all make this recommendation. Swelling of TAH agents must be considered during neurosurgical and spinal procedures, because high pressure can exercise nerve damage or paralysis. In this regard, Traumastem information asserts that the product does not increase in volume when in contact with body fluids or blood and does not expand in surrounding areas and tissues, to make unnecessary to remove the product from the areas of application. Dissolution in vitro study demonstrates absorbability of Surgicel and competitive products by phosphate-buffered solution (pH 7.3) incubation at 37°C for 120 h. Measurement of negative space areas by optical microscope was the method to evaluate degree of swelling. Surgicel was fully dissolved in 24 h, while both Curacel and Gelitacel small fibers were observed after 120 h. Compared to Gelitacel—that resulted in a very rigid form—Surgicel and Curacel showed more flexibility and drapability. To evaluate water solubility, products were left in contact with saline solution to establish absorption rapidity during operation procedures. None of them resulted soluble, but each swelled by absorption of water. Traumastem sample became swollen in both saline and phosphate-buffered solutions: fiber diameters increased at least 200% in 25 min.

14.3.5 Bactericidal Activity

Surgicel has a bactericidal activity thanks to the properties of ORC to decrease pH. Physiological blood pH range (7.2–7.4) gives to microorganism a kindly environment to survive. Acid environment ($pH < 7.0$) reduces bacterial activity; also many of pathogenic agents aren't able to survive at $pH < 4.4$ level. Surgicel drives pH level beneath 4.0, arresting bacterial proliferations and survival, allowing host's natural defenses to break down the organism. ORC has a potent action against a lot of pathogenic organism associated with surgical lesions, especially methicillin-resistant *Staphylococcus aureus* (MRSA), methicillin-resistant *Staphylococcus epidermidis* (MRSE), vancomycin-resistant *Enterococcus* (VRE), penicillin-resistant *Streptococcus pneumoniae* (PRSP), and nonresistant ATCC strains of *S. aureus* and *Pseudomonas aeruginosa*. Data indicate that antibiotic-resistant microorganisms remain susceptible to the antimicrobial activity of ORC. Spangler et al. exposed Surgicel Original, Fibrillar, and Nu-Knit to nine different types of bacteria in vitro. One hour later, there was no survival of pathogenic agents in all three types of Surgicel. Curtailment to the third power has been looked in 24 h observation. Conversely, in control group, bacteria has been increased.[16]

Bactericidal properties have been tested on experimental wounds. Kuchta et al. discovered that Surgicel family products act significantly on *Klebsiella pneumonia*,[20] and also all of them reduce and control strictly *S. aureus* infections.[21]

A recent study in vivo supports those results: Surgicel Fibrillar has been matched with iodine gauze on 98 patients submitted to non-sterile surgery. Crops from swabs drawing first and third days came out negative, and contamination turned into 66% of the patients. In contrast, contamination decreased 25% in iodinate gauze patients.[22] Testing methods on Curacel, GELITACEL, and TRAUMASTEM demonstrated bacteriostatic activity, illustrating their ability to prevent growing and multiplying of bacteria but not the killing effect. In the evaluation of bactericidal efficacy against top five pathogens isolated from surgical site infections listed on National Nosocomial Infections Surveillance System (MRSA, MRSE, VRE, PRSP, *Escherichia coli*, and *P. aeruginosa* ATCC), 10^4–10^5 CFUs of each micro-organism were inoculated in a Trypticase soy broth dilution and incubated at 35°C–37°C for 48 h. pH was measured for each product at time points 0, 4, 24, and 48 h. Among ten competitive products tested (Surgicel Original, BLOODCARE, CURACEL, Equitamp, Gelitacel, OKCEL H-T, Oxycel, Reoxcel, Traumastem, and ResoCell), only Surgicel Original reduced 4-log bacteria concentration from initial inoculums. With the exception of Equitamp, all the products acted against *P. aeruginosa* and MRSA. Equitamp reduced bacterial count less than 1-log from initial inoculum and failed to achieve at pH < 4. Only Oxycel and Surgicel played a significant role against VRE.[23]

14.3.6 Comparison to Other Hemostatic Agents

In addition to ORC, there are different methods to reduce blood loss during surgery, as patches, flowable agents, and fibrin sealants.

Main of patches is Tachosil, a hemostatic sponge with human thrombin and fibrinogen, used by direct application on bleeding side. It's available in different sizes (5 × 5 and 10 × 5 cm patches). Hemostasis is achieved with approximately TTH of 3 min.

14.3.6.1 Gelatin Matrix Hemostats

Floseal (Baxter) is a bovine gelatin matrix including human thrombin, whose components have been reconstructed, transferred, and mixed. Available in different volume and size, it achieves hemostasis with TTH inferior at 2 min. It needs to be used in 2 h after mixing. The granules swell by 10%–20% upon contact with blood or body fluids.

Surgiflo (Johnson & Johnson) is the new competitor of Floseal. Floseal and Surgiflo differ only in the source of collagen, coming from bovine and porcine derivatives, respectively. The flowable gelatin matrix of Surgiflo provides an environment for platelets to adhere to and to aggregate within, building on the patient's natural coagulation cascade. The patient's endogenous thrombin is activated, and the patient's thrombin converts fibrinogen into an insoluble fibrin clot. When exogenous thrombin is used as the additional fluid for mixing Surgiflo, it provides an ancillary effect to the innate hemostatic property of the flowable gelatin matrix. When used in appropriate amounts, Surgiflo Haemostatic Matrix is absorbed completely within 4–6 weeks. In a retrospective evaluation comparing the use of bovine (Floseal) and porcine (Surgiflo Haemostatic Matrix) gelatin matrix thrombin sealants for controlling hemostasis in a consecutive series of 35 patients undergoing laparoscopic partial nephrectomy each product was successful in all cases, achieving hemostatic efficacy with no associated complications. The authors concluded that when utilized with oxidized nitrocellulose bolster, bovine (Floseal Haemostatic Matrix) or porcine (Surgiflo Haemostatic Matrix) gelatin matrix thrombin sealants provided equivalent perioperative hemostatic efficacy and safety profiles.[24,25]

14.3.6.2 Fibrin Sealant

As fibrin sealant, Tisseel (Baxter) and Evicel (Johnson & Johnson) are both used for surgical hemostasis in the United States and Europe. Evicel is composed by frozen human fibrinogen and thrombin restrained in two different syringes. When defrosting happens, the two solutions are mixed by a specific device, and dripped or sprayed on the bleeding site.

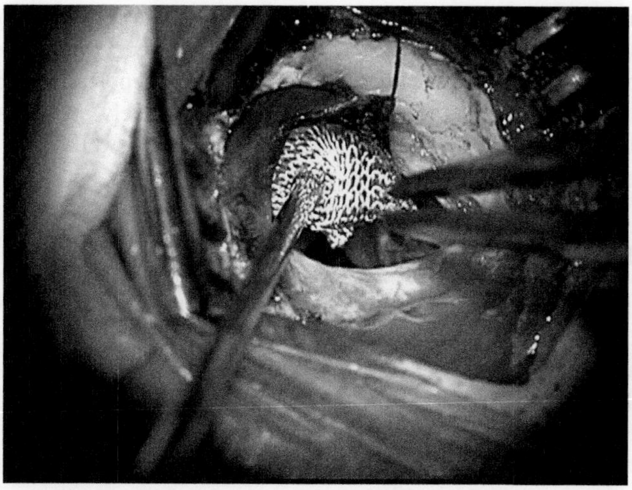

FIGURE 14.5 After removal of a vestibular schwannoma, during a retrosigmoid approach to the posterior fossa, Surgicel Original is inserted on the dural walls and tentorium to stop venous bleeding.

Its TTH is 4 min. Once opened, components are stable at room temperature for 24 h if not mixed: if not used during the surgical procedure, it can be stored in fridge for extra 30 days. The safety and effectiveness of fibrin sealants have been demonstrated in clinical trials. A prospective randomized controlled trial compared the hemostatic effectiveness of a fibrin sealant (Evicel®) in 75 patients to manual compression in 72 patients undergoing the insertion of polytetrafluoroethylene arterial anastomoses. The results of this study demonstrated that a higher percentage of patients who received fibrin sealant achieved hemostasis at 4 min (i.e., 85% versus 39% respectively) versus patients upon whom manual compression was used; likewise, a higher percentage of patients who received the fibrin sealant achieved hemostasis at 7 and 10 min. Treatment failure was lower in the fibrin sealant group, while the rate of complications potentially related to bleeding was similar; 64% of patients who received fibrin sealant experienced at least one adverse event, compared with 7% in the manual compression group (Figure 14.5).[26]

Tisseel is a fibrin sealant with fibrinogen and thrombine, available in freeze-dried kit or prefilled frozen syringe. Applications work by numerous steps: warm defrosting, reconstitution of two vials, and finally transfer to delivery device by oozing or vaporizing. Once the components are mixed, thrombin catalyzes conversion of fibrinogen to fibrin, making a clot that adheres to the tissue. In adjunction, it contains ionic calcium to activate Factor XIII and create insoluble fibrin polymers that helps to increase stability and strength of the fibrin clot. On the other hand, fibrinogen components contain unnecessary[27] and potentially deleterious antifibrinolytic–tranexamic acid or bovine-derived aprotinin to delay degradation of fibrin clot[28]: application in vivo of tranexamic acid in central nervous system blocked inhibition played by γ-aminobutyric acid inducing hyperexcitability.[29] Available in different sizes, freeze-dried kit must be used in 4 h as warmed prefilled syringe (while unopened purse can be stored at room temperature for 48 h). In neurosurgery, injection of glue has been used with positive results and without complications to treat hemangioma into the anterior cavernous sinus, prevent cerebrospinal fluid leakage and fluid collection in the subdural and epidural space, and reinforce hemostasis from the vertebral venous plexus.

14.3.6.3 Hemostatic "Sponges"

Gelatin-based Spongostan (Ethicon), Gelfoam (Pharmacia), Surgifoam (Johnson & Johnson), and other gelatin-based local hemostatic agents have been used in surgery for decades. They can be of bovine, porcine, or equine origin and are available in multiple presentations: sponge, powder, foam, etc. They can be used alone or soaked with thrombin. Their mechanism of action is still not completely clear but appears to be more physical, by "surface effect," than through any action on the blood-clotting mechanism. Gelatin-based devices have been reported to induce a better quality clot than collagen-based products. The substance has been widely used in spine surgery, as it is considered safe to leave it in the spinal canal because it does not swell. Some authors have even suggested that gelatin reduces scar adhesion.

14.4 USE IN NEUROSURGERY

Electrical and mechanical systems are traditional options for bleeding control in neurosurgery. However, these techniques have many limitations: mechanical methods as direct pressure and ligature have restrained action because of anatomical structure immovability, bone restrictions, and deepness. Bipolar cautery minimizes drift diffusion to adjacent tissues. Still, close structures remains exposed to thermal lesion by heat dispersion and compromise neuronal perfusion if blood provision came from cauterized vessel. Furthermore, it has a very few actions against widespread capillary bleeding or venous weep.

So, topical absorbable haemostatic agents became popular as operative help to avoid vessel occlusion, keeping safe distal perfusion.[1] Particularly, Surgicel Fibrillar is an adequate hemostatic choice for intrinsic and extrinsic tumor resection, surgery in close or penetrating skull-cerebral lesion.

14.4.1 Use in Conventional Brain Surgery

Despite ORC is not the best choice for the treatment of arteriolar bleeding during surgery, this product contributes to an early hemostasis in capillary and venous drain that frequently occurs in the removal of tumor or intracerebral hemorrhage (Figure 14.5). From the beginning of the surgical procedure to the end of the extradural hemostasis after dura mater closure, Surgicel may be used along all the steps of the procedure, to protect the brain and to complete local hemostasis (Figure 14.6). In brain tumors, oxidized cellulose is widely used, during the ablation of the tumor and at the end of the procedure to prevent and to stop any bleeding in the remaining cavity whatever the type of tumor. If little, persistent oozing from the cavity walls is perfectly controlled in most cases with the application of one layer of ORC (Figure 14.7). The application of Surgicel Original among the dura and craniotomy lack is very common to prevent epidural hematoma, meanwhile helping to

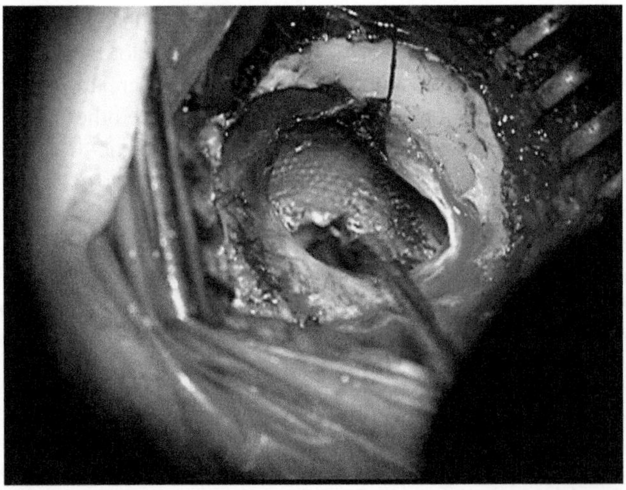

FIGURE 14.6 Surgicel adheres well on the meningeal surface to stop blood oozing.

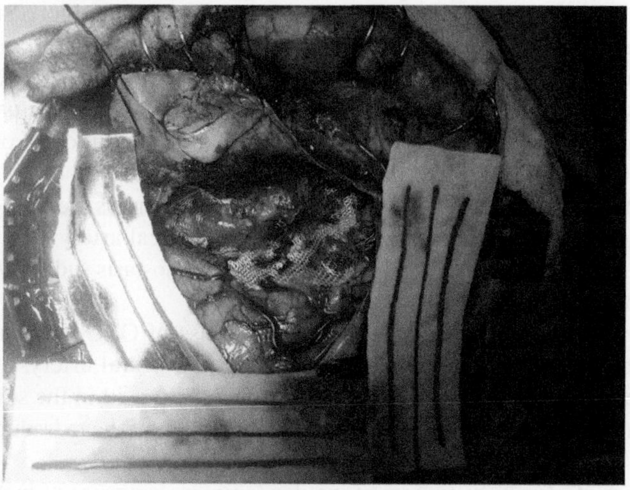

FIGURE 14.7 Oxidized regenerated cellulose adheres strongly on the walls of the surgical cavity after removal of an anterior cranial fossa meningioma.

stop filtering from the same space. Surgicel Fibrillar should be preferred due to its ability to adhere precisely to the cavity wall. If the bleeding is close to the vault, the suspension of the dura mater to the bone with interposition oxidized cellulosis is the solution. Successful use of Surgicel Original has been reported in neuroendoscopic procedures to remove extended intracranial hematomas.[30]

For endoscopic use, the ORC is cut in the desired size, then grasp and pull until the hemostat is enclosed at the end of the endoscope; after insertion of the endoscope into the surgical area, the hemostat is pushed into the cavity and, using grasping instruments, is placed over the bleeding site. Literature describes as these procedures lead an important turning into deep brain control bleeding. Thrombin-soaked gel sponges usually catch on instruments and don't adhere adequately to the tissue: these problems have not been verified with Surgicel products. Particularly, Surgicel Fibrillar does not require the use of cottonoids during suction, giving to the surgeon a better view of the site. In case of continuous bleeding, like moyamoya-type vessels and arteriovenous malformations, electrocoagulation of saturated oxidized cellulose is indeed possible.

14.4.2 Use in the Ventricular System

In case of lesions involving lateral ventricles or areas in contact with fourth ventricular chamber, it is very helpful to use Surgicel Original to promote hemostasis with both surgical sponges and electrocoagulation. Until now, no cases of postoperative hydrocephalus or pseudomeningocele have been reported after leaving Surgicel in those areas. In transcortical approaches to subdural hygroma, use of Surgicel Original flanked to tissue glue may prevent postoperative complications.[31]

14.4.3 Use in Approaches to the Skull Base

Approach to the skull base requires fast and scrupulous hemostasis; academic literature has proven how ORC has the right characteristics for hemostasis in different types of surgical procedures. In dissections of cavernous sinus lesions, it is necessary to manipulate and mobilize the dura to obtain a right shapely operative corridor, so it is not uncommon that venous bleeding occurs. Thin layers of ORC can directly dab and form a coagulum achieving hemostasis. It is necessary to remove anterior clinoid extradurally during an orbitozygomatic approach: because of anterior clinoid incorporation in siphon angle at the anteromedial triangle of the cavernous sinus, it is not a surprise to incur in massive bleeding during this procedure. This area is surrounded by a lot of critical and pressure-sensitive structure: medially the carotid and the optic nerve, and laterally two cavernous membranes and oculomotor nerve. It is very important to prevent any injury to these structures, packing generously, and use cautiously bipolar electrocoagulation. During the exposition of posterior cavernous sinus, in the area of the foramen ovale, massive bleeding occurs by sphenoid emissary veins or connection veins between lateral cavernous sinus and pterygoid venous plexus. In the dissection of the posterior cavernous region of the middle fossa, after meningeal artery electrocoagulation, use of both bipolar electrocoagulation and ORC is very helpful. Hemostasis suddenly acts packing with ORC all the cavernous sinus triangular corridors access.

Another case in which hemostasis may be achieved by use of ORC in conjunction with bipolar electrocoagulation and irrigation is during dissection of vertebral artery, with bleeding from vertebral venous plexus after manipulation of the vertebral artery within the suboccipital triangle. Use of ORC is not appropriate for bleeding during the dissection of the extradural vertebral artery component.

Sometimes, in case of glomus or tumors at jugular foramen, exposure of jugular bulb is necessary in lateral suboccipital approach; tunneling between the jugular bulb and the C-1 condyle will enable for skeletonization of the hypoglossal canal and the condylar triangle; in these cases, ORC guarantees an efficient treatment of venous ooze.[31]

14.4.4 Use in Cerebrovascular Surgery

ORC, especially the woven forms, holds characteristics required for the manipulation of aneurismal dome and refinement of the corridor for a correct clip emplacement. The use of oxycellulose insertion between the aneurysm neck and the neighboring perforators may avoid inclusion of the latter at the time of neck clipping. If an intraoperative rupture occurs in the site of dissection with ORC, the surgeon can use suction, cottonoid compression, and copious irrigation to keep the view free and treat the lesions. If appropriate surgical sponges are available, oxidized regenerate cellulose remains the second choice; it's recommended to avoid use of oxidized regenerate cellulose to bypass principles of intervention in case of cerebrovascular abnormalities.[31]

14.5 USE IN SPINAL SURGERY

Traditional bleeding control system results useless in spinal surgery, because a complete vessel occlusion can compromise neural tissue perfusion and heat dispersion can thermally damage nervous roots or neural structure.[2]

Bone wax is a well-known topical hemostatic agent composed of beeswax and Vaseline. Its biochemical proprieties allow clot formation on damaged vessels to prevent blood flow into the bone.[3]

Gelatin Foam (a.k.a. absorbable gelatin sponge) is made of animal-skin gelatin foam: thanks to its animal delivery, it is an antigenic agent. It has a strong adherence to any surfaces. Gelatin foam paste is an offshoot that, if soaked in thrombin, acts on coagulation cascade with a low-pressure mechanical bleeder.[32]

Microfibrillar collagen (MFC) gives a complete and immediate hemostasis: blood rarely leaks through it, thanks to the ability to adhere strongly to vessel surfaces that remain dry. In opposition to Gelatin foam, it doesn't swell. Both in vitro[33] and in vivo study demonstrated that MFC increases platelet aggregation; MFC worked well in case of heparinization, less in thrombocytopenia.[34] Benefits of collagen are fast induction of hemostasis and absorption and low tissue reaction as non-antigenic product.[35] At the same time, difficult manipulation during surgery acts as a disadvantage.

Intraosseous implantation of ORC promotes lamellar bone formation with the same quality of collagen-based implants.[36] Thanks to its bactericidal activity against mainly pathogen implicated in osteomielitys, Surgicel is preferred over bone wax for stop bleeding in bone procedure.[16]

Gelfoam also can be used in both skull base and spine surgery, resulting plain to apply and bereaved of impact on surgeon's view. Vertebral plexus are better controlled with local hemostatic agents as Surgicel. Spinal cord tumors must be approached through laminotomy. After retraction of the posterior arch flap, the extradural hemostasis must be perfect sometimes difficult due to epidural veins. Bipolar coagulation of the veins should be completed by appliance of small fragments of Surgicel and bone wax on bone section. Surgicel application will help for hemostasis, the coagulation use being as restricted as possible to avoid thermal injury of the nerves and spinal cord.

14.6 CONCLUSIONS

All Surgicel products have multiple neurosurgical applications in hemostasis. Furthermore, in addition to standard hemostatic procedures, they promote a faster hemostasis and guarantee a wide bactericidal activity against both common and antibiotic-resistant microorganisms, as *S. pneumoniae*, *S. aureus*, *S. epidermidis*, and *P. aeruginosa*. Thanks to its manageability, the product can be applied precisely on numerous varieties of critical bleeding areas, as foramina in bone, spinal cord, or optic nerve. Also, during approaches to the skull base or removal of intracerebral hemorrhages, both Surgicel Original and Fibrillar may well control venous oozing. Likewise, intrinsic or extrinsic tumor resections and cerebrovascular rupture find in ORC the most valid help for rapid interventions.

REFERENCES

1. Levy, M.L., Amar, A.P. 1998. The use of oxidized regenerated cellulose in neurosurgical procedure. *Surgical Technology International* VII: 467–471.
2. Sabel, M., Stummer, W. 2004. The use of local agents: Surgicel and surgifoam. *European Spine Journal* 13(Suppl. 1): S97–S101. doi:10.1007/s00586-004-0735-z.
3. Shonauer, C., Tessitore, E., Barbagallo, G., Albanese, V., Moraci, A. 2004. The use of local agents: Bone wax, collagen, oxidized cellulose. *European Spine Journal* 13(Suppl. 1): S89–S96. doi:10.1007/s00586-004-0727-z.
4. Guyton, A.C., Hall, J.E. 2006. *Textbook of Medical Physiology*, XI edn. London, U.K.: Elsevier.
5. Hess, J.R., Brohi, K., Dutton, R.P. et al. 2008. The coagulopathy of trauma: A review of mechanisms. *Journal of Trauma* 65: 748–754.
6. Rubin, E., Gorstein, F., Rubin, R., Schwarting, R., Strayer, D. 2005. *Rubin's Pathology: Clinicopathologic Foundations of Medicine*. Baltimore, MD: Lippincott Williams & Wilkins.
7. Franchini, M., Lippi, G. 2010. Factor V Leiden and hemophilia. *Thrombosis Research* 125: 119–23.
8. Stilwell, R.L., Marks, G.M., Saferstein, L., Wiseman, D.M. 1997. Oxidized cellulose. In *Handbook of Biodegradable Polymers*, Chapter 15, pp. 291–306. Reading, U.K.: Harwood Academic Publishers.
9. Zhu, L., Kumar, V., Banker, G.S. July 31, 2001. Examination of oxidized cellulose as a macromolecular prodrug carrier: preparation and characterization of an oxidized cellulose-phenylpropanolamine conjugate. *International Journal of Pharmaceutics* 223(1-2): 35–47.
10. Frantz, V.K. 1945. New methods of hemostasis. *Surgical Clinics of North America* 25: 338–349.
11. Alpaslan, C., Alpaslan, G.H., Oygur, T. April 1997. Tissue reaction to three subcutaneously implanted local hemostatic agents. *British Journal of Oral and Maxillofacial Surgery* 35(2): 129–32.
12. Voormolen, J.H., Ringers, J., Bots, G.T. et al. 1987. Haemostatic agents: Brain tissue reaction and effectiveness. A comparative animal study using collagen fleece and oxidized cellulose. *Neurosurgery* 20: 702–709.
13. Levy, M.L., Day, J.D., Fukushima, T., Batjer, H.H., Gamache, F.W. Jr. 1997. Surgicel Fibrillar absorbable oxidized regenerated cellulose. *Neurosurgery* 41(3): 701–702.
14. Masova, L., Rysava, J., Krizova, P. et al. 2003. Hemostyptic effect of oxidized cellulose on blood platelets. *Sbornik Lekarsky* 104(2): 231–236.
15. Wagner, W.R., Pachence, J.M., Ristich, J., Johnson, P.C. 1996. Comparative in vitro analysis of topical hemostatic agents. *Journal of Surgical Research* 66: 100–108.
16. Spangler, D., Rothenburger, S., Nguyen, K., Jampani, H., Weiss, S., Bhende, S. 2003. In vitro antimicrobial activity of oxidized regenerated cellulose against antibiotic-resistant microorganisms. *Surgical Infections (Larchmt)* 4: 255–262.

17. Sandhu, G.S., Elexpuru-Camiruaga, J.A., Buckley, S. 1996. Oxidized cellulose (Surgicel) granulomata mimicking tumour recurrence. *British Journal of Neurosurgery* 10: 617–619.
18. Kothbauer, K.F., Jallo, G.I., Siffert, J., Jimenez, E., Allen, J.C., Epstein, F.J. 2001. Foreign body reaction to hemostatic materials mimicking recurrent brain tumor. Report of three cases. *Journal of Neurosurgery* 95(3): 503–506.
19. Henry, M.C.W., Tashjian, D.B., Kasowski, H., Duncan, C., Moss, R.L. 2005. Postoperative paraplegia secondary to the use of oxidized cellulose (Surgicel). *Journal of Pediatric Surgery* 40(4): E9–E11.
20. Kuchta, N., Dineen, P. 1983. Effects of absorbable hemostats on intra abdominal sepsis. *Infections in Surgery* 15: 441–444.
21. Dineen, P. 1977. The effect of oxidized regenerated cellulose on experimental infected splenotomies. *Journal of Surgical Research* 23(2): 114–116.
22. Alfieri, S., Di Miceli, D., Menghi, R., Quero, G. et al. 2011. The role of oxidized regenerated cellulose in preventing infections at the surgical site: Prospective, randomized study in 98 patients affected by a dirty wound. *Minerva Chirurgica* 66(1): 55–62.
23. Bhende, S. 2012. Competitive assessment of topical absorbable hemostats (TAH) for bactericidal activity. *Ethicon* RDCF 25/2-52851; Competitive assessment of topical absorbable hemostats (TAH) for bactericidal activity (Phase II). *Ethicon* RDCF25/2-52852.
24. Gazzeri, R., Galarza, M., Alfier, A. 2012. The safety and biocompatibility of gelatin hemostatic matrix (Floseal and Surgiflo) in neurosurgical procedures. *Surgical Technology International* XXII 22: 49–54. doi:pii: sti 22/3.
25. Gazzeri, R., Galarza, M., Neroni, M., Alfieri, A., Giordano, M. 2011. Hemostatic matrix sealant in neurosurgery: A clinical and imaging study. *Acta Neurochirurgica* (Wien) 153(1): 148–154.
26. Chalmers, R.T.A., Darling, III R.C., Wingard, J.T. et al. 2010. Randomized clinical trial of tranexamic acid-free fibrin sealant during vascular surgical procedures. *British Journal of Surgery* 97(12): 1784–1789.
27. Kheirabadi, B.S., Pearson, R., Tuthill, D., Rudnicka, K., Holcomb, J.B., Drohan, W., MacPhee, M.J. 2002. Comparative study of the hemostatic efficacy of a new human fibrin sealant: Is an antifibrinolytic agent necessary? *Journal of Trauma* 52: 1107–1115.
28. Longstaff, C. 1994. Studies on the mechanisms of action of aprotinin and tranexamic acid as plasmin inhibitors and antifibrinolytic agents. *Blood Coagulation and Fibrinolysis: An International Journal in Hemostasis and Thrombosis* 5(4): 537–542.
29. Furtmuller, R., Schlag, M.G., Berger, M. et al. 2002. Tranexamic acid, a widely used antifibrinolytic agent, causes convulsions by a gamma-aminobutyric acid(A) receptor antagonistic effect. *Journal of Pharmacology and Experimental Therapeutics* 301: 168–173.
30. Bakshi, A., Bakshi, A., Banerji, A.K. 2004. Neuroendoscope-assisted evacuation of large intracerebral hematomas: Introduction of a new, minimally invasive technique. Preliminary report. *Neurosurgical Focus* 16(6): e9.
31. Keshavarz, S., MacDougall, M., Lulic, D., Kasasbeh, A., Levy, M. 2013. Clinical experience with the surgicel family of absorbable hemostats (oxidized regenerated cellulose) in neurosurgical applications: A review. *Wounds* 25(6): 160–167.
32. McCulloch, J.A., Young, P.H. 1998. Control of bleeding in microsurgery. In *Essentials of Spinal Microsurgery*, McCulloch, J.A. and Young, P.H. (eds.), pp. 69–87. Philadelphia, PA: Lippincott.
33. Zucker, W.H., Mason, R.G. 1976. Ultrastructural aspects of interactions of platelets with microcrystalline collagen. *American Journal of Pathology* 82(1): 129–142.
34. Abbott, W.M., Austen, W.G. 1974. Microcrystalline collagen as a topical hemostatic agent for vascular surgery. *Surgery* 75: 925–933.
35. Alpaslan, C., Alplaslan, G.H., Oygur, T. 1977. Tissue reaction to three subcutaneously implanted local hemostatic agents. *British Journal of Oral Maxillofacial Surgery* 35: 129–132.
36. Dias, G.J., Peplow, P.V., Teixeira, F. 2003. Osseous regeneration in the presence of oxidized cellulose and collagen. *Journal of Material Science: Materials in Medicine* 14(9): 739–745.

15 Hydroxypropyl Methyl Cellulose Grafted with Poly(Acrylamide)

Application as Novel Polymeric Material as Flocculant as well as Adsorbent

Sagar Pal, Raghunath Das, and Soumitra Ghorai

CONTENTS

15.1 POLYSACCHARIDES

Polysaccharides are polymeric carbohydrates that are created by replicating units bonded together by glycoside linkages (stereoregular polymer of monosaccharide) and consist of various degrees of branching. These are the most ecofriendly materials accessible on this planet. They are renewable (are agricultural commodities), less expensive, and hydrophilic biopolymers. They also exhibit biological and chemical properties, for instance, nontoxic (most are edible), biocompatible, biodegradable, polyfunctional characteristics, high chemical reactivity, chirality, and chelation capacities.[1] They are found in various tissues of seeds, stems, and leaves of plants, body fluids of animals, in the cell walls and extra cellular fluids of bacteria, yeast, etc.[2] Water-soluble polysaccharides (e.g., hydroxypropyl methyl cellulose (HPMC), xanthan gum, guar gum, amylopectin, dextrin, starch) have diverse industrial and agricultural applications as viscosifiers,[3,4] drag reducers,[5] flocculants,[6–8] controlled drug delivery agents,[9,10] adsorbent polymers,[11] responsive polymers, stabilizers, dispersants, water-borne polymer coatings, food additives, etc.

15.2 HYDROXYPROPYL METHYL CELLULOSE

HPMC, which comprises both hydrophobic and hydrophilic structural units,[12] is a pharmaceutically significant natural polymer. HPMC (Figure 15.1) is a modified cellulose, developed by reacting cellulose with chloromethane and epoxy propane. HPMC is having a number of hydroxypropyl groups, which promote its water solubility. Formation of superabsorbent hydrogel based on HPMC is a suitable candidate from biomaterial viewpoint because of its water solubility. It is one of the most important hydrophilic carriers used for the preparation of oral controlled drug delivery systems.[13] Because of nontoxic and excellent mechanical properties, HPMC is also used in the food industry to progress the quality of baked products,[14,15] in gluten-free breads,[16] for pioneering battered food manufacturing,[17] low-fat edible coatings,[18,19] etc., and printing technology.

However, so far, the extensive use of polysaccharides as adsorbents as well as flocculant has been inhibited because of their poor specific surface area, comparative low hydrodynamic volume, and limited potential to form H-bonding with adsorbate through extensive intramolecular chain interactions.[11] To overcome these inadequacies, recently, many attempts have been made to develop modified biopolymers in order to establish the combined functionality of the constituents.[20]

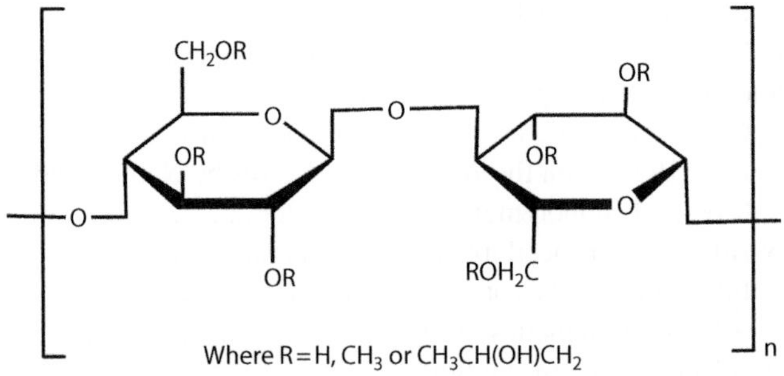

FIGURE 15.1 Structure of hydroxypropyl methyl cellulose.

Hydroxyl groups of the polysaccharide unit offer the reactive sites for the modification of biopolymer. Specifically, the grafting of long and flexible synthetic polymer chains (for instance, polyacrylamide, polyacrylonitrile, polyacrylic acid) onto natural polysaccharide backbones was found to be effective, as the developed graft copolymers may provide the advantages of both constituents.

15.3 POLYSACCHARIDE-BASED GRAFT COPOLYMERS

One of the effective techniques of modifying polysaccharide for producing functional polymeric materials is "grafting." Grafting is the branching of one type of polymer chain (usually a monomer) to the backbone of a preformed polymer (Figure 15.2). An important advantage of graft copolymerization is that the natural polymeric backbone and grafted polymeric chains (synthetic polymer) are held together by chemical bonding, permitting the two polymers to be closely connected rather than as simple physical mixtures. This increases the compatibility of new materials with hybrid characteristics. Through chemical reactions, especially crosslinking and grafting reactions, the modified polysaccharides can be used in different applications.

Different types of vinylic monomers, for example, acrylamide,[21] acrylic acid,[22] acrylonitrile,[23] methyl methacrylate,[24] and *N-tert*-butylacrylamide,[25] have been grafted to several natural polysaccharides for optimizing their commercial utilization. Grafting of vinyl monomers on natural polymer backbone improves the flocculating characteristics, in which the flexible grafted chains are able to approach the contaminants more easily. On the contrary, by introducing several hydrophobic functional groups either onto the backbone of network structure of modified polysaccharide matrix or as pendant groups through grafting technique, it is possible to develope materials with high adsorption characteristics.[1]

15.4 TECHNIQUES OF GRAFT COPOLYMERIZATION

Various grafting modification techniques onto polysaccharide backbone have been reported such as (1) the "grafting through" route, (2) the "grafting onto" route, and (3) the "grafting from" route.[26] The "grafting through" method commonly deals with copolymerizing premade vinyl functionalized polysaccharide with comonomers. The "grafting onto" method involves the presynthesis of end-functionalized linear chains, which is consequently covalently attached to the polysaccharides. But this technique generally stands with low grafting density (owing to steric hindrance) and monotonous polymerization procedures that considerably restrain its growth. In contrast, the "grafting from" technique is the most significant method where the growth of polymer chains arises directly from the polysaccharide backbone that has been widely investigated in combination with a conventional free radical procedure. Specifically, radicals can be conveniently created along with polysaccharide backbones in the existence of chemical initiators or by high-energy irradiation method. This type of copolymerization provides the opportunity of creating novel polymeric systems that eternally merge the properties of both polymer chains.[27]

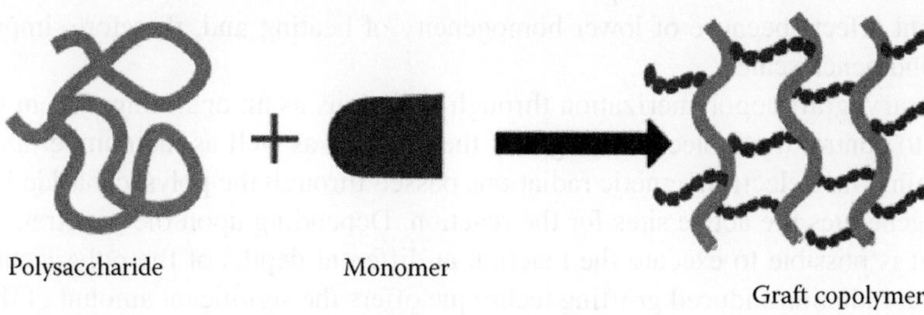

FIGURE 15.2 Schematic representation of polymer grafting.

15.4.1 Conventional Chemical Grafting Method

The conventional chemical grafting method involves the formation of graft copolymer through free radical mechanism where "grafting from" technique has been employed. In this process, the role of initiator is exceptionally critical as it determines the path of the grafting process. Here the radicals are fabricated because of the decomposition of thermal initiator (e.g., potassium persulfate (PPS), ammonium persulfate, ceric ammonium nitrate, ceric ammonium sulfate, azodiisobutyronitrile) or the oxide-redox action of redox initiator (i.e., benzoyl peroxide/dimethylaniline, $K_2S_2O_4$/ascorbic acid, H_2O_2/Fe^{+2}). In these systems, the free radicals are generated from the initiators and shifted to the substrate to form macro radicals on the polysaccharide backbone, and these radical reactive sites could initiate the vinyl groups of monomers for the chain propagation and finally form the graft copolymer.

15.4.1.1 Redox-Induced Grafting

The most frequently used initiation system is redox system as the activation energy for the redox initiation is relatively low, and it can activate the reaction under ambient state, and the reaction rate is faster.[28] Fenton's reagent (H_2O_2/Fe^{+2}) is a distinctive redox initiator used for the initiation of graft copolymerization of different monomers onto polysaccharide backbone. Though hydrogen peroxide itself acts as an initiator for graft copolymerization, the presence of reducing agent Fe^{+2} significantly enhanced the yield of graft copolymer at lower temperature because of the chelating effects of the polysaccharide with the metal ions, which promote the formation of $^{\cdot}OH$ radical in the polysaccharide backbone and accordingly reduced the opportunity for homopolymer formation, which considerably increased the purity of the grafted product.[29]

15.4.1.2 Persulfate-Induced Grafting

PPS is normally used as free radical initiator in conventional chemical grafting method since it is soluble in water and cheap as well as it is an efficient initiator for hydrogen abstraction.[30] When aqueous solution of persulfate was heated, it decomposed to create the sulfate ion radical with other radical species. In authors' laboratory, in conventional chemical grafting method using persulfate as the radical initiator via "grafting from" route, a series of polysaccharide-based graft copolymers have been synthesized.[31,32] Recently, HPMC/persulfate/acrylamide coordination system has been proposed by Das et al.,[31] where free radical sites were generated on HPMC backbone in the presence of $SO_4^{-\cdot}$ radical to form macro radicals. These active free radical sites on the backbone of HPMC react with the monomer to form graft copolymer.[31]

15.4.2 Radiation-Initiated Graft Copolymerization

Conventional chemical grafting procedures have limited potential to control the molecular weight distribution of graft copolymer. Additionally, the percentage of grafting ratio of the copolymer synthesized by this method has low reproducibility and exhibits more reaction time and suffering thermal gradient effects because of lower homogeneity of heating and, therefore, improper to be scaled up beyond bench scale.

On the contrary, graft copolymerization through radiations as an operating system permits the higher degree to control the molecular weight of the polymer as well as the number and length of the grafted chain. Once electromagnetic radiations passed through the polysaccharide backbone, it automatically generates the active sites for the reaction. Depending upon the penetrating power of the radiation, it is possible to execute the reaction at different depths of the polysaccharide backbone. Therefore, radiation-induced grafting technique offers the significant amount of the purity of grafted product because of the lack of contamination.[33]

15.4.2.1 Low-Energy Radiation-Induced Grafting

Owing to the benefits of low operation cost and mild reaction conditions, low-energy irradiations like UV and visible light via homolytic fission process (i.e., free radical formation on the polysaccharide backbone) have been broadly studied for the surface graft polymerization with the support of photo-initiator or photosensitizer like benzophenone.[34,35] Thaker and Trivedi[36] investigated photo grafting reaction of methylacrylate onto the partially carboxymethylated guar gum in solution phase by means of UV radiation along with ceric ammonium nitrate photo-initiator. However, low penetration capability of UV rays leads to nonuniform and low grafting yield.

15.4.2.2 High-Energy Radiation-Induced Grafting

High-energy radiations such as x-rays, γ-rays, or electron beam are extensively used for commercial/bulk production of the graft copolymer.[37–39] Radical formation mechanism by γ-ray irradiation has the subsequent features: for instance, radicals are generated with the aid of electron abstraction to form radical cations, in particular radical formation is concerted along the path of the incident radiation beam, and radical formation is comparatively unselective.[40] This technique exhibits a number of disadvantages in terms of its lack of specificity and complex equipment arrangement along with safety problem. Moreover, it can cause random radiation damage (radiolysis) of the backbone polymer (particularly if the backbone polymer is polysaccharide). This results the graft copolymer structure to collapse.[41–43] The methods of high-energy radiation-induced graft copolymerization are especially appropriate for fluorinated polymers, because of their exceptional stability.[44–46]

15.4.2.3 Microwave Irradiation-Induced Grafting

Microwave irradiation-based grafting has revolutionized in the field of green chemistry. Green chemistry (also known as sustainable chemistry) has appeared as a novel philosophy with the intention of diminishing (1) the utilization of nonrenewable resources and organic solvents, (2) the creation of toxic secondary products, and (3) the expenses of energy and the release of gases.[47,48] This objective might be fulfilled with the assistance of microwave irradiation-based synthesis. Microwave irradiation technique drastically decreased the exploit of toxic solvents, with shorter reaction time, higher reproducibility, promising improved yields, product selectivity (lower side reactions) compared to their conventional synthesized counterparts.[49] Moreover, microwave irradiations are capable of quickly transferring the energy into the bulk of the reaction mixture without suffering thermal gradient effects (homogeneous and selective manner), which caused the rapid interaction of the electromagnetic irradiation with the molecule in the reaction mixture, thus leading to a prospective industrial importance in the large-scale synthesis.[50] Microwave-assisted syntheses are derived from the capability of electromagnetic irradiation to excite polar molecules because of their dipolar character (dipolar polarization) or to perform charged particles, which is originating from the difference in the solvent and reactant dielectric constants.[51,52] Polysaccharides are macromolecules having numerous polar functional groups (specifically, hydroxyl, amino, carboxylic acid, and uronic acid groups) in combination with the non polar bond (C–C sequence of polymer backbone), and they could be charged or electrically neutral, depending upon the polysaccharide. Therefore, microwave irradiations affect the "selective excitation" of the polar bonds, compared to the nonpolar bonds, which in turn results to the cleavage/breakage of the polar bonds, producing the free radical active sites on the polysaccharide backbone. In lieu of the "selective excitation" properties of polysaccharide toward microwave irradiation, recently, microwave-assisted grafting technology via "grafting from" route has growing and motivated research area to the synthetic chemist. In the last few years, lots of efforts have been performed by several researchers towards graft copolymerization onto natural polymer through microwave irradiation technique, for example, polyacrylamide onto chitosan[53] and xanthan gum[54]; amino acid–based monomers onto starch[55]; methyl methacrylate onto sodium alginate,[56] acrylic acid onto Artemisia seed gum,[57] and so on. In authors' laboratory, recently, comparative investigation of microwave-assisted as well as conventional synthesis of graft copolymers based on tamarind kernel polysaccharide-*graft*-polyacrylamide[58] and carboxymethyl guar gum-*graft*-polyacrylamide[59] have been performed. In this scenario, the present chapter reflects the comparative evaluation of the application of HPMC and polyacrylamide-based graft copolymers synthesized by conventional[31] [denoted as HPMC-*g*-PAM (C)] and microwave-assisted synthesis [denoted as HPMC-*g*-PAM (M)] methods.

15.5 APPLICATION OF POLYSACCHARIDE-BASED GRAFT COPOLYMER IN WATER PURIFICATION

The global population is increasing while the accessibility of potable water is declining. In the growing world, approximately 900 million people do not have the access to safe drinking water and adequate sanitation. Worldwide, requirement of freshwater is expanding because of the mounting population, rapidly budding economic and social system, faster urbanization, and developments.[60] Removal of hazardous industrial and municipal waste, and agricultural wastes has polluted the environment. This necessitates the recycling of wastewaters and industrial effluents on a massive scale.[61] Various processes have been proposed for the removal of toxic contaminants from wastewaters and industrial effluents before its possible reuse, which includes flocculation, coagulation, adsorption processes, and so on.

15.5.1 Application in Flocculation

15.5.1.1 General Considerations on Coagulation and Flocculation

Wastewater contains solid particles along with various chemical and microbiological contaminants. Specific properties of these particles influence their behavior in liquid phases—and thus their removal abilities. Thus, the separation of suspended solids along with chemical and microbiological contaminants from aqueous environments is extremely important in the field of wastewater treatment, mineral processing, sludge dewatering, pulp and paper production, as well as in the pharmaceutical, cosmetics, metal working industries, and so on.[62,63] Among various physicochemical methods, coagulation–flocculation is an effective and widely used technique for purification and recycling of wastewater where chemical reagents are involved in a solid–liquid separation by an aggregation process of colloidal particles and regulate the stability of the disperse system.[64,65]

Coagulation of dissolved and colloidal materials in wastewater is fundamentally associated in the origin of Derjaguin–Landau–Verwey–Overbeek theory (DLVO theory) whereby coagulation refers to the process of defeating the interparticle repulsive energy barrier of the colloidal particles by increasing its ionic strength via multivalent metal ion incorporation.[66] The addition of ordinary inorganic coagulant, for example, aluminum- and iron-based materials (alum, polyaluminum chloride, ferric chloride, ferrous sulfate), plays the key role in neutralizing the surface charge of suspended particles or colloidal systems and supports the particle aggregation and settling under gravity because of the electrical double-layer compression.[67] However, this method is entirely pH dependent and reduced the alkalinity of water.[68] Besides, large quantity of the inorganic coagulants is essential to reach effective settling rate. Accordingly, large volume of metal hydroxide sludge is formed, which creates disposal problem.[69] Excluding this disposal crisis, the utilization of inorganic salts, for example, alum and polyaluminum chloride, is extremely doubtful owing to the probable impact of residual aluminum in the recycled water on Alzheimer's disease.[70]

15.5.1.2 Brief Review on Flocculation Using Synthetic, Natural, and Modified Polymers

The shortcomings of inorganic coagulants can be overcome by using synthetic flocculants,[71] which are available in various forms, that is, cationic, anionic, and nonionic. Examples of the important synthetic polymers used as flocculants are polyacrylamide, poly acrylic acid, poly(styrene sulfonic acid), and poly(diallyl dimethyl ammonium chloride) (DADMAC). These flocculants neutralized the surface charge of the hydrated colloidal particles; subsequently, interparticle repulsive forces between the approaching particles have been weakened via the formation of particle–polymer–particle bridging. Water-soluble synthetic flocculants, mainly polyacrylamide-based flocculants, with different molecular weights and charge densities showed excellent effectiveness in industries owing to the economic benefits and easy tailorability.[72] However, these synthetic polymers are not biodegradable, shear resistant, and their degraded products are considered to be harmful for health due to the discharge of toxic monomers.[73]

In view of the increasing demand for ecofriendly and healthy technologies, natural polymer-based flocculants might be applied as an alternative candidate of inorganic and synthetic polymer-based flocculants because of their biodegradability, wide range of molecular weight, renewability, wide availability, and environment-friendly nature.[74] Natural polymer-based flocculants have been even complimented as "green flocculants of the twenty-first century."[75] However, one of the main advantages of natural polysaccharide, that is, their biodegradability, appears to be a disadvantage, since it compresses their shelf-life.[72] Additionally, more dosage requirement and lower floc stability restrict the extensive utilization of natural polymers as flocculants.

Therefore, it is obvious that all polymers, be it natural or synthetic, have several drawbacks. In the last few years, lots of efforts have been made in order to combine the best properties of both natural and synthetic polymers via grafting of synthetic polymer chains onto the natural polysaccharide backbone through "grafting from" technique.[58,72,76,77] In comparison with natural or synthetic organic/inorganic flocculants, these graft copolymer–based flocculants showed controlled biodegradability, fairly shear stability, and improved functional properties.[78,79] As a tailor-made material, the dangling synthetic polymer chains of the graft copolymer have straightforward approachability in the direction of metallic and nonmetallic pollutants, and therefore they are bestowed with extremely efficient attributes.[80] In recent times, in authors' laboratory, many efforts have been focused on several grafted polysaccharide-based flocculants including amylopectin,[32] tamarind kernel polysaccharide,[58] carboxymethyl guar gum,[59] carboxymethyl starch,[81] sodium alginate,[82] chitosan,[83] and dextrin[84] for the treatment of industrial wastewaters as well as synthetic effluents. Though HPMC is an important polysaccharide from pharmaceutical standpoint, until now, without our recent investigation,[85] there is no report regarding the use of this novel hydrogel as high-performance flocculant for the treatment of synthetic effluents and industrial wastewater. Therefore, in this chapter, special attention has been focused for the comparative flocculation characteristics of HPMC-*g*-PAM synthesized by conventional and microwave-assisted technique.

15.5.1.3 Flocculation Procedure

The flocculation efficacy of the polymeric flocculant has been studied using standard jar test and settling test method. To elucidate the flocculation mechanism as well as for comparative flocculation investigation of HPMC and modified HPMCs, two different synthetic effluents (kaolin suspension and iron ore) were used.

15.5.1.3.1 Jar Test

One of the most ordinary pieces of bench test equipment observed in water treatment laboratories to identify probable coagulation–flocculation conditions in liquid suspensions is the jar test apparatus. The test is used to optimize the coagulant/flocculant dosage. A conventional jar test apparatus consists of a flocculator (Make: Gon Engineering Works, Dhanbad, India) and a turbidity meter (Digital Nephelo-Turbidity Meter 132, Systronics, India). Suspensions (0.25 wt%) of iron ore and kaolin (prepared by dispersing 1 g in 400 mL of distilled water) were utilized for the flocculation study. The suspensions were kept in 1 L beaker, and the required amount of flocculant dosage were added in solution form. The flocculant dosage was varied from 0.25 to 3 ppm. The following procedure was consistently applied: after the addition of flocculant, the suspension was stirred at a constant speed of 75 rpm for 2 min, followed by low stirring at 25 rpm for 3 min. The flocs were then allowed to settle for 15 min. Finally, after the settling period, fresh supernatant liquid was withdrawn from the top layer, and its turbidity was determined with the help of turbidity meter. The lower the turbidity, the better would be the flocculant. Distilled water was used as reference.

15.5.1.3.2 Settling/Column Test

Settling test employs a 100 mL stoppered graduated cylinder (height, 40 cm; inner diameter, 2 cm) and stopwatch. Initially, the required amount of suspension sample was taken in the cylinder, and the polymer solution was added. The cylinder was inverted 10 times for thorough mixing. After that, the cylinder was set upright, and the height of interface between supernatant water and settling solid bed was measured as a function of time.

15.5.1.4 Flocculation Study in Synthetic Wastewater

Kaolin clay is mainly used in the manufacture of cement, ceramics, paint, paper filler, chemicals, coating pigments, and rubber. Wastewater having kaolin particles is complicated to settle because of its colloidal size, anisotropic form, and repulsive interactions between negatively charged basal faces.[86] Thus, elimination of kaolinite turbidity from industrial effluent before discharge into the water bodies is a challenging issue. In contrast, hematite is the most plentiful and crucial iron-bearing mineral related to iron and steel industries. So, ecofriendly as well as safe and sound removal of these ultrafines and negatively surface-charged iron ore is another demanding topic for mining industries. In view of the growing industrial application of iron ore and kaolin suspension, we have selected these synthetic effluents for comparative flocculation study using HPMC-*g*-PAM (C) and HPMC-*g*-PAM (M) flocculants.

The flocculation efficiency of HPMC and graft copolymers synthesized by conventional and microwave-assisted methods was investigated in iron ore (Figure 15.3a) and kaolin (Figure 15.3b) suspensions with jar test method. Figure 15.3 describes the relation between flocculant dosages onto residual turbidity of the supernatant liquid. It has been observed that at low flocculant doses, the turbidity of the supernatant liquid is considerably high because limited number flocculant molecules took part in bridging the particles to form flocs. With moderate flocculant doses, additional

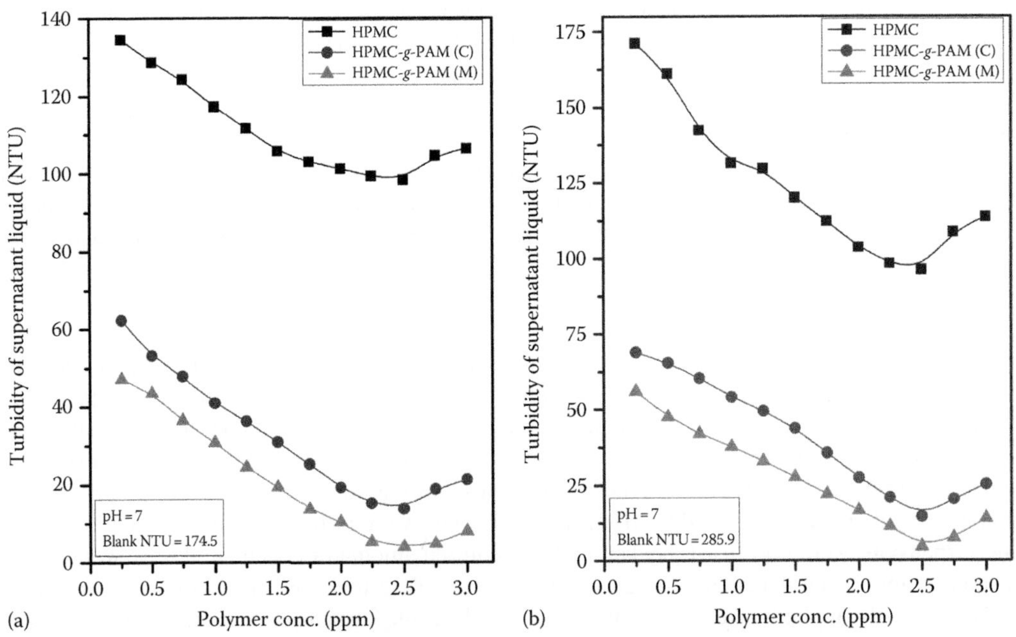

FIGURE 15.3 Effect of flocculant dosage on residual turbidity in (a) iron ore and (b) kaolin suspensions.

particles bridge together to form flocs, and consequently the turbidity of the supernatant liquid was decreased.[87] Conversely, in the overdosage region, residual turbidity of the supernatant liquid again rises owing to the steric stabilization and electrostatic repulsion.[88]

The flocculation performance of the natural and modified polymers is further verified by the settling/column test method. Settling curves (Figure 15.4) represent that in both suspensions, the fall of the interface is linear for a considerable height before it turns into retarded. The initial settling rate of the kaolin and iron ore with the addition of various flocculants was measured from the slope of the suitable linear portion (20 cm fall of the interface) of the settling curves. It has been observed that the flocculation efficacy of the polymeric flocculant is linearly associated with the settling velocity, which has been tabulated in Figure 15.4.

It is obvious from Figures 15.3 and 15.4 that in iron ore and kaolin suspensions, the graft copolymers HPMC-*g*-PAM (C) and HPMC-*g*-PAM (M) exhibit much improved flocculation properties compared to pure HPMC. The depleting flocculation behavior of HPMC could be clarified with the help of its hydrophilic nature. Hydrophilicity of HPMC retards the colloidal particle to form bridges with the noninteracting polymeric flocculant molecules.[89] In contrast, dangling flexible polyacrylamide chains on the rigid polysaccharide backbone of graft copolymers are efficient to come closer to the colloidal particles, which results in better flocculation efficiency. In addition, it is remarkable to note that graft copolymer HPMC-*g*-PAM (M) showed superior turbidity removal efficiency and better settling characteristics compared to HPMC-*g*-PAM (C). It has been scrutinized that the HPMC-*g*-PAM synthesized by microwave-assisted method exhibits enhanced% GE, higher molecular weight, superior hydrodynamic volume, and hydrodynamic radius compared to their conventional synthesized counterpart, which influence their flocculation performances. In turn, for effective bridging to arise, the polymers with longer chains would be more realistic than that with shorter chains, so that they are able to extend from one particle to another.[80] The logic behind the outstanding flocculation efficacy of the microwave-assisted graft copolymer is that "microwave dielectric effect" prevents to break the relatively nonpolar polysaccharide backbone unit; therefore, rigidity of the polysaccharide chain is preserved giving higher grafting yields selectively.

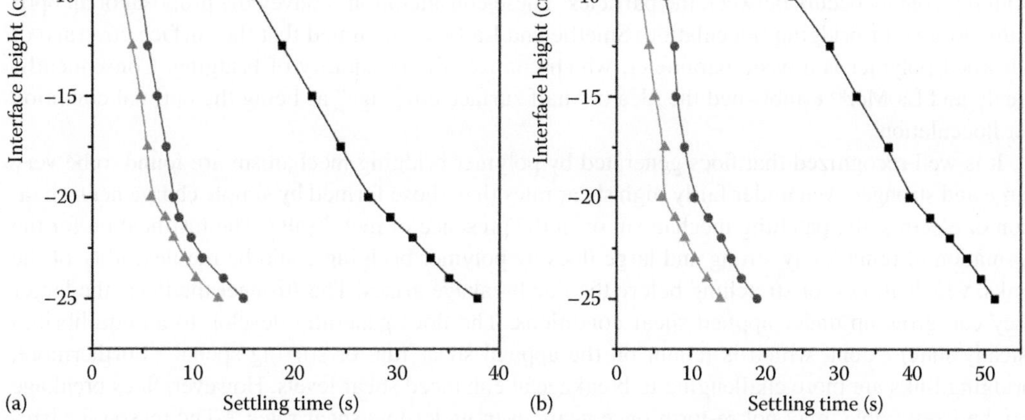

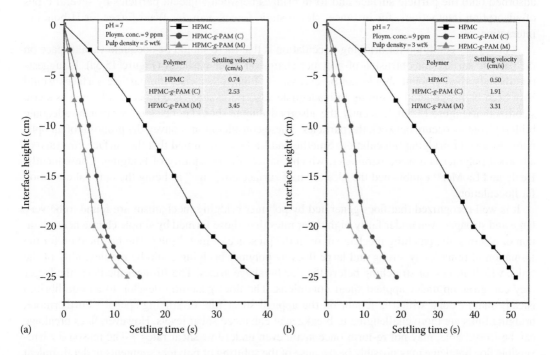

FIGURE 15.4 Settling characteristics of (a) iron ore and (b) kaolin suspensions using various flocculants.

The higher rigidity lengthens the polymer chain, and thus the pendant flexible PAM chains will be proficient to bridges with the more colloidal particles compared to the conventional one where the rigidity of the polysaccharide unit has been broken. This experimental observation again agrees with the earlier developed model (Brostow, Pal and Singh's flocculation model),[90] which highlighted that with increase in the radius of gyration, the settling rate increased, which results in better flocculation efficiency.

15.5.1.5 Flocculation Mechanism

The stability of the colloidal suspension extensively depends on the number, size, density, and surface properties of solid particles of the dispersed phase and the density of the dispersion media along with the potential difference between the stern layer and diffuse layer.[80] So, for the flocculation of colloidal stable suspension, the kinetic energy of the particles must be high enough to overcome the potential energy barrier. This potential energy barricade could be reduced via surface charge neutralization with the addition of polymeric flocculant. This interesting phenomenon of colloidal particles might be explained in light of polymer bridging mechanism (adsorption of flocculant onto the particle surface) and charge neutralization including electrostatic patch mechanism (compression of double layer).

15.5.1.5.1 Polymer Bridging Mechanism

Ruehrwein and Ward first proposed the fundamental principle of bridging flocculation in 1952.[91] They represented a model where long polymer chains were bridging between two or more particles in such a way that the loops and tails of the adsorbed polymer structure on one particle attached into solution and get connected to a second particle. The size of the tails and loops and therefore the effective thickness of the adsorbed polymer layer depend extremely on the interaction of polymer fragments with the solvent (water) and with the surface. Normally, if the interactions with the surface are moderately weak, fragments of the adsorbed chain extend further into the solution.[6] In polymer bridging, the high-molecular-weight dangling polymer chains are adsorbed onto the particle surface and form bridges between adjacent particles by several types of adsorption interactions, for instance, electrostatic forces, van der Waal forces, or H-bonding interaction.

A necessary condition for bridging flocculation is that there should be adequate vacant space on the particle surface for obtrusion of polymer chains on other particles (Figure 15.5a). It suggests that the adsorbed amount should not be excessively high; otherwise, the particle surfaces would have been highly covered, resulting in inadequate adsorption sites. The process is known as steric stabilization (Figure 15.5b). Evidently, the adsorbed amount should not be too low; then no adequate bridging contact occurs between the particles. These considerations convey the proposal of an optimum dosage for bridging flocculation. Smellie and La Mer[92] assumed that the surface coverage of adsorbed polymer is a basic parameter, which controls the possibility of bridging. Consequently, Healy and La Mer[93] established the idea of "half surface coverage" as being the optimal condition for flocculation.

It is well recognized that flocs generated by polymer bridging mechanism are found to be very large and stronger even under fairly high shear rates than those formed by simple charge neutralization or electrostatic patching mechanism or in the presence of metal salts. The justification for the formation of remarkably strong and large flocs by polymer bridging could be the flexibility of the links, which allows for stretching before the floc breakage arises. The stronger the flocs, the larger they can grow up under applied shear conditions. The flocs generally develop to an equilibrium (steady-state) extent, which is reliant on the applied shear rate or stirring speed.[94] Furthermore, bridging links are more challenging to breakage at enhanced shear levels. However, flocs breakage can be irreversible, may not re-form once again even under low shear rates.[95] The reason for irreversible floc breakage may possibly be because of the splitting of polymer segments under turbulent

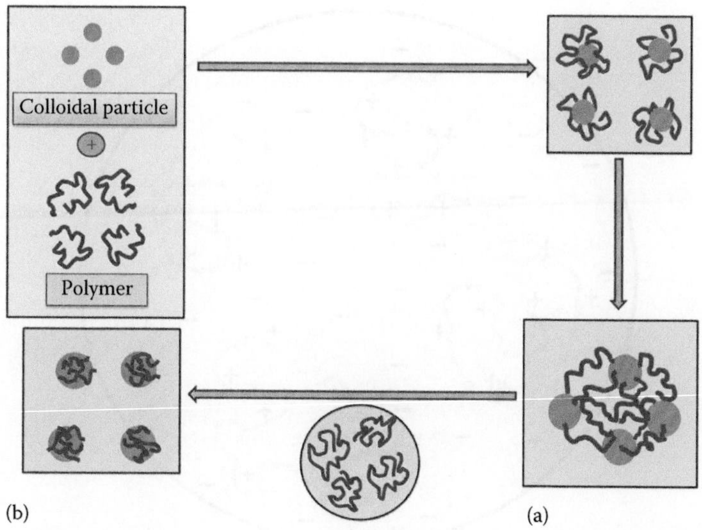

FIGURE 15.5 A schematic representation of (a) bridging flocculation and (b) restabilization by adsorbed polymer chain.

situation or the disentanglement of adsorbed polymer segments followed by re-adsorption due to the less favorable bridging interactions.[6]

It has been observed that high molecular weights of longer grafted chains are the most effective nonionic polymers for bridging. However, in case of polyelectrolytes, charge density (CD) plays a crucial role for bridging efficiency. Some degree of CD is constructive for bridging effects because of the repulsion between charged fragments, which results in the expansion and straightening of the grafted chain, and hence the better approachability towards the contaminant particles.[6] On the contrary, if the CD is extremely high, there would be complexity in adsorbing particles of the same sign of charge by the polymeric segments due to the loss of flexibility as well as rigidity behavior of the grafted chain.[72] Therefore, optimum CD for bridging flocculation is a crucial topic.

15.5.1.5.2 Charge Neutralization Mechanism

Although the bridging mechanism is effective for the flocculation of colloidal particles using nonionic and anionic polymers, this mechanism is not predominating in the case of cationic flocculants on negatively charged particles. It has been observed that electrostatic interaction between cationic polyelectrolytes and anionic colloidal particles provides strong adsorption that neutralizes the surface charge of the particles as well as decrease the electrostatic repulsion between them. High CD cationic polyelectrolytes have a tendency to adsorb in a relatively rigid configuration; therefore, there is minute possibility for bridging interaction.[6] Thus, the flocculation may probably occur by simple charge neutralization mechanism. Basically, the charge neutralization phenomenon is explained by the comparison of zeta potential measurements with flocculation results. It has been studied that optimum flocculation occurs at a particular polyelectrolyte dosages where the zeta potential is close to zero.[96] However, with further addition of polyelectrolytes, the charge reversal can occur due to the contribution of electrostatic repulsion between the particles.

15.5.1.5.3 Electrostatic Patch Mechanism

Generally, it has been investigated that quite low-molecular-weight but high CD polyelectrolytes are moderately efficient flocculants for anionic colloidal particles. For highly cationic polymers/anionic colloidal suspension coordination system, the high interaction energy supports a flattened

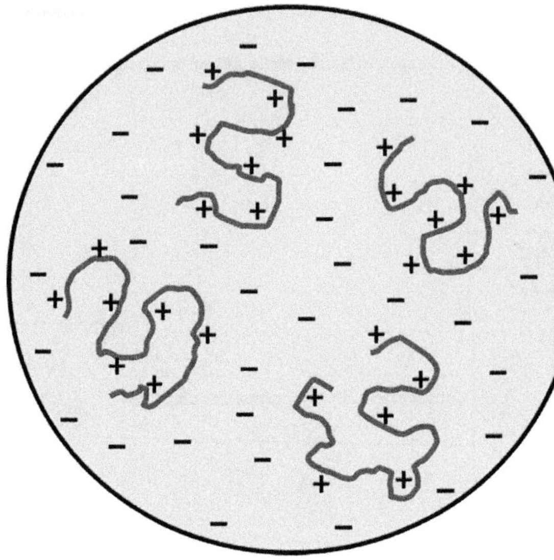

FIGURE 15.6 Schematic representation of electrostatic patch mechanism.

adsorbed configuration that decreased the construction of loops and tails for bridging the suspended particles. In such cases, surface charge particles are not neutralized individually with oppositely charged polymer segments. The charges on the polymer first create "island" patches of charges, enclosed with areas of opposite charges. Particles with polyelectrolytes adsorbed in this "patch-wise" manner can interact in such a way that oppositely charged particles of different regions come in contact, giving rise to strong electrostatic attraction, as represented schematically in Figure 15.6. Flocs formed in this process are weaker compared to bridging mechanism, but stronger than flocs produced by simple charge neutralization or in the existence of metal salts. However, in the case of "electrostatic patch" mechanism after floc breakage, re-flocculation occurs more rapidly relative to bridging mechanism.[95] Another crucial factor is ionic strength, which drastically influences the repulsive forces between charge particles via the compression of double-layer thickness, and it has been studied that higher ionic strength considerably increased the flocculation rate through polymer bridging mechanism whereas the reverse is applicable for "electrostatic patch" mechanism.

In this point of view, the major mechanistic path of flocculation by HPMC-*g*-PAM-based flocculants may possibly be explained with the help of either the charge neutralization including electrostatic patch mechanism or polymer bridging mechanism. To clarify the basic origin of flocculation mechanism, we have analyzed the zeta potential value (Figure 15.7) of HPMC-*g*-PAM (M) as well as HPMC-*g*-PAM (M)-treated synthetic effluent as a function of pH and polymer dosage. Figure 15.7a represents that both iron ore and kaolin suspensions are negatively charged over the entire pH region, while HPMC-*g*-PAM (M) has an isoelectric point at pH ~6.1. Interestingly, it has been observed that with the addition of the HPMC-*g*-PAM (M) flocculant onto colloidal suspensions (kaolin and iron ore), zeta potential value reduced, and the isoelectric point shifted towards lower pH range. However, at pH>6.1 (pHzpc), the zeta potential of the treated suspension moves toward more negative region. In the acidic pH range (below pHzpc ~6.1), the existence of CD on polymer segments creates electrostatic attraction between the positively charged graft copolymer and negatively charged colloidal particles, and hence controlling factor is the charge neutralization coupled with the "electrostatic patch" effect, which leads to the lowering of zeta potential value with better flocculation characteristics. On the other hand, in the pH range above the isoelectric point, the net charge transforms to negative and consequently strong electrostatic repulsion between the polymeric segments, and the suspended particles enhanced the negative value of zeta potential.

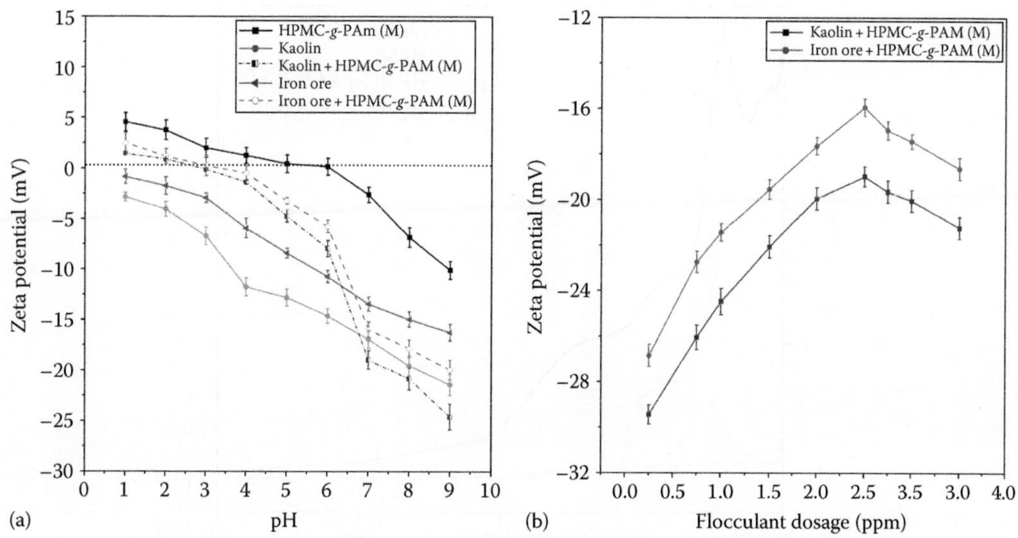

FIGURE 15.7 Effect of (a) pH and (b) flocculant dosage on zeta potential values.

Under the neutral and alkaline conditions, the morphology of the polymer chains became extensive, and more polymer loops and tail can enlarge beyond the influence of the electrical double-layer repulsion, which is cooperative for the bridging flocculation mechanism.[97] One of the important postulations of the bridging mechanism is the presence of sufficient unoccupied surface on a particle for the attachment of polymer segments. Our experimental observation also supports this demand of bridging flocculation. Figure 15.7b reflects the variation of zeta potential of suspended particles as a function of HPMC-*g*-PAM (M) flocculant dosage, at neutral pH. It has been found that the magnitude of zeta potential decreased up to optimized concentration (2.5 ppm), beyond which it was increased again. The number of active binding sites present for effective bridging on particle surface is higher at moderate polymer concentration when compared to lower concentration. In contrast, in the overdosage region, steric stabilization occurs because of the higher surface coverage and strong electrostatic repulsion between the similarly charged polymer and colloidal particles, which reduced the number of tails and loops available for bridging and hence retards the flocculation efficiency.[98] The negative zeta potential value at the optimum polymer dosage (2.5 ppm) also supports that the predominating flocculation mechanism is bridging in neutral condition.

15.5.1.6 Flocculation Study in Industrial Wastewater

Sustainable development is an idea that efforts to link the interaction between the environment and civilization. In recent years, sustainable development is gaining increased interest in recycling/reuse of industrial wastewaters with the intention of reaching the dual function of reducing economic burden as well as environmental pollution.[99] The treatment of industrial wastewaters to make them suitable for subsequent utilization required physical, chemical, and biological processes. In this perspective, the present chapter highlights the primary treatment of textile, mining, and paper industry wastewaters using modified HPMC-based graft copolymers.

15.5.1.6.1 Treatment of Textile Industry Wastewater

Textile sectors are one of the largest consumers of water and complex chemicals throughout textile processing at various processing phases. A major environmental concern connected to such a relevant economic sector is the production and release of huge amount of highly toxic wastewater. Effluent from textile industries comprised of various kinds of dyes, which are due to its high molecular weight and complex chemical structures, showed very low biodegradability and high

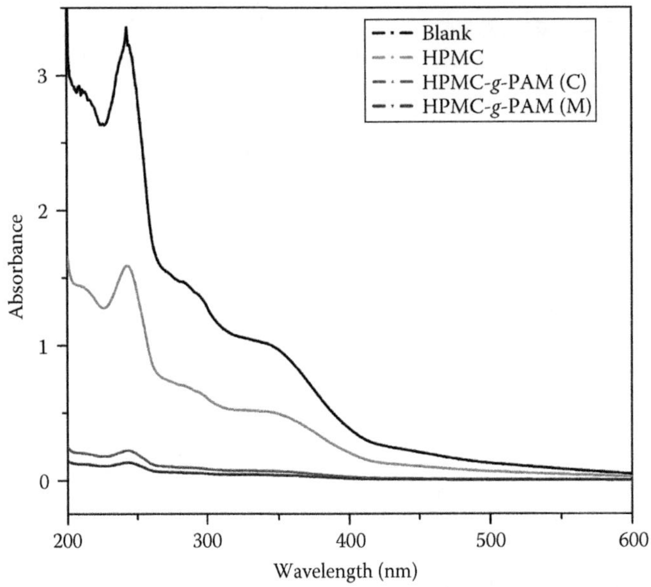

FIGURE 15.8 Comparative study of the efficiency of various flocculants in color removal from textile industry wastewater.

intensity in color.[100] Therefore, before discharging this industrial effluent into the water bodies or for possible industrial reuse, it is very crucial to remove its color by using an ecofriendly technique. From the experimental observation (Figure 15.8), it has been observed that synthesized graft copolymer HPMC-*g*-PAM (M) is a prospective candidate for the removal of color from textile industry wastewater.

15.5.1.6.2 Treatment of Paper Industry Wastewater

The paper and pulp industry is the sixth biggest industry (subsequent to oil, cement, leather, textile, and steel industries), which liberates a variety of gaseous, liquid, and solid wastes into the atmosphere.[101] Wastewater from pulp and paper mills is the major representative for aquatic pollution as it contains large amount of organic substances producing high biochemical oxygen demand and chemical oxygen demand (COD), resin acids, chlorinated organic, tannins, lignin and its derivatives,

TABLE 15.1
Effect of Flocculants for the Treatment of Paper Industry and Mine Wastewater

Flocculant	Turbidity (NTU)	TS (ppm)	TDS (ppm)	TSS (ppm)	COD (ppm)
Paper wastewater					
Without flocculant	85	798	397	401	242
HPMC	64.8	475	245	208	189
HPMC-*g*-PAM (C)	18.95	141.5	114.8	62.9	59.7
HPMC-*g*-PAM (M)	**8.65**	**84.6**	**65.5**	**32.95**	**25.65**
Mine wastewater					
Without flocculant	386.5	928.7	390.4	583.3	364.2
HPMC	281.0	599.5	325.8	273.7	304.3
HPMC-*g*-PAM (C)	25.3	167.5	129.7	37.8	112.6
HPMC-*g*-PAM (M)	**11.8**	**102.5**	**70.65**	**25.48**	**39.45**

fatty acids, suspended solids, metals, etc.[102] It is well recognized that some of these pollutants are sensitive or even chronic toxic, for instance, chlorinated organic compounds that contain dioxins and furans are the origin of genetic changes in exposed organisms.[101] Considering the adverse effects on aquatic biota and public health, we tried to find out whether HPMC-based graft copolymers can reduce the pollutant contents from paper effluent considerably or not. It is obvious that (Table 15.1) HPMC-*g*-PAM (M) notably reduces the overall pollutant content from paper industry effluent (i.e., turbidity, TS, TDS, TSS, COD).

15.5.1.6.3 Treatment of Mine Wastewater

Mine wastewater comprises a major part of the total industrial wastewaters from different sources. If discharged without proper treatment, acid mine drainage waters from mining operations can pollute the aquatic system due to the liberation of high contents of sulfate, soluble iron, and other metals and metalloids.[103] In addition, suspended and dissolved solids in mine water can obstruct the natural ecosystems by rising turbidity and decreasing light penetration.[104] These fine solids, commonly few micrometers in diameter, are enormously difficult to separate from the wastewater. This difficulty of ultrafine particle separation could be achieved by the use of HPMC-*g*-PAM (M)-based polymeric flocculant since it drastically decreased the turbidity, TS, TDS, TSS, and COD (Table 15.1) from mine wastewater.

15.5.2 Application in the Adsorption of Reactive Dyes

15.5.2.1 General Considerations on Dye Adsorption

Dyes and pigments have been an interested subject in modern years from industrial perspective. Out of various industries (for instance, textile, printing and dying, cosmetic, petroleum, and leather), an enormous amount of dyes is released by textile industries due to improper processing.[105,106] The World Bank assessed that 17%–20% of industrial water pollution occurs from textile dyeing and treatment. Water pollution with these toxic dyes is responsible for serious environmental hazard and initiates the potential danger of bioaccumulation[107,108] specifically for aquatic biosystems, where symbiotic processes might be influenced by sinking the photosynthetic activity.[109] Therefore, removal of toxic dyes from wastewaters before discharge into the water bodies appears as a foremost challenge from an ecological point of view.

Dyes are generally classified as anionic (direct, acid, and reactive dyes), cationic (basic dyes), and nonionic (dispersive dyes) in nature.[110] Reactive dyes are naturally azo-based chromophores, coupled with various kinds of reactive groups and are extensively used due to their high solubility in water, complex chemical structure, and bright colors.[111] However, most of the reactive dyes are nonbiodegradable, stable toward light, toxic to environments even at very low concentration, and human carcinogens and mutagens, as well as direct contact to this dye can cause some allergic problems.[112]

Thus, recently, the efficient decontamination of dye pollutants via reliable, straightforward, and ecofriendly techniques has acquired significant interest.[113] Conventional biological wastewater treatment method is not suitable for the dye removal because of the nonbiodegradable nature of reactive dyes. Various physicochemical techniques like electrochemical method,[114] reverse osmosis,[115] and photocatalytic degradation of dyes[116] have also been applied for the treatment of dye containing wastewater. However, these methods are often ineffective, economically unfavorable, and/or technically complicated. Out of different chemical, physical, and biological treatment processes, adsorption is a simple, economically feasible, and effective method for dye removal.[105,113]

15.5.2.2 Brief Review on the Adsorption of Dyes by Natural and Modified Biopolymers

The utilization of inexpensive and biodegradable adsorbents could be a resourceful tool from an economic as well as environmental perspective.[117,118] Therefore, particular attention has been focused on various materials like tree fern,[119] mesoporous carbon,[120] almond shell,[121] and sunflower seed hull[122] for the removal of dyes. Among those, readily accessible naturally occurring polymers, for instance, polysaccharides, are suitable alternatives as adsorbents due to its low-cost, nontoxic, and ecofriendly nature.[117] However, until now, the use of polysaccharides as adsorbents was restricted due to their poor specific surface area, comparatively low hydrodynamic volume, and limited potential to form H-bonding with dyes owing to widespread intramolecular chain interactions.[11] To compensate these inadequacies, recently, many attempts have been performed to develop modified natural polymer-based adsorbents that incorporate the combined functionality of both components.[123,124] Especially, the grafting of elongated and flexible synthetic polyacrylamide chains onto polysaccharide backbones was favorable, since the resultant graft copolymers could merge the benefits of both ingredients.[125] These polyacrylamide-modified natural polymers represent a remarkable and attractive alternative as adsorbents due to their macromolecular superstructure and flexibility of polymer chains, potential physicochemical characteristics, high chemical stability and reactivity of the functional group, as well as outstanding selectivity toward aromatic compounds because of the existence of dye chelating polyfunctionality ($-CONH_2$/–OH) behavior.

Considering these versatile properties of polyacrylamide and natural polymer-based graft copolymers, several attempts have been carried out in the past by various researchers in the field of adsorption, for instance, microwave-enhanced synthesis of chitosan-*graft*-polyacrylamide for the removal of Ca^{+2} and Zn^{+2} by Singh et al.,[53] graft copolymerization of acrylamide onto chitosan through conventional route for Cu^{+2} adsorption from water by Al-Karawi et al.,[126] and persulfate/ascorbic acid–initiated synthesis of chitosan-*graft*-poly(acrylamide) for azo dye removal from aqueous solutions by Singh et al.[125] have been studied recently. It has been mentioned before the significance of HPMC as a polysaccharide in biomedical application; however, so far by using this polysaccharide, no attempt has been performed towards the application in adsorption. Therefore, the modification of HPMC-based graft copolymer in adsorption purpose has been carried out. In the present chapter, special attention has been focused on the comparative adsorption study of the reactive blue 4 (RB 4) and reactive black 5 (RB 5) dyes from aqueous solution using conventional and microwave-assisted HPMC-*g*-PAM graft copolymer. It has been observed that HPMC-*g*-PAM (M) showed much better adsorption efficiency for the uptake of RB 4 and RB 5 than that of HPMC-*g*-PAM (C). The detailed investigation of the effect of adsorption parameters, adsorption kinetics, isotherm, thermodynamics, and reusability study of HPMC-*g*-PAM (M) has been executed. Furthermore, the origin of high adsorption properties of dyes on the HPMC-*g*-PAM (M) adsorbent is clarified on the basis of H-bonding interactions.

15.5.2.3 Adsorption Procedure

RB 4 is an anthraquinone-based chlorotriazine dye (Figure 15.9a), which is significant in the dyeing of cellulosic fabrics.[127] On the other hand, reactive RB 5 is a black bisazo reactive vinylsulfonyl dye (Figure 15.9b), specifically applied to dye urea- and sodium bicarbonate-padded cotton using steam or dry heat for fixing.[128] The formula, molecular weight, and λ_{max} of the RB 4 and RB 5 dyes are $C_{23}H_{14}N_6O_8Cl_2S_2$, 637 g mol^{-1}, and 592 nm; and $C_{26}H_{21}N_5Na_4O_{19}S_6$, 991 g mol^{-1}, and 598 nm, respectively.

The adsorption experiments of aqueous solution of RB 4 and RB 5 dyes were performed on a thermostated orbital shaker (Rivotek, Kolkata, India). The experimental parameters (e.g., solution pH, temperature, contact time, initial concentration of dye, and adsorbent dosage) were varied to achieve the optimized adsorption condition. A stock solution of 1000 mg L^{-1} dyes was prepared in double-distilled deionized water. In all typical batch study, required amount of adsorbent was thoroughly mixed with 25 mL of dye solution, whose concentration was known formerly. The samples were collected from the shaker at certain time intervals, and the dye solution was separated from the adsorbent by centrifugation (centrifuge make: REMI; model R-24) at 10,000 rpm for 10 min, and the absorbance was determined using a UV–Vis spectrophotometer (Make: Shimadzu, Japan; Model: UV 1800).

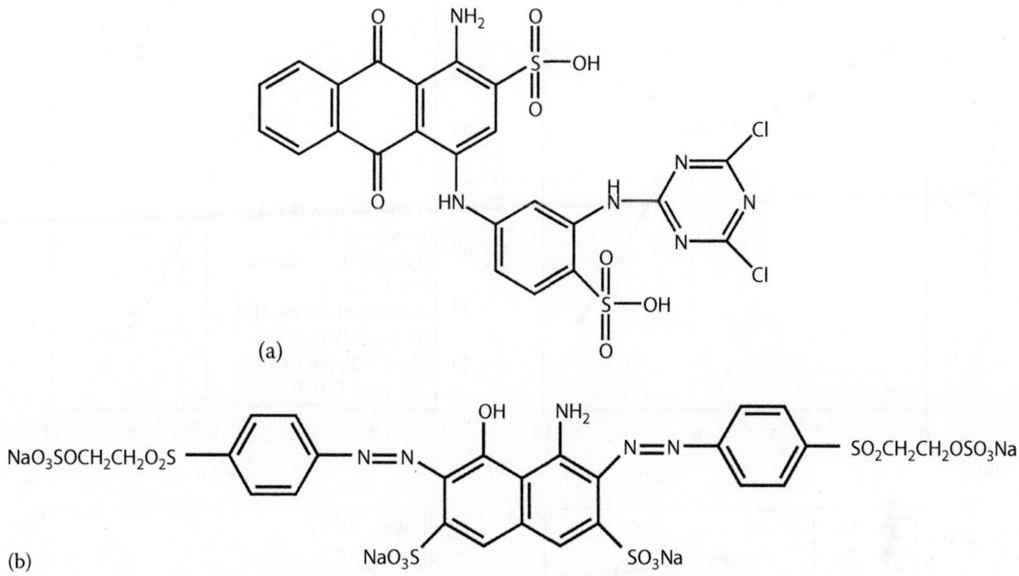

FIGURE 15.9 Chemical structure of (a) reactive blue 4 and (b) reactive black 5 dyes.

The percentage adsorption of dye was calculated using the following equation:

$$\%\,\text{Adsorption} = \frac{C_0 - C_e}{C_0} \times 100 \tag{15.1}$$

And the equilibrium uptake was calculated using the following equation:

$$q_e = (C_0 - C_e) \times \frac{V}{W} \tag{15.2}$$

where

q_e is the equilibrium capacity of dye on the adsorbent (mg g^{-1})
C_0 is the initial concentration of dye solution (mg L^{-1})
C_e is the equilibrium concentration of dye solution (mg L^{-1})
V is the volume of dye solution used (L)
W is the weight of adsorbent (g) used

All the batch experiments were performed in triplicate, and results represented here are the average of three readings.

15.5.2.4 Influence of Adsorption Parameters

The efficiency of dye adsorption from aqueous solution using an adsorbent depends on pH, equilibrium time of adsorption, temperature of the solution, amount of adsorbent dosage, and initial concentration of the dye. The details of the effect of various parameters on percentage adsorption have been explained in Figure 15.10.

The optimized adsorption condition for maximum specific removal (Q_{max} = 103.09 mg g^{-1}) of RB 4 dye was pH, 1; time, 50 min; temperature, 313 K; adsorbent dosage, 50 mg/25 mL; and initial dye concentration, 100 ppm; and for RB 5 dye (Q_{max} = 149.25 mg g^{-1}), the optimized condition was pH, 2; time, 60 min; temperature, 318 K; adsorbent dosage, 40 mg/25 mL; and initial dye concentration, 150 ppm. Here it is worth to mention that point to zero charge of HPMC-*g*-PAM (M) was 6.1.

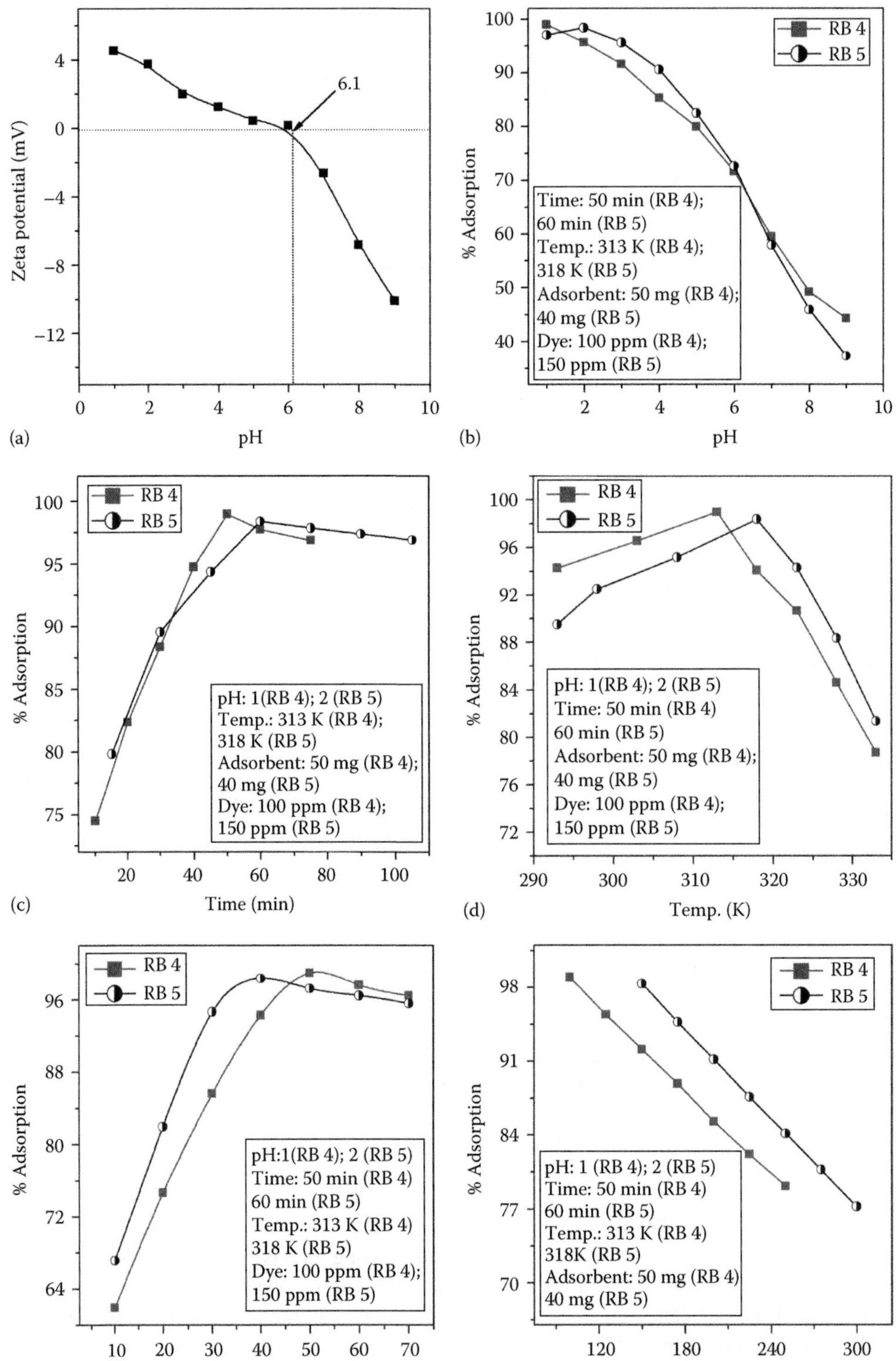

FIGURE 15.10 (a) Effect of pH on the zeta potential of HPMC-*g*-PAM (M) and effect of (b) pH, (c) time, (d) temperature, (e) adsorbent dosage, and (f) initial dye concentration on the adsorption efficiency of RB 4 and RB 5 from aqueous solution using HPMC-*g*-PAM (M).

15.5.2.5 Adsorption Kinetics Study

An excellent adsorbent should exhibit a rapid adsorption rate. Therefore, the rate of adsorption is another crucial issue for the selection of the adsorbent, and adsorption kinetics is important since it described how fast the adsorption takes place and also provides the idea about controlling factors of the adsorption rate. The rate of dye adsorption is controlled by the contact time of the solid and liquid phase and diffusion processes. During the adsorption process, adsorbate molecules passed through several stages like migration of adsorbate molecules to the external surface of adsorbent particles, molecular diffusion in the boundary layer, and solute movement from the particle surface into the internal site via pore diffusion.[129] Hence, to investigate the adsorption kinetics and realize the mechanism of adsorption, pseudo first order,[130] pseudo second order,[131] second order,[132] and intraparticle diffusion[133] kinetics models were studied.

The Legergren pseudo-first-order rate equation is given as follows:

$$\log(q_e - q_t) = \log q_e - \frac{K_1}{2.303}t \tag{15.3}$$

where

q_e and q_t (mg g^{-1}) refer to the dye adsorbed at equilibrium and t (time), respectively

K_1 (min^{-1}) indicates the rate constant

Figure 15.11a illustrates the result of the plots of log $(q_e - q_t)$ vs. t, and the parameters K_1, q_e, and correlation coefficient (R^2) are reported in Table 15.2.

The linear form of the pseudo-second order kinetic rate equation is expressed as

$$\frac{t}{q_t} = \frac{1}{K_2 q_e^2} + \frac{t}{q_e} \tag{15.4}$$

where K_2 (g mg^{-1} min^{-1}) is the pseudo-second-order rate constant. Figure 15.11b shows the plot of t/q_t vs. t, and the parameters K_2, q_e, and R^2 are listed in Table 15.2.

The third model is the second-order rate equation and is represented as

$$\frac{1}{(q_e - q_t)} = \frac{1}{q_e} + K_3 t \tag{15.5}$$

where K_3 is the second-order rate constant (g mg^{-1} min^{-1}). Figure 15.11c demonstrates the plot of $1/(q_e - q_t)$ vs. t, and the parameters K_3, q_e, and R^2 have been reported in Table 15.2.

The intraparticle diffusion kinetics model of Weber and Morris has been represented in Figure 15.11d, and the linear form of this equation is

$$q_t = K_4 t^{1/2} + C \tag{15.6}$$

where

K_4 (mg g^{-1} min$^{-1/2}$) is an intraparticle diffusion rate constant

C is the boundary layer thickness

the parameters $K_4 q_e$, and R^2 has been given in Table 15.2

The fits of the experimental results (Table 15.2) showed that the pseudo-second-order model possesses a higher correlation coefficient (R^2), compared to the pseudo-first-order and second-order models. This indicates that adsorption kinetic process might follow a pseudo-second-order model

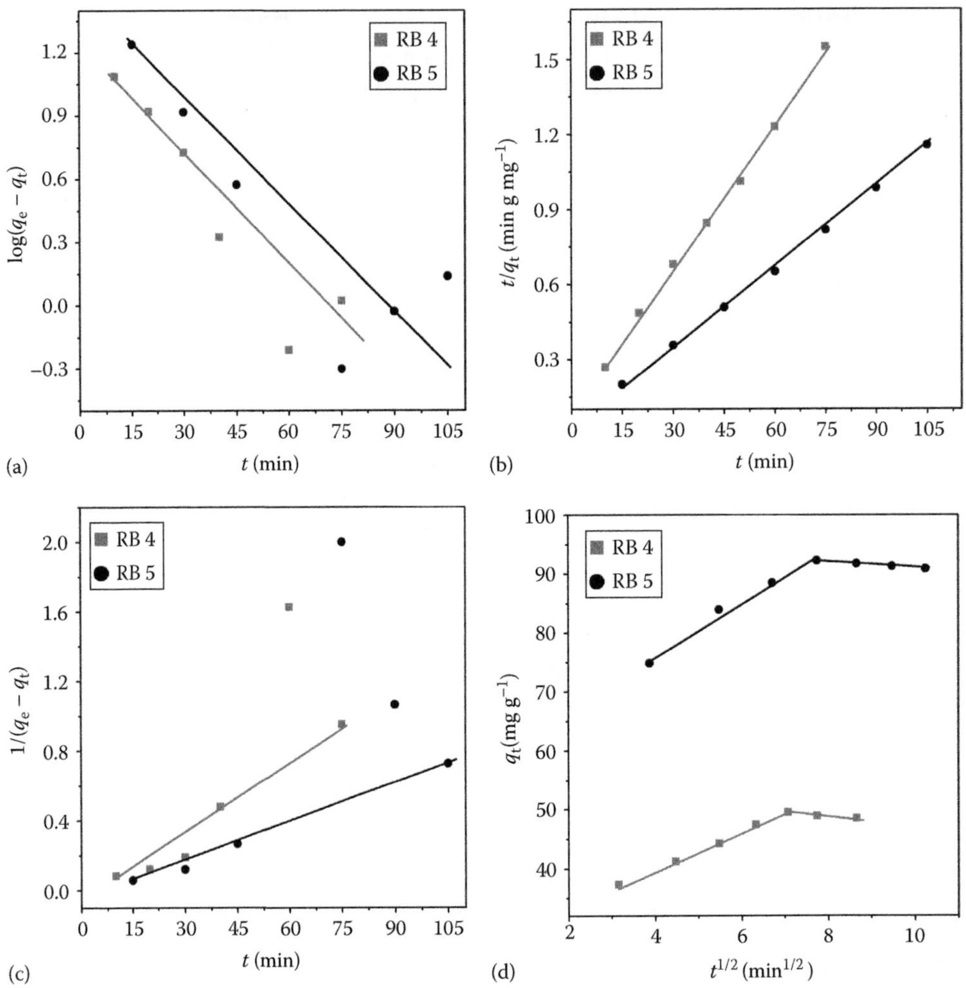

FIGURE 15.11 Modeling of the adsorption kinetics of RB 4 (100 ppm) and RB 5 (150 ppm) dyes using (a) pseudo first order, (b) pseudo second order, (c) second order, and (d) intraparticle diffusion models onto HPMC-*g*-PAM (M) adsorbent.

and is dependent on the amount of solute adsorbed on the surface of adsorbent and the amount adsorbed at equilibrium. This also signifies that the adsorption of dye possibly occurs via surface exchange reactions until the surface functional sites are completely engaged. On the contrary, the plots of q_t vs. $t^{1/2}$ (Figure 15.11d) are multilinear, including at least two linear segments. The first sharp phase represents boundary layer diffusion due to the mass transfer from the dye solution to the external surface of graft copolymer. The second portion indicates a gradual adsorption step, corresponding to intraparticle diffusion of dye molecules.[134] Actually two types of diffusion mechanisms, that is, pore diffusion (diffusion inside the pore volume) and surface diffusion (diffusion along the surface of the pores) occur in parallel within the adsorbent particle throughout adsorption process. However, if the plot of q_t vs. $t^{1/2}$ is passed through the origin, then intraparticle diffusion is the only rate-limiting step.[135] Besides, the plots have an intercept value (Table 15.2), which indicates about the thickness of the boundary layer. Therefore, the presence of multilinearity and boundary layer thickness suggests that in combination with intraparticle diffusion model, some other mechanism

TABLE 15.2
Kinetic Parameters for the Adsorption of RB 4 (100 ppm) and RB 5 (150 ppm) Dye Using HPMC-*g*-PAM (M) Adsorbent

		Dye	
Order of Reaction	**Parameter**	**RB 4**	**RB 5**
Pseudo first order	K_1 (min^{-1})	4.52×10^{-2}	3.32×10^{-2}
	q_e (mg g^{-1})	17.63	19.52
	R^2	0.8419	0.6938
Pseudo second order	K_2 (g mg^{-1} min^{-1})	4.39×10^{-3}	3.19×10^{-3}
	q_e (mg g^{-1})	52.03	94.79
	R^2	0.9973	0.9989
Second order	K_3 (g mg^{-1} min^{-1})	2.05×10^{-2}	1.34×10^{-2}
	q_e (mg g^{-1})	43.67	54.67
	R^2	0.6063	0.2632
Intraparticle diffusion	K_4 (mg g^{-1} min$^{0.5}$)	2.26	2.44
	C (mg g^{-1})	31.43	69.41
	R^2	0.8523	0.7199

could also contribute a significant role in the adsorption process. Therefore, it is believed that both surface adsorption and intraparticle diffusion took place simultaneously.

15.5.2.6 Adsorption Isotherm Study

Equilibrium data, generally identified as adsorption isotherm, are fundamentally significant to optimize the design of adsorption systems. Adsorption isotherm is the equilibrium relationship between the concentration of adsorbate in the bulk and concentration of the adsorbent particles in the surface at a given temperature. The adsorption isotherm shows how the adsorbate molecules are distributed between the liquid phase and the solid phase, and provides a comprehensive understanding of the nature of interaction. Therefore, to disclose the interactive behavior between the adsorbent and adsorbate molecules, the Langmuir and Freundlich isotherm models (Figure 15.12) have been applied in this study. The parameters obtained from these models (Table 15.3) provide essential information on the surface properties of the adsorbent and its affinity toward the adsorbate.

The Langmuir model assumes uniform energies of adsorption on structurally homogeneous surface of adsorbent with identical specific binding sites, and no transmigration between the adsorbed species occurs.[136] The linear expression of the Langmuir model is

$$\frac{C_e}{q_e} = \frac{1}{b \cdot Q_0} + \frac{C_e}{Q_0} \tag{15.7}$$

where

C_e is the equilibrium concentration of adsorbate (mg L^{-1})
q_e is the amount of dye adsorbed by the modified polymer at equilibrium (mg g^{-1})
Langmuir constant Q_0 (mg g^{-1}) signifies the maximum adsorption capacity
b (L mg^{-1}) is related to the free energy and affinity of adsorption

Figure 15.12a and c shows the linear plot of C_e/q_e against C_e for Langmuir isotherm, and the parameters Q_{max}, b, and R^2 are listed in Table 15.3.

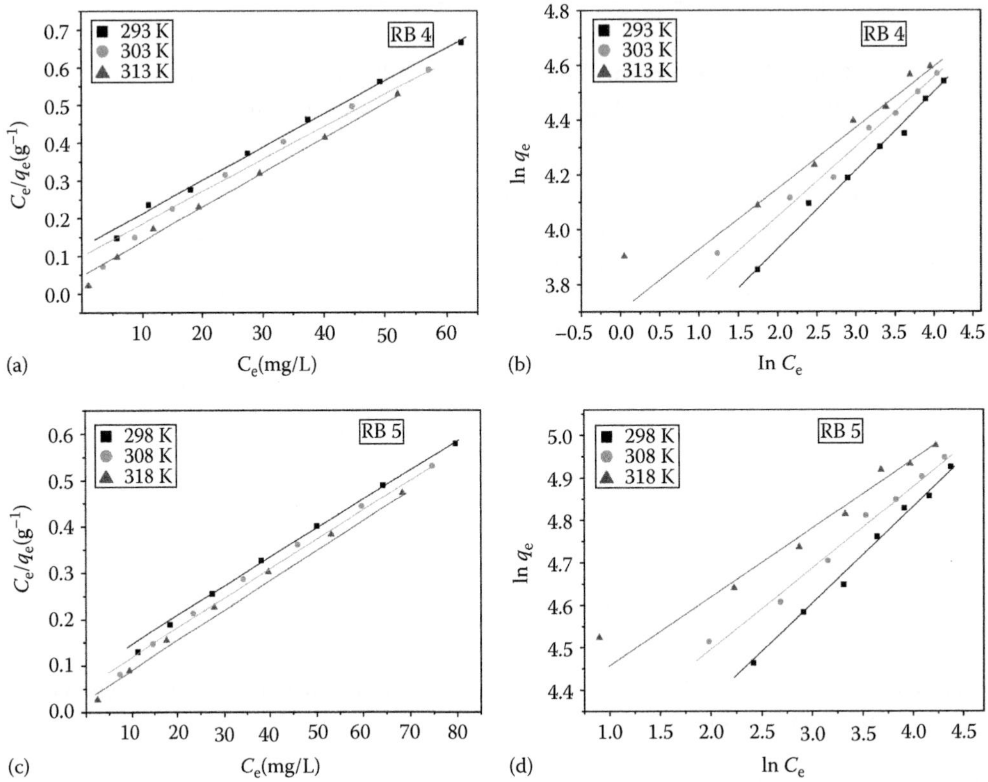

FIGURE 15.12 (a) Langmuir model for RB 4, (b) Freundlich model for RB 4, (c) Langmuir model for RB 5, and (d) Freundlich model for RB 5 using HPMC-*g*-PAM (M) at different temperatures.

TABLE 15.3
Parameters for Langmuir and Freundlich Isotherms for RB 4 and RB 5 Dyes Using HPMC-*g*-PAM (M) Adsorbent

		Langmuir Model			Freundlich Model		
Dye	**Temperature (K)**	Q_{max} (mg g^{-1})	b (L mg^{-1})	R^2	K_f (mg g^{-1})	n	R^2
Reactive blue 4	293	103.09	0.1054	0.9862	28.45	3.46	0.8475
	303	104.17	0.1429	0.9885	34.65	4.01	0.8949
	313	105.26	0.1987	0.9915	46.46	5.55	0.8028
Reactive black 5	298	149.25	0.0967	0.9939	48.89	4.20	0.8728
	308	151.52	0.1323	0.9949	59.38	5.02	0.8629
	318	153.85	0.1982	0.9968	78.65	7.21	0.8094

The feasibility of the adsorption process is calculated by the dimensionless constant, called separation factor (R_L),[137] which is defined by the following equation:

$$R_L = \frac{1}{1 + b \cdot C_0} \tag{15.8}$$

where C_0 is the initial dye concentration (mg L^{-1}). The value of R_L indicates the category of the isotherm to be either unfavorable ($R_L > 1$), linear ($R_L = 1$), irreversible ($R_L = 0$), or favorable ($0 < R_L < 1$).

The Freundlich model is based on the assumption of heterogeneous adsorption surface with energetically different sorption sites of multilayer sorption process. The linear form of the Freundlich model is[138]

$$\ln q_e = \ln K_f + \frac{1}{n} \ln C_e \tag{15.9}$$

where K_f (mg g^{-1}) and n are the Freundlich constants related to the capacity of sorption and favorability of sorption, respectively. Figure 15.12b and d represents the linear plots of ln q_e vs. ln C_e for Freundlich isotherm, and the parameters n, K_f, and R^2 are listed in Table 15.3. Generally, as the K_f value increased, the adsorption capacity of the adsorbent was enhanced. The values in the range of $0 < n < 10$ indicates favorable adsorption process. If "n" is close to 1, the surface heterogeneity might be less important, and as "n" approached to 10, the surface heterogeneity became more significant.

It is evident from Figure 15.12 that Langmuir isotherm proved to be a better mathematical fit for equilibrium data compared to Freundlich model (based on the higher correlation coefficient, i.e., R^2 value as reported in Table 15.3). Also, investigation has been performed at various temperatures, which shows that the adsorption is unilayer. The Freundlich constant values increased with increasing temperature, suggesting that dye adsorption process is endothermic in nature. The value of Langmuir constant "b" also increased with temperature, which suggests the stronger affinity between the active sites of the adsorbent and adsorbate, and also between the adjacent molecules of the adsorbed phase at higher temperature in contrast to lower temperature. At an RB 4 dye concentration of 100 mg L^{-1}, R_L was calculated to be 0.0479 at 313 K, and in the case of 150 mg L^{-1} RB 5 dye concentration, the value of R_L was found to be 0.0325. This further supports the Langmuir adsorption isotherm model. From Langmuir equation, for RB 4, Q_{max} was found to be 105.26 mg g^{-1} at 313 K, and in the case of RB 5, Q_{max} = 153.85 mg g^{-1} at 318 K (Table 15.3). This indicates that the HPMC-*g*-PAM (M) exhibits high adsorption capacity to remove the reactive dye molecules from aqueous solution.

15.5.2.7 Adsorption Thermodynamics Study

In order to realize the spontaneity of RB 4 and RB 5 adsorption on HPMC-*g*-PAM (M), the thermodynamic parameters were measured using Van't Hoff's equation as

$$\ln b = \frac{\Delta S^0}{R} - \frac{\Delta H^0}{RT} \tag{15.10}$$

$$\Delta G^0 = \Delta H^0 - T\Delta S^0 \tag{15.11}$$

where

ΔG^0 is the change in standard Gibbs free energy (J mol^{-1})
ΔH^0 is the change in enthalpy (J mol^{-1})
ΔS^0 is the change in entropy (J mol^{-1} K^{-1})
R is the universal gas constant (8.314 J K^{-1} mol^{-1})
b is the Langmuir constant at temperature T (K)

The values of ΔS^0 and ΔH^0 have been evaluated from the intercept and slope of plot between ln b vs. $1/T$ (Figure 15.13), and the parameters are reported in Table 15.4. Evaluation of these parameters provides an insight into the probable mechanisms of the adsorption process. Negative values of ΔG^0 exhibit the practicability and spontaneous nature of the adsorption process. It may be noted that for reactive dyes (RB 4 and RB 5), with enhancement in temperature, the ΔG^0 values gradually decreased, which suggests the stronger adsorptive force between adsorbent and adsorbate molecules as well as higher degree of spontaneity at elevated temperature. The positive

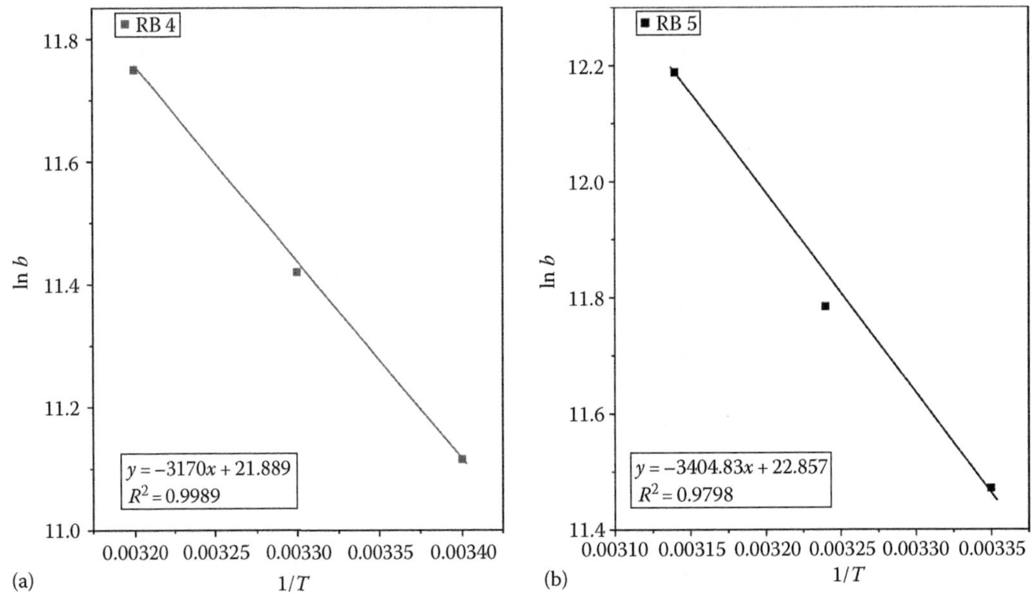

FIGURE 15.13 Thermodynamic study for the adsorption of (a) RB 4 dye and (b) RB 5 dye using HPMC-*g*-PAM (M) adsorbent.

TABLE 15.4
Thermodynamic Parameters for Adsorption of RB 4 and RB 5 Dye Using HPMC-*g*-PAM (M) Adsorbent

Dye	Temperature (K)	ΔG^0 (kJ mol^{-1})	ΔH^0 (kJ mol^{-1})	ΔS^0 (kJ mol^{-1} K^{-1})
Reactive blue 4	293	−26.991	26.335	0.182
	303	−28.811		
	313	−30.631		
Reactive black 5	298	−28.313	28.307	0.190
	308	−30.213		
	318	−32.113		

value of enthalpy change (ΔH^0) confirmed the endothermic nature of the dye sorption process.[139] The positive values of ΔS^0 reveal the increased randomness (higher degree of freedom) at the solid–liquid interface during the adsorption of reactive dye molecules on the specific active sites of HPMC-*g*-PAM (M).[123]

15.5.2.8 Regeneration Study

An efficient adsorbent should not only acquire superior adsorption capacity, but also possess excellent desorption characteristics, which would make the process economically viable. Desorption of adsorbate from the adsorbent is of paramount significance, because (1) it allows the reusability of adsorbent, (2) it permits the recovery of pollutants, (3) it minimizes the production of secondary wastes, (4) it decreases the process cost, and (5) it lets understand the mechanism of adsorption process.[140] Therefore, to determine the reusability of the HPMC-*g*-PAM (M) as an adsorbent, desorption experiment was executed with 25 mL of 100 ppm RB 4 solution mixed with 50 mg of HPMC-*g*-PAM (M) for 50 min at 313 K temperature, and for RB 5, the desorption condition

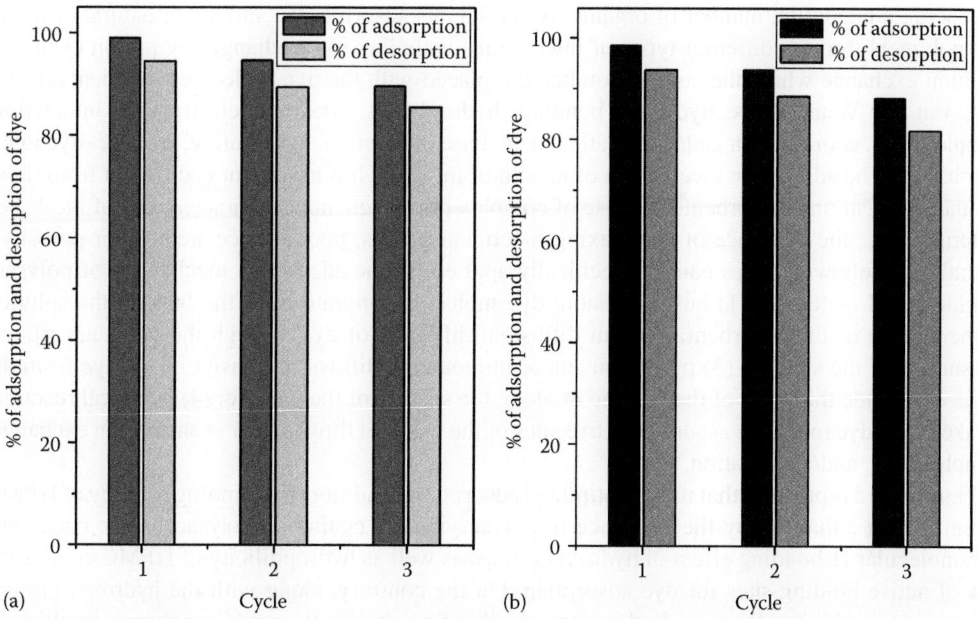

FIGURE 15.14 Reusability study of HPMC-*g*-PAM (M) adsorbent using (a) RB 4 and (b) RB 5 dyes.

was followed as given: dye concentration, 150 ppm; adsorbent dosage, 40 mg/25 mL; contact time, 60 min; and temperature, 318 K. The dye-loaded samples were separated by centrifugation followed by filtration and washed gently with a small amount of distilled water to remove any unadsorbed dye. The samples were dried entirely and utilized for the desorption study. The percentage desorption was calculated using the following equation[141]:

$$\% \text{ Desorption} = \frac{\text{Concentration desorbed (mg L}^{-1}\text{)}}{\text{Concentration adsorbed (mg L}^{-1}\text{)}} \times 100 \tag{15.12}$$

pH 2, pH 7, and pH 10 media were used to find out the maximum desorption percentage of dye from the modified HPMC-based material. Out of three solutions, maximum percent desorption was achieved in an alkaline environment (pH = 10, 94.45% for RB 4 and 93.65% for RB 5), and minimum percent desorption was observed in an acidic environment (pH = 2, 33.95% for RB 4 and 30.28% for RB 5). This explains that the opposite trend of the adsorption process with pH was followed, as should be the case. Hence, to determine the reusability of the adsorbent, three consecutive adsorption–desorption cycles were performed with pH 10 as the stripping solution. It has been found that 85.48% of RB 4 and 81.67% of RB 5 were desorbed after the third cycle (Figure 15.14). Hence, it can be concluded that HPMC-*g*-PAM (M) adsorbent showed excellent recycling ability for the treatment of reactive RB 4 and RB 5 dyes from aqueous solution.

15.5.2.9 Mechanism of Adsorption Study

A major challenge in the field of adsorption is to clearly recognize the mechanism by which target contaminants are adsorbed by the adsorbent, specifically the interactions which occur at the adsorbent/adsorbate interface. It is reported by different researchers that various factors influence the dye adsorption mechanism, for instance, functional behavior and structure of adsorbate molecule, textural properties and surface of the adsorbent, and specific interaction of adsorbent with adsorbate. In addition, adsorption mechanism was extensively controlled by wide range of factors such as solution pH, salt concentrations, and the nature of the functional groups present on the adsorbent.

In general, a maximum number of organic dye pollutants adsorb to the surface of natural or modified polymers through different types of interactions including ion exchange (by proton exchange or anion exchange where the counter ion being replaced with the dye molecule), physical adsorption, van der Waal forces, hydrogen bonding, hydrophobic attraction, electrostatic interaction, complexation, coordination and/or chelation, acid–base interaction, aggregation, and dye–dye interaction.[117,140] The adsorption mechanism of natural or modified bio-adsorbent is different from those of other conventional adsorbents because of complex physicochemical characteristics of bio-based materials (e.g., the existence of complexing functional groups, poor surface area, lower porosity). Overall, the following steps can be specifically applied for the adsorption mechanism of polysaccharide-based materials: (1) bulk diffusion: dye molecules migrate from the bulk of the solution to the surface of the adsorbent; (2) film diffusion: diffusion of dye through the boundary film to the surface of the sorbent; (3) pore diffusion or intraparticle diffusion: transfer of the dye from the surface to inside the pores of the particle or along the surface of the particle; (4) chemical reaction: uptake of the dye molecule at surface active sites of the material through, for example, ion exchange, complexation, and/or chelation.[117]

Figure 15.15 represents that under optimized adsorption condition, dye binding efficacy of HPMC is remarkably enhanced by the existence of polyacrylamide chains on polysaccharide backbone. Intramolecular H-bonding effect of hydroxyl groups as well as hydrophilicity of HPMC creates the lack of active binding sites for dye adsorption. On the contrary, along with the hydroxyl groups, amide groups additionally provide the active dye binding sites in the graft copolymer resulting in higher adsorption effectiveness. Further, the HPMC-*g*-PAM (M) exhibits superior adsorption characteristics for the RB 4 and RB 5 compared to graft copolymer synthesized by conventional grafting method. This phenomenon can be explained by the higher selectivity as well as higher percentage grafting efficiency and superior hydrodynamic radius of the microwave-synthesized product. This also further confirmed the role of flexible and elongated PAM chains toward dye adsorption.

On the basis of experimental results, we proposed a probable schematic representation of the interaction of reactive dye molecules with polyacrylamide-grafted HPMC (Figure 15.16). Thus, it is believed that H-bonding interaction between the polysaccharide hydroxyl groups, amide groups

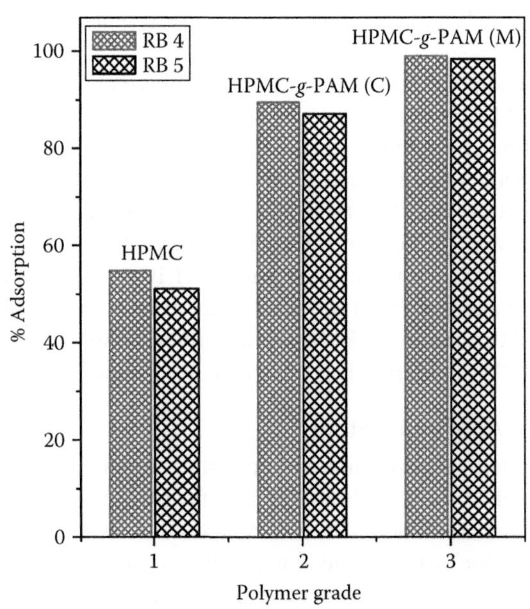

FIGURE 15.15 RB 4 and RB 5 dye adsorption efficiency of different-grade polymers.

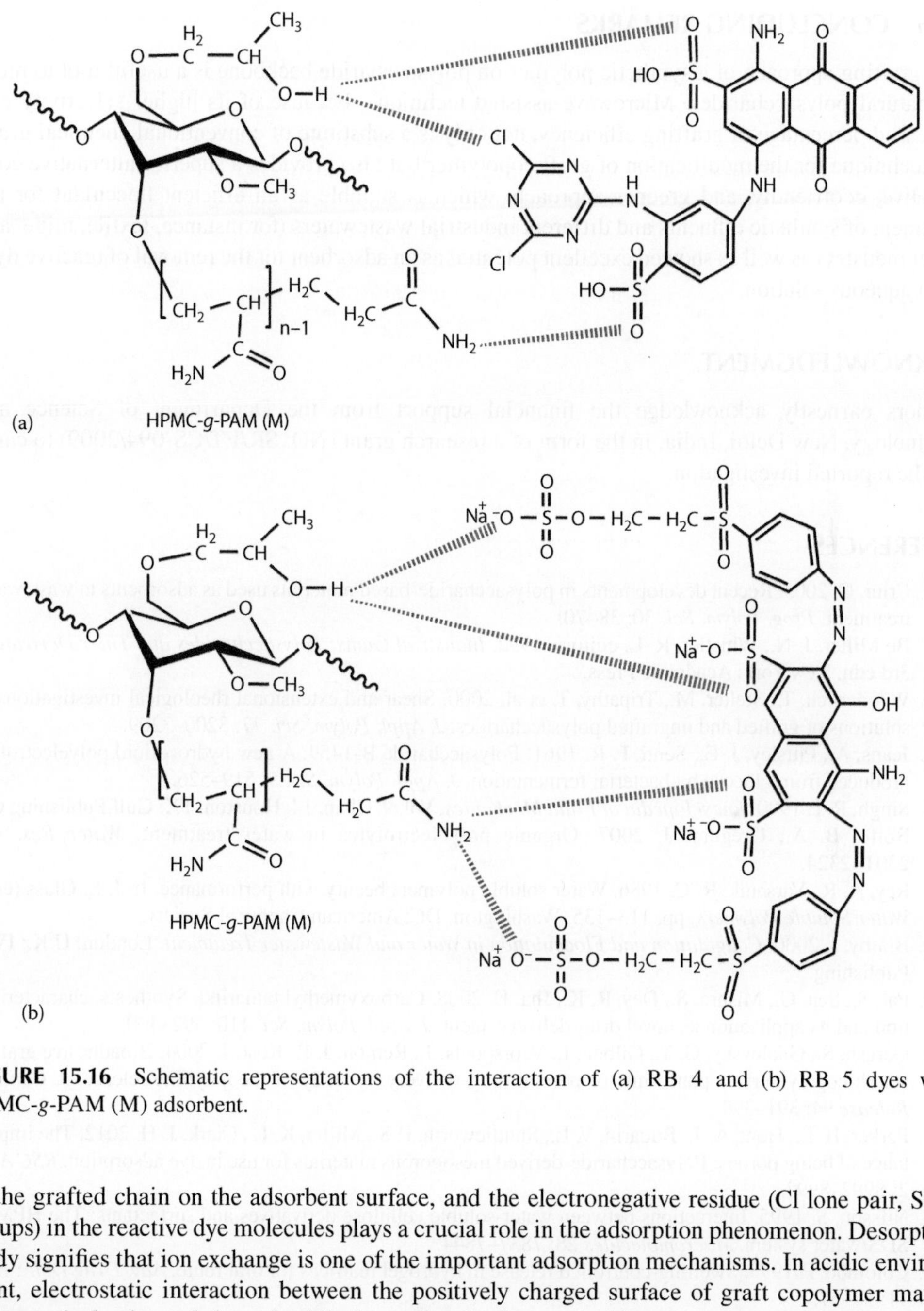

FIGURE 15.16 Schematic representations of the interaction of (a) RB 4 and (b) RB 5 dyes with HPMC-*g*-PAM (M) adsorbent.

of the grafted chain on the adsorbent surface, and the electronegative residue (Cl lone pair, SO_3^- groups) in the reactive dye molecules plays a crucial role in the adsorption phenomenon. Desorption study signifies that ion exchange is one of the important adsorption mechanisms. In acidic environment, electrostatic interaction between the positively charged surface of graft copolymer matrix and negatively charged sites of acidic dye molecule plays a vital function toward adsorption. It has been observed that the uptake of RB 4 and RB 5 is rapid primarily, and consequently, it reached equilibrium. This indicates that initially rapid dye uptake raised through surface adsorption procedure. The hydrophilic nature of the adsorbent is mainly responsible for fast adsorption process due to surface mass transport. However, the entangled network of longer polyacrylamide chains present in graft copolymer facilitates the fast diffusion process of dyes. Therefore, the overall findings suggest that HPMC-*g*-PAM (M) has a complex adsorption mechanism; basically, surface adsorption and intraparticle diffusion (pore diffusion and surface diffusion) mechanism might also take place simultaneously and control the adsorption phenomenon.

15.6 CONCLUDING REMARKS

The grafting approach of a synthetic polymer on polysaccharide backbone is a useful tool to modify natural polysaccharides. Microwave-assisted technique, because of its higher selectivity and increased percentage of grafting efficiency, not only is a substitute of conventional chemical grafting technique for the modification of graft copolymer but also provides a superior alternative cost-effective, ecofriendly, and greener approach, which is suitable as an efficient flocculant for the treatment of synthetic effluents and different industrial wastewaters (for instance, textile, mine, and paper industry) as well as showed excellent potential as an adsorbent for the removal of reactive dyes from aqueous solution.

ACKNOWLEDGMENT

Authors earnestly acknowledge the financial support from the Department of Science and Technology, New Delhi, India, in the form of a research grant (NO: SR/FT/CS-094/2009) to carry out the reported investigation.

REFERENCES

1. Crini, G. 2005. Recent developments in polysaccharide-based materials used as adsorbents in wastewater treatment. *Prog. Polym. Sci.* 30: 38–70.
2. Be Miller, J. N., Whistler, R. L. editors. 1992. *Industrial Gums: Polysaccharides and Their Derivative*, 3rd edn. New York: Academic Press.
3. Wunderlich, T., Stelter, M., Tripathy, T. et al. 2000. Shear and extensional rheological investigations in solutions of grafted and ungrafted polysaccharides. *J. Appl. Polym. Sci.* 77: 3200–3209.
4. Jeans, A., Pittsley, J. E., Senti, F. R. 1961. Polysaccharide B-1459: A new hydrocolloid polyelectrolyte produced from glucose by bacterial fermentation. *J. Appl. Polym. Sci.* 5: 519–526.
5. Singh, R. P. 1990. *Encyclopedia of Fluid Mechanics*, Vol. 9, Chap. 14. Houston, TX: Gulf Publishing Co.
6. Bolto, B. A., Gregory, J. 2007. Organic polyelectrolytes in water treatment. *Water Res.* 41: 2301–2324.
7. Rey, A. R., Varsanik, R. C. 1986. Water soluble polymers beauty with performance. In J. E. Glass (ed.), *Water Soluble Polymers*, pp. 113–135. Washington, DC: American Chemical Society.
8. Bratby, J. 2006. *Coagulation and Flocculation in Water and Wastewater Treatment*. London, U.K.: IWA Publishing.
9. Pal, S., Sen, G., Mishra, S., Dey, R. K., Jha, U. 2008. Carboxymethyl tamarind: Synthesis, characterization and its application as novel drug-delivery agent. *J. Appl. Polym. Sci.* 110: 392–400.
10. Geresh, S., Gdalevsky, G. Y., Gilboa, I., Voorspoels, J., Remon, J. P., Kost, J. 2004. Bioadhesive grafted starch copolymers as platforms for peroral drug delivery: A study of theophylline release. *J. Control. Release* 94: 391–399.
11. Parker, H. L., Hunt, A. J., Budarin, V. L., Shuttleworth, P. S., Miller, K. L., Clark, J. H. 2012. The importance of being porous: Polysaccharide-derived mesoporous materials for use in dye adsorption. *RSC Adv.* 2: 8992–8997.
12. Nilsson, S. 1995. Interactions between water-soluble cellulose derivatives and surfactants: The HPMC/SDS/water system. *Macromolecules* 28: 7837–7844.
13. Colombo, P. 1993. Swelling-controlled release in hydrogel matrices for oral route. *Adv. Drug Deliv. Rev.* 11: 37–57.
14. Bell, D. A. 1990. Methylcellulose as a structure enhancer in bread baking. *Cereal Foods World* 35: 1001–1006.
15. Rosell, C. M., Rojas, J. A., Benedicto de Barber, C. 2001. Influence of hydrocolloids on dough rheology and bread quality. *Food Hydrocoll.* 15: 75–81.
16. Toufeili, I., Dagher, S., Shaderivian, S., Noureddine, A., Sarakavi, M., Farran, M. T. 1994. Formulation of gluten-free pocket-type flat breads: Optimization of methylcellulose, gum arabic and egg albumen levels by response surface methodology. *Cereal Chem.* 71: 594–601.
17. Sanz, T., Salvador, A., Fiszman, S. M. 2004. Innovative method for preparing a frozen battered food without a prefrying step. *Food Hydrocoll.* 18: 227–231.

18. Balasubramaniam, V. M., Chinnan, M. S., Mallikarjunan, P., Phillips, R. D. 1997. The effect of edible film on oil uptake and moisture retention of a deep-fat fried poultry product. *J. Food Process. Eng.* 20: 17–29.
19. Albert, S., Mittal, G. S. 2002. Comparative evaluation of edible coatings to reduce fat uptake in a deep fried cereal product. *Food Res. Int.* 35: 445–458.
20. Xu, Y., Zhang, Y., Feng, Q. 2013. The dynamic adsorption performance of the cross-linked starch/acrylonitrile graft copolymer for copper ions in water. *Colloids Surf. A: Physicochem. Eng. Aspects* 430: 8–12.
21. Da Silva, D. A., De Paula, R. C. M., Feitosa, J. P. A. 2007. Graft copolymerisation of acrylamide onto cashew gum. *Eur. Polym. J.* 43: 2620–2629.
22. Singh, V., Singh, S. K., Maurya, S. 2010. Microwave induced poly(acrylic acid) modification of *Cassia javanica* seed gum for efficient Hg(II) removal from solution. *Chem. Eng. J.* 160: 129–137.
23. Ikhuoria, E. U., Folayan, A. S., Okieimen, F. E. 2010. Studies in the graft copolymerization of acrylonitrile onto cassava starch by ceric ion induced initiation. *Int. J. Biotechnol. Mol. Biol. Res.* 1: 10–14.
24. Sharma, B. R., Kumar, V., Soni, P. L. 2003. Ce(IV)-ion initiated graft copolymerization of methyl methacrylate onto guar gum. *J. Macromol. Sci. A* 40: 49–60.
25. Fares, M. M., El-faqeeh, A. S., Osman, M. E. 2003. Graft copolymerization onto starch-I: Synthesis and optimization of starch grafted with *N-tert*-butylacrylamide copolymer and its hydrogels. *J. Polym. Res.* 10: 119–125.
26. Tizzotti, M., Charlot, A., Fleury, E., Stenzel, M., Bernard, L. 2010. Modification of polysaccharides through controlled/living radical polymerization grafting—Towards the generation of high performance hybrids. *Macromol. Rapid Commun.* 31: 1751–1772.
27. Jenkins, D. W., Hudson, S. M. 2001. Review of vinyl graft copolymerization featuring recent advances toward controlled radical-based reactions and illustrated with chitin/chitosan trunk polymers. *Chem. Rev.* 101: 3245–3273.
28. Odian, G. 1981. *Principle of Polymerization*, 2nd edn. New York: Wiley.
29. Lagos, A., Reyes, J. 1988. Grafting onto chitosan. I. graft copolymerization of methyl methacrylate onto chitosan with Fenton's reagent (Fe^{2+}–H_2O_2) as a redox initiator. *J. Polym. Sci. Part A: Polym. Chem.* 26: 985–991.
30. Liu, S., Sun, G. 2008. Radical graft functional modification of cellulose with allyl monomers: Chemistry and structure characterization. *Carbohydr. Polym.* 71: 614–625.
31. Das, R., Panda, A. B., Pal, S. 2012. Synthesis and characterization of a novel polymeric hydrogel based on hydroxypropyl methyl cellulose grafted with polyacrylamide. *Cellulose* 19: 933–945.
32. Sarkar, A. K., Mandre, N. R., Panda, A. B., Pal, S. 2013. Amylopectin grafted with poly (acrylic acid): Development and application of a high performance flocculant. *Carbohydr. Polym.* 95: 753–759.
33. Nasef, M. M., Guven, O. 2012. Radiation grafted copolymers for separation and purification purposes: Status, challenges and future directions. *Prog. Polym. Sci.* 37, 1597–1656.
34. Shanmugharaj, A. M., Kim, J. K., Ryu, S. H. 2006. Modification of rubber surface by UV surface grafting. *Appl. Surf. Sci.* 252: 5714–5722.
35. Ma, H., Davis, R. H., Bowman, C. N. 2001. Principal factors affecting sequential photoinduced graft polymerization. *Polymer* 42: 8333–8338.
36. Thaker, M. D., Trivedi, H. C. 2005. Ultraviolet radiation induced graft copolymerization of methyl acrylate onto the sodium salt of partially carboxymethylated guar gum. *J. Appl. Polym. Sci.* 97: 1977–1986.
37. Huang, R. Y. M., Immergut, B., Immergut, E. H., Rapson, W. H. 1963. Grafting vinyl polymers onto cellulose by high energy radiation-I. High energy radiation-induced graft copolymerization of styrene onto cellulose. *J. Polym. Sci. Part A: Polym. Chem.* 1: 1257–1270.
38. Shiraishi, N., Williams, J. L., Stannett, V. 1982. The radiation grafting of vinyl monomers to cotton fabrics—I. Methacrylic acid to terry cloth to welling. *Radiat. Phys. Chem.* 19: 73–78.
39. Wang, J. P., Chen, Y. Z., Zhang, S. J., Yu, H. Q. 2008. A chitosan based flocculant prepared with gamma irradiation induced grafting. *Bioresour. Technol.* 99: 3397–3402.
40. Fossey, J., Lefort, D., Sorba, J. 1995. *Free Radicals in Organic Chemistry*, p. 106. Chichester, U.K.: John Wiley & Sons.
41. Pietraner, M. S. A., Narvaiz, P. 2001. Examination of some protective conditions on technological properties of irradiated food grade polysaccharides. *Radiat. Phys. Chem.* 60: 195–201.
42. Kim, B. N., Lee, D. H., Han, D. H. 2008. Thermal, mechanical and electrical properties on the styrene grafted and subsequently sulfonated FEP film induced by electron beam. *Polym. Degrad. Stab.* 93: 1214–1221.

43. Edimecheva, I. P., Kisel, R. M., Shadyro, O. I., Kazem, K., Murase, H., Kagiya, T. 2005. Homolytic cleavage of the O-glycoside bond in carbohydrates: A steady state radiolysis study. *J. Radiat. Res.* 46: 319–324.
44. Dargaville, T. R., George, G. A., Hill, D. J. T., Whittaker, A. K. 2003. High energy radiation grafting of fluoropolymers. *Prog. Polym. Sci.* 28: 1355–1376.
45. Farquet, P., Padeste, C., Solak, H. H., Gürsel, S., Ascherer, G. G., Wokaun, A. 2008. Extreme UV radiation grafting of glycidyl methacrylate nanostructures onto fluoropolymer foils by RAFT mediated polymerization. *Macromolecules* 41: 6309–6316.
46. Guilmeau, I., Esnouf, S., Betz, N., Le, M. A. 1997. Kinetics and characterization of radiation induced grafting of styrene on fluoropolymers. *Nucl. Inst. Methods Phys. Res. B: Beam Interact. Mater. Atoms* 131: 270–275.
47. Tucker, J. L. 2010. Green chemistry: Cresting a summit toward sustainability. *Org. Process Res. Dev.* 14: 328–331.
48. Erdmenger, T., Guerrero-Sanchez, C., Vitz, J., Hoogenboom, R., Schubert, U. S. 2010. Recent developments in the utilization of green solvents in polymer chemistry. *Chem. Soc. Rev.* 39: 3317–3333.
49. Kalia, S., Sabba, M. W. editors. 2013. *Polysaccharide Based Graft Copolymers*, Chap. 1, pp. 1–347. New York: Springer.
50. Deshayes, S., Liagre, M., Loupy, A., Luche, J. L., Petit, A. 1999. Microwave activation in phase transfer catalysis. *Tetrahedron* 55: 10851–10870.
51. Wiesbrock, F., Hoogenboom, R., Schubert, U. S. 2004. Microwave-assisted polymer synthesis: State of the art and future perspectives. *Macromol. Rapid Commun.* 25: 1739–1764.
52. Galema, S. A. 1997. Microwave chemistry. *Chem. Soc. Rev.* 26: 233–238.
53. Singh, V., Tiwari, A., Tripathi, D. N., Sanghi, R. 2006. Microwave enhanced synthesis of chitosan-*graft*-polyacrylamide. *Polymer* 47: 254–260.
54. Kumar, A., Singh, K., Ahuja, M. 2009. Xanthan-*g*-poly (acrylamide): Microwave-assisted synthesis, characterization and in vitro release behavior. *Carbohydr. Polym.* 76: 261–267.
55. Alfaifi, A. Y. A., El-Newehy, M. H., Abdel-Halim, E. S., Al-Deyab, S. S. 2014. Microwave-assisted graft copolymerization of amino acid based monomers onto starch and their use as drug carriers. *Carbohydr. Polym.* 106: 440–452.
56. Rani, P., Mishra, S., Sen, G. 2103. Microwave based synthesis of polymethyl methacrylate grafted sodium alginate: Its application as flocculant. *Carbohydr. Polym.* 91: 686–692.
57. Zhang, J., Zhang, S., Yuan, K., Wang, Y. 2007. Graft copolymerization of artemisia seed gum with acrylic acid under microwave and its water absorbency. *J. Macromol. Sci. Part A: Pure and Appl. Chem.* 44: 881–885.
58. Ghosh, S., Sen, G., Jha, U., Pal, S. 2010. Novel biodegradable polymeric flocculant based on polyacrylamide grafted tamarind kernel polysaccharide. *Bioresour. Technol.* 101: 9638–9644.
59. Pal, S., Ghorai, S., Dash, M. K., Ghosh, S., Udayabhanu, G. 2011. Flocculation properties of polyacrylamide grafted carboxymethyl guar gum (CMG-*g*-PAM) synthesised by conventional and microwave assisted method. *J. Hazard. Mater.* 192: 1580–1588.
60. Cheng, H. 2009. Meeting China's water shortage crisis: Current practices and challenges. *Environ. Sci. Technol.* 43: 240–244.
61. Shannon, M. A., Bohn, P. W., Elimelech, M., Georgiadis, J. G., Mariñas, B. J., Mayes, A. M. 2008. Science and technology for water purification in the coming decades. *Nature* 452: 301–310.
62. Zou, J., Zhu, H., Wang, F., Sui, H., Fan, J. 2011. Preparation of a new inorganic–organic composite flocculant used in solid–liquid separation for waste drilling fluid. *Chem. Eng. J.* 171: 350–356.
63. Schwarz, S., Jaeger, W., Paulke, B. R., Bratskaya, S., Smolka, N., Bohrisch, J. 2007. Cationic flocculants carrying hydrophobic functionalities: Applications for solid/liquid separation. *J. Phys. Chem. B* 111: 8649–8654.
64. Csempesz, F. 2000. Enhanced flocculation of colloidal dispersions by polymer mixtures. *Chem. Eng. J.* 80: 43–49.
65. Natalia, M., Olli, D. 2006. Environmental implications of aggregations phenomena: Current understanding. *Curr. Opin. Colloid Interface Sci.* 11: 246–266.
66. Lee, K. E., Morad, N., Teng, T. T., Poh, B. T. 2012. Development, characterization and the application of hybrid materials in coagulation/flocculation of wastewater: A review. *Chem. Eng. J.* 203: 370–386.
67. Addai-Mensah, J., Prestidge, C. A. 2005. Structure formation in dispersed system. In H. Stechemesser, B. Dobias (eds.), *Coagulation and Flocculation*, 2nd edn., pp. 135–216. Boca Raton, FL: Taylor & Francis.
68. Lee, S. H., Shin, M. C., Choi, S. J., Park, I. S. 1998. Improvement of flocculation efficiency of water treatment by using polymer flocculants. *Environ. Technol.* 19: 431–437.

69. Joo, D. J., Shin, W. S., Choi, J. K., Choi, S. J., Kim, M. C., Han, M. H., Ha, T. W., Kim, Y. H. 2007. Decolorization of reactive dyes using inorganic coagulants and synthetic polymer. *Dyes Pigm.* 73: 59–64.
70. Schintu, M., Meloni, P., Contu, A. 2000. Aluminum fractions in drinking water from reservoirs. *Ecotoxicol. Environ. Saf.* 46: 29–33.
71. Zahrim, A. Y., Tizaoui, C., Hilal, N. 2010. Evaluation of several commercial synthetic polymers as flocculant aids for removal of highly concentrated C.I. acid black 210 dye. *J. Hazard. Mater.* 182: 624–630.
72. Singh, R. P., Tripathy, T., Karmakar, G. P., Rath, S. K., Karmakar, N. C., Pandey, S. R., Kannan, K., Jain, S. K., Lan, N. T. 2000. Novel biodegradable flocculants based polysaccharides. *Curr. Sci.* 78: 798–803.
73. Roussy, J., Vooren, M. V., Dempsey, B. A., Guibal, E. 2005. Influence of chitosan characteristics of the coagulation and the flocculation of bentonite suspensions. *Water Res.* 39: 3247–3258.
74. Renault, F., Sancey, B., Badot, P. M., Crini, G. 2009. Chitosan for coagulation/flocculation processes: An eco-friendly approach. *Eur. Polym. J.* 45: 1337–1348.
75. Xiao, J., Zhou, Q. 2005. *Natural Polymer Flocculants*. Beijing, China: Chemical Industry Press.
76. Deshmukh, S. R., Singh, R. P. 1991. Drag-reduction efficiency, shear stability, and biodegradation resistance of carboxymethyl cellulose-based and starch-based graft copolymers. *J. Appl. Polym. Sci.* 43: 1091–1101.
77. Biswal, D. R., Singh, R. P. 2004. Characterisation of carboxymethyl cellulose and polyacrylamide graft copolymer. *Carbohydr. Polym.* 57: 379–387.
78. Singh, R. P., Karmakar, G. P., Rath, S. K., Karmakar, N. C., Pandey, S. R., Tripathy, T., Panda, J., Kannan, K., Jain, S. K., Lan, N. T. 2000. Biodegradable drag reducing agents and flocculants based on polysaccharides: Materials and applications. *Polym. Eng. Sci.* 40: 46–60.
79. Tripathy, T., Bhagat, R. P., Singh, R. P. 2001. The flocculation performance of grafted sodium alginate and other polymeric flocculants in relation to iron ore slimes. *Eur. Polym. J.* 37: 125–130.
80. Singh, R. P., Nayak, B. R., Biswal, D. R., Tripathy, T., Banik, K. 2003. Biobased polymeric flocculants for industrial effluent treatment. *Mater. Res. Innov.* 7: 331–340.
81. Sen, G., Kumar, R., Ghosh, S., Pal, S. 2009. A novel polymeric flocculant based on polyacrylamide grafted carboxymethylstarch. *Carbohydr. Polym.* 77: 822–831.
82. Sen, G., Singh, R. P., Pal, S. 2000. Microwave-initiated synthesis of polyacrylamide grafted sodium alginate: Synthesis and characterization. *J. Appl. Polym. Sci.* 115: 63–71.
83. Ali, S. K., Pal, S., Singh, R. P. 2010. Flocculation performance of modified chitosan in an aqueous suspension. *J. Appl. Polym. Sci.* 118: 2592–2600.
84. Pal, S., Nasim, T., Patra, A., Ghosh, S., Panda, A. B. 2010. Microwave assisted synthesis of polyacrylamide grafted dextrin (Dxt-*g*-PAM): Development and application of a novel polymeric flocculant. *Int. J. Biol. Macromol.* 47: 623–631.
85. Das, R., Ghorai, S., Pal, S. 2013. Flocculation characteristics of polyacrylamide grafted hydroxypropyl methyl cellulose: An efficient biodegradable flocculant. *Chem. Eng. J.* 229: 144–152.
86. Nasim, T., Bandyopadhyay, A. 2012. Introducing different poly(vinyl alcohol)s as new flocculants for kaolinated wastewater. *Sep. Purif. Technol.* 88: 87–94.
87. Dash, M., Dwari, R. K., Biswal, S. K., Reddy, P. S. R., Chattopadhyay, P., Mishra, B. K. 2011. Studies on the effect of flocculant adsorption on the dewatering of iron ore tailings. *Chem. Eng. J.* 173: 318–325.
88. Yang, Z., Yuan, B., Huang, X., Zhou, J., Cai, J., Yang, H., Li, A., Cheng, R. 2012. Evaluation of the flocculation performance of carboxymethyl chitosan-*graft*-polyacrylamide: A novel amphoteric chemically bonded composite flocculant. *Water Res.* 46: 107–114.
89. Ghorai, S., Sarkar, A., Panda, A. B., Pal, S. 2013. Evaluation of the flocculation characteristics of polyacrylamide grafted xanthan gum/silica hybrid nanocomposite. *Ind. Eng. Chem. Res.* 52: 9731–9740.
90. Brostow, W., Pal, S., Singh, R. P. 2007. A model of flocculation. *Mater. Lett.* 61: 4381–4384.
91. Ruehrwein, R. A., Ward, D. W. 1952. Mechanism of clay aggregation by polyelectrolytes. *Soil Sci.* 73: 485–492.
92. Smellie, R. H., La Mer, V. K. 1958. Flocculation, subsidence and filtration of phosphate slimes: A quantitative theory of filtration of flocculated suspensions. *J. Colloid Sci.* 13: 589–599.
93. Healy, T. K., La Mer, V. K. 1964. The energetics of flocculation and redispersion by polymers. *J. Colloid Sci.* 19: 323–332.
94. Mühle, K. 1993. Floc stability in laminar and turbulent flow. In Dobiàs, B. (ed.), *Coagulation and Flocculation*, pp. 355–390. New York: Marcel Dekker.
95. Yoon, S. Y., Deng, Y. L. 2004. Flocculation and reflocculation of clay suspension by different polymer systems under turbulent conditions. *J. Colloid Interface Sci.* 278: 139–145.
96. Kleimann, J., Gehin-Delval, C., Auweter, H., Borkovec, M. 2005. Super-stoichiometric charge neutralization in particle polyelectrolyte systems. *Langmuir* 21: 3688–3698.

97. Das, K. K., Somasundaran, P. 2001. Ultra-low dosage flocculation of alumina using polyacrylic acid. *Colloids Surf. A: Physicochem. Eng. Aspects* 182: 25–33.
98. Runkana, V., Somasudaran, P., Kapur, P. C. 2006. A population balance model for flocculation of colloidal suspensions by polymer bridging. *Chem. Eng. Sci.* 61: 182–191.
99. Zhang, X., Qiao, P., Ji, X., Han, J., Liu, L., Weeks, B. L., Yao, Q., Zhang, Z. 2013. Sustainable recycling of benzoic acid production waste: Green and highly efficient methods to separate and recover high value added conjugated aromatic compounds from industrial residues. *ACS Sustain. Chem. Eng.* 1: 974–981.
100. Verma, A. K., Dash, R. R., Bhunia, P. 2012. A review on chemical coagulation/flocculation technologies for removal of colour from textile wastewaters. *J. Environ. Manage.* 93: 154–168.
101. Ali, M., Sreekrishnan, T. R. 2001. Aquatic toxicity from pulp and paper mill effluents: A review. *Adv. Environ. Res.* 5: 175–196.
102. Wong, S. S., Teng, T. T., Ahmad, A. L., Zuhairi, A., Najafpour, G. 2006. Treatment of pulp and paper mill wastewater by polyacrylamide (PAM) in polymer induced flocculation. *J. Hazard. Mater.* 135: 378–388.
103. Tischler, J. S., Wiacek, C., Janneck, E., Schlömann, M. 2014. Bench scale study of the effect of phosphate on an aerobic iron oxidation plant for mine water treatment. *Water Res.* 48: 345–353.
104. Mackie, A. L., Walsh, M. E. 2012. Bench-scale study of active mine water treatment using cement kiln dust (CKD) as a neutralization agent. *Water Res.* 46: 327–334.
105. Sharma, Y. C., Uma, Upadhyay, S. N. 2009. Removal of a cationic dye from wastewaters by adsorption on activated carbon developed from coconut coir. *Energy Fuels* 23: 2983–2988.
106. Ma, J., Yu, F., Zhou, L., Jin, L., Yang, M., Luan, J., Tang, Y., Fan, H., Yuan, Z., Chen, J. 2012. Enhanced adsorptive removal of methyl orange and methylene blue from aqueous solution by alkali-activated multiwalled carbon nanotubes. *ACS Appl. Mater. Interfaces* 4: 5749–5760.
107. Zhu, T., Chen, J. S., Lou, X. W. 2012. Highly efficient removal of organic dyes from wastewater using hierarchical NiO spheres with high surface area. *J. Phys. Chem. C* 116: 6873–6878.
108. Pak, D., Chang, W. 1999. Decolorizing dye wastewater with low temperature catalytic oxidation. *Water Sci. Technol.* 40: 115–121.
109. Madadrang, C. J., Kim, H. Y., Gao, G., Wang, N., Zhu, J., Feng, H., Gorring, M., Kasner, M. L., Hou, S. 2012. Adsorption behavior of EDTA graphene oxide for Pb(II) removal. *ACS Appl. Mater. Interfaces* 4: 1186–1193.
110. Mishra, G., Tripathy, M. 1993. A critical review of the treatment for decolorization of textile effluent. *Colourage* 40: 35–38.
111. Panswad, T., Luangdilok, W. 2000. Decolorization of reactive dyes with different molecular structures under different environmental conditions. *Water Res.* 34: 4177–4184.
112. Wong, Y., Yu, J. 1999. Laccase catalyzed decolorization of synthetic dyes. *Water Res.* 33: 3512–3520.
113. Liu, F., Chung, S., Oh, G., Seo, T. S. 2012. Three dimensional graphene oxide nanostructure for fast and efficient water soluble dye removal. *ACS Appl. Mater. Interfaces* 4: 922–927.
114. Bayram, E., Ayranci, E. 2010. Electrochemically enhanced removal of polycyclic aromatic basic dyes from dilute aqueous solutions by activated carbon cloth electrodes. *Environ. Sci. Technol.* 44: 6331–6336.
115. Al-Bastaki, N. 2004. Removal of methyl orange dye and Na_2SO_4 salt from synthetic wastewater using reverse osmosis. *Chem. Eng. Process. Process Intensif.* 43: 1561–1567.
116. Kabra, K., Chaudhary, R., Sawhney, R. L. 2004. Treatment of hazardous organic and inorganic compounds through aqueous phase photocatalysis: A review. *Ind. Eng. Chem. Res.* 43: 7683–7696.
117. Crini, G., Badot, P. M. 2008. Application of chitosan, a natural amino polysaccharide, for dye removal from aqueous solutions by adsorption processes using batch studies: A review of recent literature. *Prog. Polym. Sci.* 33: 399–447.
118. Crini, G. 2006. Non conventional low cost adsorbents for dye removal: A review. *Bioresour. Technol.* 97: 1061–1085.
119. Ho, Y. S., Chiang, T. H., Hsueh, Y. M. 2005. Removal of basic dye from aqueous solution using tree fern as a biosorbent. *Process Biochem.* 40: 119–124.
120. Zhuang, X., Wan, Y., Feng, C., Shen, Y., Zhao, D. 2009. Highly efficient adsorption of bulky dye molecules in wastewater on ordered mesoporous carbons. *Chem. Mater.* 21: 706–716.
121. Duran, C., Ozdes, D., Gundogdu, A., Senturk, H. B. 2011. Kinetics and isotherm analysis of basic dyes adsorption onto almond shell (*Prunus dulcis*) as a low cost adsorbent. *J. Chem. Eng. Data* 56: 2136–2147.
122. Hameed, B. H. 2008. Equilibrium and kinetic studies of methyl violet sorption by agricultural waste. *J. Hazard. Mater.* 154: 204–212.
123. Zhou, Y., Zhang, M., Hu, X., Wang, X., Niu, J., Ma, T. 2013. Adsorption of cationic dyes on a cellulose based multicarboxyl adsorbent. *J. Chem. Eng. Data* 58: 413–421.

124. Zhang, W., Yang, H., Dong, L., Yan, H., Li, H., Jiang, Z., Kan, X., Li, A., Cheng, R. 2012. Efficient removal of both cationic and anionic dyes from aqueous solutions using a novel amphoteric straw based adsorbent. *Carbohydr. Polym.* 90: 887–893.
125. Singh, V., Sharma, A. K., Sanghi, R. 2009. Poly(acrylamide) functionalized chitosan: An efficient adsorbent for azo dyes from aqueous solutions. *J. Hazard. Mater.* 166: 327–335.
126. Al-Karawi, A. J. M., Al-Qaisi, Z. H. J., Abdullah, H. I., Al-Mokaram, A. M. A., Al-Heetimi, D. T. A. 2011. Synthesis, characterization of acrylamide grafted chitosan and its use in removal of copper(II) ions from water. *Carbohydr. Polym.* 83: 495–500.
127. Binupriya, A. R., Sathishkumar, M., Ku, C. S., Yun, S. 2010. Sequestration of reactive blue 4 by free and immobilized bacillus subtilis cells and its extracellular polysaccharides. *Colloids Surf. B: Biointerfaces* 76: 179–185.
128. Gibbs, G., Tobin, J. M., Guibal, E. 2004. Influence of chitosan preprotonation on reactive black 5 sorption isotherms and kinetics. *Ind. Eng. Chem. Res.* 43: 1–11.
129. Ghorai, S., Sarkar, A., Raoufi, M., Panda, A. B., Schönherr, H., Pal, S. 2014. Enhanced removal of methylene blue and methyl violet dyes from aqueous solution using a nanocomposite of hydrolyzed polyacrylamide grafted xanthan gum and incorporated nanosilica. *ACS Appl. Mater. Interfaces* 6: 4766–4777.
130. Legergren, S. 1898. About the theory of so-called adsorption of soluble substances. *K. Sven. Vetenskapsakad. Handl. Band* 24: 1–39.
131. Ho, Y. S., McKay, G. 1999. Pseudo second order model for sorption processes. *Process Biochem.* 34: 451–465.
132. Ho, Y. S. 2006. Second order kinetic model for the sorption of cadmium onto tree fern: A comparison of linear and non linear methods. *Water Res.* 40: 119–125.
133. Weber, W. J., Morris, J. C. 1963. Kinetics of adsorption on carbon from solution. *J. San. Eng. Div. ASCE* 89: 31–59.
134. Ai, L., Zhang, C., Meng, L. 2011. Adsorption of methyl orange from aqueous solution on hydrothermal synthesized Mg–Al layered double hydroxide. *J. Chem. Eng. Data* 56: 4217–4225.
135. Ai, L., Li, M., Li, L. 2011. Adsorption of methylene blue from aqueous solution with activated carbon/cobalt ferrite/alginate composite beads: Kinetics isotherms and thermodynamics. *J. Chem. Eng. Data* 56: 3475–3483.
136. Langmuir, I. 1916. The constitution and fundamental properties of solids and liquids. *J. Am. Chem. Soc.* 38: 2221–2295.
137. Ayad, M. M., El-Nasr, A. A. 2010. Adsorption of cationic dye (methylene blue) from water using polyaniline nanotubes base. *J. Phys. Chem. C* 114: 14377–14383.
138. Freundlich, H. M. F. 1906. Über die adsorption in Lösungen. *Z. Phys. Chem.* 57: 385–470.
139. Rahchamani, J., Mousavi, H. Z., Behzad, M. 2011. Adsorption of methyl violet from aqueous solution by polyacrylamide as an adsorbent: Isotherm and kinetic studies. *Desalination* 267: 256–260.
140. Reddy, D. H. K., Lee, S. M. 2013. Application of magnetic chitosan composites for the removal of toxic metal and dyes from aqueous solutions. *Adv. Colloid Interface Sci.* 201–202: 68–93.
141. Sajab, M. S., Chia, C. H., Zakaria, S., Jani, S. M., Ayob, M. K., Chee, K. L., Khiew, P. S., Chiu, W. S. 2011. Citric acid modified kenaf core fibres for removal of methylene blue from aqueous solution. *Bioresour. Technol.* 102: 7237–7243.

16 Preparation of Graft Copolymers of Cellulose Derivatives and Their Use in Recovery Processes

Nursel Pekel Bayramgil

CONTENTS

16.1 INTRODUCTION

With the advancing technology, the area of usage of synthetic polymer materials has expanded. While it takes 3 months for a paper tissue, 6 months for an apple garbage, and 10 years for a coke bottle to be destroyed, a synthetic polymer material may last up to 1000 years. Left in the environment as waste after their usage, these materials cause water, air, and soil pollution since they remain there for long. Now, they threaten our health as a result of the release of toxic gases due to degradation caused by ultraviolet (UV) lights, and also the discharge of toxic materials into the waters that resulted by their disintegration by acids. In modern civilizations, synthetic polymer materials give way to the natural or modified natural polymers day by day. Natural polymers that are and obtained from biorenewable resources and that are biodegradable are known as environmentally friendly polymers, since, with the attack of microorganisms, they transform into two harmless products, that is, CO_2 and H_2O, when left to the environment. On the other hand, it is proven inevitable for the modified natural polymers to be produced by means of reaction with synthetic polymers, since the materials derived from pure natural polymers fall short of the features that they are supposed to show such as resistance to light, heat, moisture, and chemicals, and mechanical endurance. In order to modify natural polymers, the methods of blending, curing, and grafting are used [1]. Blending is an important method that is used in order either to enhance the original physical features of one or more polymers or to develop new materials that differ from their own features. Curing is a method by which a coating produced with polymerization is attached, by means of physical forces, to a surface where oligomer mixture is applied. Thus, a smoother and homogeneous surface is obtained on polymer-based materials. When it comes to the method of grafting, monomers/monomer mixtures are chemically linked into the main chain of the natural polymer [2]. Thus, the physical and chemical features of the natural polymer are permanently changed.

When literature is reviewed, it can be seen that the most commonly studied natural polymers are cellulose and its derivatives. Cellulose was discovered in 1838 by the French chemist Anselme Payen [3], who isolated it from plant matter and determined its chemical formula. Cellulose is an important structural component of the primary cell wall of green plants and other organisms like algae and oomycetes. Linen, cannabis, and elder essence are quite pure cellulose (~90%). Wood contains at least 50% cellulose [4]. It can be microfibrils with a radius of 2–20 nm and a length of 100–40,000 nm. It is a white, odorless, and tasteless material. It burns with a release of carbon dioxide (CO_2) and water vapor (H_2O), and it leaves char. Cellulose, which is shown with the general formula of $(C_6H_{12}O_6)_n$, is the most abundantly existent organic polymer on earth. It has a linear structure consisting of glucopyranose rings linked with up to 10 thousands of β (1→4) ether (glucosidic) bonds [5] (Figure 16.1).

Although widely used in the industries of textile, paper, food, cosmetic, and pharmacy, cellulose lacks some of the features that synthetic polymers show. For this reason, many researchers are focused on the enhancement of the physical and chemical features of cellulose, that is, biorenewable and biodegradable. Cellulose can be chemically modified via the hydroxyl (–OH) groups in its structure. Small organic molecules (ether, ester, nitrate, acetate groups) can be added, or polymers can be grafted. With chemical modification, its hydrophilic/hydrophobic character, elasticity, water absorption capacity, adhesive features, adsorption or ion exchange ability, resistance to microbial attacks, and heat, light, and mechanical resistance can be enhanced [6]. For the last 30 years, there are researches on the changing of the features of cellulose by means of grafting acrylic or vinyl monomers on it. A variety of methods of grafting have been developed [7], such as graft copolymerizations initiated with chemicals, high-energy radiation, photosensitizer, plasma, and enzymes. In these methods, grafting is carried out not only by using the known (free radical, ionic) mechanisms but also by using different (chain breaking polymerization, controlled/"living" free radical polymerization) mechanisms.

In this chapter, the graft copolymers that contain cellulose derivatives as the environmentally friendly natural polymer will be the subject matter. The grafting methods used for cellulose and its derivatives will be explained, and specifically, the grafting method by which high-energy radiations are used will be elaborated. The characterization and the area of usage of copolymers obtained by grafting will be presented to capture the reader's attention. Some examples related with the usage of cellulose and its derivatives for recovery purposes will be given from both literature and our own studies.

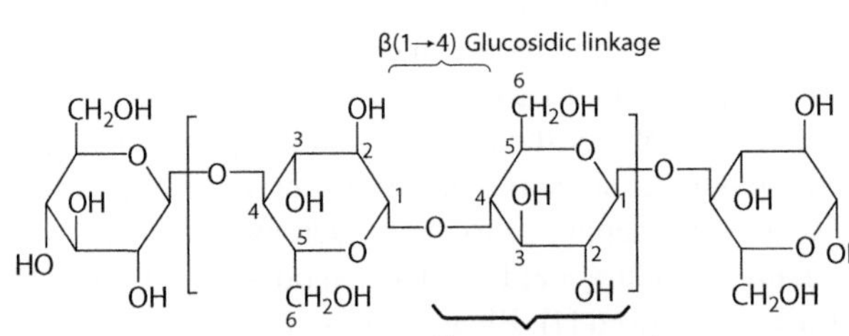

FIGURE 16.1 The structure of cellulose, which consists of repeated glucose units.

16.2 CELLULOSE AND CELLULOSE DERIVATIVES

In industry, cellulose is used in the production of paper, the preparation of nitrocellulose and its products, the production of artificial silk, the food industry (stabilizer), the pharmaceutical industry (release agent/film coating/densifier), and cosmetics (densifier) [8]. With the features of biodegradability, biocompatibility, renewability, and cheapness, it is an attractive substance. Cellulose is far more superior to synthetic polymers in terms of its biodegradable character (environmentally friendly polymer), that is, when it interacts with microorganisms, it converts into CO_2 and H_2O, which do not produce secondary pollution. In order to make the most of these outstanding features of cellulose in various and useful areas, it needs to be chemically modified.

In terms of chemical structure, cellulose is a linear and a quite rigid natural polymer consisting of D-anhydroglucopyranose units. These units are linked together with β (1→4) glucosidic bonds that occur between C atoms in positions 1 and 4 in two adjacent glucose components. Successive glucopyranose units are rotated 180° around polymer main chain axis with respect to the last repeated unit [9]. This arrangement of glucopyranose units underlies many features that cellulose has. In each glucopyranose unit in the cellulose molecule, there are three hydroxyl (–OH) groups (Figure 16.1). The one in position 6 is the primary hydroxyl group ($-CH_2OH$), and the ones that are directly linked to the chain in positions 2 and 3 are secondary hydroxyl groups (–OH). The hydroxyl group in position 2, contrary to the ones in positions 3 and 6, is located in a different place of the plane [8]. As a result of the orientation of the hydroxyl groups to the different sides of the plane, H-bonds occur, which are not only the ones made between each other by the hydroxyl groups that are located in the same rings of the chain but also those made by the hydroxyl groups of glucopyranose units located in different chains. In cellulose, the linear structure composed of covalent bonds reaches to a structure that is 3D and difficult to dissolve with the occurrence of intramolecular and intermolecular H-bonds (Figure 16.2).

Cellulose is a largely crystalline material because of the intramolecular and intermolecular H-bonds in its structure. The stable crystalline regions with a ratio of 65% (linear structures with covalent bonds form crystalline regions like parallel concatenated plaque bundle with the effect of intermolecular H-bonds) are linked to the unstable amorphous areas with a ratio of 35% [11].

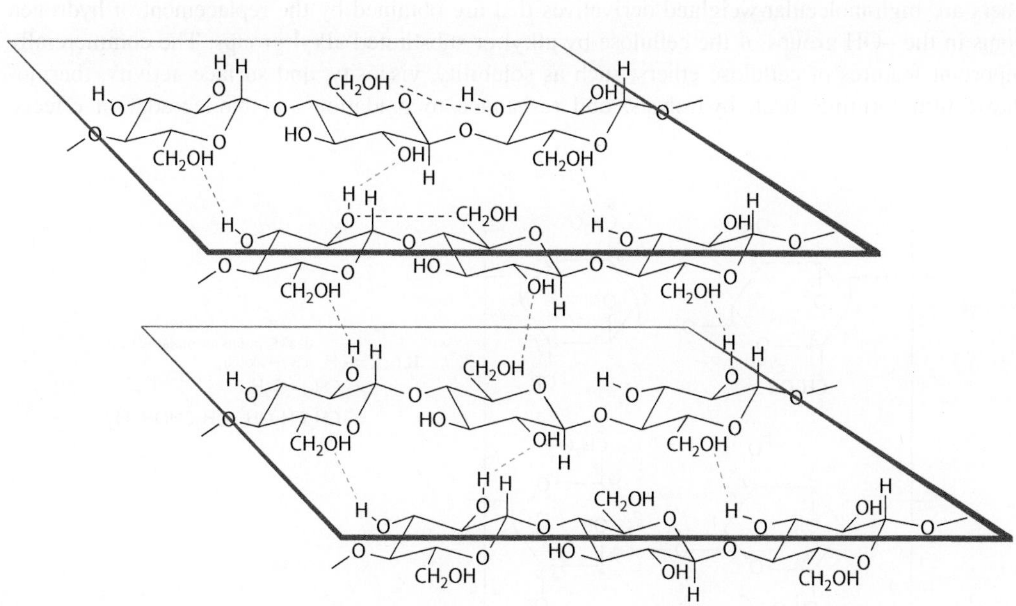

FIGURE 16.2 Intramolecular and intermolecular H-bonds in the cellulose molecule. (From https://s10.lite.msu.edu/res/msu/botonl/b_online/e26/26a.htm.)

These crystalline regions make cellulose resistant to water and chemical agents. On the other hand, in chemical reactions that cellulose is involved, in order for cellulose to get into interaction with chemical agents, the separation of the plaques that form crystalline regions, or in other words making it more prone to reaction by the breaking of some of its intramolecular or intermolecular H-bonds, is an important issue.

The replacement of the three hydroxyl groups in the glucopyranose ring seen in Figure 16.1 by other groups is called degree of substitution (DS). It is possible for DS to be between the rates of 0 (cellulose itself) and 3 (all the hydroxyl groups replaced by others). Sometimes, the one replaced by a hydroxyl group can also contain a hydroxyl group (such as $-OCH_2CH_2OH$ for –OH). New groups give reactions easier than –OH groups of cellulose itself. Degree of molar substitution (MS), on the other hand, signifies the total number of the moles of the reactant that is attached to the ring and gets reacted with such groups that contain hydroxyl groups [8]. In the cellulose molecule, the H atoms of –OH groups of glucopyranose units are partially or completely replaced by other groups such as acetate, butyrate, methyl, ethyl, hydroxyethyl, and hydroxypropyl; as a result, the commercially valuable ethers and esters of cellulose are obtained. In Figure 16.3, the groups that take the place of the three hydroxyl groups of glucopyranose ring and produce cellulose ethers are shown.

In this figure, which shows that different R groups can be attached to the same glucopyranose ring, cellulose molecule itself is obtained if all the R groups represented with different colors are H atoms. In that case, strong H-bonds take place between adjacent hydroxyl groups and the hydroxyl groups in other glucopyranose units. The replacement of the H atoms in the cellulose molecule by R groups (derivatization) ($0 < DS < 3$) means that some of these strong H-bonds have been broken. Thus, the molecule becomes more accessible to water and chemical agents, and it takes place in chemical reactions easily.

Cellulose, which has a narrow area of usage because of its highly crystalline structure, becomes more amorphous after it gets derivatized, and becomes more controllable, and much more convenient for use. It can be used as a fiber, coating, optic film, and sorption medium; also, it can be used as a chemical agent in construction materials, pharmaceutics, food additives, and cosmetics.

The major commercially important derivatives of cellulose are its ethers and esters. Cellulose ethers are high-molecular-weighted derivatives that are obtained by the replacement of hydrogen atoms in the –OH groups of the cellulose by alkyl or substituted alkyl groups. The commercially important features of cellulose ethers, such as solubility, viscosity, and surface activity, thermoplastic film forming, heat, hydrolysis, and resistance to oxidation and biodegradation effects,

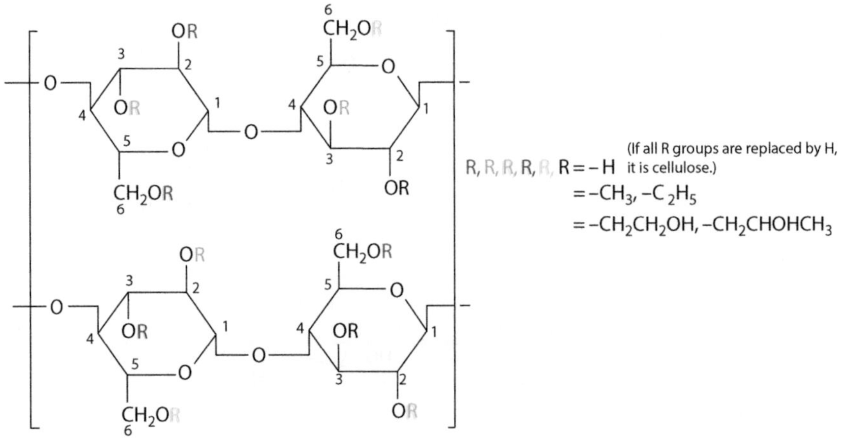

FIGURE 16.3 Groups that are replaced by H atoms in –OH groups in cellulose.

are determined by their molecular weight, their chemical structures and their distribution on the main chain of the substitute groups, and their substitution and MS degrees [12].

The following are some examples of commercially important cellulose ethers:

"Methylcellulose (MC)" is obtained by the reaction of cellulose with methyl chloride in basic medium. The R groups shown in Figure 16.3 are replaced by –H or $-CH_3$ groups (Figure 16.4). Commercially available MC is between the range of DS = 0.1–2.8. While it is soluble in water between DS = 1.4 and 2.0, it is soluble in organic solvents between DS = 2.4 and 2.8 [8]. Its features that determine its areas of usage are its solubility in cold water, compatibility with solutions containing heavy metals, independence from pH, surface activity, and gelling depending upon heating or salt addition. It works as a stabilizer and colloid preservative. It is used in ceramic, paper, and battery industries, in agriculture, and in cosmetics [13].

"Ethyl cellulose (EC)" is obtained by the reaction of cellulose with ethyl chloride in basic medium. The R groups shown in Figure 16.3 are replaced by –H or $-CH_2CH_3$ groups (Figure 16.5). Commercially available MC is between the range of DS = 0.6 and 2.8. It is the only cellulose derivative that is insoluble in water. It has a high stability in relation to light, heat, aerobic environment, humidity, and chemicals. It is soluble in organic solvents such as alcohol, ether, ketone, ester, aromatic hydrocarbon, and halohydrocarbon [8]. EC is used as coating on the surface of drug tablets and as food additive in the form of emulsifiers [14]. In addition to these, it is also used in isolation, bonding materials, and dyestuffs.

"Hydroxyethylcellulose (HEC)" is obtained by the reaction of cellulose with ethylene oxide in basic medium. The R groups shown in Figure 16.3 are replaced by –H or $-CH_2CH_2OH$ groups (Figure 16.6). Commercially available HEC is between the range of MS = 0.05 and 4.1. While its solubility in water is in the foreground between MS = 1.0 and 3.0, its solubility in basic solvents is between MS = 0.05 and 0.4 [8]. Its features that determine its area of usage are its nonionic character, its absence of gel point, and its tolerance against cations. It works as stabilizer and colloid preservative. It is used in ceramic, glass, paper, and dye industries, in coating technology by electrolysis, and in cosmetics [15].

"Hydroxypropyl methylcellulose (HPMC)" is obtained by the reaction of cellulose with propylene oxide in basic medium. The R groups shown in Figure 16.3 are replaced by –H, $-CH_3$, or $-CH_2CHOHCH_3$ groups (Figure 16.7). For HPMC, MS lies between 0.15 and 0.25 [8]. It has a lot of hydroxypropyl groups that increase its dissolution in water. HPMC is used in food, dye, and

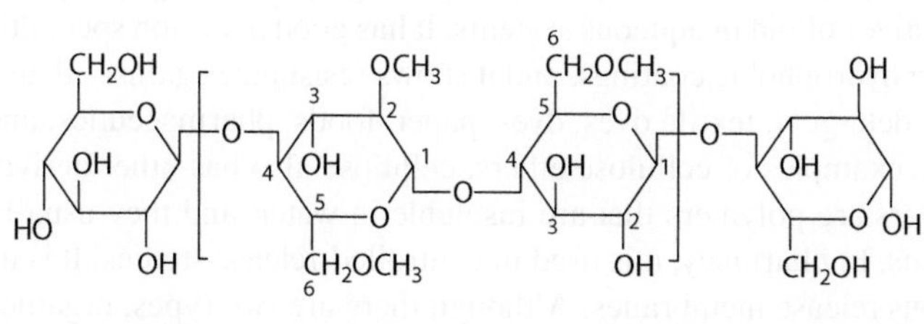

FIGURE 16.4 The structure of MC.

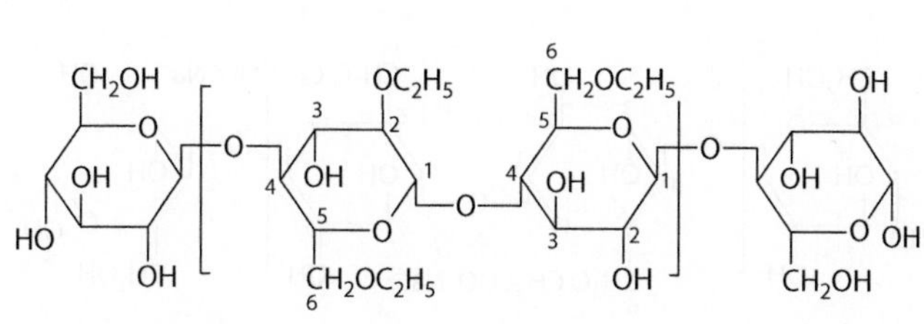

FIGURE 16.5 The structure of EC.

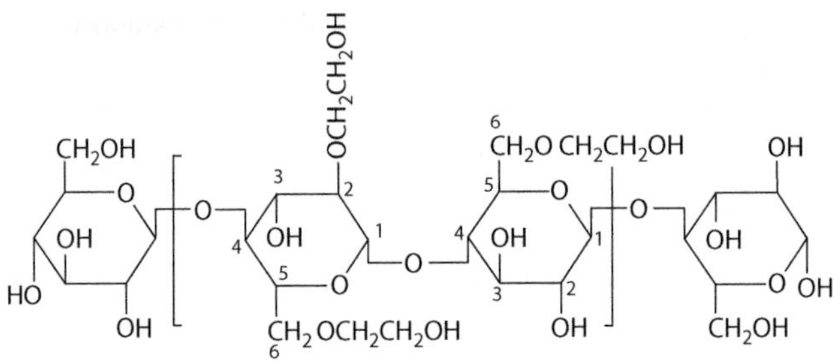

FIGURE 16.6 The structure of HEC.

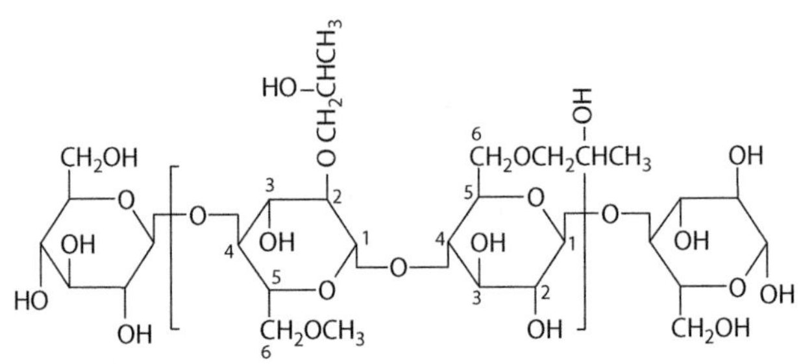

FIGURE 16.7 The structure of HPMC.

construction industries, in cosmetics, and especially in pharmaceutical tablets. At the same time, it is an alternative to animal gelatin. In the medical area, it is used in the production of plaster bandages. Due to its advantages such as attainability and low cost, it is used in various researches [16,17].

"Sodium carboxymethylcellulose (CMC)" is obtained by the reaction of cellulose with sodium chloroacetate in basic medium. The R groups shown in Figure 16.3 are replaced by –H or $-CH_2COO^-Na^+$ groups (Figure 16.8). Commercially available CMC is between the range of DS=0.4 and 1.4. While DS grows to 1.4, CMC's dissolution in water and its processability increase [8]. It shows a polyelectrolyte behavior due to the acetate groups in its structure. It works as stabilizer and protective colloid in aqueous systems. It has good adhesion specialties in film applications, it forms strong hydrophobic coatings, and it shows resistance against oil and grease. It is used in the production of detergent, textile dyes, dyes, paper, foods, pharmaceutics, and cosmetics [18].

Apart from these examples of cellulose ethers, cellulose also has other derivatives, particularly esters. Cellulose esters are polymers that are insoluble in water, and they usually have the feature of forming good films. In pharmacy, it is used in controlled-release studies. It is used with cellulose ethers in microporous release membranes. Although there are two types, organic (cellulose acetate [CA], CA phthalate, and cellulose triacetate) and inorganic (cellulose nitrate and cellulose sulfate), organic cellulose esters are more commonly used in pharmacy applications.

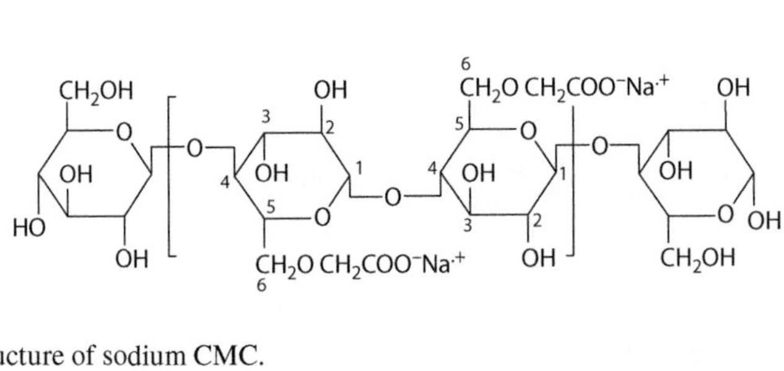

FIGURE 16.8 Structure of sodium CMC.

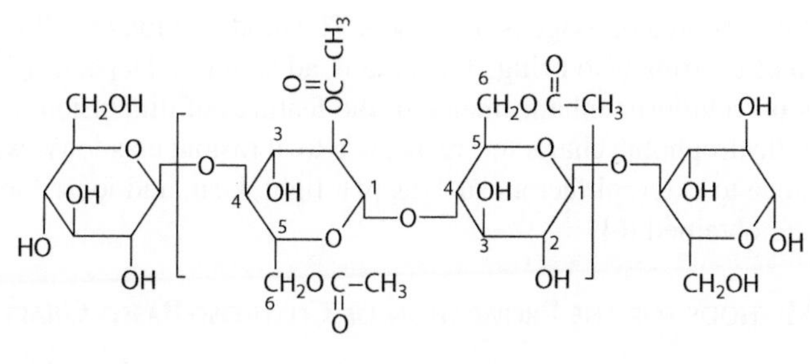

FIGURE 16.9 Structure of CA.

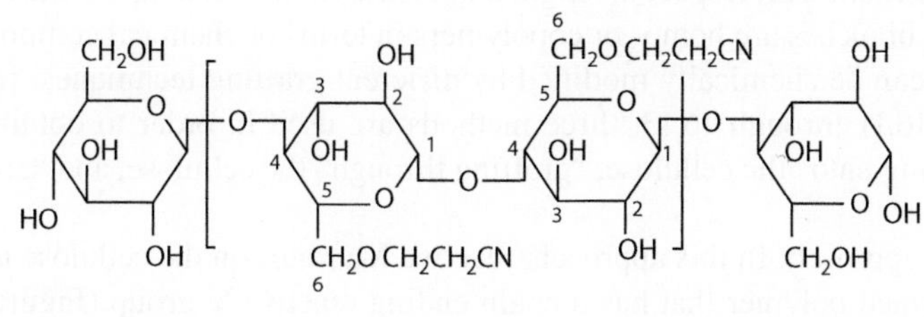

FIGURE 16.10 Structure of CEC.

The following are two examples of other cellulose derivatives that are most widely used:

"CA" is obtained by the reaction of cellulose with acetic anhydride in acetic acid medium. Almost all of the hydrogen atoms in cellulose molecules are replaced with $-COCH_3$ groups (Figure 16.9). For CA, DS is between the range of 0.8 and 2.9 [19]. It dissolves in various organic solvents and water. It is used in textiles because it provides a silky appearance, in film applications due to its features of permeability, and also in cigarette filters, osmosis applications, and production of molded articles and plastics, wound dressings, and hygiene products [20].

Cyanoethylcellulose (CEC) is obtained by the reaction of cellulose with acrylonitrile (AN) in basic medium. The R groups shown in Figure 16.3 are replaced by $-H$ or $-CH_2CH_2CN$ groups (Figure 16.10). When DS = 0.2–0.3, it dissolves in alkaline medium; when 0.7–1.0, it dissolves in water; and while DS grows, it becomes soluble in organic solvents [8]. It is used in the paper industry for making paper resistant against thermal degradation and for providing high dimensional stability and in the production of cotton resistant to microorganisms and acids, and CEC having high DS is used in electroluminescent lamps as phosphorus resin matrix due to its high dielectric constant [21].

As shown in these examples, the limited usage area of cellulose, which has high crystallinity, is expanded after derivatization with ether, ester, and other functional groups. In literature, it is remarkable that most of them also involve copolymers when the studies on cellulose and its other commercially important derivatives are taken into account. Although derivatizations are made, cellulose and its derivatives still lack some features required in various important applications. For that reason, as a result of the chemical modification of cellulose and its derivatives in the presence of a monomer or polymer, their hydrophilic/hydrophobic character, elasticity, water absorption capacities, adsorption or ion exchange ability, and resistance to the effects of microorganisms, heat, light, etc., can be improved [6]. In the next chapter, graft copolymers of cellulose and its derivatives will be the subject matter.

16.3 CELLULOSE-BASED GRAFT COPOLYMERS

Another important and successful method used in order to enhance the physical and chemical features of cellulose is grafting. By grafting acrylic or vinyl monomers into the main chain of cellulose, different features of natural polymer cellulose and synthetic polymers are gathered together in the same structure, and thus, its area of usage is increased. The modification of cellulose and its derivatives with the method of grafting also brings forth many advantages. Depending on the features of the grafted polymers on cellulose, enhancements in the features of dimensional stability; biocompatibility; hydrophilic/hydrophobic character; resistance to abrasion; elasticity; water and ion holding capacities; resistance to external factors such as pH, light, heat, and ionic force; and resistance to microbial effects are obtained [6].

16.3.1 Various Methods for the Preparation of Cellulose-Based Graft Copolymers

Graft copolymers are composed of a main polymer chain (the backbone) to which one or more side chains (the branches) are chemically connected through covalent bonds. Branches can show homogeneity on the main chain with respect to length and distribution or can be arbitrarily arranged. The main chain and the branches are homo- or copolymers in terms of chemical composition. Cellulose and its derivatives can be chemically modified by different grafting techniques. In the techniques shown in Figures 16.11 through 16.13, three methods are used in order to obtain cellulose graft copolymers: "grafting onto" the cellulose, "grafting through" the cellulose, and "grafting from" the cellulose.

"Grafting onto" approach: In this approach, reactive **X** groups on the cellulose main chain combines with a preformed polymer that has a chain ending reactive **Y** group (Figure 16.11). Mostly, the addition of **X** groups onto the cellulose is performed by the chemical modification of the main chain [22].

In the reactions realized with this approach, it is more appropriate for cellulose and the polymer having reactive **Y** group to occur in a dissolved form in a common solvent for a homogeneous reaction medium. The structures of graft copolymers can be analyzed in detail since the main chain and the branches can be separately formed and separately characterized. It is possible for the number of the grafts on a chain and the distance between two adjacent grafts to be evaluated when the molecular weights of cellulose and the polymer and the general composition of the graft copolymer. The main problem in the application of this method is the complexity that naturally arises from the polymer chains on the surface. In this complexity of chains, the polymers that have **Y** reactive groups are hindered from diffusing more onto the cellulose surface (steric hindrance), and as a result, low graft densities are obtained [23]. The grafting of thermosensitive amine-terminated statistical polymers onto the surface of cellulose nanocrystals with the "grafting onto" approach is performed by the peptidic coupling reaction [24]. Extraordinary features such as colloidal stability at high ionic power, structure activity, and thermoreversible aggregation are observed in the obtained modified cellulose nanocrystals, and in addition, it is seen that they remain stable even in high electrolyte concentrations.

The "grafting through" approach: In this approach, the cellulose main chain on which the vinyl group is attached (macromonomer of cellulose) is linked to a low-molecular-weight comonomer (Figure 16.12). Since the polymerization of a monomer takes place in the presence of cellulose containing unsaturated vinyl group, a cross-linked product can arise by the combination of the growing chain with two or more unsaturated groups to the cellulose main chain [7].

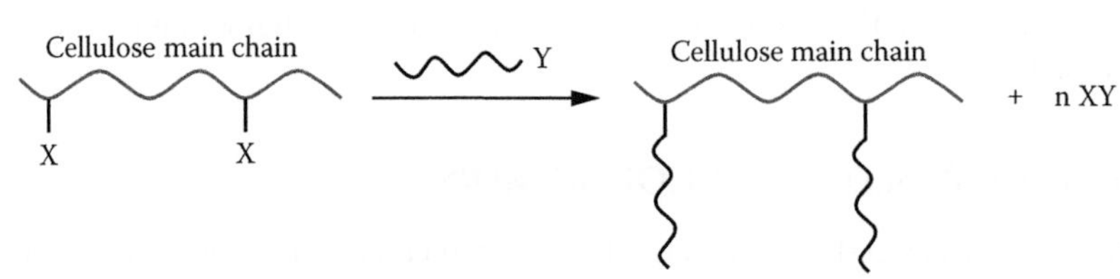

FIGURE 16.11 A schematic representation of the "grafting onto" approach.

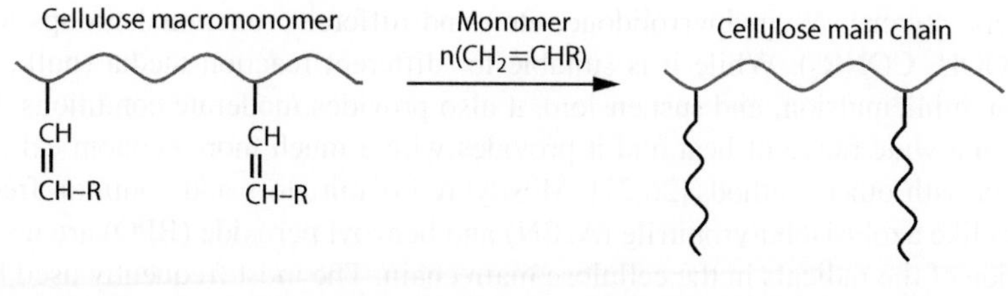

FIGURE 16.12 A schematic representation of the "grafting through" approach.

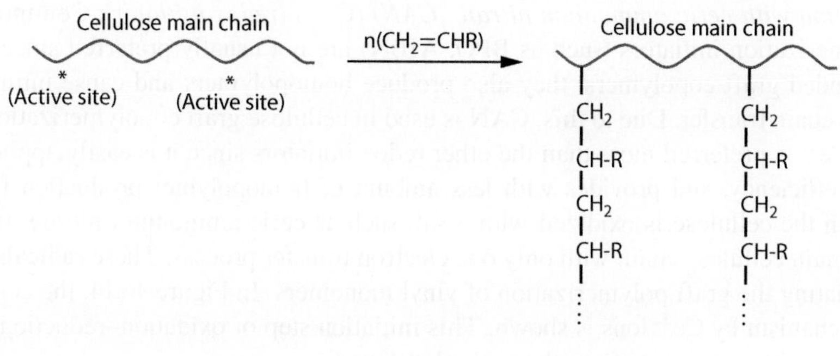

FIGURE 16.13 A schematic representation of the "grafting from" approach.

Although the "grafting through" approach is quite convenient for the preparation of graft copolymers, primarily, the previous phase of the synthesis of the macromonomers of cellulose and its derivatives must be completed successfully.

The "grafting from" approach: In this approach, active centers that will start polymerization are prepared by chemical modification of the main cellulose chain. These active centers on the main chain can be in the sort of free radicals, anionic, cationic, or Ziegler–Natta [25]. The number of the grafted chains is controlled with the number of the active centers that arise on the main chain of the cellulose, and each of which is regarded responsible for the growth of a graft (Figure 16.13). However, differences in length may arise due to kinetic and steric effects.

In order to prepare modified cellulose, the method of "grafting onto," and more frequently "grafting from," is used. One of the important advantages of "grafting from" approach is that a high graft density can be obtained since reactive monomers can easily reach the edge of the polymer chain growing on cellulose.

Now here, let's have a look at the grafting methods realized chemically, with high-energy radiation, photochemically, or enzymatically.

16.3.1.1 Grafting Initiated by Chemicals

Grafting initiated by chemicals can be performed in three different ways: (1) free radical polymerization, (2) ionic and ring-opening polymerization (ROP), and (3) controlled/"living" free radical polymerization [7]. In the grafting initiated by chemicals, the role of the "initiator" is very important since it determines the grafting mechanism. The initiator produces free radicals, and it is transferred onto the cellulose in order for it to get together with the monomer that will initiate the graft copolymerization.

1. "Free radical polymerization" is a method in which, typically, only about 60% of the available polymers are produced. There are good reasons for its wide usage. It can be in a wide range, applied to a variety of monomers (acrylate-type monomers, water-soluble

monomers, styrene, *N*-vinylpyrrolidone, etc.) and different functional groups (e.g., OH, NR_2, COOH, $CONR_2$). While it is suitable for different reaction media (bulk, solution, emulsion, miniemulsion, and suspension), it also provides moderate conditions. It can be applied in a wide range of heat and it provides with a much more economical operation compared with other methods [26,27]. Mostly, redox initiators and common free radical initiators like azobisisobutyronitrile (AIBN) and benzoyl peroxide (BPO) are used for the production of the radicals in the cellulose main chain. The most frequently used free radical initiators in the preparation of cellulose graft copolymers via the chemicals are ceric ammonium nitrate, potassium persulfate, and Fenton's reagent.

Direct oxidation with ceric ammonium nitrate (CAN) (Ce^{4+}) (redox initiator): Common-type free radical polymerization initiators (such as BPO, AIBN) are not usually preferred since while they produce intended graft copolymers, they also produce homopolymers and cause unintended side effects in the chain transfer. Due to this, CAN is used in cellulose graft copolymerization. Grafting initiated by Ce^{4+} is preferred more than the other redox initiators since it is easily applicable, gives higher graft efficiency, and provides with less amount of homopolymer production [28]. In this method, when the cellulose is oxidized with a salt such as ceric ammonium nitrate, free radicals arise on the main cellulose chain with only one electron transfer process. These radicals are convenient for initiating the graft polymerization of vinyl monomers. In Figure 16.14, the cellulose graft initiating mechanism by Ce^{4+} ions is shown. This initiation step of oxidation–reduction minimizes the production of homopolymer from the grafted chain.

Using this mechanism, it has been possible to graft monomers such as vinyl acetate, ethyl acrylate, methyl methacrylate, methyl acrylate, styrene, acrylamide (AAm), and AN on cellulose [29]. In literature, other oxidizing species that work similar to the mechanism of Ce^{4+} (Mn^{3+}, Mn^{4+}, Co^{3+}, V^{5+}, IO_4^-) are also reported [22].

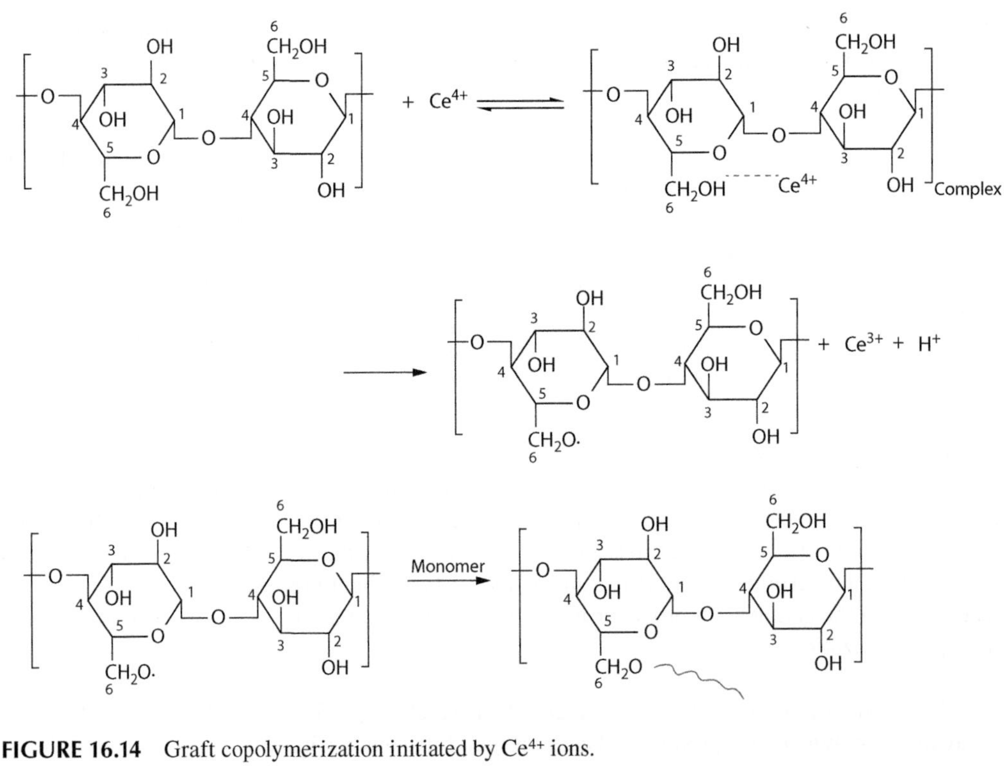

FIGURE 16.14 Graft copolymerization initiated by Ce^{4+} ions.

$$Fe^{2+} + H_2O_2 \longrightarrow Fe^{3+} + OH^- + HO\cdot$$

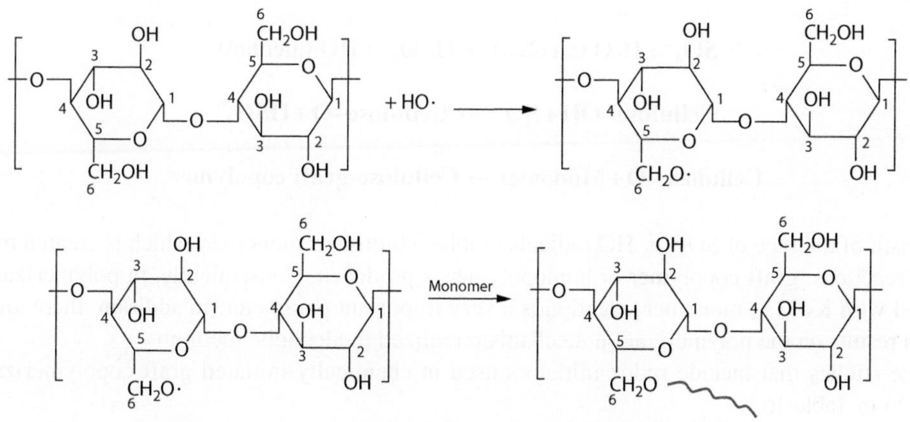

$$M + HO\cdot \longrightarrow \text{Homopolymer}$$

FIGURE 16.15 Graft copolymerization initiated with Fenton's reagent.

Initiation with Fenton's (Fe^{2+}–H_2O_2) reagent (redox initiator): Because it is cheap and easy to apply, grafting can be initiated with Fenton's reagent. There are studies in which acrylate-type monomers are grafted on the cellulose main chain by using Fenton's reagent [30]. In those studies, the decomposition reaction of H_2O_2 by Fe^{2+} is proposed as a typical redox reaction that creates OH radicals that will initiate grafting. When H_2O_2 and Fe^{2+} diffuse into cellulose in high initiation concentrations, there occur various grafting centers (macroradicals). First, Fe^{2+} adsorbs on cellulose. Then, OH radicals are produced as a result of the contact of cellulose with aqueous H_2O_2. Those radicals create cellulose macroradicals by removing one hydrogen molecule from cellulose. In the areas where macroradicals exist, grafting occurs with the participation of acrylic or vinyl monomers. Here, homopolymerization can be seen also by the addition of radicals to monomers. As it can be seen in the mechanism in Figure 16.15, it is required for types in which Fe^{3+} can easily make reactions with, such as ascorbic acid, which can be added to the reaction medium in order to remove the negative effects of Fe^{3+} ions present in the grafting medium [31].

Initiation with potassium persulfate ($K_2S_2O_8$) (redox initiator): Potassium persulfate ($K_2S_2O_8$, KPS) is the best radical initiator for abstracting hydrogen from a monomeric or polymeric structure in a polymerization process. It is cheap and soluble in water. There are studies in which persulfate redox systems are used as initiator of the graft copolymerization to the cellulose main chain [32]. Ghosh and Das [33] modified cotton cellulose by grafting acrylic acid (AA) in the presence of potassium persulfate as free radical initiator. Suo et al. [34] applied this initiation technique for the graft copolymerization of AA and AAm monomers onto CMC, to make cellulose-based superabsorbent polymers. Similarly, Aliouche et al. [35] synthesized cellulose substrates with improved absorption and retention via the graft copolymerization of AA and AN using KPS as the initiator.

Kolthoff and Miller [36] showed that persulfate ions, due to heating in an aqueous solution with or without a catalyzer, disintegrate into sulfate radical ions:

$$S_2O_8^{2-} \rightarrow 2SO_4^{-}$$

$$S_2O_8^{2-} + Fe^{2+} \rightarrow Fe^{3+} + SO_4^{2-} + SO_4^{-}$$

Sulfate radicals can create hydroxyl radicals in water (alcohol). Thus, OH or SO_4^- radicals can initiate polymerization:

$$\mathbf{SO_4^- + H_2O\ (alcohol) \rightarrow HSO_4^- + HO\ (alcohol)}$$

$$\mathbf{Cellulose{-}OH + SO_4^- \rightarrow Cellulose{-}O + HSO_4^-}$$

$$\mathbf{Cellulose{-}O + Monomer \rightarrow Cellulose\text{-}graft\ copolymer}$$

As a result of the race of SO_4^- or HO radicals to join cellulose or monomer, which is created by the earlier reactions, graft copolymer or homopolymer is produced. Consequently, in polymerizations initiated with $K_2S_2O_8$, monomer selection is a very important parameter. In addition, there are not enough results on the polymerization mechanism realized in alcoholic medium.

Some studies that include redox initiators used in chemically initiated graft copolymerization are given in Table 16.1.

2. Ionic polymerization and ROP: There are very few studies about ionic graft polymerization based on "cationic" or "anionic" mechanism, since it requires very challenging reaction conditions (low temperature, highly pure reagents, inert atmosphere, anhydrous condition, etc.). In "anionic" grafting, alkali metal alkoxides from the cellulose main chain are used as initiators. Polymerization is made in low temperatures in liquid ammonia or other inert solvents. Since the desired results are not obtained with the approaches of anionic "grafting onto" or "grafting from" and unwanted side effects occurred, it did not became to be a preferred choice of method [48]. For example, in propylene sulfide's anionic graft copolymerization on cellulose, it has been observed that in high monomer concentration, more homopolymer is obtained [49]. On the other hand, when grafting proceeds on a "cationic" [22] mechanism, easy and effective preparation of some unique graft copolymers (exhibit extraordinary physicochemical and mechanical properties) became possible. In cationic grafting, a Lewis acid such as $AlBr_3$, $TiCl_4$, and BF_3 make complexes with the OH groups

TABLE 16.1
Some Studies That Include Redox Initiators Used in Chemically Initiated Graft Copolymerization

Cellulose or Derivative	Monomer	Initiator	Reference
Cellulose	Acrylic acid	CAN	[37]
Cellulose	Acrylamide	CAN	[38]
Cellulose	Vinyl acetate	CAN	[39]
Carboxymethylcellulose	Acrylamide	CAN	[40]
Cellulose	Acrylonitrile	CAN	[41]
Cellulose	Vinyl acetate	Fe^{2+}–H_2O_2	[42]
Cellulose	Ethyl acrylate	Fe^{2+}–H_2O_2	[43]
Cellulose	Methyl methacrylate	Fe^{2+}–H_2O_2	[42]
Cellulose	Ethyl acrylate	Fe^{2+}–H_2O_2	[43]
Ethyl cellulose	Methyl methacrylate	$K_2S_2O_8$	[44]
Ethyl cellulose	Acrylamide	$K_2S_2O_8$	[45]
Methylcellulose	Acrylamide	$K_2S_2O_8$	[46]
Cellulose	Acrylic acid	$K_2S_2O_8$	[33]
Cellulose	Itaconic acid	$K_2S_2O_8$	[47]

of cellulose. Thus, the cationic centers created on cellulose join monomer and initiate graft copolymerization. The grafting of isobutylene on cellulose can be given as an example of cationic graft polymerization [50].

"ROP," although there are not many studies in literature, is a method that introduces cyclic monomer's polymerization mechanism such as lactose and lactides with all of their details [51]. Since hydroxyl groups are used as initiators in this method, cellulose itself is taken as a natural multifunctional initiator. It is not a coincidence that in literature there are studies about cellulose copolymers that are obtained with cyclic monomers by ROP. In a study by Hafren and Cordova, [52] graft copolymers of ε-caprolactone (CL) on cellulose in the presence of tartaric acid catalyzer were obtained by ROP, and very high graft yields were achieved. The most important advantage of ROP in the preparation of cellulose graft copolymers is that there is no need for cellulose to be modified chemically in advance. In addition, by changing monomer/cellulose rates, it is possible to control copolymer molecular weight.

3. Controlled/"living" free radical polymerization: In recent years, "living" free radical polymerization methods are also used in grafting on cellulose. Szwarc [53] used the definition of "living polymer" for polymer that "keeps the activity of polymerization for a long time and is able to come to the desired size when termination or chain transfer reactions are not important." Controlled/"living" free radical polymerization shows both free radical and ionic polymerization characteristics together. Methods of controlled/"living" radical polymerization are nitroxide-mediated polymerization [54], atom transfer radical polymerization (ATRP) [55], and reversible addition–fragmentation chain transfer polymerization [56]. These methods provide opportunity to the living polymer, which has controllable molecular weights and low polydispersity.

The most used controlled/"living" radical polymerization to change cellulose and its derivatives' surface properties is ATRP. In a study by Nystrom et al. [57], using ATRP initiator, polyglycidylmethacrylate (PGMA) was grafted on modified cellulose, and superhydrophobic surfaces were obtained. The polymerization was performed by epoxy units of PGMA, which hydrolyzed under acidic conditions. It showed that when functionalization is made by using different agents, surface properties can be changed.

16.3.1.2 Grafting Initiated with High-Energy Radiation

Grafting with high-energy radiation (γ rays or accelerated electrons) is known as a method that makes functional groups join inorganic materials and various polymers [58]. In copolymerization process made with high-energy γ rays, thanks to adjustable dose speed, the most appropriate dose speed is determined, and a monomer makes copolymerization with another monomer/polymer without the need for a catalyzer. Since high-energy radiations corrupt cellulose's glucopyranose ring structure, it could not be used successfully at the beginning. When late years' studies are seen, in polymerizations in which monomers' access to cellulose is controlled, cellulose copolymers that have high graft yield were obtained successfully [22].

The "preirradiation" method and the "mutual irradiation" method are the two major approaches to the grafting of cellulose by radiation. The cellulose substrate in the former [59], which comes before the introduction of monomers and swelling agents, is irradiated first. As a result, although the degradation of the cellulose backbone is usually greater especially in grafting in the presence of air and oxygen, significantly less amount of homopolymer occurs compared with the mutual irradiation method. In the latter method, [60] in the presence of the monomers or monomer–solvent mixtures, the cellulose substrate is irradiated directly. This approach usually leads to a considerable amount of homopolymer occurrence resulting from the direct radiolysis of the monomer. Badawy et al. [61], in the mutual irradiation-induced graft copolymerization of AN onto cellulosic filter paper, found that the amount of homopolymer could be reduced by the introduction of a small amount of styrene monomer. However, the mutual irradiation method results in less degradation of cellulose fiber, as a result of protective action of the vinyl and acrylic monomers during the actual irradiation.

The grafting of a monomer to cellulose using high-energy radiation has some clear advantages, including the fact that the processes can be speedy and relatively simple to operate. This is partly because there is no "synthesis" step to modify the cellulose substrate prior to polymerization. Grafting takes place in lower temperatures compared to polymerization initiated with chemicals. In addition, because there is no initiator or catalyzer used for grafting, the resulting product does not include residue materials [62]. However, radical formation occurs mainly along the path of the incident radiation beam, and therefore the radical generation process is unselective. In addition, the radiation degrades cellulose in a disproportionation reaction via the splitting of glycosidic linkages, resulting in a loss of mechanical strength of the cellulose fibers.

16.3.1.3 Grafting Initiated with Photochemicals

If a monomer medium includes photosensitizing agent irradiated with lower-energy photons (UV radiation), polymerization can be initiated. In studies by Geacintov [63,64], by using anthraquinoid-type dyes as photosensitizers, methyl methacrylate or styrene polymerizations are carried out successfully with UV radiation.

The grafting of various vinyl and acrylic monomers to cellulose using low-energy UV radiation causes less degradation of the backbone polymer and gives an option for better control over the grafting reaction than that achieved by the high-energy γ-radiation method. This process is usually carried out in the presence of photoinitiators, which accelerate the process by forming additional radicals when exposed to UV radiation. These radicals can enhance grafting by creating sites in the backbone polymer via abstraction reactions. The use of UV radiation for the grafting of glycidyl methacrylate (GMA), 2-hydroxyethyl methacrylate, styrene, and AN onto cotton cellulose in the presence of various photoinitiators such as uranyl nitrate, ceric ammonium nitrate, and benzoin ethyl ether has been studied [22]. In a study by Hong and coworkers [65], AAm was grafted in cellulose by using benzophenone as photoinitiator via UV radiation. Grafting yield is increased by increasing the amount of benzophenone. The thermal stability of grafted cotton fabrics was increased, and its excellent antibacterial ability was obtained after treatment by simple chlorination process.

16.3.1.4 Enzymatic Grafting

This type of grafting is quite new. It is a method in which chemical/electrochemical grafting reaction starts via enzymes. In 2004, Martinelle et al. [66] used a lipase for the ROP of CL in close proximity to cellulose fibers in a filter paper. In the first step, the enzyme was immobilized on the filter paper used as substrate, and in the second step, the polymerization was performed. This did not create covalently bonded grafts, but the polycaprolactone still coated the cellulose surface, as determined by FTIR spectroscopy and contact angle (CA) measurements.

As it can be seen from all of those methods, the search for improving/changing the features of cellulose graft copolymers is continuously going on. Correct characterization of cellulose graft copolymers after they have been prepared is also an important matter to be dwelled upon.

16.3.2 Characterization Methods for Cellulose-Based Graft Copolymers

In order for the determination of the physical and chemical features of cellulose graft copolymers prepared by choosing the appropriate methods from that given earlier, true characterization is required for the average molecular weight, average composition, distribution of branches on cellulose main chain, and heterogeneity between grafting points and branches [25]. Since no method became perfect in the preparation of synthetic polymers, the obtained final polymer is a complex structure. In this complex structure, along with the desired graft copolymers, there can also be unwanted types such as cellulose and synthetic polymer chains not yet connected as graft copolymer and copolymeric types having different architectural structures. They should be isolated from resulting graft copolymers and must be characterized. For this reason, by extracting the complex structure, after grafting, with appropriate solvent or solvent mixtures, homopolymer/different polymer structures are completely removed from graft copolymers. On the basis of initial mass of the cellulose (m_0), the increase in the mass (m) after grafting and extraction is taken as the apparent grafting yield [31]:

$$\text{Grafting yield}(\%) = \frac{\text{mass of grafted polymer}}{\text{original mass of cellulose}} \times 100 = \frac{m - m_0}{m_0} \times 100 \qquad (16.1)$$

Grafting yield can be calculated with simple laboratory processes, that is, gravimetric [67] and volumetric [68]; it can also be decided by using elemental analysis [69] over the heteroatoms on polymer grafted on the cellulose main chain. There are different methods used in order to determine the average molecular weight of graft copolymers. For graft polymers having low molecular weight, since there will be no dissolution problems, molecular weight can be determined correctly by using spectroscopic methods in solution. NMR spectroscopy provides both quantitative and qualitative information about comonomer composition and the stereochemistry of polymer chains [25]. FTIR spectroscopy is used to monitor chemical, structural, and conformational changes. Oxidative depolymerization products of cellulose are also among the macrocellulosic radicals made with the "grafting from" approach. Consequently, the increases in the intensities of carbonyl (C=O) and carboxyl (COOH) groups are followed by FTIR spectroscopy [31].

It is important to determine the average molecular weight of graft polymers since it directly affects the features of copolymer. For this reason, there are several methods used to decide the molecular weight of copolymers whose average molecular weights vary in a wide range. The branches obtained after grafting can be separated from the main chain by the hydrolyzing of cellulose main chain, and thus, the molecular weights of the main chain and the branches can be found separately. Apart from viscometry [70], membrane osmometry [71], and light scattering [72], the methods of proton nuclear magnetic resonance (^{1}H-NMR) [73] and gel permeation chromatography/size exclusion chromatography (SEC) [74] are also used. In detailed studies conducted with light scattering, the molecular size of the main chain and branches can be calculated separately. With SEC, the molecular weights of graft copolymers can be determined, and the molecular mass distribution and composition in copolymer can be determined. If the molecular weight of the graft polymer should be calculated in an appropriate solution medium, the methods of dynamic and static light scattering [75], small-angle neutron scattering (SANS) [76], and small-angle x-ray scattering (SAXS) [77] are used. While static light scattering, SAXS, and SANS are used in order to determine the gyration radius of the polymers separated from the main chain, the methods of dynamic light scattering and viscometry give important clues about the hydrodynamic radius.

The end products obtained by the grafting of acrylic or vinyl monomers on cellulose and its derivatives show alterations from the original cellulose structures with regard to surface properties, microbial decomposition resistance, chemical reactivity, water absorption features, and thermal and mechanical features. The morphological and supramolecular structure of graft copolymers are their most easily affected features from monomer's interaction with the cellulose main chain. Change in the surface properties before and after grafting is measured with the methods of light microscopy [78], scanning electron microscopy (SEM) [79], transmission electron microscopy (TEM) [80], atomic force microscopy (AFM) [81], and contact angle (CA) [79]. As a result of the interaction of monomer solution with cellulose, monomer breaks some of the intra- and intermolecular H-bonds by diffusing into the crystalline areas of cellulose. Thus, it causes cellulose plates to separate partially; in other words, it causes a reduction in crystallinity. To determine these alterations, x-ray diffraction (XRD) [82] method is used. By using x-ray photoelectron spectroscopy (XPS), information about graft copolymer chain and its branches and its composition is gathered. Again, SEM simultaneously used with energy-dispersive x-ray spectroscopy (EDX) gives information about the chemical structure of graft copolymers, and loosely about their composition. The thermal behaviors of cellulose graft copolymers are monitored with TGA, DTA, and DSC [74,83,84]. Their mechanical features such as the modulus of elasticity, tensile strength, and failure strain are determined by calculating from obtained stress–strain curves [85,86]. Apart from these, it is possible to use other characterization methods suitable for the cellulose and synthetic monomer/polymer features, preparation method, and the purpose of use.

16.3.3 Possible Applications of Cellulose-Based Graft Copolymers

Cellulose and its derivatives are very convenient because of the fact that they can be chemically modified with respect to the intended area of usage. Since they are biodegradable, biorenewable, and biocompatible, it is not wrong at all to call them "the materials of the future." The features that determine their area of usage are the chemical structure of the synthetic monomer grafted on cellulose and its derivative and the architectural structure of such copolymer. The manipulable modified cellulose derivatives are widely used in the areas of pharmaceutics and biomedicals, which require controlled wetting, encapsulation, and release of an active matter [23]. The cellulose and derivative surfaces, which are grafted with bioactive polymers, are used in the preparation of biosensors [87], active packaging [80], bioreactors [88], wound dressings, and antimicrobial surfaces [89]. In filtration systems [90], they are used as controllable membranes with the features of porosity and permeability. For outdoor applications, they are used in textile industry as the raw material of superhydrophobic and dirt-proof fabric [91]. If the monomer used in grafting is a structure showing the electrical properties [92], then cellulose graft copolymers convenient for electrical applications are prepared.

CMC is the most important water-soluble ionic derivative of cellulose. It is widely used in the industries of pharmaceutics, cosmetics, food, paper, and textile. However, it needs to be modified with grafting for special applications. In literature, there are a lot of studies on this subject. Polymethacrylamide (PMAm) is grafted on CMC in the presence of initiator CAN/water, and the obtained graft copolymers are characterized with FTIR and TGA [93]. The efficiency of grafting, the initiator, the amounts of cellulose and monomer, and their temperature and dissolution effects are studied. In another study, *N*-vinyl-2-pyrrolidone (VP) and AA mixtures are grafted on CMC/HEC mixtures in order to prepare membranes that have special biological features [94]. In a study [95], polyacrylamide (PAAm) is grafted on CMC surface in the presence of a cross-linker, *N,N'*-methylene bisacrylamide (MBA), and initiator ammonium persulfate, and the usability of the obtained graft copolymers as membranes in desalination is examined. Structural, thermal, and surface characterizations were studied with FTIR, TGA, and SEM methods. While the original PAAm was at a water uptake value of 37 g/g, it has reached to 158 g/g after being grafted on CMC.

There are, again, a lot of studies in which cellulose is used in biomedicine and pharmaceutics. Since they are biocompatible, biodegradable, and easily modifiable, cellulose derivatives such as hydroxypropylcellulose, HPMC, HEC, and CMC are expected to be the most widely used controlled-release systems in the future. Wang et al. [96], having prepared HPMC and EC graft copolymers, studied the characterization of these structures and the changes that take place in these structures after grafting. HPMC has a wide area of usage in the applications of controlled release since it has features such as having a nontoxic structure, independence from pH, and high-level medication carrying capacity [97]. It is the most important hydrophilic carrier that is used in the preparation of oral controlled drug release systems [98]. The reason why it is that important in controlled release is its high swelling degree. In case of contact with water or biological fluids, polymer chains are opened, and extension in its volume occurs. Thus, the drug placed in the polymer is easily released [99].

Cellulose acetate (CA) is widely used since it is a cellulose ester that can make good film forming. It is used efficiently in membrane separation processes, photographic films, cigarette filters, cosmetic products, and pharmaceutical formulations. However, its high glass transition temperature (~190°C), rigidity, and relative hydrophobic character narrow its area of usage. Grafting of methyl diethylene glycol methacrylate is carried out on the surface of CA with the method of controlled radical polymerization/ATRP [100]. It is found that the chain elasticity of graft copolymers characterized with the methods of SAXS, WAXS, ^{1}H-NMR, ^{13}C-NMR, SEC, and MALLS is increased, their hydrophilic/hydrophobic character can be controlled, and they can be used as a strong membrane in the membrane separation processes. In another study, AAm and styrene are grafted on the surface of CA with UV, and the obtained graft copolymers are characterized with the methods of FTIR, TGA, and DSC. It is shown that they can be used in reverse osmosis processes as graft membranes having a high-level salt-repellant property [101]. Acyclic halamine cotton has been prepared with a chlorination process following the grafting of amid monomers on the surface of cellulose [102]. It is found that acrylic halamines produced with free radical polymerization using AAm and methacrylamide have durable and chargeable biocidal functions, but they are easily affected by hydrolysis compared with cyclic halamines. In a study conducted in order to increase the sensitivity of cellulose to humidity [103], polyaniline (PANi) is grafted on the surface of cellulose in $CuSO_4$/HCl medium, and the graft copolymers are characterized by the methods of FTIR, XRD, TGA, and SEM. It is found that the humidity sensitivity of cellulose, which has a nonconducting and nonionic character, has increased after PANi has been grafted.

Graft copolymers of polyester/cotton blend fabric with PAA and PMAA were prepared by Hebeish et al. [29] using mutual gamma irradiation and Fenton's reagent. The obtained copolymers were treated with durable-press finishes with cross-linking agent, and their sensitivity to aqueous and nonaqueous oily soiling and soil-releasing ability were examined. The result was that, especially after cross-linking, the hydrophilization of the fabric surface obtained by grafting enhanced the resistance to soiling. The soil release with oily soil is also found to be capable of improvement.

Maulik and Banerjee [104] modified the cotton fabric by presoaking with $K_2S_2O_8$, subsequent application of AAm monomer by padding technique, followed by drying and curing, and dying the modified fabric with pigment colors. They found that prior modification produced good colorfastness to wash, light, and dry rubbing. The modification also resulted in increased color values with increase in bending length. Rowland and Mason [105] studied the simultaneous finishing of cotton with dimethylol dihydroxy ethylene urea and a polymerizable zinc salt of acrylic, methacrylic, and itaconic acid. They ended up not only with a good performance of durable press but also with a strength preservation and abrasion resistance above average. In this study, various degrees of improvement in the release of oily soil are observed, and a higher antibacterial performance compared with conventional durable-press cotton fabrics is obtained.

Franklin et al. [106] carried out combined acrylic polymerization and methylol cross-linking reaction to make durable-press cotton fabrics. Continuous grafting with low-cost commercial reagents is the gist of this operation. In this study, using dimethylol dihydroxyethyleneurea, AA, and persulfate–bisulfite redox-initiating catalyst, pad bath is obtained, and pad-care process is followed. The resulting fabric was found to show high wrinkle recovery angles with good creasability.

Graft copolymers can also be used in composite materials. It is difficult to get wood materials and plastics together and make them compatible. However, if this is performed successfully, the area of usage of the newly obtained materials will be wider. In a study on the adhesive applications [107], in order to make polystyrene and wood compatible with themselves, copolymers that are polystyrene grafted made compatible wood and plastic by making polystyrene branches stick to plastic and cellulose main chain to wood. The obtained composite structures made the preparation of mechanically more resistant but biodegradable materials possible, to be used in the industries such as molded objects, packaging, and furniture.

Apart from all these areas of usage, there is also a considerable amount of studies on cellulose and its derivatives grafted with polymers having appropriate functional group, aiming to avoid the aqueous systems due to the harmful effects of heavy metals and organic pollutants to environment. Examples from literature about such applications are given further in text.

Cellulose derivatives such as EC and HPMC, or other natural polymers, are used in many areas widely, especially in the adsorption studies, due to their advantageous features. Lin and Juang [108] discussed the technical feasibility of the subject of the removal of phenol and its derivatives from waters with low-cost natural adsorbents, and they concluded that these adsorbents promise hope for the future for commercial purposes.

In another study, monomer of dimethylamino ethylacrylate (DMAEA) is grafted on the surface of cellulose in the presence of CAN–HNO_3, and the obtained graft copolymers are characterized with the methods of FTIR, SEM, and TGA. It is emphasized that DMAEA-grafted cellulose can be used in the textile industry as a raw material of fabric whose hydrophobic/hydrophilic feature is controllable [109]. It is shown that the graft copolymers obtained by grafting functional monomers such as AAm [110], AA [111], AN [112], and 2-acrylamidomethylpropane sulfonic acid [113] on the surface of cellulose and its derivatives successfully removed the heavy metals and anionic, organic, and colorant pollutants, which are known to be harmful for the environment, from aqueous solutions.

16.3.4 Use of Cellulose-Based Graft Copolymers for Recovery Purposes

The leading problem at the present time is the environmental pollution due to industrial and other pollutants. Heavy metals, which belong to the industrial pollutants, are an important source of pollution of soil, air, and water. These areas, which are polluted by various pollutants, especially heavy metals, pose a high danger to the living organisms within them. Thus, the efforts for providing a permanent solution to environmental pollution, which occurred due to the industrialization contributing to our development and dramatic rise of population, are going on increasingly. Since cleaning the polluted environment requires long-lasting efforts with quite expensive and complex systems, the measures to prevent water, soil, and air pollution are gaining importance more and more.

The materials that create soil and air pollution are transferred to water in time by the factors of rain and snow. The heavy metals contained in water become more toxic, interacting with inorganic or organic wastes. The toxic materials received by the body create many health problems [114]. The most known harmful metals in industrial wastewaters are copper, cadmium, lead, nickel, chromium, and zinc. Among these pollutants, there are not only cationic but also anionic pollutants such as arsenic, cyanide, pesticides, dyes, and phosphates. Among these, there are also economically valuable pollutants like lead recovered from wastewaters and uranium recovered from seawater or wastewaters [115,116]. The decreasing of the toxic effects of heavy metals in aqueous systems and the recovery of the economically important heavy metals for reuse are important subjects that need attention [117,118]. The leading method for the removal of the pollutants from water is "adsorption" due to its flexible working conditions, less initial cost, smaller land investment, simple design, easy usage, and nontoxicity.

In the adsorption systems, the interest in the usage of the low-cost biomasses such as clay, active carbon, tea leaves, agricultural waste, cellulose, wool fiber, fly ash, animal bones, and pineapple shell is growing increasingly. Another important thing about these examples is that they are degradable in nature in a short period of time, and the released CO_2 and H_2O are environmentally friendly end products.

The water uptake capacity, adsorption, and ion exchange features of cellulose can be enhanced by modifying it with graft copolymerization [6]. For the last 30 years, the studies on the subject of the enhancement of its features by grafting acrylic and vinyl monomers on cellulose are going on widely. Liu et al. [41,119] have grafted AN on cellulose using CAN as initiator and examined the Cu(II) and Co(III) adsorption capacity by converting nitrile groups to amide (–$CONH_2$) and carboxylate (–COONa) groups. For the removal of heavy metal ions from aqueous solutions, scientists used cellulose graft copolymers having thermosensitive graft chains, such as poly(*N*-isopropylacrylamide) or poly(*N*,*N*-diethylacrylamide). In this process, the method of temperature swing adsorption is used, and this method differs from the removal of metal ions by complexation or ion exchange [120].

There are also studies aiming at removing water pollutants due to agricultural activities (pesticides, phosphates, and nitrates). The prevention of threats to living organisms caused by phosphates and nitrates by reducing the oxygen in water with eutrophication is possible with the removal of these ions from water. In a study related to the removal and the recovery of phosphate because of its biological importance [121], epichlorohydrin and high-density cationic charged polyethyleneimine (PEI) mixture is grafted on cellulose. In the free radical graft copolymerization performed using cross-linker MBA and initiator AIBN at 30°C, the end product is characterized with the methods of FTIR, TGA, DSC, SEM, and XRD. Phosphate is successfully removed with $q_e = 100$ mg/g adsorption value at pH = 6, as a result of the electrostatic interaction of the PEI branches of the graft copolymer with phosphate anions.

GMA is grafted on cellulose in the presence of cross-linker MBA and initiator BPO; the graft copolymers functionalized with $NH(CH_3)_2$ are used in removing vanadium (V) ions [122]. In the adsorption conducted with AAS, the adsorption value of 178 mg/g is reached at pH = 6. It is claimed that the interaction had taken place between the amine groups and $V_3O_9^{3-}$ ions. Diaminomaleonitrile is grafted on the surface of cellulose in the initiator medium of dilute HNO_3–CAN, [123] and the graft copolymers are used in the recovery of Pb^{2+}, Cd^{2+}, Zn^{2+}, Fe^{3+}, Cu^{2+}, Ni^{2+}, and Co^{2+} ions. For all the ions, 95% recovery is achieved.

AAm-grafted cellulose copolymer is used in the removal of Hg(II) [110]. Amide groups are selective for Hg(II) ion since it holds this ion covalently. In this study, Ce(IV) sulfate is used as initiator, and the adsorption capacity of 3.55 mmol/g is reached.

Apart from the studies on the removal of heavy metal ions from water, the recovery of the economically valuable uranium, thorium, and vanadium from water is, again, performed on the basis of adsorption. Thorium can be found in the earth's crust with rare earth elements and uranium, and naturally in the oceans. It is a primarily important radioactive metal in nuclear fuel plants since its waste problem is in a minimum level. In a study aiming at the recovery of thorium [124], polymethacrylic acid is grafted on TiO_2-densified cellulose by using cross-linker MBA and initiator Mn^{4+}/citric acid, and the adsorption capacity of 95 mg Th^{4+}/g is obtained with the batch adsorption using graft copolymers. Among the methods developed for changing the physical and chemical features of cellulose, grafting with radiation is also preferred frequently. In this method, a monomer is copolymerized with another, with the adjustment of dose rate, by means of high-energy γ rays without the need of an additive or a catalyst. The functional groups that occur on copolymer are sometimes modified for their high metal ion selectivity.

GMA is grafted on the surface of cellulose with γ rays, and the epoxy ring of GMA is modified with amine groups [125]. Amine-functionalized cellulose graft copolymers are used in the removal of acid red dye, Co(II) cation, and dichromate anion. Adsorption capacities are 18 mg/g at pH = 3 for Co(II), 3 mg/g at pH = 9 for dichromate, and 13 mg/g at pH = 9 for acid red dye.

The grafting of 2-hydroxyethyl methacrylate phosphoric acid monomer on nonwoven cotton fabric is performed via γ rays [126]. Zirconium (V), which is bound to the phosphoric acid groups, is used in the removal of As (V). The adsorption capacity of 0.1 mmol/g is obtained at pH = 2.

GMA-*co*-MAAc is grafted on cotton fabric with ^{60}Co-γ rays, and the epoxy ring of GMA is modified with triethylamine groups [127]. Thus, graft copolymers having amine and carboxyl functionality are used in the removal of Co(II) and nitrate. The adsorption capacity of 38.5 mg/g is obtained at pH = 5 for Co(II), and that of 11 mg/g is obtained at pH = 3 for nitrate.

Badawy et al. [61], for the purpose of uranium recovery, grafted AN on cotton cloth filter with the method of grafting with radiation and then converted the nitrile groups to chelating amidoxime (AO) groups. On the other hand, Goswami and Das [128] used the fly ash that they modified for the removal of uranium and thorium in Indian monazite sand, and they concluded that the resulting resin can also be used in the removal of uranium and thorium in aqueous solutions.

In Table 16.2, some examples are shown from the studies in which graft copolymers prepared with different methods are used in the removal of heavy metal ions [129].

Our research group also contributed to these various heavy metal removal and valuable metal recovery studies. EC, which is the only cellulose derivative that is insoluble in water, and cross-linked HPMC films are modified for the uranium recovery from aqueous systems, having grafted

TABLE 16.2
Cellulose and Cellulose-Type Materials Grafted for Metal Ion Adsorption

Metal/Polymer	Monomer	Initiating Method	Recovery mol dm^{-3}	Capacity mg g^{-1}	Reference
Cd(II)					
Paper stock, amylum	AAc	γ-radiation		4	[130]
Cellulose dust	AAc	Chemical	HCl, 1	30	[111]
Banana shell	AAm, carboxylate	Chemical	HCl, 0.2	66	[131]
Paper stock	NVP	γ-radiation		362	[132]
Cr(III)					
Paper stock, amylum	AAC	γ-radiation		7	[130]
Cr(IV)					
Cellulose	GMA + comonomers	Chemical	NaCl, 0.5		[133]
Cu(II)					
Cellulose	AAm + AAc	Microwave	8 v/v NH_4OH	49.6	[134]
Cellulose dust	AAc	Chemical		17	[111]
Cellulose	GMA imidazole	Chemical	HCl, 1	68.5	[135]
Cellulose	Amidoxime	Photo		51	[136]
Cellulose	GMA + comonomer	Chemical			[133]
Cellulose	St + AN, MAA	γ-radiation		100–200	[137]
Hg(II)					
Banana shell	AAm, modified	Chemical	HCl, 0.2	138 (30°C) 210 (60°C)	[131]
Cotton	AAm	Chemical	Acetic acid	12.5	[110]
Ni(II)					
Cellulose	GMA imidazole	Chemical	HCl, 0.1	48.5	[135]
Pb(II)					
Paper stock, amylum	AAc	γ-radiation		6	[130]
Cellulose powder	AAc	Chemical	HCl, 1	56	[111]
Cellulose	GMA imidazole	Chemical	HNO_3	75.8	[135]
Banana shell	AAm, carboxylate	Chemical	HCl, 0.2	185	[131]
Paper stock	NVP	γ-radiation		323	[132]
U(VI)					
Cotton cloth	AN/MAAc, amidox	γ-radiation	HCl, 1–5		[116]
V(V)					
Cellulose	GMA, MBA	Chemical	NaOH, 0.1	198	[122]
Zn(II)					
Porous cellulose	GMA modified	Chemical		30	[138]

with ^{60}Co-γ rays in the presence of AN [79,83]. Since HPMC powder is insoluble in AN monomer, it has been used in the form of cross-linked film. Grafting of AN on the surface of film has been performed in a dimethylformamide (DMF). On the other hand, since EC mixed with AN homogeneously, irradiation has been performed using EC–AN–DMF solutions containing various amounts of AN monomer. Grafting efficiency has been calculated using Equation 16.1 gravimetrically and found to be 60% for HPMC [79] and 90% for EC [83]. Here, an important point is that grafting in a heterogeneous medium in the form of film or fiber is advantageous, since the separation of the graft copolymer obtained in a homogeneous medium (as it is such with EC–AN–DMF mixture) from homopolymer is very time consuming, and the end product contains inextractable homopolymer chains. In our study too, although grafting efficiencies have been found high, there exist unextracted PAN chains in the EC-*g*-AN polymer; in other words, the copolymer is not as pure as HPMC-*g*-AN copolymer. The nitrile (C≡N) groups in both graft copolymers are converted to amidoxime groups in a medium with hydroxylamine hydrochloride (neutralized with NaOH) at 50°C. In Figure 16.16, the FTIR spectra taken for the structure analysis of HPMC-*g*-AN copolymers are shown. In the spectra,

1. At 3443 cm^{-1}, the wide peak belongs to the reactive –OH groups in the C_2, C_3, and C_6 positions of cellulose
2. At 2924 cm^{-1}, the peak belongs to $-CH_2$ groups of cellulose
3. At 1453 cm^{-1}, the peak belongs to the bending of the –CH groups of cellulose
4. At 947 cm^{-1}, the peak belongs to –CH groups in the glucopyranose ring of cellulose
5. At 1062 cm^{-1}, the peak belongs to –C–O groups of cellulose
6. At 2242 cm^{-1}, the peak belongs to –C≡N groups of poly AN, and at 1450 cm^{-1}, the peak belongs to the bending of the $-CH_2$ groups

The intensity of the peak seen at 2242 cm^{-1} belonging to the hydrophobic C≡N group is observed to decrease as the amidoximation time increases, and after 72 h, it is seen to be almost disappearing. This situation is an evidence for the conversion of nitrile groups in the structure of copolymer to hydrophilic amidoxime groups. In the same manner, the peak seen at around 1450 cm^{-1}, caused by AN groups and belonging to $-CH_2$ bendings, is observed to decrease in relation to amidoxime conversion. The characteristic peaks at 1660 and 900 cm^{-1}, which are observed to be sharper in relation to the amidoximation duration, belong, respectively, to the stretching of C=N and N–O, which

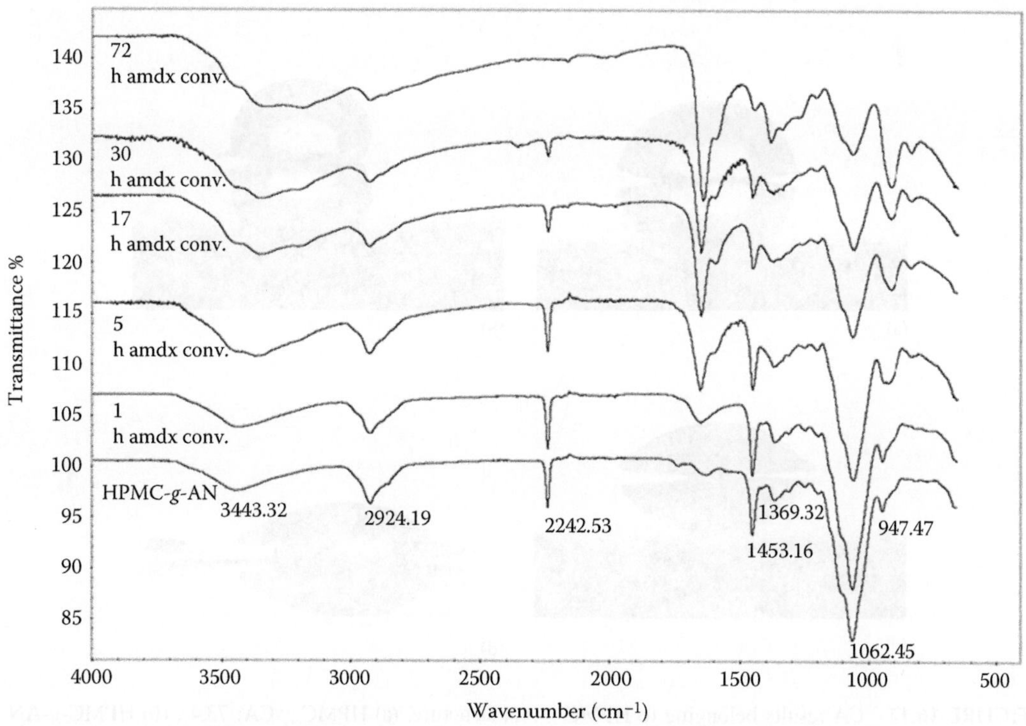

FIGURE 16.16 FTIR/ATR spectra taken for HPMC-*g*-AN copolymers after amidoximation reaction.

occur in the newly obtained amidoxime groups. And the characteristic absorption bands at around 1065 cm^{-1} and 1614 cm^{-1} are due to C–N stretchings.

Similar results are obtained for EC-*g*-AN copolymers [83]. The thermal stabilities of graft copolymers are determined using TGA. In Table 16.3, the degradation temperatures and percent weight losses belonging to HPMC-*g*-AN polymers are shown [79].

The surface characterizations of HPMC-*g*-AN and EC-*g*-AN copolymers are performed with CA, SEM, AFM, and EDX methods. The measurements of CAs of HPMC-*g*-AN copolymers are done in a noncontact mode using water as solvent (Figure 16.17).

In the second photograph, the increase in the angle value with the grafting of hydrophobic AN groups on HPMC and, after 72 h of amidoxime conversion, the decrease in the angle value with the existence of hydrophilic amidoxime groups in the structure are very interesting.

Since all of the features of high magnification (>100,000×), wider focus depth, and high resolution make more detailed analyses possible in the studies of polymer and biochemistry, they make

TABLE 16.3
Temperatures Corresponding to Degradation Peak Maxima for HPMC-*g*-AN

	Degradation Temperature Range (°C) (Peak Maxima)					Weight
Polymer	**0–200**	**200–300**	**300–400**	**400–500**	**500–700**	**Loss (%)**
Irradiated AN		278.6				65
$HPMC_{org}$			357			90
HPMC-*g*-AN		264	385.6	452.3		45
HPMC-*g*-AO after amidox.		288.2	363.3			60

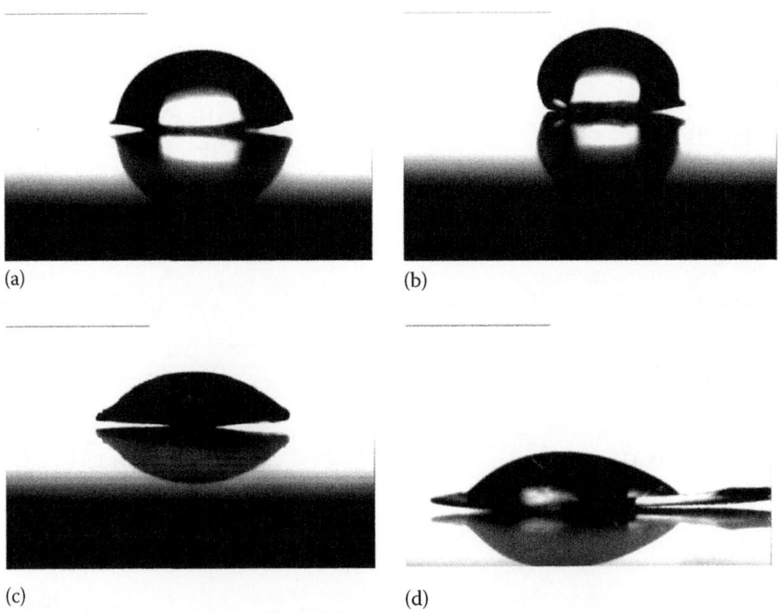

FIGURE 16.17 CA results belonging to HPMC-*g*-AN structure. (a) $HPMC_{org}$ CA: 73.4°, (b) HPMC-*g*-AN CA: 92.9°, (c) HPMC-*g*-AO (5 h) CA: 48.5°, and (d) HPMC-*g*-AO (72 h) CA: 45°. (From Başarır, S.S. and Bayramgil, N.P., *Cellulose*, 20, 1511, 2013.)

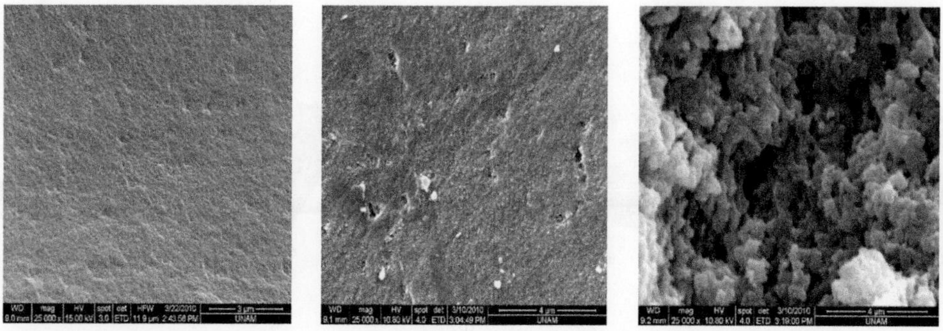

(a) (b) (c)

FIGURE 16.18 SEM images for EC-*g*-AN copolymers. (a) EC_{org}, (b) EC-*g*-AN, and (c) EC-*g*-AO. (From Başarır, S.S. and Bayramgil, N.P., *Radiochimica Acta*, 100, 893, 2012.)

SEM quite useful [1]. Among the research areas in which SEM is most widely used, microscopic feature measurement, fracture-break characterization, microstructure analysis, thin film coating studies, determination of structure pollution, and the damage assessment of electronic circuits in semiconductors might be taken into account. Furthermore, it is possible to do composition analysis by using SEM device equipped with EDX.

In Figure 16.18, SEM images for EC powder, and also grafted and amidoximation conversion-completed AN copolymers taken between 10,000× and 50,000× magnification are given.

While no roughness seems to stand out on the EC surfaces due to their crystalline structure, the increase in the roughness on the surface and pore formation after the grafting and amidoximation indicate the corruption of the crystalline structure and increase in amorphous structures.

By doing structure analysis with AFM, polymers can be seen in two or three dimensions clearly, observation about the quality of polymer modification can be performed either in nanometer or in micrometer levels, and it is possible to estimate the amount of grafting on polymers from roughness parameters [1]. As shown in Figure 16.19, the roughness has increased (R_a=33.672 nm) with the grafting of AN having hydrophobic C≡N groups on the surface of HPMC film (R_a=3.684 nm). And the R_a value calculated for the AFM image belonging to HPMC-*g*-amidoxime copolymer is 26.855 nm [79]. As a result of the replacement of hydrophobic C≡N groups with amidoxime groups having hydrophilic character, due to the possible H-bonds the amidoxime groups made between themselves, it is observed that the surface roughness value R_a has decreased.

Thus, HPMC-*g*-AO and EC-*g*-AO copolymers whose structure analyses have been performed detailed and whose amidoxime conversion has been completed are used for uranium ion recovery. Batch adsorption values and uranium uptake capacities for HPMC-*g*-AO and EC-*g*-AO are found to be 765 mg/g [79,112] and 240 mg/g [83], respectively. These values are quite high compared with those in literature.

As a result of our studies, it is found that the copolymers that are obtained by the grafting of AN monomers on cellulose and its derivatives using ^{60}Co-γ rays adsorb uranium ions with a high capacity after the completion of amidoxime conversion in hydroxylamine hydrochloride. Detailed analyses of grafting, amidoxime conversion, and adsorption have been done using various methods such as gravimetry, FTIR, TGA, SEM, AFM, and CA.

16.4 CONCLUSION

Since it is biodegradable and biorenewable, cellulose has the potential of being a material we will use frequently in the future. Cellulose is used in many fields such as textile, paper, food, cosmetics, and pharmaceutics; however, it lacks some features that synthetic polymers show.

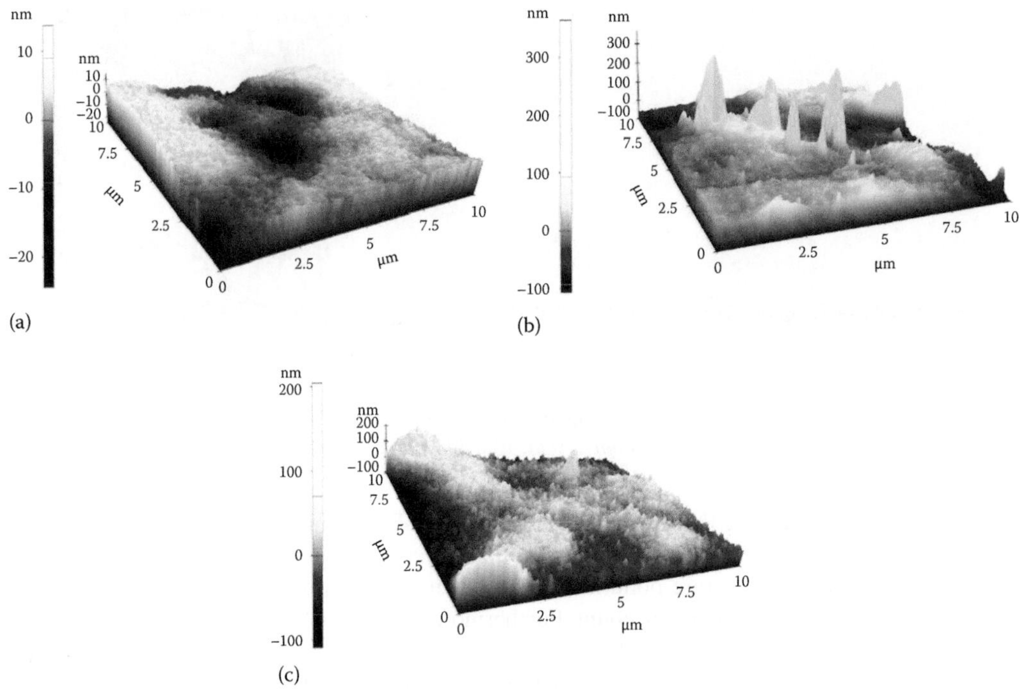

FIGURE 16.19 AFM images for HPMC-*g*-AN copolymers. (a) $HPMC_{org}$, (b) HPMC-*g*-AN, and (c) HPMC-*g*-AO. (From Başarır, S.S. and Bayramgil, N.P., *Cellulose*, 20, 1511, 2013.)

Many researches are done to improve and enhance the physical and chemical features of cellulose. In its grafting, acrylic and vinyl polymers are bound to the cellulose main chain with covalent bond. Cellulose graft copolymers can be prepared with polymerizations initiated by chemicals, high-energy radiation, UV rays, and enzymes. By using FTIR, elemental analysis, NMR, SEM, TEM, AFM, XRD, XPS, TGA, and mechanical test analysis methods, copolymers are characterized with regard to chemical composition, graft length, and graft frequency. Cellulose and its derivatives are used successfully in the industries of biotechnology, pharmaceutics, environment, food, paper, textile, and construction and electricity with its altered/improved features as a result of grafting, such as its hydrophilic/hydrophobic character, elasticity, water absorption capacity, adhesive features, adsorption or ion exchange skills, resistance to microbial attacks, and thermal, optical, and mechanical resistance. Studies aiming at the diversity of the area of usage of cellulosic polymers, which are converted into environmentally friendly end products such as CO_2 and H_2O by natural microbial decomposition in a short period of time, will continue to be conducted in the future.

REFERENCES

1. Bhattacharya, A., Rawlins, J.W., and Ray, P. 2009. *Polymer Grafting and Crosslinking*. John Wiley & Sons, Inc., Hoboken, NJ, p. 3.
2. Blacha, A., Krukiewicz, K., and Zak, J. 2011. The covalent grafting of polymers to the solid surface. *Chemik* 65: 11–9.
3. Habibi, Y. and Dufresne, A. 2011. Nanocrystals from natural polysaccharides. In *Handbook of Nanophysics: Nanoparticles and Quantum Dots*, K.D. Sattler (ed.), vol. 10. CRC Press, Taylor & Francis Group, Boca Raton, FL, pp. 1–14.
4. Sjostrom, E. 1993. *Wood Chemistry. Fundamentals and Applications*, 2nd edn. Academic Press, San Diego, CA, p. 292.

5. Kamide, K. 2005. *Cellulose and Cellulose Derivatives*. Elsevier B.V. Amsterdam, the Netherlands, pp. 1–3.
6. Qiu, X. and Hu, S. 2013. "Smart" materials based on cellulose: A review of the preparations, properties, and applications. *Materials* 6: 738–781.
7. Bhattacharya, A. and Misra, B.N. 2004. Grafting: A versatile means to modify polymers techniques, factors and applications. *Progress in Polymer Science* 29: 767–814.
8. Savage, A.B. 1965. C-Cellulose ethers. In Bikales, N.M. (ed.), *Encyclopedia of Polymer Science and Technology*, vol. 3. John Wiley & Sons, Inc., Hoboken, NJ, pp. 459–548.
9. Saxena, I.M. and Brown, R.M. 2005. Cellulose biosynthesis: Current views and evolving concepts. *Annals of Botany* 96: 9–21.
10. Bergfeld, A., Bergmann, R., and Sengbusch, P.V. November 25, 2005. Cellulose. https://s10.lite.msu.edu/res/msu/botonl/b_online/e26/26a.htm.
11. Rowell, R.M., Petterso, R., Han, J.S. et al. 2005. Cell wall chemistry. In *Handbook of Wood Chemistry and Wood Composites*, R.M. Rowell (ed.), vol. 3. CRC Press, Boca Raton, FL, pp. 35–74.
12. Patural, L., Marchal, P., Govin, A. et al. 2011. Cellulose ethers influence on water retention and consistency in cement-based mortars. *Cement and Concrete Research* 41: 46–55.
13. Varshney, V.K. and Naithani, S. 2011. Chemical functionalization of cellulose derived from nonconventional sources. In *Bio- and Nano-Polymer Composites*, S. Kalia et al. (eds.). Springer-Verlag, Berlin, Germany, pp. 43–60.
14. Koch, W. 1937. Properties and uses of ethylcellulose. *Industrial and Engineering Chemistry* 29: 687–690.
15. *Natrosol-Hydroxyethylcellulose*. 2001. Aqualon, Hercules Plaze, Hercules Incorporated, Wilmington, DE, Hercules Incorporated, 2001.
16. Gafourian, T., Safari, A., Adibkia, K., Parviz, F., and Nokhodchi, A. 2007. A drug release study from hydroxypropylmethylcellulose (HPMC) matrices using QSPR modeling. *Journal of Pharmaceutical Sciences* 96: 3334–3351.
17. Fatimi, A., Tassin, J.F., Quillard, S., Axelos, M.A.V., and Weiss, P. 2008. The rheological properties of silated hydroxypropylmethylcellulose tissue engineering matrices. *Biomaterials* 29: 533–543.
18. Heydarzadeh, H.D., Najafpour, G.D., and Moghaddam, A.A.N. 2009. Catalyst-free conversion of alkali cellulose to fine carboxymethyl cellulose at mild conditions. *World Applied Sciences Journal* 6: 564–569.
19. Morgado, D.L., Rodrigues, B.V.M., Almeida, E.V.R., El Soud, O.A., and Frollini, E. 2013. Bio-based films from linter cellulose and its acetates: Formation and properties. *Materials* 6: 2410–2435.
20. Fischer, S., Thümmler, K., Volkert, B., Hettrich, K., Schmidt, I., and Fischer, K. 2008. Properties and applications of cellulose acetate. *Macromolecular Symposia* 262: 89–96.
21. Pastýr, J. and Kuniak, L. 1972. Cyanoethylation of powdered cross-linked cellulose. *Chemicke Zvesti* 26: 84–88.
22. Roy, D., Semsarilar, M., Guthrie, J.T., and Perrier, S. 2009. Cellulose modification by polymer grafting: A review. *Chemical Society Reviews* 38: 2046–2064.
23. Malmström, E. and Carlmark, A. 2012. Controlled grafting of cellulose fibres—An outlook beyond paper and cardboard. *Polymer Chemistry* 3: 1702–1713.
24. Azzam, F., Heux, L., Putaux, J.L., and Jean, B. 2010. Preparation by grafting onto, characterization and properties of thermally responsive polymer-decorated cellulose nanocrystals. *Biomacromolecules* 11: 3652–3659.
25. Mark, H.F. 2007. G-Graft copolymers. In Mark, H.F. (ed.), *Encyclopedia of Polymer Science and Technology, Concise*. John Wiley & Sons, Inc., Hoboken, NJ, pp. 526–531.
26. Moad, G. and Solomon, D.H. 2006. *The Chemistry of Radical Polymerization*, 2nd edn. Elsevier Ltd, Oxford, U.K.
27. Moad, G., Rizzardo, E., and Thang, S.H. 2005. Living radical polymerization by the RAFT process. *Australian Journal of Chemistry* 58: 379–410.
28. Tosh, B. and Routray, C.R. 2011. Homogeneous grafting of PMMA onto cellulose in presence of Ce^{4+} as initiator. *Indian Journal of Chemical Technology* 18: 234–243.
29. Sheikh, J.N. 2013. Performance enhancement of fibrous polymers. Chapter 2. *Literature Survey*. *Indian ETD Repository*. Institute of Chemical Technology, Mumbai, India.
30. Kubota, H. and Ogiwara, Y. 1980. Cellulose peroxides derived from carboxylated cellulose and hydrogen peroxide. *Journal of Applied Polymer Science* 25: 683–689.
31. Gürdağ, G. and Sarmda, S. 2013. Cellulose graft copolymers: Synthesis, properties, and applications. In *Polysaccharide Based Graft Copolymers*, S. Kalia and M.W. Sabaa (eds.). Springer-Verlag, Berlin, Germany, pp. 15–57.

32. Sankalia, S.M., Chaudhuri, D.K.R., and Hermans, J.J. 1962. Studies on the mechanism of persulphate-initiated grafting onto cellulose. *Canadian Journal of Chemistry* 40: 2249–2255.
33. Ghosh, P. and Das, D. 2000. Modification of jute by some low molecular weight glycols and a polyol under thermal treatment. *European Polymer Journal* 36: 2147–2157.
34. Suo, A., Qian, J., Yao, Y., and Zhang, W. 2007. Synthesis and properties of carboxymethyl cellulose-graft-poly(acrylic acid-co-acrylamide) as a novel cellulose-based superabsorbent. *Journal of Applied Polymer Science* 103: 1382–1388.
35. Aliouche, D., Sid, B., and Ait-Amar, H. 2006. Graft-copolymerization of acrylic monomers onto cellulose. Influence on fibre swelling and absorbency. *Annalesde Chimie Science des Matériaux* 31: 527–540.
36. Kolthoff, I.M. and Miller, I.K. 1951. The chemistry of persulfate. I. The kinetics and mechanism of the decomposition of the persulfate ion in aqueous medium. *Journal of the American Chemical Society* 73: 3055–3059
37. Gürdağ, G., Yaşar, M., and Gürkaynak, M.A. 1997. Graft copolymerization of acrylic acid on cellulose: Reaction kinetics of copolymerization. *Journal of Applied Polymer Science* 66: 929–934.
38. Gupta, K.C. and Khandekar, K. 2006. Graft copolymerization of acrylamide onto cellulose in presence of comonomer using ceric ammonium nitrate as initiator. *Journal of Applied Polymer Science* 101: 2546–2558.
39. Borbély, É. and Erdélyi, J. 2004. Grafting of industrial cellulose pulp with vinyl acetate monomer by ceric ion redox system as initiator. *Acta Polytechnica Hungarica* 1: 86–95.
40. Tame, A., Ndikontar, M.K., Ngamveng, J.N. et al. 2011. Graft copolymerisation of acrylamide on carboxymethyl cellulose (CMC). *Rasayan Journal of Chemistry* 4: 1–7.
41. Bhatt, N., Gupta, P.K., and Naithani, S. 2011. Ceric-induced grafting of acrylonitrile onto alpha cellulose isolated from *Lantana camara*. *Cellulose Chemistry and Technology* 45: 321–327.
42. Misra, B.N., Dogra, R., Kaur, I., and Jassal, J.K. 1979. Grafting onto cellulose. IV. Effect of complexing agents on Fenton's reagent (Fe^{2+}–H_2O_2)—Initiated grafting of poly(vinylacetate). *Journal of Polymer Science: Polymer Chemistry Edition* 17: 1861–1863.
43. Misra, B.N., Dogra, R., and Mehta, I.K. 1980. Grafting onto cellulose. V. Effect of complexing agents on Fenton's reagent (Fe^{2+}–H_2O_2)—Initiated grafting of poly(ethyl acrylate). *Journal of Polymer Science: Polymer Chemistry Edition* 18: 749–752.
44. Abdel-Razik, E.A. 1997. Aspects of thermal graft copolymerization of methyl methacrylate onto ethyl cellulose in homogeneous media. *Polymer Plastics Technology and Engineering* 36: 891–903.
45. Abdel-Razik, E.A. 1990. Homogeneous graft copolymerization of acrylamide onto ethylcellulose. *Polymer* 31: 1739–1744.
46. Bardhan, K., Mukhopadhyay, S., and Chatterjee, S.R. 1977. Grafting of acrylamide onto methyl cellulose by persulfate ion. *Journal of Polymer Science: Polymer Chemistry Edition* 15: 141–148.
47. Sabaa, M.W. and Mokhtar, S.M. 2002. Chemically induced graft copolymerization of itaconic acid onto cellulose fibers. *Polymer Testing* 21: 337–343.
48. Kennedy, J.P. 1978. Free radical and ionic grafting. *Journal of Polymer Science: Polymer Symposium* 64: 117–124.
49. Cohen, E., Avny, Y., and Zilkha, A. 2003. Anionic graft polymerization of propylene sulfide on cellulose. I. *Journal of Polymer Science Part A-1: Polymer Chemistry* 9: 1469–1479.
50. Hebeish, A. and J. T. Guthrie. 1981. *The Chemistry and Technology of Cellulosic Copolymers*. Springer-Verlag, New York.
51. Carlmark, A., Larsson, E., and Malmström, E. 2012. Grafting of cellulose by ring-opening polymerization—A review. *European Polymer Journal* 48: 1646–1659.
52. Cordova, A. and Hafren, J. 2005. Direct organic acid-catalyzed polyester derivatization of lignocellulosic material. *Nordic Pulp and Paper Research Journal* 20: 477–480.
53. Szwarc, M. 1956. Living polymers. *Nature* 178: 1168–1169.
54. Solomon, D.H. 2005. Genesis of the CSIRO polymer group and the discovery and significance of nitroxide-mediated living radical polymerization. *Journal of Polymer Science: Polymer Chemistry* 43: 5748–5764.
55. Wang, J.S. and Matyjaszewski, K. 1995. Controlled/"living" radical polymerization. Atom transfer radical polymerization in the presence of transition-metal complexes. *Journal of American Chemical Society* 117: 5614–5615.
56. Matyjaszewski, K. 2000. Controlled/living radical polymerization: Progress in ATRP, NMP and RAFT. In *ACS Symposium Series*, K. Matyjaszewski (ed.), vol. 768. American Chemical Society, Washington, DC, pp. 2–25.

57. Nystrom, D., Lindqvist, J., Ostmark, E., Hult, A., and Malmstrom, E. 2006. Superhydrophobic bio-fibre surfaces via tailored grafting architecture. *Chemical Communications* 34: 3594–3596.
58. Okamoto, J., Sugo, T., Katakakai, A., and Omichi, H. 1985. Amidoxime-group-containing adsorbents for metal ions synthesized by radiation-induced grafting. *Journal of Applied Polymer Science* 30: 2967–2977.
59. Takacs, E., Wojnarovits, L., Borsa, J., Papp, J., Hargittai, P., and Korecz, L. 2005. Modification of cotton-cellulose by preirradiation grafting. *Nuclear Instruments and Methods in Physics Research Section B* 236: 259–265.
60. Stannett, V.T. and Hopfenberg, H.B. 1971. In *Cellulose and Cellulose Derivatives*, N.M. Bikales and L. Segal (eds.), vol. 5. John Wiley & Sons, New York, pp. 907–936.
61. Badawy, S.M., Sokker, H.H., Othman, S.H., and Hashem, A. 2005. Cloth filter for recovery of uranium from radioactive waste. *Radiation Physics and Chemistry* 73: 125–130.
62. Jenkins, D.W. and Hudson, S.M. 2001. Review of vinyl graft copolymerization featuring recent advances toward controlled radical-based reactions and illustrated with chitin/chitosan trunk polymers. *Chemical Reviews* 101: 3245–3273.
63. Geacintov, N. 1961. Thesis. State University College of Forestry, Syracuse, New York.
64. Geacintov, N., Stannett, V., Abrahamson, E.W., and Hermans, J.J. 1960. Grafting onto cellulose and cellulose derivatives using ultraviolet irradiation. *Journal of Applied Polymer Science* 3: 54–60.
65. Hong, K.H., Liu, N., and Sun, G. 2009. UV-induced graft polymerization of acrylamide on cellulose by using immobilized benzophenone as a photo-initiator. *European Polymer Journal* 45: 2443–2449.
66. Malin, T.G., Per, V.P., Iversen, T., Hult, K., and Martinelle, M. 2004. Polyester coating of cellulose fiber surfaces catalyzed by a cellulose-binding module-Candida antarctica lipase B fusion protein. *Biomacromolecules* 5: 106–112.
67. Soleimani, F., Sadeghi, M., and Shahsavari, H. 2012. Graft copolymerization of gelatin-g-poly (acrylic acid-co-acrylamide) and calculation of grafting parameters. *Indian Journal of Science and Technology* 5: 2041–2046.
68. Nishioka, N. and Kosai, K. 1981. Homogeneous graft copolymerization of vinyl monomers onto cellulose in a dimethyl sulfoxide-paraformaldehyde solvent system I. Acrylonitrile and methyl methacrylate. *Polymer Journal* 13: 1125–1133.
69. Gupta, K.C. and Sahoo, S. 2001. Graft copolymerization of acrylonitrile and ethyl methacrylate comonomers on cellulose using ceric ions. *Biomacromolecules* 2: 239–247.
70. Gupta, K.C. and Khandekar, K. 2006. Ceric(IV) ion-induced graft copolymerization of acrylamide and ethyl acrylate onto cellulose. *Polymer International* 55: 139–150.
71. Ikada, Y., Nishizaki, Y., and Sakurada, I. 1972. Chemical structure of cellulose-styrene graft copolymer. *Bulletin of the Institute for Chemical Research, Kyoto University* 50: 20–26.
72. Liu, W., Liu, R., Li, Y. et al. 2009. Self-assembly of ethyl cellulose-graft-polystyrene copolymers in acetone. *Polymer* 50: 211–217.
73. Yan, L. and Tao, W. 2008. Graft copolymerization of *N,N*-dimethylacrylamide to cellulose in homogeneous media using atom transfer radical polymerization for hemocompatibility. *Journal of Biomedical Science and Engineering* 1: 37–43.
74. Lönnberg, H., Fogelström, L., Berglund, M.A.S.A.S.L., Malmström, E., and Hult, A. 2008. Surface grafting of microfibrillated cellulose with poly(e-caprolactone)—Synthesis and characterization. *European Polymer Journal* 44: 2991–2997.
75. Lima, M.M.D. and Borsali, R. 2002. Static and dynamic light scattering from polyelectrolyte microcrystal cellulose. *Langmuir* 18: 992–996.
76. Tosh, B. and Routray, C.R. 2013. Graft copolymerization of methyl methacrylate onto cellulose in homogeneous medium—Effect of solvent and initiator. *World Academy of Science, Engineering and Technology, International Journal of Chemical, Materials Science and Engineering* 7: 89–96.
77. El Seoud, O.A., Nawaz, H., and Arêas, E.P.G. 2013. Chemistry and applications of polysaccharide solutions in strong electrolytes/dipolar aprotic solvents: An overview. *Molecules* 18: 1270–1313.
78. Kan, K.H.M., Li, J., Wijesekera, K., and Cranston, E.D. 2013. Polymer-grafted cellulose nanocrystals as pH-responsive reversible flocculants. *Biomacromolecules* 14: 3130–3139.
79. Başarır, S.S. and Bayramgil, N.P. 2013. The uranium recovery from aqueous solutions using amidoxime modified cellulose derivatives. III. Modification of hydroxypropylmethylcellulose with amidoxime groups. *Cellulose* 20: 1511–1522.
80. Xin, T-T., Yuan, T., Xiao, S., and He, J. 2011. Synthesis of cellulose-graft-poly(methyl methacrylate) via homogeneous ATRP. *Bioresources* 6: 2941–2953.

81. Lönnberg, H., Zhou, Q., Brumer, H. 3rd, Teeri, T.T., Malmström, E., and Hult, A. 2006. Grafting of cellulose fibers with poly(epsilon-caprolactone) and poly(L-lactic acid) via ring-opening polymerization. *Biomacromolecules* 7: 2178–2185.
82. Chauhan, A. and Kaith, B. 2011. X-ray diffraction studies and assessment of roselle graft-copolymers. *Malaysian Polymer Journal* 6: 155–164.
83. Başarır, S.S. and Bayramgil, N.P. 2012. The uranium recovery from aqueous solutions using amidoxime modified cellulose derivatives. I. Preparation, characterization and amidoxime conversion of radiation grafted ethyl cellulose-acrylonitrile copolymers. *Radiochimica Acta*, 100: 893–899.
84. Hiltunen, M. 2013. Cellulose based graft copolymers prepared via controlled radical polymerization methods. Academic Dissertation for the Degree of Doctor of Philosophy, Faculty of Science of the University of Helsinki, Finland.
85. Shukla, S.R., Rao, G.V.G., and Athalye, A.R. 1992. Mechanical and thermal behavior of cotton cellulose grafted with hydroxyethyl methacrylate using photoinitiation. *Journal of Applied Polymer Science* 44: 577–580.
86. El-Khouly, A.S., Takahashi, Y., Takada, A. et al. 2010. Characterization and mechanical properties of cellulose-graft-polyacrylonitrile prepared by using $KMnO_4$/different acids as redox system. *Nihon Reoroji Gakkaishi* 38: 133–140.
87. Kang, H., Liu, R., and Huang, Y. 2013. Cellulose derivatives and graft copolymers as blocks for functional materials. *Polymer International* 62: 338–344.
88. Sarvi, F., Yue, Z., Hourigan, K., Thompson, M.C., and Chan, P.P.Y. 2013. Surface-functionalization of PDMS for potential micro-bioreactor and embryonic stem cell culture applications. *Journal of Materials Chemistry B* 1: 987–996.
89. Czaja, W.K., Young, D.J., Kawecki, M., and Brown, R.M. Jr. 2007. The future prospects of microbial cellulose in biomedical applications. *Biomacromolecules* 8: 1–12.
90. Tyagi, C., Tomar, L.K., and Singh, H. 2009. Surface modification of cellulose filter paper by glycidyl methacrylate grafting for biomolecule immobilization: Influence of grafting parameters and urease immobilization. *Journal of Applied Polymer Science* 111: 1381–1390.
91. Teisala, H. 2013. Multifunctional superhydrophobic nanoparticle coatings for cellulose-based substrates by liquid flame spray. Thesis for the degree of Doctor of Science in Technology, Tampere University of Technology, Finland. Publication 1169.
92. Shukla, S.K. 2013. Synthesis and characterization of polypyrrole grafted cellulose for humidity sensing. *International Journal of Biological Macromolecules* 62: 531–536.
93. Sadeghi, M., Ghasemi, N., and Soliemani, F. 2012. Graft copolymerization methacrylamide monomer onto carboxymethyl cellulose in homogeneous solution and optimization of effective parameters. *World Applied Sciences Journal* 16: 119–125.
94. Flefel, E.M., Ibrahim, M.M., El-Zawawy, W.K., and Ali, A.M. 2002. Graft copolymerization of *N*-vinylpyrrolidone and acrylamide on cellulose derivatives: Synthesis, characterization and study of their biological effect. *Polymers for Advanced Technologies* 13: 541–547.
95. Eldin, M.S. Mohy, Omer, A.M., Soliman, E.A., and Hassan, E.A. 2013. Superabsorbent polyacrylamide grafted carboxymethyl cellulose pH sensitive hydrogel: I. Preparation and characterization. *Desalination and Water Treatment* 51: 16–18.
96. Wang, L., Dong, W., and Xu, Y. 2007. Synthesis and characterization of hydroxypropyl methylcellulose and ethyl acrylate graft copolymers. *Carbohydrate Polymers* 68: 626–636.
97. Amaral, M.H, Lobo, J.M., and Ferreira, D.C. 2001. Effect of HPMC and hydrogenated castor oil on naproxen release from sustained-release tablets. *Pharmaceutical Science and Technology* 2: 1–8.
98. Colombo, P., Bettini, R., Santi, P., and Peppas, N.A. 2000. Swellable matrices for controlled drug delivery: Gel-layer behaviour, mechanisms and optimal performance. *PSTT* 3: 198–204.
99. Siepmann, J. and Peppas, N.A. 2001. Modelling of drug release from delivery systems based on hydroxypropyl methylcellulose (HPMC). *Advanced Drug Delivery Reviews* 48: 139–157.
100. Billy, M., Da Costa, A.R., Lochon, P. et al. 2010. Cellulose acetate graft copolymers with nano-structured architectures: Synthesis and characterization. *European Polymer Journal* 46: 944–957.
101. Choudhury, J.P., Ghosh, P., and Guha, B.K. 1988. Styrene-grafted cellulose acetate reverse osmosis membrane for ethanol separation. *Journal of Membrane Science* 35: 301–310.
102. Liu, S. and Sun, G. 2008. Biocidal acyclic halamine polymers: Conversion of acrylamide-grafted-cotton to acyclic halamine. *Journal of Applied Polymer Science* 108: 3480–3486.
103. Shukla, S.K. 2012. Synthesis of polyaniline grafted cellulose suitable for humidity sensing. *Indian Journal of Engineering and Materials Sciences* 19: 417–420.

104. Maulik, S.R. and Banerjee, A. 2009. Dyeing of cotton fabric with pigment colour. *Asian Dyer* 6: 24–29.
105. Rowland, S.P. and Mason, J.S. 1978. Enhanced DP finishing of cotton with dimethylol dihydroxyethyleneurea and a metal acrylate-type monomer. *Textile Research Journal* 48: 625–632.
106. Franklin, W.E., Madasci, and J.P., Rowland, S.P. 1976. Creasable durable press cotton fabrics by polymerization and crosslinking. *Textile Chemist and Colorist* 8: 28–33.
107. Narayan, R., Biermann, J., Hunt, M.O., and Horn, D.P. 1989. Cellulose graft copolymers for potential adhesive applications, bonding of plastics to wood. In *Adhesives from Renewable Resources*, R.W. Hemingway and A.H. Conner (eds.). American Chemical Society, Washington, DC, ACS Symposium Series No. 385, pp. 337–354.
108. Lin, S.H. and Juang, R.S. 2009. Adsorption of phenol and its derivatives from water using synthetic resins and low-cost natural adsorbents: A review. *Journal of Environmental Management* 90: 1336–1349.
109. Kathirvelan, D., Senthivel, S., and Reddy, B.S.R. 2011. Graft copolymerization of 2-(dimethylamino) ethyl acrylate onto cellulose (Alkali scoured cotton) material. *International Journal of Fiber and Textile Research* 1: 31–38.
110. Biçak, N., Sherrington, D.C., and Filiz Senkal, B. 1999. Graft copolymer of acrylamide onto cellulose as mercury selective sorbent. *Reactive and Functional Polymers* 41: 69–76.
111. Güçlü, G., Gürdağ, G., and Özgümüş, S. 2003. Competitive removal of heavy metal ions by cellulose graft copolymers. *Journal of Applied Polymer Science* 90: 2034–2039.
112. Başarır, S.S. and Bayramgil, N.P. 2013. The uranium recovery from aqueous solutions using amidoxime modified cellulose derivatives. IV. Recovery of uranium by amidoximated hydroxypropyl methylcellulose. *Cellulose* 20: 827–839.
113. Ali, A.E-H. 2012. Removal of heavy metals from model wastewater by using carboxymethyl cellulose/2-acrylamido-2-methyl propane sulfonic acid hydrogels. *Journal of Applied Polymer Science* 123: 763–769.
114. Rainbow, P.S. and Blackmore, G. 2001. Barnacles as biomonitors of trace metal availabilities in Hong Kong coastal waters: Changes in space and time. *Marine Environmental Research* 51: 441–463.
115. Seko, N., Tamada, M., and Yoshii, F. 2005. Current status of adsorbent for metal ions with radiation grafting and crosslinking techniques. *Nuclear Instruments Methods Physics Research B* 236: 21–29.
116. Othman, S.H., Sohsah, M.A., and Ghoneim, M.M. 2009. The effects of hazardous ions adsorption on the morphological and chemical properties of reactive cloth filter. *Radiation Physics and Chemistry* 78: 976–985.
117. Chang, D.J. and Hwang, S.J. 1996. Removal of metal ions from liquid solutions by cross flow microfiltration. *Separation Science and Technology* 31: 1831–1842.
118. Takeda, T., Saito, K., Uezu, K., Furusaki, S., Sugo, T., and Okamoto, J. 1991. Adsorption and elution in hollow-fiber-packed bed for recovery of uranium from seawater. *Industrial Engineering and Chemical Research* 30: 185–190.
119. Khullar, R., Varshney, V.K., Naithani, S., and Soni, P.L. 2008. Grafting of acrylonitrile onto cellulosic material derived from bamboo (*Dendrocalamus strictus*). *eXPRESS Polymer Letters* 2: 12–18.
120. Tokuyama, H. and Ishihara, N. 2010. Temperature-swing adsorption of precious metal ions onto poly(2-(dimethylamino)ethylmethacrylate) gel. *Reactive and Functional Polymers* 70: 610–615.
121. Anirudhan, T.S., Rauf, T.A., and Rejeena, S.R. 2012. Removal and recovery of phosphate ions from aqueous solutions by amine functionalized epichlorohydrin-grafted cellulose. *Desalination* 285: 277–284.
122. Anirudhan, T.S., Jalajamony, S., and Divya, L. 2009. Efficiency of amine-modified poly(glycidyl methacrylate)-grafted cellulose in the removal and recovery of vanadium(V) from aqueous solutions. *Industrial and Engineering Chemistry Research* 48: 2118–2124.
123. Abdel-Razik, H.H., El-Asmar, A.M., and Abbo, M. 2013. Heavy metal adsorbents based on chelating amidoximated grafted cellulose. *International Journal of Basic and Applied Chemical Sciences* 3: 1–8.
124. Anirudhan, T.S., Sreekumari, S.S., and Jalajamony, S. 2013. An investigation into the adsorption of thorium(IV) from aqueous solutions by a carboxylate-functionalised graft copolymer derived from titanium dioxide-densified cellulose. *Journal of Environmental Radioactivity* 116: 141–147.
125. Sokker, H.H., Badawy, S.M., Zayed, E.M., Nour Eldien, F.A., and Farag, A.M. 2009. Radiation-induced grafting of glycidyl methacrylate onto cotton fabric waste and its modification for anchoring hazardous wastes from their solutions. *Journal of Hazardous Materials* 168: 137–144.
126. Hoshina, H., Takahashi, M., Kasai, N., and Seko, N. 2012. Adsorbent for arsenic(V) removal synthesized by radiation-induced graft polymerization onto nonwoven cotton fabric. *International Journal of Organic Chemistry* 2: 173–177.

127. Sokker, H.H., Gad, Y.H., and Ismail, S.A. 2012. Synthesis of bifunctional cellulosic adsorbent by radiation induced graft polymerization of glycidyl methacrylate-*co*-methacrylic acids. *Journal of Applied Polymer Science* 126: E54–E62.
128. Goswami, D. and Das, A.K. 2003. Preconcentration and recovery of uranium and thorium from Indian monazite sand by using a modified fly ash bed. *Journal of Radioanalytical and Nuclear Chemistry* 258: 249–254.
129. Wojnárovits, L., Földváry, Cs.M., and Takács, E. 2010. Radiation-induced grafting of cellulose for adsorption of hazardous water pollutants: A review. *Radiation Physics and Chemistry* 79: 848–862.
130. Abdel-Aal, S.E., Gad, Y., and Dessouki, A.M. 2006. The use of wood pulp and radiation modified starch in wastewater treatment. *Journal of Applied Polymer Science* 99: 2460–2469.
131. Shibi, I.G. and Anirudhan, T.S. 2002. Synthesis, characterisation, and application as a mercury(II) sorbent of banana stalk-polyacrylamide grafted copolymer bearing carboxyl groups. *Industrial Engineering and Chemical Research* 41: 5341–5352.
132. Aly, A.S., Sokker, H.H., Hashem, A., and Hebeish, A. 2005. Preparation of cellulosic membrane containing pyrrolidone moiety via radiation induced grafting and its application in wastewater treatment. *American Journal of Applied Sciences* 2: 508–513.
133. Chauhan, G.S., Guleria, L., and Sharma, R. 2005. Synthesis, characterization and metal ion sorption studies of graft copolymers of cellulose with glycidyl methacrylate and some comonomers. *Cellulose* 12: 97–110.
134. Zhou, D., Zhang, L., Zhou, J., and Guo, S. 2004. Cellulose/chitin beads for adsorption of heavy metals in aqueous solution. *Water Research* 38: 2643–2650.
135. O'Connell, D.W., Birkinshaw, C., and Dwyer, T.F. 2008. Heavy metal adsorbents prepared from the modification of cellulose: A review. *Bioresource Technology* 99: 6709–6724.
136. Kubota, H. and Shigehisa, Y.J. 1995. Introduction of amidoxime groups into cellulose and its ability to adsorb metal ions. *Journal of Applied Polymer Science* 56: 147–151.
137. Chauhan, G.S., Chauhan, S., and Guleria, L.K. 2001. Polymers from renewable sources: Effects of zinc chloride on kinetics of gamma-radiation induced grafting of styrene and acrylonitrile onto extracted cellulose. *Polymers and Polymer Composites* 9: 483–485.
138. Navarro, R.R., Sumi, K., and Matsumura, M., 1999. Improved metal affinity of chelating adsorbents through graft polymerization. *Water Research* 33: 2037–2044.

17 Grafting of Cellulose-Based Materials

Techniques, Factors, and Applications of the Grafted Products

Biranchinarayan Tosh

CONTENTS

17.1 INTRODUCTION

The chemical modification of cellulose and its derivatives by graft copolymerization has generated interest among researchers, because few comonomer molecules significantly change a number of characteristics of the original natural polymer. In the polymeric age, it is essential to modify the properties of a polymer according to tailor-made specifications designed for target applications. There are several means to modify the properties of a polymer, viz., blending, curing, grafting, and derivatization. Blending is the physical mixture of two (or more) polymers to obtain the requisite properties. In curing, the polymerization of an oligomer mixture forms a coating that adheres to the substrate by physical forces, whereas in grafting, the monomers are covalently bonded and polymerized onto the polymer chain. The process of grafting can take minutes, hours, or even days for completion, whereas curing is a very rapid process and occurs in a fraction of second. In derivatization, simple molecules are substituted with the reactive groups of the polymer chain. The most common derivatization reactions of cellulose are esterification and etherification. The schematic presentation of the polymer modification is presented in Figure 17.1.

In this review, different techniques of grafting of cellulose and cellulose derivatives have been discussed in the first part. The second part consists of the discussion about the primary factors that control grafting. Following that, the third part mainly deals with the application of cellulose-grafted and cellulose ester–grafted products.

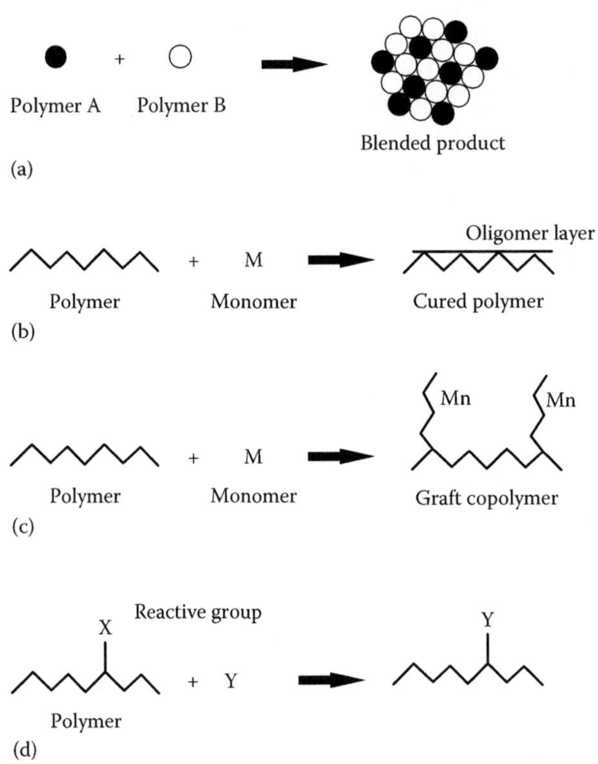

FIGURE 17.1 Methods for polymer modification. (a) Blending, (b) curing, (c) grafting, and (d) derivatization.

17.2 TECHNIQUES OF GRAFTING

Considerable work has been carried out on the techniques of graft copolymerization of different monomers on cellulose backbone. These techniques include chemical, radiation, photochemical, and enzymatic grafting.

17.2.1 Grafting Initiated by Chemical Means

This type of grafting can proceed along two major paths, viz., free radical and ionic. In this process, the role of initiator is very important as it determines the path of the grafting process. Apart from the general free radical grafting, grafting by atom transfer radical polymerization (ATRP) is also an interesting technique to carry out grafting.

17.2.1.1 Initiators Used for Grafting of Cellulosic Materials

It is known that the type of initiator has an important effect on grafting, and it determines the grafting percentage depending on the monomer to be grafted. In the grafting of vinyl monomers onto cellulose or cellulose derivatives, the initiation can be performed by chemical initiators or by irradiation. The grafting of non-vinyl monomers is performed by the reaction of monomer with the reactive functional groups of cellulose. As chemical initiators, redox initiators such as ceric(IV) ion (ceric ammonium nitrate: $(NH_4)_2Ce(NO_3)_6$) (CAN)[1–7] or cerium(IV) sulfate,[8] ceric ammonium sulfate (CAS),[9] iron(II)–hydrogen peroxide (Fe^{2+}–H_2O_2: Fenton reagent), cobalt(III) acetylacetonate complex salts,[10] Co(II)–potassium monopersulfate,[11] and sodium sulfite–ammonium persulfate,[12] and free radical generators such as azobisisobutyronitrile ($C_8H_{12}N_4$: AIBN),[13] potassium persulfate ($K_2S_2O_8$: KPS),[14–17] ammonium persulfate ($(NH_4)_2S_2O_8$: APS),[14,15] and benzoyl peroxide ($C_{14}H_{10}O_4$: BPO)[3–5,14,15] can be used.

17.2.1.1.1 Fe(II)–H_2O_2

Iron(II)–hydrogen peroxide system (Fenton reagent) is a cheap and easily available redox initiator, and the grafting with that initiator may be carried out in low temperatures.[18] The mechanism for the creation of ˙OH radicals by one electron transfer by the reaction of Fe(II) ion with hydrogen peroxide is given as follows:

$$Fe^{2+} + H_2O_2 \rightarrow {}^{\bullet}OH + OH^- + Fe^{3+}$$

$${}^{\bullet}OH + Fe^{2+} \rightarrow OH^- + Fe^{3+}$$

$${}^{\bullet}OH + H_2O_2 \rightarrow H_2O + {}^{\bullet}OOH$$

$${}^{\bullet}OOH + H_2O_2 \rightarrow {}^{\bullet}OH + O_2 + H_2O$$

The hydrogen peroxide molecules react with ferrous (Fe^{2+}) ions, and thus, ferric (Fe^{3+}) ions and primary hydroxyl radicals are created. Then, the primary hydroxyl radicals abstract a hydrogen atom from cellulose resulting in a secondary cellulose radical, and the grafting is initiated from these hydrogen-abstracted sites on the cellulose backbone. When the molar ratio of Fe^{2+}/H_2O_2 is higher than 1, some of the ˙OH radicals created in the aforementioned equations are consumed by Fe^{2+}, and Fe^{3+} ions affect the grafting adversely and lead to a decrease in the grafting percentage. H_2O_2 alone does not lead to the formation of radicals, and it can only create radicals together with metal impurities that are considered as reducing agent. In order to avoid the negative effect of Fe^{3+} ions on grafting, grafting has been carried out in the presence of some complexing agents with Fe^{3+} ions such as ascorbic acid, potassium fluoride (KF), and ethylenediaminetetraacetic acid (EDTA).[18] In order to minimize the formation of homopolymer and the wastage of primary hydroxyl (˙OH) radicals by Fe^{3+} ions, Fe^{2+} ions are adsorbed on the lignocellulose by contacting it with an Fe^{2+} salt solution in a given time period (15 min), and then the Fe^{2+} ion–adsorbed cellulose is separated from the solution containing excess Fe^{2+} ions by filtration. Then, methyl methacrylate (MMA) is grafted onto that Fe^{2+} salt–pretreated lignocellulose.[19]

17.2.1.1.2 Ceric Ion

Among the various types of redox initiators, ceric ion offers many advantages because of its high grafting efficiency and lower amount of homopolymer formation. When Ce^{4+} salts such as cerium sulfate or CAN is used as initiator in the grafting of vinyl monomers onto cellulose, at first, a ceric ion–cellulose complex occurs, and then it decomposes to cerous (Ce^{3+}) ion, and cellulose radicals are created by hydrogen abstraction from cellulose.[2–7] Thus, the initiation sites for grafting are created on the cellulose backbone. The radical formation on the cellulose backbone may occur on the oxygen atom of methylol ($-CH_2OH$) group.

$$Ce^{4+} + \text{Cell} - \text{OH} \rightarrow \text{Complex} \rightarrow \text{Cell} - \text{O}^{\bullet} + Ce^{3+} + H^{+}$$

The grafting may also be initiated on C_2 carbon by the ring opening of cellulose backbone as given in Figure 17.2.

It is also proposed that grafting occurs mainly at the C_2–C_3 glycol unit and, to a lesser amount, at the C_6-hydroxyl in the grafting of acrylonitrile onto Cassia tora gum, which is a common herbaceous annual weed growing in India.[20]

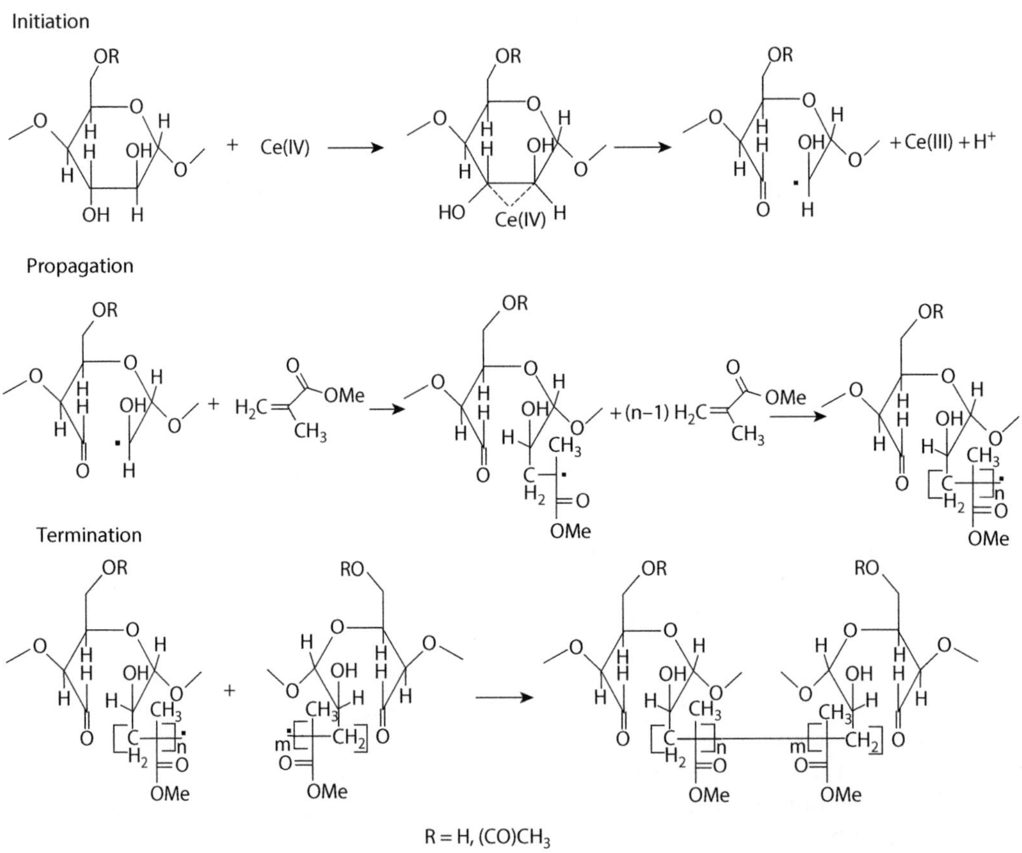

FIGURE 17.2 Mechanism of grafting of PMMA onto cellulose/CA using CAN as the initiator.

Although Ce^{4+} is an efficient initiator for the grafting of vinyl monomers onto cellulose, it requires the use of an acid together in order to create initiation sites (radicals) on graft substrate since the ceric ion undergoes hydrolysis in neutral medium[21] through $Ce(OH)^{3+}$ finally to $[Ce–O–Ce]^{6+}$ ion, which has no or low activity[20] for the creation of radicals via the reactions as shown in the following:

$$Ce^{4+} + H_2O \rightarrow \left[Ce\left(OH\right)\right]^{3+} + H^+$$

$$2\left[Ce\left(OH\right)\right]^{3+} \rightarrow \left[Ce-O-Ce\right]^{6+} + H_2O$$

In the absence of acid, no grafting on wool was determined most probably because $[Ce–O–Ce]^{6+}$, which is the hydrolysis product of Ce^{4+} ions, could not form a complex with wool.[22] Since the grafting efficiency of Ce^{4+} ion in neutral medium is low,[23] it is used together with an acid, mostly nitric acid (HNO_3). In order to reduce the formation of homopolymer accompanying grafting, the reaction has been carried out in the absence of the excess of ceric ions. For that reason, ceric ion solution has been contacted with cellulose in acidic medium for a predetermined time duration, and ceric ions are adsorbed on the cellulose, and then the excess of ceric ions in the mixture (non-adsorbed ceric ions) are removed from the ceric ion–adsorbed cellulose by filtration.[23–25] The rate of disappearance of ceric ions during the grafting of binary monomers (acrylamide (AM) and ethyl acrylate (EA)) onto cellulose[26] was found to be very high in the initial 1 h period of grafting, and the disappearance of ceric ions was attributed to their consumption for the creation of active sites on cellulose. After that initial 1 h period, no significant change in the concentration of ceric ions has been observed. In homogeneous grafting conditions, where HNO_3 forms gel in cellulose solution, CAN can be used with dimethyl sulfoxide (DMSO) to initiate the graft copolymerization reaction.[2–7]

17.2.1.1.3 Persulfates

When KPS/cobalt sulfate ($K_2S_2O_8/CoSO_4$) system was used as the redox initiator,[16] at first, the primary radicals, $SO_4^{\bullet-}$ and $^{\bullet}OH$, are generated by the decomposition of $K_2S_2O_8$ in the presence of $CoSO_4$, and then these primary SO4•− and •OH radicals abstract a hydrogen atom from cellulose backbone and create the secondary C- or O-centered cellulose radicals. The growth of graft chains carries on these hydrogen-abstracted active sites. KPS is the best radical initiator for hydrogen abstraction, and it is cheap and soluble in water. In the investigation of the grafting site via oxidative hydrogen abstraction by KPS without monomer, the carbon atoms of C3 and C4 on saccharide ring are reported to be probable grafting sites.[17] Besides these, there are other initiators that will be discussed in the forthcoming sections.

17.2.1.2 Free Radical Grafting

To promote grafting reaction and avoid homopolymerization of the monomers, radical initiators should preferably react with cellulose instead directly reacting with monomers. Radical initiators can undergo two different paths, addition to vinyl monomers or hydrogen abstraction from weak C–H sites on cellulose. Alkoxide radicals prefer to abstract hydrogen atoms from weak C–H bonds rather than addition to vinyl monomers, different from other initiator radicals.[27]

In the chemical process, free radicals are produced from the initiators and transferred to the substrate to react with monomer to form the graft copolymers. In general, one can consider the generation of free radicals by indirect or direct methods.

An example of free radicals produced by an indirect method is the production through redox reaction, viz., M^{n+}/H_2O_2, persulfates.[18,28–32]

$$Fe^{2+} + H_2O_2 \rightarrow Fe^{3+} + OH^- + OH$$

$$Fe^{2+} + {}^-O_3S\ \ OO\ \ SO_3^- \rightarrow Fe^{3+} + SO_4^{2-} + SO_4^{\bullet-}$$

It may be observed that the active species in the decomposition of H_2O_2 and KPS induced by Fe^{2+} are $^{\bullet}OH$ and $SO_4^{\bullet-}$, respectively.

There are different views regarding the activity of $SO_4^{\bullet-}$. Some authors reported that initially formed $SO_4^{\bullet-}$ reacts with water to form $^{\bullet}OH$, subsequently producing free radicals on the polymeric backbone.

Grafting process of MMA onto wood fiber was also studied using SB/KPS pair as the initiator. The sulfate radical ($SO_4^{\bullet-}$) was formed according to the following reaction[33]:

$$H_2O + HSO_3^- + 2S_2O_8^{2-} \rightarrow 3HSO_4^- + 2SO_4^{\bullet-}$$

The $SO_4^{\bullet-}$ formed reacts directly with the polymeric backbone (cellulose) to produce the requisite radicals.

$$SO_4^{\bullet-} + \text{Cell} - OH \rightarrow HSO_4^- + \text{Cell} - O^{\bullet}$$

However, it is established that during grafting of vinyl monomers onto wool/cellulose, $^{\bullet}OH$ is more reactive than $SO_4^{\bullet-}$. It was also reported that the decrements in grafting were attributed to increments in the initiator concentration, but also to deactivation of the free radicals due to side reactions when bisulfite is used as follows[29]:

$$SO_4^{\bullet-} + H_2O \rightarrow HSO_4^- + HO^{\bullet}$$

$$2SO_4^{\bullet-} + 3HSO_3^- \rightarrow 2HSO_4^- + 3SO_3^{2-} + H^+$$

$$2HO^{\bullet} + HSO_3^- \rightarrow SO_4^{2-} + H_2O + H^+$$

At a temperature of 60°C–80°C, KPS can produce $KSO_4^{\bullet}$ radical, which can induce the grafting reaction of EA to hydroxyl propyl methyl cellulose,[34] itaconic acid to cellulose fibers,[35] and acrylic acid to cellulose microfibers using an epoxide[36] according to the following reactions:

$$\text{Cell} - OH + KSO_4^{\bullet} \rightarrow KSO_4^- + \text{Cell} - O^{\bullet} + H^+$$

Hydroperoxides and Fe^{2+} comprise another important redox system, with free radicals generated by the interaction between them via thermal decomposition.[37] By analog with Fenton's reagent (Fe^{2+}–H_2O_2), the activity of tertiary butyl hydroperoxide (TBHP)–Fe^{2+} system is attributed to the formation of *t*-butoxy radical arising from one electron transfer between TBHP and Fe^{2+}:

$$t\text{-BuOOH} + Fe^{2+} \rightarrow t\text{-BuO}^{\bullet} + OH^- + Fe^{3+}$$

The resulting *t*-BuO• radical may participate in hydrogen abstraction reaction to generate HO• and the macro-radical on polymeric backbone.

$$\text{With monomer: } t\text{-BuO}^{\bullet} + M \rightarrow t\text{-BuO} - M^{\bullet} \rightarrow t\text{-BuO} - M_n - M^{\bullet}$$

$$\text{With polymer: } t\text{-BuO}^{\bullet} + PH \rightarrow t\text{-BuOH} + P^{\bullet}$$

$$\text{With water: } t\text{-BuO}^{\bullet} + H_2O \rightarrow t\text{-BuOH} + HO^{\bullet}$$

CAN in the presence of nitric acid can be used as an efficient initiator for graft copolymerization of acrylic monomers onto cellulose.[38–44] The ceric(IV) ion initiation offers great advantages of forming radicals at cellulose backbone through a single-electron-transfer process to promote grafting of monomer onto cellulose. However, the ceric(IV) ion–initiated grafting depends on the pH of the medium and the type of acid used for graft copolymerization. The proposed mechanism for such a process has been ascribed to the intermediate formation of a metal ion–polymer chelate complex, viz., ceric ion is known to form a complex with hydroxyl groups on a polymeric backbone, which can be dissociated via one-electron transfer to give free radicals.[45–48]

$$Ce^{4+} + Cell-OH \rightarrow Complex \rightarrow Cell-O^{\bullet} + Ce^{3+} + H^{+}$$

$$Cell-O^{\bullet} + M \rightarrow Cell-OM^{\bullet} \rightarrow Cell-OMM^{\bullet}$$

In place of CAN, ceric sulfate ($Ce(SO_4)_2 \cdot 4H_2O$) can also be used.[8]

Another reaction mechanism of graft copolymerization of cellulosic materials, initiated by Ce(IV) ion, is proposed by various workers,[2–7,49–51] in which the complex is formed at C_2 and C_3 of the anhydroglucose unit of cellulose, as shown in Figure 17.2.

Accordingly, cerium salt (Ce^{4+}) functioned as a powerful oxidizing agent, while cellulose itself acted as a reducing component in the redox system. The active centers are directly produced on the cellulose backbone, and no charge transfer mechanism is necessary to initiate the cellulose graft copolymer formation. Cerium(IV) ions in the acidic medium or in the presence of DMSO form chelates with the hydroxyl groups of carbons C_2 and C_3 of the anhydroglucose unit of cellulose. Transfer of electrons from cellulose to the Ce(IV) gives Ce(III), which dissociates from the chelate. The anhydroglucose ring is scissioned between C_2 and C_3, and a short living radical is formed. In the presence of the monomer, grafting reactions are initiated to produce the copolymer.

MnO^{4-} dissolves in the acid medium to give rise to Mn^{3+} ions via Mn^{4+}. These highly reactive Mn^{3+} ions are responsible for initiating graft copolymerization and homopolymerization.[52]

$$PH + Mn(III) \rightarrow PH\text{-}Mn(III)\,[Complex]$$

$$PH + Mn(III) \rightarrow P^{\bullet} + Mn(II) + H^{+}$$

$$P^{\bullet} + M \rightarrow PM^{\bullet}$$

$$Mn(III) + M \rightarrow M^{\bullet} + Mn(II) + H^{+}$$

$$PM^{\bullet} + nM \rightarrow PM^{\bullet}{}_{n+1}$$

$$M^{\bullet} + nM \rightarrow M^{\bullet}{}_{n+1}$$

$$PM_{n+1} + M(III) \rightarrow PM_{n+1} + Mn(II) + H^{+}$$

$$P^{\bullet} + Mn(II) \rightarrow Oxidized\ product + Mn(II)$$

where PH refers to polymer.

Apart from the initiators discussed earlier, BPO and AIBN are also effective in grafting reactions.[3–5,53–57] This is important to note that the grafting efficiency is low with BPO and AIBN, compared with that obtained using one-electron-transfer agents. For example, not all of the radical species contribute toward grafts of poly(MMA) on cellulose. Moreover, between the two, BPO is more reactive than AIBN, since the effects of resonance stabilization reduce the efficiency of the primary radical (I) from AIBN in generating active sites on the backbone.

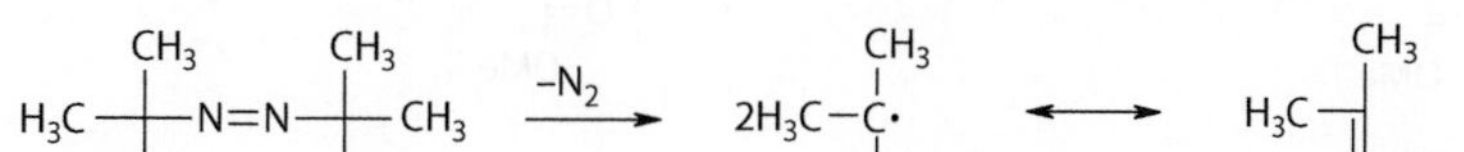

(I)

Chemical pretreatment (e.g., ozonation) of the polymer backbone[58–60] may also generate free radical sites upon reaction with Fe^{2+}, which can provide sites for grafting.

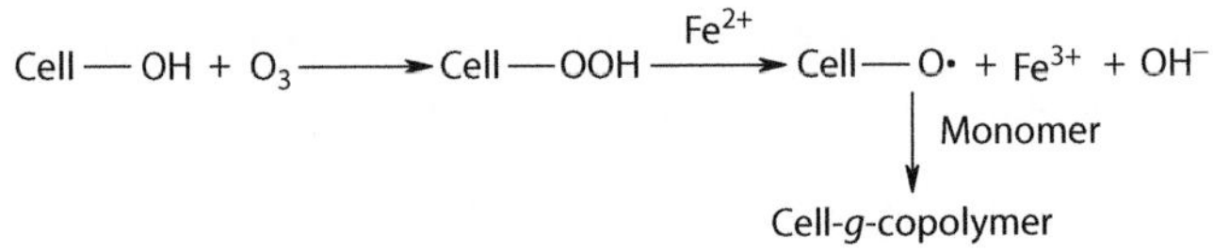

17.2.1.3 Ionic Grafting

Grafting can also proceed through an ionic mode. Alkali metal suspensions in a Lewis base liquid, organometallic compounds, and sodium naphthalenide are useful initiators in this purpose. Alkyl aluminum (R_3Al) and the backbone polymer in the halide form (ACl) interact to form carbonium ions along the polymer chain, which leads to copolymerization. The reaction proceeds through cationic mechanism.

$$ACl + R_3Al \rightarrow A^+R_3AlCl^-$$

$$A^+ + M \rightarrow AM^+ + M \rightarrow \text{Graft copolymer}$$

BF_3 can also be used as a cationic catalyst.

Grafting can also proceed through an anionic mechanism. Sodium-ammonia or methoxide of alkali metals form the alkoxide of polymer (PO^-Na^+), which reacts with the monomer to form the graft copolymer.

$$P-OH + NaOR \rightarrow PO^-Na^+ + ROH$$

$$PO^- + M \rightarrow POM^- + M \rightarrow \text{Graft copolymer}$$

In the presence of tin-bis(2-ethyl hexanoate) as an initiator, ε-caprolactone and MMA can be grafted onto cellulose and cellulose acetate.[3–5,61,62] The mechanism of polymerization when tin-bis(2-ethyl hexanoate) is used as the initiator is still in dubious. The most promising mechanism is a coordination–insertion mechanism where the hydroxyl group is thought to coordinate to $Sn(Oct)_2$, forming the tin alkoxide complex[63] and is given in Figure 17.3.[3]

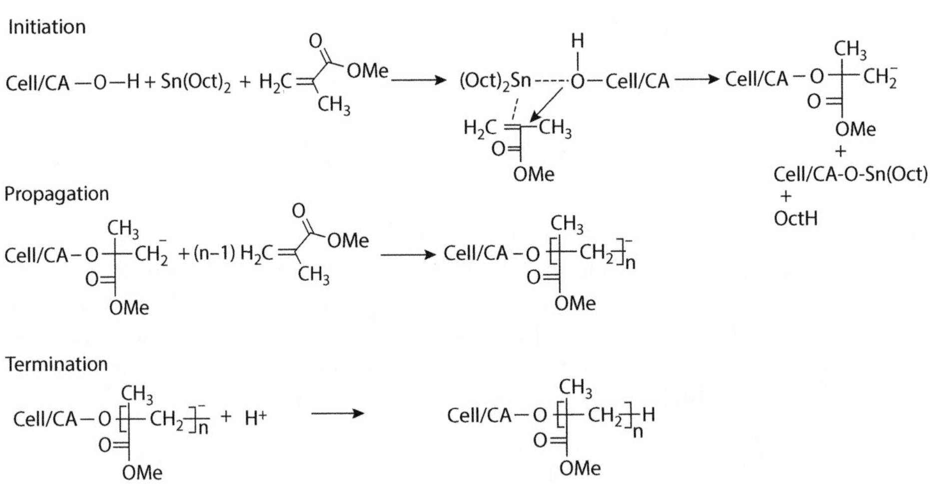

FIGURE 17.3 Mechanism of grafting of PMMA onto cellulose/CA using $Sn(Oct)_2$ as the initiator.

17.2.1.4 Grafting through Living Polymerization

In recent years, methods of "living polymerization" have developed to provide a potential for grafting reactions. The definition of living polymer is "that retains their ability to propagate for a long time and grow to a desired maximum size while their degree of termination or chain transfer is still negligible."[64] Controlled free radical polymerizations combine features of conventional free radical and ionic polymerizations. Conventional free radical polymerization requires continuous initiation, with termination of the growing chain radicals in coupling or disproportionation reactions and, as a result, leads to unreactive ("dead") polymers and essentially time-invariant degree of polymerization and broad molecular weight distribution. In case of living polymerization, it provides living polymers with regulated molecular weights and low polydispersities.[65–72]

Controlled free radical polymerization may be effective through ATRP. In recent years, a couple of papers have been appeared reporting on controlled grafting of cellulose using ATRP. First, the grafting can be performed in heterogeneous system, that is, on the surface of cellulose fibers or particles, giving surface-modified cellulose, which could be used, for instance, as a filler in appropriate polymer composites.[73,74] Thus, cellulose fibers (filter paper) were in the first step surface acylated with 2-bromoisoburyryl bromide, giving the fibers with chemically anchored initiating sites, which are subsequently used for ATRP grafting of methyl acrylate by immersing the modified filter paper into a reaction mixture containing MA, Cu(I)Br, tris-2-(dimethyl amino) ethylamine (Me_6-TREN), sacrificial initiator, and ethyl acetate.[75] Further, these fibers with the anchored poly MA brush were used as macroinitiators of ATRP of 2-hydroxy ethyl methacrylate (HEMA), leading to poly(MA-b-HEMA) surface-anchored polymer.[76] It is also reported that cellulose powder can be surface-acylated with chloroacetic acid chloride, and the anchored chloroacetyl groups then used as initiating sites for ATRP grafting of styrene, MMA, methacrylamide, or 4-acryloyl morpholine.[77] Cellulose diacetate was also acylated with 2-bromoisobutyryl bromide or dichloro acetyl chloride in the presence of triethylamine (TEA) and 4-(dimethylamino) pyridine (DMAP) for ATRP grafting copolymerization of MMA, styrene, and butyl acrylate under CuCl, $CuCl_2$, Cu powder/hexamethyl triethylene tetraamine, pentamethyl diethylene triamine catalyst[78] as shown in Figure 17.4.

In another report, cellulose acetate was acylated with 2-bromoisobutyryl bromide in the presence of TEA in tetrahydro furan to form the macroinitiator, which was then grafted by methyl diethylene glycol methacrylate (MDEGMA) by ATRP mechanism[79] as shown in Figure 17.5.

Hydroxyethyl cellulose-*graft*-polyacrylamide (HEC-*g*-PAM) was synthesized by using ATRP, in which the macroinitiator for ATRP was synthesized first by reacting HEC with 2-bromoisobutyryl bromide in the presence of TEA and DMAP. Then, AM was grafted from this macroinitiator in the presence of $CuBr/CuBr_2$ catalyst and 5,5,7,12,12,14-hexamethyl-1,4,8,11-tetra azomacro-cyclo tetradecane (Me_6[14]ane N_4) ligand.[80]

Due to poor solubility of cellulose in common organic solvents, the graft copolymerization of cellulose by ATRP reported earlier occurs only on the surface of cellulose fiber due to heterogeneous process, or otherwise cellulose derivatives are taken for grafting by ATRP. Homogeneous grafting of cellulose dissolved in DMAc/LiCl solvent system has also been carried out through ATRP[81] in which the macroinitiator was synthesized first by the reaction of cellulose with 2-bromoisobutyryl bromide in the presence of pyridine. The macroinitiator was then reacted with *N,N*-dimethylacrylamide in the presence of CuBr and 2,2′-bipyridine in DMSO to get the graft copolymer as shown in Figure 17.6.

Reversible addition–fragmentation chain transfer (RAFT) polymerization, another "living"/controlled radical polymerization method, is of promising and particular interest, over other "living"/controlled process, as a wider range of functional monomers can be used under the mild-demanding reaction conditions. Using the controlled RAFT technique, a number of different functional monomers like MMA, MA, and styrene were grafted onto the surface of cellulose.[82–84]

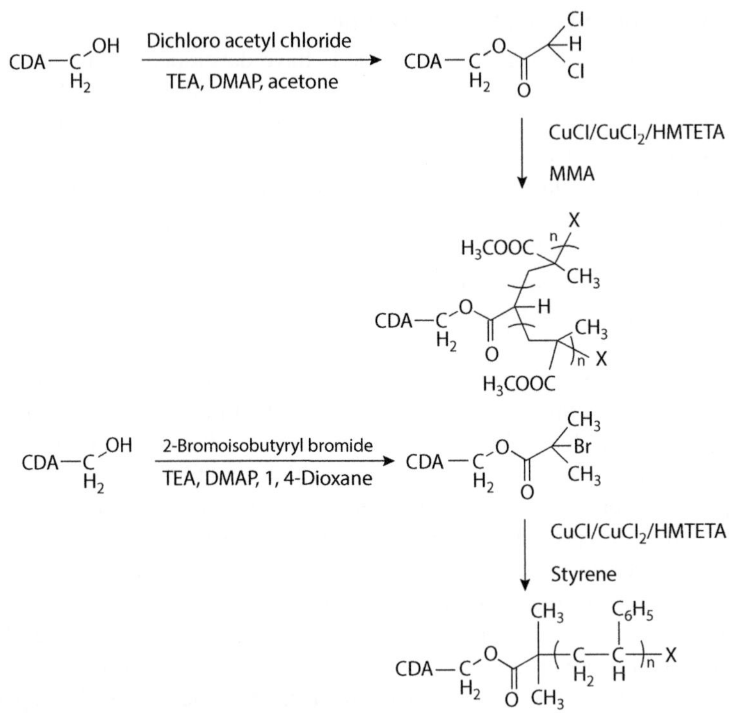

FIGURE 17.4 ATRP of MMA onto cellulose diacetate.

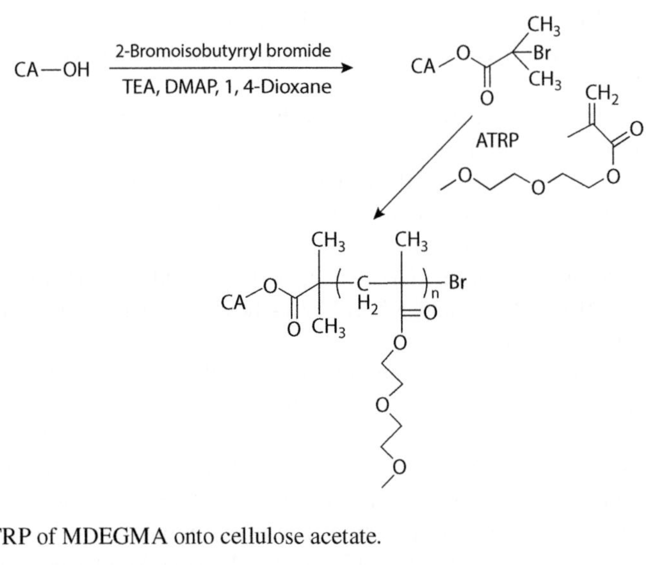

FIGURE 17.5 ATRP of MDEGMA onto cellulose acetate.

17.2.1.5 Ring-Opening Polymerization

Ring-opening polymerization (ROP) is a well-established technique to polymerize cyclic monomers such as lactones and lactides. An alcohol (or hydroxyl group) is generally used as the initiator for ROP, which makes it especially interesting to utilize ROP of cyclic monomers for the polymer modification of cellulose or cellulose derivatives.[85]

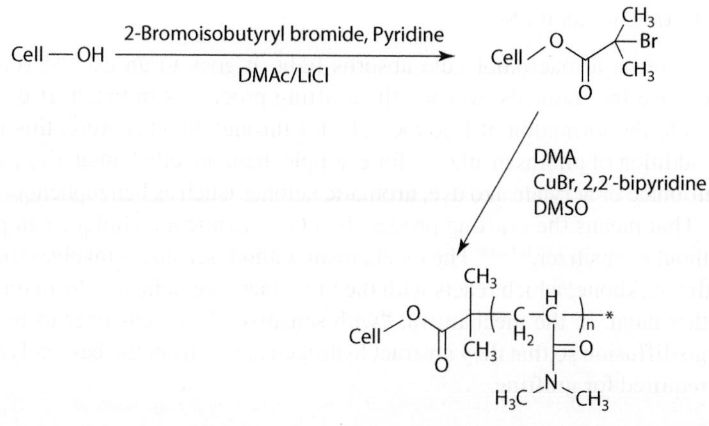

FIGURE 17.6 Homogeneous grafting of *N*,*N*-dimethylacrylamide onto cellulose through ATRP.

ROP operates through different mechanisms depending on the monomer, initiator, and catalytic system that are utilized. Tin(II) 2-ethyl hexanoate ($Sn(Oct)_2$) is a commonly used catalyst for the polymerization of monomers such as ε-caprolactone, lacide, and *p*-dioxanone. Several different mechanisms have been hypothesized for this system, but the most commonly accepted mechanism for the initiation is that $Sn(Oct)_2$ is converted into tin alkoxide, the actual initiator, by reaction with alcohols, that is, the "coordination–insertion" mechanism.[85–87]

$$\mathrm{Sn(Oct)_2 + R\text{-}OH \rightarrow Oct\text{-}Sn\text{-}OR + OctH}$$

$$\mathrm{Oct\text{-}Sn\text{-}OR + ROH \rightarrow Sn(OR)_2 + OctH}$$

17.2.2 Grafting Initiated by Radiation Technique

The irradiation of macromolecules can cause homolytic cleavage and thus form free radicals on the polymer. In the radiation technique, the presence of an initiator is not essential. The medium is important in this case, for example, if irradiation is carried out in air, peroxides may be formed on the polymer. The lifetime of the free radical depends upon the nature of the polymer backbone. Grafting proceeds in three different ways: (1) pre-irradiation, (2) peroxidation, and (3) mutual irradiation techniques. In pre-irradiation technique, the polymer backbone is first irradiated in vacuum or in the presence of an inert gas to form free radicals. The irradiated polymer substrate is then treated with the monomer in liquid of vapor state or as a solution in a suitable solvent.[88–92]

In the peroxidation grafting method, the trunk polymer is subjected to high-energy irradiation in the presence of air or oxygen to form hydroperoxides or diperoxides, depending on the nature of the polymeric backbone and the irradiation conditions. The stable peroxy products are then treated with the monomer at high temperature, whence the peroxides undergo decomposition to radicals, which then initiate grafting. The advantage of this technique is that, the intermediate peroxy products can be stored for long periods before performing the grafting step. On the other hand, with the mutual irradiation technique, the polymer and the monomers are irradiated simultaneously, to form free radicals and subsequent addition.[93–100] Since the monomers are not exposed in pre-irradiation technique, the obvious advantage is that the method is relatively free from homopolymer formation, which occurs with the simultaneous technique. However, the decided disadvantage of the pre-irradiation technique is scission of the base polymer due to its direct irradiation, which can result in the formation of block copolymer.

17.2.3 Photochemical Grafting

When a chromophore on a macromolecule absorbs light, it goes to an excited state, which may dissociate into reactive free radicals, whence the grafting process is initiated. If the absorption of light does not lead to the formation of free radical sites through bund rupture, this process can be promoted by the addition of photosensitizers, for example, benzoin ethyl ether, dyes such as Na-2,7-anthraquinone sulfonate or acrylate azo dye, aromatic ketones (such as benzophenone, xanthone), or metal ion UO_2^{2+}. That means the grafting process by photochemical technique can proceed in two ways: with or without a sensitizer.[101–104] The mechanism without sensitizer involves the generation of free radicals on the backbone, which reacts with the monomer free radical to form the grafted copolymer. On the other hand, in the mechanism, "with sensitizer," the sensitizer forms free radicals, which can undergo diffusion so that they abstract hydrogen atoms from the base polymer, producing the radical sites required for grafting.

17.2.4 Enzymatic Grafting

The enzymatic grafting of cellulose is quite new, and only two reports in which enzymes are used to catalyze ROP from cellulose surface have been published.[105,106] Lipase is used for the ROP of ε-caprolactone in close proximity to cellulose fibers in a filter paper. In the first step, the enzyme was immobilized on the filter paper used as substrate, and in the second step, the polymerization was performed. This did not create covalently bonded grafts, but the polycaprolactone formed is coated on the cellulose surface.

17.3 CONTROLLING FACTORS OF GRAFTING

The factors that control the grafting reactions onto cellulosic materials will be discussed in the following sections. These factors include nature of the backbone, monomer, solvent, initiator, additives, and temperature.

17.3.1 Nature of the Backbone

As grafting involves covalent attachment of a monomer to a preformed polymeric backbone, the nature of the backbone (physical nature and chemical composition) plays an important role in the process. It is reported that crystallinity decreases with increasing degree of substitution of cellulose derivatives, affecting the grafting of AM on acetylated wood pulp.[107] As the crystallinity decreases, it is less ordered, facilitating the grafting reaction.

There are various reports regarding the role of chemical composition on grafting. For example, the presence of lignin (phenolic –OH) in straw affects the grafting of 2-methyl vinyl pyridine, since lignin is a good scavenger of radicals.[108] This phenomenon has also been observed in EA grafted to a sisal fiber system; sisal fiber contains 8% lignin. The grafting rate is higher when NaOH is used as a lignin remover, but the reverse has also been reported, that is, the presence of lignin increases the graft yield if the backbone is ozonized and grafted using Fe^{2+}–H_2O_2 as initiator. In that case, lignin is oxidized with ozone, as a result of which the carboxylic group is formed in the lignin structure, favoring the free radical formation, which influences grafting.[109] This phenomenon has also been observed in acrylonitrile grafted on pulp by xanthation method. In cases in which lignin is present in the cellulose structure, chain transfer may occur to lignin from the $^{\bullet}OH$ radical, giving rise to less reactive lignin radical.[110]

The presence of functional groups in the backbone also influences grafting. Styrene is grafted relatively with high efficiency on cellulose acetate-*p*-nitro benzoate. This result indicates that the pendant aromatic nitro group is more effective in obtaining a graft copolymer.[111] Replacement of –OH by –SH groups in a cellulose substrate increases the level of grafting as initiation by Ce^{4+} ion occurs by H-abstraction from C-atom having –OH groups. But in case of MMA grafting on holocellulose (comprising a mixture of α-cellulose and hemicellulose), H-abstraction is not the mode of initiation, and –SH group is associated with a marked decrease in the level of grafting.[112]

17.3.2 Effect of Monomer

As with the nature of backbone, the reactivity of the monomer is also important in grafting. The reactivity of monomer depends upon the various factors, viz., polar and steric nature, swellability of backbone in the presence of the monomers, and concentration of monomers. The difference in the grafting of vinyl acetate (2.6%) and EA (60.8%) on wool can be explained on these monomers. Since vinyl acetate acts as electron-donating monomer, it is extremely susceptible to monomer concentration, whereas EA is highly reactive to free radicals.[113] Thus, the percentage of grafting of EA is higher because the loss of EA in side reaction is minimal. On the other hand, being less reactive to radicals, vinyl acetate is reduced in side reactions.

In case of grafting of acrylonitrile, EA, and MMA onto starch, it is observed that the reactivity is in order AN > EA ≈ MMA. In this case, grafted polyethylacrylate forms gel over the starch granules, acting as a barrier to monomer diffusion to the vicinity of starch.[114] The order of the monomers on wool in terms of grafting is MA>EA>MMA>VAc>AAc. The reactivity of first three monomers is explained by steric considerations. Thus, MMA, being a highly crowded monomer, forms complex with Ce^{4+} less readily and affords minimum grafting. By contrast, VAc is susceptible to monomer transfer reaction and tends to terminate the growing grafted chain by that process, resulting in poor grafting efficiency. Since AAc and its polymer are soluble in water, AAc tends to undergo homopolymerization preferentially, resulting in poor grafting efficiency. The order of grafting of the substituted acrylamides onto cellulose acetate is AM > methylacrylamide > *N,N*-dimethylacrylamide.[88] The methyl group in methylacrylamide may reduce the mobility of the monomer, thus suppressing grafting. The low grafting with methylacrylamide may also be due to the stability of the polymer radical, which is tertiary, whereas polymer radical from AM is secondary. The secondary radicals are more reactive than the tertiary. With *N,N*-dimethylacrylamide, two methyl groups play a key role on the extent of grafting. Due to the steric effect of the two methyl groups, the easy approach of the monomer to the backbone is maximally hindered, and thus the extent of grafting is the least. Earlier workers also observed this phenomenon in case of substituted acrylates. The grafting order on cellulose by means of a Ce^{4+} initiation is methyl acrylate > EA > butyl acrylate > MMA. They offered an explanation of reactivity in terms of steric and polar effects. It was also proposed that grafting depends upon the stability of the radical. The polymer radical that is formed in case of MMA is relatively stable, whereas in case of MMA, which is the most reactive, the corresponding polymer radical is probably stable.

17.3.3 Effect of Solvent

In grafting mechanisms, the solvent is the carrier by which monomers are transported to the vicinity of the backbone. The choice of the solvent depends upon several parameters, including the solubility of monomer in solvent, the solubility or swelling properties of the backbone, the miscibility of the solvents if more than one is used, and the generation of free radical in the presence of the solvent.

The solubility of the monomer depends on the nature of the solvent and the polymer, for example, alcohols are useful solvents for grafting styrene onto cellulose or cellulose acetate.[115–117] This is because alcohols can swell the backbone effectively and can dissolve the styrene so that the monomer can easily diffuse in the cellulosic structure. The extent of grafting, however, decreases progressively when the alcohol is changed from methanol to ethanol to isopropanol and to *t*-butanol; this decrease in grafting is due to the gradually decreased swelling properties of the alcohol, known to be corroborated by the bulkiness of the alcohol molecules. The grafting of styrene is suppressed by the addition of water to alcohol in the grafting medium. Incidentally, although cellulose acetate has a greater affinity for water than MeOH, grafting from the alcohol–water mixture is affected by the decreased solubility of styrene in the solvent.[115]

Homogeneous graft copolymerization of MMA onto cellulose and cellulose acetate is carried out in 1,4-dioxane, DMSO, DMSO/PF, and DMAc/LiCl solvent systems.[2–7] The molecular weight and graft yield of the cellulose-grafted product are higher in DMSO/PF solvent system concluding as a better solvent in comparison to DMAc/LiCl for graft copolymerization of MMA onto cellulose. Dissolution of cellulose in DMSO/PF solvent system forms methylol cellulose, whereas in DMAc/LiCl, it forms a complex the structure of which hinders the reaction sites for the formation of free radicals for grafting and thereby decreases the graft yield.[118,119]

17.3.4 Effect of Initiator

As discussed earlier, apart from the radiation technique, all chemical grafting reactions require an initiator, and its nature, concentration, solubility, as well as function need to be considered. Grafting percentage can be increased either by increasing the number of grafts (grafting frequency) per substrate chain or by increasing the molecular weight of grafted chains at constant number of graft. It is apparent that the initiator concentration affects both the number of grafts per cellulose chain and the molecular weights of graft chains. Radicalic sites may be created on cellulose by some transition metals such as Ce^{4+}, Co^{3+}, and Cr^{6+}. The number of active sites created on the cellulose backbone depends on the initiator concentration, namely, the ratio of initiator/cellulose. It is observed in the grafting of *N*-vinyl pyrrolidone (NVP) onto cellulose with $Co(acac)_3$–$HClO_4$ as the initiator, the amount of grafted NVP and the conversion of cellulose to graft copolymer first increased with the increase in the initiator concentration and then decreased with further increase in initiator concentration.[10] The similar finding, first the increase in grafting with the initiator and then the decrease with further increase in initiator, has also been determined in the grafting reactions performed by the initiators CAN–HNO_3,[20,21,23,26,120,121] ceric ammonium sulfate,[9] persulfates,[122,123] and $KHSO_3$–$CoSO_4$.[11] In the grafting of AAm–MA onto cellulose by CAN–HNO_3 initiator system, it is determined that the disappearance rate of Ce^{4+} ions did not change with the variation of monomer concentration from 0.1 to 0.5 M and concluded from this finding that the Ce^{4+} ions do not directly create active radicals on the monomers.[120] The high efficiency of grafting with Ce^{4+} ions was attributed to the creation of active radicals by CAN initiator preferentially on the cellulose backbone than the monomers.[26] In addition, it is also observed that true grafting percentage (GT%) increased with the increase in Ce^{4+} concentration from 1.5×10^{-3} to 7.5×10^{-3} M, but the higher concentrations of CAN than 7.5×10^{-3} M led to a decrease in GT% due to hydrolysis of CAN and being the hydrolysis product inactive for the creation of active sites in the absence of sufficient amount of nitric acid (HNO_3). The increase in CAN concentration leads to a decrease in grafting yield, but an increase in homopolymer formation.[21] CAN prefers to form complex with cellulose over the monomer. However, at higher concentrations of CAN, Ce^{4+} ions form complex with the monomer in addition to that with cellulose, and homopolymer formation can also occur. The termination of growing polymer radicals is also accelerated with Ce^{4+} concentration, and it leads to a decrease in grafting yield. When CAN is used as an initiator, the acid, mostly HNO_3, has an important effect on the efficiency of initiator for grafting. As known, the reaction of CAN with aqueous HNO_3 occurs as follows:

$$Ce^{4+} + H_2O \rightleftarrows Ce(OH)^{3+} + H^+$$

As known, ceric ion in CAN exists as the species of Ce^{4+}, $Ce(OH)^{3+}$, and $(Ce–O–Ce)^{6+}$ in its aqueous solution. It was reported that the efficiency of Ce^{4+} and $Ce(OH)^{3+}$ species to form radical sites on cellulose backbone is higher than that of $(Ce–O–Ce)^{6+}$ since the size of the former is smaller than that of the latter,[121] and the former is more mobile than the latter. At high acid concentrations, Ce^{4+} and $Ce(OH)^{3+}$ species affect the grafting adversely, namely, the termination reaction dominates over the propagation. A possible explanation for this adverse effect of high acid concentration on the grafting may be the difficulty in hydrogen abstraction from graft substrate. The concentration of these species depends on the amount of acid present in the medium. At high nitric acid concentrations, this equilibrium reaction shifts to the left, and ceric ions in CAN occur in the form of Ce^{4+}, which is responsible for the creation of active radicals preferably on the cellulose than monomer. In the case of low acid concentrations, the equilibrium shifts to the right, and the formation of high amount of $Ce(OH)^{3+}$ led to the formation of considerable amount of $(Ce–O–Ce)^{6+}$, which is not active for the creation of radical sites.

$$2Ce\left(OH\right)^{3+} \rightleftarrows \left(Ce-O-Ce\right)^{6+} + H_2O$$

For that reason, CAN or another ceric salt should be used together with an acid (i.e., HNO_3). The increase in the concentration of HNO_3 from 0.3 to 0.5 M led to 20% increase in grafting percentage of NVP onto cellulose by CAN initiator, and further increase in HNO_3 concentration resulted in 10% decrease in grafting percentage. The decrease in grafting with the increase in acid concentration beyond the optimum value was attributed to the effect of excess H^+ ions as free radical terminator.[21] The effect of complexing agent such as KF, ascorbic acid, and EDTA on the grafting of EA onto cellulose by Fenton reagent ($Fe^{2+}–H_2O_2$) is investigated.[18] In order to avoid the negative effect of Fe^{3+} ions on the grafting, namely, the wastage of $^{\bullet}OH$ radicals by reaction with Fe^{3+} ions, the grafting was carried out in the presence of some complexing agents with Fe^{3+} ions such as ascorbic acid, KF, and EDTA.[18] At low concentration (81×10^{-4} M), KF gave highest amount of grafting among the complexing agents, but its increase to 166×10^{-4} M reduced the grafting of EA significantly. The similar behavior was observed for the grafting of VAc under the same conditions. KF makes complex with Fe^{3+} ions and favors the grafting. The decrease in grafting percentage with KF attributed to the oxidation of KF to elemental fluorine (F), which reacts with vinyl monomer giving as an addition product, and it leads to a decrease in grafting. Both EDTA and ascorbic acid reduced the grafting of both EA and vinyl acetate (Vac) at all concentrations investigated. In the grafting of MMA onto stone ground wood by Fenton reagent, it is determined that graft yield increases with the molar ratio of $Fe^{2+}–H_2O_2$ up to 0.085, and after that concentration, the graft yield decreased slightly.[19] It is concluded that only a low molar ratio of $Fe^{2+}–H_2O_2$ is enough to succeed the grafting. The similar trend (first increase and then decrease) for the grafting with the concentration is also observed for various persulfates such as KPS,[16] and APS[122–124] is observed for AIBN[124] and BPO[122] too. The effects of various redox initiators, viz., APS, KPS, and BPO, in the grafting of AAm onto ethyl cellulose (EC) in DMSO/toluene solution have been studied.[15] It is determined that APS is a suitable initiator for the grafting of AAm onto EC because it leads no degradation in EC chains. Again, the increase in APS concentration led to a decrease in grafting parameters such as grafting percentage or grafting yield due to termination of primary radicals, but the use of KPS in the same reaction increased the same grafting parameters. The opposite effects of the concentration of redox initiators APS and KPS on the grafting are attributed to the difference in the decomposition rates of initiators.[125] It is also determined that BPO is not a suitable initiator since it leads to degradation of EC, and for that reason, BPO gave considerably lower grafting yield and efficiency in comparison to APS and KPS. Grafting of AN and MMA separately onto cellulose in DMSO/PF system (in homogeneous medium) using two types of initiators, APS and BPO, has been investigated.[124] It is known that DMSO/PF system is a nondegrading solvent for cellulose. The nature of the initiator has an important effect on the grafting. AIBN is known to show resonance stabilization, but no such resonance exists in the peroxide initiators. For that reason, it is reported that higher grafting yield is obtained with APS, 87.3% for AN and 52% for MMA, in comparison to those with AIBN, that is, 10% for AN and 48% for MMA. The number of grafts per cellulose chain by APS and AIBN initiator were found to be 3.9 and 0.5 for AN and 3.4 and 1.3 for MMA monomers. From the results, it is suggested that, grafting occurred in higher parts of cellulose chain in homogeneous medium than heterogeneous medium in which the number of grafts per cellulose chain rarely exceeds the unity. It is also found that the grafting onto cellulose hardly proceeded with AN–AIBN system, but appreciably in MMA–AIBN system.

17.3.5 Role of Additives on Grafting

Graft yield or the extent of graft copolymerization depends on the presence of additives such as metal ions, acids, and inorganic salts. Thus, the reaction between the monomer and the backbone must compete with any reactions between the monomer and additives. Although some additives may enhance the monomer/backbone reaction to augment the grafting efficiency, the reverse will be true if the reaction between the monomer and the additive is dominant.

The addition of acids and alkali can affect the nature of the backbone, solvent, as well as the initiator, so that it can influence the grafting. For example, when EA and styrene are co-grafted on sisal fiber, the presence of sulfuric acid or alkali controls the grafting yield.[126] The increase in crystallinity due to the alkali treatment will result in reduction in the sorption capacity of the fiber. As a result, the amount of monomer solution sorbed in the fiber during the grafting process will be reduced. This accounts for a decrease in the grafting efficiency for sisal fibers subjected to alkali treatment. By contrast, when the fibers are subjected to the combined treatment, fibrillation due to intracrystallite swelling by the acid facilitates the subsequent penetration of NaOH solution, resulting in better grafting onto cellulose. Moreover, the combined treatment may result in an increase in the ordering of the fibers in addition to an increase in the crystalline regions. These effects are reflected in a slight decrease in the grafting yield of fibers subjected to the combined treatment, compared to that of the fibers subjected to the alkali treatment alone.

In case of Ce^{4+}, taken as the initiator for the grafting of MMA onto cellulose, maximum grafting takes place in the presence of sulfuric acid.[126,127] In aqueous medium, initiator Ce^{4+} is believed to combine with water according to the reaction discussed in Section 17.3.4. It is also clear that $[Ce^{+4}]$ facilitates the formation of complex with the base polymer with increasing the concentration of H_2SO_4, as the equilibrium shifts toward formation of more and more of $Ce(OH)^{3+}$ and Ce^{4+}. Having smaller size, these species facilitate the formation of a complex between Ce^{4+} ion and cellulose, resulting in an increase in the percentage of grafting[128].

The effect of amines upon ceric ion–initiated grafting of poly(methyl acrylate) onto wool has been explained by assuming a complex formation between wool and the ceric ion[129] in the following manner:

$$Ce^{4+} + RNH_2 \rightleftarrows \text{Complex} \rightarrow Ce^{3+} + H^+ + RN^{\bullet}H$$

The ceric amine complex decomposes to give free radical species, which at lower concentration generate more active sites on wool by H-abstraction. However, there exists a critical concentration of amines that promotes grafting. With a further increase in concentration, the percentage of grafting decreases owing to the termination of growing grafted chain-by-chain transfer with the amine. The reactivity of amines followed the order diethylamine > dipropylamine > ammonia > triethylamine > triethanolamine > pyridine.[130] The grafting percentage increases linearly with an increase in the basicity of amines. Though diethylamine is as nucleophilic as dipropylamine, only DEA enhances grafting rate tremendously, while in the presence of DPA, no accelerating effect upon grafting efficiency is observed. This is explained by the steric factor, such that DEA, having a smaller steric requirement than DPA, easily forms a complex with Ce^{4+}. Ammonia, having a smaller steric requirement than TEA, forms a complex with Ce^{4+} more easily than does TEA. With triethanolamine and pyridine, all three factors, that is, basicity, nucleophilicity, and steric size, are responsible for giving a low grafting efficiency.

The addition of $NaNO_3$ or NaCl in the grafting of vinyl acetate and methyl acrylate on cellulose acetate affects the graft copolymerization by enhancing the oxidation of cellulose by the transition metal ions (viz., Ce^{4+}), initiates the formation of free radicals for grafting, but it left the homopolymerization almost unaffected.[131]

17.3.6 Effect of Temperature

Temperature is one of the important factors that controls the kinetics of graft copolymerization. In general, graft yield increases with an increase in reaction temperature until a limit is attained, and then it decreases for persulfates.[14,15,122,124] Similar results have also been reported in the literature for Ce^{4+} initiator.[2–7,15,22,24] For example, Nishioka et al.[122,123] found in the grafting in homogeneous medium by persulfate initiators that with an increase in temperature, the molecular weight of graft chains decreased, but the number of grafts increased up to a certain amount and then leveled off. The optimum temperature for highest grafting depends on the initiator used. In the grafting of HEMA onto cellulose in DMSO/PF solvent system using various initiators,[125] it is determined that the optimum temperatures are 40°C for APS, 50°C for KPS, and 60°C for both AIBN and BPO. In the grafting of AA onto cellulose in a heterogeneous medium by CAN–HNO_3 initiator,[132] nearly the same grafting percentages were obtained at 30°C, 50°C, and 70°C, but three to four times lower grafting percentages were obtained at 90°C than those at former temperatures. The graft copolymer prepared at 30°C had highest water absorption capacity probably due to a difference in their grafting frequencies and graft lengths. Therefore, the optimum grafting temperature was determined as 30°C for the grafting of AA onto cellulose by CAN–HNO_3 initiator.[132] It was also determined that the rate constants for the disappearance of AA during the grafting increased from 0.018 to 0.033 min^{-1} with an increase in temperature from 30°C to 90°C, and the increase in temperature favored the formation of homopolymer poly(acrylic acid) (PAA).

17.4 APPLICATIONS

Modified polymers are very much useful as they can be tailored to the requirements of particular applications. The applications of cellulose graft copolymers change with the structure of polymer grafted on cellulose. There are in fact many applications of grafted cellulosic materials, but here the discussion is limited to four areas, viz., heavy metal absorption, hydrogels, coating applications, and membranes.

17.4.1 Heavy Metal Adsorption

"Heavy metals" is a collective term applying to the group of metals and metalloids with an atomic density greater than 6 g cm^{-3}. Although it is only a loosely defined term, it is widely recognized and usually applied to the elements such as cadmium (Cd), chromium (Cr), copper (Cu), mercury (Hg), nickel (Ni), lead (Pb), and zinc (Zn), which are commonly associated with pollution and toxicity problems.[133] Industrial usage of metals and domestic processes like burning of fossil fuels, incineration of wastes, automobile exhausts, smelting processes, and the use of sewage sludge as landfill material and fertilizer have introduced substantial amount of potentially toxic heavy metals into the atmospheric, aquatic, and terrestrial environments. While many of the heavy metals are needed by plants at micronutrient level, higher concentrations are known to produce a range of toxic effects. Hence, it is necessary to remove these heavy metals from the environment for a healthy life process.

Among all the treatment processes, adsorption using sorbent is one of the most popular and effective processes for the removal of heavy metals. There are a lot of adsorbents that are used for the removal of heavy metals, out of which cellulose-grafted product is one.

Introduction of amidoxime or triethylenetetraamine groups to cellulose using photo-grafting technique produces cellulose amidoximated or triethylenetetraaminated products, which adsorb Cu(II) with a maximum adsorption capacity of 51 and 30 mg g^{-1}, respectively. Initially, acrylonitrile was grafted to cellulose surface; subsequently, the cyano groups were amidoximated or triethylenetetraaminated by reaction with hydroxylamine or triethylenetetraamine, respectively.[134]

It is also reported that graft copolymerization of acrylic acid or AM by radiation grafting onto cellulose or wood pulp gives the grafted product that adsorbs Cu(II) from wastewater[135] and removed Fe(III), Cr(III), Pb(II), and Cd(II) from aqueous solution.[99,136]

AM-grafted cellulose materials produced by redox initiation system, after aminated by reacting the product with ethylenediamine or without amination[8] can be used for adsorption of Cr(II),[137] Hg(II).[8,138] Amidoximation product of the acrylonitrile-grafted sunflower stalks, by reacting with hydroxylamine hydroxide, can be used for the adsorption of Cu(II).[139] Acrylonitrile-grafted regenerated cellulose beads are saponified using sodium hydroxide, which converts the cyano groups to both amide ($–CONH_2$) and carboxylate (–COONa) groups.[140,141] Adsorption of trivalent chromium on the amide functionalized compound reached 73.5 mg g^{-1}, whereas Cu(II) uptake on the carboxylate functionalized compound was 70.5 mg g^{-1}.

Cellulose powder has been grafted with acrylic acid, *N,N′*-methylene bisacrylamide, 2-acrylamido-2-methyl propane sulfonic acid ($AASO_3H$), and a mixture of acrylic acid and 2-acrylamido-2-methyl propane sulfonic acid using CAN as the initiator.[142] All four grafted cellulose materials were compared in the adsorption of Pb(II), Cu(II), and Cd(II) under competitive conditions. It is seen that cellulose-*g*-PAA is the most efficient adsorbent under these conditions with its carboxyl groups responsible for chelating the divalent metal ion. The sawdust-grafted PAA has also high adsorption capacity for Cu(II) (104 mg g^{-1}), Ni(II) (97 mg g^{-1}), and Cd(II) (169 mg g^{-1}).[143]

In addition, the cellulose graft copolymers obtained by grafting of vinyl monomers with functional groups such as acrylamide,[8] acrylic acid,[140,144–146] acrylonitrile, and 2-acrylamido-methylpropane sulfonic acid[140] have been used in the adsorption of hazardous contaminants such as heavy metal ions or dyes[75] from aqueous solutions.[17,147] In recent years, cellulose graft copolymers with thermosensitive graft chains such as poly(*N*-isopropylacrylamide or poly(*N,N*-diethylacrylamide) have been used in the removal of heavy metal ions from aqueous solutions by temperature swing adsorption, which is different from the removal of metal ions by complexation or ion exchange.[148–153]

17.4.2 pH and Thermosensitive Hydrogels

Stimuli-responsive hydrogels are cross-linked hydrophilic polymeric networks that exhibit various swelling properties depending on environmental variables such as, pH, temperature, ionic strength, and electric current. Such hydrogels are utilized by the human body, for example, where the muscle function is controlled by gels that are expanded and contracted as a result of electrical nerve signals. The other applications of hydrogels are in the field of drug delivery and molecular separation.

pH-sensitive cellulose fiber-supported hydrogels are prepared by ozone-induced graft polymerization of acrylic acid using cotton linters and wood pulp fiber substrates.[59,60] A cross-linked grafted poly acrylic chain around the pulp fibers has been prepared by replacing various amounts of acrylic acid monomer with ethylene glycol dimethacrylate monomer, which is a typical cross-linker for hydrogels. These fibers are found to exhibit a stimuli-responsive swelling behavior depending on the pH level in the environment.

Temperature-sensitive polymer, poly(*N*-isopropyl acrylamide), has been grafted on the surface of cotton cellulose fabric by pre-irradiation-induced grafting,[90] to produce environmental-sensitive hydrogel. The product has been found to be temperature sensitive having lower critical solution temperature of 35.4°C.

A wide spectrum of reactive networks and graft copolymers of AM and acrylic acid, alone or with some binary monomers with cellulose, have been synthesized, using BPO as the initiator and glutaraldehyde as the cross-linker to get the cellulose-based hydrogels.[54] By this method, cell-*g*-polyacrylamide, cell-*g*-poly(AM-*co*-glycidyl methacrylate), cell-*g*-poly(AM-*co*-acrylic acid), cell-*g*-poly(AM-*co*-HEMA), cell-*g*-poly(AM-*co*-acrylonitrile), cell-*g*-poly(acrylic acid), and cell-*g*-poly(acrylic acid comonomers with all of the monomers given earlier) have been prepared, and their swelling behavior has been studied. Higher water uptake by the grafted products is observed as the cellulose matrix opens up by grafting due to loss of crystallinity, where diffusion of the solvent takes place and leads to an increase in the liquid retention volume. Since AM and acrylic acid are hydrophilic monomers, their grafting increases the water retention character of the graft copolymer.

pH-responsive poly(2-diethylamino) ethyl methacrylate grafted-ethyl cellulose (EC-*g*-PDEAEMA) has been synthesized by ATRP, which can be used in the pH-responsive release of rifampicin (RIF).[154]

17.4.3 UV-Curable Coatings

Radiation curing is now being increasingly used in various sectors of applications, mainly in coating industry, graphic arts, and micro-electronics replacing conventional solvent-based coatings, inks, and adhesives. They have other advantages such as fast cure speed, room temperature operation, high-quality end products, less rejection rates, less energy consumption, and requirement of less floor space.[50,155]

The introduction of pendant branches that provide cross-linkable functionality to cellulose derivatives aids in the formation of a hard, scratch-resistant, and solvent-resistant surface following radiation curing. The presence of cellulose ester produces a quick drying, workable lacquer that is easily buffed, sanded, or removed with solvent as needed prior to cross-linking.[156]

With a view to develop UV-curable surface coatings, glycidyl methacrylate has been grafted to carboxymethyl cellulose in homogeneous medium to introduce photoreactive epoxide groups onto the cellulose chain.[50] Acrylate groups are involved in the grafting reaction, while the glycidyl groups remain as pendant groups for a subsequent reaction introduced by cationic photoinitiators and UV light. Triarylsulfonium hexafluorophosphate has been used as the photoinitiator.

In the other report, *N*-methylol acrylamide has been grafted to cellulose acetate in a homogeneous medium to get acrylamidomethylated cellulose acetate (AMCA). The UV surface coating formulation has been prepared by mixing AMCA, trimethylol propane triacrylate, epoxy acrylate oligomer, and 1-hydroxy-cyclohexyl-phenyl ketone as the photoinitiator and is coated onto a glass plate and then cured by UV radiation.[155]

17.4.4 Membranes

For use in the separation technologies, membrane may be considered to be a phase that acts as a barrier to prevent mass movement in general, but allows restricted and/or regulated passage of one or more species through it, that is, it controls the selective transfer of molecules or ions. There are a number of membrane-based separation techniques, varying in the driving forces employed including concentration, pressure, and electric potential. For example, osmosis and dialysis, useful in the separation of solutes involving large molecules, are concentration driven. Microfiltration, ultrafiltration, nanofiltration, and reverse osmosis are pressure-driven techniques by which solutes of different sizes are separated. Pervaporation especially suitable for the separation of azeotropic mixtures is a vacuum-driven technique, in which volatile small molecules pass through the membrane. Thus, a nonvolatile solute can be separated from the volatile solvent. Electrodialysis is an electric potential—driven separation technique useful to separate ionized molecules.

Graft copolymers could form micelles with less number of chains compared with block copolymers. Even unimolecular micelles could often be formed by intramolecular association. Graft copolymer solutions should also have higher sieving ability than linear polymer solutions, since grafted points could prevent the polymer chains from sliding away from each other and thus could form relatively more stable pore sizes. Therefore, design and synthesis of low-viscosity graft copolymer solution with high sieving ability and self-coating ability is an important portion of DNA separation media.[80] In this report, the acrylamide has been grafted to hydroxyl ethyl cellulose to get the grafted product HEC-*g*-PAM by ATRP and is applied as a medium for the separation of double-stranded DNA in the bare fused-silica capillaries by electro-osmosis. The HEC-*g*-PAM copolymer has dynamic coating properties due to the HEC coieties and thus effectively suppresses interactions of the analytes with the capillary wall and unwanted electro-osmosis.

MDEGMA has been grafted to cellulose acetate by ATRP[79] to get the graft copolymer having very good film-forming property and is used for the separation of alcohol/ether mixtures by pervaporation and purification of ethyl-tert-butyl ether.

In another report, grafting of AM onto cellulose acetate powder and membranes has been carried out, followed by activation with glutaraldehyde, in order to provide supports for enzyme immobilization.[53] The enzyme bonding is favored by small grafting degrees, probably due to steric impediments.

Protein fouling is a critical factor governing membrane performance in various filtration processes. In this report, a new surface modification technique is carried out to modify mixed cellulose ester membranes to reduce protein fouling.[102] The first step of this modification involves coating of the membrane with a monolayer of allyl dimethylchlorosilane. The silanized membrane is then covalently linked to a triblock copolymer of polyethylene oxide and polypropylene oxide (PEO-PPO-PEO) by UV irradiation. The membrane has been used for filtration of bovine serum albumin.

17.4.5 Miscellaneous

Cellulose graft copolymers with poly(acrylic acid), *N*-vinyl-2-pyrrolidone, or polyacrylamide grafts that are hydrophilic in structure have high water absorption capacity.[132] For that reason, they could be used as body fluid absorbent in medical applications.[36] For example, the water and saline absorbencies of polyacrylamide-grafted Ce^{4+}-treated wood pulp were found to be 2500–2700 g g^{-1} and 40–60 g g^{-1}, respectively.[23] The grafting of water-soluble vinyl monomers onto amine-treated cotton fiber gave a graft copolymer with enhanced moisture sorption ability that can be used in fabrics, such as underwear and athletic wear.[16] Cellulose-thiocarbamate-*g*-PAN had high antimicrobial activity. It is reported that *N*-isopropyl acrylamide and methyl acrylate-grafted cellulose as template in the crystallization of $CaCO_3$ has better nucleating property than cellulose.[157] The product of poly(4-vinyl pyridine)-grafted cellulose with sodium borohydride has been used as reducing agents for various carbonyl compound such as benzaldehyde, cyclohexanone, crotonaldehyde, acetone, and furfural.[21] In addition, another graft product obtained by ATRP, which is a graft copolymer of EC with azobenzene-containing polymethacrylates, was reported to be used in some applications such as sensors and optical materials.[158]

17.5 CONCLUSIONS

The discussions in this chapter show that through grafting, one may implement a beautiful level of control of both structure and function of cellulosic materials. In this chapter, I have sketched different mechanistic approaches for grafting by chemical method, radiation technique, photochemical, and enzymatic techniques. Apart from the conventional grafting process, living radical polymerization and ROP are also focused. Different factors that control grafting, like the nature of the backbone, initiator, and monomer, have also been discussed. Application of the grafted cellulosic materials in heavy metal adsorption, as hydrogels, UV-curable coatings, and membranes, is also discussed.

ACKNOWLEDGMENTS

The author acknowledges his wife Puspa, daughter Adyasha, and son Anshuman for their constant inspiration to complete this work.

REFERENCES

1. Okieimen, E. F. and Ebhoaye, J. E. 1986. Grafting acrylic acid monomer on cellulosic materials. *J Macromol Chem A* 23: 349–353.
2. Tosh, B. and Routray, C. R. 2011. Homogeneous grafting of MMA onto cellulose in presence of Ce^{+4} initiator. *Indian J Chem Technol* 18: 234–243.
3. Routray, C. R. and Tosh, B. 2012. Controlled grafting of MMA onto cellulose and cellulose acetate. *Cellulose* 19: 2115–2139.
4. Tosh, B. and Routray, C. R. 2012. Study of the effect of solvent and initiator on grafting parameters during homogeneous grafting of methyl methacrylate onto cellulose. *Chem Sci Rev Lett* 1(3): 120–132.
5. Routray, C. R. and Tosh, B. 2013. Graft copolymerization of methyl methacrylate (MMA) onto cellulose acetate in homogeneous medium; effect of solvent, initiator and homopolymer inhibitor. *Cellulose Chem Technol* 47(3–4): 171–190.
6. Routray, C. R.; Tosh, B.; and Nayak, N. 2013. Grafting of polymethyl methacrylate onto cellulose acetate in homogeneous medium using ceric(IV) ion as initiator. *Indian J Chem Technol* 20(3): 202–209.
7. Tosh, B. and Routray, C. R. 2013. Graft copolymerization of methyl methacrylate onto cellulose in homogeneous medium—Effect of solvent and initiator. *Int J Chem Sci Eng* 7(1): 1253–1260.
8. Bicak, N.; Sherrington, D. C.; and Senkal, B. F. 1999. Graft copolymer of acrylamide onto cellulose as mercury selective sorbent. *Reactive Funct Polym* 41: 69–76.
9. Ibrahim, M. M.; Flefel, E. M.; and El-Zawawy, W. K. 2002. Cellulose membranes grafted with vinyl monomers in homogeneous system. *J Appl Polym Sci* 84: 2629–2638.
10. Gupta, K. C. and Sahoo, S. 2001. Co(III) acetylacetonate-complex-initiated grafting of *N*-vinyl pyrrolidone on cellulose in aqueous media. *J Appl Polym Sci* 81: 2286–2296.
11. Sahoo, P. K.; Samantaray, H. S.; and Samal, R. K. 1986. Graft copolymerization with new class of acidic peroxo salts as initiators. I. Grafting of acrylamide onto cotton-cellulose using potassium monopersulfate, catalyzed by Co(II). *J Appl Polym Sci* 32: 5693–5703.
12. Yang, F.; Li, G.; He, Y. G.; Ren, F. X.; and Wang, J. X. 2009. Synthesis, characterization, and applied properties of carboxymethyl cellulose and polyacrylamide graft copolymer. *Carbohydr Polym* 78: 95–99.
13. Ouajai, S.; Hodzic, A.; and Shanks, R. A. 2004. Morphological and grafting modification of natural cellulose fibers. *J Appl Polym Sci* 94: 2456–2465.
14. Abdel-Razik, E. A. 1997. Aspects of thermal graft copolymerization of methyl methacrylate onto ethyl cellulose in homogeneous media. *Polym Plast Technol Eng* 36: 891–903.
15. Abdel-Razik, E. A. 1990. Homogeneous graft copolymerization of acrylamide onto ethylcellulose. *Polymer* 31: 1739–1744.
16. Ibrahim, M. D.; Mondal, H.; Uraki, Y.; Ubukata, M.; and Itoyama, K. 2008. Graft polymerization of vinyl monomers onto cotton fibres pretreated with amines. *Cellulose* 15: 581–592.
17. Liu, S. and Sun, G. 2008. Radical graft functional modification of cellulose with allyl monomers: Chemistry and structure characterization. *Carbohydr Polym* 71: 614–625.
18. Misra, B. N.; Dogra, R.; and Mehta, I. K. 1980. Grafting onto cellulose V. Effect of complexing agents on Fenton's reagent (Fe^{2+}–H_2O_2) initiated grafting of poly(ethyl acrylate). *J Polym Sci Polym Chem* 18: 749–752.
19. Huang, Y.; Zhao, B.; Zheng, C.; He, S.; and Gao, J. 1992. Graft copolymerization of methyl methacrylate on stone ground wood using the H_2O_2–Fe^{2+} method. *J Appl Polym Sci* 45: 71–77.
20. Sharma, B. R.; Kumar, V.; and Soni, P. L. 2003. Graft copolymerization of acrylonitrile onto *Cassia tora* gum with ceric ammonium nitrate-nitric acid as a redox initiator. *J Appl Polym Sci* 90: 129–136.
21. Dhiman, P. K.; Kaur, I.; and Mahajan, R. K. 2008. Synthesis of a cellulose-grafted polymeric support and its application in the reductions of some carbonyl compounds. *J Appl Polym Sci* 108: 99–111.
22. Fanta, G. F.; Burr, R. C.; and Doane, W. M. 1987. Graft polymerization of acrylonitrile onto wheat straw. *J Appl Polym Sci* 33: 899–906.
23. Kim, B. S. and Mun, S. P. 2009. Effect of Ce^{4+} pretreatment on swelling properties of cellulosic superabsorbents. *Polym Adv Technol* 20: 899–906.

24. Gurdag, G.; Guclu, G.; and Ozgumus, S. 2001. Graft copolymerization of acrylic acid onto cellulose: Effects of pretreatments and crosslinking agent. *J Appl Polym Sci* 80: 2267–2272.
25. Fernandez, M. J.; Casinos, I.; and Guzman, G. M. 1990. Grafting of a vinyl acetate/methyl acrylate mixture onto cellulose. Effect of temperature and nature of substrate. *Makromol Chem* 191: 1287–1299.
26. Gupta, K. C. and Khandekar, K. 2006. Ceric(IV) ion-induced graft copolymerization of acrylamide and ethyl acrylate onto cellulose. *Polym Int* 55: 139–150.
27. Moad, G. and Solomon, D. H. 1995. *The Chemistry of Free Radical Polymerization*. Oxford, U.K.: Pergamon.
28. Pepenzhik, M. A.; Virnik, A. D.; and Rogovin, Z. A. 1969. Synthesis of graft cellulose copolymers and calcium salt of poly(acrylic acid). *Vysokomol Soedin Ser B* 11: 245–250.
29. Misra, B. N.; Mehta, I. K.; and Khetrapal, R. C. 1984. Grafting onto cellulose VIII. Graft copolymerization of poly(ethyl acrylate) onto cellulose by use of redox initiators. Comparison of initiator reactivities. *J Polym Sci Polym Chem* 22: 2767–2775.
30. Prasanth, K. V. H. and Tharanathan, R. N. 2003. Studies on graft copolymerization of chitosan with synthetic monomers. *Carbohydr Polym* 54(3): 43–51.
31. Xie, W.; Xu, P.; Wang, W.; and Liu, Q. 2002. Preparation and antibacterial activity of a water-soluble chitosan derivative. *Carbohydr Polym* 50: 35–40.
32. Lin, M. S. and Chen, A. J. 1993. Preparation and characterization of water soluble and crosslinkable cellulose acrylate. *Polymer* 34(2): 389–393.
33. Roman-Aguirre, M.; Marquez-Lucero, A.; and Zaragoza-Contreras, E. A. 2004. Elucidating the graft copolymerization of methyl methacrylate onto wood-fiber. *Carbohydr Polym* 55: 201–210.
34. Wang, L.; Dong, W.; and Xu, Y. 2007. Synthesis and characterization of hydroxyl propyl methyl cellulose and ethyl acrylate graft copolymers. *Carbohydr Polym* 68: 626–636.
35. Sabaa, M. W. and Mokhtar, S. M. 2002. Chemically induced graft copolymerization of itaconic acid onto cellulose fibers. *Polym Testing* 21: 337–343.
36. Toledano-Thompsom, T.; Loria-Bastarrchea, M. I.; and Aguilar-Vega, M. J. 2005. Characterization of henequen cellulose microfibers treated with an epoxide and grafted with poly(acrylic acid). *Carbohydr Polym* 62: 67–73.
37. Misra, B. N. and Sood, D. S. 1981. Graft co-polymerization of vinyl monomers onto wool by use of TBHP-FAS system as redox initiators. In *Physiochemical Aspects of Polymer Surfaces*, K. L. Mittal (ed.), pp. 881–891. New York: Plenum Press.
38. Gupta, K. C.; Sahoo, S.; and Khandekar, K. 2002. Graft copolymerization of ethyl acrylate onto cellulose using ceric ammonium nitrate as initiator in aqueous medium. *Biomacromolecules* 2: 1087–1094.
39. Gupta, K. C. and Sahoo, S. 2001. Graft copolymerization of acrylonitrile and ethyl methacrylate comonomers on cellulose using ceric ions. *Biomacromolecules* 2: 239–247.
40. Gupta, K. C. and Khandekar, K. 2003. Temperature-responsive cellulose by ceric(IV) ion-initiated graft copolymerization of *N*-isopropyl acrylamide. *Biomacromolecules* 4: 758–765.
41. Egboh, S. H. O. and Akonwu, L. N. 1991. Graft polymerization of acrylamide onto cellulose acetate initiated by ceric ion. *Acta Polym.* 42(6): 279–281.
42. Chand, N.; Bajpai, S. K.; Joshi, R.; and Mary, G. 2010. Thermomechanical behavior of sisal fibers grafted with poly(acrylamide-*co*-*N*-vinyl-2-pyrrolidone) and loaded with silver ions or silver nanoparticles. *BioResources* 5(1): 372–388.
43. Khullar, R.; Varshney, V. K.; Naithani, S.; and Soni, P. L. 2008. Grafting of acrylonitrile onto cellulose material derived from bamboo (*Dendrocalamus strictus*). *eXPRESS Polym Lett* 2(1): 12–18.
44. Saikia, C. N. and Ali, F. 1999. Graft copolymerization of methyl methacrylate onto high α-cellulose pulp extracted from *Hibscus sabdariffa* and *Gmelina arborea*. *Bioresour Technol* 68: 165–171.
45. Zhang, J.; Yuan, Z.; Yuan, Y.; Shen, J.; and Lin, S. 2003. Chemical modification of cellulose membrane with sulfoammonium zwitterionic vinyl monomer to improve haemocompatibility. *Colloids Surf B: Biointerface* 30: 249–257.
46. Han, T. L.; Kumar, R. N.; Rozman, H. D.; and Md Noor, M. A. 2003. GMA grafted sago starch as a reactive component in ultraviolet radiation curable coatings. *Carbohydr Polym* 54(4): 509–516.
47. Zhang, J.; Youling, Y.; Kehua, W. K.; Shen, J.; and Lin, S. 2003. Surface modification of segmented poly(ether urethane) by grafting sulfoammonium zwitterionic monomer to improve haemocompatibilities. *Colloids Surf B: Biointerface* 30(3): 249–257.
48. Zhang, J.; Youling, Y.; Shen, J.; and Lin, S. 2003. Synthesis and characterization of chitosan grafted poly(*N*,*N*-dimethyl-*N*-methacryloxy ethyl-*N*-3-sulfopropyl ammonium) initiated by Ce(IV) ion. *Eur Polym J* 39(4): 847–850.

49. Nada, A. M. A.; Alkady, M. Y.; and Fekry, H. M. 2007. Synthesis and characterization of grafted cellulose for use in water and metal ion sorption. *BioResources* 3(1): 46–59.
50. Lin, O. H.; Kumar, R. N.; Rozman, H. D.; Azemi, M.; and Noor, M. 2005. Grafting of sodium carboxy methyl cellulose (CMC) with glycidyl methacrylate and development of UV curable coatings from CMC-*g*-GMA induced by cationic photoinitiators. *Carbohydr Polym* 59: 57–69.
51. Halab-Kessira, L. and Ricard, A. 1999. Use of trial and error method for the optimization of the graft copolymerization of cationic monomer onto cellulose. *Eur Polym J* 35: 1065–1071.
52. Moharana, S.; Mishra, S. B.; and Tripathy, S. S. 1991. Chemical modification of jute fibers. I. Permanganate-initiated graft copolymerization of methyl methacrylate onto jute fibers. *J Appl Polym Sci* 40(4/5): 345–357.
53. Sarbu, A.; de Pinho, M. V.; Freixo, M. R.; Goncalves, F.; and Udrea, I. 2006. New method for the covalent immobilization of a xylanase by radical grafting of acrylamide on cellulose acetate membranes. *Enzyme Microb Technol* 39: 125–130.
54. Chauhan, G. S. and Lal, H. 2003. Novel grafted cellulose-based hydrogels for water technologies. *Desalination* 159: 131–138.
55. Das, P. and Saikia, C. N. 2003. Homogeneous graft copolymerization of acrylonitrile onto high α-cellulose in a dimethyl acetamide and lithium chloride solvent system. *J Appl Polym Sci* 89: 630–637.
56. Bianchi, E.; Marsano, E.; Ricco, L.; and Russo, S. 1998. Free radical grafting onto cellulose in homogeneous conditions 1. Modified cellulose-acrylonitrile system. *Carbohydr Polym* 36: 313–318.
57. Bianchi, E.; Bonazza, A.; Marsano, E.; and Russo, S. 2000. Free radical grafting onto cellulose in homogeneous conditions 2. Modified cellulose-methyl methacrylate system. *Carbohydr Polym* 41: 47–53.
58. Yun, Y.; Zhang, J.; Di, F.; Yuan, J.; Zhou, J.; Shen, J.; and Lin, S. 2003. Surface modification of SPEU films by ozone induced graft copolymerization to improve haemocompatibility. *Colloids Surf B: Biointerface* 29(4): 247–256.
59. Karlsson, J. O. and Gatenholm, P. 1999. Cellulose fibre-supported pH-sensitive hydrogels. *Polymer* 40: 379–387.
60. Karlsson, J. O.; Henriksson, A.; Michalek, J.; and Gatenholm, P. 2000. Control of cellulose-supported hydrogel microstructures by three-dimensional graft polymerization of glycol methacrylate. *Polymer* 41: 1551–1559.
61. Videki, B.; Klebert, S.; and Pukanszky, B. 2005. Grafting of caprolactone to cellulose acetate by reactive processing. *Eur Polym J* 41: 1699–1707.
62. Szamel, G.; Domjan, A.; Klebert, S.; and Pukanszky, B. 2008. Molecular structure and properties of cellulose acetate chemically modified with caprolactone. *Eur Polym J* 44: 357–365.
63. Stridsberg, K. M.; Ryner, M.; and Albertsson, A. 2000. Controlled ring-opening polymerization: Polymers with designed macromolecular architecture. *Adv Polym Sci* 157: 41–65.
64. Szware, M. 1998. Living polymers. Their discovery, characterization and properties. *J Polym Sci Part A: Polym Chem* 36: IX–XV.
65. Russel, K. E. 2002. Free radical graft polymerization and copolymerization at high temperatures. *Prog Polym Sci* 27: 1007–1038.
66. Stehling, U. M.; Malmstrom, E. E.; Waymouth, R. M., and Hawker, C. J. 1998. Synthesis of poly(olefin) graft copolymers by a combination of metallocene and living free radical polymerization techniques. *Macromolecules* 31: 4396–4398.
67. Percea, V. and Barboiu, B. 1995. 'Living' radical polymerization of styrene initiated by arenesulfonyl chloride and $CuI(bpy)_nCl$. *Macromolecules* 28: 7970–7972.
68. Wang, J. S. and Matyjaszewski, K. 1995. Controlled 'living' radical polymerization. Atom transfer radical polymerization in the presence of transition metal complexes. *J Am Chem Soc* 117: 5614–5615.
69. Matyjaszewski, K. and Xia, J. 2001. Atom transfer radical polymerization. *Chem Rev* 101: 2921–2990.
70. Matyjaszewski, K. 1999. Transition metal catalysis in controlled radical polymerization: Atom transfer radical polymerization. *Chem Eur J* 5: 3095–3102.
71. Coessens, V.; Pintauer, T.; and Matyjaszewski, K. 2001. Functional polymers by atom transfer radical polymerization. *Prog Polym Sci* 26: 337–377.
72. Kato, M.; Kamigaito, M.; Sawamoto, M.; and Higashimura, T. 1995. Polymerization of methyl methacrylate with the carbon tetrachloride/dichloro tris (triphenylphosphine) ruthenium (II)/methyl aluminum bis(2,6-di-tert-butyl phenoxide) initiating system: Possibility of living radical polymerization. *Macromolecules* 28: 1721–1723.

73. Cai, X. L.; Riedl, B.; and Bouaziz, M. 2005. Lignocellulosic composites with grafted polystyrene interfaces. *Compos Interface* 12: 25–39.
74. Bledzki, A. K. and Gassan, J. 1999. Composites reinforced with cellulose based fibres. *Prog Polym Sci* 24(2): 221–274.
75. Calmark, A. and Malmstrom, E. 2002. Atom transfer radical polymerization from cellulose fibers at ambient temperature. *J Am Chem Soc* 124: 900–901.
76. Calmark, A. and Malmstrom, E. E. 2003. ATRP grafting from cellulose fibers to create block-copolymer grafts. *Biomacromolecules* 4(6): 1740–1745.
77. Coskun, M. and Temuz, M. M. 2005. Grafting studies onto cellulose by atom-transfer radical polymerization. *Polym Int* 54(2): 342–347.
78. Vleck, P.; Janata, M.; Latalova, P.; Kriz, J.; Cadova, E.; and Toman, L. 2006. Controlled grafting of cellulose diacetate. *Polymer* 47: 2587–2595.
79. Billy, M; Ranzani Da Costa, A.; Lochon, P.; Clement, R.; Dresch, M.; Etienne, S.; Hiver, J. M.; David, L.; and Johquieres, A. 2010. Cellulose acetate graft copolymers with nano-structured architectures: Synthesis and characterization. *Eur Polym J* 46: 944–957.
80. Yang, R.; Wang, Y.; and Zhou, D. 2007. Novel hydroxyethyl cellulose-*graft*-poly acrylamide copolymer for separation of double-stranded DNA fragments by CE. *Electrophoresis* 28: 3223–3231.
81. Yan, L. F. and Tao, W. 2008. Graft copolymerization of *N,N*-dimethyl acrylamide to cellulose in homogeneous media using atom transfer radical polymerization for haemocompatibility. *J Biomed Sci Eng* 1: 37–43.
82. Roy, D.; Guthrei, J. T.; and Perrier, S. 2005. Graft polymerization: Grafting poly(styrene) from cellulose via reversible addition-fragmentation chain transfer (RAFT) polymerization. *Macromolecules* 38: 10363–10372.
83. Roy, D.; Knapp, J. S.; Guthrie, J. T.; and Perrier, S. 2008. Antibacterial cellulose fiber via RAFT surface graft polymerization. *Biomacromolecules* 9: 91–99.
84. Chen, J.; Yi, J.; Sun, P.; Liu, Z. -T.; and Liu, Z. -W. 2009. Grafting from ramie fiber with poly(MMA) or poly(MA) via reversible addition-fragmentation chain transfer polymerization. *Cellulose* 16: 1133–1145.
85. Jeroma, C. and Lecomte, P. 2008. Recent advances in the synthesis of aliphatic polyesters by ring-opening polymerization. *Adv Drug Deliv Rev* 60(9): 1056–1076.
86. Teramoto, Y.; Ama, S.; Higeshiro, T.; and Nishio, Y. 2004. Cellulose acetate-*graft*-poly(hydroxyl alkanoates): Synthesis and dependence of the thermal properties on copolymer composition. *Macromol Chem Phys* 205: 1904–1915.
87. Lonnberg, H.; Fogelstrom, L.; Berglund, M. A. S. A. S. L.; Malmstrom, E.; and Hult, A. 2008. Surface grafting of microfibrillated cellulose with poly(ε-caprolactone)—Synthesis and characterization. *Eur Polym J* 44: 2991–2997.
88. Bhattacharya, A.; Das, A.; and De, A. 1998. Structural influence on grafting of acrylamide based monomers on cellulose acetate. *Indian J Chem Technol* 5: 135–138.
89. Garnett, J. L.; Ng, L.-T.; Viengkhou, V.; Hennessy, I. W.; and Zilic, E. F. 2000. Significance of grafting in curing process initiated by UV, excimer and ionizing radiation sources. *Radiat Phys Chem* 57: 355–359.
90. Jianqin, L.; Maolin, Z.; and Hongfei, H.1999. Pre-irradiation grafting of temperature sensitive hydrogel on cotton cellulose fabric. *Radiat Phys Chem* 55: 55–59.
91. Mazzei, R. O.; Smolko, E.; Torres, A.; Tadey, D.; Rocco, C.; Gizzi, L.; and Strangis, S. 2002. Radiation grafting studies of acrylic acid onto cellulose triacetate membranes. *Radiat Phys Chem* 64: 149–160.
92. Yamagashi, H.; Saito, K.; and Furusaki, S. 1990. Permeability of methyl methacrylate grafted cellulose triacetate membrane. *Chem Mater* 2: 705–708.
93. Kaur, I.; Misra, B. N.; Barsola, R.; and Singla, K. 1993. Viscometric studies of starch-*g*-polyacrylamide composites. *J Appl Polym Sci* 47: 1165–1174.
94. Basu, S.; Bhattacharya, A.; Mondal, P. C.; and Bhattacharyya, S. N. 1994. Spectroscopic evidence for grafting of *N*-vinyl carbazole on cellulose acetate film. *J Polym Sci, Polym Chem* 32: 2251–2255.
95. Aich, S.; Bhattacharya, A.; and Basu, S. 1997. Fluorescence polarization of *N*-vinyl carbazole on cellulose acetate film and electron transfer with 1,4-dicyanobenzene. *Radiat Phys Chem* 50(4): 347–354.
96. Aich, S.; Sengupta, T.; Bhattacharya, A., and Basu, S. 1999. Magnetic field effect on an exciplex between *N*-vinyl carbazole grafted on cellulose acetate film and 1,4-dicyanobenzene. *J Polym Sci, Polym Chem* 37: 3910–3915.

97. Badway, S. M.; Dessouki, A. M.; and El-Din H. M. N. 2001. Direct pyrolysis mass spectroscopy of acrylonitrile-cellulose graft copolymer prepared by radiation-induced graft polymerization in presence of styrene as homopolymer suppresser. *Radiat Phys Chem* 61: 143–148.
98. Hassanpour, S. 1999. Radiation grafting of styrene and acrylonitrile to cellulose and polyethylene. *Radiat Phys Chem* 55: 41–45.
99. Feng, H.; Li, J.; and Wang, L. 2010. Preparation of biodegradable flax shive cellulose-based super absorbent polymer under microwave irradiation. *BioResources* 5(3): 1484–1495.
100. Wan, Z.; Xiong, Z.; Ren, H.; Huang, Y.; Liu, H.; Xiong, H.; Wu, Y.; and Han, J. 2011. Graft copolymerization of methyl methacrylate onto bamboo cellulose under microwave irradiation. *Carbohydr Polym* 83: 264–269.
101. Kubota, H.; Suka, I. G.; Kuroda, S.; and Kondo, T. 2001. Introduction of stimuli-responsive polymers into regenerated film by means of photografting. *Eur Polym J* 37: 1367–1372.
102. Rajam, S. and Ho, C.-C. 2006. Graft coupling of PEO to mixed cellulose esters microfiltration membranes by UV radiation. *J Membr Sci* 281: 211–218.
103. Princi, E.; Vicini, S.; Proietti, N.; and Capitani, D. 2005. Grafting polymerization on cellulose based textiles: A ^{13}C solid state NMR characterization. *Eur Polym J* 41: 1196–1203.
104. Princi, E.; Vicini, S.; Pedemonte, E.; Mulas, A.; Franceschi, E.; Luciano, G.; and Trefiletti, V. 2005. Thermal analysis and characterization of cellulose grafted with acrylic monomers. *Thermochim Acta* 425: 173–179.
105. Li, J.; Xie, W.; Cheng, H. N.; Nickol, R. G.; and Wang, P. G. 1999. Polycaprolactone-modified hydroxyl ethyl cellulose films prepared by lipase-catalyzed ring-opening polymerization. *Macromolecules* 32(8): 2789–2792.
106. Gustavsson Malin, T.; Persson Per, V.; Iversen, T.; Hult, K.; and Martinelle, M. 2004. Polyester coating of cellulose fiber surfaces catalyzed by a cellulose-binding module—*Candida antarctica* lipase B fusion protein. *Biomacromolecules* 5(1): 106–112.
107. Ibrahem, A. A. and Nada, A. M. A. 1985. Grafting of acrylamide onto cotton linters. *Acta Polym* 36(6): 320–322.
108. Tyuganova, M. A.; Galbraikh, L. S.; Ulmasove, A. A.; Tsarevskaya, I. Y.; and Khidoyator, A. A. 1985. Use of rice straw as cellulosic raw material for ion exchanger production. *Cell Chem Technol* 19(5): 557–568.
109. Kokta, B. V.; Valade, J. L.; and Daneault, C. 1981. Modification of mechanical and thermomechanical pulps by grafting with synthetic polymers. II. Effect of ozonation on polymerization parameters and pulp properties. *Transactions* 7: TR5–TR10.
110. Hornof, V.; Kokta, B. V.; and Valade, J. L. 1976. The xanthate method of grafting. IV. Grafting of acrylonitrile onto high yield pulp. *J Appl Polym Sci* 20: 1543–1554.
111. Nakamura, S.; Yoshikawa, E.; and Matsuzuki, K. 1980. Graft copolymerization of styrene onto cellulose acetate *p*-nitrobenzoate by chain transfer reaction. *J Appl Polym Sci* 25: 1833–1837.
112. Okieima, E. F. and Idehem, I. K. 1987. Graft copolymerization of acrylonitrile, methyl methacrylate and vinyl acetate on bleached holocellulose by use of ceric ion. *J Macromol Sci Chem A* 24(11): 1381–1391.
113. Misra, B. N.; Sharma, R. K.; and Mehta, I. K. 1982. Grafting onto wool. XV. Graft copolymerization of MA and MMA by use of $Mn(acac)_3$ as initiator. *J Macromol Sci Chem A* 17(3): 489–500.
114. Nagaty, A.; Abd-El-Mouti, F.; and Mansour, O. Y. 1980. Graft polymerization of vinyl monomers onto starch by use of tetravalent cerium. *Eur Polym J* 16: 343–346.
115. Bhattacharyya, S. N. and Maldas, D. 1982. Radiation induced graft copolymerization of mixtures of styrene and acrylamide onto cellulose acetate. I. Effect of solvents. *J Polym Sci Polym Chem* 20: 939–950.
116. Yasukawa, T.; Sasaki, Y.; and Marukami, K. 1973. Kinetics of radiation induced grafting reaction. II. Cellulose acetate-styrene system. *J Polym Sci Polym Chem* 11(10): 2547–2556.
117. Dilli, S. and Garnett, J. L. 1967. Radiation induced reactions with cellulose. III. Kinetics of styrene copolymerization in methanol. *J Appl Polym Sci* 11(6): 859–870.
118. Tosh, B.; Saikia, C. N.; and Dass, N. N. 2000. Homogeneous esterification of cellulose in the lithium chloride-*N*,*N*-dimethylacetamide solvent system: Effect of temperature and catalyst. *Carbohydr Res* 327: 345–352.
119. Tosh, B. 1999. Studies on the kinetics of homogeneous esterification of prepolymers like fractionated cellulose and polyvinyl alcohol of different molecular weights. PhD thesis, Dibrugarh University, Assam, India.
120. Gupta, K. C. and Khandekar, K. 2002. Graft copolymerization of acrylamide-methylacrylate comonomers onto cellulose using ceric ammonium nitrate. *J Appl Polym Sci* 86: 2631–2642.

121. Goyal, P.; Kumar, V.; and Sharma, P. 2008. Graft copolymerization of acrylamide onto tamarind kernel powder in the presence of ceric ion. *J Appl Polym Sci* 108: 3696–3701.
122. Nishioka, N.; Minami, K.; and Kosai, K. 1983. Homogeneous graft copolymerization of vinyl monomers onto cellulose in a dimethyl sulfoxide-paraformaldehyde solvent system III. Methyl acrylate. *Polym J* 15: 591–596.
123. Nishioka, N.; Matsumoto, K., and Kosai, K. 1983. Homogeneous graft copolymerization of vinyl monomers onto cellulose in a dimethyl sulfoxide-paraformaldehyde solvent system II. Characterization of graft copolymers. *Polym J* 15: 153–158.
124. Nishioka, N. and Kosai, K. 1981. Homogeneous graft copolymerization of vinyl monomers onto cellulose in a dimethyl sulfoxide-paraformaldehyde solvent system I. Acrylonitrile and methyl methacrylate. *Polym J* 13: 1125–1133.
125. Nishioka, N.; Matsumoto, Y.; Yumen, T.; Monmae, K.; and Kosai, K. 1986. Homogeneous graft copolymerization of vinyl monomers onto cellulose in a dimethyl sulfoxide-paraformaldehyde solvent system IV. 2-hydroxyethyl methacrylate. *Polym J* 18: 323–330.
126. Zaharan, A. H. and Zhoby, M. H. 1986. Effect of radiation chemical treatment on sisal fibers. I. Radiation induced grafting of ethyl acrylate. *J Appl Polym Sci* 31: 1925–1934.
127. Misra, B. N.; Chauhan, G. S.; and Rawat, B. R. 1991. Grafting onto wool. XXVIII. Effects of acids on gamma radiation induced graft copolymerization of methyl methacrylate onto wool fiber. *J Appl Polym Sci* 42: 3223–3227.
128. Misra, B. N.; Mehta, I. K.; Rathore, M. P. S.; and Lakhanpal, S. 1993. Effect of L(–) threonine, 5-hydroxy tryptophan and 5-hydroxy tryptamine on the ceric-ion-initiated grafting of methyl acrylate onto cellulose. *J Appl Polym Sci* 49: 1979–1984.
129. Misra, B. N. and Chandel, P. S. 1980. Grafting onto wool. IV. Effect of amines upon ceric ion-initiated grafting of poly(methyl methacrylate). *J Polym Sci Polym Chem* 18: 1171–1176.
130. Misra, B. N. and Mehta, I. K. 1980. Grafting onto wool. Graft copolymerization of methyl methacrylate (MMA) by use of Ce^{4+}-amine system as redox initiator. *J Polym Sci Polym Chem* 18: 1911–1918.
131. Fernandez, H. J.; Casino, I.; and Guzman, G. M. 1991. Grafting of vinyl acetate-methyl acrylate mixture onto cellulose. Effects of inorganic salts. *J Appl Polym Sci* 42: 767–778.
132. Gurdag, G.; Yasar, M.; and Gurkaynak, M. A. 1997. Graft copolymerization of acrylic acid on cellulose: Reaction kinetics of copolymerization. *J Appl Polym Sci* 66: 929–934.
133. O'Connell, D. W.; Birkinshaw, C.; and O'Dwyer, T. F. 2008. Heavy metal adsorbents prepared from the modification of cellulose: A review. *Bioresour Technol* 99(15): 6709–6724.
134. Kubota, H. and Suzuki, S. 1995. Comparative examinations of reactivity of grafted celluloses prepared by ultra violet and ceric salt-initiated grafting. *Eur Polym J* 31(8): 701–704.
135. Bao-Xiu, Z.; Peng, W.; Tong, Z.; Chun-yun, C.; and Jing, S. 2006. Preparation and adsorption performance of a cellulose adsorbent resin for copper(II). *J Appl Polym Sci* 99: 2951–2956.
136. Abdel-Aal, S. E.; Gad, Y.; and Sessouki, A. M. 2006. The use of wood pulp and radiation modified starch in waste water treatment. *J Appl Polym Sci* 99: 2460–2469.
137. Raji, C. and Anirudhan, T. S. 1998. Batch Cr(IV) removal by polyacrylamide grafted sawdust: Kinetics and thermodynamics. *Water Res* 32(12): 3772–3780.
138. Shibi, I. G. and Anirudhan, T. S. 2002. Synthesis, characterization, and application as a mercury(II) sorbent of banana stalk-polyacrylamide grafted co-polymer bearing carboxylic groups. *Ind Eng Chem* Res 41: 5341–5352.
139. Hashem, A. 2006. Amidoximated sunflower stalks (ASFS) as a new adsorbent for removal of Cu(II) from aqueous solution. *Polym Plastics Technol Eng* 45: 35–42.
140. Liu, M.; Deng, Y.; Zhan, H.; and Zhang, X. 2002. Adsorption and desorption of copper (II) from solutions on new spherical cellulose adsorbent. *J Appl Polym Sci* 84: 478–485.
141. Liu, M.; Deng, Y.; Zhan, H.; Zhang, X.; Liu, W.; and Zhan, H. 2001. Removal and recovery of chromium(III) from aqueous solutions by spheroidal cellulose adsorbent. *Water Environ Res* 73(3): 322–328.
142. Guclu, G.; Gurdag, G.; and Ozgumus, S. 2003. Competitive removal of heavy metal ions by cellulose graft copolymers. *J Appl Polym Sci* 90: 2034–2039.
143. Gaey, M.; Marchetti, V.; Clement, A.; Loubinoux, B.; and Gerardin, P. 2000. Decontamination of synthetic solutions containing heavy metals using chemically modified sawdust bearing polyacrylic acid chains. *J Wood Sci* 46: 331–333.
144. Lin, C. X.; Zhan, H. U.; Liu, M. H.; Fu, S. U.; and Huang, L. H. 2010. Rapid homogeneous preparation of cellulose graft copolymer in BMIMCL under microwave irradiation. *J Appl Polym Sci* 118: 399–404.

145. Cavus, S.; Gurdag, G.; Yasar, M.; Guclu, K.; and Gurkaynak, M. A. 2006. The competitive heavy metal removal by hydroxyethyl cellulose-*g*-poly(acrylic acid) copolymer and its sodium salt: The effect of copper content on the adsorption capacity. *Polym Bull* 57: 445–456.
146. Wen, O. H.; Kuroda, S. I.; and Kubota, H. 2001. Temperature-responsive character of acrylic acid and *N*-isopropylacrylamide binary monomers-grafted celluloses. *Eur Polym J* 37: 807–813.
147. O'Connell, D. W.; Birkinshaw, C.; and O'Dwyer, T. F. 2006. A modified cellulose adsorbent for the removal of nickel(II) from aqueous solutions. *J Chem Technol Biotechnol* 81: 1820–1828.
148. Xie, J. and Hsieh, Y. L. 2003. Thermosensitive poly(*n*-isopropylacrylamide) hydrogels bonded on cellulose supports. *J Appl Polym Sci* 89: 999–1006.
149. Ifuku, S. and Kadla, J. 2008. Preparation of a thermosensitive highly regioselective cellulose/*n*-isopropylacrylamide copolymer through atom transfer radical polymerization. *Biomacromolecules* 9: 3308–3313.
150. Esen, E.; Ozbas, Z.; Kasgoz, H.; and Gurdag, G. 2011. Thermoresponsive cellulose-*g*-*N,N'*-diethyl acrylamide copolymers. *Curr Opin Biotechnol* 22(1): S61–S62.
151. Csoka, G.; Marton, S.; Gelencser, A.; and Klebovich, I. 2005. Thermoresponsive properties of different cellulose derivatives. *Eur J Pharm Sci* 25: S74–S75.
152. Bokias, G.; Mylonas, Y.; Staikos, G.; Bumbu, G. G.; and Vasile, C. 2001. Synthesis and aqueous solution properties of novel thermoresponsive graft copolymers based on a carboxymethylcellulose backbone. *Macromolecules* 34: 4958–4964.
153. Li, Y. X.; Liu, R. G.; Liu, W. Y.; Kang, H. L.; Wu, M.; and Huang, Y. 2008. Synthesis, self-assembly, and thermosensitive properties of ethyl cellulose-*g*-p(PEGMA) amphiphilic copolymers. *J Polym Sci Part A: Polym Chem* 46: 6907–6915.
154. Wang, D.; Tan, J.; Kang, H.; Ma, L.; Jin, X.; Liu, R.; and Huang, Y. 2011. Synthesis, self-assembly and drug release behaviors of pH-responsive copolymers ethyl cellulose-*graft*-PDEAEMA through ATRP. *Carbohydr Polym* 84: 195–202.
155. Kumar, R. N.; Po, P. L.; and Rozman, H. D. 2006. Studies on the synthesis of acrylamidomethyl cellulose ester and its application in UV curable surface coatings induced by free radical photoinitiator. Part 1: Acrylamidomethyl cellulose acetate. *Carbohydr Polym* 64: 112–126.
156. Edgar, K. J.; Buchanan, C. M.; Debenham, J. S.; Randquist, P. A.; Seiler, B. D.; Shelton, M. C.; and Tindall, D. 2001. Advances in cellulose ester performance and application. *Prog Polym Sci* 26: 1605–1688.
157. Matahwa, H.; Ramiah, V.; Jarrett, W. L.; McLeary, J. B.; and Sanderson, R. D. 2007. Microwave assisted graft copolymerization of *n*-isopropyl acrylamide and methyl acrylate on cellulose: solid state NMR analysis and $CaCO_3$ crystallization. *Macromol Symp* 255: 50–56.
158. Tang, X.; Gao, L.; Fan, X.; and Zhou, Q. 2007. Controlled grafting of ethyl cellulose with azobenzene-containing polymethacrylates via atom transfer radical polymerization. *J Polym Sci, Part A Polym Chem* 45: 1653–1660.

18 Preparation, Self-Assembly, and Application of Amphiphilic Cellulose-Based Graft Copolymers

Xiaohui Wang, Yanzhu Guo, Haoquan Zhong, Meiwan Chen, and Runcang Sun

CONTENTS

18.1 INTRODUCTION

In recent years, the self-assembled nanomicelles of amphiphilic cellulose-based graft copolymers have emerged as a new generation of value-added functional nanostructures (Li et al. 2008, Yan et al. 2009a). The amphiphilic cellulose micelles were found able to solubilize and encapsulate poorly soluble drugs and functional materials for improved applications in versatile fields including drug delivery, bioimaging, sensing, and catalysis. Compared with the synthetic amphiphilic block copolymers, the cellulose-based graft copolymer amphiphiles have many promising properties, for example, renewability, good biocompatibility, biodegradability, nontoxicity, and non-immunogenicity (Hassani et al. 2012). As the most abundant biomass in nature, cellulose is especially advantageous due to its large availability and low price.

To date, many amphiphilic cellulose-based graft copolymers and their self-assembled nanomicelles have been developed. These amphiphilic celluloses can be prepared by grafting hydrophobic side chains (e.g., long-chain alkyl or ester segments) onto the backbone of cellulose's water-soluble derivatives (e.g., hydroxypropyl cellulose (HPC), hydroxyethyl cellulose (HEC), cellulose sulfate (CS), carboxymethyl cellulose (CMC), cellulose acetate, and cationic cellulose) (Landoll 1982b, Charpentier et al. 1997, Taylor and Nasr-El-Din 1998, Shi and Burt 2003, Sroková et al. 2004, Kang et al. 2006, 2008, Wei and Cheng 2007, Li et al. 2008, Yang et al. 2008b, Berthier et al. 2011, Jiang et al. 2011, Song et al. 2011b). In another way, the amphiphilic cellulose derivatives can also be synthesized by grafting hydrophilic segments (e.g., poly(poly(ethylene glycol), poly(2-hydroxyethyl methacrylate) (PHEMA), poly(acrylic acid) (PAA), and methyl ether methacrylate) onto the organosoluble cellulose derivatives, for example, ethyl cellulose (EC; Kang et al. 2006, 2008). Many techniques, such as ring-opening polymerization (ROP) (Habibi and Dufresne 2008, Lonnberg et al. 2008, Labet and Thielemans 2011), atom transfer radical polymerization (ATRP) (Carlmark and Malmström 2003), reversible addition–fragmentation chain transfer (RAFT) polymerization (Liu et al. 2010), and click chemistry (Krouit et al. 2008), have been applied to cellulose modification. More and more new structures of amphiphilic cellulose graft copolymers are being reported in the recent a few years.

In this chapter, the latest progress on the synthesis, self-assembly of amphiphilic cellulose-based graft copolymers, and their cutting-edge applications will be reviewed. The scientific mechanisms behind the molecular self-assembly of amphiphilic cellulose graft copolymers will be discussed.

18.2 AMPHIPHILIC COPOLYMERS

18.2.1 General Information of Amphiphilic Copolymers

Amphiphilic copolymers refer to those compounds composed of two or more types of monomers that contain both hydrophilic and hydrophobic segments. Most of amphiphilic copolymers have linear chains, and random or ordered mixture of different monomers. Amphiphilic polymer can be broadly classified into block, random, star, graft polymers, etc. (Figure 18.1) (Alexandridis 1996). Block copolymers comprise two or more distinct blocks linked by covalent bonds. Graft copolymers are constituted by the main chain of one polymer with covalently bonded side chains of another polymer. And star polymers consist of several linear polymer chains connected at one point. Random copolymers refer to a special type of copolymer in which the probability of finding a special monomer residue at a particular point in the chain is equal to the mole fraction of that monomer residue in the chain.

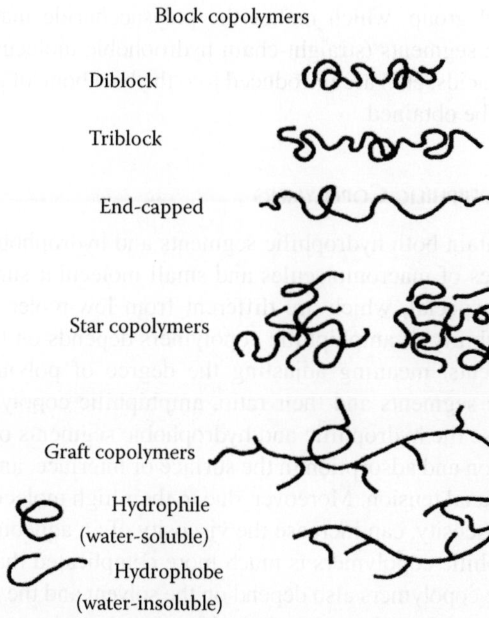

FIGURE 18.1 Schematic of various copolymer architectures that could lead to macromolecules exhibiting amphiphilic nature. (From Alexandridis, P., *Curr. Opin. Colloid Interface Sci.*, 1, 490, 1996.)

Over the past decades, natural amphiphilic polymers have been developed to combine the features of natural productions and the special functions of amphiphilic polymers. Compared to synthetic polymers, natural amphiphilic polymer materials have the favor of good biocompatibility and biodegradability, which make them have an extremely wide range of applications in the field of biomedicine, biological imaging, and biological materials (Alexandridis 1996). Currently, researches on natural amphiphilic polymer are focusing on natural polysaccharides, including chitosan, cellulose, starch, dextran, cyclodextrin, and sodium alginate (Lapasin and Pricl 1995, He and Zhao 2005). As shown in Table 18.1, most polysaccharides contain a large amount of hydrophilic

TABLE 18.1
Polysaccharides Commonly Used in the Preparation of Amphiphiles

Polysaccharide	Functional Groups
Chitosan	$-NH_3^+$, –OH
Starch	–OH
Alginate	–OH, –COO–
Hyaluronic acid	–OH, –COO–
Heparin	–OH, $-OSO_3-$
Chondroitin sulfate	–OH, –COO–, $-OSO_3-$
Pectin	–OH, –COO–
Pullulan	–OH
Amylose	–OH
Cyclodextrins	–OH
Dextran	–OH

hydroxyl, amino, or carboxyl group, which makes the polysaccharide main chains hydrophilic. Therefore, if the hydrophobic segments (straight-chain hydrophobic molecules, small hydrophobic molecules, cyclic polyacrylic acids, etc.) are introduced into the backbone of polysaccharide, natural amphiphilic polymers would be obtained.

18.2.2 Properties of Amphiphilic Copolymers

Amphiphilic copolymers contain both hydrophilic segments and hydrophobic segments, thus they have the combined advantages of macromolecules and small molecular surfactants. Properties of amphiphilic copolymers are special, which are different from low-molecular-weight surfactants and ionic polymers. The solubility of amphiphilic copolymers depends on the ratio of hydrophilic segments/hydrophobic segments, meaning adjusting the degree of polymerization (DP) of the hydrophilic and hydrophobic segments and their ratio, amphiphilic copolymers can be dissolved both in water and oil. Because the hydrophilic and hydrophobic segments of amphiphilic polymer chain have a certain orientation and adsorption in the surface or interface, amphiphilic polymer can reduce the surface and interfacial tension. Moreover, due to their high molecular weight, their water solution, usually with high viscosity, can increase the viscosity of an aqueous system.

The dissolution of amphiphilic copolymers is much more complicated than other polymers. The dissolution properties of these copolymers also depend on the solvent and the structure of the copolymers. For example, in some low-polar solvents (such as chloroform), the hydrophobic segments would be extended, and the hydrophilic segments would be curly. On the contrary, in high-polar solvents, the hydrophilic segments would be extended, and the hydrophobic segments would be curly. Once placed in an aqueous environment, some amphiphilic copolymers can aggregate into spherical, core-shell-like nanoparticles above their critical micelle concentration (CMC). In this situation, the core is formed by the hydrophobic segments, while the shell is formed by the hydrophilic segments (Otsuka et al. 2001). However, the converse structure is formed in an organic solvent, called "reverse micelles."

18.2.3 Application of Amphiphilic Copolymers

Amphiphilic copolymers used for surfactant have attracted considerable attention because they can reduce the surface and interfacial tension. However, their ability to reduce the surface and interfacial tension is weaker than low-molecular-weight surfactants. Moreover, their surfactivity would reduce sharply with increasing molecular weight. Due to their high molecular weight, they have excellent film-forming resistance, adhesion, water retention, and foam-stabilizing effect. Comparing with the low molecular surfactants, the amphiphilic polymeric surfactants are advantageous at their significantly improved colloidal stability due to their low CMC.

In recent decades, the demand for amphiphilic copolymers for use in targeted drug delivery (Rösler et al. 2012), gene therapy, sensing, etc., has increased tremendously. In a selective solution, amphiphilic copolymers tend to self-assemble into micelles, with the hydrophobic core and hydrophilic shell. The hydrophobic core can serve as a nano-container of hydrophobic functional molecules, which was wrapped inside the core, to increase its solubility in aqueous solution, and meanwhile the hydrophilic shell can separate hydrophobic molecules from the external environment, to increase its stability in aqueous solution. What's more, targeting micelles, drug delivery system has been developed to decrease the side effect of drugs.

18.3 AMPHIPHILIC CELLULOSE

18.3.1 Cellulose

Cellulose is the most abundant organic polymer in the world, and it has been widely studied during the past decades because it is a biodegradable material and a renewable resource. This polymer

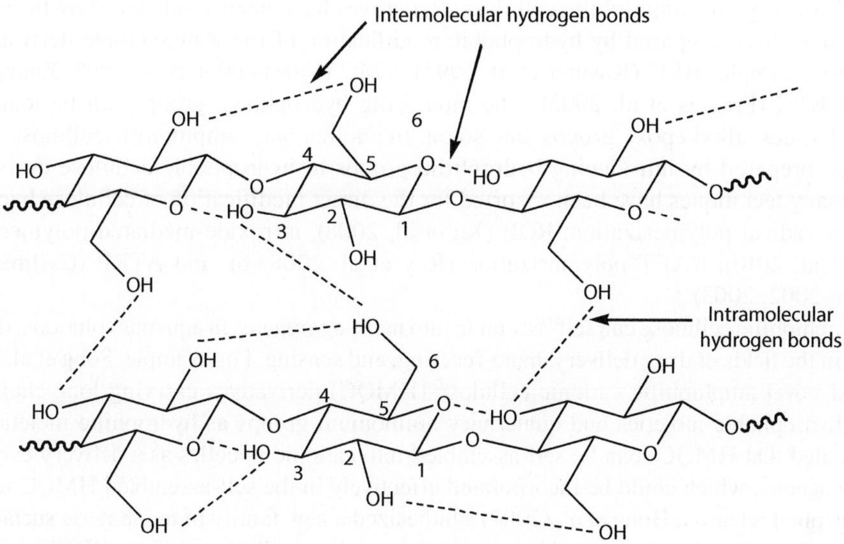

FIGURE 18.2 Inter- or intramolecular hydrogen bonds of cellulose.

makes up about 45% of the dry weight of wood, which is the main structural component of the primary cell walls of plants. Although wood pulp remains the most important raw material for cellulose, it can also be extracted from algae, bacteria, and annual crops.

Structurally, cellulose is composed of D-glucose subunits linked by β-1,4-glycosidic bonds. These long chains are bonded together by hydrogen bonds and van der Waals forces. As shown in Figure 18.1, these pyranose rings have been found to be in the chair conformation 4C1, with the hydroxyl groups in an equatorial position. Each glucose unit of cellulose contains three free alcoholic hydroxyl groups, successively linked in C2, C3, and C6 (O'Sullivan 1997). These groups form many intramolecular and intra-strand hydrogen bonds with –OH groups on adjacent chains, bundling the chains together (Figure 18.2). On the one hand, it endows cellulose high crystallinity, stable physical properties, and high glass transition temperature, thus cellulose is insoluble in water and most organic solvents, which limits the application of cellulose. In the past few decades, several new solvents have been reported to dissolve cellulose, such as 4-N methylmorpholine-oxide (NMMO), lithium chloride/dimethylacetamide (LiCI/DMAc), sodium hydroxide (NaOH)/urea, and ionic liquids.

Cellulose usually appears in hemi-crystalline form, in which a small percentage of nonorganized cellulose chains form amorphous cellulose. In crystalline form, all hydroxyl groups formed hydrogen bonds, and molecules are arranged neatly, resulting in high density. Several different crystalline structures of cellulose (I, II, III1, III11, IV1, and IV11) can be interconverted in the determined conditions. Among these crystalline structures, cellulose I is natural cellulose, which has been found to be a mixture of two polymorphs (Iα and Iβ), and the other crystalline structures are called "man-made" crystalline structures. For the cellulose in amorphous form, only a part of hydroxyl groups formed hydrogen bonds, and the density is lower.

18.3.2 Amphiphilic Cellulose

Amphiphilic cellulose is a kind of novel cellulose-based functional derivatives, which has special chemical structures composed of hydrophilic cellulose chains and hydrophobic segments (Yang et al. 2008a, Qiu and Hu 2013). Amphiphilic cellulose derivatives are mostly prepared by grafting modification, which show different structure with most block copolymer-based amphiphilic polymers. Basically, the amphiphilic cellulose derivatives have been synthesized by three ways. First, they have been prepared by hydrophobic modification of the water-soluble derivatives of cellulose, for example, HEC (Kästner et al. 1994), CMC (Charpentier et al. 1997, Zhang et al. 2000), and HPC (Francis et al. 2003). The modifying hydrophobic groups can be long-chain alkyl, acyl halides, alkyl epoxy groups, and so on. In another way, amphiphilic cellulose derivatives can be prepared by introducing hydrophilic groups to hydrophobic cellulose derivatives. Recently, many techniques have been reported for the direct modification of cellulose backbone, such as free radical polymerization, ROP (Xu et al. 2008), nitroxide-mediated polymerization (Tizzotti et al. 2010), RAFT polymerization (Roy et al. 2008a,b), and ATRP (Carlmark and Malmström 2002, 2003).

Since amphiphilic cellulose can self-assemble into nano-aggregates in aqueous solutions, they can be applied in the fields of drug delivery, nano-reacting, and sensing. For example, Song et al. (2011a) synthesized novel amphiphilic cationic cellulose (HMQC) derivatives carrying long-chain alkyl groups as hydrophobic moieties and quaternary ammonium groups as hydrophilic moieties. The results revealed that HMQCs can be self-assembled into cationic micelles as a delivery carrier for prednisone acetate, which could be incorporated effectively in the self-assembled HMQC micelles and be controlled released. Hong et al. (2007) synthesized a new family of amphoteric surfactant—2-hydroxy-3-(*N*,*N*-dimethyl-*N*-dodecyl-ammonium)-propyloxy cellulose sulfate (GDCS)—through etherification of CS. Rheological measurements of GDCS indicated that the solution first behaved like a pseudoplastic fluid, the apparent viscosity decreased sharply, and then exhibited a Newtonian property, and the apparent viscosity did not change obviously anymore. Moreover, amphiphilic cellulose can be used as an environmentally friendly nanosized reaction vessel for in situ synthesizing functional nanoparticles like nano-Ag, quantum dots (Dubertret et al. 2002), and nano-Fe_3O_4 (Liu et al. 2002, Lee et al. 2005).

18.4 SYNTHESIS AND CHARACTERIZATION OF AMPHIPHILIC CELLULOSE DERIVATIVES

Based on the properties of starting materials, amphiphilic cellulose derivatives have been synthesized by different pathways that can be generally classified into three major groups: (1) direct hydrophobic modification of cellulose main chain, (2) amphiphilic modification of cellulose water-soluble derivatives, and (3) amphiphilic graft copolymerization of the oil-soluble derivatives of cellulose. These amphiphilic modifications are based on one or more kinds of chemical reactions of hydroxyl groups, including the esterification or etherfication, the grafting copolymerization such as ATRP, and ROP.

18.4.1 Direct Amphiphilic Modification of Cellulose Main Chain

It was well known that there were three hydroxyl groups present in each glucose residue of cellulose. The hydroxyl groups at 2 and 3 positions behave as secondary alcohols, while the hydroxyl at the 6 position acts as a primary alcohol. Due to these abundant contents of hydrophilic hydroxyl groups, cellulose main chain presents hydrophilic nature. But it lacks hydrophobic segments to form amphiphilic structure. Thus, partial substitution of hydroxyl groups with hydrophobic chains would impart amphiphilic properties to cellulose.

18.4.1.1 Direct Amphiphilic Modification of Cellulose Main Chain in Heterogeneous System

It has been established that cellulose has crystalline structure and strong inter/intramolecular hydrogen bonds, which make it not soluble in water or common organic solvents, such as ethanol and acetone. So the direct amphiphilic modification of cellulose main chain was initially carried out in a heterogeneous system. The grafting of hydrophobic polymers, such as methyl acrylate (MA),

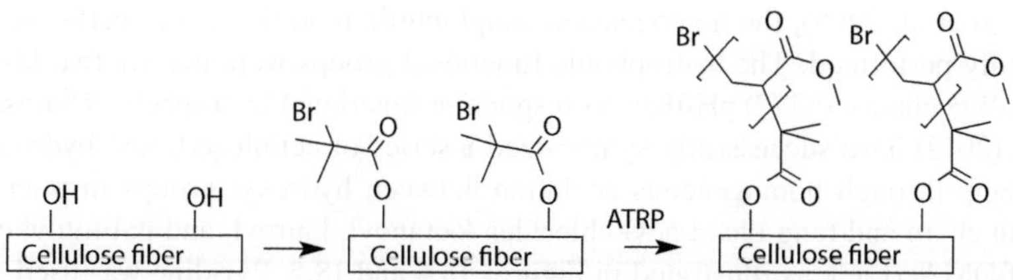

FIGURE 18.3 Synthetic pathway for the preparation of the PMA-grafted filter papers. (From Carlmark, A. and Malmström, E., *J. Am. Chem. Soc.*, 124, 900, 2002; Carlmark, A. and Malmström, E., *Biomacromolecules*, 4, 1740, 2003.)

methyl methacrylate, and 2-(dimethylamino) ethyl methacrylate (DMAEMA) greatly enhanced the hydrophobic property of cellulose fiber surfaces.

Carlmark and Malmström (2002, 2003) successfully grafted hydrophobic functional groups of poly(methyl acrylate) (PMA) onto the surface hydroxyl groups of filter paper fibers using ATRP method, mediated by tris(2-(dimethylamino)ethyl)amine (Me_6–TREN) and Cu(I)Br. The initiator was immobilized by reacting 2-bromoisobutyrylbromide with the hydroxyl groups, whereupon MA was grafted from the surface by immersing the initiator-modified paper into the reaction mixture containing MA, Cu(I)Br, Me_6–TREN, sacrificial initiator, and ethyl acetate. The synthetic pathway for the preparation of PMA-grafted filter papers was outlined in Figure 18.3.

The hydrophobic poly(methyl methacrylate) (PMMA) was also grafted onto surface of ramie fiber through ATRP by Liu et al. (2008b). The initiator was also immobilized by reacting 2-bromoisobutyrylbromide with the hydroxyl groups. The optimal reaction conditions for preparing the macroinitiated ramie fiber were determined to be at the temperature of 60°C and a reaction time of 24 h.

Lindqvist et al. (2008) obtained a novel thermo-responsive cellulose (filter paper) surfaces of *N*-isopropylacrylamide (NIPAAm) and pH-responsive cellulose surfaces of 4-vinylpyridine (4VP) through surface-initiated ATRP. To enable grafting via ATRP, the hydroxyl groups on the surface of filter paper were first esterified by the reaction with 2-chloropropionyl chloride to yield covalently linked ATRP initiators on the surface. Grafting of 4VP or NIPAAm was conducted by immersing the initiator-modified cellulose substrates into a reaction mixture containing monomer, copper salt, ligand, and solvent. Deactivating Cu(II)Cl_2 was added to achieve control over the reaction by efficient deactivation of the propagating radicals on the surface. The graft length was controlled by varying the reaction time. With changes in pH and temperature, the surfaces of filter paper fiber can be tailored from high hydrophilicity to high hydrophobicity.

The pH-responsive hydrophobic functional groups of DMAEMA was grafted onto cellulosic filter paper surfaces via RAFT polymerization by Roy et al. (2008a,b). The initiator used in this reaction was 2,2-azobis-(isobutyronitrile) (AIBN), while the reaction was conducted in the system of toluene or ethanol at 60°C. The parameters during this chemical process, such as monomer concentration, polymerization time, DP, solvent amount, and free chain-transfer agent, had a pronounced effect on the graft ratios of PDMAEMA onto cellulose fibers.

However, the heterogeneous amphiphilic modification to cellulose main chain had obvious disadvantages such as low accessibility and chemical reactivity of the hydroxyl groups, low grafting ratio of hydrophobic functional groups, high difficulty to achieve the desired chemical reaction, and complex systems for reaction.

18.4.1.2 Direct Amphiphilic Modification of Cellulose Main Chain in Homogeneous System

With the advent of cellulose solvents, such as DMAc/LiCl (Dawsey and McCormick 1990), ionic liquids (Heinze et al. 2005, Zhang et al. 2005), and NaOH/carbamide (Zhang et al. 2002, Cai and

Zhang 2005, Qi et al. 2008), the homogeneous amphiphilic modification of cellulose main chain was successfully performed. The hydrophobic functional groups were mainly two kinds: (1) long hydrophobic alkyl chains and (2) pH/thermo-responsive functional hydrophobic chains.

Guo et al. (2012) have successfully synthesized a series of cellulose-based hydrophobic associating polymers through homogeneous acylation between hydroxyl groups in microcrystalline cellulose main chain and long-chain acyl chlorides (octanoyl, lauroyl, and palmitoyl chlorides) in the solvent of DMAc/LiCl, as illustrated in Figures 18.4 and 18.5. Pyridine was used as a catalyst and an acid scavenger in this reaction. Their chemical structure and property were systematically characterized by elemental analysis, FT-IR, CP/MAS ^{13}C-NMR, x-ray diffraction, and the thermogravimetry analysis. Through controlling the chain length of fatty acyl chlorides and the molar ratio of acyl chlorides versus anhydroglucose unit, the hydrophobic cellulose derivatives with degrees of substitution (DSs) in the range of 0.02–1.75 were obtained. Because these polymers had both long hydrophobic alkyl chains and hydrophilic hydroxyl groups in their molecules, they exhibited excellent amphiphilic ability and could self-assemble into spherical nanoparticles in aqueous solution.

The comb-shaped amphiphilic *O*-(2-hydroxy-3-butoxypropyl) cellulose (HBPC) was prepared by a homogeneous reaction of cellulose with butyl glycidyl ether (BGE) in the LiCl/DMAc system (Nishimura et al. 1997). The molar substitutions (MSs) of water-soluble HBPC that range from 0.4 to 1.0 were adjusted by the added amount of BGE. All these polymers showed good solubility both in aqueous water and in organic solvent.

In the late years, the FDA-approved aliphatic polyesters, such as poly(ε-caprolactone) (PCL), poly(L-lactide) (PLA), and poly(*p*-dioxanone) (PPDO), had also been successfully grafted onto cellulose main chain via the ring-opening grafting polymerization (ROP) of ε-caprolactone, L-lactide, and *p*-dioxanone by our group (Guo et al. 2012, 2013a,b). The obtained cellulose-*g*-PLA, cellulose-*g*-PCL, and cellulose-*g*-PPDO polymers not only have self-associating ability but also have biodegradable and compatible properties. The solvents for this reaction were (1-*n*-butyl-3-methylimidazolium chloride (BmimCl) (ILs) ionic liquids, which are often regarded as intrinsically "green" due to their negligible vapor pressure. Two kinds of catalysts, metal-based catalyst (e.g., stannous octanoate $Sn(Oct)_2$) and organic catalyst (e.g., *N,N*-dimethylamino-4-pyridine (DMAP)), were used in the reaction. Both of the two catalysts do not require additional co-initiator or activated precursor to catalyze the ROP of monomers onto cellulose, whereas the hydroxyl groups of cellulose play important roles as the initiators. The raw materials we used were microcrystalline cellulose and dissolving pulp cellulose, respectively. The microstructures of these three kinds of copolymers, such as the DP of polyesters, the MS of polyesters, the DS of polyesters, and the weight content of polyesters side chains, were analyzed in detail through calculations based on the peak intensity in

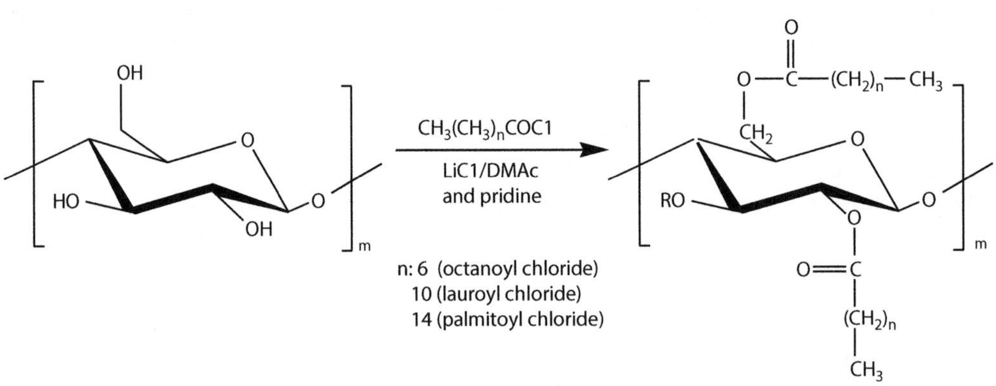

FIGURE 18.4 Synthetic procedure of cellulose-based hydrophobically associating polymers. (From Guo, Y. et al., *Polym. Bull.*, 69, 389, 2012.)

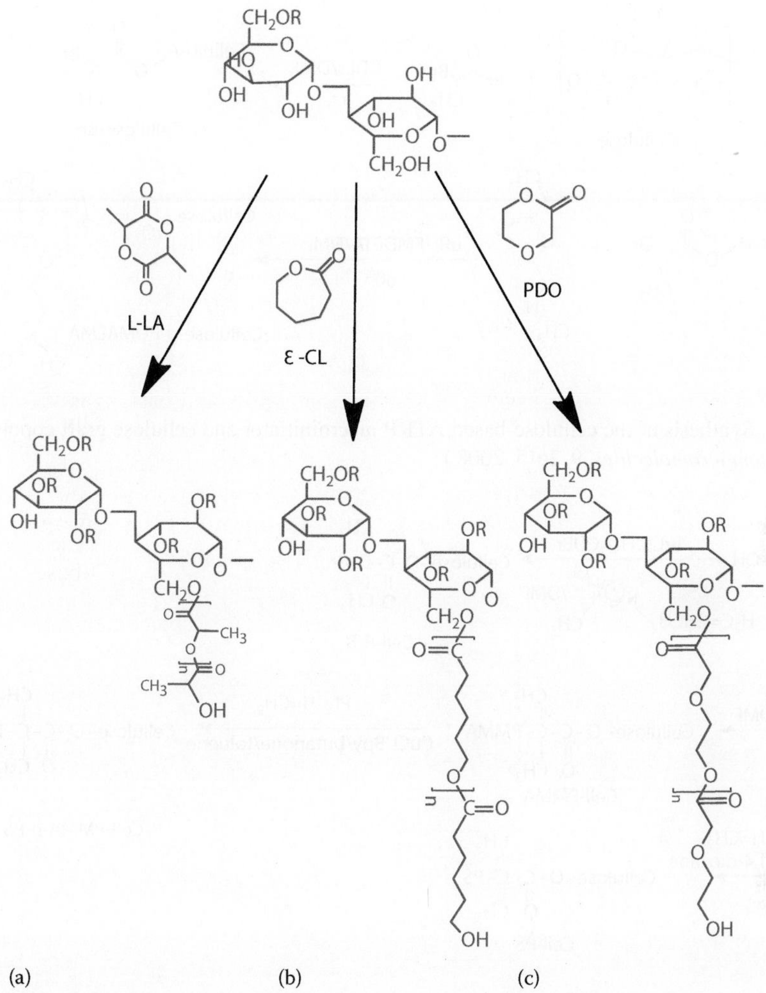

FIGURE 18.5 The synthetic routes for (a) cellulose-*g*-PLA, (b) cellulose-*g*-PCL, and (c) cellulose-*g*-PPDO polymers. (From Guo, Y. et al., *J. Agric. Food Chem.*, 60, 3900, 2012; Guo, Y. et al., *Cellulose*, 20, 873, 2013a; Guo, Y. et al., *Carbohydr. Polym.*, 92, 77, 2013b.)

^{1}H NMR spectra. The highest values of DS of PLA, PCL, and PPDO in the resultant copolymers are varied in a wide range up to 2.00, 2.41, and 2.30, respectively. It was also concluded that increase in the feed ratio of monomers was in favor to graft copolymerization of cellulose with monomers. We also found that with all the other conditions kept same, the copolymers synthesized using DMAP as catalyst show significantly higher grafting amount of PCL (in terms of MS, DS, W_{PCL}) than those synthesized using $Sn(Oct)_2$ as catalyst. Dong et al. (2008) have also synthesized two cellulose-*g*-PLA copolymers obtained by different weight ratios of L-LA to cellulose (2:1 and 1:1) with stannous octanoate as catalyst in ILs of 1-*N*-alkyl-3-methylimidazolium chloride (AmimCl). The MS values of two samples were 1.27 and 1.45, respectively.

A stimuli-responsive poly(*N*,*N*-dimethylamino-2-ethyl methacrylate) (PDMAEMA) side chain was successfully grafted onto cellulose backbone via ATRP (Figure 18.6) reaction by Sui et al. (2008). The whole preparing process was divided into two parts as depicted in Figure 18.7. Cellulose macroinitiators were initially obtained by direct acylation of cellulose with 2-bromopropionyl bromide in a room temperature ionic liquid (RTIL) of AmimCl. The obtained macroinitiator

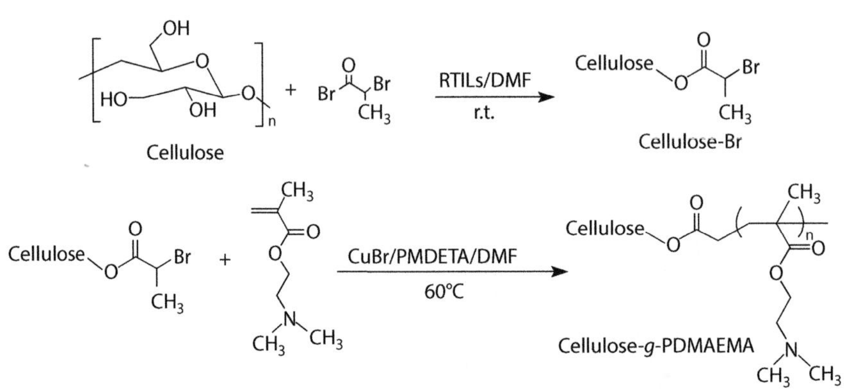

FIGURE 18.6 Synthesis of the cellulose-based ATRP macroinitiator and cellulose graft copolymer. (From Sui, X. et al., *Biomacromolecules*, 9, 2615, 2008.)

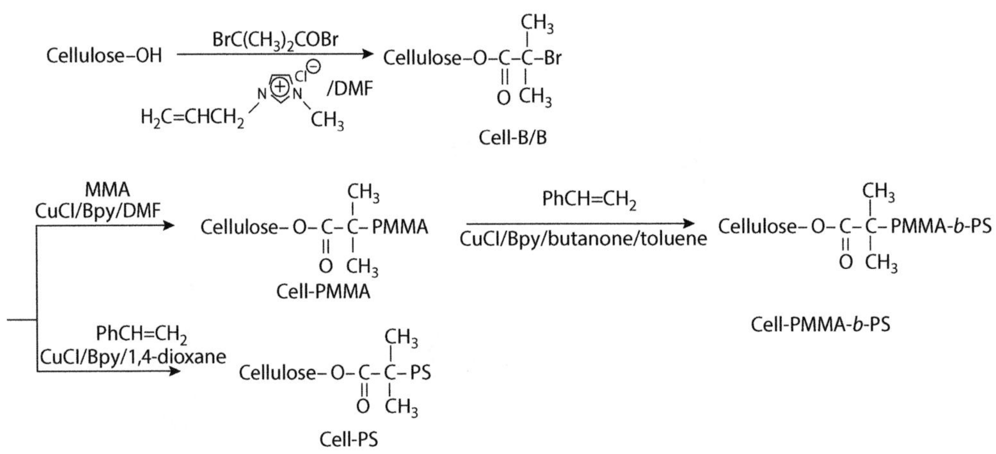

FIGURE 18.7 Synthesis procedure of macroinitiator Cell-BiB and cellulose graft PMMA/PS copolymers. (From Meng, T. et al., *Polymer*, 50, 447, 2009.)

cellulose-Br exhibited good solubility in organic solvents. And then, cellulose-*g*-PDMAEMA copolymer was synthesized via ATRP with DMAEMA as monomer and CuBr/pentamethyldiethylenetriamine (PMDETA) as catalyst in the solvent of *N*,*N*-dimethylformamide (DMF). The whole process was conducted in a homogeneous system at 60°C, which ensured the uniform distribution of grafting polymer chains in the cellulose macromolecules.

The hydrophobic side chains of PMMA or poly(styrene) (PS) were grafted onto cellulose main chain via ATRP (Meng et al. 2009) as shown in Figure 18.8. Cellulose-based macroinitiator was synthesized by partially converting hydroxyl groups into tertiary bromoester groups through homogeneous reaction with 2-bromoisobutyryl bromide (BrBiB) in ionic liquid AmimCl without analyst. ATRP of PMMA or/and PS onto cellulose was initiated by these tertiary bromoester groups and catalyzed by CuCl.

A series of novel amphiphilic cellulose derivatives carrying a pyrene group regioselectively at the reducing end, that is, *N*-(1-pyrenebutyloyl)-4-*O*-(*b*-D-glucopyranosyl)-*b*-D-glucopyranosylamine, *N*-(15-(1-pyrenebutyloylamino)-pentadecanoyl)-4-*O*-(*b*-D-glucopyranosyl)-*b*-D-glucopyranosylamine, *N*-(1-pyrenebutyloyl)-*b*-cellulosylamine, were prepared by Rogers groups (Enomoto-Rogers et al. 2006, 2011). As the pyrene was a common fluorescent probe, these copolymers could be applied in a wide range of bioimaging and bioprobe.

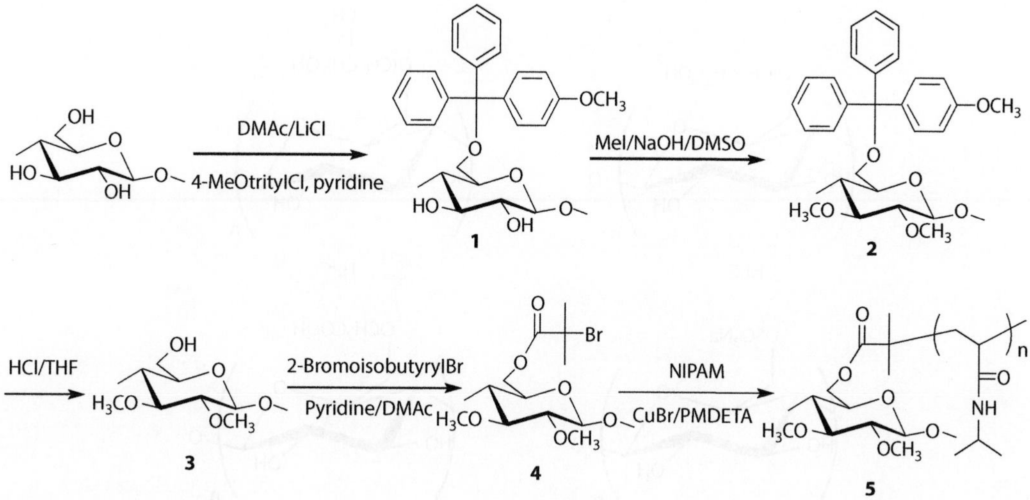

FIGURE 18.8 Synthetic scheme for the preparation of 6-*O*-PolyNIPAM cellulose copolymers. (From Ifuku, S. and Kadla, J.F., *Biomacromolecules*, 9, 3308, 2008.)

Ifuku and Kadla (2008) had prepared and thoroughly characterized a highly regioselective cellulose macroinitiator derivative of 6-*O*-bromoisobutyryl-2,3-di-*O*-methyl cellulose. ATRP of the cellulose macroinitiators was performed with NIPAM, and copolymers with poly(NIPAM) side chains of DP up to 46.3 were synthesized.

18.4.2 Amphiphilic Modification of Cellulose Water-Soluble Derivatives

Currently, water-soluble cellulose derivatives used for the synthesis of amphiphilic cellulose derivatives were mainly divided into three kinds: (1) nonionic water-soluble cellulose derivatives: HEC, HPC; (2) anionic water-soluble cellulose derivatives: CMC, CS; (3) cationic water-soluble cellulose derivatives: quaternary ammoniation of cellulose, etc. Their typical structures were depicted in Figure 18.9. Due to the limited content of hydrophobic groups in their molecular structure, the surface activity of these derivatives was very poor. So if we want to get amphiphilic polymers from water-soluble cellulose derivatives, the introduction of functional groups with hydrophobic property was necessary. Up to now, the amphiphilic polymers based on water-soluble cellulose derivatives have been successfully synthesized via basically two routes: long-chain hydrophobic modification and amphiphilic grafting copolymerization.

18.4.2.1 Long-Chain Hydrophobic Modification for Cellulose Water-Soluble Derivatives

The long-chain alkyl hydrophobic groups can be attached to cellulose water-soluble substrates via an ether, ester, or urethane linkage. The linkages were formed through nucleophilic substitution reaction between hydroxyl groups in cellulose main chain, and hydrophobic long-chain modifiers include epoxide, acyl halide, halide, isocyanate, and acid anhydride. The typical reactions were listed in Figure 18.10. Although the hydrophobic groups obtained through this method were referred to "long-chain alkyl groups," it should be pointed out that except in the case where cellulose water-soluble derivatives were hydrophobically modified with an alkyl halide, the modifier was not limited to the long-chain alkyl group. The group can actually be an alphahydroxy alkyl radical in the case of an epoxide, a urethane radical in the case of an isocyanate, or an acyl radical in the case of an acid or acyl chloride. Furthermore, among all the linkages, the ether linkage was preferred because that the commonly used etherification reagents were readily obtained and more easily handled than

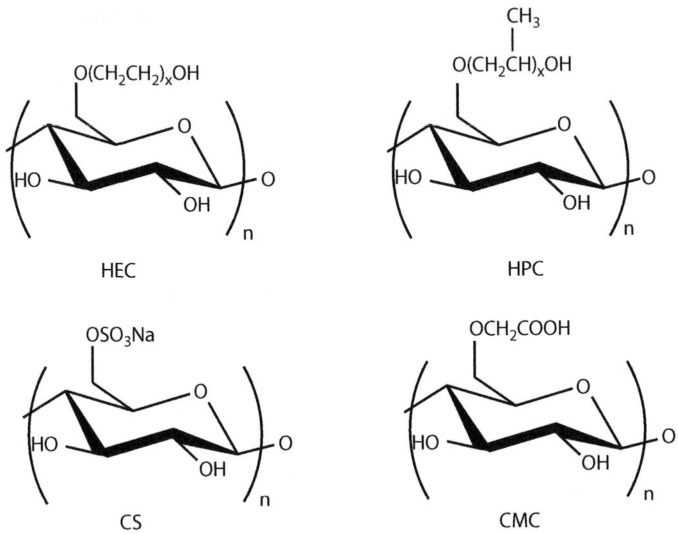

FIGURE 18.9 Typical structure of cellulose water-soluble derivatives.

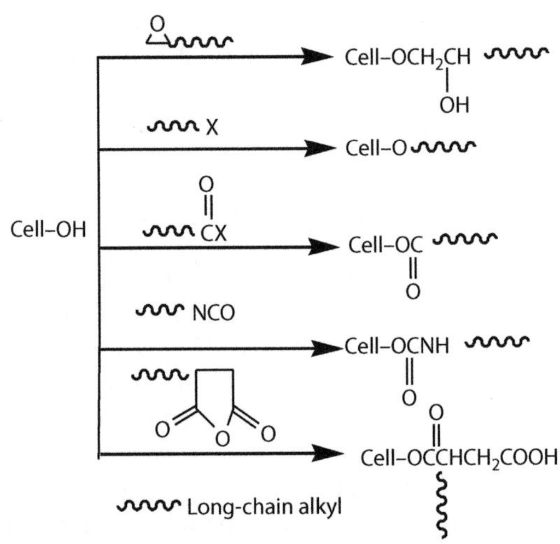

FIGURE 18.10 Typical synthesis pathways of long-chain hydrophobically modified water-soluble cellulose derivatives.

the others employed for the modification via other linkages. Above all, the obtained linkage was also usually more resistant to further reactions.

Landoll (1982a) has first prepared long-chain alkyl hydrophobic modified polymers from nonionic water-soluble cellulose derivatives, such as HEC and HPC, via ether linkage in 1982. The common reagents used were C10–C24 epoxides, halides, or halohydrides. Briefly, the preparing procedures were compromising slurred nonionic cellulose derivatives in an inert organic solvent such as a lower aliphatic alcohol, ketone, or hydrocarbon and added an aqueous solution of sodium hydroxide to the resultant slurry at a low temperature. When the ether was thoroughly wetted and swollen by the sodium hydroxide solution, the long-chain alkyl hydrophobic modifiers were added, and the reaction was continued under stirring. Residual sodium hydroxide was then neutralized, and the product was recovered, washed with inert diluents, and dried. The efficiency of hydrophobic etherification with halides or halohydrides was sometimes less than that with epoxides. The etherification without sodium hydroxide slurry pretreatment was ineffective. In the late years, lots of cellulose-based amphiphilic polymers through long-chain alkyl hydrophobic modifying for nonionic water-soluble cellulose derivatives have been reported. HPC had been hydrophobically modified through esterification between hydroxyl groups and palmitoyl chloride in THF/acetone solution by López-Velázquez et al. (2004). Ye et al. (Dai et al. 2006, Li et al. 2006, Ye et al. 2006) had successfully synthesized a series amphiphilic polymers from HEC by the macromolecular reaction of HEC with 1,2-epoxyhexadecane, or bromododecane or 4-isopropylbenzyl chloride. Bagheri and Shateri (2012a,b) have obtained two new series of cholesteryl-modified HPC amphiphilic derivatives by performing reactions involving HPC, a cholesterol-based mesogenic dimer (HPC-G1-Chol), or cholesteryl chloroformate (HPC-Chol), all with different DSs of hydrophobic groups. Wang et al. (2012) also prepared cellulose-based amphiphilic derivatives through the etherification of HEC with bromododecane. The solvent we used in this part was isopropanol/sodium hydroxide aqueous solution.

Anionic water-soluble derivatives of cellulose such as CMC and CS were also hydrophobic modified through esterification and etherification of hydroxyl groups with long-chain alkyl modifiers. Srokova et al. (1998, 2004) prepared water-soluble partially hydrophobized derivatives from CMC in its gel suspension. Before esterification, carboxylate groups in CMC main chain were activated and protonated by stirring it in mixtures of DMSO/water-free 4-toluenesulfonic acid under elevated temperatures. The reactions used were parted into three kinds: classical esterification method using stearoyl chloride/pyridine and two unconventional methods based on reaction with mixed anhydrides and transesterification with vinyl laurate, respectively. Cholesteryl-bearing CMC (CCMC) amphiphilic derivatives were systematically prepared and characterized by Yang et al. (2008a). Briefly, purified CMC was partly protonated by stirring it in the solvents of water/DMSO for 30 min. Then, cholesterol, DCC, and DMAP were added, and the reaction was allowed to proceed at room temperature for 24 h.

Wei et al. (Hong et al. 2007, Wei and Cheng 2007, Wei et al. 2008) reported a novel synthetic route for long-chain hydrophobically associating water-soluble CS derivatives. The new pathway is shown in Figure 18.11. Different from other synthetic route, the procedure is as follows: hydrophobic side chain is introduced in the backbone of cellulose, then hydrophilic groups. Hydrophobic modified cellulose derivative: cellulose octaonate could be easily synthesized by the reaction between cellulose with octanoyl in homogeneous LiCl/DMAc solution, and the degree of substitution (DS) was well controllable. The obtained cellulose octaonate could swell and even be dissolved in DMF. The amphiphilic cellulose-based copolymers could be obtained by a sulfonatin modification with chlorosulfonic acid in DMF. Cheng et al. (2003) also synthesized amphiphilic cellulose adsorbents with different ratios of sulfonic ligand to cholesterol ligand through this pathway.

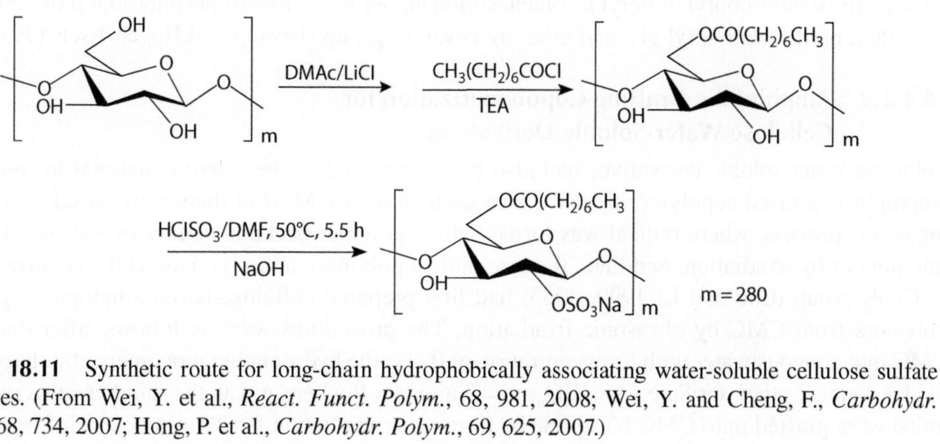

FIGURE 18.11 Synthetic route for long-chain hydrophobically associating water-soluble cellulose sulfate derivatives. (From Wei, Y. et al., *React. Funct. Polym.*, 68, 981, 2008; Wei, Y. and Cheng, F., *Carbohydr. Polym.*, 68, 734, 2007; Hong, P. et al., *Carbohydr. Polym.*, 69, 625, 2007.)

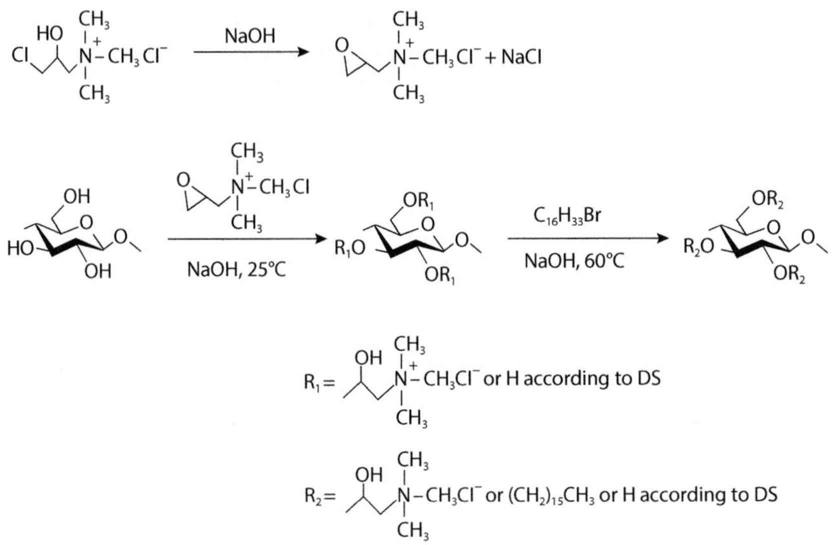

FIGURE 18.12 Synthesis of hydrophobically modified quaternized cellulose (HMQC). (From Song, Y. et al., *Colloids Surf. B: Biointerfaces*, 83, 313, 2011b.)

A novel hydrophobically modified quaternized cellulose (QC) derivative had been successfully synthesized by a two-step process as illustrated in Figure 18.12 (Song et al. 2011b). First, a water-soluble cationic derivative (QC) with N content of 3.85% and DS value of 0.76 were homogeneously prepared in NaOH/urea aqueous solutions direct from cellulose. And then, HMQC was obtained through etherification between hexadecyl bromide and the residue hydroxyl groups of cellulose in NaOH aqueous solutions. The 2-hydroxypropyl trimethylammonium chloride and long alkyl chain (hexadecyl) in the molecular of derived polymers were acted as hydrophilic and hydrophobic groups respectively.

The amphiphilic polymers carrying a long fluorocarbon chain had been synthesized since 1890s. Compared with the long hydrocarbon groups, long fluorocarbon groups had favorable properties such as high surface activity and excellent chemical and thermal stability. Additionally, due to their strong hydrophobic ability, the CMC and surface tension of fluorocarbon-modified cellulose surfactants were usually very low. Grafting fluorocarbon chain onto cellulose backbone was very meaningful. 1,1-Dihydroperfluorobutyl and 1-dihydroperfluorooctyl derivatives of HEC were prepared through reaction of the Na salt of HEC in isopropyl alcohol/aqueous solution with 1,1-dihydroperfluorobutyl or octyl *p*-toluenesulfonate, with 1,1-dihydroperfluorobutyl or octyl glycidyl ether, or/and with octyl glycidyl ether by Hwang's group (Hwang and Hogen-Esch 1993).

18.4.2.2 Amphiphilic Grafting Copolymerization for Cellulose Water-Soluble Derivatives

Cellulose water-soluble derivatives had also been employed as the starting material for preparing amphiphilic grafted copolymer by using various techniques. Most of them were based on a "grafting-from" process, where radical was formed along polymer backbone either by various chemical initiators or by irradiation, and then, the free radical polymerization such as ATRP occurred.

Cao's group (Cao and Li 1999, 2003) had first prepared cellulose-based amphiphilic grafting polymers from CMC by ultrasonic irradiation. The procedures were as follows: after dissolving CMC into aqueous water with a concentration of 0.6%, the hydrophobic monomers of poly(ethylene oxide) dodecyl ether acrylate ($AR_{12}EO_n$, n = 7 and n = 9 where n was the number of oxyethylene units) were grafted onto CMC backbone by ultrasonic irradiation for 20 min at 25°C. The reaction mixture was dried and extracted by a Soxhlet apparatus with acetone for 36 h to remove unreacted macromonomers. The hydrophobic molecular contents in amphiphilic polymers could be regulated through varying ultrasound irradiation power.

The amphiphilic CMC-*graft*-poly(*N*,*N*-hexyl acrylamide) was prepared by Vidal's group (Vidal et al. 2008) via successive radical polymerization using potassium persulfate redox system as initiator and sodium dodecyl sulfate as hydrophobic monomer. Dou et al. (2003) prepared the pH-sensitive amphiphilic HEC-*graft*-PAA (HEC-*g*-PAA) via free radical polymerization, which were initiated by cerium(IV) salt.

Hydrophobic side chain of poly(4-vinyl pyridine) (P4VP) with pH and thermosensitivity was grafted onto HPC backbone via ATRP by Ma's group (Ma et al. 2010a). The synthesis route of the graft copolymers was shown in Figure 18.13. Macroinitiator HPC-Br for ATRP copolymerization had been first synthesized in pyridine/THF solution at 30°C. The DS of bromide groups (DS-Br) could be controlled by varying the feeding molar ratio of 2-bromoisobutylrylbromide (BriB) and HPC. The ATRP reaction was well controlled by using CuCl/Me_6–TREN as the catalyst complex in the 2-propanol solvent at 30°C. The use of CuCl catalyst could achieve good control and narrow molecular weight distribution of the polymers. The Me_6–TREN was a more reactive ligand that could form a strong complex with the alky halide. Subsequently, Ma et al. (2010b) also synthesized dual-stimuli sensitivities (pH and thermosensitivity) of HPC-*graft*-poly(*N*,*N*-dimethyl aminoethyl methacrylate) (HPC-*g*-PDMAEMA) copolymers via ATRP in isopropanol solvent with macroinitiator HPC-Br as initiator and CuCl/1,1,4,7,10,10-hexamethyl-triethylenetetramine as catalyst.

Biodegradable and compatible hydrophobic polyester of PCL was grafted onto HEC main chain via ROP using trimethylsilyl protection method by Jiang's group (Jiang et al. 2011). As depicted in Figure 18.14, the synthesis of HEC-*g*-PCL copolymers was divided into three steps. In the first step, HEC was trimethyl silylated using hexamethyldisilazane (HMDS) and trimethylsilyl chloride as silylated agent in the solvent of DMSO. The obtained trimethyl silylated HEC could be dissolved in common organic solvents such as toluene, xylene, chloroform, and acetone. In the second step, PCL chain was grafted onto HEC through ROP between monomer ε-caprolactone and residual hydroxyl groups catalyzed by $Sn(Oct)_2$ in homogeneous solution. Finally, HEC-*g*-PCL copolymers were obtained by deprotecting trimethyl silylation in 1.0 M HCl aqueous solution.

Both hydrophobic PMMA and hydrophilic PAA functional groups were together associated with the main chain of HPC via ATRP by Östmark et al. (2007). As illustrated in Figure 18.15, the hydroxyl groups of HPC was either allowed to react with 2-bromoisobutyryl anhydride or the

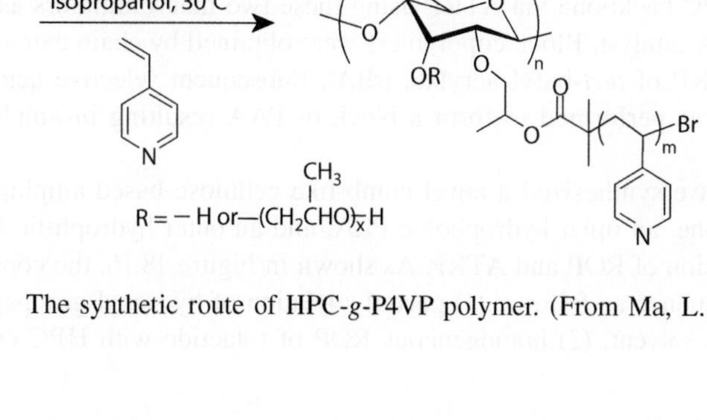

FIGURE 18.13 The synthetic route of HPC-*g*-P4VP polymer. (From Ma, L. et al., *Langmuir*, 26, 18519, 2010a.)

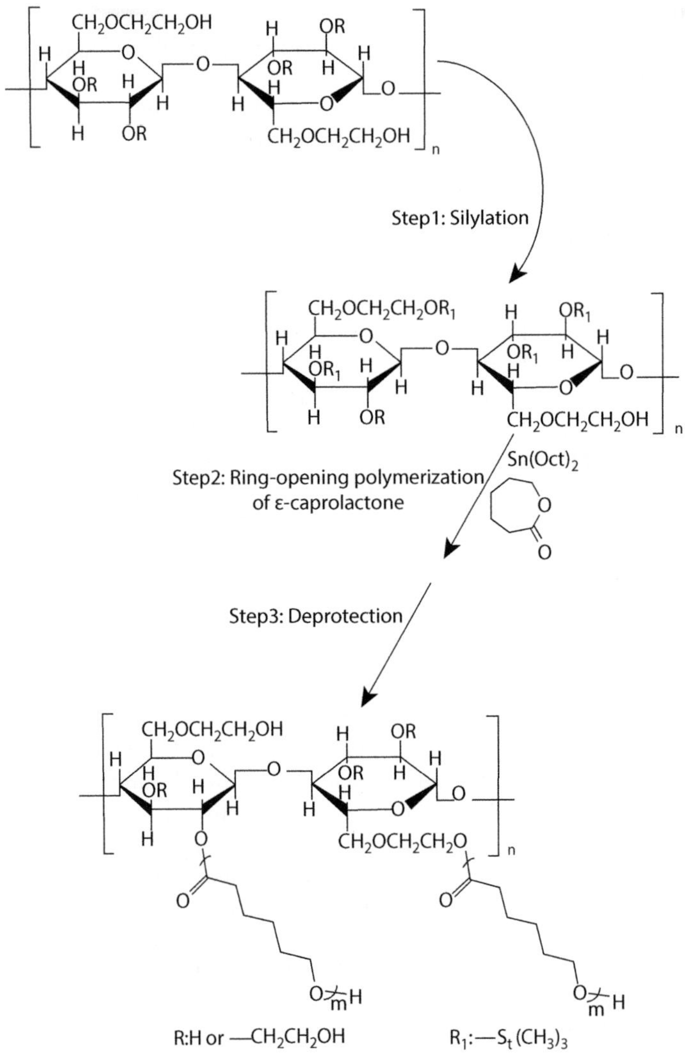

FIGURE 18.14 The synthetic route of HEC-*g*-PCL copolymers. (From Jiang, C. et al., *Int. J. Biol. Macromol.*, 48, 210, 2011.)

first-generation initiator-functionalized 2,2-bis(methylol)propionic acid dendron to create macroinitiators of HPC-1 and HPC-G1-1, respectively. Both of these two kinds of macroinitiators had high degrees of functionality. The monomers of methyl methacrylate (MMA) or hexadecyl methacrylate were then grafted onto HPC backbone via ATRP using these two macroinitiators as initiator and Cu(I or II)Br_2/PMDETA as catalyst. Block copolymers were obtained by chain extending PMMA-grafted HPCs via the ATRP of *tert*-butyl acrylate (*t*BA). Subsequent selective acidolysis of the *tert*-butyl ester moieties was performed to form a block of PAA resulting in amphiphilic block copolymer grafts.

Berthier et al. (2011) have synthesized a novel comb-like cellulose-based amphiphilic copolymers with an HPC backbone, an inner hydrophobic PLA, and an outer hydrophilic PAA block in combination with the reaction of ROP and ATRP. As shown in Figure 18.16, the copolymers were prepared in a five-step sequence as follows: (1) partial silylation of hydroxyl groups of HPC with HMDS in dry acetonitrile solvent, (2) homogeneous ROP of L-lactide with HPC catalyzed with

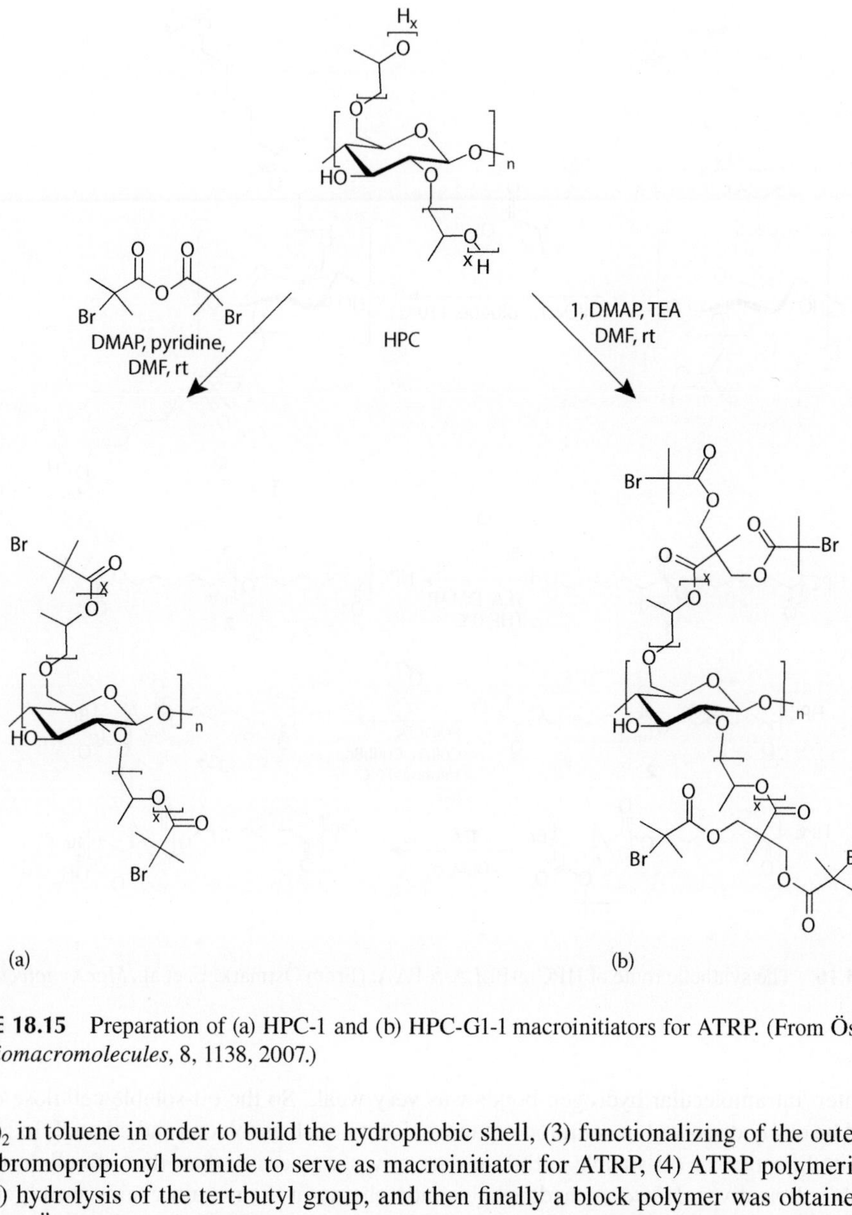

FIGURE 18.15 Preparation of (a) HPC-1 and (b) HPC-G1-1 macroinitiators for ATRP. (From Östmark, E. et al., *Biomacromolecules*, 8, 1138, 2007.)

$Sn(Oct)_2$ in toluene in order to build the hydrophobic shell, (3) functionalizing of the outer surface with 2-bromopropionyl bromide to serve as macroinitiator for ATRP, (4) ATRP polymerization of *t*BA, (5) hydrolysis of the tert-butyl group, and then finally a block polymer was obtained. In the late years, Östmark et al. (2008) also synthesized the amphiphilic HPC-*g*-PLLA-*b*-PAA polymers through this method.

Wan's group (Wan et al. 2007) had successfully prepared a new binary graft copolymer HEC-*g*-PNIPAAm-PAA, which was composed of biodegradable material (HEC) as the backbone and a pair of complementary sensitive polymers, PAA and PNIPAAm, as the two grafts through successive cerium(IV)-initiated free radical copolymerization. This graft copolymer can dissolve in water and self-assemble into three forms of micelles by tuning pH and temperature based on the thermosensitivity of PNIPAAm, the pH sensitivity of PAA.

18.4.3 Amphiphilic Modification of Oil-Soluble Cellulose Derivatives

The oil-soluble cellulose derivatives such as EC and methyl cellulose (MC) mainly had a certain amount of hydrophobic side chains in their main chains. Compared with cellulose, their ability of

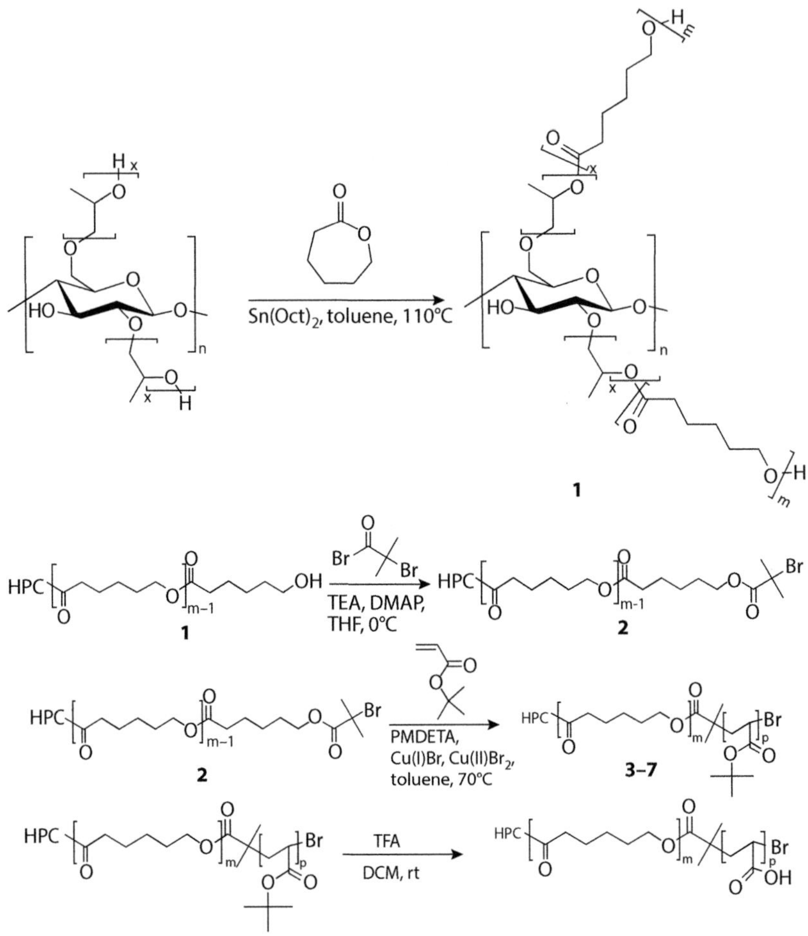

FIGURE 18.16 The synthetic route of HPC-*g*-PLLA-*b*-PAA. (From Östmark, E. et al., *Macromolecules*, 41, 4405, 2008.)

forming inter-/intramolecular hydrogen bonds was very weak. So the oil-soluble cellulose derivatives could be easily dissolved in common organic solvents, such as toluene and ethanol. In general, chemical modification of oil-soluble cellulose derivatives was easier than that of cellulose or its water-soluble derivatives. However, hydrophobic side chains in their main chains were generally alkyl groups. The alkyl groups mainly contained one to three carbons, and their hydrophobic ability was not as good as that of the long chains. Therefore, introducing hydrophobic long chains or hydrophilic functional groups into oil-soluble cellulose molecules through chemical modification was one of the key ways of alleviating this problem. The graft polymerization reactions, for example, ATRP and ROP, were mostly used.

Among the oil-soluble cellulose derivatives (Figure 18.17), EC possessed high mechanical strength, good heat resistance, cold resistance, and stability. Thus, it was a potential material for practical use. In the present investigation, the amphiphilic derivation of EC with styrene through ATRP had been first studied by Shen et al. (2005, 2006). In the synthesis of EC-grafting-polystyrene (EC-*g*-PSt) copolymers, an EC-based macroinitiator had been homogeneously prepared through the reaction of the residual hydroxyl groups of EC with 2-bromoisobutyrylbromide in the solvent of pyridine/THF. The obtained EC macroinitiators were successfully used to initiate ATRP of styrene in toluene with CuBr/PMDETA as catalyst at 110°C. A series of EC-*g*-PSt graft copolymers with

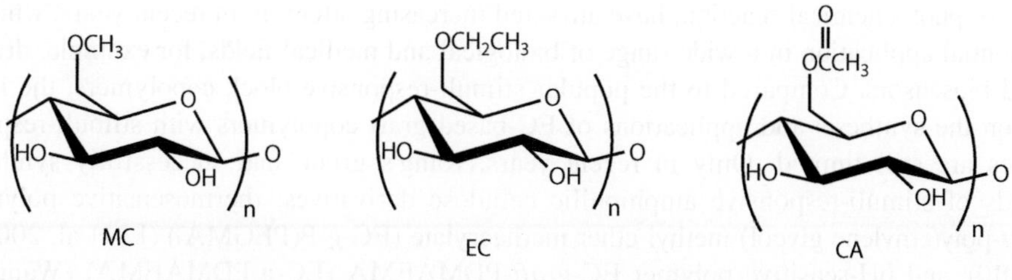

FIGURE 18.17 The molecular structures of typical oil-soluble cellulose derivatives.

varied length of side chains had been prepared. Kinetic study indicated that the grafting polymerization is living/controlled. Liu et al. (2009) also synthesized amphiphilic EC-*g*-PSt copolymers by this method.

Hydrophilic PAA was one of the most useful blocks in amphiphilic block polymer. If the hydrophilic PAA chains are grafted onto the hydrophobic EC backbone, an amphiphilic grafting copolymer could be obtained. Kang et al. (2006) first synthesized EC-*g*-PAA copolymers via ATRP (Figure 18.18). The preparation of macroinitiators was same as initiators synthesized by Shen. *t*BA was polymerized by ATRP using CuBr/PMDETA as the catalyst and EC-Br macroinitiator as the initiator in toluene/cyclohexanone mixed solvent. EC-*g*-PAA was obtained by the hydrolysis of the *tert*-butyl group on the PtBA block in CF_3COOH/CH_2Cl_2 solvents.

A typical hydrophilic vinyl side chain of PHEMA was also grafted onto EC backbone via ATRP using EC-Br as the macroinitiator and $CuI[bpy]_2$ as the catalyst in methanol by Kang et al. (2008). Stimuli-responsive side chains with environmental sensitivities, such as pH, temperature, ionic

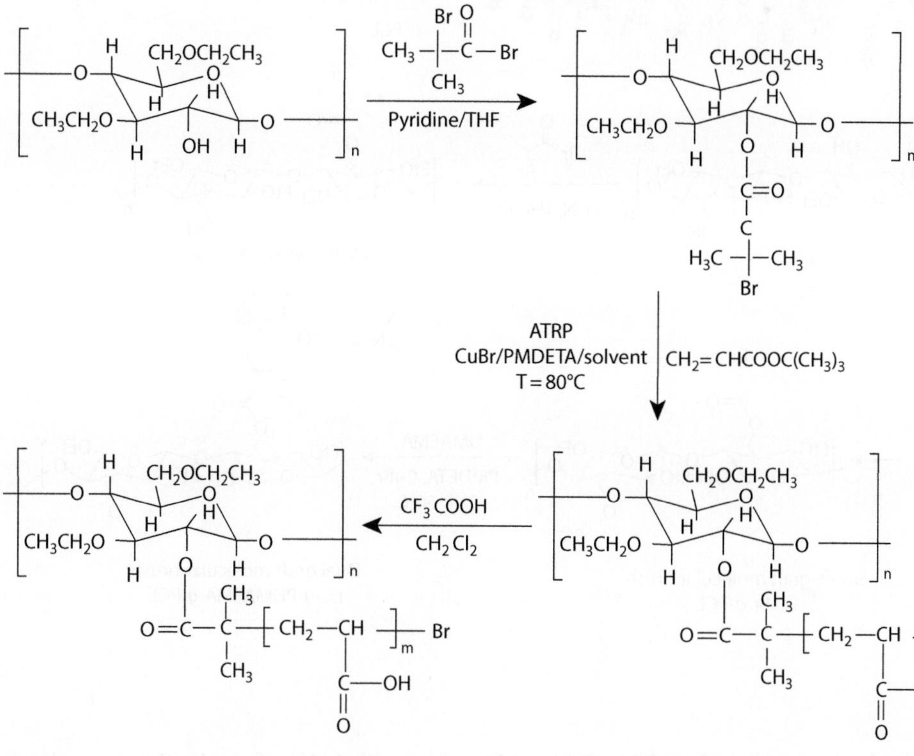

FIGURE 18.18 Synthesis of the EC-*g*-PAA copolymer. (From Kang, H. et al., *Polymer*, 47, 7927, 2006.)

strength, or photochemical reaction, have attracted increasing attention in recent years, which had high potential application in a wide range of biological and medical fields, for example, drug carriers and biosensors. Compared to the popular stimuli-responsive block copolymers, the investigations on the synthesis and applications of EC-based graft copolymers with stimuli-responsive properties are still limited. Only in recent years, Kang's group had successfully synthesized two kinds of stimuli-responsive amphiphilic cellulose derivatives, thermosensitive polymer of EC-*graft*-poly(ethylene glycol) methyl ether methacrylate (EC-*g*-P(PEGMA)) (Li et al. 2008, Tan et al. 2010), and pH-sensitive polymer EC-*graft*-PDMAEMA (EC-*g*-PDMAEMA) (Wang et al. 2011), respectively.

Yan et al. (2009b) combined the ROP and ATRP processes to graft two different chains (PDMAEMA and PCL, respectively) onto the EC backbone and obtained a well-defined cellulose-based dual graft molecular brushes, EC-*g*-PDMAEMA-*g*-PCL polymers as shown in Figure 18.19. The preparing process was divided into three stages: (1) preparation of EC-Br macroinitiator for ATRP through the acrylation between 2-bromopropionyl bromide and residual hydroxyl groups in EC molecule; (2) single graft polymerization of ε-CL with EC-Br in the presence of $Sn(Oct)_2$ as catalyst and xylene as solvent to afford the EC-Br-*g*-PCL copolymers; and (3) synthesis of the target EC-*g*-PDMAEMAg-PCL dual graft molecular brushes using EC-Br-*g*-PCL macroinitiator in the presence of CuBr/PMDETA catalyst in THF at 60°C. Unlike other brush copolymers, the new

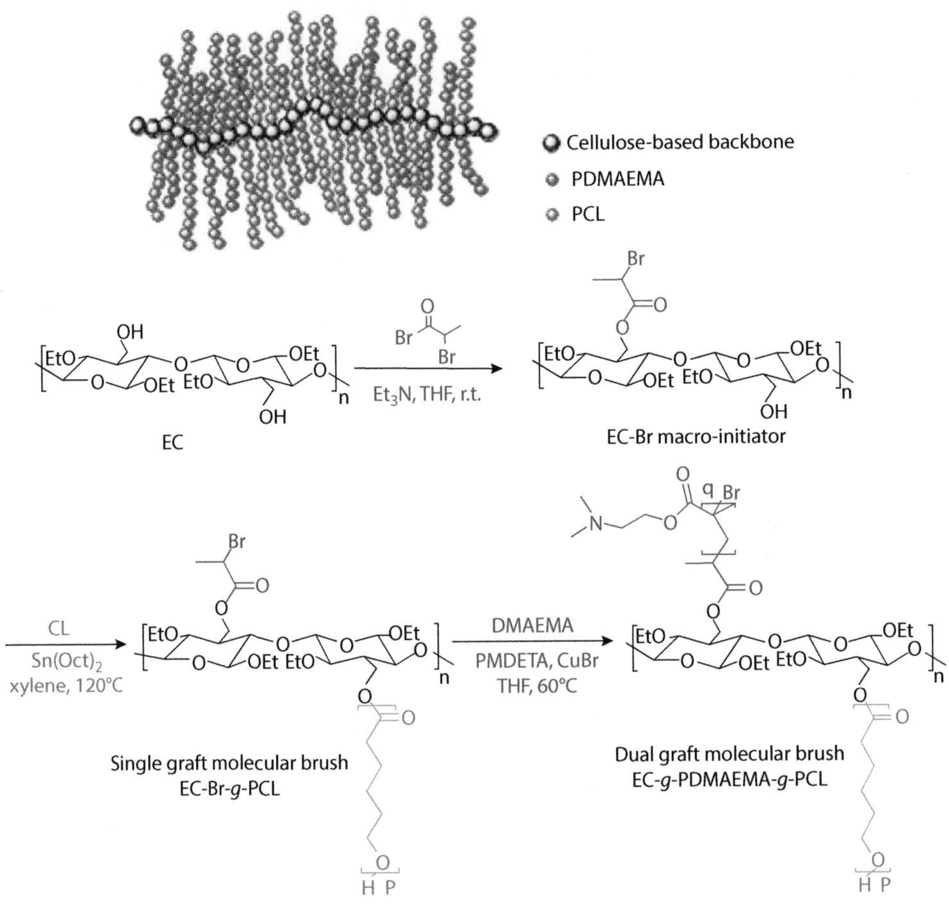

FIGURE 18.19 Synthesis of EC-*g*-PDMAEMA-*g*-PCL polymer. (From Yan, Q. et al., *Biomacromolecules*, 10, 2033, 2009b.)

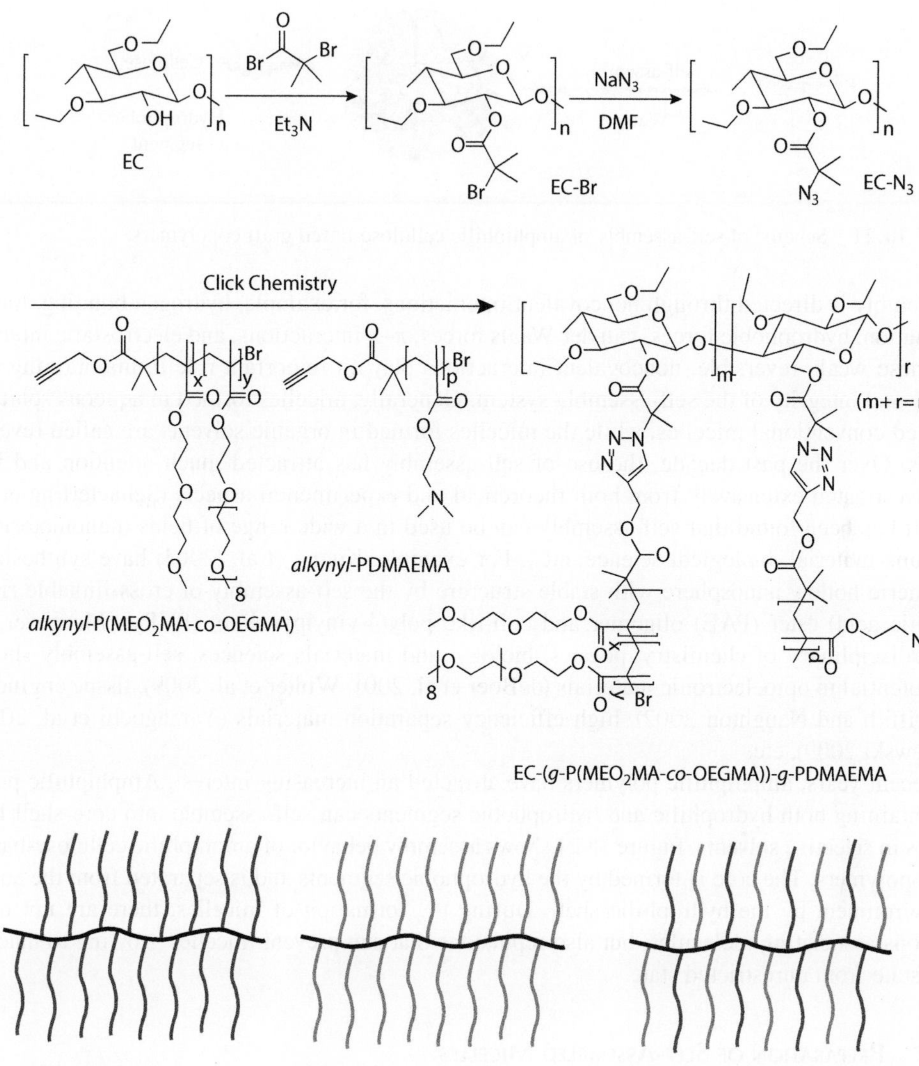

FIGURE 18.20 Synthesis of EC brush polymers with mono and dual side chains of P(MEO$_2$MA-*co*-OEGMA) and PDMAEMA. (From Yuan, W.Z. et al., *Polymer*, 53, 956, 2012.)

molecular brushes show some unique physicochemical properties and multifunction due to their unique topological structures.

A novel amphiphilic EC brush polymer with mono and dual side chains of poly(2-(2-methoxyethoxy)ethyl methacrylate)-*co*-oligo(ethylene glycol) methacrylate) (P(MEO$_2$MA-*co*-OEGMA)) (Figure 18.20) and PDMAEMA were synthesized by the combination of ATRP and click chemistry (Yuan et al. 2012).

18.5 SELF-ASSEMBLY OF AMPHIPHILIC CELLULOSE GRAFT COPOLYMERS

18.5.1 General Information of Self-Assembly

Self-assembly is a type of process in which a number of components spontaneously form special structure and morphology without guidance or management from an outside source. Molecular

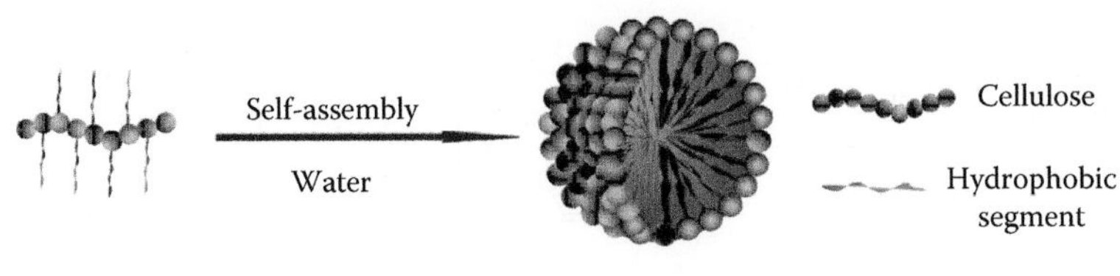

FIGURE 18.21 Scheme of self-assembly of amphiphilic cellulose-based graft copolymers.

self-assembly is directed through noncovalent interactions, for example, hydrogen bonding, metal coordination, hydrophobic forces, van der Waals forces, π–π interactions, and electrostatic interaction. These weak, reversible, noncovalent interactions play an important role in maintaining the stability and integrity of the self-assembly system. Generally, micelles formed in aqueous solution are called conventional micelles, while the micelles formed in organic solvents are called reverse micelles. Over the past decade, the use of self-assembly has attracted much attention and has been investigated extensively from both theoretical and experimental aspects (Schaeferling et al. 2002). It has been found that self-assembly can be used in a wide range of fields (nanomaterials, membrane material, biological science, etc.). For example, Kuang et al. (2003) have synthesized a polymeric hollow nanosphere with stable structure by the self-assembly of cross-linkable rigid poly(amic acid) ester (PAE) oligomer and coil-like poly(4-vinylpyridine) (PVPy). Moreover, as an interdisciplinary of chemistry, physics, biology, and materials sciences, self-assembly shows great potential in optoelectronic materials (deBoer et al. 2001, Winter et al. 2009), tissue engineering (Griffith and Naughton 2002), high-efficiency separation materials (Yamaguchi et al. 2004, Wasielewski 2009), etc.

In recent years, amphiphilic polymers have attracted an increasing interest. Amphiphilic polymer containing both hydrophilic and hydrophobic segments can self-assemble into core-shell like particles in selective solvents. Figure 18.21 shows assembly behavior of amphiphilic cellulose-based graft copolymers. The core is formed by the hydrophobic segments and is separated from the aqueous environment by the hydrophilic shell. During the formation of micelles, there are not only attractions associating molecules, but also repulsions that can prevent micelles growing to macroscopic state from unrestricted state.

18.5.2 Preparation of Self-Assembled Micelles

Methods for the preparation of polymeric micelles vary from different characteristics of amphiphilic polymers. Dissolution induction is the most commonly used technique in the preparation of amphiphilic polymer micelles. And it is based on the selective dissolution behavior of segments in different solvents. According to the difference of the solvent, two main methods can be followed for the preparation of micelles by dissolution induction. The first approach is to dissolve the amphiphilic polymer in a nonselective solvent, that is, a common solvent for both blocks. In some cases, the desired micellar structure can be obtained through ultrasound, heating, and stirring treatments. In other cases, selective solvents are usually added to dissolve amphiphilic polymers and then removed via dialysis (Leventis et al. 2008, Liu et al. 2008a). Another approach to prepare micelles consists of introducing the copolymer into a low-boiling-point organic solvent, followed by slow drop-wise addition into water with vigorous stirring. Hydrophobic segment will gather into the core, while hydrophilic segments will slowly enter into the aqueous phase (Liu et al. 2006).

In addition, some water-soluble polymers such as polyvinyl methyl ether and poly(*N*-isopropylacrylamide) (PNIPAM) (Butun et al. 1998) have a lower critical solution temperature behavior in an aqueous solution, that is, temperature-sensitive properties. Amphiphilic polymers containing these segments can self-assemble into micelles by temperature induction method. If an amphiphilic polymer contains protonatable groups or functional groups that is capable of providing a proton, such as poly(2-vinylpyridine)-*b*-polyethylene oxide (Martin et al. 1996), the polymer can self-assemble by adjusting the pH value.

18.5.3 Characterization of Micelles

In order to characterize a micellar system, several parameters have to be considered, including the equilibrium constant, the quality of the solvent, the critical micelle temperature and the CMC, the overall molar mass (Mw) of the micelle, and its morphology (Rodríguez-Hernández et al. 2005). Several methods have been utilized for the characterization of typical micelle parameters given earlier, such as light scattering, electron microscopy, fluorescent probe, viscosity method, and NMR spectroscopy. Table 18.2 lists some common methods to characterize amphiphilic polymer micelles.

18.5.3.1 Particle Size

Particle size and its distribution are important parameters to evaluate the stability of polymer micelles. They are mainly measured by light scattering (dynamic light scattering (DLS) and static light scattering (SLS)) (Xu et al. 1991, Brown et al. 1992). SLS is a powerful technique to estimate average molar masses of self-assembled structures (Rodríguez-Hernández et al. 2005) and their radius of gyration (R_G). DLS can be used to evaluate average particle size and distribution of an amphiphilic polymeric micellar system through the determination of its diffusion coefficient (Gebhardt et al. 2006). Small-angle x-ray scattering has also been employed in the analysis of micellar solutions to obtain overall and internal sizes from differences in electron density of the solvent and the solute.

18.5.3.2 Morphology

Morphology is an important parameter to exhibit the size, shape, or internal structure of the micelles. It is usually observed by electron microscopy including transmission electron microscopy (TEM), scanning electron microscopy (SEM), and atomic force microscopy (AFM). TEM and SEM can show the morphology of micelles directly (Denker et al. 2002, Martin et al. 2006). For carbohydrate polymer micelles, samples should be dyed by stains like phosphotungstic acid and uranyl acetate by TEM, while samples should be sprayed gold on the surface to improve their conductivity by SEM. AFM gathers surface morphology image by a probe scanning the micellar surface (Gebhardt et al. 2006). Figure 18.22 shows the TEM micrograph of micelles of cellulose derivatives (Guo et al. 2013b).

TABLE 18.2
Methods to Characterize Amphiphilic Polymer Micelles

Methods	Micellar Information
Dynamic light scattering	Average particle size and its distribution
Static light scattering	Overall molar mass (M_w) and the radius of gyration (R_G)
Small-angle x-ray scattering	M_w and R_G
Electron microscopy	Size and shape
Gel filtration chromatography	Dynamic equilibrium
Fluorescent probe	CMC of amphiphilic polymers
NMR spectroscopy	Dynamics
Dilute solution capillary viscometry	Hydrodynamic
Surface tension	CMC

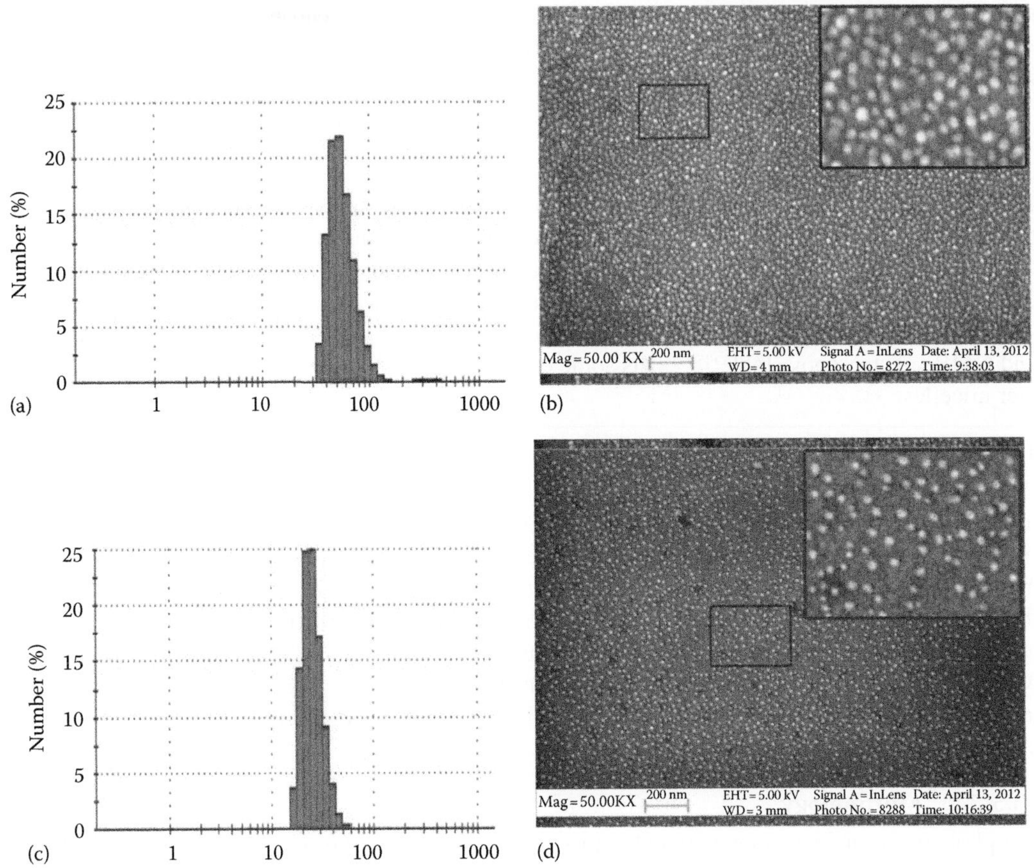

FIGURE 18.22 (a, c) The size histogram of cellulose-*g*-PCL micelles with different degree of substitution determined by DLS and (b, d) their SEM images. (From Guo, Y. et al., *Carbohydr. Polym.*, 92, 77, 2013b.)

18.5.3.3 CMC

CMC is the minimum required concentration for amphiphilic polymers to form micelles in selected solvent through self-assembling. Thus, the value of CMC is a vital parameter exhibiting the self-assembly ability of amphiphilic polymers. It is usually determined by fluorescent probes, UV-absorption spectroscopy (Dominguez et al. 1997), and surface tension. In recent years, fluorescent probe technique is the most commonly used method for the determination of CMC, which is easy to operate and has low interference and high sensitivity. It is based on the fluorescence of fluorescent probes, which can reflect the change in polarity of the solvent environment. Fluorescent probe, for example, pyrene, is water insoluble and shows weak fluorescence intensity in polar solvent such as water, while its fluorescence intensity is high in nonpolar solvents. Fluorescence emission spectrum of pyrene shows five peaks, and the ratio of first peak and the third peak, that is, I1/I3 will change as the polarity of the solvent changes. When the polymer concentration is below CMC, amphiphilic polymer will exist as molecular chains, then the fluorescence probe will present in the water. When the polymer concentration is higher than CMC, amphiphilic polymer will form micelles, and pyrene will be packaged in the micelles, where it will change to nonpolar environment from polar environment spontaneously, leading to the change in fluorescence emission spectra and the diminution of I1/I3. As amphiphilic polymer concentration increases, the number of micelles in solution increase, and more pyrene is coated in the hydrophobic core of micelles, while I1/I3 will

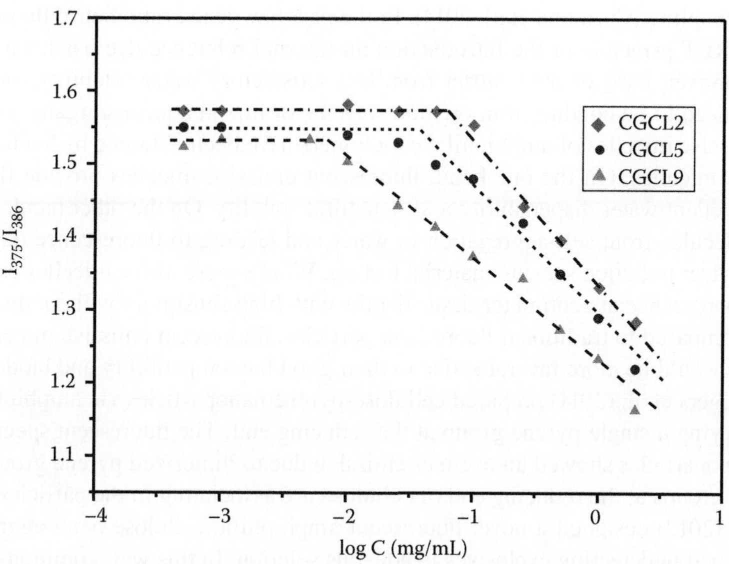

FIGURE 18.23 Experimental determination of CMC from fluorescence measurements with pyrene as a probe. Plots of the I1/I3 ratio of pyrene emission spectra in water as a function of the log concentration of cellulose-*g*-PCL copolymers. (From Guo, Y. et al., *Carbohydr. Polym.*, 92, 77, 2013b.)

reduce gradually. I1/I3 can be plotted as a function of concentration; the crossover value represents the CMC (seen in Figure 18.23) (Guo et al. 2013b).

18.6 APPLICATIONS OF AMPHIPHILIC CELLULOSE MICELLES

18.6.1 Drug Delivery

Amphiphilic copolymer micelles used for drug delivery have received widespread attention over the past decades. Micelles have been demonstrated to improve the apparent water solubility of hydrophobic drugs, including anticancer drugs (Hsieh et al. 2008). Moreover, with sizes ranging from tens of nanometers to several hundred nanometers, polymeric micelles can provide both passive targeting capabilities (usually through tumors' enhanced permeability and retention effect) and active targeting (usually using ligands, such as folic acid, and antibodies) (Tyrrell et al. 2010). In other words, it permits drugs to be steadily transported through the bloodstream, delivered to the tumor location, thereby decreasing side effects (Rösler et al. 2001). Dong et al. (2008) designed and synthesized a new biodegradable copolymer comprised of hydrophobic poly(L-lactide) (PLLA) segments and hydrophilic cellulose segment (cellulose-*g*-PLLA). The cellulose copolymer-self-assembled micelles can be carriers for the encapsulation of prednisone acetate. The drug-loading micelles show sustained drug release, which indicates potential applicability of its micelles in drug carrier. Bagheri and Shateri (2012b) prepared naproxen-loaded thermo-responsive self-assembled polymeric micelles composed of different cholesterol-based side chain and HPC. In vitro drug release study indicated that naproxen release from these micelles was thermosensitive as expected.

18.6.2 Fluorescent Sensing

Fluorescence resonance energy transfer (FRET) refers to a donor chromophore, initially in its electronic excited state, that may transfer energy to an acceptor chromophore through nonradiative dipole–dipole coupling (Carmona et al. 2014). In the past few years, ratiometric fluorescent probes based on the FRET principle or the introduction an internal reference dye has been reported (Hu et al. 2011). However, most of them suffer from less satisfactory water solubility, and the sensing measurements need to be conducted in organic solvents or mixed aqueous/organic solution. Thus, fluorescent emissive micelles of amphiphilic copolymers have been obtained by loading fluorescent probes into the micelles. On the one hand, fluorescent emissive micelles provide the fluorescent probes with excellent water dispersibility and structural stability. On the other hand, it can prevent fluorescent molecules from self-aggregation in water and leading to fluorescence quench, thereby can realize the river pollution sensing material testing. What's more, these micelles can be detected in vivo with fluorescence at centimeter tissue depths with high sensitivity without disturbing cellular function. Compared to traditional fluorescent particles, fluorescent emissive micelles of amphiphilic cellulose would be more favorable due to their good biocompatibility and biodegradability.

Enomoto-Rogers et al. (2011) prepared cellulose-pyrene nanoparticles via amphiphilic cellulose derivatives carrying a single pyrene group at the reducing end. The fluorescent spectrum of cellulose-pyrene nanoparticles showed an excimer emission due to dimerized pyrene groups, indicating that the pyrene groups at the reducing end of cellulose are associating in the particles.

Wang et al. (2012) designed a novel fluorescent amphiphilic cellulose nano-aggregate sensing system and applied in detecting explosives in aqueous solution. In this way, common commercially available light-emitting CPs are easily dispersed in water by encapsulating them in the amphiphilic cellulose nanocarriers, and their fluorescence properties are well kept.

18.6.3 Nanocontainer for Biological Probes

Recently, biological probes including quantum dot semiconductor materials, organic fluorescent polymers, and nano-Fe_3O_4 particles have showed good prospects in medical diagnosis and treatment. However, oil-soluble quantum dots have poor water solubility, and water-soluble quantum dots have obviously toxicity. Most organic fluorescent polymers are hydrophobic with low quantum efficiency in water. Similarly, nano-Fe_3O_4 particles are not stable and would self-aggregate together. These shortcomings greatly limit their clinical application as biological probes.

Since amphiphilic cellulose could self-assemble into nanocapsules in aqueous solution, they may be environmentally friendly when used as nanocontainers for biological probes like quantum dots and nano-Fe_3O_4. The hydrophobic biological probes are introduced into the core of micelles, which is protected by a hydrophilic shell with excellent biocompatibility and biodegradability. Therefore, amphiphilic cellulose micelles can not only protect the luminescent properties or paramagnetic of biological probes, but improve their biocompatibility and water solubility as well.

18.7 CONCLUSION

Recent years have seen great progress made in the study of amphiphilic cellulose-based graft copolymers. The amphiphilic cellulose-based graft copolymers with various molecular structures could be obtained either heterogeneously or homogeneously. Many new polymerization techniques including ATRP, ROP, and RAFT have been applied in the synthesis of amphiphilic cellulose-based graft copolymers. The amphiphilic cellulose-based graft copolymers mostly have brush-like molecular structures and show different crystalline properties and improved solubilities both in water and in organic solvents. The self-assembly of amphiphilic cellulose-based graft copolymers has been studied and reported by many groups, most of which revealed that their self-assembling behaviors correlated with the molecular structures. The size, size distribution, morphology, and CMC of the self-assembled nanoparticles of amphiphilic cellulose can be characterized by DLS, TEM, SEM, AFM, photoluminescence, etc. Exciting application potentials of the self-assembled amphiphilic cellulose nanomicelles in drug delivery and fluorescent sensing, and as container of bioprobes have been established.

REFERENCES

Alexandridis, P. 1996. Amphiphilic copolymers and their applications. *Current Opinion in Colloid and Interface Science*, 1, 490–501.

Bagheri, M. and Shateri, S. 2012a. Synthesis and characterization of novel liquid crystalline cholesteryl-modified hydroxypropyl cellulose derivatives. *Journal of Polymer Research*, 19, 1–13.

Bagheri, M. and Shateri, S. 2012b. Thermosensitive nanosized micelles from cholesteryl-modified hydroxypropyl cellulose as a novel carrier of hydrophobic drugs. *Iranian Polymer Journal*, 21, 365–373.

Berthier, D. L., Herrmann, A., and Ouali, L. 2011. Synthesis of hydroxypropyl cellulose derivatives modified with amphiphilic diblock copolymer side-chains for the slow release of volatile molecules. *Polymer Chemistry*, 2, 2093–2101.

Brown, W., Schillen, K., and Hvidt, S. 1992. Triblock copolymers in aqueous solution studied by static and dynamic light scattering and oscillatory shear measurements: Influence of relative block sizes. *The Journal of Physical Chemistry*, 96, 6038–6044.

Butun, V., Billingham, N. C., and Armes, S. P. 1998. Synthesis of shell cross-linked micelles with tunable hydrophilic/hydrophobic cores. *Journal of the American Chemical Society*, 120, 12135–12136.

Cai, J. and Zhang, L. 2005. Rapid dissolution of cellulose in LiOH/urea and NaOH/urea aqueous solutions. *Macromolecular Bioscience*, 5, 539–548.

Cao, Y. and Li, H. 1999. Synthesis of a novel family of polymeric surfactants with low interfacial tension by ultrasonic method. *Polymer Journal*, 31, 920–923.

Cao, Y. and Li, H. 2003. Micellar solutions of amphipathic copolymers based on carboxymethyl cellulose. *Polymer International*, 52, 869–875.

Carlmark, A. and Malmström, E. 2002. Atom transfer radical polymerization from cellulose fibers at ambient temperature. *Journal of the American Chemical Society*, 124, 900–901.

Carlmark, A. and Malmström, E. 2003. ATRP grafting from cellulose fibers to create block-copolymer grafts. *Biomacromolecules*, 4, 1740–1745.

Carmona, F., Munoz-Robles, V., Cuesta, R., Galvez, N., Capdevila, M., Marechal, J. D., and Dominguez-Vera, J. M. 2014. Monitoring lactoferrin iron levels by fluorescence resonance energy transfer: A combined chemical and computational study. *Journal of Biological Inorganic Chemistry*, 19, 439–447.

Charpentier, D., Mocanu, G., Carpov, A., Chapelle, S., Merle, L., and M Ller, G. 1997. New hydrophobically modified carboxymethylcellulose derivatives. *Carbohydrate Polymers*, 33, 177–186.

Cheng, Y., Wang, S., Yu, Y., and Yuan, Y. 2003. In vitro, in vivo studies of a new amphiphilic adsorbent for the removal of low-density lipoprotein. *Biomaterials*, 24, 2189–2194.

Dai, S., Ye, L., and Huang, R. 2006. A study on the solution behavior of IPBC-hydrophobically-modified hydroxyethyl cellulose. *Journal of Applied Polymer Science*, 100, 2824–2831.

Dawsey, T. R. and Mccormick, C. L. 1990. The lithium chloride/dimethylacetamide solvent for cellulose: A literature review. *Journal of Macromolecular Science, Part C*, 30, 405–440.

de Boer, B., Stalmach, U., Van Hutten, P. F., Melzer, C., Krasnikov, V. V., and Hadziioannou, G. 2001. Supramolecular self-assembly and opto-electronic properties of semiconducting block copolymers. *Polymer*, 42, 9097–9109.

Denker, U., Dashiell, M. W., Jin-Phillipp, N. Y., and Schmidt, O. G. 2002. Trenches around and between self assembled silicon/germanium islands grown on silicon substrates investigated by atomic force microscopy. *Materials Science and Engineering: B*, 89, 166–170.

Dominguez, A., Fernandez, A., Gonzalez, N., Iglesias, E., and Montenegro, L. 1997. Determination of critical micelle concentration of some surfactants by three techniques. *Journal of Chemical Education*, 74, 1227.

Dong, H., Xu, Q., Li, Y., Mo, S., Cai, S., and Liu, L. 2008. The synthesis of biodegradable graft copolymer cellulose-*graft*-poly(L-lactide) and the study of its controlled drug release. *Colloids and Surfaces B: Biointerfaces*, 66, 26–33.

Dou, H. J., Jiang, M., Peng, H. S., Chen, D. Y., and Hong, Y. 2003. pH-dependent self-assembly: Micellization and micelle-hollow-sphere transition of cellulose-based copolymers. *Angewandte Chemie-International Edition*, 42, 1516–1519.

Dubertret, B., Skourides, P., Norris, D. J., Noireaux, V., Brivanlou, A. H., and Libchaber, A. 2002. In vivo imaging of quantum dots encapsulated in phospholipid micelles. *Science*, 298, 1759–1762.

Enomoto-Rogers, Y., Kamitakahara, H., Takano, T., and Nakatsubo, F. 2006. Synthesis of diblock copolymers with cellulose derivatives. 3. Cellulose derivatives carrying a single pyrene group at the reducing-end and fluorescent studies of their self-assembly systems in aqueous NaOH solutions. *Cellulose*, 13, 437–448.

Enomoto-Rogers, Y., Kamitakahara, H., Yoshinaga, A., and Takano, T. 2011. Synthesis of diblock copolymers with cellulose derivatives 4. Self-assembled nanoparticles of amphiphilic cellulose derivatives carrying a single pyrene group at the reducing-end. *Cellulose*, 18, 1005–1014.

Francis, M. F., Piredda, M., and Winnik, F. M. 2003. Solubilization of poorly water soluble drugs in micelles of hydrophobically modified hydroxypropylcellulose copolymers. *Journal of Controlled Release*, 93, 59–68.

Gebhardt, R., Doster, W., Friedrich, J., and Kulozik, U. 2006. Size distribution of pressure-decomposed casein micelles studied by dynamic light scattering and AFM. *European Biophysics Journal*, 35, 503–509.

Griffith, L. G. and Naughton, G. 2002. Tissue engineering—Current challenges and expanding opportunities. *Science*, 295, 1009–1014.

Guo, Y., Liu, Q., Chen, H., Wang, X., Shen, Z., Shu, X., and Sun, R. 2013a. Direct grafting modification of pulp in ionic liquids and self-assembly behavior of the graft copolymers. *Cellulose*, 20, 873–884.

Guo, Y., Wang, X., Shen, Z., Shu, X., and Sun, R. 2013b. Preparation of cellulose-*graft*-poly(ε-caprolactone) nanomicelles by homogeneous ROP in ionic liquid. *Carbohydrate Polymers*, 92, 77–83.

Guo, Y., Wang, X., Shu, X., Shen, Z., and Sun, R.-C. 2012. Self-assembly and paclitaxel loading capacity of cellulose-*graft*-poly(lactide) nanomicelles. *Journal of Agricultural and Food Chemistry*, 60, 3900–3908.

Guo, Y., Wang, X., Shu, X., Shen, Z., and Sun, R.-C. 2012. Synthesis and characterization of hydrophobic long-chain fatty acylated cellulose and its self-assembled nanoparticles. *Polymer Bulletin*, 69, 389–403.

Habibi, Y. and Dufresne, A. 2008. Highly filled bionanocomposites from functionalized polysaccharide nanocrystals. *Biomacromolecules*, 9, 1974–1980.

Hassani, L. N., Hendra, F., and Bouchemal, K. 2012. Auto-associative amphiphilic polysaccharides as drug delivery systems. *Drug Discovery Today*, 17, 608–614.

He, F. and Zhao, D. 2005. Preparation and characterization of a new class of starch-stabilized bimetallic nanoparticles for degradation of chlorinated hydrocarbons in water. *Environmental Science and Technology*, 39, 3314–3320.

Heinze, T., Schwikal, K., and Barthel, S. 2005. Ionic liquids as reaction medium in cellulose functionalization. *Macromolecular Bioscience*, 5, 520–525.

Hong, P., Fa, C., Wei, Y., and Sen, Z. 2007. Surface properties and synthesis of the cellulose-based amphoteric polymeric surfactant. *Carbohydrate Polymers*, 69, 625–630.

Hsieh, M. F., Cuong, N. V., Chen, C. H., Chen, Y. T., and Yeh, J. M. 2008. Nano-sized micelles of block copolymers of methoxy poly(ethylene glycol)-poly(epsilon-caprolactone)-*graft*-2-hydroxyethyl cellulose for doxorubicin delivery. *Journal of Nanoscience and Nanotechnology*, 8, 2362–2368.

Hu, J., Dai, L., and Liu, S. 2011. Analyte-reactive amphiphilic thermoresponsive diblock copolymer micelles-based multifunctional ratiometric fluorescent chemosensors. *Macromolecules*, 44, 4699–4710.

Hwang, F. S. and Hogen-Esch, T. E. 1993. Fluorocarbon-modified water-soluble cellulose derivatives. *Macromolecules*, 26, 3156–3160.

Ifuku, S. and Kadla, J. F. 2008. Preparation of a thermosensitive highly regioselective cellulose/*N*-isopropylacrylamide copolymer through atom transfer radical polymerization. *Biomacromolecules*, 9, 3308–3313.

Jiang, C., Wang, X., Sun, P., and Yang, C. 2011. Synthesis and solution behavior of poly(ε-caprolactone) grafted hydroxyethyl cellulose copolymers. *International Journal of Biological Macromolecules*, 48, 210–214.

Kang, H., Liu, W., He, B., Shen, D., Ma, L., and Huang, Y. 2006. Synthesis of amphiphilic ethyl cellulose grafting poly(acrylic acid) copolymers and their self-assembly morphologies in water. *Polymer*, 47, 7927–7934.

Kang, H., Liu, W., Liu, R., and Huang, Y. 2008. A novel, amphiphilic ethyl cellulose grafting copolymer with poly(2-hydroxyethyl methacrylate) side chains and its micellization. *Macromolecular Chemistry and Physics*, 209, 424–430.

Kästner, U., Hoffmann, H., Donges, R., and Ehrler, R. 1994. Hydrophobically and cationically modified hydroxyethyl cellulose and their interactions with surfactants. *Colloids and Surfaces A: Physicochemical and Engineering Aspects*, 82, 279–297.

Krouit, M., Bras, J., and Belgacem, M. N. 2008. Cellulose surface grafting with polycaprolactone by heterogeneous click-chemistry. *European Polymer Journal*, 44, 4074–4081.

Kuang, M., Duan, H., Wang, J., Chen, D., and Jiang, M. 2003. A novel approach to polymeric hollow nanospheres with stabilized structure. *Chemical Communications*, 496–497.

Labet, M. and Thielemans, W. 2011. Improving the reproducibility of chemical reactions on the surface of cellulose nanocrystals: ROP of epsilon-caprolactone as a case study. *Cellulose*, 18, 607–617.

Landoll, L. M. 1982a. Nonionic polymer surfactants. *Journal of Polymer Science: Polymer Chemistry Edition*, 20, 1649–1649.

Landoll, L. M. 1982b. Nonionic polymer surfactants. *Journal of Polymer Science: Polymer Chemistry Edition*, 20, 443–455.

Lapasin, R. and Pricl, S. 1995. The polysaccharides: Sources and structures. *Rheology of Industrial Polysaccharides: Theory and Applications*. Blackie Academic and Professional. Springer.

López-Velázquez D., Bello, A., and Pérez, E. 2004. Preparation and characterisation of hydrophobically modified hydroxypropylcellulose: Side-chain crystallisation. *Macromolecular Chemistry and Physics*, 205, 1886–1892.

Lee, Y., Lee, J., Bae, C. J., Park, J. G., Noh, H. J., Park, J. H., and Hyeon, T. 2005. Large-scale synthesis of uniform and crystalline magnetite nanoparticles using reverse micelles as nanoreactors under reflux conditions. *Advanced Functional Materials*, 15, 503–509.

Leventis, N., Mulik, S., Wang, X. J., Dass, A., Patil, V. U., Sotiriou-Leventis, C., Lu, H. B., Chum, G., and Capecelatro, A. 2008. Polymer nano-encapsulation of templated mesoporous silica monoliths with improved mechanical properties. *Journal of Non-Crystalline Solids*, 354, 632–644.

Li, Q., Ye, L., Cai, Y., and Huang, R. 2006. Study of rheological behavior of hydrophobically modified hydroxyethyl cellulose. *Journal of Applied Polymer Science*, 100, 3346–3352.

Li, Y., Liu, R., Liu, W., Kang, H., Wu, M., and Huang, Y. 2008. Synthesis, self-assembly, and thermosensitive properties of ethyl cellulose-*g*-P(PEGMA) amphiphilic copolymers. *Journal of Polymer Science Part A: Polymer Chemistry*, 46, 6907–6915.

Lindqvist, J., Nystrom, D., Östmark, E., Antoni, P., Carlmark, A., Johansson, M., Hult, A., and Malmström, E. 2008. Intelligent dual-responsive cellulose surfaces via surface-initiated ATRP. *Biomacromolecules*, 9, 2139–2145.

Liu, J., Lee, H., and Allen, C. 2006. Formulation of drugs in block copolymer micelles: Drug loading and release. *Current Pharmaceutical Design*, 12, 4685–4701.

Liu, L., Guo, K., Lu, J., Venkatraman, S. S., Luo, D., Ng, K. C., Ling, E.-A., Moochhala, S., and Yang, Y.-Y. 2008a. Biologically active core/shell nanoparticles self-assembled from cholesterol-terminated PEG-TAT for drug delivery across the blood-brain barrier. *Biomaterials*, 29, 1509–1517.

Liu, S., Weaver, J. V. M., Save, M., and Armes, S. P. 2002. Synthesis of pH-responsive shell cross-linked micelles and their use as nanoreactors for the preparation of gold nanoparticles. *Langmuir*, 18, 8350–8357.

Liu, W., Liu, R., Li, Y., Kang, H., Shen, D., Wu, M., and Huang, Y. 2009. Self-assembly of ethyl cellulose-*graft*-polystyrene copolymers in acetone. *Polymer*, 50, 211–217.

Liu, X., Chen, J., Sun, P., Liu, Z.-W., and Liu, Z.-T. 2010. Grafting modification of ramie fibers with poly(2,2,2-trifluoroethyl methacrylate) via reversible addition-fragmentation chain transfer (RAFT) polymerization in supercritical carbon dioxide. *Reactive and Functional Polymers*, 70, 972–979.

Liu, Z. T., Sun, C., Liu, Z. W., and Lu, J. 2008b. Adjustable wettability of methyl methacrylate modified ramie fiber. *Journal of Applied Polymer Science*, 109, 2888–2894.

Lonnberg, H., Fogelstrom, L., Berglund, M. A. S. A. S. L., Malmström, E., and Hult, A. 2008. Surface grafting of microfibrillated cellulose with poly(epsilon-caprolactone)—Synthesis and characterization. *European Polymer Journal*, 44, 2991–2997.

Ma, L., Kang, H., Liu, R., and Huang, Y. 2010a. Smart assembly behaviors of hydroxypropylcellulose-*graft*-poly(4-vinyl pyridine) copolymers in aqueous solution by thermo and pH stimuli. *Langmuir*, 26, 18519–18525.

Ma, L., Liu, R., Tan, J., Wang, D., Jin, X., Kang, H., Wu, M., and Huang, Y. 2010b. Self-assembly and dual-stimuli sensitivities of hydroxypropylcellulose-*graft*-poly(*N*,*N*-dimethyl aminoethyl methacrylate) copolymers in aqueous solution. *Langmuir*, 26, 8697–8703.

Martin, A. H., Douglas Goff, H., Smith, A., and Dalgleish, D. G. 2006. Immobilization of casein micelles for probing their structure and interactions with polysaccharides using scanning electron microscopy (SEM). *Food Hydrocolloids*, 20, 817–824.

Martin, T. J., Procházka, K., Munk, P., and Webber, S. E. 1996. pH-dependent micellization of poly(2-vinylpyridine)-*block*-poly(ethylene oxide). *Macromolecules*, 29, 6071–6073.

Meng, T., Gao, X., Zhang, J., Yuan, J. Y., Zhang, Y. Z., and He, J. S. 2009. Graft copolymers prepared by atom transfer radical polymerization (ATRP) from cellulose. *Polymer*, 50, 447–454.

Nishimura, H., Donkai, N., and Miyamoto, T. 1997. Preparation and properties of a new type of comb-shaped, amphiphilic cellulose derivative. *Cellulose*, 4, 89–98.

Östmark, E., Harrisson, S., Wooley, K. L., and Malmström, E. 2007. Comb polymers prepared by ATRP from hydroxypropyl cellulose. *Biomacromolecules*, 8, 1138–1148.

Östmark, E., Nystr M. D., and Malmström, E. 2008. Unimolecular nanocontainers prepared by ROP and subsequent ATRP from hydroxypropylcellulose. *Macromolecules*, 41, 4405–4415.

O'Sullivan, A. 1997. Cellulose: The structure slowly unravels. *Cellulose*, 4, 173–207.

Otsuka, H., Nagasaki, Y., and Kataoka, K. 2001. Self-assembly of poly(ethylene glycol)-based block copolymers for biomedical applications. *Current Opinion in Colloid and Interface Science*, 6, 3–10.
Qi, H., Chang, C., and Zhang, L. 2008. Effects of temperature and molecular weight on dissolution of cellulose in NaOH/urea aqueous solution. *Cellulose*, 15, 779–787.
Qiu, X. and Hu, S. 2013. "Smart" materials based on cellulose: A review of the preparations, properties, and applications. *Materials*, 6, 738–781.
Rodr Guez-Hern Ndez, J., Ch Cot, F., Gnanou, Y., and Lecommandoux, S. 2005. Toward 'smart' nano-objects by self-assembly of block copolymers in solution. *Progress in Polymer Science*, 30, 691–724.
Rösler, A., Vandermeulen, G. W. M., and Klok, H.-A. 2001. Advanced drug delivery devices via self-assembly of amphiphilic block copolymers. *Advanced Drug Delivery Reviews*, 53, 95–108.
Rösler, A., Vandermeulen, G. W. M., and Klok, H.-A. 2012. Advanced drug delivery devices via self-assembly of amphiphilic block copolymers. *Advanced Drug Delivery Reviews*, 64(Supplement), 270–279.
Roy, D., Guthrie, J. T., and Perrier, S. 2008a. Synthesis of natural-synthetic hybrid materials from cellulose via the RAFT process. *Soft Matter*, 4, 145–155.
Roy, D., Knapp, J. S., Guthrie, J. T., and Perrier, S. 2008b. Antibacterial cellulose fiber via RAFT surface graft polymerization. *Biomacromolecules*, 9, 91–99.
Schaeferling, M., Schiller, S., Paul, H., Kruschina, M., Pavlickova, P., Meerkamp, M., Giammasi, C., and Kambhampati, D. 2002. Application of self-assembly techniques in the design of biocompatible protein microarray surfaces. *Electrophoresis*, 23, 3097–3105.
Shen, D., Yu, H., and Huang, Y. 2005. Densely grafting copolymers of ethyl cellulose through atom transfer radical polymerization. *Journal of Polymer Science Part A: Polymer Chemistry*, 43, 4099–4108.
Shen, D., Yu, H., and Huang, Y. 2006. Synthesis of graft copolymer of ethyl cellulose through living polymerization and its self-assembly. *Cellulose*, 13, 235–244.
Shi, R. and Burt, H. M. 2003. Synthesis and characterization of amphiphilic hydroxypropylcellulose-*graft*-poly(ε-caprolactone). *Journal of Applied Polymer Science*, 89, 718–727.
Song, Y., Zhang, L., Gan, W., and Zhou, J. 2011a. Self-assembled micelles based on hydrophobically modified quaternized cellulose for drug delivery. *Colloids and Surface B: Biointerfaces*, 83, 313–320.
Song, Y., Zhang, L., Gan, W., Zhou, J., and Zhang, L. 2011b. Self-assembled micelles based on hydrophobically modified quaternized cellulose for drug delivery. *Colloids and Surfaces B: Biointerfaces*, 83, 313–320.
Srokova, I., Talaba, P., Hodul, P., and Balazova, A. 1998. Emulsifying agents based on *O*-(carboxymethyl)cellulose. *Tenside Surfactants Detergents*, 35, 342–344.
Srokova, I., Tomanova, V., Ebringerova, A., Malovikova, A., and Heinze, T. 2004. Water-soluble amphiphilic *O*-(carboxymethyl)cellulose derivatives—Synthesis and properties. *Macromolecular Materials and Engineering*, 289, 63–69.
Sui, X., Yuan, J., Zhou, M., Zhang, J., Yang, H., Yuan, W., Wei, Y., and Pan, C. 2008. Synthesis of cellulose-*graft*-poly(*N,N*-dimethylamino-2-ethyl methacrylate) copolymers via homogeneous ATRP and their aggregates in aqueous media. *Biomacromolecules*, 9, 2615–2620.
Tan, J., Li, Y., Liu, R., Kang, H., Wang, D., Ma, L., Liu, W., Wu, M., and Huang, Y. 2010. Micellization and sustained drug release behavior of EC-*g*-PPEGMA amphiphilic copolymers. *Carbohydrate Polymers*, 81, 213–218.
Taylor, K. C. and Nasr-El-Din, H. A. 1998. Water-soluble hydrophobically associating polymers for improved oil recovery: A literature review. *Journal of Petroleum Science and Engineering*, 19, 265–280.
Tizzotti, M., Charlot, A., Fleury, E., Stenzel, M., and Bernard, J. 2010. Modification of polysaccharides through controlled/living radical polymerization grafting—Towards the generation of high performance hybrids. *Macromolecular Rapid Communications*, 31, 1751–1772.
Tyrrell, Z. L., Shen, Y., and Radosz, M. 2010. Fabrication of micellar nanoparticles for drug delivery through the self-assembly of block copolymers. *Progress in Polymer Science*, 35, 1128–1143.
Vidal, R. R. L., Balaban, R., and Borsali, R. 2008. Amphiphilic derivatives of carboxymethylcellulose: Evidence for intra-and intermolecular hydrophobic associations in aqueous solutions. *Polymer Engineering and Science*, 48, 2011–2026.
Wan, S., Jiang, M., and Zhang, G. 2007. Dual temperature- and pH-dependent self-assembly of cellulose-based copolymer with a pair of complementary grafts. *Macromolecules*, 40, 5552–5558.
Wang, D. Q., Tan, J. J., Kang, H. L., Ma, L., Jin, X., Liu, R. G., and Huang, Y. 2011. Synthesis, self-assembly and drug release behaviors of pH-responsive copolymers ethyl cellulose-*graft*-PDEAEMA through ATRP. *Carbohydrate Polymers*, 84, 195–202.
Wang, X., Guo, Y., Li, D., Chen, H., and Sun, R.-C. 2012. Fluorescent amphiphilic cellulose nanoaggregates for sensing trace explosives in aqueous solution. *Chemical Communications*, 48, 5569–5571.

Wasielewski, M. R. 2009. Self-assembly strategies for integrating light harvesting and charge separation in artificial photosynthetic systems. *Accounts of Chemical Research*, 42, 1910–1921.

Wei, Y. and Cheng, F. 2007. Synthesis and aggregates of cellulose-based hydrophobically associating polymer. *Carbohydrate Polymers*, 68, 734–739.

Wei, Y., Cheng, F., Hou, G., and Sun, S. 2008. Amphiphilic cellulose: Surface activity and aqueous self-assembly into nano-sized polymeric micelles. *Reactive and Functional Polymers*, 68, 981–989.

Winter, A., Friebe, C., Chiper, M., Hager, M. D., and Schubert, U. S. 2009. Self-assembly of π-conjugated bis(terpyridine) ligands with zinc(II) ions: New metallosupramolecular materials for optoelectronic applications. *Journal of Polymer Science Part A: Polymer Chemistry*, 47, 4083–4098.

Xu, Q., Kennedy, J. F., and Liu, L. 2008. An ionic liquid as reaction media in the ring opening graft polymerization of ε-caprolactone onto starch granules. *Carbohydrate Polymers*, 72, 113–121.

Xu, R., Winnik, M. A., Hallett, F. R., Riess, G., and Croucher, M. D. 1991. Light-scattering study of the association behavior of styrene-ethylene oxide block copolymers in aqueous solution. *Macromolecules*, 24, 87–93.

Yamaguchi, A., Uejo, F., Yoda, T., Uchida, T., Tanamura, Y., Yamashita, T., and Teramae, N. 2004. Self-assembly of a silica-surfactant nanocomposite in a porous alumina membrane. *Nature Materials*, 3, 337–341.

Yan, C., Zhang, J., Lv, Y., Yu, J., Wu, J., Zhang, J., and He, J. 2009a. Thermoplastic cellulose-*graft*-poly(L-lactide) copolymers homogeneously synthesized in an ionic liquid with 4-dimethylaminopyridine catalyst. *Biomacromolecules*, 10, 2013–2018.

Yan, Q., Yuan, J., Zhang, F., Sui, X., Xie, X., Yin, Y., Wang, S., and Wei, Y. 2009b. Cellulose-based dual graft molecular brushes as potential drug nanocarriers: Stimulus-responsive micelles, self-assembled phase transition behavior, and tunable crystalline morphologies. *Biomacromolecules*, 10, 2033–2042.

Yang, L., Kuang, J., Li, Z., Zhang, B., Cai, X., and Zhang, L.-M. 2008a. Amphiphilic cholesteryl-bearing carboxymethylcellulose derivatives: Self-assembly and rheological behaviour in aqueous solution. *Cellulose*, 15, 659–669.

Yang, L., Kuang, J., Wang, J., Li, Z., and Zhang, L.-M. 2008b. Loading and in vitro controlled release of indomethacin using amphiphilic cholesteryl-bearing carboxymethylcellulose derivatives. *Macromolecular Bioscience*, 8, 279–286.

Ye, L., Li, Q., and Huang, R. 2006. Study on the rheological behavior of the hydrophobically modified hydroxyethyl cellulose with 1,2-epoxyhexadecane*. *Journal of Applied Polymer Science*, 101, 2953–2959.

Yuan, W. Z., Zhang, J. C., Zou, H., Shen, T. X., and Ren, J. 2012. Amphiphilic ethyl cellulose brush polymers with mono and dual side chains: Facile synthesis, self-assembly, and tunable temperature-pH responsivities. *Polymer*, 53, 956–966.

Zhang, H., Wu, J., Zhang, J., and He, J. 2005. 1-Allyl-3-methylimidazolium chloride room temperature ionic liquid: A new and powerful nonderivatizing solvent for cellulose. *Macromolecules*, 38, 8272–8277.

Zhang, J., Zhang, L.-M., and Li, Z.-M. 2000. Synthesis and aqueous solution properties of hydrophobically modified graft copolymer of sodium carboxymethylcellulose with acrylamide and dimethyloctyl(2-methacryloxyethyl)ammonium bromide. *Journal of Applied Polymer Science*, 78, 537–542.

Zhang, L., Ruan, D., and Gao, S. 2002. Dissolution and regeneration of cellulose in NaOH/thiourea aqueous solution. *Journal of Polymer Science Part B: Polymer Physics*, 40, 1521–1529.

19 Hydroxypropyl Cellulose-Based Graft Copolymers

Structure, Properties, and Application

Massoumeh Bagheri

CONTENTS

19.1 INTRODUCTION

Cellulose is the most abundant biopolymer in nature and has attracted increasing attention in both scientific and industrial aspects [1]. It is produced by plants, algae, tunicates, and some bacterial cultures [2]. The currently growing interest in the study of cellulose and its derivatives is due to the tendency toward rational use of renewable sources as a basis for the production of new products for science, medicine, and engineering. Cellulose is colorless and odorless and possesses some promising properties, such as superior mechanical strength, biocompatibility, nontoxicity, biodegradability, accessibility, hydrophilicity, relative thermostabilization, high sorption capacity, and alterable optical appearance [3].

Cellulose is a linear polymer of β (1 → 4)-linked D-glucose unit with three hydroxyl groups on each anhydroglucose unit of cellulose, enabling strong cooperative intra- and intermolecular hydrogen bond patterns, stiffening the chain and forming mechanically stable and insoluble fibrils

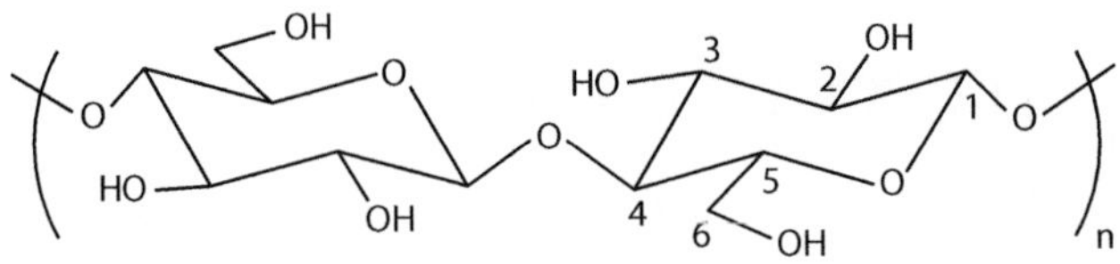

FIGURE 19.1 Chemical structure of cellulose.

and fibers (Figure 19.1). The molecular size of cellulose can be defined by its average degree of polymerization (DP). The DP values of cellulose samples differ widely, depending on origin and pretreatment. It is insoluble in water and most other common solvents. In addition, the β-acetal linkage in cellulose makes it indigestible in humans [2].

Owing to a number of earlier-mentioned valuable properties, high-quality cellulose is a required multipurpose product and the original basis for producing a wide spectrum of new materials, including nanomaterials [4], for use in various fields of science and industry: pharmaceutical, biomedical, electronic, food, wood pulp and paper, textile, etc. [5]. Due to the three hydroxyl groups within one anhydroglucose and due to the polymeric character of the cellulose, a great variety of structural modifications of cellulose and combinations are possible to prepare cellulose derivatives with desired properties for specific applications in industry, coatings, pharmaceutics, and domestic commodities. The primary hydroxyl group at C-6 and the two secondary ones at C-2 and C-3 (Figure 19.1) can participate in all the classical reactions as the alcoholic hydroxyl group does, including esterification, etherification, oxidation reactions, nucleophilic substitution, grafting copolymerization, and regioselective introduction of functional groups [6].

19.1.1 Cellulose Ethers

Cellulose ethers are still the most important and significant cellulose derivatives. These cellulose derivatives, particularly those that are water soluble, constitute a class of polymers that have attracted considerable interest for certain conservation applications. Cellulose ethers are generally synthesized by etherification of cellulose or Michael addition in heterogeneous or homogeneous media (Figure 19.2) [7,8].

Due to the high crystallinity, modification of cellulose is commonly performed in heterogeneous processes, in which chemical reactions occur only at the surface. In homogeneous conditions, the crystallinity of the cellulose tends to be destroyed by treatment with alkali, and in the ideal case, all glucose residues should become equally accessible. Thus, well-defined cellulose materials can be obtained through chemical modifications in homogeneous conditions [9]. The properties of a modified cellulose depend on several factors, such as the modification reaction, the nature of the substitution group, the degree of substitution (DS), and the distribution of the substitution groups. DS is defined as the average number of substituted hydroxyl groups of glucose residue and is thus in the range of 0–3 as long as end groups can be neglected. For modifications, including tandem reactions, a molar degree of substitution (MS) is additionally defined as the average number of substituent groups linked to glucose residues, that is, in the DS range of up to a theoretically unlimited level.

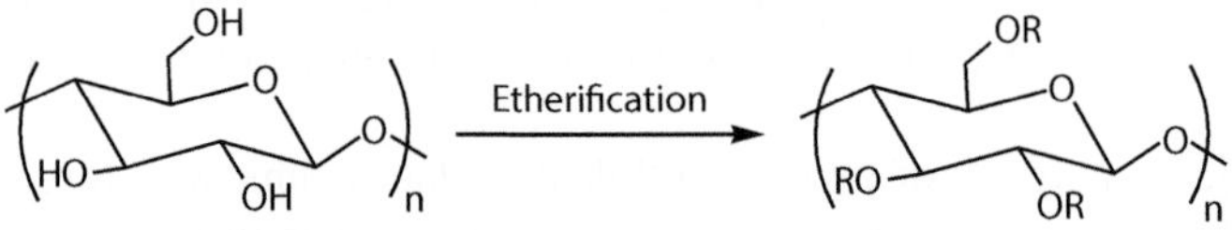

FIGURE 19.2 Synthesis of cellulose ethers. Cellulose ether: R = H, alkyl, hydroxyalkyl, sulfoalkyl, aralkyl, silyl, etc., groups.

TABLE 19.1
Cellulose Ethers

Substitution Group	Abbreviations of Commercial Product	Etherifying Agent	By-Products	Field of Application
Methyl	MC, HPMC	CH_3Cl	Methanol, dimethyl ether	Building materials, paint removers
Ethyl	EC, EHEC	C_2H_5Cl	Ethanol, diethyl ether	Paints, lacquers
Hydroxyethyl	HEC, EHEC	Ethylene oxide	Ethylene glycol and polymers thereof	Paints, emulsions, drilling mud
Hydroxypropyl	HPC, HPMC	Propylene oxide	Propylene glycol and polymers thereof	Building materials, paints, tablets
Carboxymethyl	CMC	$Cl\text{-}CH_2\text{-}COOH$	Glycolic acid	Detergents, textiles, food products

The chemical modification of cellulose fibers with the etherifying agent results in the introduction of side chains into the polymeric backbone of cellulose. This chemical modification is mainly done to convert the water-insoluble cellulose to water-soluble derivative (cellulose ether) [10]. In general, an excess of etherifying agent over the minimum required for the desired DS must be used because organic by-products are formed. Table 19.1 provides a list of some typical reagents, co-products, and by-products.

No major co-product such as NaCl is formed in etherification with ethylene oxide or propylene oxide because the sodium hydroxide is only a catalyst [11]. The most widespread ethers are the sodium salt of carboxymethyl cellulose, hydroxypropyl cellulose (HPC), and methyl cellulose.

The interest of researchers to cellulose ethers has remained, and their modification has been studied to improve their water solubilities and to study the effect of substituents and the DS on their properties.

19.2 HYDROXYPROPYL CELLULOSE

19.2.1 Chemical Structure, Preparation, and Properties

Among the cellulose ethers, HPC has the unique advantages of considerable hydrophilicity, special phase behavior, ease of production, and thermal sensitivity and has been widely applied in the pharmaceutical, food, and biomedical fields [12]. It has been approved by the US Food and Drug Administration in biomedical and pharmaceutical applications for its nontoxicity, biocompatibility, and biodegradability [13].

Water-soluble HPC has been produced through the modification of hydroxyl group in the 2-, 3-, and 6-positions of anhydroglucose ring unit of cellulose with very reactive propylene oxide reagent (Figure 19.3). In this substitution reaction, the cellulose molecule should first be activated to make the O–H bond nucleophilic and to facilitate the formation of alkali cellulose

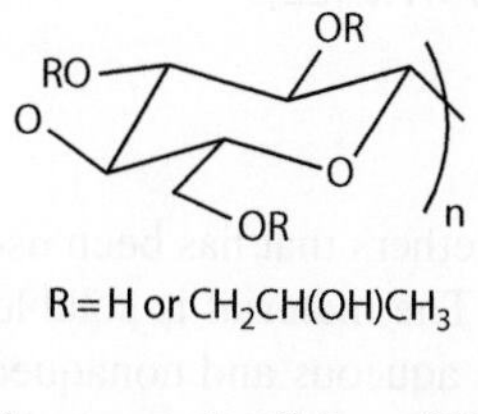

FIGURE 19.3 Chemical structure of hydroxypropyl cellulose (HPC).

(cellulose-O⁻). Alkaline reagents in this regard are excellent as catalysts for the formation of alkali cellulose. This alkalization step is to be followed by the reaction of cellulose-O– with propylene oxide, which results in the formation of HPC through bimolecular substitution reaction. The efficiency of hydroxypropylation reaction is greatly influenced by the reagents used as well as the reaction conditions [14]. This chemical modification significantly increases the solubility of the biopolymer in organic solvents, but its reactivity is maintained because the number of hydroxyl side groups is unaffected. The low solubility of HPC in organic solvents has been attributed to the hydrogen bonding interactions present in this system, involving the hydroxyl functionalities along the polymer chains [15].

The average number of substituted hydroxyl groups per glucose unit is referred to as the degree of substitution (DS_{HP}). Complete substitution would provide a DS_{HP} of 3. Because the hydroxypropyl group added contains a hydroxyl group, this can also be etherified during the preparation of HPC. When this occurs, the number of moles of hydroxypropyl groups per glucose ring, moles of substitution (MS_{HP}), can be higher than 3. Because cellulose is very crystalline, HPC must have an MS_{HP} about 4 in order to reach a good solubility in water. The average molecular weight, MS_{HP}, and distribution of substituent determine the properties of the prepared HPC [14,16].

HPC is a temperature-responsive derivative of natural macromolecules and exhibits a lower critical solution temperature (LCST) in aqueous solution in the range of 41°C–45°C [17] and a remarkable hydration–dehydration change in aqueous solution in response to relative changes in temperature around the LCST [5]. At temperatures below the LCST, HPC is readily soluble in water, and therefore, the solution becomes turbid on heating above LCST. The DS on HPC influences the intermolecular interactions so the onset of turbidity during heating. This phenomenon has been studied in dilute HPC solutions using various experimental techniques like turbidimetry, viscometry, rheology, laser light scattering, and differential scanning calorimetry (DSC) from a macroscopic scale [18]. Carotenuto et al. found that concentrated HPC solution (20 wt%) would subject to another sol–gel transition at even higher temperature using rheological method [19]. Jing and Wu [20] reported that during the heating process from 35°C to 63°C, HPC concentrated aqueous solution (20 wt%) would first go through coil-to-globule transition and then sol–gel transition with temperature elevation. Both the coil-to-globule transition and the sol–gel transition at different temperatures in the same HPC solution (20 wt%) were well studied using both middle- and near-infrared spectroscopy. They discovered that the driving force of the coil-to-globule transition process in micro-dynamics could only be the dehydration and hydrophobic interactions of C–H groups. However, in the sol–gel transition, the system cross-linked to form a physical network with no mobility. The driving force of this process in micro-dynamics was primarily the self-assembly behavior of O–H groups in HPC "active molecules." The total transition mechanism and the sol–gel transition process are vividly depicted in Figure 19.4.

Additionally, HPC and its derivatives are of specific interest because they are representative liquid crystalline cellulose derivative, and they can form either cholesteric lyotropic (the type of mesomorphic state in a variety of common solvents) or thermotropic LC phases (in the melt) [15,21]. Obviously, the helical structure in cholesteric mesophases most probably originates from the chiral carbons on the cellulose main chain. Cholesteric mesophases often impart a color because of selective light reflection, when the pitch in the supramolecular helical structure is comparable to wavelengths of visible light. HPC solutions in water exhibit such a typical optical character at polymer concentrations of approximately 50–70 wt% [22].

19.2.2 Applications

HPC belongs to the group of cellulose ethers that has been used already for a year by paper of conservators as glue and sizing material. The material is soluble in water as well as in polar organic solvents (makes it possible to combine aqueous and nonaqueous conservation methods) [23]. HPC is used as a topical ophthalmic protectant and lubricant. In pharmaceuticals, HPC is used as a

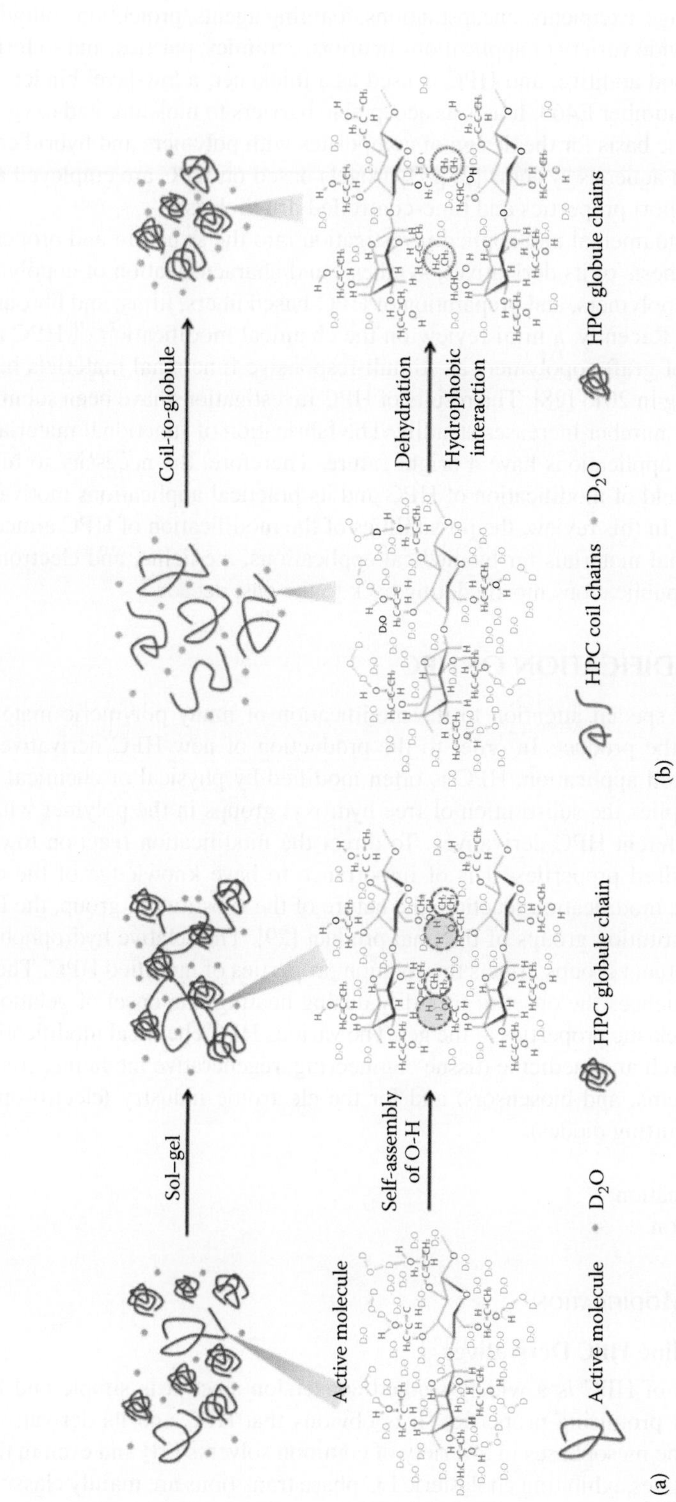

FIGURE 19.4 Micro-dynamics of the HPC molecules in 20 wt% HPC D_2O solution in the (a) coil-to-globule and (b) sol–gel transition process. (D_2O can be substituted by H_2O). (From Jing, Y. and Wu, P., *Cellulose*, 20, 67, 2013.)

disintegrant and is a commonly used binder for the wet granulation method of making tablets [24]. It is also employed as coatings, excipients, encapsulations, foaming agents, protection colloids, flocculants, and so forth, for a wide variety of applications in drugs, ceramics, plastics, and so forth [25]. HPC films are used as a food additive, and HPC is used as a thickener, a low-level binder, and an emulsion stabilizer with E number E463. It acts as acceptable barriers to moisture and oxygen [26].

Moreover, HPC forms the basis for the design of composites with polymers and hybrid composites formed by hydrogels in aqueous systems [27]. Hydrogels based on HPC are employed as drug carriers with targeted transport properties and time-controlled drug release.

In recent years, both fundamental and applied investigation into the structure and properties of HPC, methods for the synthesis of its derivatives, synthesis and characterization of copolymers of HPC and various synthetic polymers, and preparation of HPC-based fibers, films, and fibrous materials have been developed. Recently, a mini-review on the chemical modification of HPC accompanied by the fabrication of graft copolymers as stimuli-responsive functional materials has been published by Liu and Huang in 2013 [28]. The results of HPC investigations have been submitted in numerous papers, and their number increases steadily. The fabrication of functional materials with cellulosic blocks and their applications have a bright future. Therefore, the necessity to highlight the state of the art in the field of modification of HPC and its practical applications motivated the author to write this review. In this review, the possibilities of the modification of HPC aimed at the production of new functional materials for biomedical applications, medicine, and electronics are considered on the basis of publications mostly dating back to the past decade.

19.3 CHEMICAL MODIFICATION OF HPC

Researchers have directed special attention to the modification of many polymeric materials to impart new properties to the product. In order to the production of new HPC derivative–based materials to suit the required application, HPC is often modified by physical or chemical means. Chemical modification implies the substitution of free hydroxyl groups in the polymer with functional groups, yielding different HPC derivatives. To direct the modification reaction toward the HPC product with the desired properties, it is of importance to have knowledge of the correlations that exist between the modification reaction, the nature of the substitution group, the DS, and the distribution of the substitution groups of the final product [29]. The relative hydrophobicity or hydrophilicity of the substituent groups affects the solution properties of modified HPC. The DS on HPC and temperature influences the onset of turbidity during heating, the onset of gelation, drug release rates, and the viscoelastic properties of the gel. The various HPC chemical modifications are useful in biomedical research and medicine (tissue engineering, regenerative medicine, controlled-release drug delivery systems, and biosensors) and for the electronic industry (electro-optic elements and organic light emitting diodes):

1. Hydrophobic modification
2. Graft copolymerizaion

19.3.1 Hydrophobic Modification

19.3.1.1 Liquid Crystalline HPC Derivatives

Hydrophobic modification of HPC is a widely studied conversion since it is simple and leads to products with a variety of promising properties. It is obvious that HPC and its derivatives form cholesteric liquid crystalline mesophases in a variety of common solvents [21] and even in the melt. Thermotropic HPC derivatives exhibiting cholesteric LC phase transitions are mainly classified into two groups, that is, one is ester derivative and the other ether one. No difference in the type of liquid crystalline phase and the helical sense of mesophases formed by the ester and ether derivatives has been observed.

Liquid crystalline materials based on HPC often impart a color because of selective light reflection, when the pitch in the supramolecular helical structure is comparable to wavelengths of visible light. HPC solutions in water exhibit such a typical optical character at polymer concentrations of approximately 50–70 wt% [30]. At lower polymer concentrations and at ambient temperature, an aqueous solution of HPC forms an isotropic phase. As the concentration of HPC increases, the semirigid HPC molecules converge into a cholesteric mesophase. HPC derivatives such as trimethylsilyl hydroxypropylcellulose (TMS-HPC) in concentrated acetone solution with approximately 36% critical concentration showed the lyotropic liquid crystalline behavior [31]. Therefore, liquid crystalline properties of HPC in electro-optic applications open new horizons for HPC derivatives.

Huang et al. [32] synthesized a series of aliphatic acid esters of HPC (CnPC) to understand the side chain effect on the formation of thermotropic cholesteric LC phases and phase transitions as well as their unique selectivity for color reflections and the pitch distance in the cholesteric LC phases. The molecular structure of CnPC on the basis of the idealized molecular structure is shown in Figure 19.5. They found that increasing the number of methylene units in the side chains narrows the thermotropic phase transition window (between T_g and isotropization temperature (T_i)) and increases the layer spacing of the cholesteric liquid crystals in the series of CnPC polymers. Besides, the maximum selective reflection peak wavelength and the corresponding pitch distance of the cholesteric LC phases (CnPC) were strongly dependent on the number of methylene units in the side chains.

El-Wakil et al. [33] reported the synthesis of a series of 4-alkoxybenzoyloxypropy cellulose (ABPC-n) samples via the esterification of HPC with 4-alkoxybenzoic acid (see Figure 19.6). The sample with n = 7, 8, 12 exhibited both lyotropic and thermotropic (cholesteric) liquid crystalline behavior. While the ABPC-n samples with n = 1–4 showed only lyotropic behavior. Their study showed that the side chain participates in thermal properties and in enhancing the liquid crystalline properties of the HPC.

Recently, we have reported two series of cholesteryl-modified HPC derivatives (CHDs) with different degrees of substitution (D_{Chol}) (see Figure 19.7) [15]. First series was synthesized by performing reactions involving HPC and a preformed cholesterol-based mesogenic dimer (HPC-G1-Chol). In the second series, the hydroxyl groups of HPC reacted with cholesteryl chloroformate to form HPC-Chol. All of the synthesized polymers formed thermotropic liquid crystalline phases. Polymers with a mesogenic side chain (i.e., the HPC-G1-Chol series) had wider mesophases than HPC and polymers that were derived from HPC-Chol.

The ΔH values and the transition temperatures determined from the first DSC scan and POM observations are listed in Table 19.2. The melting temperatures (T_m), isotropization temperatures (T_i), and the T_g values of both series of CHDs were lower than those for HPC, indicating that both

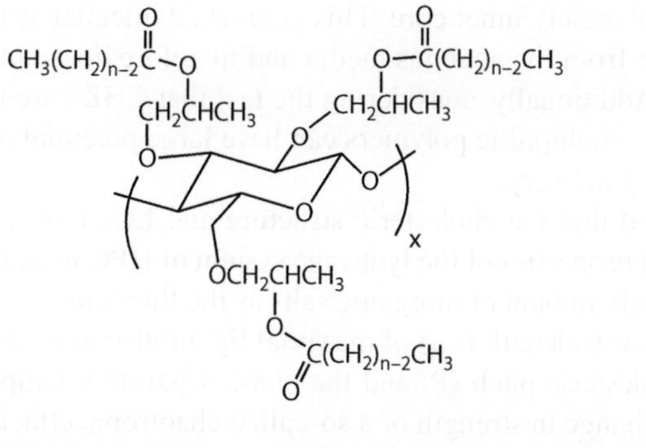

FIGURE 19.5 An idealized chemical structure of CnPC with three substituents. (From Huang, B. et al., *Polymer*, 48, 264, 2007.)

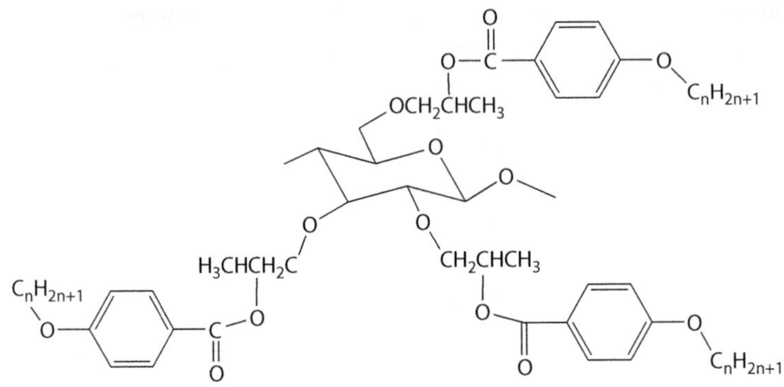

FIGURE 19.6 Chemical structure for a substituted anhydroglucose unit of 4-alkoxybenzoyloxypropyl cellulose; degree of etherification = 3, degree of esterification = 3. (From El Wakil, N.A. et al., *BioResources*, 5, 1834, 2010.)

the backbones and the side chains are involved in the formation of the LC phases and the phase transitions [15].

The optical textures of the samples were studied via POM with a hot stage, as displayed in Figure 19.8. The HPC-Chol polymers showed the color texture of a cholesteric phase. The results also showed that the D_{Chol} of each cellulose derivative significantly influences the properties of its thermotropic mesophases.

19.3.1.2 Thermoresponsive HPC-Based Materials

Thermoresponsive polymers tend to self-associate above the LCST and/or below the upper critical solution temperature (UCST) via intra- and/or intermolecular interactions [34]. HPC is attractive thermoresponsive polymers due to its wide and tunable LCST and can be adjusted by grafting HPC with a more hydrophobic side chain. Aqueous HPC solutions also show a phase-separation behavior with the LCST usually in the range of 41°C–45°C [17], which is known as the coil-to-globule transition, and therefore they become turbid on heating.

For reported CHDs (HPC-G1-Chol and HPC-Chol) [35], the respective value was 38.7°C, while the unmodified HPC in aqueous solution exhibited an LCST of more than 41°C. The incorporation of hydrophobic moieties into HPC promoted the LCST shift to a lower temperature than the corresponding pure HPC, because the incorporation of the hydrophobic moieties facilitated chain aggregation. However, there was no obvious change in the LCST for HPC-G1-Chol and HPC-Chol polymers, that is, cholesteryl moieties show little hydrophobic contribution to LCST. This indicated that the hydrophobic terminals of the polymers self-assemble into a phase-separated inner core under hydrophobic affinity. Hydrated HPC chains remain dispersed surrounding the aggregated hydrophobic cholesterol moiety inner core. This core–shell micellar structure of CHDs isolates the hydrophobic inner core from the aqueous media and therefore does not influence the LCST of the HPC outer shell [35]. Additionally, considering the fact that CHDs are body temperature–sensitive polymers, the resultant amphiphilic polymers can have large potential application as a drug carrier for thermosensitive drug delivery.

Nishio [36] indicated that the cholesteric structure and LCST-type phase-separation behavior, and the ensuing optical properties of the lyotropic system of HPC in water are significantly affected by the addition of a small amount of inorganic salts as the third component. As a universal rule, the optical parameters, the wavelength (λ_M) of maximal light reflectance, and the cloud point (T_c) shift and, therefore, the cholesteric pitch (P) and the phase-separation temperature were found to vary systematically with a change in strength of a so-called chaotropic effect of the ions constituting the additive salts. Generally, an increase in ionic chaotropicity weakens the hydrophobic interaction of (the side chains of) water-soluble polymers. From a practical point of view, this result implies that

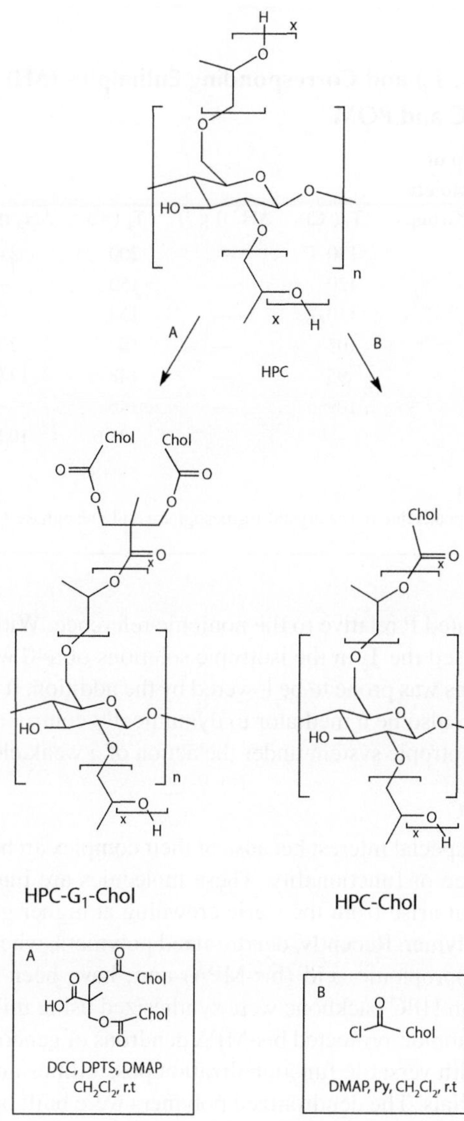

FIGURE 19.7 Synthetic route for the cholesteryl-modified HPC derivatives. (From Bagheri, M. and Shateri, Sh., *J. Polym. Res.*, 19, 9842, 2012.)

the coloration and turbidity of the aqueous HPC lyotropic system can be controlled desirably by selecting the combination of cation and anion species of the added salt.

Meanwhile, recently, much attention has been paid to the usefulness of low-temperature molten organosalts, that is, the so-called ionic liquids, as solvents to dissolve and functionalize unmodified cellulose and related natural polysaccharides [37,38]. Representative examples of the conventionally used ionic liquids are salts with *N*,*N*′-dialkylimidazolium, *N*-alkylpyridinium, alkylammonium, and alkylphosphonium as the cationic moiety. In an extension study by Chiba et al. [39], the effects of *N*-alkyl-substituted imidazolium salts also described as a new series of additives on the cholesteric mesophase formation and ensuing optical properties of HPC aqueous solutions, in comparison with the previous case using alkali metallic salts to control the structure and properties of the cellulosic liquid crystalline system. In the cholesteric mesophase formation, at concentrations of more than 50 wt% HPC, P was confirmed to shift upward according to the chaotropic strength of X^-.

TABLE 19.2
Transition Temperatures (T_1, T_2) and Corresponding Enthalpies (ΔH) for HPC and Modified HPCs Determined from DSC and POM

Sample	Molar Ratio of Cholesteryl Moiety per Hydroxyl Groups	T_1 (°C)	ΔH_1 (J g^{-1})	T_2 (°C)	ΔH_2 (J g^{-1})	T_3 (°C)	ΔH_3 (J g^{-1})
HPC	—	130	—	200	2.46	—	—
HPC-G1-Chol (a)	0.05	120[a]	—	150	—	184	4.32
HPC-G1-Chol (b)	0.1	110.6	—	157	—	197	3.62
HPC-G1-Chol (c)	0.2	105	—	184	2.15	200	3.77
HPC–Chol (a)	0.1	95[a]	—	148	19.90	—	—
HPC–Chol (b)	0.2	109[a]	—	146	—	—	—
HPC–Chol (c)	0.4	—[b]	—	131.6	10.8	—	—

[a] Determined from POM observation.
[b] Significant overlapping of the two peaks due to the crystal-to-mesophase and mesophase-to-isotropic transitions.

Organocations generally elevated P relative to the nonionic reference. With regard to LCST behavior, imidazolium additives raised the T_c in the isotropic solutions of ≤40 wt% HPC, whereas the T_c value of mesomorphic solutions was prone to be lowered by the addition. It was preliminarily shown that the imidazolium salts can also be a mediator to dynamically control the cholesteric coloration and optical turbidity of this lyotropic system under the action of a weak electric field.

19.3.1.3 Dendronized HPC

Dendronized polymers are of special interest because of their complex architecture, highly branched with a presumably high degree of functionality. These molecules are interesting because of their unique physical properties that arise from the steric crowding at higher generations, which results in an extended rod-shaped polymer. Recently, dendronized polymers, where the dendritic part constitutes the 2,2-bis (methylol)propionic acid (bis-MPA) unit, have been thoroughly studied [40]. Dendronized polymers with an HPC backbone were synthesized using mild esterification reactions at ambient temperature of acetonide-protected bis-MPA dendrons of generation with the aim of producing complex molecules with versatile functionalization possibilities and high molecular weight from bio-based starting materials. The dendronized polymers were built by attaching premade acetonide-protected 2,2-bis(methylol)propionic acid functional dendrons of generation 1–3 to a HPC backbone. Deprotection or functionalization of the end groups of the first-generation dendronized polymer to hydroxyl groups and long alkyl chains was performed, respectively. They found that the molecules were in the size range of tens of nanometers and that they were apt to undertake a more elongated conformation on the HOPG surfaces when long alkyl chains were attached as the dendron end groups (Figure 19.9).

19.3.2 Graft Copolymerization

Graft copolymers have been extensively studied from both synthetic and theoretical points of view [41–47]. They belong to the general class of segmented copolymers and generally consist of a linear backbone of one composition and randomly distributed branches of a different composition (Figure 19.10). In common graft copolymers, the branches are randomly distributed along the backbone. The backbone and the branches may be homo- or copolymers, but they differ in chemical nature or composition. Graft copolymers in which the side chains and backbone are of the same chemical nature are generally referred to as comb-shaped polymers, in reference to their

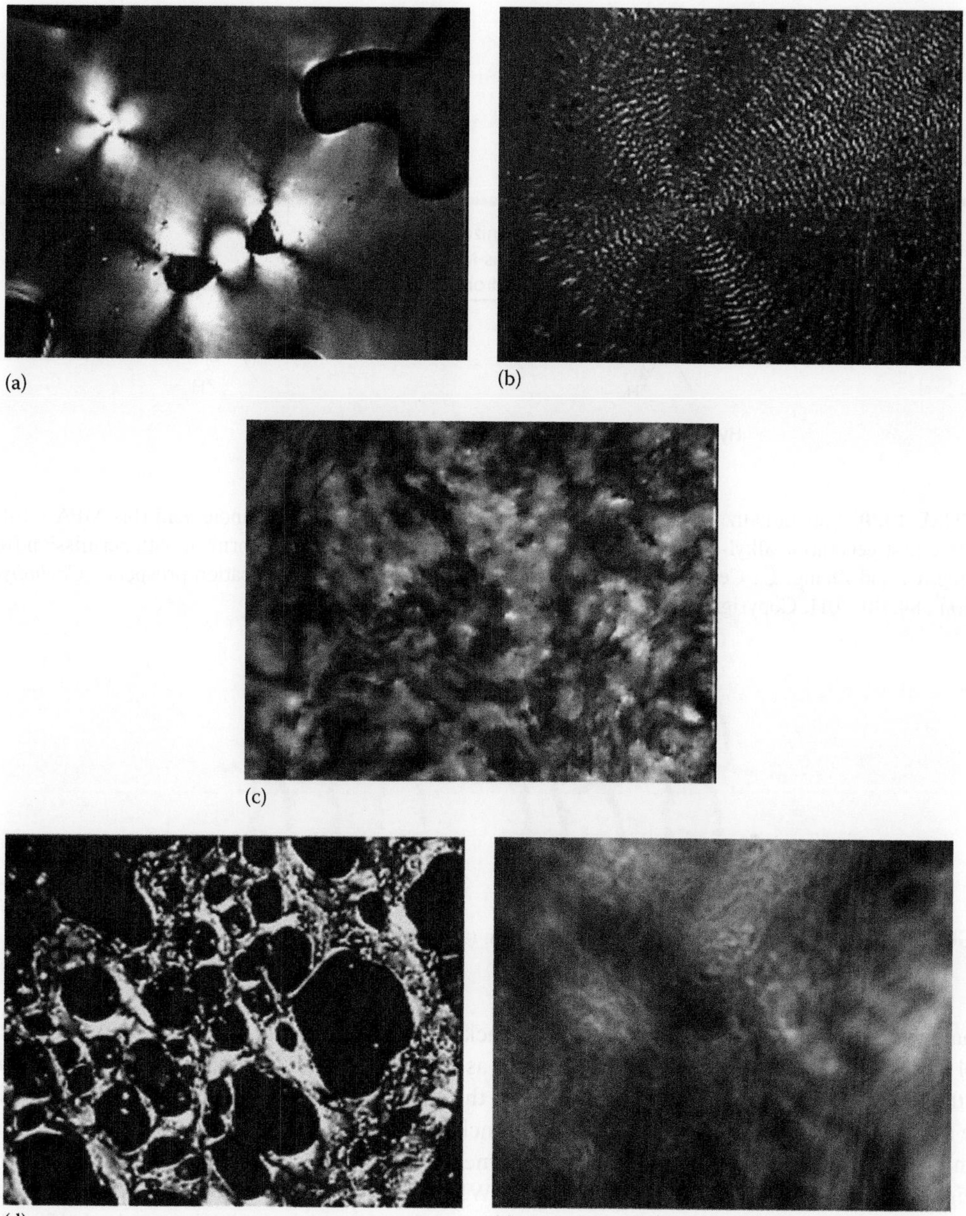

FIGURE 19.8 Polarizing optical photomicrographs: (a) focal conic smectic phase texture of HPC-G1-Chol (a) upon heating to 130°C; (b) cholesteric finger texture of HPC-G1-Chol (a) upon heating to 170°C; (c) cholesteric phase texture of HPC-Chol (a) upon heating to 135°C; (d) lyotropic texture of HPC-G1-Chol (a) in 40 wt% acetone at room temperature; and (e) lyotropic texture of HPC-Chol (a) in 40 wt% acetone at room temperature (magnification 200×). (From Bagheri, M. and Shateri, Sh., *J. Polym. Res.*, 19, 9842, 2012.)

structure. The synthetic methodologies of graft copolymers have been extensively studied and reviewed in several articles over the years [48].

Graft copolymers are of increasing interest as surface-modifying agents, emulsifiers, coating materials, or compatibilizers for polymer blends to improve the interfacial interaction between two polymers or of polymers and other materials [49]. The interest in graft polymers arises also in part

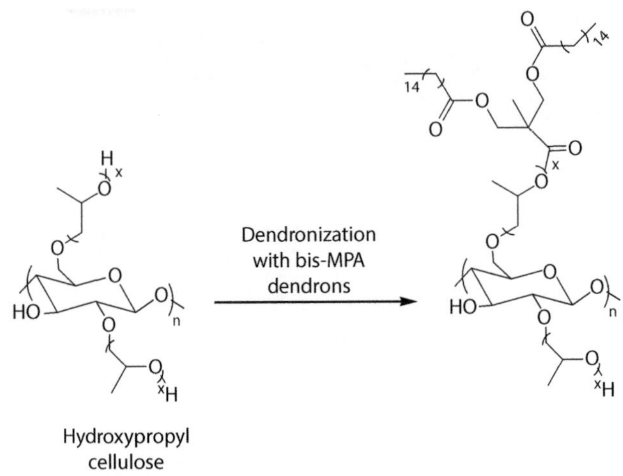

FIGURE 19.9 Functionalization of HPC with 2,2-bis(methyl palmitate)propanoic acid (bis-MPA-C16) to achieve first-generation alkyl-terminated dendronized HPC (HPC-G1-C16). (Reprinted with permission from Chang, C. and Zhang, L., Cellulose-based hydrogels: Present status and application prospects, *Carbohydr. Polym.*, 84, 40, 2011. Copyright 2014 American Chemical Society.)

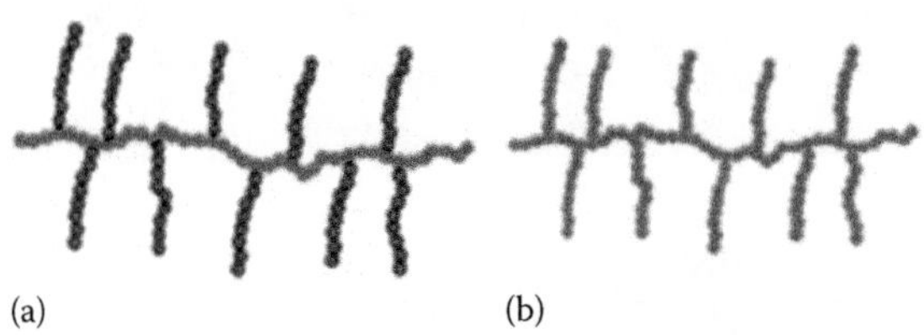

FIGURE 19.10 Schematic of branched architectures: (a) graft copolymer and (b) comb-shaped polymer.

from the protection exerted by the grafts on the backbone. All these studies revealed that a good control of macromolecular architecture has emerged as a very important parameter in the manipulation of the graft copolymer properties and prompted the development of efficient approaches allowing the synthesis of well-defined graft copolymers including graft copolymers of controlled composition. The structural parameters of graft copolymers, such as the chemical nature, the molecular weight and the molecular weight distribution (MWD) of backbone and grafts, and the graft density along the backbone can be well controlled by means of various polymerization methods [50]. The most important methods to design graft copolymers have been reviewed by Lutz and Peruch, and their advantages and drawbacks will be discussed [48]. Provided appropriate polymerization methods are used, tailor-made graft copolymers can be obtained.

Graft copolymers can be synthesized by "graft to," "graft from," and "graft through" approaches, among which "graft from" is the most commonly used approach. In the "grafting onto" method, functional polymeric side chains (the grafts) are attached to an existing backbone containing, in most cases, randomly distributed antagonist functions. In a "grafting from" process, initiating sites, or functions capable of generating such sites, are attached to a polymeric backbone. The polymerization of a second monomer can then be initiated from the sites present on the backbone chain to yield the grafts, provided that initiation occurs by addition of the incoming monomer. The macromonomer-based "grafting through" method involves first the synthesis and the determination of the structural parameters of the α- or ω-functional macro-monomers. In the

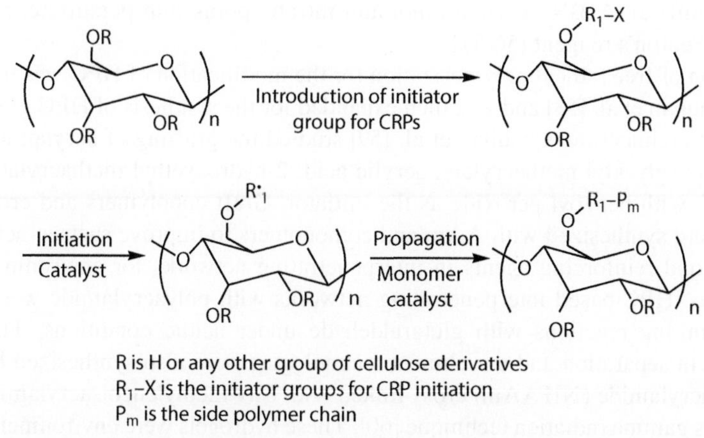

FIGURE 19.11 Synthesis route to cellulose graft copolymers via CRP, R can be H (cellulose itself) or other groups (cellulose derivatives). R_1–X is the initiator groups for CRP initiation; P_m is the side polymer chain. (From Hawker, C.J. et al., *Chem. Rev.*, 101, 3661, 2001.)

second step, the backbone chain is formed upon copolymerization of a low-molecular-weight monomer with the macromonomer [51].

Besides the three grafting processes extensively described before, a number of ways of synthesizing graft copolymers have been developed that are not easy to classify unambiguously such as graft copolymerization initiated by chemical treatment, photo-irradiation, or high-energy radiation technique and surface grafting of various polymer films and fibers [50].

Due to their structural diversity and water solubility, natural polysaccharides could be interesting starting materials for the synthesis of graft copolymers [52]. This fascinating technique may be considered as an approach to achieve novel polysaccharide-based materials with improved properties including all the expected usefulness of these biomaterials. Properties such as melting point, glass transition temperature, solubility, permeability, chemical reactivity, and elasticity can be modified through graft copolymerization as per the specific requirements [53,54]. Polysaccharides and their graft copolymers find extensive applications in diversified fields. Applications of modified polysaccharides include drug delivery devices, controlled release of fungicides, selective water absorption from oil–water emulsions, and purification of water [41–46].

In recent years, modification of chemical and physical properties of natural polymers and their derivatives through graft copolymerization has attracted much attention [50]. Graft copolymerization of various vinyl monomers onto different polysaccharides has been reported by various workers [41–47]. Graft copolymerization for the synthesis of HPC graft copolymers is a typical "graft from" approach, which is generally classified into free radical polymerization, ionic and ring-opening polymerization, and controlled/living radical polymerization (CRP). The strategy for the synthesis of HPC graft copolymers by CRP is illustrated schematically in Figure 19.11. Typical CRPs are nitroxide-mediated polymerization (NMP), atom transfer radical polymerization (ATRP), and reversible addition–fragmentation chain transfer (RAFT) polymerization. Briefly, initiator groups for CRP are first introduced onto the cellulose backbone via esterification or etherification. Then, graft copolymerization is carried out in the presence of monomers and catalyst [55].

19.3.2.1 Grafting via Free Radical Polymerization

Graft copolymers are prepared by first generating free radicals on the biopolymer backbone and then allowing these radicals to serve as macroinitiators for the vinyl or acrylic monomer. Free radical grafting of vinyl monomers onto polymeric backbones has been accomplished by using a range of free radical initiators and redox systems like dibenzoyl peroxide, azobis(isobutyronitrile) (AIBN), ceric ammonium nitrate, potassium persulfate, potassium permanganate, and Fenton's reagent [56,57].

The application of free radical polymerization for the modification of HPC was first reported in the 2000s by Chauhan et al. [58] and was then expanded for the synthesis of HPC graft copolymers with well-defined architecture. Chauhan et al. [59] studied the grafting of acrylamide (AAm) and some comonomers (glycidyl methacrylate, acrylic acid, 2-hydroxyethyl methacrylate, and acrylonitrile) onto HPC with benzoyl peroxide as the initiator. Graft copolymers and cross-linked networks of HPC were synthesized with AAm and comonomers to improve surface-active properties and to provide good reinforcing agents in interpenetrating networks for environmental management technologies. HPC-based interpenetrating networks with polyacrylamide were also synthesized by cross-linking reactions with glutaraldehyde under acidic conditions. Thermosensitive networks for use in separation and enrichment technologies were also synthesized based on HPC and *N*-isopropylacrylamide (NIPAAm) cross-linked with *N*,*N*-methylenebisacrylamide (MBAAm) by a simultaneous gamma radiation technique [60]. These hydrogels were environmentally sensitive and responded to changes in their thermal and ionic environment and have potential applications in diverse fields such as drug delivery, enzyme technology, and environmental management.

19.3.2.2 Grafting via Controlled Radical Polymerization

The synthesis of graft copolymers with well-defined architectures has been a focus of many research activities since the introduction of the CRP techniques. CRPs for the synthesis of HPC graft copolymers with well-defined architecture have attracted interest in recent years [61–63].

Complex architectures, such as comb polymers with a high grafting density, were not realistic synthetic goals until techniques providing more control were established; these techniques have since had a tremendous impact on the development of novel predesigned materials [64]. Comb polymers, grafted from HPC, were synthesized by NMP of styrene using Barton ester intermediates (esters or carbonates of *N*-hydroxypyridines-2-thine) [61]. Treatment of Barton carbonate modified HPC with styrene in the presence of TEMPO afforded corresponding TEMPO adduct, which could be used to promote the controlled radical graft polymerization of styrene (Figure 19.12).

Water-soluble polysaccharides, such as starch, dextran, and pullulan were widely used as main chain polymers with hydrophobic poly(ε-caprolactone) (PCL), polylactide, and polyglycolide as side chains. Graft copolymerizations have been initiated by the hydroxyl groups of the polysaccharides and catalyzed by stannous 2-ethylhexanoate [65–67]. Brush-like graft polymers of hydrophobic ε-caprolactone (CL) were reported with HPC as the backbone by ring-opening bulk polymerization of CL by without a catalyst [68] or by homogeneous graft polymerization with the partial protecting technique of the hydroxyl group via the trimethylsilyl group as a protecting group and deprotection [69]. The synthesis of a graft copolymer of HPC with hydrophobic PCL side chains increased the hydrophobicity of the resulting copolymer and potentially made it a more suitable carrier for hydrophobic drugs.

RAFT polymerization is a very versatile route that allows the synthesis of star-, comb-, or block copolymers with good control over molecular weight [70]. Control over molecular weight and MWD can be achieved using thio-containing compounds such as thioester, thiocarbonates, dithiocarbamates, or xanthates. The detailed mechanism of the RAFT process can be found elsewhere [71]. Comb polymers, grafted from HPC, have been synthesized via RAFT polymerization of styrene [62]. The polymers obtained were, despite their rather broad distribution, found to be suitable for the preparation of porous films with regular arrays. The prepared regular porous honeycomb-structured films from HPC-based polystyrenes showed great versatility of this method for preparing porous films for a range of applications.

Among these techniques, ATRP is one of the most popular CRP methods for the synthesis of HPC graft copolymers in a living/controllable way. HPC was found to be a versatile multifunctional biopolymer that was readily converted into an ATRP macroinitiator. The backbones of HPC graft copolymers can be HPC or its derivatives and can be hydrophobic or hydrophilic. The properties

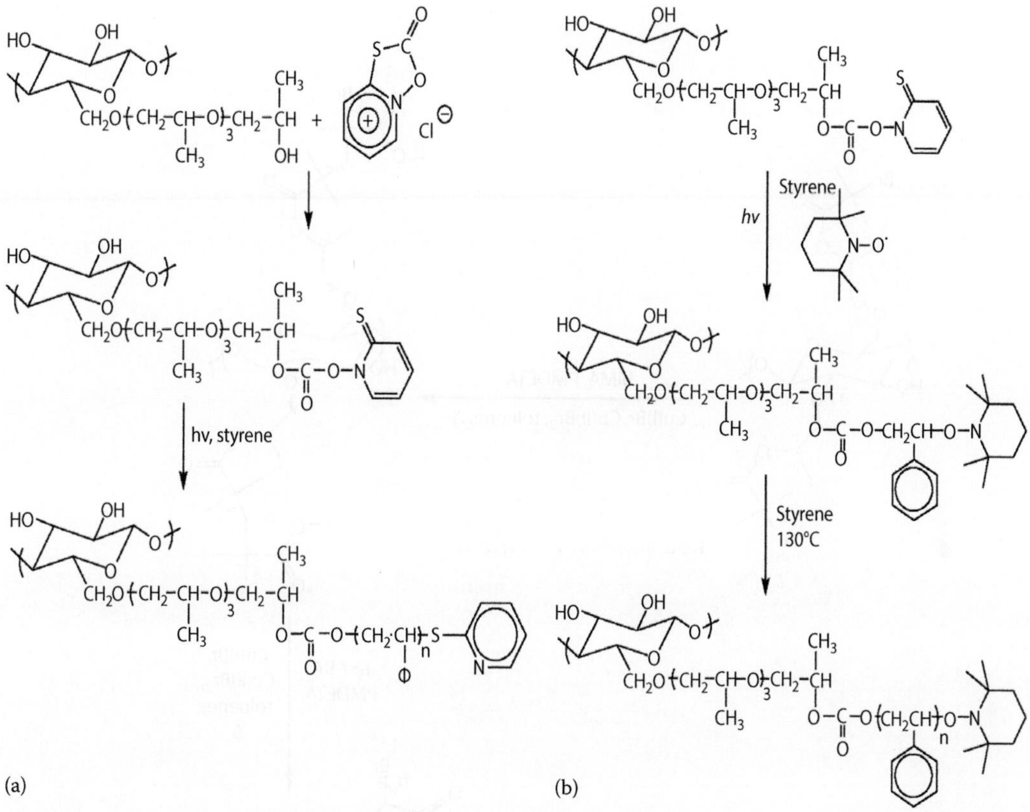

FIGURE 19.12 (a) Grafting styrene to HPC using Barton ester intermediate (b) controlled radical grafting from HPC. (From Daly, W.H. et al., *Macromol. Symp.*, 174, 155, 2001.)

of the side chains can be tailored by selecting desired monomers and controlling the length of the side chains [28].

Dendronized polymers (a subclass of comb polymers) are one of the new architectures that have gained increasing attention during the latest years [40,64]. These molecules are interesting because of their unique physical properties that arise from the steric crowding at higher generations, which results in an extended rod-shaped polymer. Several appealing applications for dendronized polymers have been suggested based upon their size and versatile post-functionalization possibilities. Östmark et al. [64] reported a controlled grafting of monomers by ATRP using HPC as a core molecule for the synthesis of amphiphilic comb copolymers. HPC was allowed to react either with an ATRP initiator or with the first-generation initiator-functionalized 2,2-bis (methylol) propionic acid dendron to create macroinitiators having high degrees of functionality (HPC-I and HPC-G1, respectively). Dendronized HPCs of different generations as macroinitiators were then "grafted from" using ATRP of methyl methacrylate (MMA) (HPC-PMMA and HPC-G1-PMMA, respectively). The "livingness" of HPC-PMMA and HPC-G1-PMMA was confirmed by polymerization of a second block using *tert*-butyl acrylate as outlined in Figure 19.13. Subsequent selective acidolysis of the *tert*-butyl ester moieties was performed to form a block of poly(acrylic acid) (PAA) resulting in amphiphilic block copolymer grafts. It was found that the comb (co)polymers were in the nanometer size range and that the dendronization had an interesting effect on the rheological properties. The advantage of using HPC is the available hydroxyl groups, which show high reactivity with bis-MPA derivatives combined with the improved solubility HPC exhibits as compared to native cellulose. Furthermore, bis-MPA and

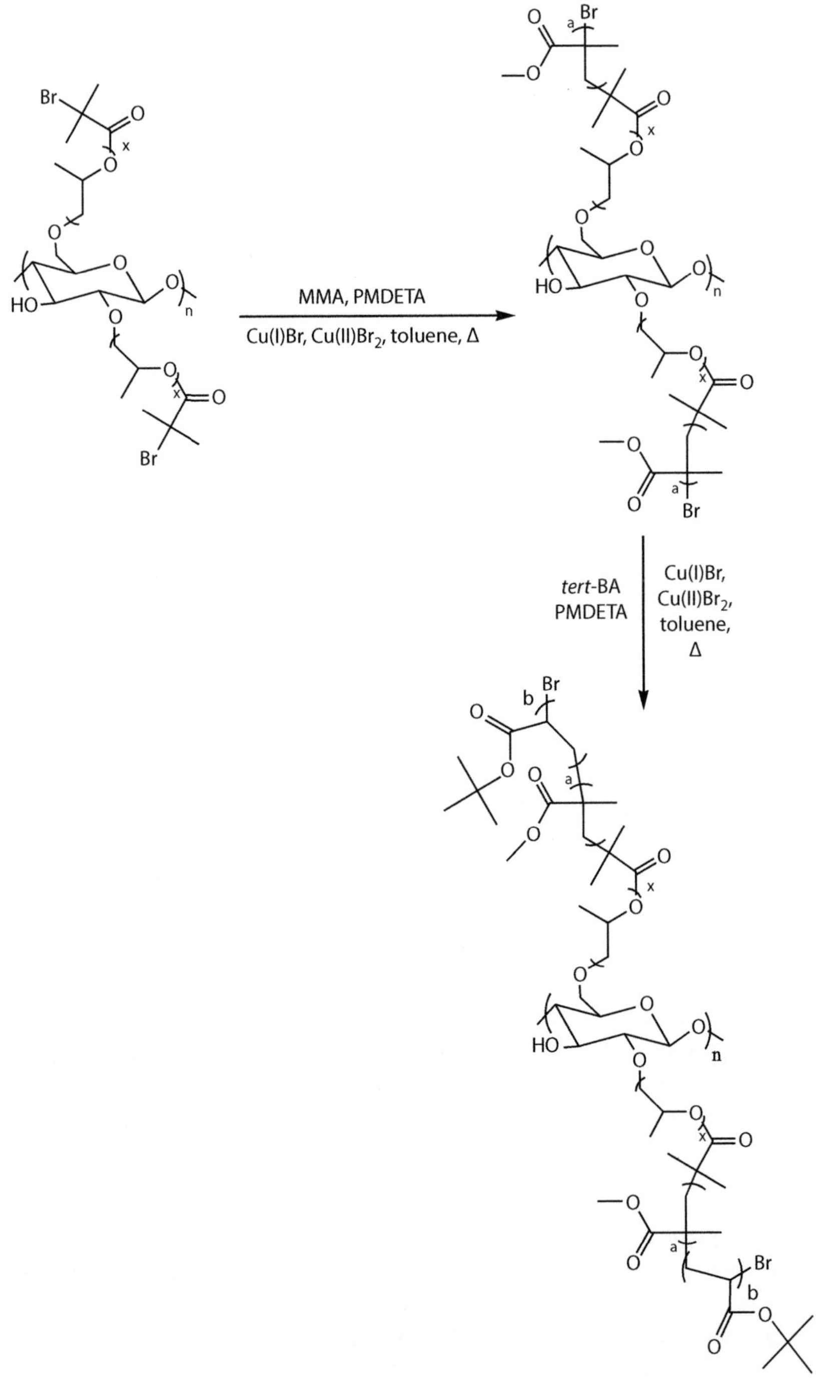

FIGURE 19.13 Polymerization of MMA, initiated by the macroinitiator HPC-I, under ATRP conditions. (From Östmark, E. et al., *Biomacromolecules*, 8, 1138, 2007.)

HPC are both biocompatible, which could make these dendronized polymers promising candidates for biomedical applications.

Recently, amphiphilic grafted HPC containing polycholesteryl methacrylate (PCMA) side chains was reported by our group to prepare the new biodegradable and biocompatible nanocarriers [72]. The hydrophobic polymethyl methacrylate (PMMA) and PCMA side chains were grafted from an HPC under ATRP conditions (Figure 19.14). The prepared homo- and random-copolymers, HPC-*g*-PMMA and HPC-*g*-(PMMA-*ran*-PCMA)s achieved solubility's in a variety of organic solvents. The formation of nanoparticles was carried out in water/ethyl acetate using the emulsion–diffusion technique and polyvinyl alcohol as the emulsifier. DLS and TEM results showed that the length of the chains (monomer/initiator ratio) of copolymers has a big influence on the stability and polydispersity of nanoparticles.

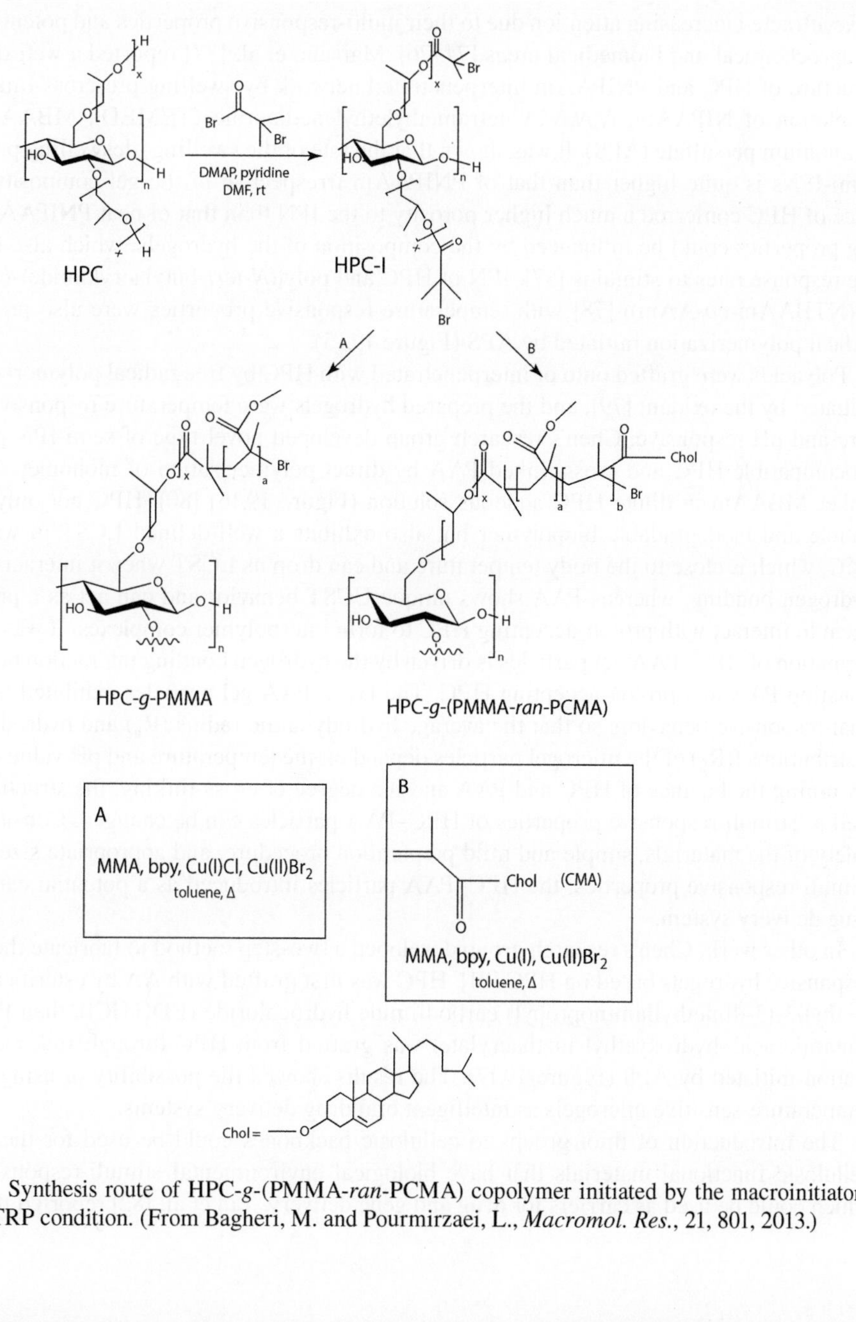

FIGURE 19.14 Synthesis route of HPC-*g*-(PMMA-*ran*-PCMA) copolymer initiated by the macroinitiator HPC-I, under ATRP condition. (From Bagheri, M. and Pourmirzaei, L., *Macromol. Res.*, 21, 801, 2013.)

19.3.3 Stimuli-Responsive HPC-Based Graft Copolymers: Properties and Applications

"Smart" materials based on HPC are also intensively studied these years because of its solubility in water and temperature-responsive property. Depending on the properties of both HPC backbones and side chains, HPC graft copolymers can have stimuli-responsive properties.

Stimuli-responsive hydrogels, which are able to swell or shrink as a function of external stimuli, have recently gained a great deal of attention, especially for their use in biomedical applications due to their unique properties such as biocompatibility, biodegradability, and biological functionality [73]. The mechanism of hydrogels' swelling and shrinking is similar to that of aggregate assembly: stimulus-induced intermolecular and intramolecular hydrogen bonding changes. Loaded drugs in the hydrogels can be released while they swell to looser structures due to environmental changes in the vicinity.

Microgel and nanogel particles with the full interpenetrating polymer network (IPN) structure have attracted increasing attention due to their multi-responsive properties and potential application in agrochemical and biomedical areas [74–76]. Marsano et al. [77] reported a well-defined porous structure of HPC and PNIPAAm interpenetrated network by swelling pre-cross-linked HPC with a solution of NIPAAm, *N,N,N′,N′*-tetramethylethylenediamine (TEMED), MBAAm (BIS), and ammonium persulfate (APS). It was shown that the rate of the swelling–deswelling process of these semi-IPNs is quite higher than that of PNIPAAm irrespective of the gel composition. The presence of HPC conferred a much higher porosity to the IPN than that of neat PNIPAAm. The swelling properties could be influenced by the composition of the hydrogels, which also had effects on the response rates to stimulus [57]. IPN of HPC and poly[(*N-tert*-butylacrylamide)-*co*-acrylamide] (P(NTBAAm-*co*-AAm)) [78] with temperature-responsive properties were also prepared by free radical polymerization initiated by APS (Figure 19.15).

Polyacids were grafted onto or interpenetrated with HPC by free radical polymerization in water initiated by the oxidant [79], and the prepared hydrogels were temperature responsive, or temperature and pH responsive. Chen's research group developed novel type of semi-IPN particles using biocompatible HPC and cross-linked PAA by direct polymerization of monomer AA and cross-linker MBAAm in dilute HPC aqueous solution (Figure 19.16) [80]. HPC not only is a biocompatible and biodegradable biopolymer but also exhibits a well-defined LCST in water at around 41°C, which is close to the body temperature and can drop its LCST when it interacts with PAA by hydrogen bonding, whereas PAA shows unique UCST behavior and can act as a proton-donating agent to interact with proton-accepting HPC to form interpolymer complexes. It was found that the formation of HPC–PAA gel particles is driven by the hydrogen bonding interaction between proton-donating PAA and proton-accepting HPC. The HPC–PAA gel particles exhibited thermo and pH dual-responsive behaviors so that the average hydrodynamic radius (R_h) and hydrodynamic radius distributions $f(R_h)$ of the microgel particles depend on the temperature and pH value (Figure 19.16). By tuning the balance of HPC and PAA and the degree of cross-linking, the structure and size as well as stimuli-responsive properties of HPC–PAA particles can be changed. Considering the biosafety of the materials, simple and mild preparation procedure, and appropriate size as well as the stimuli-responsive properties, the HPC–PAA particles introduced as a potential candidate for the drug delivery system.

In other work, Chen's research group developed a two-step method to fabricate thermo- and pH-responsive hydrogels based on HPC [81]. HPC was first grafted with AA by esterification, by using 1-ethyl-3-(3-dimethyllaminopropyl) carbodiimide hydrochloride (EDC·HCl), then PAA or poly(L-glutamic acid–hydroxyethyl methacrylate) was grafted from HPC through free radical polymerization initiated by APS (Figure 19.17). The results showed the possibility of using such pH- and temperature-sensitive microgels as intelligent oral drug delivery systems.

The introduction of thiol groups to cellulosic backbones could be used for the fabrication of cellulosic functional materials that have biological environmental stimuli-responsive properties, which could be used as carriers for drug and gene delivery. Tan et al. [82] reported the synthesis of

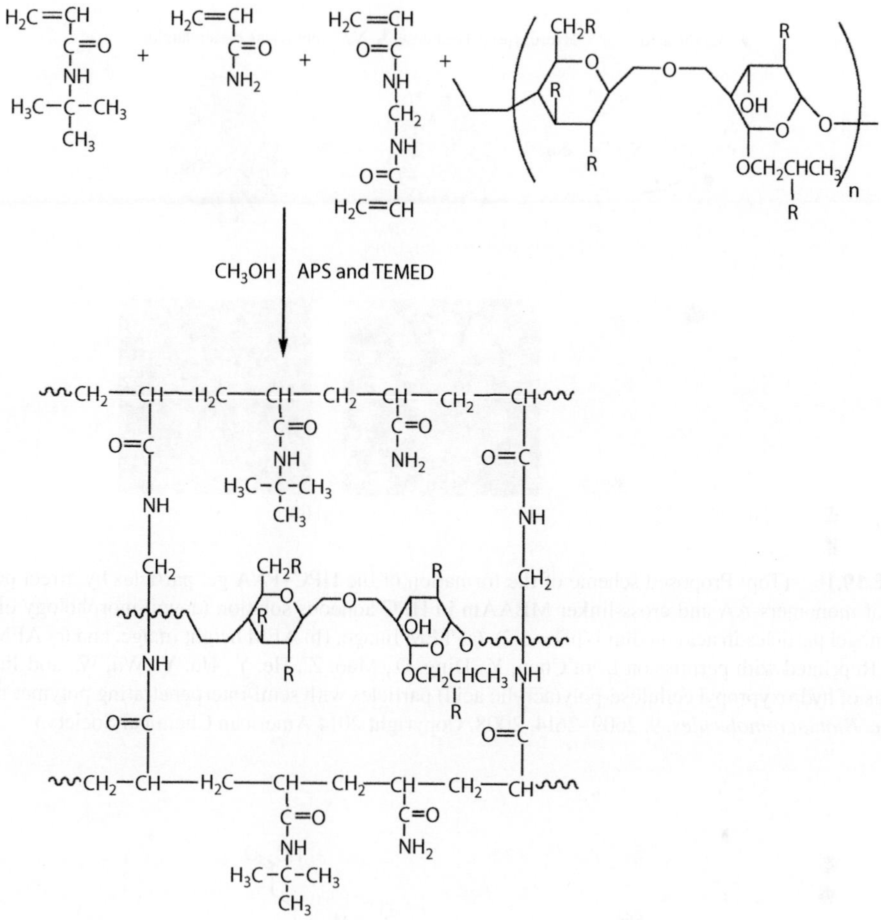

FIGURE 19.15 Preparation of the semi-IPN P(NTBAAm-*co*-AAm)/HPC hydrogels. (From Çaykara, T. et al., *Macromol. Mater. Eng.*, 291, 1044, 2006.)

thiolated HPC (HPC-SH) and the fabrication of a thermo- and redox-sensitive nanogel therefrom and then oxidation of thiol groups to disulfide bonds to stabilize the associated structure. HPC was first activated by 4-nitrophenyl chloroformate. Then, the modified HPC was converted to HPC-SH in the presence of cysteamine. On heating a dilute solution of HPC-SH to a temperature above the LCST of HPC, the HPC-SH will collapse to form a nanogel, which can be cross-linked by disulfide bonds formed by oxidation of thiol groups. The cross-linked nanogel shows both thermal and redox stimuli-responsive properties (Figure 19.18).

Regulation of the LCST to body temperature region was reported by Jin et al. [83] through graft copolymerization of PNIPAAm from HPC by controlling the PNIPAAm side chains to a proper length. HPC-*g*-PNIPAAm copolymers were synthesized by single-electron transfer living radical polymerization through "grafting from" approach in water and THF mixture solvent. They found that the thermo-responsive property of HPC-*g*-PNIPAAm copolymers in aqueous solution depends on the length of the graft chains (Figure 19.19). The shorter side PNIPAm chains correlate to a relatively lower LCST of the copolymers in aqueous solution.

A promising group of thermo-responsive polymers is thus poly(ethylene glycol) methacrylates (PEGMAs), which have shown to be nontoxic and biocompatible [84]. Furthermore, the LCST of these polymers can be tailored by changing the length of the ethylene glycol segment in the side chain.

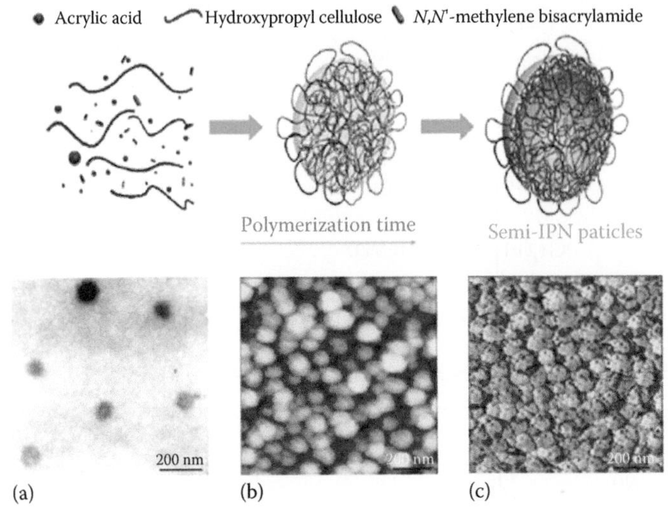

FIGURE 19.16 (Top) Proposed scheme of the formation of the HPC–PAA gel particles by direct polymerization of monomers AA and cross-linker MBAAm in HPC aqueous solution (down) morphology of HPC–PAA nanogel particles in acid medium (pH = 3.2). (a) TEM image, (b) AFM height image, and (c) AFM phase image. (Reprinted with permission from Chen, Y., Ding, D., Mao, Z., He, Y., Hu, Y., Wu, W., and Jiang, X., Synthesis of hydroxypropyl cellulose-poly(acrylic acid) particles with semi-interpenetrating polymer network structure, *Biomacromolecules*, 9, 2609–2614, 2008. Copyright 2014 American Chemical Society.)

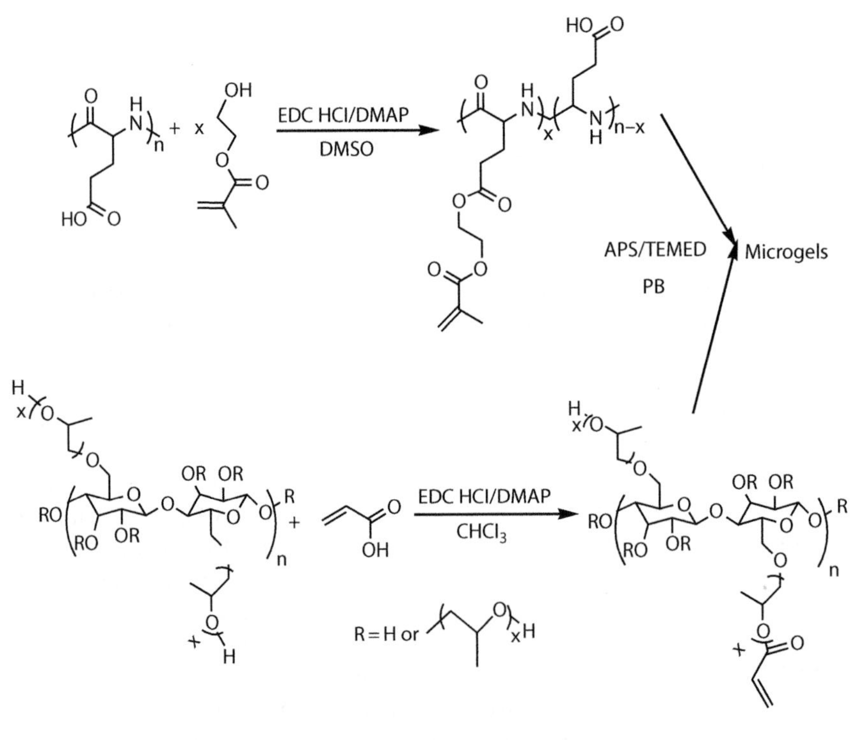

FIGURE 19.17 Synthesis route of microgels prepared from HPC. (From Baia, Y. et al., *Carbohydr. Polym.*, 89, 1207, 2012.)

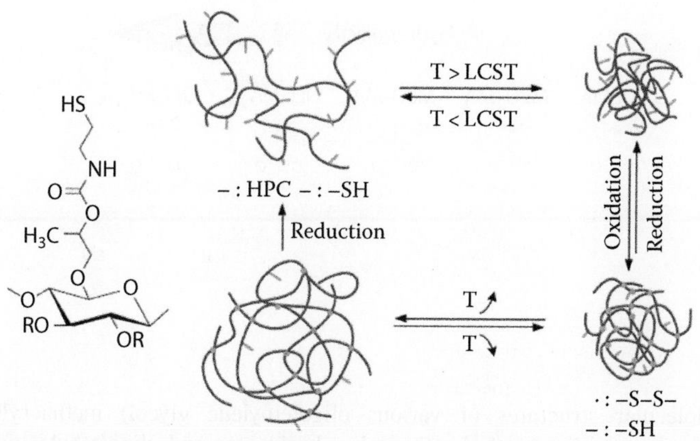

FIGURE 19.18 Schematic of the fabrication of dual-stimuli-responsive nanogels from HPC-SH and their stimuli-responsive properties. (From Tan, J. et al., *Polym. Chem.*, 2, 672, 2011.)

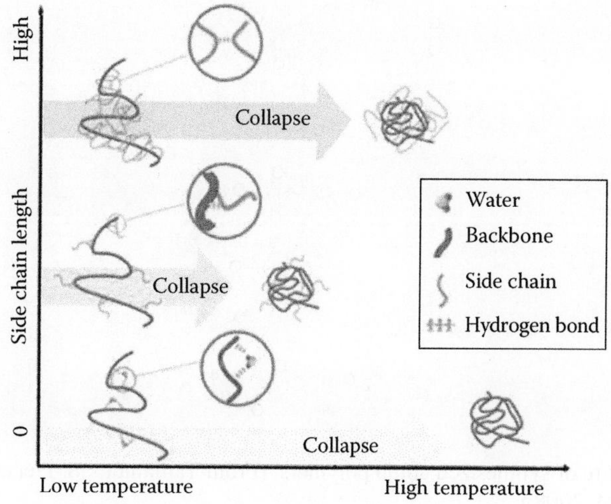

FIGURE 19.19 Mechanism for regulating LCST of HPC-*g*-PNIPAAm by the side chain length. (From Jin, X. et al., *Carbohydr. Polym.*, 95, 155, 2013.)

Longer ethylene glycol segments result in a more hydrophilic nature of the polymer, thus increasing the LCST (Figure 19.20). As a result, the LCST can be tuned in the range of 26°C–90°C by the appropriate choice of monomer [85,86]. For example, random copolymers of MEO_2MA and $OEGMA_{475}$ exhibit LCST values in between 26°C and 90°C, which can be precisely adjusted by varying the comonomer composition [87]. However, none of the available PEGMAs shows an LCST close to the physiological temperature. In 2011, Porsch et al. [87] employed ARGET ATRP as a straightforward technique for the preparation of thermo-responsive copolymers of $OEGMA_{300}$ and MEO_2MA with tunable LCSTs. Furthermore, they reported comb copolymers of HPC and the thermoresponsive copolymers employing surface-initiated ARGET ATRP (Figure 19.21). The grafting of the thermo-responsive polymers from HPC resulted in a consistent decrease in the LCST compared to the linear analogs; however, interestingly, the ability to tune the transition temperature remained. Consequently, these advanced architectures combine the favorable properties of HPC with the interesting thermo-responsive and stealth properties of PEGMAs.

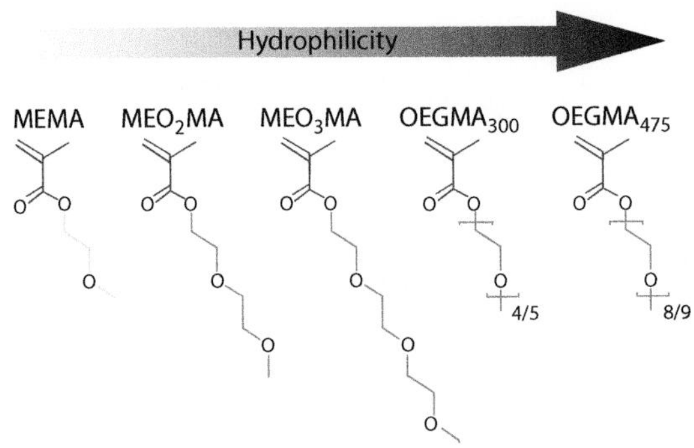

FIGURE 19.20 Molecular structures of various oligo(ethylene glycol) methacrylates. Hydrophobic and hydrophilic molecular regions are the methacrylate backbones and oligo(ethylene glycol) side chains, respectively.

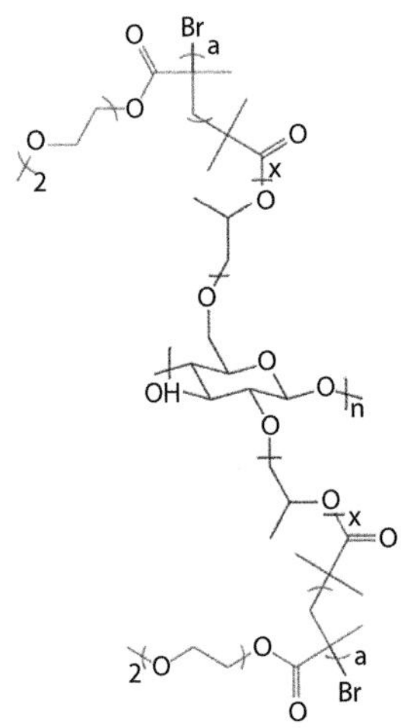

FIGURE 19.21 Structure of synthesized comb polymers. (From Yamamoto, S.-I. et al., *J. Polym. Sci., Part A: Polym. Chem.*, 46, 194, 2008.)

Considering the properties of cellulosic backbone and graft chains, HPC graft copolymers may have thermal-, pH-, or dual-stimuli responsive properties, by which the HPC graft copolymers can self-assemble into micelles with different architectures. Double-hydrophilic copolymers with HPC as backbone and PNIPAAm and PAA as graft chains were prepared by free radical polymerization initiated by ceric ammonium nitrate [88]. The results showed that the hydrophilicity of copolymers improves as the pH increases, whereas the hydrophobicity of copolymers enhances as the temperature increases. It showed different micellizing behavior at acidic and basic conditions when temperature increases. The micelles also enhanced pH sensitivity in the release process.

Amphiphilic graft copolymers are used as emulsifiers, surface modifiers, adhesives, moisturizers, or water repellents. The cellulose derivative graft copolymers have a range of potential applications. The applications of amphiphilic graft copolymers in the design of drug delivery systems and for surface modification of materials aimed to be used in biomedical applications have also to be highlighted. Over the years, increasing interest has been devoted to studies on the micellization behavior of graft copolymers or more complex structures. Micellar-type conformations, especially in the presence of a solvent exhibiting preference for the grafts, can exist for graft copolymers. The backbone is then collapsed and surrounded by the solvated grafts that protect it from precipitation by coacervation. If the grafts and the backbone exhibit different solubilities, they are of special interest. In particular, amphiphilic graft copolymers with water-soluble grafts have become the focus of much research because of the ability to undergo microphase separation and micellization. HPC graft copolymers can self-assemble into micelles in selected solvents. The morphology of the resultant micelles depends on the properties of both backbone and graft chains and on the properties of the solvents [89]. Ma et al. first reported the synthesis of dual pH- and temperature-sensitive HPC graft poly(*N*,*N*-dimethyl aminoethyl methacrylate) (HPC-*g*-(PDEMAEMA)) [90] and poly(4-vinyl pyridine) (HPC-*g*-P4VP) [91]. These copolymers can self-assemble into a trinity of micelles with different structures by combined pH- and temperature-stimuli of the complementary grafts. HPC was first esterified by 2-bromoisobutyryl bromide (BriB), and then PDMAEMA and/or P4VP [54] were grafted from HPC backbones via ATRP in homogeneous conditions. Figure 19.22 shows the synthetic route of HPC-*g*-P4VP by graft ATRP using CuCl and Me_6-TREN as the catalyst complex as an example.

The pH-induced micellization is due to the deprotonation and collapsing of P4VP graft chains at pH above the pK_a of P4VP side chains (pH > 4), by which micelles with a P4VP core stabilized with HPC shell are formed. The temperature-induced micellization is due to the HPC backbone becoming hydrophobic and collapsing to form the core of micelles stabilized with P4VP graft chains as the shell upon heating. They illustrated the intermolecular/intramolecular interaction changes with temperature and/or pH changes of HPC-*g*-P4VP using ^{1}H NMR spectroscopy with samples in D_2O (Figure 19.23). At low pH value, for example, pH 1.1, the protonated P4VP side chains and HPC were both well soluble in aqueous solution, and the characteristic peaks of both P4VP side chains (8.3, 6.6, and 1.5 ppm) and HPC backbones (3.0–5.0 and 1.1 ppm) appeared in the ^{1}H NMR spectrum of the HPC-*g*-P4VP graft copolymers. The peaks at 8.3, 6.6, and 1.5 ppm became quite weak at pH = 4.8 and totally disappeared at pH = 7.4, indicating that P4VP side chains are deprotonated and aggregated. Similarly, the peaks of the HPC backbone at 3.0–5.0 and 1.1 ppm disappeared, and the peaks of P4VP graft chains (8.3, 6.6, and 1.5 ppm) remained unchanged at a temperature above the LCST of HPC. An increase in both pH and temperature led to an increase in $\langle R_h \rangle$, of the graft copolymer, which indicates pH- or temperature-induced micellization. Moreover, the

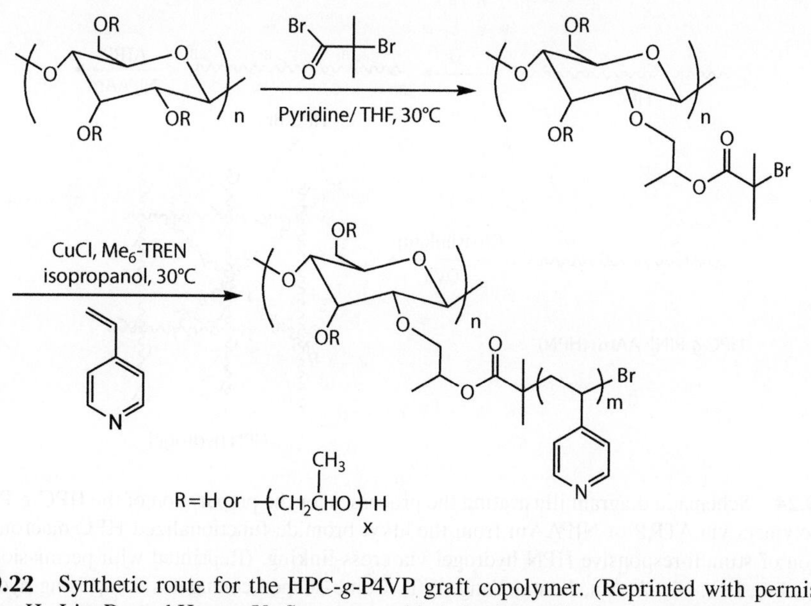

FIGURE 19.22 Synthetic route for the HPC-*g*-P4VP graft copolymer. (Reprinted with permission from Ma, L., Kang, H., Liu, R., and Huang, Y., Smart assembly behaviors of hydroxypropylcellulose-*graft*-poly(4-vinyl pyridine) copolymers in aqueous solution by thermo and pH stimuli, *Langmuir*, 26, 18519–18525, 2010. Copyright 2014 American Chemical Society.)

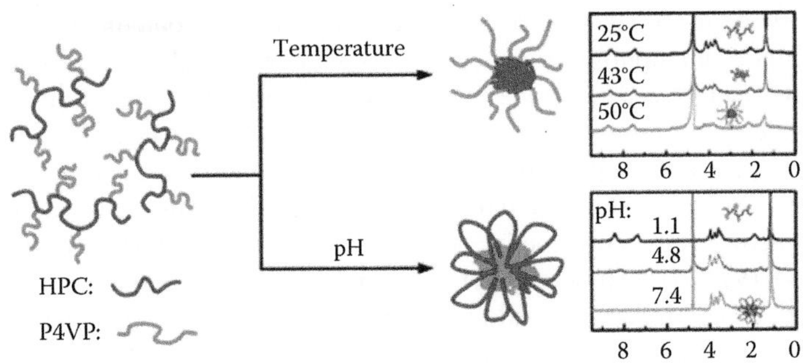

FIGURE 19.23 ^{1}H NMR spectra of HPC$_{0.05}$-*g*-P4VP$_{35}$ aqueous solutions (top, right) at 25°C at the pH values indicated and (bottom, right) at pH = 7.4 at the temperatures indicated. (Reprinted with permission from Ma, L., Kang, H., Liu, R., and Huang, Y., Smart assembly behaviors of hydroxypropylcellulose-*graft*-poly(4-vinyl pyridine) copolymers in aqueous solution by thermo and pH stimuli, *Langmuir*, 26, 18519–18525, 2010. Copyright 2014 American Chemical Society.)

results of transmittance and R$_h$ conformed to the ^{1}H NMR results. The ^{1}H NMR results for HPC-*g*-PDMAEMA showed similar changes according to the pH or temperature [90].

The low-molecular-weight PNIPAAm side chains were grafted via ATRP from the bromoisobutyryl-functionalized HPC backbones similarly. The obtained comb-shaped copolymer conjugates (HPC-*g*-PNIPAAm) or HPN) were further modified by cross-linking with divinylsulfone for the preparation of stable HPN hydrogels (Figure 19.24) [92]. Prepared hydrogel was thermoresponsive. By changing the composition ratio of HPC and PNIPAAm, the LCSTs of HPNs could be adjusted to be lower than the body temperature. In comparison with the HPC hydrogels, the resultant cross-linked HPN hydrogels possess interconnected pore structures and higher swelling ratios. The in vitro release kinetics of fluorescein isothiocyanate–labeled dextran and BSA

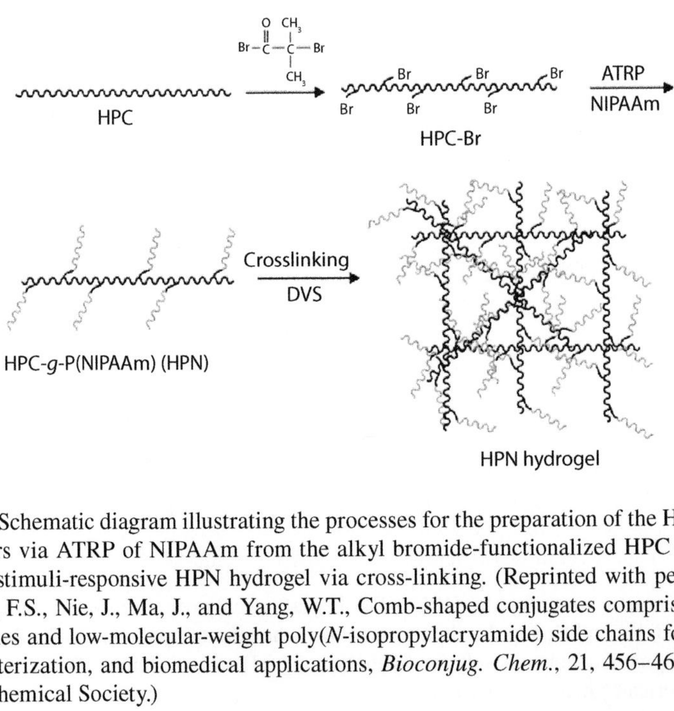

FIGURE 19.24 Schematic diagram illustrating the processes for the preparation of the HPC-*g*-P(NIPAAm) (HPN) copolymers via ATRP of NIPAAm from the alkyl bromide-functionalized HPC macroinitiator and the formation of stimuli-responsive HPN hydrogel via cross-linking. (Reprinted with permission from Xu, F.J., Zhu, Y., Liu, F.S., Nie, J., Ma, J., and Yang, W.T., Comb-shaped conjugates comprising hydroxypropyl cellulose backbones and low-molecular-weight poly(*N*-isopropylacryamide) side chains for smart hydrogels: Synthesis, characterization, and biomedical applications, *Bioconjug. Chem.*, 21, 456–464, 2010. Copyright 2014 American Chemical Society.)

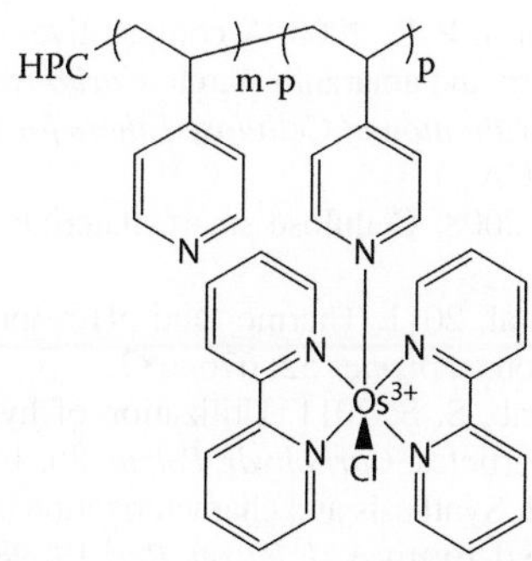

FIGURE 19.25 The structure of HPC-*g*-P4VP-Os(bpy) copolymer used as biosensors. (From Kang, H.L. et al., *J. Phys. Chem. B*, 116, 55, 2012.)

(or dextran-FITC and BSA-FITC) as model hydrophilic drugs from the hydrogels showed that the HPN hydrogels are suitable for long-term sustained release of macromolecular drugs at body temperature.

Moreover, cellulose graft copolymers can be used as biosensors. Examples for this application are HPC-*g*-P4VP copolymers, which further conjugated with Os (bipyridine) (Os (bpy)) to yield HPC-*g*-P4VP-Os (bpy) (Figure 19.25). The HPC-*g*-P4VP-Os (bpy) copolymers have pH-dependent redox properties and have a wide working window, which can be used for the decoration of electrodes for application in biosensors. Electrodes co-decorated with HPC-*g*-P4VP-s (bpy), and glucose oxidase can be used for the detection of glucose [93].

ACKNOWLEDGMENTS

The author would like to thank Ms. Akram Golshan Hosseini and Ms. Shaghayegh Shateri for their helpful assistance. The author's warm thanks are also extended to Ms. Veghar Barri, whose suggestions on the English language used in parts of the chapter.

REFERENCES

1. Kim, J., Yun, S., and Ounaies, Z. 2006. Discovery of cellulose as a smart material. *Macromolecules* 39: 4202–4206.
2. Matyjaszewski, K. and Möller, M. 2012. Polysaccharides. In *Polymer Science: A Comprehensive Reference*, E.-H. Song, J. Shang, and D. M. Ratner (eds.), vol. 9, pp. 137–155, Elsevier, Amsterdam, the Netherlands.
3. Klemm, D., Philipp, B., Heinze, T., Heinze, U., and Wagenknecht, W. 1998. *Comprehensive Cellulose Chemistry, Volume 1: Fundamentals and Analytical Methods*. Wiley-VCH Verlag GmbH, Weinheim, Germany.
4. Moon, R. J., Martini, A., Nairn, J., Simonsen, J., and Youngblood, J. 2011. Cellulose nanomaterials review: Structure, properties and nanocomposites. *Chem. Soc. Rev*. 40: 3941–3994.
5. Tkacheva, N. I., Morozov, S. V., Grigor'ev, I. A., Mognonov, D. M., and Kolchanov, N. A. 2013. Modification of cellulose as a promising direction in the design of new materials. *Polym. Sci., Ser. B* 55(7–8): 409–429.
6. Qiu, X. and Hu, S. 2013. "Smart" materials based on cellulose: A review of the preparations, properties, and applications. *Materials* 6: 738–781.
7. Nagel, M. C. V. and Heinze, T. 2010. Esterification of cellulose with acyl-1 *H*-benzotriazole. *Polym. Bull.* 65: 873–881.
8. Fischer, S., Thummler, K., Pfeiffer, K., Liebert, T., and Heinze, T. 2002. Inorganic molten salts as solvents for cellulose. *Cellulose* 9: 293–300.
9. Petra, M. and Dane, M. Chemical structure analysis of starch and cellulose derivatives. 2010. *Adv. Carbohydr. Chem. Biochem.* 64: 117–210.

10. Pal, J., Singhal, R. S., and Kulkarni, P. R. 2000. A comparative account of conditions of synthesis of hydroxypropyl derivative from corn and amaranth starch. *Carbohydr. Polym.* 43: 155–162.
11. Feller, R. L. and Wilt, M. 1990. *Evaluation of Cellulose Ethers for Conservation*, second printing, p. 13. J. Paul Getty Trust, Los Angeles, CA.
12. Kim, J., Yun, S., and Lee, S.-K. 2008. Cellulose smart material: Possibility and challenges. *J. Intell. Mater. Syst. Struct.* 19: 417–422.
13. Zhang, Z., Chen, L., Zhao, C. et al. 2011. Thermo- and pH-responsive HPC-*g*-AA/AA hydrogels for controlled drug delivery applications. *Polymer* 52: 676–682.
14. Abdel-Halima, E. S. and Al-Deyab, S. S. 2011. Utilization of hydroxypropyl cellulose for green and efficient synthesis of silver nanoparticles. *Carbohydr. Polym.* 86: 1615–1622.
15. Bagheri, M. and Shateri, Sh. 2012. Synthesis and characterization of novel liquid crystalline cholesteryl-modified hydroxypropyl cellulose derivatives. *J. Polym. Res.* 19: 9842.
16. Mark, J. E. 1999. *Polymer Data Handbook*. Oxford University Press, Inc., Oxford, U.K.
17. Fortin, S. and Charlet, G. 1989. Phase diagram of aqueous solutions of (hydroxypropyl) cellulose. *Macromolecules* 22: 2286–2292.
18. Chevillard, C. and Axelos, M. A. V. 1997. Phase separation of aqueous solution of methylcellulose. *Colloid Polym. Sci.* 275(6): 537–545.
19. Carotenuto, C. and Grizzuti, N. 2006. Thermoreversible gelation of hydroxypropylcellulose aqueous solutions. *Rheol. Acta* 45(4): 468–473.
20. Jing, Y. and Wu, P. 2013. Study on the thermoresponsive two phase transition processes of hydroxypropyl cellulose concentrated aqueous solution: From a microscopic perspective. *Cellulose* 20: 67–81.
21. Yamagishp, T.-A., Guittard, F., Godinho, M. H., Martins, A. F., Cambon, A., and Sixou, P. 1994. Comparison of thermal and cholesteric mesophase properties among the three kind of hydroxypropylcellulose (HPC) derivatives. *Polym. Bull.* 32: 47–54.
22. Shimamura, K., White, J. A., and Fellers, J. F. 1981. Hydroxypropyl cellulose, a thermotropic liquid crystal: Characteristics and structure development in continuous extrusion and melt spinning. *J. Appl. Polym. Sci.* 26: 2165–2180.
23. Hofenk-de Graaff, J. 1981. Central Research Laboratory for Objects of Art and Science. Hydroxy propyl cellulose, a multipurpose conservation material, Gabriel Metsustroat and 1071 EA, Amsterdam, the Netherlands.
24. Ishikawa, T., Mukai, B., Shiraishi, S., Utoguchi, N., Fuji, M., Matsumota, M., and Watanabe, Y. 2001. Preparation of rapidly disintegrating tablet using new types of micro-crystalline cellulose (PH-M series) and low substituted-hydroxypropylcellulose or spherical sugar granules by direct compression method. *Chem. Pharm. Bull.* 49: 134–139.
25. Cascone, M. G., Silvio, L. Di, Sim, B., and Downes, S. 1994. Collagen and hyaluronic acid based polymeric blends as drug delivery systems for the release of physiological concentrations of growth hormone. *J. Mater. Sci.* 5(9–10): 770–774.
26. Hagenmaier, R. D. and Shaw, P. E. 1990. Moisture permeability of edible films made with fatty acid and (hydroxypropyl) methylcellulose. *J. Agric. Food Chem.* 38(9): 1799–1803.
27. Chang, C. and Zhang, L. 2011. Cellulose-based hydrogels: Present status and application prospects. *Carbohydr. Polym.* 84: 40.
28. Kang, H., Liu, R., and Huang, Y. 2013. Cellulose derivatives and graft copolymers as blocks for functional materials. *Polym. Int.* 62: 338–344.
29. Richardsonl, S. and Gorton, L. 2003. Characterisation of the substituent distribution in starch and cellulose derivatives. *Anal. Chim. Acta* 497: 27–65.
30. Werbowyj, R. S. and Gray, D. G. 1980. Ordered phase formation in concentrated hydroxypropyl cellulose solutions. *Macromolecules* 13: 69–73.
31. Wang, C., Dong, Y., and Tan, H. 2003. Study on lyotropic liquid-crystalline properties of trimethylsilyl hydroxypropyl cellulose, *Carbohydr. Res.* 338: 535–540.
32. Huang B., Jason, J., Ge, J. J., Li, Y., and Hou, H. 2007. Aliphatic acid esters of (2-hydroxypropyl) cellulosed effect of side chain length on properties of cholesteric liquid crystals. *Polymer* 48: 264–269.
33. El-Wakil, N. A., Fahmy, Y., Abou-Zeid, R. E., Dufresne, A., and El-Sherbiny, S. 2010. Liquid crystalline behavior of hydroxypropyl cellulose esterified with 4-alkoxybenzoic acid. *BioResources* 5(3): 1834–1845.
34. Mori, H., Kato, I., Saito, S., and Endo, T. 2010. Proline-based block copolymers displaying upper and lower critical solution temperatures. *Macromolecules* 43(3): 1289–1298.
35. Bagheri, M. and Shateri, Sh. 2012. Thermosensitive nanosized micelles from cholesteryl-modified hydroxypropyl cellulose as a novel carrier of hydrophobic drugs. *Iran Polym. J.* 21: 365–373.

36. Nishio, Y. 2006. Material functionalization of cellulose and related polysaccharides via diverse microcompositions. *Adv. Polym. Sci.* 205: 97–151.
37. El Seoud, O. A., Koschella, A., Fidale, L. C., Dorn, S., and Heinze, T. 2007. Applications of ionic liquids in carbohydrate chemistry: A window of opportunities. *Biomacromolecules* 8: 2629–2647.
38. Fukaya, Y., Hayashi, K., Wada, M., and Ohno, H. 2008. Cellulose dissolution with polar ionic liquids under mild conditions; required factors for anions. *Green Chem.* 10: 44–46.
39. Chiba, R., Ito, M., and Nishio, Y. 2010. Addition effects of imidazolium salts on mesophase structure and optical properties of concentrated hydroxypropyl cellulose aqueous solutions. *Polym. J.* 42: 232–241.
40. Östmark, E., Lindqvist, J., Nyström, D., and Malmström, E. 2007. Dendronized Hydroxypropyl cellulose: Synthesis and characterization of biobased nanoobjects, *Biomacromolecules* 8: 3815–3822.
41. Meshram, M. W., Patil, V.V., Mhaske, S. T., and Thorat, B. N. 2009. Graft copolymers of starch and its application in textiles. *Carbohydr. Polym.* 75: 71–78.
42. Dhiman, P. K., Kaur, I., and Mahajan, R. K. 2008. Synthesis of a cellulose-grafted polymeric support and its application in the reductions of some carbonyl compounds. *J. Appl. Polym. Sci.* 108: 99–111.
43. Maiti, S., Ranjit, S., and Sa, B. 2010. Polysaccharide-based graft copolymers in controlled drug delivery. *Int. J. Pharm. Tech. Res.* 2(2): 1350–1358.
44. Chauhan, G. S., Singh, B., and Kumar, S. 2005. Synthesis and characterization of *N*-vinyl pyrrolidone and cellulosics based functional graft copolymers for use as metal ions and iodine sorbents. *J. Appl. Polym. Sci.* 98: 373–382.
45. Guo,Y., Wang, X., Shu, X., Shen, Z., and Sun, R.-C. 2012. Self-assembly and paclitaxel loading capacity of cellulose-*graft*-poly(lactide) nanomicelles. *J. Agric. Food Chem.* 60: 3900–3908.
46. Gref, R., Rodrigues, J., and Couvreur, P. 2002. Polysaccharides grafted with polyesters: Novel amphiphilic copolymers for biomedical applications, *Macromolecules* 35: 9861–9867.
47. Rakutyte, V. and Makuska, J. R. 2008. Synthesis and properties of chitosan-*N*-dextran graft copolymer. *React. Funct. Polym.* 68 (3): 787–796.
48. Lutz, P. J. and Peruch, F. 2012. Graft copolymers and comb-shaped homopolymers. *Polymer Science: A Comprehensive Reference*, 6: 511–542.
49. Neugebauer, D. 2007. Graft copolymers with hydrophilic and hydrophobic polyether side chains. *Polymer* 48(17): 4966–4973.
50. Kalia, S., Sabaa, M. W., and Kango, S. 2013. Chapter 1, Polymer grafting: A versatile means to modify the polysaccharides. In *Polysaccharide Based Graft Copolymers*, S. Kalia and M.W. Sabaa (eds.), pp. 1–14. Springer-Verlag, Berlin, Germany.
51. Lutz, P. J. 2012. Graft copolymers and comb-shaped homopolymers. *Polym. Sci.: Comprehen. Ref.* 6: 511–542.
52. Athawale, V. D. and Rathi, S. C. 1999. Graft polymerization: Starch as a model substrate. *J. Macromol. Sci.-Rev. Macromol. Chem. Phys.* C39: 445–480.
53. Fares, M. M., El-faqeeh, A. S., and Osman, M. E. 2003. Graft copolymerization onto starch–I. Synthesis and optimization of starch grafted with *N-tert*-butylacrylamide copolymer and its hydrogels. *J. Polym. Res.* 10: 119–125.
54. Kaith, B. S. and Kalia, S. 2008. A study of crystallinity of graft copolymers of flax fiber with binary vinyl monomers. *E-Polymers* 2: 1–6.
55. Hawker, C. J., Bosman, A. W., and Harth, E., 2001. New polymer synthesis by nitroxide mediated living radical polymerizations. *Chem. Rev.* 101: 3661–3688.
56. Cho, C. G. and Lee, K. 2002. Preparation of starch graft copolymer by emulsion polymerization. *Carbohydr. Polym.* 48: 125–130.
57. Misra, B. N. and Dogra, R. 1980. Grafting onto starch. IV. Graft copolymerization of methylmethacrylate by use of AIBN as radical initiator. *J. Macromol. Sci. Chem. A* 14: 763–770.
58. Chauhan, G. S., Dhiman, S. K., Guleria, L. K., Misra, B. N., and Kaur, I. 2000. Polymers from renewable resources: Kinetics of 4-vinyl pyridine radio chemical grafting onto cellulose extracted from pine needles. *Radiat. Phys. Chem.* 58: 181–190.
59. Chauhan, G. S., Sharma, R., and Lal, H. 2004. Synthesis and characterization of graft copolymers of hydroxypropyl cellulose with acrylamide and some comonomers. *J. Appl. Polym. Sci.* 91: 545–555.
60. Chauhan, G. S., Lal, H., and Mahajan, S. 2004. Synthesis, characterization, and swelling responses of poly(*N*-isopropylacrylamide)- and hydroxypropyl cellulose-based environmentally sensitive biphasic hydrogels. *J. Appl. Polym. Sci.* 91: 479–488.
61. Daly, W. H., Evenson, T. S., Iacono, S. T., and Jones, R. W. 2001. Recent developments in cellulose grafting chemistry utilizing Barton ester intermediates and nitroxide mediation. *Macromol. Symp.* 174: 155–163.

62. Stenzel, M. H., Davis, T. P., and Fane, A. G. 2003. Honeycomb structured porous films prepared from carbohydrate based polymers synthesized via the RAFT process. *J. Mater. Chem.* 13: 2090–2097.
63. Meng, T., Gao, X., Zhang, J., Yuan, J., Zhang, Y., and He, J. 2009. Graft copolymers prepared by atom transfer radical polymerization (ATRP) from cellulose. *Polymer* 50: 447–454.
64. Östmark, E., Harrisson, S., Wooley, K. L., and Malmström, E. E. 2007. Comb polymers prepared by ATRP from hydroxypropyl cellulose. *Biomacromolecules* 8: 1138–1148.
65. Choi, S. W., Choi, S. Y., Jeong, B., Kim, S. W., and Lee, D. S. 1999. Thermoreversible gelation of poly(ethylene oxide) biodegradable polyester block copolymers. II. *J. Polym. Sci. Part A: Polym. Chem.* 37(13): 2207–2218.
66. Donabedian, D. H. and McCarthy, S. P. 1998. Acylation of pullulan by ring-opening of lactones. *Macromolecules* 31: 1032–1039.
67. Lendlein, A. and Sisson, A. 2011. *Handbook of Biodegradable Polymers: Synthesis, Characterization and Applications*. Wiely-VCH Verlag GmbH&Co.KGaA, Weinheim, Germany.
68. Shi, R. and Burt, H. M. 2003. Synthesis and characterization of amphiphilic hydroxypropylcellulose-*graft*-poly(ε-caprolactone). *J. Appl. Polym. Sci.* 89: 718–727.
69. Wang, K., Dong, Y., and Tan, H. 2003. Biodegradable brushlike graft polymers. I. Polymerization of ε-caprolactone onto water-soluble hydroxypropyl cellulose as the backbone by the protection of the trimethylsilyl group. *J. Polym. Sci., Part A: Polym. Chem.* 41: 273–280.
70. Stenzel-Rosenbaum, M., Davis, T. P., Fane, A. G., and Chen, V. 2001. Star-polymer synthesis via radical reversible addition–fragmentation chain-transfer polymerization. *Polym. Sci., Part A: Polym. Chem.* 39: 2777–2783.
71. Hernandez-Guerrero, M., Davis, T. P., Barner-kKowollik, C., and Stenzel, M. H. 2005. Polystyrene comb polymers built on cellulose or poly(styrene-*co*-2-hydroxyethyl-methacrylate) backbones as substrates for the preparation of structured honeycomb films. *Eur. Polym. J.* 41(10): 2264–2277.
72. Bagheri, M. and Pourmirzaei, L. 2013. Synthesis and characterization of cholesteryl-modified graft copolymer from hydroxypropyl cellulose and its application as nanocarrier. *Macromol. Res.* 21(7): 801–808.
73. Prabaharan, M. and Mano, J. F. 2006. Stimuli-responsive hydrogels based on polysaccharides incorporated with thermo-responsive polymers as novel biomaterials. *Macromol. Biosci.* 6: 991–1008.
74. Owens, D. E., Jian, Y., Fang, J. E., Slaughter, B. V., Chen, Y. H., and Peppas, N. A. 2007. Thermally-responsive swelling properties of polyacrylamide/poly(acrylic acid) interpenetrating polymer network nanoparticles. *Macromolecules* 40: 7306–7310.
75. Feil, H., Bae, Y. H., Feijen, J., and Kim, S. W. 1991. Molecular separation by thermosensitive hydrogel membranes. *J. Membr. Sci.* 64: 283–294.
76. Recum, H. V., Okano, T., and Kim, S. W. 1998. Growth factor release from thermally reversible substrates to improve growth and attachment. *J. Control. Release* 55: 121–130.
77. Marsano, E., Bianchi, E., and Viscardi, A. 2004. Stimuli responsive gels based on interpenetrating network of hydroxyl propylcellulose and poly(*N*-isopropylacrylamide). *Polymer* 45: 157–163.
78. Çaykara, T., Şengül, G., and Birlik, G. 2006. Preparation and swelling properties of temperature-sensitive semi-interpenetrating polymer networks composed of poly[(*N-tert*-butylacrylamide)-coacrylamide] and hydroxypropyl cellulose. *Macromol. Mater. Eng.* 291: 1044–1051.
79. Liao, Q., Shao, Q., Qiu, G., and Lu, X. 2012. Methacrylic acid-triggered phase transition behavior of thermosensitive hydroxypropylcellulose. *Carbohydr. Polym.* 89: 1301–1304.
80. Chen, Y., Ding, D., Mao, Z., He, Y., Hu, Y., Wu, W., and Jiang, X. 2008. Synthesis of hydroxypropyl cellulose-poly(acrylic acid) particles with semi-interpenetrating polymer network structure. *Biomacromolecules* 9: 2609–2614.
81. Baia, Y., Zhanga, Z., Zhanga, A. et al. 2012. Novel thermo- and pH-responsive hydroxypropyl cellulose- and poly(L-glutamic acid)-based microgels for oral insulin controlled release. *Carbohydr. Polym.* 89: 1207–1214.
82. Tan, J., Kang, H., Liu, R. et al. 2011. Dual-stimuli sensitive nanogels fabricated by self-association of thiolated hydroxypropyl cellulose. *Polym. Chem.* 2: 672–678.
83. Jin, X., Kang, H., Liu, R., and Huang, Y. 2013. Regulation of the thermal sensitivity of hydroxypropyl cellulose by poly(*N*-isopropylacryamide) side chains. *Carbohydr. Polym.* 95: 155–160.
84. Lutz, J.-F. 2008. Polymerization of oligo(ethylene glycol) (meth)acrylates: Toward new generations of smart biocompatible materials. *J. Polym. Sci., Part A: Polym. Chem.* 46: 3459–3470.
85. Becer, C. R, Hahn, S., Fijten, M. W. M., Thijs, H. M. L., Hoogenboom, R., and Schubert, U. S. 2008. Libraries of methacrylic acid and oligo (ethylene glycol) methacrylate copolymers with LCST behavior. *J. Polym. Sci., Part A: Polym. Chem.* 46: 7138–7147.

86. Yamamoto, S.-I., Pietrasik, R., and Matyjasewski, K. 2008. The effect of structure on the thermoresponsive nature of well-defined poly(oligo(ethylene oxide) methacrylates) synthesized by ATRP. *J. Polym. Sci., Part A: Polym. Chem.* 46: 194–202.
87. Porsch, C., Hansson, S., Nordgren N., and Malmström, E. 2011. Thermo-responsive cellulose-based architectures: Tailoring LCST using poly(ethylene glycol) methacrylates. *Polym. Chem.* 2: 1114–1123.
88. Li, X., Yin, M., Zhang, G., and Zhang, F. 2009. Synthesis and characterization of novel temperature and pH responsive hydroxylpropyl cellulose-based graft copolymers. *Chin. J. Chem. Eng.* 17(1): 145–149.
89. Mourya V. K., Inamdar, N., Nawale, R. B., and Kulthe, S. S. 2011. Polymeric micelles: General considerations and their applications. *Ind. J. Pharm. Educ. Res.* 45(2): 128–138.
90. Ma, L., Liu, R., Tan, J. et al. 2010. Self-assembly and dual-stimuli sensitivities of hydroxypropylcellulose-*graft*-poly(*N,N*-dimethyl aminoethyl methacrylate) copolymers in aqueous solution. *Langmuir* 26: 8697–8703.
91. Ma, L., Kang, H., Liu, R., and Huang, Y. 2010. Smart assembly behaviors of hydroxypropylcellulose-*graft*-poly(4-vinyl pyridine) copolymers in aqueous solution by thermo and pH stimuli. *Langmuir* 26: 18519–18525.
92. Xu, F. J., Zhu, Y., Liu, F. S., Nie, J., Ma, J., and Yang, W. T. 2010. Comb-shaped conjugates comprising hydroxypropyl cellulose backbones and low-molecular-weight poly(*N*-isopropylacryamide) side chains for smart hydrogels: Synthesis, characterization, and biomedical applications. *Bioconjug. Chem.* 21: 456–464.
93. Kang, H. L., Liu, R. G., Sun, H. F., Zhen, J. M., Li, Q. M., and Huang, Y. 2012. Osmium bipyridine-containing redox polymers based on cellulose and their reversible redox activity. *J. Phys. Chem. B* 116: 55–62.

20 Intelligent Responsive Copolymers Based on Cellulose

Structure, Properties, and Applications

Xiuli Chen, Yajia Huang, Haixiang Zhang, Mario Gauthier, and Guang Yang

CONTENTS

20.1 INTRODUCTION

Cellulose is one of the most common natural polymers produced by plants, certain bacteria, algae, fungi, and so on (Klemm et al. 2005, 2011). As the most abundant renewable biomacromolecule, cellulose is a linear homopolymer generated from repeating anhydroglucose units that are joined together by β-1,4-glycosidic bonds (Figure 20.1a; Roy et al. 2009; Yokota et al. 2007). This inexpensive, renewable, and biodegradable material has attracted considerable attention because of its excellent physical and chemical properties. This is mainly due to its molecular structure, leading to a large number of hydroxyl groups on the surface of cellulose fibers (Klemm 1999).

The good mechanical stability, biocompatibility, hydrophilicity, and chemical reactivity of cellulose have led to applications for that biopolymer in many areas, including biomaterials (Bledzki and Gassan 1999; Fu et al. 2013; Kim et al. 2006), textiles (Dall Acqua et al. 2004), food products (Okiyama et al. 1992), drug delivery systems (Kamel 2008; Pal et al. 2006),

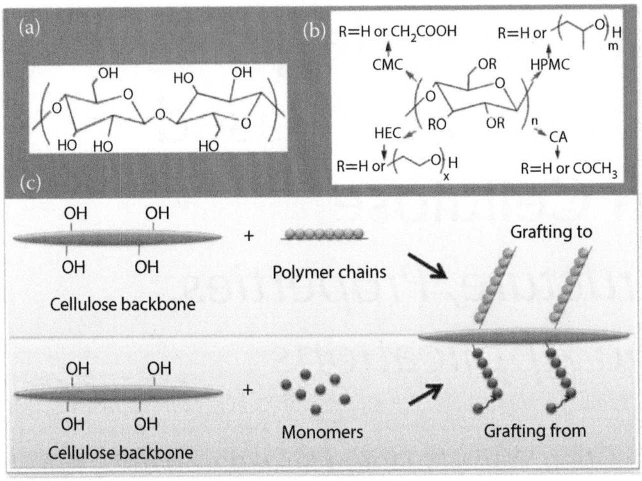

FIGURE 20.1 (a) Molecular structure of cellulose, (b) structure of cellulose derivatives, and (c) schematic representation of cellulose grafting.

TABLE 20.1
Some Applications of Cellulose in Different Forms

Cellulose Forms	Size	Application
Film/membrane	—	Adsorption, separation, packaging, water treatment, biomembranes
Hydrogel	—	Biomaterials, drug delivery, conductive materials, implants
Microcrystalline	1–1000 μm	Food products, reinforced materials, carrier membranes
Nanowhisker	5–1000 nm	Biomaterials, drug delivery, reinforced materials, conductive materials, adhesion, biomedical materials

films (Kontturi et al. 2006), and personal care products (Czaja et al. 2007). Table 20.1 (Klemm et al. 2005, 2011; Moon et al. 2011) summarizes the main application of cellulose in its different forms.

It is well known that many physiological actions arise from feedback-controlled interactions between biomacromolecules (nucleic acids, proteins, and polypeptides) and their surroundings (Duncan 2003). Responsive polymers also have responsive behaviors following changes in their environment such as temperature, pH, and ionic strength (Gil and Hudson 2004). The interest in responsive polymers has grown for many years, and many investigations have shown that environment-responsive polymers could be used as smart materials (Shanmuganathan et al. 2010). Stimuli-responsive polymers are defined as polymers that undergo relatively large and abrupt physical or chemical changes in response to small external changes in the environmental conditions (Jin et al. 2011). The applications of responsive polymers include drug delivery (Delcea et al. 2011), biomaterials (Prabaharan and Mano 2006), and sensors (Fleige et al. 2012).

A simple way to generate "intelligent" responsive polymers based on cellulose is by introducing an "intelligent" responsive polymer or side chains by graft copolymerization. These stimuli-responsive copolymers can render the modified cellulose responsive to environmental stimuli including pH or temperature variations, light, electricity, magnetic fields, moisture, and mechanical forces (Prabaharan and Mano 2006). Intelligent copolymers based on cellulose own their unique properties to the biocompatibility and strong mechanical strength contributed by the cellulose component and are expected to find a wide range of applications in drug delivery, as biomaterials, sensors, etc. (Sannino et al. 2009).

In view of the considerable increase in research activity on stimulus-responsive cellulose-based copolymers over the last decade, this chapter reviews the current state of knowledge on the synthesis, the structure, and the applications of these smart materials. We will focus our attention on intelligent cellulose copolymers obtained by chemical polymerization and their applications.

20.2 STRUCTURE AND PREPARATION

"Intelligent" materials derived from cellulose include thermo-, pH-, and other stimuli- and doubly or multiply stimuli-responsive copolymers. The properties of the cellulose derivatives depend on the smart responsive polymers grafted on the cellulose backbone. As mentioned earlier, cellulose is very easy to modify by traditional chemical methods such as etherification (Fox et al. 2011), esterification (Edgar et al. 2001), and oxidation reactions (Abdul Khalil et al. 2012). The synthesis of cellulose copolymers is different from traditional means and has extended the applications of cellulose even further (Edgar 2006). Graft copolymerization offers the possibility to introduce a variety of functional groups on cellulose by many different methods and modifies its properties depending on the polymer type used, the degree of polymerization, the grafting density, etc. (Roy et al. 2009). The synthesis of copolymers is an important method to modify the physical and chemical properties of cellulose. Cellulose graft copolymerization mainly includes "grafting to," "grafting from," and "grafting through" strategies, the "grafting to" and "grafting from" techniques being most useful (Habibi et al. 2010). The cellulose serves as backbone or substrate in graft copolymerization, and the polymer side chains contribute their specific properties to the cellulose (Figure 20.1c).

20.2.1 CELLULOSE AND DERIVATIVES

Cellulose is a reactive chemical due to the three hydroxyl groups present on each anhydroglucose residue. It has been confirmed that the hydroxyl groups in the 2- and 3-positions behave like secondary alcohols, while the one in the 6-position is similar to a primary alcohol. In general, the relative reactivity of these three hydroxyl groups varies in the order $C_6-OH \gg C_2-OH > C_3-OH$ (Klemm 1999; Roy et al. 2009). Cellulose is very difficult to dissolve because of its high crystallinity. There are a limited number of solvents that can be used for that purpose such as *N,N*-dimethylacetamide/LiCl and N_2O_4/dimethylformamide (Qiu and Hu 2013).

Common cellulose derivatives (Figure 20.1b) include carboxymethyl cellulose (CMC), hydroxypropyl cellulose (HPC), hydroxyethyl cellulose (HEC), and cellulose acetate (Doelker 1993; Zhang 2001). The cellulose derivatives are easier to dissolve in water and/or common organic solvents, so their chemical modification is easier to achieve under homogeneous conditions. Furthermore, at sufficiently high degrees of substitution (DS), CMC displays pH-responsive properties, and its pK_a is around 3–4 (Tan et al. 2010). HPC is a temperature-responsive polymer exhibiting an obvious change in solubility in aqueous solution around 41°C, which is called the lower critical solution temperature (LCST) for thermoresponsive polymers (Bai et al. 2012; Zhang et al. 2011). In other words, some cellulose derivatives (CMC and HPC) can exhibit intelligent stimuli-responsive behavior even without grafting with polymers.

20.2.2 THERMORESPONSIVE COPOLYMERS

It is as early as 1967 that Scarpa et al. reported the temperature-dependent behavior of poly(*N*-isopropylacrylamide) (PNIPAM); this is the earliest report on a thermoresponsive polymer (Schild 1992). The specific or critical temperature at which a phase transition is observed for thermoresponsive polymers is either defined as an LCST or an upper critical solution temperature (UCST; Savitskaya et al. 2000). If a thermoresponsive polymer displays LCST-type behavior in aqueous solution, it becomes soluble in water below the critical temperature due to hydrogen bonding between the polymer and the water molecules, while intermolecular hydrogen bonding between the

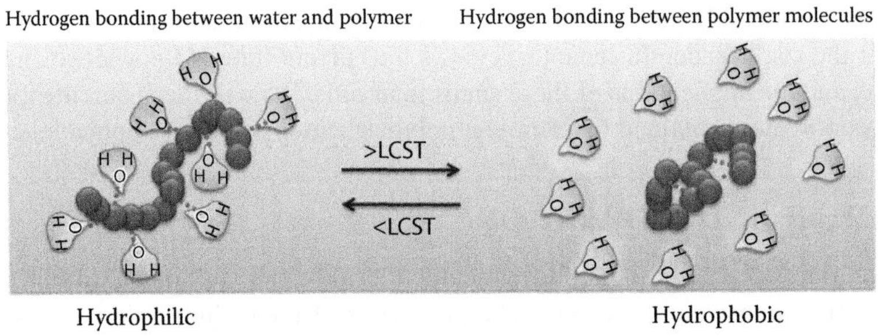

FIGURE 20.2 Intelligent behavior of thermoresponsive polymers.

polymer molecules is weak. At temperatures beyond the LCST, hydrogen bonding with the water molecules is disrupted and the formation of intermolecular hydrogen bonding between polymer molecules is favored, so the water is excluded from the polymer that forms a gel. Figure 20.2 shows the phase transition of thermoresponsive polymers (de Las Heras Alarcón et al. 2005). In contrast to the LCST, some thermoresponsive polymers display the opposite phase transition behavior with temperature known as a UCST.

PNIPAM, the best known and most studied thermoresponsive polymer, exhibits a sharp coil-to-globule transition in water at about 32°C (Schild 1992). The LCST of a thermoresponsive polymer is the most important parameter of interest for the application of thermoresponsive polymers under most conditions (Roy et al. 2013). Many thermoresponsive polymers have been reported that have potential applications in the biomedical field because their phase transition temperature lies between room temperature and body temperature (37°C), similarly to PNIPAM (Tang et al. 2006). This includes poly(*N*,*N*-diethylacrylamide) (PDEAM), poly(*N*-vinylcaprolactam) (PVCL), and poly(diethylene glycol methyl ether methacrylate) ($PMEO_2MA$), all potentially useful as biomaterials. Other polymers such as poly(ethylene oxide) (PEO) are soluble in water up to much higher temperatures (85°C in this specific case), but their copolymers with other components like poly(propylene oxide) (PPO) may also find a wide range of applications (Guan and Zhang 2011; Hansson et al. 2012; Roy et al. 2013). The chemical structure of some of the common thermoresponsive polymers is provided in Table 20.2.

The graft polymerization of a thermoresponsive monomer is necessary to impart thermoresponsive behavior to cellulose without loss of any of its desirable properties, in contrast to random substitution with small functional groups like cellulose ether derivatives. The result from this combination of properties is that thermoresponsive copolymers based on cellulose have a wider range of applications. Cellulose grafting can be achieved under either heterogeneous or homogeneous conditions. Since cellulose is very difficult to dissolve in the usual solvents due to its high crystallinity (Klemm et al. 2005), cellulose grafting was initially achieved with more soluble cellulose derivatives.

HPC has been intensively studied because of its solubility in water and its thermoresponsive behavior. It is a derivative of cellulose in which some of the hydroxyl groups have been hydroxypropylated with propylene oxide to become more hydrophobic (Harsh and Gehrke 1991). Due to the presence of both hydrophobic and hydrophilic groups, HPC is a thermoresponsive polymer with an LCST of >40°C, that is, higher than the body temperature (Harsh and Gehrke 1991; Schagerlöf et al. 2006). HPC is widely used as coating, excipient, for encapsulation, as binding material, foaming agent, protective colloid, and flocculant for a wide range of materials such as food products, drugs, paper, ceramics, and plastic materials. Several families of sequential networks based on HPC and PNIPAM were found to have much faster rates of swelling and deswelling than PNIPAM homopolymer gels (Marsano et al. 2000). Free radical polymerization has often been used to form interpenetrating polymer networks (IPNs) of two cross-linked polymers.

TABLE 20.2
Chemical Structure of Common Thermoresponsive Polymers

Polymer	LCST/UCST (°C)
Poly(*N*-isopropylacrylamide) (PNIPAM) 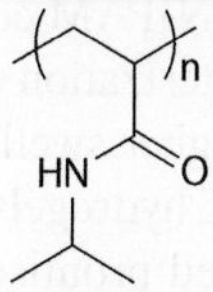	32
Poly(*N*,*N*-diethylacrylamide) (PDEAM) 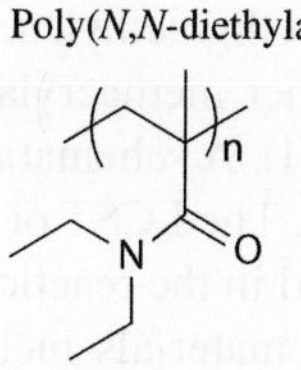	33
Poly(*N*-vinylcaprolactam) (PVCL) 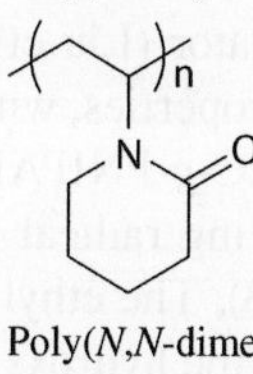	32
Poly(*N*,*N*-dimethylaminoethyl methacrylate) (PDMAEMA) 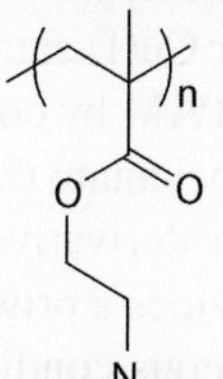	14–50
Poly(2-(2-methoxyethoxy)ethyl methacrylate) (PMEO$_2$MA) 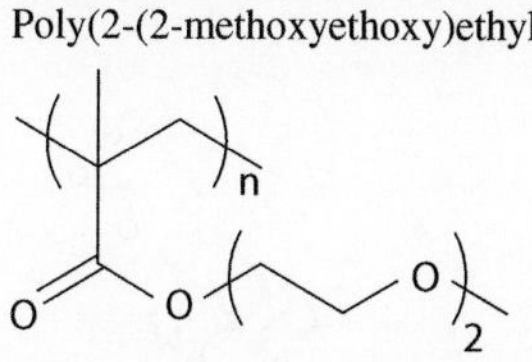	26
Poly(oligo(ethylene glycol) methacrylate) (POEGMA) 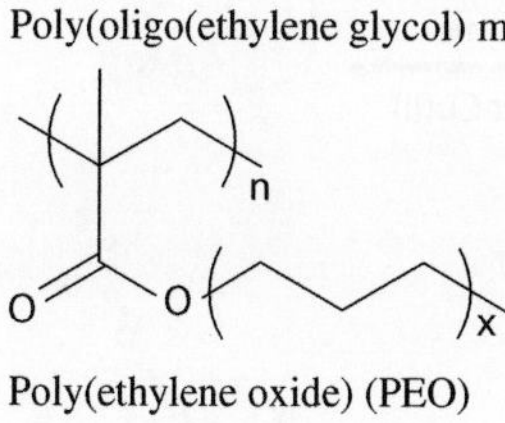	60–90
Poly(ethylene oxide) (PEO) 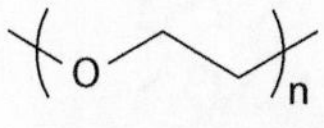	85
Poly(propylene oxide) (PPO) 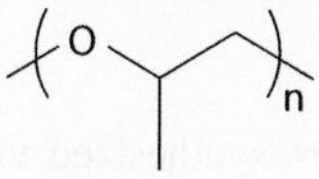	0–50

Poly[(*N-tert*-butylacrylamide)-*co*-acrylamide] [P(NTBA-*co*-AAm)]/HPC semi-IPN hydrogels have also been prepared by free radical cross-linking copolymerization using an ammonium persulfate (APS)—*N,N,N′,N′*-tetramethylethylenediamine (TEMED) redox initiator system (Çaykara et al. 2006). The LCST of HPC copolymers can also be decreased below body temperature via grafting of a low LCST thermoresponsive polymer. Xu et al. (2010) thus reported the synthesis of comb-shaped copolymers obtained by grafting low-molecular-weight PNIPAM side chains on an HPC backbone via atom transfer radical polymerization (ATRP). The HPC-*g*-PNIPAM copolymers with a PNIPAM content above 53 wt% exhibited a LCST below 37°C. Characterization of the hydrogel by SEM showed the presence of an interconnected pore structure, and higher swelling ratios were observed for the cross-linked HPC-*g*-PNIPAM hydrogels than for the HPC hydrogels. Furthermore, thermoresponsive polymers of poly(ethylene glycol) methacrylates showed promise as responsive materials in many fields due to their biocompatibility and nontoxicity. Oligo(ethylene glycol) methyl ether methacrylate (OEGMA300) and di(ethylene glycol) methyl ether methacrylate also formed comb copolymers by grafting from HPC via ATRP (Porsch et al. 2011). A schematic illustration of the comb polymers synthesized via ATRP is provided in Figure 20.3a. The LCST of different copolymers could be controlled by changes in the monomer feed ratio used in the reaction.

Other cellulose derivatives also used to synthesize "intelligent" materials include methylcellulose (MC), due to its thermoreversible gelation behavior in water at 60°C–80°C. PNIPAM was thus grafted to MC in various ratios using APS and TEMED as initiator (Liu et al. 2004). The PNIPAM-*g*-MC hydrogels displayed strongly temperature-responsive properties, with LCST values increasing as the MC content increased. Ethyl cellulose-*g*-PNIPAM (EC-*g*-PNIPAM) copolymers were likewise synthesized, in this case by single-electron transfer living radical polymerization (SET-LRP) in a THF/methanol mixed solvent system (Kang et al. 2013). The ethyl cellulose macroinitiators (EC-Br) for SET-LRP were synthesized by esterification of the hydroxyl groups on EC with 2-bromoisobutyryl bromide, and EC-*g*-PNIPAM was obtained under Cu(I) catalysis. The thermoresponsive hydrogels were also prepared from modified HEC and PNIPAM by copolymerization (Peng and Chen 2010). The HEC was first modified with 2,4-toluenediisocyanate (2,4-TDI).

For reactions carried out under homogeneous conditions on soluble derivatives, the original supramolecular structure of crystalline cellulose is destroyed, which provides a product with a uniform composition. The situation is completely different under heterogeneous conditions, when the

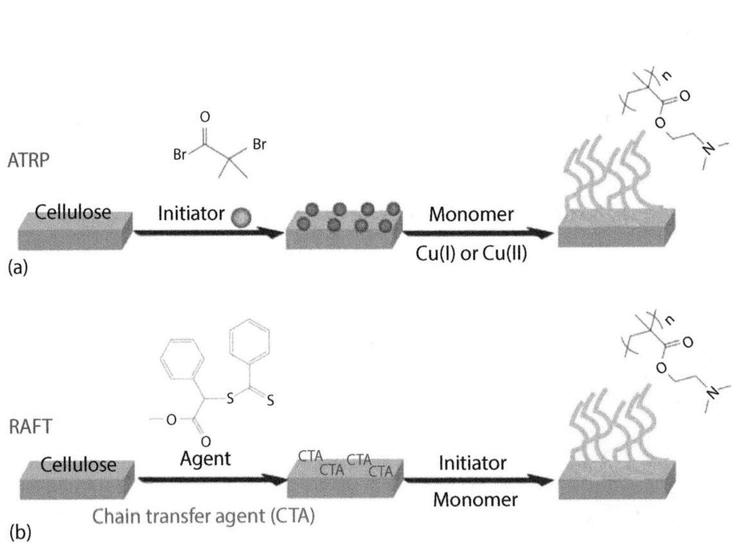

FIGURE 20.3 Schematic illustration of the PDMAEMA comb polymers synthesized via (a) ATRP and (b) RAFT. (From Sui, X. et al., *Biomacromolecules*, 9, 2615, 2008; Roy, D. et al., *Aust. J. Chem.*, 59, 737, 2006.)

insoluble crystalline superstructures are chemically modified. Since the chemical reactions occur only at the surface layer under heterogeneous conditions, the bulk structure of the cellulose sample can be largely maintained.

Temperature-responsive cellulose was thus obtained by graft polymerization of the NIPAM monomer using ceric ammonium nitrate (CAN) as initiator in acidic media (Gupta and Khandekar 2003). The rate of polymerization depended on the concentration of NIPAM and on the relative concentrations of ceric (IV) ions and nitric acid in the reaction mixture. The thermal stability, water absorbency, and degree of swelling of the PNIPAM-grafted cellulose materials were thus markedly increased. Hebeish et al. (2014) also reported that the preparation of PNIPAM hydrogel grafted onto lyocell (regenerated cellulose (RC)) fibers was performed in aqueous acidic media with cerium (IV).

Modification strategies used recently more frequently for cellulose in heterogeneous conditions are controlled/living radical polymerization (CRP) methods, especially ATRP (Figure 20.3a) and reversible addition–fragmentation chain transfer (RAFT, Figure 20.3b), which can provide controlled composition, architecture, and molecular weight distribution for the polymers (Matyjaszewski and Xia 2001). For example, thermoresponsive RC membranes were synthesized via surface-initiated atom transfer radical polymerization (SI-ATRP) (Pan et al. 2010). The RC membranes were first modified by reacting the hydroxyl groups on their surface with 2-bromoisobutyrylbromide, to serve initiator in the ATRP reaction. PNIPAM brushes were likewise grafted from cotton fabric surfaces by SI-ATRP in methanol/water mixtures (Yang et al. 2012). In this case, aminopropyl trimethoxysilane (ATMS) was first reacted with the cotton surface to provide amine groups (Cotton-ATMS). 2-Bromoisobutyryl bromide was then reacted with the amino-functionalized cotton to form the surface-grafted initiator (Cotton-ATMS-Br). The initiation of surface polymerization yielded PNIPAM brushes (Cotton-*g*-PNIPAM). A two-step "green" grafting process using cold plasma was also proposed to modify cellulose/chitin (CC) mixed fibers with NIPAM and obtain fibers responsive to external stimuli (Sdrobiş et al. 2012). The CC fibers were activated for 15 min in a high-frequency plasma operated at 0.4 mbar (40 Pa) pressure. Furthermore, 2-(dimethylamino) ethyl methacrylate (DMAEMA) was successfully grafted from the surface of the ramie fibers via ATRP polymerization using a brominated initiator and the CuCl/1,10-phenanthroline catalyst system (Liu et al. 2009).

RAFT polymerization (Figure 20.3b) was likewise used to modify different solid substrates with monomers such as DMAEMA (Roy et al. 2006). A free radical chain transfer agent was used to achieve better control over the grafting density, the length of the grafted polymer chains, and the monomer conversion. The cellulose substrate was first modified to form a cellulose-based chain transfer agent for the polymerization.

Microcrystalline cellulose (MCC) and cellulose nanocrystals (CNCs) or nanowhiskers are very different in form and size from cellulose films. CNCs or nanowhiskers are produced by the hydrolysis of cellulose fibers from different sources including wood and bacterial cellulose (BC) with sulfuric acid. Hao et al. (2009) studied the modification of MCC in ionic liquids via radiation-induced grafting. The synthesis of MCC-*g*-PNIPAM was successful when using 1-butyl-3-methylimidazolium chloride ([Bmim]Cl) as ionic liquid with γ-ray irradiation.

The synthesis of CNC-*g*-PNIPAM was achieved via surface-initiated single-electron transfer living radical polymerization (SI-SET-LRP) under various conditions at room temperature (Zoppe et al. 2010). The PNIPAM side chains on the surface of CNCs conferred thermoresponsiveness to the nanocrystals, and it was determined that the molar mass of the chains could be controlled by varying the initiator and monomer concentrations used in the reactions. Temperature-responsive PDMAEMA-grafted CNCs were also synthesized by SI-ATRP (Yi et al. 2009). The graft copolymers exhibited a "fingerprint" liquid crystalline texture when investigated by polarizing optical microscopy in the lyotropic state.

Finally, Kloser and Gray (2010) prepared PEO-grafted nanocrystalline cellulose (PEO-grafted NCC) to demonstrate the use of steric rather than electrostatic stabilization for these systems.

This was achieved by treating NCC suspensions, obtained by sulfuric acid hydrolysis, with epoxy-terminated poly(ethylene oxide) (PEO epoxide) macromonomers under alkaline conditions, to induce coupling of the chains on the surface.

20.2.3 pH-Responsive Copolymers

Different pH values exist in several body tissues such as the stomach (pH 2), the intestine (pH 5–8), and the blood (pH 7.35–7.45), as well as in different intracellular organelles such as lysosomes (pH 4.5–5.0) and the Golgi apparatus (pH 6.4), and cancer tissue is also reported to be extracellularly acidic (Gupta et al. 2002). Similar to thermoresponsive polymers, pH-responsive polymers exhibit a change in the ionization state of their pendant groups upon variation in the pH. Following the change in pH, a conformation change for soluble polymers or a change in swelling behavior for hydrogels takes place (Schmaljohann 2006). Polymers synthesized from ionizable monomer units can also display phase transitions and solubility changes depending on the pH of the medium.

The pH, as one of the most important biochemical signals in the human body, can be targeted by pH-responsive materials due to the wide range of pH encountered in vivo. The pH response of ionizable polymers ranges from 3 to 10 (Siegel 1993). The corresponding pH-responsive copolymers derived from cellulose and cellulose derivatives can be obtained using monomers like acrylic acid (AA), maleic anhydride (MA), DEAEMA, methacrylic acid (MAA), or 4-vinylpyridine (P4VP) (Schmaljohann 2006). The chemical modification of side chains is another approach to afford pH sensitivity via –COOH and $-NH_2$ moieties (Way et al. 2012).

As one of the cellulose derivatives, CMC has been widely investigated because of its high degree of substitution with carboxymethyl groups, making it a pH-responsive polyelectrolyte with a pK_a around 3–4 on the cellulose backbone (Pourjavadi et al. 2006). A report on the enzymatic degradation of CMC and PNIPAM-*g*-CMC showed that enzymatic degradation was facilitated by the presence of PNIPAM grafts (Vasile et al. 2003). The behavior of blends of CMC with PNIPAM was also compared with their graft copolymers (Vasile et al. 2004). In solution, the graft copolymers exhibited thermally induced thickening, while the corresponding mixtures exhibited Arrhenius-type behavior. In the solid state, the morphology of the copolymers was also different from the physical blends.

Kubota et al. (1998) reported a temperature-responsive copolymer in the form of PNIPAM-grafted CMC, obtained by photografting with a xanthone photoinitiator. The CMC was reacted with H_2O_2 to form peroxides, which were efficient initiators for the photografting of vinyl monomers. The temperature-sensitive PNIPAM could also be grafted on the surface of cotton fabric by pre-irradiation with γ-rays; the grafting reaction was found to be mainly located at the interface between the crystalline and amorphous regions (Jianqin et al. 1999). The CMC-*g*-PNIPAM copolymers were also prepared by a coupling reaction between CMC and PNIPAM (with a relatively low molecular weight) promoted by 1-(3-(dimethylamino)propyl)-3-ethyl-carbodiimide hydrochloride as condensing agent (Bokias et al. 2001). Due to the hydrophilic CMC backbone, turbidity measurements for the copolymer solutions showed that the temperature of the phase transition was higher than the LCST of pure PNIPAM.

Cellulose-based dual graft molecular brushes, consisting of ethyl cellulose-*graft*-poly(*N*,*N*-dimethylaminoethyl methacrylate)-*graft*-poly(ε-caprolactone) (EC-*g*-PDMAEMA-*g*-PCL), have been prepared via ring-opening polymerization (ROP) and ATRP (Yan et al. 2009). The copolymers showed unique physicochemical properties and multifunctional properties resulting from their unique topological structure: the copolymers could self-assemble into micelles in aqueous solution due to a change in pH. In this study, the ROP and ATRP were used to prepare EC-Br-*g*-PCL copolymers and EC-*g*-PDMAEMA-*g*-PCL copolymers respectively. The dual graft molecular brushes exhibited multiple functions and different properties from other brush copolymers due to their special topological structure, because PCL is a crystalline hydrophobic polymer while PDMAEMA is a common hydrophilic polyelectrolyte.

The early examples of AA-*g*-cellulose copolymers were synthesized through CAN-initiated free radical copolymerization with AA from the cellulose backbone in aqueous nitric acid solutions (Gürdağ et al. 1997). Abdel-Halim rather prepared PAA-HPC composites via the reaction of HPC with AA using a potassium bromate/thiourea redox initiator system (Abdel-Halim et al. 2008). A PAA-*g*-HEC copolymer was similarly prepared by the polymerization of AA in the presence of HEC using potassium bromate/thiourea dioxide ($KBrO_3$/TUD) redox system (Abdel-Halim 2012). Finally, neutralized AA-*g*-CMC copolymers were obtained by free radical solution polymerization in the presence of attapulgite, participating in the polymerization reaction through its active –OH groups with APS and *N,N'*-methylenebisacrylamide (MBA) as cross-linker (Wang and Wang 2010).

Poly(2-(diethylamino)ethyl methacrylate) (PDEAEMA) was used to obtain pH-sensitive ethyl cellulose-*g*-PDEAEMA copolymers through ATRP (Wang et al. 2011). Micelles of EC-*g*-PDEAEMA in aqueous solutions could be prepared by mixing the copolymer in THF with an aqueous solution at pH 3.2 with continuous stirring. The micelle solutions were then dialyzed against water at pH 3.2 for 3 days in a dialysis bag with a cutoff molecular weight of 3500, to gradually remove the organic solvent and avoid the formation of large aggregates (Wang et al. 2011). Sui et al. (2008) also reported that cellulose-*g*-PDMAEMA copolymers could be prepared by homogeneous ATRP (Figure 20.3a) under mild conditions, where the cellulose macroinitiator was synthesized by direct acylation of cellulose with 2-bromopropionyl bromide in a room temperature ionic liquid. In the synthesis of the cellulose-*g*-PDMAEMA copolymer, the cellulose-Br substrate served as macroinitiator for the polymerization of DMAEMA using CuBr/PMDETA as catalyst. The cellulose-*g*-PDMAEMA copolymers showed pH-responsive behavior due to the protonation/deprotonation of the *N,N*-dimethylaminoethyl groups in PDMAEMA component: at low pH, the PDMAEMA chains are expected to be entirely protonated and stretched along the radial direction, due to geometrical constraints and electrostatic repulsion between the polymer chains. As the pH was changed from 2 to 12, the PDMAEMA chains gradually shrink and precipitate from solution due to the deprotonation of the amine groups. The cellulose-*g*-PDMAEMA copolymers were thus soluble in acidic solutions and precipitated in alkaline solutions, illustrating how the pH-sensitive behavior can be used to prepare new biomaterials with desired properties.

20.2.4 Other Responsive Copolymers

Biomaterial can be modified to provide "intelligent" copolymers not only responsive to environmental stimuli including pH or temperature variations, but also light, electricity, magnetic fields, moisture, or mechanical forces. Responsive properties typically arise when stimuli-responsive polymers are chemically grafted onto a cellulose substrate. While temperature- and pH-responsive polymers are most widely used in many fields, the other types of responsive polymers derived from cellulose have been less investigated. These and other copolymers displaying pH or temperature responsiveness, synthesized from cellulose and more exotic monomers, have also been reported.

PVCL chains were thus grafted from the surface of RC membranes using ATRP (Himstedt et al. 2013). The grafting density of PVCL chains depended on the ATRP initiator immobilization time. PVCL is a thermoresponsive polymer with an LCST depending on the concentration of salt ions in solution but is above room temperature when the ionic concentration is low enough. The LCST lies below room temperature in 1.8 M $(NH_3)_2SO_4$, however, and the polymers exhibit more hydrophobic/collapsed behavior under these conditions.

Cellulose may be modified not only with organic molecules, but also with inorganic particles. For example, Peng et al. (2012) synthesized novel interfacially active and magnetically responsive nanoparticles (NPs) by grafting bromoesterified ethyl cellulose (EC-Br) onto the surface of amino-functionalized magnetite (Fe_3O_4) NPs for multiphase separation applications. The magnetic response of EC-*g*-Fe_3O_4 was determined in room temperature magnetization measurements.

This was the first report on the synthesis of interfacially active and magnetically responsive NPs, containing a magnetic core and an interfacially active polymer layer.

Photocleavable polymeric chains were also grafted from CNCs using the ATRP method (Morandi and Thielemans 2012). The synthesis of NPs based on these materials had two main steps. Grafting of a photosensitive moiety bearing an ATRP initiating site onto the surface of CNC with toluene diisocyanate (TDI) was followed by the surface-initiated ATRP growth of polystyrene (PS) chains from the modified surface outward to form CNCs-*g*-photolinker-PS NPs. UV irradiation of the NPs led to the cleavage of an important fraction of the PS chains.

The piezoelectric effect was first observed in wood by Bazhenov in the 1960s (Bazhenov 1961). The asymmetric crystalline structure of cellulose causes it to display inhomogeneous deformation associated with piezoelectric response when subjected to an electric field (Csoka et al. 2012). Cellulose has many advantages including large strains in response to an electric stimuli, ease of processing, good mechanical properties, low density, low cost, biodegradability, low actuation voltage, and low power consumption as sensors and actuators, usually identified as electro-active paper (EAPap) (Csoka et al. 2012; Kim et al. 2010). Hu et al. (2011) also reported novel conductive polyaniline (PANI)/BC nanocomposite membranes synthesized in situ by oxidative polymerization. The PANI/BC nanocomposites displayed excellent electrical conductivity, sensitive to strain, and good mechanical properties.

Zhao et al. (2010) prepared a novel electrolyte-responsive membrane, RC-*g*-PSBMA, by grafting sulfobetaine methacrylate (SBMA), a zwitterionic monomer, on the surface of RC membranes via surface-initiated ATRP (SIP). The degree of polymerization of the PSBMA chains grafted on the surface of the RC membranes could be controlled through the ATRP reaction conditions. The permeability of the RC-*g*-PSBMA membranes showed a clear dependence on NaCl concentration in the solutions. Membranes with such electrolyte-responsive properties have great potential in protein purification as well as for many other separation applications.

20.2.5 Dual or Multiple Stimuli-Responsive Copolymers

These polymers can be classified as responding to physical or chemical stimuli (Chuang et al. 2010). Chemical stimuli include the pH, ionic strength, and chemical agents, and physical stimuli include temperature, electric, or magnetic stimuli. Some researchers have developed polymers that have two or more stimuli-response mechanisms combined into one polymer system. As illustrated in Figure 20.4 for dual-responsive polymers, a temperature-responsive polymer may also respond to pH changes. Meanwhile, it has also been reported that more than two signals could be applied simultaneously to induce response in so-called multiple responsive polymer systems.

Wan et al. (2007) reported that dual temperature- and pH-responsive cellulose-based copolymers, HEC-*g*-PNIPAM-PAA (CNipAa), synthesized via successive cerium (IV) initiated free radical copolymerization of NiPAM and AA from an HEC substrate. The CNipAa copolymers were able to self-assemble into three different micellar structures controlled by pH and temperature changes. Micelles with a PNIPAM/PAA complex core and a solvated HEC shell were obtained below pH 4.6, while the PNIPAM and PAA chains grafted from the HEC backbone formed the PNIPAM-*g*-HEC-*g*-PAA branched-like copolymers when at pH 12 and $T = 30°C$. The CNipAa copolymers in solution at pH > 4.6 self-assembled into micelles with PNIPAM grafts as the core and HEC/PAA as shell when the temperature was elevated above the LSCT of PNIPAM. When the pH of the micellar solution was decreased while the temperature was maintained at 45°C, protonation of the PAA chains in the shell led to the formation of a complex with the PNIPAM chains. As a result, a new inner shell composed of PAA and PNIPAM chains was generated.

The amphiphilic EC brush polymers with side chains of poly(2-(2-methoxyethoxy)ethyl methacrylate)-*co*-oligo(ethylene glycol) methacrylate) (P(MEO_2MA-*co*-OEGMA)) and poly(2-(*N,N*-dimethylamino)ethyl methacrylate) (PDMAEMA) were synthesized by a combination of ATRP and click chemistry (Yuan et al. 2012). The brush polymers could self-assemble into

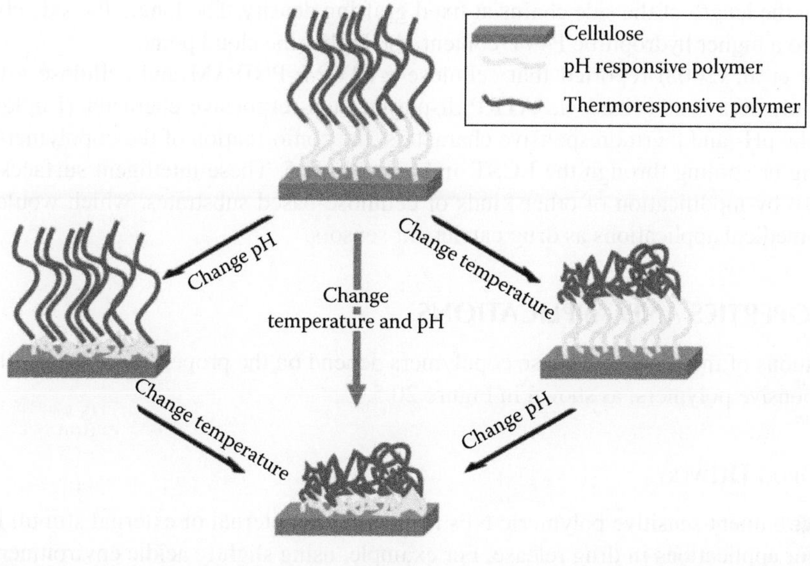

FIGURE 20.4 Dual-responsive polymers responding to pH and temperature changes. Upon a rise in temperature above the LCST, the thermoresponsive part of the polymer will collapse on the surface. Following a change in pH, the pH-responsive part will behave the same way. The same result is obtained when a change in pH is followed by a change in temperature.

spherical micelles/aggregates with tunable temperature- and pH-responsive properties that could be tuned with variations in the EC chains and the ratio of P(MEO_2MA-*co*-OEGMA) and PDMAEMA side chains, to be applied as biomedical or intelligent materials. P(MEO_2MA-*co*-OEGMA) is a temperature-responsive polymer that has a critical phase transition temperature in water, while PDMAEMA is a pH- and temperature-responsive polymer that has a phase transition temperature in water and a pH-triggered phase transition point.

Membranes of PNIPAAM-*co*-PDEAEMA-*g*-(cross-linked-cellulose) copolymer were prepared via surface-initiated ATRP grafting of PNIPAAM and PDEAEMA from the cross-linked cellulose substrate (Qiu et al. 2013). The cross-linked cellulose membrane (CCM) was prepared via drying on a Teflon plate of a solution of MCC in DMAc/LiCl mixed with TDI. A BriB-grafted CCM macroinitiator was prepared by grafting the excess BriB on the CCM with NIPAAm and DEAEMA through RGET ATRP.

Kubota et al. (2001) prepared xanthone-photoinitiated MAA-*N*-isopropylacrylamide (NIPAM)-cellulose copolymers in aqueous reaction media. The photografting reaction was carried out in a Pyrex glass tube containing the cellulose film with AA and NIPAM monomers in solution, by irradiation with a 400 W high-pressure mercury lamp for 24 h. The MAA-*g*-cellulose-*g*-PNIPAM copolymers obtained shrank in acidic media and swelled in alkaline solutions, thus showing pH-responsive properties, while PNIPAM grafting led to temperature-responsive character, with swelling and shrinking in water below and above about 30°C, respectively.

Ma et al. (2010) obtained the thermo- and pH-sensitive graft copolymers HPC-*g*-poly(4-vinylpyridine) (P4VP) via HPC-Br-initiated ATRP using CuCl and Me_6-TREN as catalyst complex. The thermally and pH-induced micellization of the HPC-*g*-P4VP copolymers in aqueous solutions was investigated by different methods including transmittance, ^{1}H NMR, and dynamic light scattering measurements. For pH-induced micellization, the P4VP side chains collapsed to form the core of the micelles when the pH increased above the pK_a of the P4VP side chains, while the HPC backbone formed the shell to stabilize the micelles. Upon heating, the HPC backbone collapsed to form the core of the micelles, and the P4VP side chains stabilized the micelles as the shell in thermally induced micellization. The cloud point of the HPC-*g*-P4VP copolymers in aqueous solution depended on the length of the side chains at fixed grafting density. The longer the side chains, corresponding to a higher hydrophilic P4VP content, the higher the cloud point.

Lindqvist et al. (2008) reported that cellulose-*g*-P4VP-*b*-PNIPAM and cellulose-*g*-PNIPAM-*b*-P4VP copolymers synthesized via ATRP displayed dual-responsive character (Lindqvist et al. 2008). For the pH- and thermoresponsive characters, the conformation of the copolymers changed when heating or cooling through the LCST and around pH 5. These intelligent surfaces could be obtained also by modification of other kinds of cellulose-based substrates, which would open up possible biomedical applications as drug carriers or sensors.

20.3 PROPERTIES AND APPLICATIONS

The applications of intelligent cellulose copolymers depend on the properties of both cellulose and stimuli-responsive polymers, as shown in Figure 20.5.

20.3.1 Drug Delivery

Various environment-sensitive polymeric NPs responding to internal or external stimuli have been developed for applications in drug release. For example, using slightly acidic environments typical of cancerous tissues (pH 6.5–7.2) as compared to the physiological pH of 7.4 in the blood and normal tissues, pH-sensitive NPs have been developed to release drugs at tumor sites (Schmaljohann 2006). The stimuli-responsive NPs offer obvious advantages in terms of spatial precision as well as dose control in drug release.

Hydrogels based on acrylamide monomer and different ratios of CMC were prepared by gamma irradiation (Nizam El-Din et al. 2010). In this work, interpenetrating networks of PAM, poly(acrylic acid) (PAAc), and PNIPAAm with CMC were synthesized by gamma irradiation in the presence of the cross-linker methylenebisacrylamide (MBA). Variations in temperature and pH showed that the degree of swelling of all the hydrogels changed within the temperature range 30°C–40°C and within the pH range 4–8. The PAM/CMC hydrogels were evaluated for possible use in drug delivery. Methylene blue (MB) indicator served as a model drug in the study; MB loading reached equilibrium after 3 h. The MTT assay using the HEK293 cell line showed that HPC-PNIPAM exhibited low cytotoxicity (Xu et al. 2010). The in vitro release kinetics from the hydrogels of fluorescein isothiocyanate-labeled dextran and BSA as model drugs showed that the hydrogels were suitable for the long-term sustained release of macromolecular drugs at body temperature.

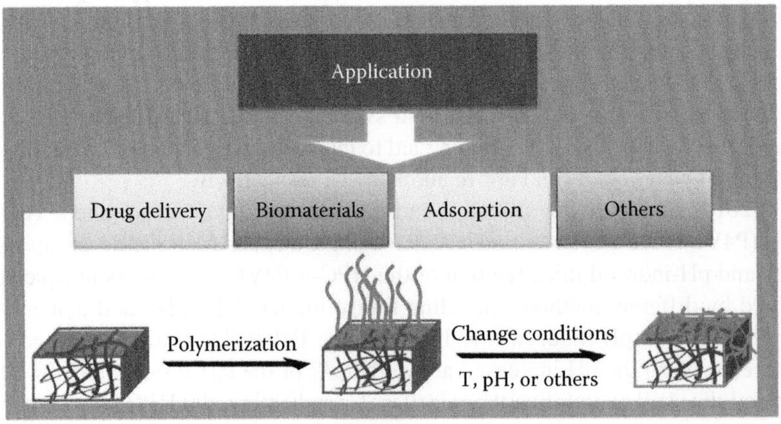

FIGURE 20.5 Applications of intelligent responsive cellulose copolymers.

The pH-responsive EC-*g*-PDEAEMA copolymers prepared by Wang at al. (2011) collapsed in the pH range of 6.0–6.9, started to aggregate at pH ≥ 6.9, and remained unchanged at pH < 6.0. To exploit this pH-responsive property in drug delivery, rifampicin was selected to investigate its release behavior in buffer solutions at pH 6.6 and 7.4. The results indicated that the loading efficiency and the rifampicin (RIF) content increased with increasing m(RIF) content. The release of RIF at pH 6.6 was higher than that at pH 7.4, due to the different response of the copolymer micelles to pH changes affecting the conformation of the copolymer chains. It was concluded that the EC-*g*-PDEAEMA copolymers can self-assemble into micelles in acidic aqueous solution, to be used in drug delivery systems due to their reversible pH sensitivity.

Hydrogels of solubilized BC/acrylamide (Am), responsive to pH and ionic strength changes, were synthesized by freezing (FM), microwave irradiation (HM), and combinations of both methods (HFM), using epichlorohydrin and *N,N′*-methylenebisacrylamide as cross-linkers for BC and Am, respectively (Pandey et al. 2013). SEM images for the hydrogels exhibited pores on the surface for the HF method that were larger than for the HFM and HM. The drug-loading capacity of the hydrogels was mainly controlled by the nature of the polymer, the pore volume per unit area, and the swelling properties. The drug-loading capacity of the HM and HFM hydrogels was better than for HF due to the presence of more polar groups available for swelling and interactions with the drug, and a higher pore density.

EC-*g*-PDMAEMA-*g*-PCL copolymers were synthesized via ROP and ATRP (Yan et al. 2009). These copolymers self-assembled into micelles in aqueous solution at pH below 4.5. When the pH was above 6.2, the PDMAEMA chains were deprotonated, and the interpolymer interactions between PDMAEMA/PCL and PDMAEMA/EC dominated. The PDMAEMA chains thus began to collapse and shrink, became more hydrophobic, and the single micelles further assembled into micellar aggregates. The pH-responsive character of these micelles in aqueous media suggests that they could act as drug nanocarriers for controlled drug release. The crystallinity and crystal morphology of the copolymers could be controlled via the length of the side chains, which was determined by the polymerization conditions used. Chlorambucil was used as a chemotherapy anticancer drug commonly applied to treat a variety of cancers (You et al. 2007). Controlled drug release by polymeric carriers could be the best way to solve cytotoxic issues when the dosage of the drug exceeds its biological carrying capacity. In addition, the length of the grafted PDMAEMA chains could be tailored to control and adjust the extent of PCL crystallization over a broad range.

BC is a kind of cellulose produced by *Gluconacetobacter xylinum* and other microorganisms such as *Agrobacterium*, *Rhizobium*, *Pseudomonas*, and *Sarcina* (Fu et al. 2013). It is widely used in different fields because of its many excellent characteristics (Gatenholm and Klemm 2010; Klemm et al. 2005). BC is a promising biomaterial as drug delivery carrier because of its nanodimensional network structure (Huang et al. 2013). Intelligent BC also has potential as drug delivery carrier not only because of its network structure, but also because of its stimuli-responsive properties. Mohd Amin et al. (2012) thus prepared BC/AA hydrogels with different proportions of AA by exposure to accelerated electron-beam irradiation at different doses. Thermal and morphological characterization showed that the thermal stability and the pore size of the hydrogels were determined by the AA content and the irradiation dose used: the pore size decreased with increasing AA content and the irradiation dose. The thermo- and pH-responsive properties of the BC/AA hydrogels were revealed by swelling and in vitro drug release studies. SEM images also suggested that the highly porous sponge-like structure of the BC/AA hydrogels was suitable as drug delivery carrier.

20.3.2 Biomaterials

Liver cancer remains a significant medical problem, and one promising therapeutic approach is to embolize the tumor to deprive it of blood nutrients (Bruix and Sherman 2005). Current embolization methods have limitations, but one emerging strategy is to use thermally responsive gel-forming materials that can be injected and gel at the tumor site (Zhao et al. 2011).

PNIPAM was thus grafted to MC using APS and TEMED as an initiator by Liu et al. (2004) to yield PNIPAM-*g*-MC hydrogels with strongly temperature-responsive behavior. At lower MC contents, the LCST of the copolymer decreased. It was observed that the phase transition of the hydrogels occurred reversibly within 1 min, and that above the LCST–near body temperature, rigid gels could be generated within a certain range of MC contents. The copolymer hydrogels hold promise as blood vessel barrier by tuning the gelation temperature, the gelation time, and the mechanical strength. The synthesis of BC nanowhisker-*g*-PNIPAM copolymers was also achieved via ATRP with a catalyst system of Cu(II) and ascorbic acid (AsAc) (Chen et al. 2014). Chemical and physical evidence for grafting was a sol–gel transition observed as the temperature was increased above the LCST. Cytotoxicity examination in human umbilical vein endothelial cells treated with the copolymer demonstrated the good biocompatibility of these copolymers for use as materials for the embolization of hepatocellular carcinoma.

20.3.3 Adsorption

IPN hydrogels show volume changes in response to environmental stimuli including pH, temperature, electric field, light, the presence of specific molecules, a magnetic field, and the ionic strength, because of the presence of the intelligent synthetic and/or natural polymers (Dadsetan et al. 2010; Satarkar and Hilt 2008). Three-dimensional IPNs are formed by homogeneous or heterogeneous polymers cross-linked in the presence of one another (Kosmala et al. 2000). Cylindrical-shaped PNIPAM-CMC IPNs, based on PNIPAm and CMC, were thus cross-linked with *N,N′*-methylenebisacrylamide (CL) (Ekici 2011). The stimuli-responsive swelling behavior of these hydrogels was investigated under different conditions, and they exhibited sensitivity to both pH and temperature. The PNIPAM-CMC IPNs were investigated for the adsorption of biomolecules by utilizing a model protein, bovine serum albumin (BSA). The adsorption of the protein molecules onto the PNIPAM-CMC IPNs mainly depended on the temperature and the pH of the environment. The maximum adsorption capacity was observed at pH 4.7, which is the isoelectric point of BSA, and at 40°C. These BSA adsorption results demonstrated the usefulness of PNIPAm-CMC sorbents through proper control of the solution pH and temperature.

20.3.4 Other Applications

Cellulose-*g*-PVCL membranes were formed via ATRP by Himstedt et al. (2013) for the adsorption and desorption of BSA and immunoglobulin G (IgG). Loading was achieved in high ionic strength buffer, and elution was operated at low ionic strength. By using a responsive PVCL copolymer that had conformation changes during loading and elution, high protein recoveries were achieved. This thermoresponsive and ionic strength-responsive copolymer thus showed promise for high-performance hydrophobic interaction chromatography. The modified membranes displayed an elution peak confirming desorption of the adsorbed BSA. The BSA-loading capacity and recovery depended on the initiator immobilization time used.

EC-*g*-Fe_3O_4 NPs displayed interfacially active and magnetically responsive properties at the oil/water interface, where they allowed the rapid separation of the water droplets from an emulsion by applying an external magnetic field (Peng et al. 2012). The interfacial activity of the EC-*g*-Fe_3O_4 NPs allowed them to effectively attach to the water droplets in the emulsions, while the strong magnetic properties of the Fe_3O_4 core allowed the quick and effective separation of the emulsified water droplets from the multiphase systems. More importantly, the magnetic response of the EC-*g*-Fe_3O_4 NPs at the oil/water interface enhanced the coalescence of emulsified water droplets in toluene stabilized by asphaltenes.

Over the last few decades, stimuli-responsive porous membranes that can change their permeation/separation properties have been prepared by the surface modification of porous membranes with intelligent polymers that can respond to external stimuli such as pH, temperature, the ionic strength, or light (Lee et al. 2006). Permeation selectivity is easy to control through changes in the condition of separation processes. For example, variation of the pore size and the surface properties of membranes through stimuli-responsive polymers could be used for the separation of biomaterials of different sizes with just one tunable membrane (Tokarev et al. 2006).

The electrolyte-responsive behavior of RC-*g*-PSBMA was evaluated in permeation experiments at different concentrations of sodium chloride (NaCl) in solution. There are different conformational states possible for the PSBMA chains on the membrane surface under different conditions. Electrostatic attractions between the cations and anions generate inter- and/or intra-chain association in water, resulting in a collapsed or contracted conformation for the PSBMA chains on the pore surface. The interactions between the ammonium and sulfonate groups of the collapsed PSBMA chains can be disrupted by the small Na^+ and Cl^- ions, which can easily penetrate the PSBMA chains, resulting in an extended conformation for the PSBMA chains and a reduced effective pore size for the membrane. Therefore, variations in flux observed for deionized water and the 0.1 M NaCl solution can be explained by the electrolyte-responsive property of RC-*g*-PSBMA. BSA as a model protein and PS NPs of different sizes (as representative impurities) were selected to examine the rejection performance of the membranes. The rejection rate for BSA was at a very low level regardless of the concentration of NaCl in the solutions; however, the rejection rates for NPs of different sizes changed remarkably with the NaCl concentration in the solutions. This investigation highlighted the potential usefulness of electrolyte-responsive membranes in protein purification.

20.4 CONCLUSIONS

Cellulose is a naturally occurring polymer with many desirable characteristics including good mechanical properties, low cost, high biocompatibility, and biodegradability; for these reasons, it has found a wide range of applications. That biomaterial can be modified to provide "intelligent" copolymers responsive to environmental stimuli including pH or temperature variations, light, electricity, magnetic fields, moisture, and mechanical forces. The responsive properties typically arise when stimuli-responsive polymers are chemically grafted onto cellulose or cellulose derivative (such as CMC, HPC, HEC, EC) substrates. Some cellulose derivatives such as CMC and HPC also display intelligent behavior. The thermoresponsive, pH-, dual-, or multiple stimuli-responsive copolymers and other responsive copolymers can be formed by many different chemical polymerization methods under homogeneous or heterogeneous conditions. Due to their intelligent behavior combined with the excellent physical properties of cellulose, these copolymers have clear advantages in applications as biomaterials, drug delivery vehicles, EAPaps, sensors, responsive membranes, shape memory materials, etc.

Thermoresponsive, pH-responsive, and other responsive polymers have been a hot research topic in recent years. It is hoped that these intelligent copolymers could find a wide range of applications worldwide, especially in the field of biology. There have already been many exciting discoveries during this decade, but we still need more work to bring these materials to real application in our everyday life.

ACKNOWLEDGMENTS

This work was supported by the National Natural Science Foundation of China; contract grant numbers: 20774033 and 21074041. The National Program on Key Basic Research Project of China (No. 2012CB932500). The Natural Science of Hubei Province for Distinguished Young Scholars; contract grant number: No. 2008CDB279. Fundamental Research Funds for the Central Universities, HUST (2010JC016).

REFERENCES

Abdel-Halim, E. S. 2012. Preparation and characterization of poly(acrylic acid)-hydroxyethyl cellulose graft copolymer. *Carbohydrate Polymers* 90: 930–936.

Abdel-Halim, E. S., Emam, H. E., and El-Rafie, M. H. 2008. Preparation and characterization of water soluble poly(acrylic acid)-hydroxypropyl cellulose composite. *Carbohydrate Polymers* 74: 783–786.

Abdul Khalil, H. P. S., Bhat, A. H., and Ireana Yusra, A. F. 2012. Green composites from sustainable cellulose nanofibrils: A review. *Carbohydrate Polymers* 87: 963–979.

Bai, Y., Zhang, Z., Zhang, A., Chen, L., He, C., Zhuang, X., and Chen, X. 2012. Novel thermo- and pH-responsive hydroxypropyl cellulose- and poly(L-glutamic acid)-based microgels for oral insulin controlled release. *Carbohydrate Polymers* 89: 1207–1214.

Bazhenov, V. A. 1961. *Piezoelectric Properties of Wood*. New York: Consultants Bureau.

Bledzki, A. K. and Gassan, J. 1999. Composites reinforced with cellulose based fibres. *Progress in Polymer Science* 24: 221–274.

Bokias, G., Mylonas, Y., Staikos, G., Bumbu, G. G., and Vasile, C. 2001. Synthesis and aqueous solution properties of novel thermoresponsive graft copolymers based on a carboxymethylcellulose backbone. *Macromolecules* 34: 4958–4964.

Bruix, J. and Sherman, M. 2005. Management of hepatocellular carcinoma. *Hepatology* 42: 1208–1236.

Çaykara, T., Şengül, G., and Birlik, G. 2006. Preparation and swelling properties of temperature-sensitive semi-interpenetrating polymer networks composed of poly[(*N-tert*-butylacrylamide)-*co*-acrylamide] and hydroxypropyl cellulose. *Macromolecular Materials and Engineering* 291: 1044–1051.

Chen, X., Huang, L., Sun, H. J., Cheng, S. Z., Zhu, M., and Yang, G. 2014. Stimuli-responsive nanocomposite: Potential injectable embolization agent. *Macromolecular Rapid Communications* 35: 579–584.

Chuang, C. Y., Don, T. M., and Chiu, W. Y. 2010. Synthesis and characterization of stimuli-responsive porous/hollow nanoparticles by self-assembly of chitosan-based graft copolymers and application in drug release. *Journal of Polymer Science Part A: Polymer Chemistry* 48: 2377–2387.

Csoka, L., Hoeger, I. C., Rojas, O. J., Peszlen, I., Pawlak, J. J., and Peralta, P. N. 2012. Piezoelectric effect of cellulose nanocrystals thin films. *ACS Macro Letters* 1: 867–870.

Czaja, W. K., Young, D. J., Kawecki, M., and Brown, R. M. 2007. The future prospects of microbial cellulose in biomedical applications. *Biomacromolecules* 8: 1–12.

Dadsetan, M., Liu, Z., Pumberger, M., Giraldo, C. V., Ruesink, T., Lu, L., and Yaszemski, M. J. 2010. A stimuli-responsive hydrogel for doxorubicin delivery. *Biomaterials* 31: 8051–8062.

Dall Acqua, L., Tonin, C., Peila, R., Ferrero, F., and Catellani, M. 2004. Performance and properties of intrinsic conductive cellulose-polypyrrole textiles. *Synthetic Metals* 146: 213–221.

de Las Heras Alarcón, C., Pennadam, S., and Alexander, C. 2005. Stimuli responsive polymers for biomedical applications. *Chemical Society Reviews* 34: 276–285.

Delcea, M., Möhwald, H., and Skirtach, A. G. 2011. Stimuli-responsive LbL capsules and nanoshells for drug delivery. *Advanced Drug Delivery Reviews* 63: 730–747.

Doelker, E. 1993. Cellulose derivatives. *Advances in Polymer Science* 107: 199–265.

Duncan, R. 2003. The dawning era of polymer therapeutics. *Nature Reviews Drug Discovery* 2: 347–360.

Edgar, K. J. 2006. Cellulose esters in drug delivery. *Cellulose* 14: 49–64.

Edgar, K. J., Buchanan, C. M., Debenham, J. S., Rundquist, P. A., Seiler, B. D., Shelton, M. C., and Tindall, D. 2001. Advances in cellulose ester performance and application. *Progress in Polymer Science* 26: 1605–1688.

Ekici, S. 2011. Intelligent poly(*N*-isopropylacrylamide)-carboxymethyl cellulose full interpenetrating polymeric networks for protein adsorption studies. *Journal of Materials Science* 46: 2843–2850.

Fleige, E., Quadir, M. A., and Haag, R. 2012. Stimuli-responsive polymeric nanocarriers for the controlled transport of active compounds: Concepts and applications. *Advanced Drug Delivery Reviews* 64: 866–884.

Fox, S. C., Li, B., Xu, D., and Edgar, K. J. 2011. Regioselective esterification and etherification of cellulose: A review. *Biomacromolecules* 12: 1956–1972.

Fu, L., Zhang, J., and Yang, G. 2013. Present status and applications of bacterial cellulose-based materials for skin tissue repair. *Carbohydrate Polymers* 92: 1432–1442.

Gatenholm, P. and Klemm, D. 2010. Bacterial nanocellulose as a renewable material for biomedical applications. *MRS Bulletin* 35: 208–213.

Gil, E. and Hudson, S. 2004. Stimuli-responsive polymers and their bioconjugates. *Progress in Polymer Science* 29: 1173–1222.

Guan, Y. and Zhang, Y. 2011. PNIPAM microgels for biomedical applications: From dispersed particles to 3D assemblies. *Soft Matter* 7: 6375–6384.

Gupta, K. C. and Khandekar, K. 2003. Temperature-responsive cellulose by ceric (IV) ion-initiated graft copolymerization of *N*-isopropylacrylamide. *Biomacromolecules* 4: 758–765.

Gupta, P., Vermani, K., and Garg, S. 2002. Hydrogels: From controlled release to pH-responsive drug delivery. *Drug Discovery Today* 7: 569–579.

Gürdağ, G., Yaşar, M., and Gürkaynak, M. A. 1997. Graft copolymerization of acrylic acid on cellulose: Reaction kinetics of copolymerization. *Journal of Applied Polymer Science* 66: 929–934.

Habibi, Y., Lucia, L. A., and Rojas, O. J. 2010. Cellulose nanocrystals: Chemistry, self-assembly, and applications. *Chemical Reviews* 110: 3479–3500.

Hansson, S., Trouillet, V., Tischer, T., Goldmann, A. S., Carlmark, A., Barner-Kowollik, C., and Malmström, E. 2012. Grafting efficiency of synthetic polymers onto biomaterials: A comparative study of grafting-from versus grafting-to. *Biomacromolecules* 14: 64–74.

Hao, Y., Peng, J., Li, J., Zhai, M., and Wei, G. 2009. An ionic liquid as reaction media for radiation-induced grafting of thermosensitive poly(N-isopropylacrylamide) onto microcrystalline cellulose. *Carbohydrate Polymers* 77: 779–784.

Harsh, D. C. and Gehrke, S. H. 1991. Controlling the swelling characteristics of temperature-sensitive cellulose ether hydrogels. *Journal of Controlled Release* 17: 175–185.

Hebeish, A., Farag, S., Sharaf, S., and Shaheen, T. I. 2014. Thermal responsive hydrogels based on semi interpenetrating network of poly(NIPAm) and cellulose nanowhiskers. *Carbohydrate Polymers* 102: 159–166.

Himstedt, H. H., Qian, X., Weaver, J. R., and Wickramasinghe, S. R. 2013. Responsive membranes for hydrophobic interaction chromatography. *Journal of Membrane Science* 447: 335–344.

Hu, W., Chen, S., Yang, Z., Liu, L., and Wang, H. 2011. Flexible electrically conductive nanocomposite membrane based on bacterial cellulose and polyaniline. *Journal of Physical Chemistry B* 115: 8453–8457.

Huang, L., Chen, X., Nguyen, T. X., Tang, H., Zhang, L., and Yang, G. 2013. Nano-cellulose 3D-networks as controlled-release drug carriers. *Journal of Materials Chemistry B* 1: 2976–2984.

Jianqin, L., Maolin, Z., and Hongfei, H. 1999. Pre-irradiation grafting of temperature sensitive hydrogel on cotton cellulose fabric. *Radiation Physics and Chemistry* 55: 55–59.

Jin, C., Yan, R., and Huang, J. 2011. Cellulose substance with reversible photo-responsive wettability by surface modification. *Journal of Materials Chemistry* 21: 1751–1759.

Kamel, S. 2008. Pharmaceutical significance of cellulose: A review. *eXPRESS Polymer Letters* 2: 758–778.

Kang, H., Liu, R., and Huang, Y. 2013. Synthesis of ethyl cellulose grafted poly(*N*-isopropylacrylamide) copolymer and its micellization. *Acta Chimica Sinica—Chinese Edition* 71: 114–120.

Kim, J., Yun, S., Mahadeva, S. K., Yun, K., Yang, S. Y., and Maniruzzaman, M. 2010. Paper actuators made with cellulose and hybrid materials. *Sensors* 10: 1473–1485.

Kim, J., Yun, S., and Ounaies, Z. 2006. Discovery of cellulose as a smart material. *Macromolecules* 39: 4202–4206.

Klemm, D., Heublein, B., Fink, H. P., and Bohn, A. 2005. Cellulose: Fascinating biopolymer and sustainable raw material. *Angewandte Chemie International Edition in English* 44: 3358–3393.

Klemm, D., Kramer, F., Moritz, S., Lindstrom, T., Ankerfors, M., Gray, D., and Dorris, A. 2011. Nanocelluloses: A new family of nature-based materials. *Angewandte Chemie International Edition* 50: 5438–5466.

Klemm, D., Philipp, B., and Heinze, T. 1999. *Comprehensive Cellulose Chemistry: Fundamentals and Analytical Methods*, Vol. 1. Chichester, U.K.: Wiley VCH.

Kloser, E. and Gray, D. G. 2010. Surface grafting of cellulose nanocrystals with poly(ethylene oxide) in aqueous media. *Langmuir* 26: 13450–13456.

Kontturi, E., Tammelin, T., and Sterberg, M. 2006. Cellulose—Model films and the fundamental approach. *Chemical Society Reviews* 35: 1287–1304.

Kosmala, J. D., Henthorn, D. B., and Brannon-Peppas, L. 2000. Preparation of interpenetrating networks of gelatin and dextran as degradable biomaterials. *Biomaterials* 21: 2019–2023.

Kubota, H., Kondo, T., Ichikawa, T., and Katakai, R. 1998. Synthesis and characteristics of cellulose peroxides of the peracid type having a temperature-responsive function. *Polymer Degradation and Stability* 60: 425–430.

Kubota, H., Suka, I. G., Kuroda, S., and Kondo, T. 2001. Introduction of stimuli-responsive polymers into regenerated cellulose film by means of photografting. *European Polymer Journal* 37: 1367–1372.

Lee, D., Nolte, A. J., Kunz, A. L., Rubner, M. F., and Cohen, R. E. 2006. pH-induced hysteretic gating of track-etched polycarbonate membranes: Swelling/deswelling behavior of polyelectrolyte multilayers in confined geometry. *Journal of the American Chemical Society* 128: 8521–8529.

Lindqvist, J., Nyström, D., Östmark, E., Antoni, P., Carlmark, A., Johansson, M., Hult, A., and Malmström, E. 2008. Intelligent dual-responsive cellulose surfaces via surface-initiated ATRP. *Biomacromolecules* 9: 2139–2145.

Liu, W., Zhang, B., Lu, W. W., Li, X., Zhu, D., De Yao, K., Wang, Q., Zhao, C., and Wang, C. 2004. A rapid temperature-responsive sol-*gel* *r*eversible poly(*N*-isopropylacrylamide)-*g*-methylcellulose copolymer hydrogel. *Biomaterials* 25: 3005–3012.

Liu, Z. T., Sun, C., Liu, Z. W., and Lu, J. 2009. Modification of ramie fiber with an amine-containing polymer via atom transfer radical polymerization. *Journal of Applied Polymer Science* 113: 3612–3618.

Ma, L., Kang, H., Liu, R., and Huang, Y. 2010. Smart assembly behaviors of hydroxypropylcellulose-*graft*-poly(4-vinylpyridine) copolymers in aqueous solution by thermo and pH stimuli. *Langmuir* 26: 18519–18525.

Marsano, E., Bianchi, E., Gagliardi, S., and Ghioni, F. 2000. Hydroxypropyl-cellulose derivatives: Phase behaviour of hydroxypropylcellulose methacrylate. *Polymer* 41: 533–538.

Matyjaszewski, K. and Xia, J. 2001. Atom transfer radical polymerization. *Chemical Reviews* 101: 2921–2990.

Mohd Amin, M. C. I., Ahmad, N., Halib, N., and Ahmad, I. 2012. Synthesis and characterization of thermo- and pH-responsive bacterial cellulose/acrylic acid hydrogels for drug delivery. *Carbohydrate Polymers* 88: 465–473.

Moon, R. J., Martini, A., Nairn, J., Simonsen, J., and Youngblood, J. 2011. Cellulose nanomaterials review: Structure, properties and nanocomposites. *Chemical Society Reviews* 40: 3941–3994.

Morandi, G. and Thielemans, W. 2012. Synthesis of cellulose nanocrystals bearing photocleavable grafts by ATRP. *Polymer Chemistry* 3: 1402–1407.

Nizam El-Din, H. M., Abd Alla, S. G., and El-Naggar, A. W. M. 2010. Swelling and drug release properties of acrylamide/carboxymethyl cellulose networks formed by gamma irradiation. *Radiation Physics and Chemistry* 79: 725–730.

Okiyama, A., Motoki, M., and Yamanaka, S. 1992. Bacterial cellulose II. Processing of the gelatinous cellulose for food materials. *Food Hydrocolloids* 6: 479–487.

Pal, K., Banthia, A. K., and Majumdar, D. K. 2006. Development of carboxymethyl cellulose acrylate for various biomedical applications. *Biomedical Materials* 1: 85–91.

Pan, K., Zhang, X., and Cao, B. 2010. Surface-initiated atom transfer radical polymerization of regenerated cellulose membranes with thermo-responsive properties. *Polymer International* 59: 733–737.

Pandey, M., Amin, M. C. I. M., Mohamad, N., Ahmad, N., and Muda, S. 2013. Structure and characteristics of bacterial cellulose-based hydrogels prepared by cryotropic gelation and irradiation methods. *Polymer-Plastics Technology and Engineering* 52: 1510–1518.

Peng, J., Liu, Q., Xu, Z., and Masliyah, J. 2012. Synthesis of interfacially active and magnetically responsive nanoparticles for multiphase separation applications. *Advanced Functional Materials* 22: 1732–1740.

Peng, Z. and Chen, F. 2010. Synthesis and properties of temperature-sensitive hydrogel based on hydroxyethyl cellulose. *International Journal of Polymeric Materials* 59: 450–461.

Porsch, C., Hansson, S., Nordgren, N., and Malmström, E. 2011. Thermo-responsive cellulose-based architectures: Tailoring LCST using poly(ethylene glycol) methacrylates. *Polymer Chemistry* 2: 1114–1123.

Pourjavadi, A., Barzegar, S., and Mahdavinia, G. R. 2006. MBA-crosslinked Na-Alg/CMC as a smart full-polysaccharide superabsorbent hydrogels. *Carbohydrate Polymers* 66: 386–395.

Prabaharan, M. and Mano, J. F. 2006. Stimuli-responsive hydrogels based on polysaccharides incorporated with thermo-responsive polymers as novel biomaterials. *Macromolecular Bioscience* 6: 991–1008.

Qiu, X. and Hu, S. 2013. "Smart" materials based on cellulose: A review of the preparations, properties, and applications. *Materials* 6: 738–781.

Qiu, X., Ren, X., and Hu, S. 2013. Fabrication of dual-responsive cellulose-based membrane via simplified surface-initiated ATRP. *Carbohydrate Polymers* 92: 1887–1895.

Roy, D., Brooks, W. L., and Sumerlin, B. S. 2013. New directions in thermoresponsive polymers. *Chemical Society Reviews* 42: 7214–7243.

Roy, D., Guthrie, J. T., and Perrier, S. 2006. RAFT graft polymerization of 2-(dimethylaminoethyl) methacrylate onto cellulose fibre. *Australian Journal of Chemistry* 59: 737–741.

Roy, D., Semsarilar, M., Guthrie, J. T., and Perrier, S. 2009. Cellulose modification by polymer grafting: A review. *Chemical Society Reviews* 38: 2046–2064.

Sannino, A., Demitri, C., and Madaghiele, M. 2009. Biodegradable cellulose-based hydrogels: Design and applications. *Materials* 2: 353–373.

Satarkar, N. S. and Hilt, J. Z. 2008. Magnetic hydrogel nanocomposites for remote controlled pulsatile drug release. *Journal of Controlled Release* 130: 246–251.

Savitskaya, T. A., Epshtein, O. L., Kulinkovich, O. G., and Tret'Yakova, S. M. 2000. Dynamic membranes based on poly(*N*-isopropylacrylamide-*co*-heptadecyl vinyl ketone): Preparation and properties. *Colloid Journal* 62: 746–750.

Scarpa, J. S., Mueller, D. D., and Klotz, I. M. 1967. Slow hydrogen-deuterium exchange in a non-.alpha.-helical polyamide. *Journal of the American Chemical Society* 89: 6024–6030.

Schagerlöf, H., Richardson, S., Momcilovic, D., Brinkmalm, G., Wittgren, B., and Tjerneld, F. 2006. Characterization of chemical substitution of hydroxypropyl cellulose using enzymatic degradation. *Biomacromolecules* 7: 80–85.

Schild, H. G. 1992. Poly(*N*-isopropylacrylamide): Experiment, theory and application. *Progress in Polymer Science* 17: 163–249.

Schmaljohann, D. 2006. Thermo- and pH-responsive polymers in drug delivery. *Advanced Drug Delivery Reviews* 58: 1655–1670.

Sdrobiş, A., Ioanid, G. E., Stevanovic, T., and Vasile, C. 2012. Modification of cellulose/chitin mix fibers with N-isopropylacrylamide and poly(*N*-isopropylacrylamide) under cold plasma conditions. *Polymer International* 61: 1767–1777.

Shanmuganathan, K., Capadona, J. R., Rowan, S. J., and Weder, C. 2010. Stimuli-responsive mechanically adaptive polymer nanocomposites. *ACS Applied Materials and Interfaces* 2: 165–174.

Siegel, R. 1993. Hydrophobic weak polyelectrolyte gels: Studies of swelling equilibria and kinetics. In *Responsive Gels: Volume Transitions I*, ed. K. Dušek, Vol. 109, pp. 233–267. Berlin, Germany: Springer.

Sui, X., Yuan, J., Zhou, M., Zhang, J., Yang, H., Yuan, W., Wei, Y., and Pan, C. 2008. Synthesis of cellulose-*graft*-poly(*N,N*-dimethylamino-2-ethyl methacrylate) copolymers via homogeneous ATRP and their aggregates in aqueous media. *Biomacromolecules* 9: 2615–2620.

Tan, J., Liu, R., Wang, W., Liu, W., Tian, Y., Wu, M., and Huang, Y. 2010. Controllable aggregation and reversible pH sensitivity of AuNPs regulated by carboxymethyl cellulose. *Langmuir* 26: 2093–2098.

Tang, Z., Wang, Y., Podsiadlo, P., and Kotov, N. A. 2006. Biomedical applications of layer-by-layer assembly: From biomimetics to tissue engineering. *Advanced Materials* 18: 3203–3224.

Tokarev, I., Orlov, M., and Minko, S. 2006. Responsive polyelectrolyte gel membranes. *Advanced Materials* 18: 2458–2460.

Vasile, C., Bumbu, G. G., Dumitriu, R. P., and Staikos, G. 2004. Comparative study of the behavior of carboxymethyl cellulose-*g*-poly(*N*-isopropylacrylamide) copolymers and their equivalent physical blends. *European Polymer Journal* 40: 1209–1215.

Vasile, C., Marinescu, C., Vornicu, R., and Staikos, G. 2003. Enzymatic degradation of thermoresponsive poly(N-isopropylacrylamide) grafted to carboxymethylcellulose copolymers. *Journal of Applied Polymer Science* 87: 1383–1386.

Wan, S., Jiang, M., and Zhang, G. 2007. Dual temperature- and pH-dependent self-assembly of cellulose-based copolymer with a pair of complementary grafts. *Macromolecules* 40: 5552–5558.

Wang, D., Tan, J., Kang, H., Ma, L., Jin, X., Liu, R., and Huang, Y. 2011. Synthesis, self-assembly and drug release behaviors of pH-responsive copolymers ethyl cellulose-*graft*-PDEAEMA through ATRP. *Carbohydrate Polymers* 84: 195–202.

Wang, W. and Wang, A. 2010. Nanocomposite of carboxymethyl cellulose and attapulgite as a novel pH-sensitive superabsorbent: Synthesis, characterization and properties. *Carbohydrate Polymers* 82: 83–91.

Way, A. E., Hsu, L., Shanmuganathan, K., Weder, C., and Rowan, S. J. 2012. pH-responsive cellulose nanocrystal gels and nanocomposites. *ACS Macro Letters* 1: 1001–1006.

Xu, F. J., Zhu, Y., Liu, F. S., Nie, J., Ma, J., and Yang, W. T. 2010. Comb-shaped conjugates comprising hydroxypropyl cellulose backbones and low-molecular-weight poly(*N*-isopropylacryamide) side chains for smart hydrogels: Synthesis, characterization, and biomedical applications. *Bioconjugate Chemistry* 21: 456–464.

Yan, Q., Yuan, J., Zhang, F., Sui, X., Xie, X., Yin, Y., Wang, S., and Wei, Y. 2009. Cellulose-based dual graft molecular brushes as potential drug nanocarriers: Stimulus-responsive micelles, self-assembled phase transition behavior, and tunable crystalline morphologies. *Biomacromolecules* 10: 2033–2042.

Yang, H., Esteves, A., Zhu, H., Wang, D., and Xin, J. H. 2012. *In-situ* study of the structure and dynamics of thermo-responsive PNIPAAm grafted on a cotton fabric. *Polymer* 53: 3577–3586.

Yi, J., Xu, Q., Zhang, X., and Zhang, H. 2009. Temperature-induced chiral nematic phase changes of suspensions of poly(*N,N*-dimethylaminoethyl methacrylate)-grafted cellulose nanocrystals. *Cellulose* 16: 989–997.

Yokota, S., Kitaoka, T., Sugiyama, J., and Wariishi, H. 2007. Cellulose I nanolayers designed by self-assembly of its thiosemicarbazone on a gold substrate. *Advanced Materials* 19: 3368–3370.

You, Y., Zhou, Q., Manickam, D. S., Wan, L., Mao, G., and Oupický, D. 2007. Dually responsive multiblock copolymers via reversible addition-fragmentation chain transfer polymerization: Synthesis of temperature-and redox-responsive copolymers of poly(*N*-isopropylacrylamide) and poly(2-(dimethylamino) ethyl methacrylate). *Macromolecules* 40: 8617–8624.

Yuan, W., Zhang, J., Zou, H., Shen, T., and Ren, J. 2012. Amphiphilic ethyl cellulose brush polymers with mono and dual side chains: Facile synthesis, self-assembly, and tunable temperature-pH responsivities. *Polymer* 53: 956–966.

Zhang, L. 2001. New water-soluble cellulosic polymers: A review. *Macromolecular Materials and Engineering* 286: 267–275.

Zhang, Z., Chen, L., Zhao, C., Bai, Y., Deng, M., Shan, H., Zhuang, X., Chen, X., and Jing, X. 2011. Thermo- and pH-responsive HPC-*g*-AA/AA hydrogels for controlled drug delivery applications. *Polymer* 52: 676–682.

Zhao, Y., Wee, K., and Bai, R. 2010. A novel electrolyte-responsive membrane with tunable permeation selectivity for protein purification. *ACS Applied Materials and Interfaces* 2: 203–211.

Zhao, Y., Zheng, C., Wang, Q., Fang, J., Zhou, G., Zhao, H., Yang, Y., Xu, H., Feng, G., and Yang, X. 2011. Permanent and peripheral embolization: Temperature-sensitive p(*N*-isopropylacrylamide-*co*-butyl methylacrylate) nanogel as a novel blood-vessel-embolic material in the interventional therapy of liver tumors. *Advanced Functional Materials* 21: 2035–2042.

Zoppe, J. O., Habibi, Y., Rojas, O. J., Venditti, R. A., Johansson, L., Efimenko, K., Osterberg, M., and Laine, J. 2010. Poly(*N*-isopropylacrylamide) brushes grafted from cellulose nanocrystals via surface-initiated single-electron transfer living radical polymerization. *Biomacromolecules* 11: 2683–2691.

21 Synthesis and Applications of Grafted Carboxymethyl Cellulose

A Review

Sumit Mishra, Gautam Sen,
Kartick Prasad Dey, and G. Usha Rani

CONTENTS

21.1 INTRODUCTION

Cellulose constitutes one of the most abundant and renewable organic materials on this planet. It is an integral part of all plants. It is estimated that by photosynthesis, 10^{11}–10^{12} tons of cellulose is synthesized annually in the world; for example, sometimes it is found combined with lignin and other polysaccharides (hemicelluloses) in the cell wall of woody plants [1]. It is the most preferred raw material for the textile, paper, and packaging industry. CMC is the most important commercial cellulose ether. It is a cellulose derivative with sodium carboxy methyl group ($-CH_2COONa$) substitution to some of the hydroxyl groups of the glucopyranose monomers that make up the cellulose backbone. The functional properties of CMC depend upon the degree of substitution (DS) of the cellulose chains. The DS indicates that the average number of hydroxyl groups of the glucose units in the cellulose chain has been substituted. The CMC has been synthesized by the base-catalyzed reaction of cellulose and chloroacetic acid [2]. Commercial water-soluble CMC usually has a DS between 0.4 and 1.2 [3].

$$\text{Cell–OH} + \text{ClCH}_2\ \text{COONa} \xrightarrow{\text{NaOH}} \text{Cell–O–CH}_2\text{–COONa} + \text{HCl}$$

CMC acts as an effective thickener, rheology control agent, binder, stabilizer, and film former [3–5]. It thus finds applications in the cosmetics, food, pharmaceutical, textile, adhesives, oil drilling fluids, cation exchange resins, and other industries. In the recent years, attempts to graft-polymerize vinyl and acryl monomers on cellulose backbone have aroused considerable interest. By the grafting of a monomer, some of the drawbacks of cellulose such as low tensile strength, high moisture transmission, and low strength against microbial degradation can be eliminated.

21.2 MOLECULAR STRUCTURE AND REACTIVITY OF CELLULOSE

The physical and chemical properties of cellulose and its derivatives depend upon its specific structure. Payen was the first to determine the elemental composition of cellulose as early in 1838 [6]. He found that cellulose contains 44%–45% carbon, 6%–6.5% hydrogen, and rest oxygen. Based on these data, the empirical formula was deduced to be $C_6H_{10}O_5$. However, the actual macromolecular structure of cellulose was still unclear. Haworth proposed a chain-like macromolecular structure in the late 1920s, whereas Staudinger delivered the final proof of the highly polymeric nature of the cellulose molecule [7–9].

Acetylation and de-acetylation reactions of cellulose were used to determine the chemical structure. The molecular structure of cellulose as a carbohydrate polymeric comprises of repeating β-(1 → 4)-D-glucopyranose units [10] (Figure 21.1), which are covalently linked through acetal

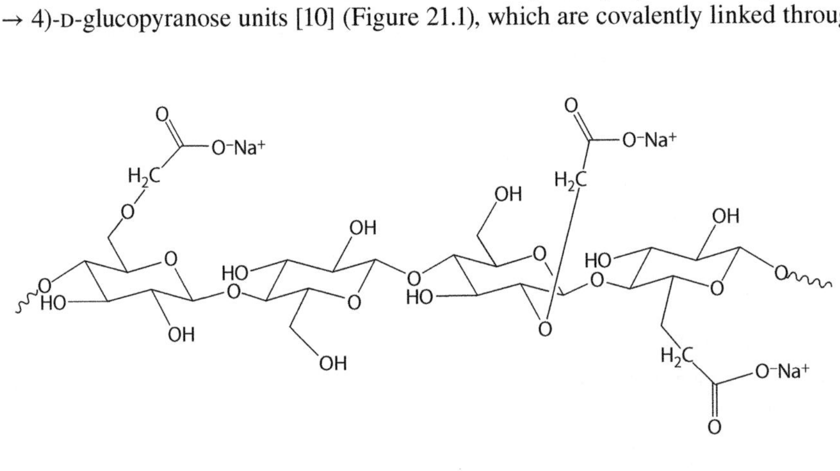

FIGURE 21.1 Chemical structure of carboxymethyl cellulose sodium salt (CMC). (From Mishra, S. et al., *Carbohydr. Polym.*, 87, 2255, 2012.)

functions between the OH group of the C_4 and C_1 carbon atoms (β-1,4-glucan). Cellulose is a large, linear-chain polymer with a large number of hydroxyl groups (three per anhydroglucose unit (AGU)) and present in the preferred C_1 conformation. To accommodate the preferred bond angles, every second AGU unit is rotated 180° in the plane. The length of the polymeric cellulose chain depends on the number of constituent AGU units, degree of polymerization, and varies with the origin and treatment of the cellulosic raw material [11].

Cellulose has a ribbon shape that allows it to twist and bend in the direction out of the plane, so that the molecule is moderately flexible. There is a relatively strong interaction between neighboring cellulose molecules in dry fibers due to the presence of the hydroxyl (–OH) groups, which stick out from the chain and form intermolecular hydrogen bonds. Regenerated fibers from cellulose contain 250–500 repeating units per chain [1]. This molecular structure gives cellulose its characteristic properties of hydrophilicity, chirality, and degradability [11].

The chemical character and reactivity of cellulose are determined by the presence of three equatorially positioned OH groups in the AGU, one primary and two secondary groups. In addition, the β-glycosidic linkages of cellulose are susceptible to hydrolytic attack [10]. The hydroxyl groups not only play a role in the typical reactions of primary and secondary alcohols that are carried out on cellulose, but also play an important role in the solubility of cellulose [9]. Cellulose is insoluble in common organic solvents and in water. This is due to the fact that the hydroxyl groups are responsible for the extensive hydrogen bonding network forming both intra- and intermolecular hydrogen bonding [10]. However, it is soluble in some selective solvents like LiCl-AMAc (lithium chloride–dimethylacetamide), NMP-LiCl (NMethylpyrrolidone-lithium chloride), and DMSO-PF (dimethyl sulfoxide paraformaldehyde) and also dissolve in strong concentrated acids such as H_2SO_4 and H_3PO_4 [12].

One of the most effective methods of chemical modification is grafting with some polymeric material. The resulting hybrid material can have tailor-made properties optimized toward required applications.

21.3 CHEMICAL MODIFICATION OF CELLULOSE BY GRAFTING TECHNIQUE

The chemical modification of these materials by grafting has received considerable attention in recent years. Among the methods of modification of polymers, grafting is one of the prevalent methods. In the past several years, there has been an increased emphasis on applications of grafted polymers. Graft copolymerization is a process in which side chain grafts are covalently attached to the main chain of polymer backbone to form branched copolymer (Figure 21.2) [13]. The extent of polymerization graft is referred to as the percentage grafting. It can be calculated by the following formula:

$$\%\ \text{Grafting} = \frac{\text{Wt. of graft copolymer} - \text{wt. of polysaccharide}}{\text{Wt. of polysaccharide}} \times 100$$

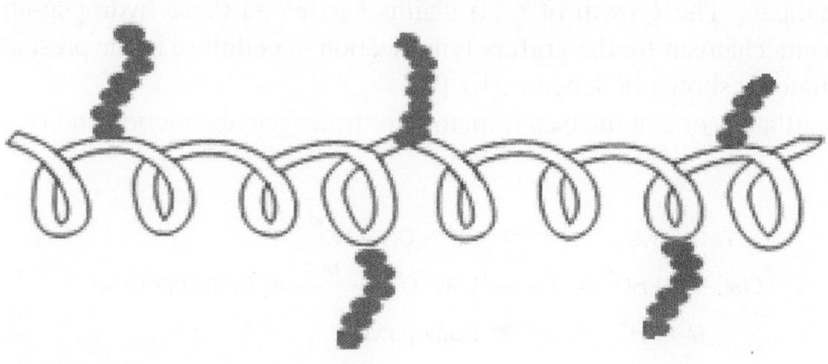

FIGURE 21.2 Schematic diagram of "grafting."

Both the backbone and side chain grafts can be either homopolymer or copolymer. Free radicals are active sites to initiate the polymerization reactions. These reactions proceed via three steps: initiation, propagation, and termination. In the initiation step, the polymer chains are initiated by the radicals derived from the initiator in the polymer chain and add to monomers. In the propagation step, the subsequent addition of monomers to polymeric radicals for propagating the reaction becomes the basis. In the termination process, the propagating radicals combine together to form the graft copolymers.

Various methodologies including conventional (chemical initiation) [14–20] and radiation-induced techniques (high energy radiation [21–25], photochemical [26–30], and microwave-based techniques [31–40]) have been used to create the free radical sites on backbone of cellulose to initiate the grafting reactions. The rate of grafting is dependent upon the free radical initiator concentration as well as the monomer, time of irradiation, and the nature of backbone of polysaccharide (cellulose).

21.3.1 Chemical Initiation Grafting

The grafting proceeds through free radical initiators such as redox reagents like Fenton's reagent (Fe^{+2}/H_2O_2), persulfate, peroxides, transition metal ions (e.g., Ce^{4+}, Cr^{6+}, V^{5+}, Co^{3+}), and metal chelates (e.g., $Fe(acac)_3$, $Zn(acac)_2$, $Al(acac)_3$, and $VO(acac)_2$). In this process, the role of initiator is very important as it determines the path of the grafting process.

21.3.1.1 Fenton's Reagent Initiator

Fenton's reagents are iron(II)-hydrogen peroxide. In the grafting reaction, it acts as a redox initiator in low temperature, because above 25°C temperature, the hydrogen peroxide decomposes, losing its reactivity. During the course of reaction, the hydroxyl ion is produced, involving a redox reaction between iron(II) ion and hydrogen peroxide by one electron transfer. This mechanism was first proposed by Haber and Weiss [14–15]. Cellulose graft copolymerization via Fenton's reagent initiation is shown in Scheme 21.1.

The hydrogen peroxide molecule reacts with ferrous ions, producing ferric ions and primary hydroxyl radicals. The hydroxyl radicals abstract one hydrogen atom from polysaccharide backbone resulting in secondary polysaccharide radicals. The grafting is initiated from the hydrogen abstract sites of the polysaccharide backbone with monomers. The hydroxyl radicals react with monomers to produce homopolymer. Merz and Waters [16] reported the formation of hydroxyl radicals in a reaction that can be used for the grafting on vinyl monomers on cellulose.

21.3.1.2 Potassium Persulfate

Potassium persulfate generates the initiating species on the polysaccharide backbone. In the reaction mixture, first the primary radicals SO_4^- are generated by the decomposition of $K_2S_2O_8$. These primary SO_4^- abstract a hydrogen atom from the polysaccharide backbone and create the O^- centered polysaccharide radicals. The growth of graft chains carries on these hydrogen-abstracted active sites. The reaction mechanism for the graft polymerization of cellulose in the presence of $K_2S_2O_8$ as a free radical initiator is shown in Scheme 21.2 [9].

Potassium persulfate is one of the best initiators for hydrogen abstraction and is soluble in water.

$$Fe^{2+} + H_2O_2 \longrightarrow Fe^{3+} + OH^- + HO^\bullet$$

$$\text{CMC–OH} + HO^\bullet \longrightarrow \text{CMC–O}^\bullet \xrightarrow{M} \text{Graft copolymer}$$

$$M + OH^\bullet \longrightarrow \text{Homopolymer}$$

SCHEME 21.1 Schematic mechanism of cellulose graft copolymerization by Fenton's reagent.

$$S_2O_8^{2-} \longrightarrow 2SO_4^{-\bullet}$$
$$CMC\text{–}OH + S_2O_8^{2-} \longrightarrow CMC\text{–}O^{\bullet} + HSO_4^{-} + SO_4^{-\bullet}$$
$$CMC\text{–}O^{\bullet} + M \longrightarrow \text{Graft copolymer}$$
$$SO_4^{-\bullet} + M \longrightarrow \text{Homopolymer}$$

SCHEME 21.2 Schematic representation of graft polymerization of cellulose in the presence of $K_2S_2O_8$ as a free radical initiator.

Suo et al. [17] reported the graft copolymerization of acrylic acid and acrylamide monomers on CMC to make superabsorbent polymers. Similarly, Aliouche et al. [18] synthesized graft copolymer of cellulose with acrylic acid and acryronitrile using potassium persulfate as an initiator. El-Hady et al. [19] reported the graft copolymer, xanthate mixture of carboxymethyl with a acrylamide monomer using sodium bisulfate-ammonium persulfate redox initiator system in water.

21.3.1.3 Transition Metal Ions

Among the various types of transition metal ion initiators in grafting reaction, ceric ion is one of the most important and effective initiators because of its advantages. The probability of competing homopolymer formation is minimum in the case of this initiator. Generally, ceric sulfate and ceric ammonium nitrate (CAN) are used as initiators of Ce^{4+} ion [20,21]. First, ceric ion–polysaccharide complex is formed, and then it decomposes to cerous (Ce^{3+}) ion and polysaccharide radicals created by the hydrogen abstraction from polysaccharide by a single-electron process. So the initiation sites are created on the polysaccharide backbone for grafting. The actual process involves oxidation of polysaccharide to form an intermediate reversible complex (chelated species) between the Ce(IV) ion and the cellulose (Scheme 21.3). Such complex formation is not restricted to all polymers especially for cellulose types, where there is a possibility of glycol groups participating in the reaction [22]. The rate of polymerization reaction by this initiator is very high at low temperatures.

Kumar et al. [23] reported the grafting of sodium carboxymethylcellulose (CMC) with glycidyl methacrylate (GMA) using CAN as an initiator for the development of UV-curable coating from CMC-*g*-GMA induced by cationic photo-initiators. Chen and Hsieh [24] used Ce(IV) ions as an initiator to graft acrylic acid on the surface of ultrafine cellulose fibers (diameter 200–400 nm) for the absorption behavior and activity of bound lipase enzymes. This method has low reproducibility, is time consuming, and requires inert atmosphere. Among the various redox-type initiators, ceric ion (Ce(IV)) has gained importance because of its high grafting efficiency [25]. With many of the aforesaid methods, the extent of ungrafted homopolymer has been high in comparison with that from ceric(IV) ion–initiated grafting, in which homopolymerization of vinyl monomers has been minimal [26]. Previously, researchers have used this ceric ion initiation method to graft

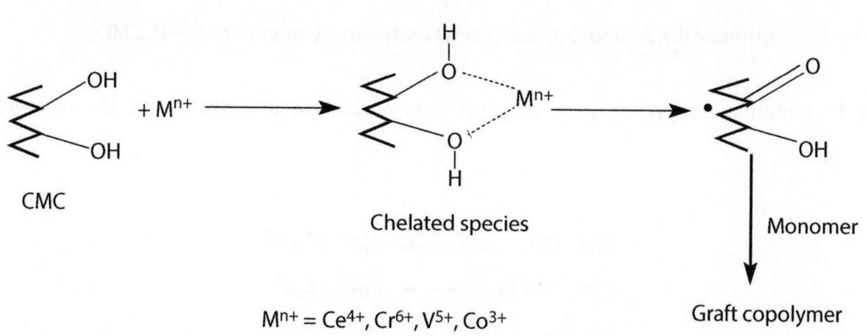

SCHEME 21.3 The mechanism of transition metal ion–induced cellulose graft copolymerization.

functional polymers to cellulose in various forms. Hence, these reactive sites are introduced for either direct chelation of metal ions or subsequent reaction with a chelating agent for the same purpose. Bicak et al. [27] grafted polyacrylamide on cotton cellulose using ceric ammonium sulfate as initiator and studied the removal of Hg(II) from aqueous solution. Liu et al. [28,29] grafted regenerated cellulose beads with arylonitrile using CAN as initiator. A saponification reaction using sodium hydroxide was subsequently carried out on this material. The saponification converts the same grafted poly(acrylonitrile) (AN) with its cyano groups as the main group to both amide (–$CONH_2$) and carboxylate (–COONa) groups. In another study, Aoki et al. [30] grafted bead cellulose with AN, again utilizing CAN as the initiator. Navarro et al. [31] modified a porous cellulose material (aquacel) for heavy metal adsorption through graft polymerization of glycidyl methacrylate using CAN as initiator. This was followed by the fictionalization of the reactive epoxy groups present in poly(glycidyl methacrylate) with polyethyleneimine to introduce nitrogenous ligands.

21.3.1.4 Metal Chelates

To avoid undesired reactions, controlling redox potential in the form of metal chelates (e.g., $Fe(acac)_3$, $Zn(acac)_2$, $Al(acac)_3$, $VO(acac)_2$) are useful in the grafting reaction [22]. The metal ion forming complex with the monomer decomposes to the free radical, which undergoes a chain transfer to the polymer. The formation of the free radical in the polymer through monomer is sketched in Scheme 21.4.

21.3.2 Radiation-Induced Grafting

In recent years, the radiation-induced graft copolymerization techniques have received interest. The accelerated electrons impart sufficient energy to induce cleavage of the chemical bonds, which initiate graft copolymerization.

21.3.2.1 High-Energy Radiation Grafting

The use of high energy radiation for the synthesis of graft polymers began in early 1960s, and since then, it has been investigated in great depth. High energy radiation (γ-rays or x-rays) [32–37] can be used to graft various functional polymers to cellulose [38,39] (Scheme 21.5). Radioactive isotopes such as Cobalt-60 (Co-60) and Cesium-137 (Cs-137) are the main sources of γ-irradiation [40].

$$M^{n-}(acac)_n \longrightarrow M^{(n-1)-}(acac)_{n-1} + {}^{\bullet}CH(COCH_3)_2$$

$$^{\bullet}CH(CH_3CO)_2 + nX \longrightarrow (CH_3CO)_2CH_2\text{-}X_{n-1}\text{-}X^{\bullet}$$

$$\sim\!\!-H + (CH_3CO)_2CH_2\text{-}X_{n-1}\text{-}X^{\bullet} \longrightarrow \sim\!\!{}^{\bullet}$$

M, metal (Fe, Al, and Zn); acac, acetyl acetonate; X, monomer; $\sim\!\!-$H, CMC

SCHEME 21.4 Schematic representation of graft polymerization of cellulose in the presence of metal chelates.

$$\text{CMC-OH} \xrightarrow{h\nu} \text{CMC-O}^{\bullet} + H^{\bullet}$$

$$\text{CMC-O}^{\bullet} + M \longrightarrow \text{CMC-O-M}^{\bullet}$$

SCHEME 21.5 Schematic representation of high energy radiation-induced graft copolymerization of cellulose.

Since radiation interacts with macromolecules to produce free radicals, cations, and anions, all three types of paths are possible.

The main advantage of the high energy radiation grafting is that the process is very fast and simple to operate. The main disadvantage of this process is the degradation of polymeric backbone via the splitting of glycosidic linkage by the disproportion reaction caused as an impact of radiation. Hence, it loses the mechanical strength of the polymer.

Huang et al. [38] used high energy radiation for the grafting of vinyl polymers on cellulose and graft copolymerization of styrene on cellulose. γ-radiation were used for "reversible addition–fragmentation chain transfer polymerization"–mediated polymerization and grafting of sodium 4-styrenesulfonate on cellulose [39].

Abdel-Aal et al. [41] used γ-irradiation for the graft copolymerization of acrylic acid on wood pulp. The parameters affecting the abilities of the grafted wood pulp for removing Fe(III), Cr(III), Pb(II), and Cd(II) from aqueous solutions were investigated.

21.3.2.2 Photografting

Photografting [42–48] is a useful means for the introduction of various vinyl monomers on cellulose materials [49]. The energy from the incident ultraviolet light is absorbed by sensitizer, monomer, and/or polymer, or by an electron band structure of the excited cellulose molecule [50]. When a chromophore on a molecule absorbs light, it goes to an excited state producing dissociation into reactive free radicals and initiating the grafting process. If the absorption of light does not lead to the formation of free radical sites through bond rupture, the process can be promoted by addition of photosensitizers, for example, benzoin ethyl ether, dyes such as acrylated azo dye, and aromatic ketones. Photochemical grafting can be achieved with or without a sensitizer. The mechanism without sensitizer involves the generation of free radicals on the cellulose backbone that react with the monomer free radical to form the graft copolymer. In the mechanism with the sensitizer, the sensitizer forms free radicals, which can undergo diffusion so that they abstract hydrogen atoms from the base polymer, producing radical sites required for grafting to take place [51] (Scheme 21.6). In the presence of vinyl monomers, these free radicals initiate growth of polymer chains from the surface of the activated cellulose and also homopolymerization of the vinyl monomers. Photografting has many advantages including readily available UV light sources, the reactions are selective, and photo energy requirements are low relative to other higher energy sources such as γ-ray and electron beam, resulting in less deterioration of polymeric materials.

The main disadvantage is that the UV radiation is not able to reach in the lower portion of the solution. So the photoinitiator is needed during the reaction for the generation of free radicals.

Kubota and Suzuki [52] introduced amidoxime groups to cellulose using a photografting technique. Initially, AN was grafted to the cellulose surface; subsequently, the cyano groups were amidoximated by reaction with hydroxylamine. The ability of these cellulose-amidoximated samples to adsorb Cu(II) were examined. Kubota and Suzuki [53] also grafted AN to cellulose using the photografting technique. The resultant AN-grafted cellulose was subjected to reactions with triethylenetetraamine (Trien). The sample containing triethylenetetraamine groups showed an ability to absorb Cu(II).

21.3.2.3 Microwave Radiation-Based Grafting Methods

Microwave-enhanced chemistry is based on the efficiency of the interaction of molecules in a reaction mixture with electromagnetic waves generated by a "microwave dielectric effect" depending

$$\text{CMC–OH} \xrightarrow{\text{UV}} \text{CMC–O}^{\bullet} + \text{H}^{\bullet}$$

$$\text{CMC–O}^{\bullet} + \text{M} \longrightarrow \text{CMC–O–M}^{\bullet}$$

SCHEME 21.6 Schematic representation of photograft copolymerization of cellulose.

upon the specific polarity of the molecules. Polysaccharide grafting reactions when performed under the influence of microwaves become more productive and selective. Conventional thermal grafting reaction usually results in low grafting yields due to the competing homopolymerization, but under microwave, copolymerization is the favored reaction [54,55].

Recently, the field of graft copolymer synthesis has been revolutionized by use of microwave radiation [56–68]. It generates free radical sites on the backbone polymer. In microwave-based method of graft copolymer synthesis, any inert atmospheric condition is not required unlike the case of conventional method of synthesis. Microwave-based methods of graft copolymer synthesis are fast, easy to operate, and highly reproducible and thus have all the qualities of being the most suitable method of synthesis.

The microwave-based techniques of graft copolymer synthesis have been classified into two types:

1. *Microwave-initiated synthesis*: This technique employs microwave radiation alone to create free radical sites on the polysaccharide, from where the graft chains are attached [5,57–63].
2. *Microwave-assisted synthesis*: This technique uses a combination of microwave radiation and a chemical free radical initiator to create the free radical sites on the polysaccharide backbone, from where the graft chains grow [64–69].

21.3.2.3.1 Microwave-Initiated Synthesis

In microwave-initiated reactions, no chemical initiators are added. In the reaction mixture, the polar molecules are irradiated by microwave; it results in the rotation of the molecules, leading to the generation of heat. However, no free radical is produce as such [60]. When a macromolecule is present, rotation of the entire molecule is not possible. So the microwave is absorbed by the polar group present in the macromolecules, which then behave as if they were anchored to an immobile raft, and its immobile localized rotations will occur in the microwave region, and consequently, the severing of bond leads to the formation of free radical sites [70–74].

However, it has been noticed [75] that the grafting in reaction mixtures without initiators does not occur under purely thermal heating. This may support the possibility of in situ formation of radicals in microwave grafting reactions, which could possibly be due to microwave effect. Mishra et al. [5] used microwave irradiation for the graft copolymerization of acrylic acid onto CMC. This material was examined as flocculant for river water clarification. FTIR spectroscopy confirmed that free radicals are formed on polysaccharide backbone by cleavage of 1°–OH bond, indicating microwave effect and not thermal decomposition as the cause of free radical generation (Scheme 21.7).

Bao-Xiu et al. [76] recently prepared an adsorbent resin by graft copolymerization of acrylic acid and acrylamide on cellulose under microwave irradiation (electromagnetic radiation). This material was examined for its adsorption capacity for Cu(II) from wastewater.

Orlando et al. [77] utilized microwave radiation to produce chelating agents from sugarcane bagasse by reaction of urea with reactive sites present in bagasse.

21.3.2.3.2 Microwave-Assisted Synthesis

It involves use of both microwave radiation and redox initiators. In grafting reactions, redox initiators produce ions, and their presence enhances the ability of the aqueous reaction mixture to convert the microwave energy to heat energy [78–81]. Under the influence of microwave dielectric heating,

$$\text{CMC–OH} \xrightarrow{\text{MW}} \text{CMC–O}^{\bullet} + \text{H}^{\bullet}$$

$$\text{CMC–O}^{\bullet} + \text{M} \longrightarrow \text{CMC–O–M}^{\bullet}$$

SCHEME 21.7 Mechanism of microwave-initiated graft copolymerization of CMC.

$$\text{CMC–OH} \xrightarrow[\text{Redox reagent}]{\text{MW}} \text{CMC–O}^{\bullet} + \text{H}^{\bullet}$$

$$\text{CMC–O}^{\bullet} + \text{M} \longrightarrow \text{CMC–O–M}^{\bullet}$$

Redox reagent: Persulphate, ceric salts, etc...

SCHEME 21.8 Mechanism of microwave-assisted graft copolymerization of CMC.

the generation of free radicals from the initiators facilitates the grafting reactions [82]. It may be postulated that localized heating of the initiator takes place at hot spot regions to generate free radicals faster than under the influence of thermal heating. Such grafting reactions have been frequently studied for producing modified polysaccharides for numerous applications (Scheme 21.8).

Rajesh et al. [83] synthesized the glycidyl methacrylate (GMA)–grafted cellulose adsorbent by the novel microwave-assisted method for the effective adsorption of mercury from a coal fly ash sample.

21.4 CONTROLLING FACTORS OF GRAFTING

The rate of grafting is dependent upon the initiator, concentration as well as the monomer, radiation irradiation time, and the nature of backbone of polysaccharide.

21.4.1 Effect of Chemical Free Radical Initiator Concentration

All chemical grafting reactions require an initiator, and its nature, concentration, solubility, as well as function need to be considered.

A low concentration of catalyst should initiate a few grafting sites, which results in longer monomer chains, compared to a high concentration of catalyst, which will initiate a larger number of grafting sites, making the average size of grafted chains shorter for the same monomer concentration. So during the grafting of monomers on polysaccharides, there are two possibilities. One can either have a small number of long monomer chains or a large number of short monomer chains in the graft copolymer. In the former case, the compact shape of the original polysaccharide would be changed, due to the presence of long monomer chains. This would result in larger hydrodynamic volume, leading to higher intrinsic viscosity. On the other hand, a large number of short monomer chains will not alter the original compact shape to a great extent, thus resulting in lower hydrodynamic volume, which should be reflected again in its lower intrinsic viscosity value [84].

21.4.2 Effect of Monomer Concentration

As with the nature of backbone, the reactivity of the monomer is also important in grafting. The reactivity of monomers depends upon the various factors, viz., polar and steric nature, swellability of backbone in the presence of the monomers, and concentration of monomers.

With an increase in the concentration of monomer, percentage grafting increased continuously and reached the maximum. Afterward, the percentage grafting decreased. This behavior can be explained by the fact that an increase in monomer concentration leads to the accumulation of monomer molecules in close proximity to the polysaccharide backbone. The decrease in the percentage grafting after optimization could be associated with the reduction in the active sites on the polysaccharide backbone as graft copolymerization proceeds. It can also be accounted for because once the graft copolymer radical has formed, the excess monomer will shield the graft copolymer, which may decrease the rate of graft copolymerization. In addition to this, with excess monomer concentration, the competing homopolymer formation reaction becomes significant, leading to depletion in the percentage of grafting [84].

21.4.3 Effect of Exposure Time

With the increase in exposure time, the percentage grafting increased (which is optimized) after which it decreased. This may be because of the fact that prolonged exposure irradiation (high energy, microwave) may have degraded the polysaccharide backbone. Hence, the percentage grafting and intrinsic viscosity decreased [84].

21.4.4 Nature of the Backbone

As grafting involves covalent attachment of a monomer to a preformed polymeric backbone, the nature of the backbone (viz., physical nature and chemical composition) plays an important role in the process.

21.5 ANALYTICAL EVIDENCE FOR GRAFTING

The modification of cellulose can be proved by various analytical tools. The mostly used techniques are spectroscopic, elemental composition, and morphography. They are discussed briefly in this review.

21.5.1 By Infrared Spectroscopy

From the FTIR spectrum of CMC (Figure 21.3a), it has been observed that a small peak at 3606.85 cm^{-1} is due to stretching vibration of 2° –O–H(Diols). The broad peak at 3126.61 cm^{-1} is due to the stretching vibrations of 1° –O–H(CH_2OH). Smaller peaks at 2879.72 cm^{-1} and 2825.72 cm^{-1} are assigned to the C–H stretching vibrations. The band at 1060.88 cm^{-1} is attributed to the C–O–C stretching vibrations. The peak at 1770.65 cm^{-1} is due to C=O stretching vibration. The peak at 1579.70 cm^{-1} is due to asymmetrical stretching vibrations of COO^- groups. Smaller peaks at 1421.54 and 1325.10 cm^{-1} are assigned to symmetrical stretching vibrations of COO^- groups.

In the case of polyacrylic acid–grafted CMC (Figure 21.3b), 1° O–H broad peak is absent. This confirms 1° O–H as the grafting site. This is the experimental proof of Scheme 21.7. If the grafting would have been thermally induced, then "C–C" bond would have cleaved to generate the free radical site for grafting (as "C–C" bond is weaker than "O–H" bond). But "microwave effect" excites the more polar "O–H" bond, leading to its cleavage resulting in the free radical site for grafting. This vanishing of 1° O–H broad peak due to grafting is the first ever experimental proof presented of the involvement of "microwave effect" (not "thermal effect") as the cause of grafting in "microwave-initiated synthesis" of graft copolymers [5].

21.5.2 By Scanning Electron Microscopy

It is evident from the scanning electron microscopy (SEM) micrographs of CMC (Figure 21.4a) and that of polyacrylic acid–grafted CMC (Figure 21.4b) that profound morphological change, in the form of transition from cylindrical structure (of CMC) to stretchy structure (of CMC-*g*-PAA), has taken place because of grafting of PAA chains onto CMC.

21.5.3 Elemental Analysis

The results of elemental analysis for CMC and that of polyacrylic acid–grafted CMC (i.e., CMC-*g*-PAA) are given in Table 21.1. The stoichiometrically calculated elemental composition of the CMC-*g*-PAA grade has been shown in bracket in Table 21.1.

As evident, the actual composition of the CMC-*g*-PAA is practically same as that of its stoichiometrically expected composition. This confirms that PAA chains have indeed got grafted on the CMC backbone.

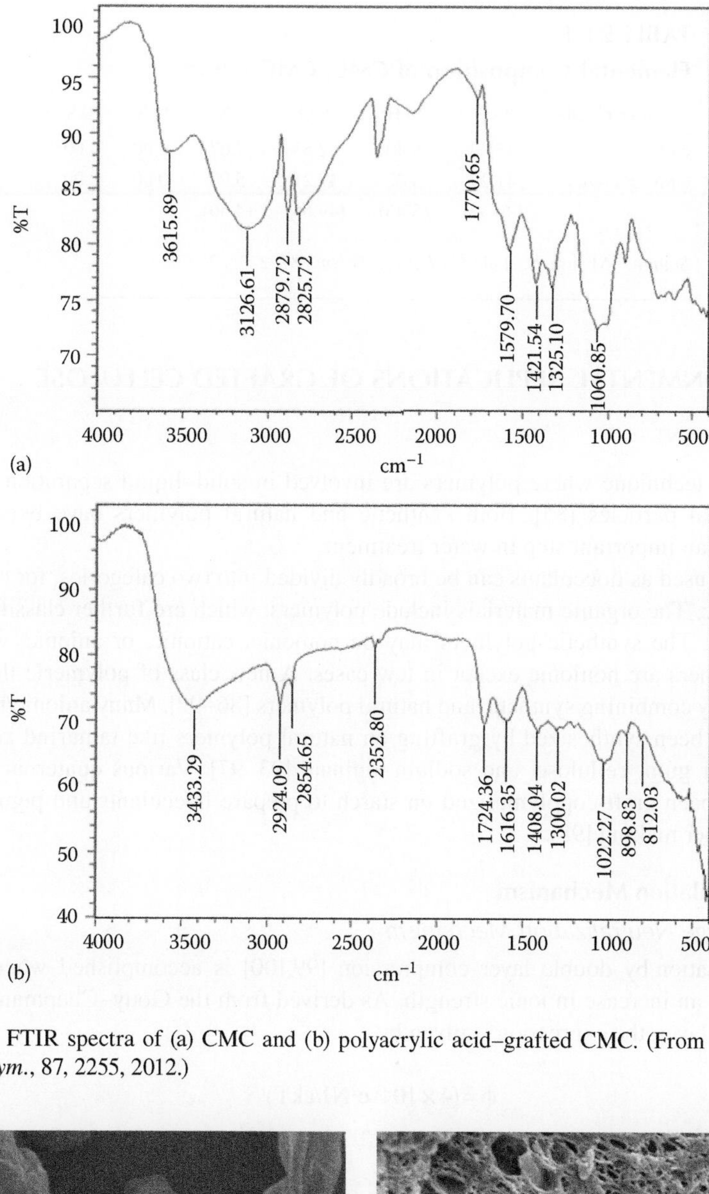

FIGURE 21.3 FTIR spectra of (a) CMC and (b) polyacrylic acid–grafted CMC. (From Mishra, S. et al., *Carbohydr. Polym.*, 87, 2255, 2012.)

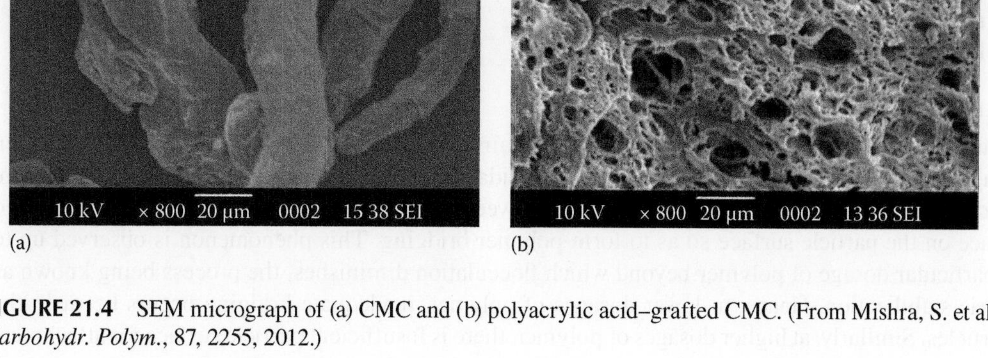

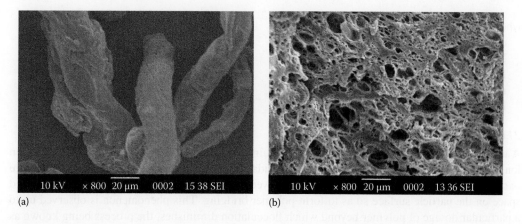

FIGURE 21.4 SEM micrograph of (a) CMC and (b) polyacrylic acid–grafted CMC. (From Mishra, S. et al., *Carbohydr. Polym.*, 87, 2255, 2012.)

TABLE 21.1
Elemental Composition of CMC, CMC-*g*-PAA

Polymer Grade	%C	%H	%O	%Na	%N	%S
CMC	35.00	5.401	52.53	7.07	0.00	0.00
CMC-*g*-PAA	41.29	5.60	47.21	5.90	0.00	0.00
	(40.32)	(5.46)	(49.64)	(4.56)		

Source: Mishra, S. et al., *Carbohydr. Polym.*, 87, 2255, 2012.

21.6 ENVIRONMENTAL APPLICATIONS OF GRAFTED CELLULOSE

21.6.1 Flocculant

Flocculation is a technique where polymers are involved in solid–liquid separation by an aggregation of colloidal particles [85]. Both synthetic and natural polymers have been utilized for flocculation. It is an important step in water treatment.

The materials used as flocculants can be broadly divided into two categories, for example, inorganic and organic. The organic materials include polymers, which are further classified into natural and synthetic. The synthetic polymers may be nonionic, cationic, or anionic, while most of the natural polymers are nonionic except in few cases. A new class of polymeric flocculants has been developed by combining synthetic and natural polymers [86–92]. Many anionic/nonionic graft copolymers have been synthesized by grafting on natural polymers like tamarind kernel powder, agar, starch, guar gum, cellulose, and sodium alginate [93–97]. Various quaternary ammonium monomers have been graft-copolymerized on starch to prepare flocculants and pigment retention aids useful in paper making [98].

21.6.1.1 Flocculation Mechanism

21.6.1.1.1 Charge Neutralization Mechanism

Charge neutralization by double layer compression [99,100] is accomplished when flocculation operates through an increase in ionic strength. As derived from the Gouy–Chapman model of the electrical double layer, the expression is given by

$$\phi = (4 \times 10^{-3}\, e^2 NI/\varepsilon kT)^{1/2}$$

where
- e is the electronic charge
- N is the Avogadro's number
- I is the ionic strength
- ε is the electrical permittivity of the solvent
- k is the Boltzmann constant

21.6.1.1.2 Bridging Mechanism

A model is presented where a single polymer chain bridges between two or more particles. When long chain polymers [99,100] are added to a colloidal suspension, they get adsorbed on two or more particle surfaces and thus form a bridge [99] between them. There should be sufficient unoccupied space on the particle surface so as to form polymer bridging. This phenomenon is observed up to a particular dosage of polymer beyond which flocculation diminishes, the process being known as steric stabilization. Hence, at lower dosages of polymer, inadequate bridging occurs between the particles. Similarly, at higher dosages of polymer, there is insufficient particle surface for attachment of the polymer segments leading to destabilization. Flocs formed by bridging mechanism are found to be large and stronger than those produced by addition of salts. However, under high shear rates, these flocs are broken and may not reform once again.

21.6.1.1.3 Electrostatic Patch Mechanism

It explains the effect of highly charged cations on negatively charged particles. For a system of high cationic charge in anionic colloidal suspensions, the high interaction energy favors a flattened adsorbed configuration. The charges on the polymer first form "island" patches of charge, surrounded by areas of opposite charge. Particles with polyelectrolytes adsorbed in this "patch-wise" manner can interact in such a way that oppositely charged areas of different particles come in contact giving rise to strong attraction [101–103].

21.6.1.1.4 Singh's Easy Approachability Model

According to this model, as the branching of a polysaccharide increases, aggregation of the contaminants on the grafted chains also increases [104–107]. Thus, the hyperbranched grafted polysaccharides will have easier accessibility to form aggregates of the contaminants, hence resulting in the best flocculation characteristics. Mishra et al. [5] reported first the polyacrylic acid–grafted CMC (CMC-*g*-PAA) synthesized by microwave. This confirms the "extension of Singh's easy approachability model" to PAA systems also.

21.6.1.1.5 Brostow, Pal, and Singh Model of Flocculation

Radius of gyration is directly proportional to flocculation efficacy; the relation is stated as [108]

$$y = a \cdot R_G^b$$

where

R_G is the radius of gyration

a and b are parameters characteristic for a given suspension medium, that is, both the dispersed phase and the majority liquid

21.6.1.2 Factors Affecting the Flocculation

The effects of molecular weight on flocculation [109–111] are best described in terms of bridging and electrostatic patch mechanisms. Optimum flocculent concentration has been found to be independent of molecular weight but dependent on ionic strength. In a flocculation involving two different molecular weight polyacrylamides, the higher-molecular-weight polymer performed best [112,113]. The degree of flocculation can be markedly affected by dosing and mixing [114] conditions. The configuration of polyelectrolytes in solution is significantly affected by ionic strength, and this effects flocculation. The importance of particle size variation with regard to flocculation has been investigated by many researchers [115].

21.6.1.3 Flocculation: Its Applications

Polymeric flocculants are employed for wastewater treatment in metals, chemicals, pulp and paper, food processing, petroleum refining, paper making, and textile industries [116–118].

Sagar Pal et al. [119] reported the flocculation performance in two different synthetic effluents, namely, kaolin and iron-ore suspensions of hydroxypropyl methyl cellulose grafted with polyacrylamide (HPMC-*g*-PAM). Yang et al. [120] reported the dye removal efficiency of polyacrylamide-grafted CMC (PAM-*g*-CMC) by flocculation process. Katsura et al. [121] reported the flocculation study of aqueous suspension of microcrystalline cellulose powder grafted with polyacrylamide in kaolin suspensions.

21.6.2 Biosorbent

Biosorbents are three-dimensional cross-linked hydrophilic polymers with the ability to absorb large quantities of water or deswell in response to changes in their external environment [122–124]. The volume phase transitions as a response to different stimuli arouse scientific interest and make this usage in advanced technologies. These changes can be induced by changing the surrounding pH, temperature, time, and ionic strength. With excellent hydrophilic properties and high swelling ratio, they are used in agriculture [125], biomedical area as antibacterial materials [126], tissue engineering [127], biosensors [128,129] and sorbents for the removal of heavy metals [130], and drug delivery [131,132].

Among many chelating agents, grafted and cross-linked synthetic or natural polymers containing functional groups (ion exchange resins and membranes, affinity adsorbents, and hydrogels) have been used for these applications [128].

Adsorption of toxic metal ions using chelating polymers has the advantages of high efficiency, easy handling, availability of different adsorbents, and cost-effectiveness. Therefore, it is of great importance, especially in environmental applications [133,134]. Several functional groups such as amino, phosphate, amido, sulfonate, carboxyl, and hydroxyl groups can be grafted on the polysaccharides to give them additional ionic characters with their stability further enhanced by cross-linking. The biosorption mechanism in these grafted and cross-linked materials is a complex process involving (1) ion exchange, (2) chelation, (3) complexation, and (4) adsorption by physical forces such as H-bonding [22,135].

Ibrahim et al. [125] synthesized cross-linked superabsorbent CMC/acrylamide hydrogels through electron beam irradiation. Rodriguez et al. [131] synthesized cationic cellulose hydrogels and studied kinetics of the cross-linking process, as pH-/ion-sensitive drug delivery systems. Mohy Eldin et al. [136] synthesized the polyacrylamide-grafted CMC, a pH-sensitive hydrogel for protein concentration. Mohy Eldin et al. [137] synthesized the polyacrylamide-grafted CMC by the radical polymerization process for pH-sensitive hydrogel. Kulkarni et al. [138] synthesized the novel pH-sensitive interpenetrating network hydrogel beads of CMC–(polyacrylamide-grafted alginate) for controlled release of ketoprofen. El-Naggar et al. [139] reported the temperature- and pH-responsive behaviors of CMC/AAc hydrogels prepared by electron beam irradiation. Chang et al. [140] synthesized the novel superabsorbent hydrogels from CMC sodium and cellulose in the NaOH/urea aqueous system by using epichlorohydrin as cross-linker for controlled delivery.

21.6.3 Membrane Filters

In the separation science, membrane plays an important role for the separation of natural gases, liquid–liquid separation, heavy metal ion separation by "membrane filter process." In general, the homogeneous membranes are not suitable for separation. So the selective separation of molecule or ion needs some kind of heterogeneity of the membrane [141,142].

Polymeric membrane is very attractive for the development of the separation property by grafting procedure. Due to the grafting, the heterogeneity of the polymeric membrane increases, that is, suitable for the selective separation of the various types of mixtures. Chowdhury et al. [143] synthesized the polystyrene-grafted cellulose acetate reverse osmosis membrane for ethanol separation.

21.7 BIOMEDICAL APPLICATIONS

Graft copolymers are used as matrix for prolonged-release of drugs via oral mode, due to its simple and low-cost manufacturing process. It is important to maintain the therapeutic level of any drug that is administered in body for treatment. Therapeutic level refers to the concentration of drug in the body tissues, blood, etc., without causing any side effects.

Controlled-release drug delivery technologies have made quantum advances in the last three decades. The therapeutic advantages of controlled drug delivery systems are release of active agent at predetermined rate, maintenance of optimal and effective drug level for prolonged duration, reduction of side effects, increase in patient's compliance, reduction in the frequency of dosing, delivery of drug in the vicinity of site of action, and more efficient utilization of active agent [144].

Basically, there are three basic modes of drug delivery:

1. Targeted delivery or spatial distribution of drug: It has the goal of delivering the drug to specific cells, tissues, or organs [144].
2. Controlled release or temporal distribution of drug: It releases drug at a predetermined rate or at specific times or with specific release profiles [144].
3. Modulated release refers to the use of a drug at a variable rate controlled by various factors [144].

In the field of controlled drug delivery, polysaccharides (such as starch, chitosan, alginate, and cellulose) and modified polysaccharides (e.g., cellulose derivatives) have earned special attention due to their high biocompatibility and hydrophilicity [145–147].

Nowadays, graft copolymers are being used as an interesting option when developing a direct compression excipient for controlled-release matrix tablets. Among the current approaches in the development of new polymeric systems, the synthesis of graft copolymers is an easy method for modifying the properties of polysaccharides. The low cost, nontoxicity, biodegradability, and biocompatibility of polysaccharides make the graft copolymers a focus of increasing attention.

Wen et al. [148] synthesized POEOMA-grafted CMC using oligo(ethylene oxide)-containing methacrylate (OEOMA)), and a disulfide-labeled dimethacrylate allows for the synthesis of dual stimuli-responsive bionanogels cross-linked with disulfide linkages for the controlled release of anticancer drug. Yuan et al. [149] synthesized the ethyl cellulose-*graft*-poly(*N,N*-dimethylamino-ethyl methacrylate)-*graft*-poly(ε-caprolactone)(EC-*g*-PDMAEMA-*g*-PCL) by ring-opening polymerization and atom transfer radical polymerization for the potential drug nanocarriers. Sadeghi et al. [150] synthesized the superabsorbent hydrogels that were prepared by grafting cross-linked poly (*N*-vinyl pyrollidin and 2-acrylamido-2-methyl propan sulfonic acid (PNVP-*co*-PAMPS) chains onto CMC backbones through a free radical polymerization for controlled released of drug.

21.8 CONCLUSION

Nowadays, researchers have great attention toward the modification of CMC by the different methods of graft copolymerization. The modern graft copolymerization methods are more effective than the earlier methods and need to be addressed from the industrial point of view. The physical and chemical properties of the CMC profoundly change due to the grafting by different monomers. The grafting product of CMC has potential application in the environmental and biomedical field. CMC-based graft copolymers will continue to remain in the forefront of cutting-edge research.

REFERENCES

1. D. Klemm, H.P. Schmauder, T. Heinze, S. De Baets, E.J. Vandamme. 2002. Cellulose. In A. Steinbuchel (Ed.), *Polysaccharides II: Polysaccharides from Eukaryotes*, Vol. 6. Wiley-VCH, Weinheim, Germany, pp. 275–320.
2. J.-L. Wertz, O. Bedue, J.P. Mercie. 2010. *Cellulose Science and Technology*, 1st edn. EPFL Press/CRC Press/Taylor & Francis Group/LLc Rdlon, Lausanne, Switzerland.
3. A.D. French, N.R. Bertoniere, R.M. Brown, H. Chanzy, D. Gray, K. Hatton, W. Glasser. 2003. *Encyclopedia of Polymer Science and Technology, Cellulose*. John Wiley & Sons Inc, New York.
4. H. Krassing. 1993. *Cellulose-Structure, Accessibility and Reactivity, Polymers Monographs*, Vol. II. Gordon & Breach Science Publishers, Amsterdam, the Netherlands.

5. S. Mishra, G.U. Rani, G. Sen. 2012. Microwave initiated synthesis and application of polyacrylic acid grafted carboxymethyl cellulose. *Carbohydrate Polymer* 87:2255–2262.
6. A. Payen. 1842. Third memoir on the development végétaux 'Extrait memories the Royal Academy of Sciences: Volumes III Scholars Éntranges. Imprimerie Royale, Paris, France.
7. W.N. Haworth. 1928. The structure of carbohydrates. *Helvetica Chimica Acta* 11:534.
8. W.N. Haworth. 1932. Die Konstitution einiger Kohlenhydrate. *Berichte der deutschen chemischen Gesellschaft* (*A*) 65(4):43–65.
9. H. Staudinger. 1960. *Die hochmolekularen organichen Verbindungen—Kautschuk und Cellulose*, 2nd edn. Springer Verlag, Berlin, Germany; D. Roy, M. Semsarilar, T.J. Guthrie, S. Perrier. 2009. Cellulose modification by polymer grafting: A review. *Chemical Society Reviews* 38:2046–2064.
10. D. Klemm, B. Philipp, T. Heinze, U. Heinze, W. Wagenknecht. 1998. *Comprehensive Cellulose Chemistry*: *Fundamentals and Analytical Methods*, Vol. 1. Wiley-VCH, Weinheim, Germany.
11. D.W. O'Connell, C. Birkinshaw, T.F. O'Dwyer. 2008. Heavy metal adsorbents prepared from the modification of cellulose: A review. *Bioresource Technology* 99(15):6709–6724.
12. E. Bianchi, A. Bonazza, E. Marsano, S. Russo. 2000. Free radical grafting onto cellulose inhomogeneous conditions. 2. Modified cellulose–methyl methacrylate system. *Carbohydrate Polymer* 41:47–53.
13. V.R. Gowariker, N.V. Viswanathan, J. Sreedhar. 1986. *Polymer Science*. New Age International (p) Ltd, New Delhi, Chapter 12.
14. F. Haber, J. Weiss. 1932. Über die Katalyse des Hydroperoxydes. *Naturwissenschaften* 20:948–950.
15. F. Haber, J. Weiss. 1934. The catalytic decomposition of hydrogen peroxide by iron salts. *Proceedings of the Royal Society A* 147:332–351.
16. J.H. Merz, W.A. Waters. 1949. Some oxidations involving the free hydroxyl radical. *Journal of the Chemical Society* S15–S25. doi:10.1039/JR9490000S15.
17. A.L. Suo, J.M. Qian, Y. Yao, W.G. Zhang. 2007. Synthesis and properties of carboxymethyl cellulose-*graft*-poly(acrylic acid-*co*-acrylamide) as a novel cellulose-based superabsorbent. *Journal of Applied Polymer Science* 103(3):1382–1388.
18. D. Aliouche, B. Sid, H. Ait-Amar. 2006. Graft-copolymerization of acrylic monomers onto cellulose: Impact on fiber swelling and absorbency. *Annales de Chimie Science des Materiaux* 31(5):527–540.
19. B.A. El-Hady, M.M. Ibrahim. 2004. Graft copolymerization of acrylamide onto carboxymethyl cellulose with the xanthate method. *Journal of Applied Polymer Science* 93:271–278.
20. G.U. Rani, S. Mishra, G. Sen, U. Jha. 2012. Polyacrylamide grafted agar: Synthesis and applications of conventional and microwave assisted technique. *Carbohydrate Polymers* 90:784–791.
21. S. Bharti, S. Mishra, G. Sen. 2013. Ceric ion initiated synthesis of polyacrylamide grafted oatmeal: Its application as flocculant for wastewater treatment. *Carbohydrate Polymers* 93:528–536.
22. A. Bhattacharya, J.W. Rawlins, P. Ray. 2008. *Polymer Grafting and Crosslinking*, John Wiley & Sons, New York.
23. O.H. Lin, R.N. Kumar, H.D. Rozman, M. Azemi, M. Noor. 2005. Grafting of sodium carboxymethyl cellulose (CMC) with glycidylmethacrylate and development of UV curable coatings from CMC-*g*-GMA induced by cationic photoinitiators. *Carbohydrate Polymers* 59:57–69.
24. H. Chen and Y. L. Hsieh. 2005. Enzyme immobilization on ultrafine cellulose fibers via poly(acrylic acid) electrolyte grafts. *Biotechnology and Bioengineering* 90(4):405–413.
25. D.N.S. Hon. 1982. Graft copolymerization of lignocellulosic fibers. *ACS Symposium Series, American Chemical Society*, Washington, DC, 1982.
26. K.C. Gupta, K. Khandehar. 2002. Graft copolymerization of acrylamide–methylacrylate co-monomers onto cellulose using ceric ammonium nitrate. *Journal of Applied Polymer Science* 86:2631–2642.
27. N. Bicak, D.C. Sherrington, B.F. Senkal. 1999. Graft copolymer of acrylamide onto cellulose as mercury selective sorbent. *Reactive and Functional Polymers* 41:69–76.
28. M. Liu, Y. Deng, H. Zhan, X. Zhang, W. Liu, H. Zhan. 2001. Removal and recovery of chromium(III) from aqueous solutions by a spheroidal cellulose adsorbent. *Water Environmental Research* 73(3):322–328.
29. M. Liu, Y. Deng, H. Zhan, X. Zhang. 2002. Adsorption and desorption of copper(II) from solutions on new spherical cellulose adsorbent. *Journal of Applied Polymer Science* 84:478–485.
30. Y. Aoki, K. Tanaka, M. Sakamoto, K. Furuhata. 1999. Sorption of metal ions by bead cellulose grafted with amidoximated polyacrylonitrile. *Sen'i Gakkaishi* 55(12):569–575.
31. R.R. Navarro, K. Sumi, M. Matsumura. 1999. Improved metal affinity of chelating adsorbents through graft polymerization. *Water Research* 33(9):2037–2044.
32. A. Hebeish, P.C. Mehta. 1968. Grafting of acrylonitrile to different cellulosic materials by high-energy radiation. *Textile Research Journal* 38:1070–1071.

33. S. Geresh, G.Y. Gdalevsky, I. Gilboa, J. Voorspoels, J.P. Remon, J. Kost. 2004. Bioadhesive grafted agar copolymers as platforms for per oral drug delivery: A study of theophylline release. *Journal of Controlled Release* 94:391–399.
34. N. Shiraishi, J.L. Williams, V. Stannett. 1982. The radiation grafting of vinyl monomers to cotton fabrics—I. Methacrylic acid to terry cloth towelling. *Radiation Physics and Chemistry* 19:73–78.
35. R.K. Sharma, B.N. Misra. 1981. Grafting onto wool. *Polymer Bulletin* 6:183–188.
36. M. Carenza. 1992. Recent achievements in the use of radiation polymerization and grafting for biomedical applications. *Radiation Physics and Chemistry* 39:485–493.
37. J.P. Wang, Y.Z. Chen, S.J. Zhang, H.Q. Yu. 2008. A chitosan-based flocculant prepared with gamma-irradiation-induced grafting. *Bioresource Technology* 99:3397–3402.
38. R.Y.M. Huang, B. Immergut, E.H. Immergu, W.H. Rapson. 2003. Grafting vinyl polymers onto cellulose by high energy radiation. I. High energy radiation-induced graft copolymerization of styrene onto cellulose. *Journal of Polymer Science Part A: General Papers* 1:1257–1270.
39. M. Barsbay, O. Guven, T.P. Davis, C.B. Kowollik, L. Barner. 2009. RAFT-mediated polymerization and grafting of sodium 4-styrenesulfonate from cellulose initiated via γ-radiation. *Polymer* 50:973–982.
40. M.M. Nasef, A.H. El-Sayed. 2004. Preparation and applications of ion exchange membranes by radiation-induced graft copolymerization of polar monomers onto non-polar films. *Progress in Polymer Science* 29:499–561.
41. S.E. Abdel-Aal, Y. Gad, A.M. Dessouki. 2006. The use of wood pulp and radiation modified starch in wastewater treatment. *Journal of Applied Polymer Science* 99:2460–2469.
42. J. Deng, L. Wang, L. Liu, W. Yang. 2009. Developments and new applications of UV-induced surface graft polymerizations. *Progress in Polymer Science* 34:156–193.
43. J. Wang, G. Liang, W. Zhao, S. Lu, Z. Zhang. 2006. Studies on surface modification of UHMWPE fibers via UV initiated grafting. *Applied Surface Science* 253:668–673.
44. H. Hua, N. Li, L. Wu, H. Zhong, G. Wu, Z. Yuan, X. Lin, L. Tang. 2008. Anti-fouling ultrafiltration membrane prepared from polysulfone-*graft*-methyl acrylate copolymers by UV-induced grafting method. *Journal of Environmental Science* (China) 20:565–570.
45. A.M. Shanmugharaj, J.K. Kim, S.H. Ryu. 2006. Modification of rubber surface by UV surface grafting. *Applied Surface Science* 252:5714–5722.
46. Z. Zhu, M.J. Kelley. 2005. Grafting onto poly(ethylene terephthalate) driven by 172 nm UV light. *Applied Surface Science* 252:303–310.
47. J. Deng, W. Yang. 2005. Grafting copolymerization of styrene and maleic anhydride binary monomer systems induced by UV irradiation. *European Polymer Journal* 41:2685–2692.
48. M.D. Thaker, H.C. Trivedi. 2005. Ultraviolet-radiation-induced graft copolymerization of methyl acrylate onto the sodium salt of partially carboxymethylated guar gum. *Journal of Applied Polymer Science* 97:1977–1986.
49. H. Kubota, Y. Shigehisa. 1995. Introduction of amidoxime groups into cellulose and its ability to adsorb metal ions. *Journal of Applied Polymer Science* 56:147–151.
50. J.A. Harris, J.C. Arthur, J.H. Carra. 1978. Photoinitiated polymerization of glycidyl methacrylate with cotton cellulose. *Journal of Applied Polymer Science* 22:905–915.
51. A. Bhattacharya, B.N. Misra. 2004. Grafting: A versatile means to modify polymers: Techniques, factors and applications. *Progress in Polymer Science* 29(8):767–814.
52. H. Kubota, S. Suzuki. 1995. Comparative examinations of reactivity of grafted celluloses prepared by ultra violet and ceric salt-initiated graftings. *European Polymer Journal* 31(8):701–704.
53. H. Kubota, S. Suzuki. 1995. Comparative examinations of reactivity of grafted celluloses prepared by ultra violet and ceric salt-initiated graftings. *European Polymer Journal* 31:701–704.
54. V. Singh, A. Tiwari, D.N. Tripathi, R. Sanghi. 2005. Microwave promoted synthesis of chitosan-*graft*-poly(acrylonitrile). *Journal of Applied Polymer Science* 95:820–825.
55. V. Singh, A. Tiwari, D.N. Tripathi, R. Sanghi. 2006. Microwave enhanced synthesis of chitosan-*graft*-polyacrylamide. *Polymer* 47:254–260.
56. V.K. Thakur, M.K. Thakur, R.K. Gupta. 2013. Graft copolymers from cellulose: Synthesis, characterization and evaluation. *Carbohydrate Polymers* 97(1):18–25.
57. S. Mishra, G. Sen. 2011. Microwave initiated synthesis of polymethylmethacrylate grafted guar (GG-*g*-PMMA), characterizations and application. *International Journal of Biological Macromolecule* 48:688–694.
58. G. Sen, S. Mishra, U. Jha, S. Pal. 2010. Microwave initiated synthesis of polyacrylamide grafted guar-gum (GG-*g*-PAM)—Characterizations and application as matrix for controlled release of 5-amino salicylic acid. *International Journal of Biological Macromolecule* 47:164–170.

59. G. Sen, R. Kumar, S. Ghosh, S. Pal. 2009. A novel polymeric flocculant based on polyacrylamide grafted carboxymethylstarch. *Carbohydrates Polymer* 77:822–831.
60. G. Sen, R.P. Singh, P. Sagar. 2010. Microwave-initiated synthesis of polyacrylamide grafted sodium alginate: Synthesis and characterization. *Journal of Applied Polymer Science* 115:63–71.
61. G. Sen, S. Mishra, G.U. Rani, P. Rani, R. Prasad. 2012. Microwavc initiated synthesis of polyacrylamide grafted *Psyllium* and its application as a flocculant. *International Journal of Biological Macromolecule* 50:369–375.
62. G. Sen, S. Pal. 2009. Microwave initiated synthesis of polyacrylamide grafted carboxymethylstarch (CMS-*g*-PAM): Application as a novel matrix for sustained drug release. *International Journal of Biological Macromolecule* 45:48–55.
63. G.U. Rani, S. Mishra, G. Pathak, U. Jha, G. Sen. 2013. Synthesis and applications of poly (2-hydroxyethylmethacrylate) grafted agar: A microwave based approach. *International Journal of Biological Macromolecule* 61:276–284.
64. S. Mishra, A. Mukul, G. Sen, U. Jha. 2011. Microwave assisted synthesis of polyacrylamide grafted starch (St-*g*-PAM) and its applicability as flocculant for water treatment. *International Journal of Biological Macromolecule* 48:106–111.
65. S. Mishra, G. Sen, G.U. Rani, S. Sinha. 2011. Microwave assisted synthesis of polyacrylamide grafted agar (Ag-*g*-PAM) and its application as flocculant for wastewater treatment. *International Journal of Biological Macromolecule* 49:591–598.
66. G. Sen, G.U. Rani, S. Mishra. 2013. Microwave assisted synthesis of poly(2-hydroxyethylmethacrylate) grafted agar (Ag-*g*-P(HEMA)) and its application as flocculant for wastewater treatment. *Frontiers of Chemical Science and Engineering* 7:312–321.
67. P. Rani, G. Sen, S. Mishra, U. Jha. 2012. Microwave assisted synthesis of polyacrylamide grafted gum ghatti and its application as flocculent. *Carbohydrate Polymers* 89:275–281.
68. P. Rani, S. Mishra, G. Sen. 2013. Microwave based synthesis of polymethyl methacrylate grafted alginate: Its application as flocculant. *Carbohydrate Polymers* 91:686–692.
69. G. Usha Rani, A.K. Konreddy, S. Mishra, G. Sen. 2014. Synthesis and applications of polyacrylamide grafted agar as a matrix for controlled drug release of 5-ASA. *International Journal of Biological Macromolecules* 65:375–382.
70. W. Xue, S. Champ, M.B. Huglin. 2000. Observations on some copolymerizations involving N-isopropylacrylamide. *Polymer* 41:7575–7581.
71. S.A. Galema. 1997. Microwave chemistry. *Chemical Society Reviews* 26:233–238.
72. D. Dallinger, C.O. Kappe. 2007. Microwave-assisted synthesis in water as solvent. *Chemical Reviews* 107:2563–2591.
73. J. Robinson, S. Kingman, D. Irvine, P. Licence, A. Smith, G. Dimitrakis, D. Obermayer, C.O. Kappe. 2010. Electromagnetic simulations of microwave heating experiments using reaction vessels made out of silicon carbide. *Physical Chemistry Chemical Physics* 12:10793–10800.
74. C. Gabriel, S. Gabriel, E.H. Grant, B.S.J. Halstead, D.M.P. Mingos. 1998. Dielectric parameters relevant to microwave dielectric heating. *Chemical Society Reviews* 27:213–223.
75. V. Singh, A. Tiwari, D.N. Tripathi, R. Sanghi. 2004. Microwave assisted synthesis of guar-g polyacrylamide. *Carbohydrate Polymers* 58:1–6.
76. Z. Bao-Xiu, W. Peng, Z. Tong, C. Chun-Yun, S. Jing. 2006. Preparation and adsorption performance of a cellulosic adsorbent resin for copper(II). *Journal of Applied Polymer Science* 99:2951–2956.
77. U.S. Orlando, A. Baes, W. Nishijima, M. Okada. 2002. Preparation of chelating agents from sugarcane bagasse by microwave radiation as an alternative ecologically benign procedure. *Green Chemistry* 4:555–557.
78. C. Gabriel, S. Gabriel, E.H. Grant, B.S.J. Halstead, D.M.P. Mingos. 1998. Dielectric parameters relevant to microwave dielectric heating. *Chemical Society Reviews* 27:213–223.
79. P. Lidstrom, J. Tierney, B. Wathey, J. Westman. 2001. Microwave assisted organic synthesis—A review. *Tetrahedron* 57:9225–9283.
80. D.M.P. Mingos, D.R. Baghurst. 1991. Applications of microwave dielectric heating effects to synthetic problems in chemistry. *Chemical Society Reviews* 20:1–47.
81. E.D. Neas, M.J. Collins. 1988. Microwave heating: Theoretical concepts and equipment design. In H.M. Kingston, L.B. Jassie (Eds.), *Introduction to Microwave Sample Preparation: Theory and Practice*. American Chemical Society, Washington, DC, pp. 7–22.
82. V. Singh, A. Tiwari, S. Pandey, S.K. Singh. 2007. Peroxydisulfate initiated synthesis of potato starch-*graft*-poly(acrylonitrile) under microwave irradiation. *Express Polymer Letters* 1:51–58.

83. A. Santhana Krishna Kumar, M. Barathi, S. Puvvada, N. Rajesh. 2013. Microwave assisted preparation of glycidyl methacrylate grafted cellulose adsorbent for the effective adsorption of mercury from a coal fly ash sample. *Journal of Environmental Chemical Engineering* 1:1359–1367.
84. G. Sen, A. Sharon, S. Pal. 2011. Grafted polysaccharides: Smart materials of future, synthesis and applications. In S. Kalia, L. Averous (Eds.), *Biopolymers: Biomedical and Environmental Applications*. Wiley-Scrivener, Hoboken, NJ, pp. 99–128.
85. M.A. Hughes. 1990. Coagulation and flocculation. In L. Svarosky (Ed.), *Solid-Liquid Separation (Part 1)*, 3rd edn. Butterworth & Co-Publishers Ltd, Belfast, UK, p. 74.
86. N. Paul. 1995. *Cheremisin Off: Handbook of Water and Wastewater Treatment Technology*. Marcel Dekker, Inc., New York, Chapter 4.
87. F.W. Pontius. 1990. *Water Quality and Treatment*, 4th edn. McGraw-Hill, Inc., New York.
88. C.A. Finch. 1983. *Chemistry and Technology of Water-Soluble Polymers*. Plenum Press, New York, p. 380.
89. R.L. Davidson, M. Sittig. 1962. *Water-Soluble Resins*, 2nd edn. Reinhold Publishing Corp, New York, pp. 69–88.
90. P. Molyneaux. 1984. *Water-Soluble Synthetic Polymers*, Vols. 1 and 2. CRC Press, Inc., Boca Raton, FL.
91. C.L. McCormic, J. Bock. 1987. Water soluble polymers. In H.F. Mark, N.M. Bikales, C.G. Overberger, G. Menges, J.I. Kroschwitz (Eds.), *Encyclopedia of Polymer Science and Engineering*, Vol. 17. John Wiley & Sons, New York, p. 730.
92. B.A. Bolt. 1995. Soluble polymers in water purification. *Progress in Polymer Science* 20:987–1041.
93. S.R. Deshmukh, R.P. Singh. 1986. Drag reduction characteristics of graft copolymers of xanthangum and polyacrylamide. *Journal of Applied Polymer Science* 32:6163–6176.
94. S.R. Deshmukh. 1986. Turbulent drag reduction effectiveness, shear stability and biodegradability of graft copolymers. PhD thesis, IIT, Kharagpur, India.
95. G.P. Karmakar. 1994. Flocculation and rheological properties of grafted polysaccharides, PhD thesis. IIT, Kharagpur, India.
96. G.F. Fanta, R.C. Burr, C.R. Russel, R.E. Rist. 1970. Graft copolymers of starch and poly (2-hydroxy-3-methycryloxy propyl trimethyl ammonium chloride) preparation and testing as flocculating agents. *Journal of Applied Polymer Science* 14:2601–2609.
97. G.F. Fanta, R.C. Burr, W.M. Doane, C.R. Russel. 1972. Graft copolymers of starch with mixtures of acrylamide and the nitric acid salt of dimethylaminomethyl methacrylate. *Journal of Applied Polymer Science* 16:2835–2845.
98. D.A. Jones, W.A. Jordan. 1971. Starch graft polymers I. Graft co-and terpolymers of starch with 2-hydroxy-3-methacryloyloxy propyltrimethyl ammonium chloride and acrylamide: Preparation and evaluation as silica depressants. *Journal of Applied Polymer Science* 15:2461–2469.
99. G.R. Rose, M.R. St. John. 1985. In J.I. Kroschwitz (Ed.), *Flocculation in Encyclopedia of Polymer Science and Engineering*. Wiley-Interscience, New York.
100. J. Gregory. 1987. Flocculation by polymers and polyelectrolytes. In T.F. Tadros (Ed.), *Solid-Liquid Dispersionsed*. Academic Press, London, U.K., Chapter 8, pp. 163–180.
101. J. Gregory. 1985. The use of polymeric flocculants. In *Proceedings of the Engineering Foundation Conference of Flocculation Sedimentation and Consolidation*, The Cloiser Seaislands, GA, p. 125.
102. P.F. Richardson, L.J. Connely. 1988. Industrial coagulants and flocculants. In P. Somasundaran and B.M. Modugil (Eds.), *Reagents in Mineral Technology*, Vol. 27. Surfactant Science Series, CRC Press, Taylor & Francis Group, p. 519.
103. F. Mabire, R. Audebert, C. Quivoron. 1984. Flocculation properties of some water soluble cationic copolymers towards silica suspension: A semi quantitative interpretation of the role of molecular weight and cationicity through a patchwork model. *Journal of Colloid and Interface Science* 97:120–136.
104. R.P. Singh. 1990. Drag reduction and shear stability mechanism. In I.P. Cheremisinoff (Ed.), *Encyclopedia of Fluid Mechanics: Polymer Flow Engineering*, Vol. 9. Gulf Publishing, Houston, TX, p. 425.
105. R.P. Singh, G.P. Karmakar, S.K. Rath, N.C. Karmakar, T. Tripathy, J. Panda, K. Kannan, S.K. Jain, N.T. Lan. 2000. Biodegradable drag reducing agents and flocculants based on polysaccharides: Materials and applications. *Polymer Engineering and Science* 40:46–60.
106. S. Pal, R.P. Singh. 2005. Investigations on flocculation characteristics of cationic polysaccharides: Novel polymeric flocculants. *Materials Research Innovation* 9:354–358.
107. S. Pal, D. Mal, R.P. Singh. 2005. Cationic starch: An effective flocculating agent. *Carbohydrate Polymers* 59:417–423.
108. W. Brostow, S. Pal, R.P. Sing. 2007. A model of flocculation. *Material Letters* 61:4381–4384.

109. L.S. Sandell, P. Luner. 1974. Flocculation of micro crystalline cellulose with cationic ionene polymers. *Journal of Applied Polymer Science* 18:2075–2083.
110. Y. Adachi, M.A. Cohen Stuart, R. Fokkink. 1995. Initial rates of flocculation of polystyrene latex with polyelectrolyte: Effect of ionic strength. *Journal of Colloid and Interface Science* 171:520–521.
111. A.S. Michaels. 1954. Aggregation of suspensions of polyelectrolytes. *Industrial and Engineering Chemistry* 46(7):1485–1490.
112. P. Somasundaran, T.V. Vasudevan, K.F. Tjipangandjara. 1994. Enhanced flocculation and dispersion of colloidal suspensions through manipulation of polymer conformation, dispersion aggregation. In B.M. Moudgil and P. Somasundaran (Eds.), *Proceedings of the Engineering Foundation Conference*, Engineering Foundation, New York.
113. X. Yu, P. Somasundaran. 1996. Kinetics of polymer conformational changes and its role in flocculation. *Journal of Colloid and Interface Science* 178:770–774.
114. R. Hogg, P. Bunnaul, H. Suharyono. 1993. Chemical and physical variables in polymer-induced flocculation. *Minerals and Metallurgical Processing* 294:81–86.
115. B. Moudgil, M.S. Behi, V. Mehta. 1994. Effect of particle size in flocculation, dispersion aggregation. In B.M. Moudgil, P. Somasundaran (Eds.), *Proceedings of the Engineering Foundation Conference*, Engineering Foundation, New York, p. 419.
116. S.A. Ravishankar, S.A. Pradip, M.G. Deo, R.A. Kulkarni, S. Gundiah. 1988. Selective flocculation of iron oxide-kaolin mixtures using a modified polyacrylamide flocculant. *Material Science* 10:423–433.
117. R.A. Pradip, S. Kulkarni, B.M. Gundiah, B.M. Moudgil. 1991. Selective flocculation of kaolinite from mixtures with tribasic calcium phosphate using hydrolysed polyacrylamides. *International Journal of Mineral Processing* 32:259–270.
118. R.A. Pradip, B.M. Moudgil. 1991. Selective flocculation of tribasic calcium phosphate from mixtures with quartz using polyacrylic acid flocculant. *International Journal of Mineral Processing* 32:271–281.
119. R. Das, S. Ghorai, S. Pal. 2013. Flocculation characteristics of polyacrylamide grafted hydroxypropyl methyl cellulose: An efficient biodegradable flocculant. *Chemical Engineering Journal* 229:144–152.
120. T. Cai, Z. Yang, H. Li, H. Yang, A. Li, R. Cheng. 2013. Effect of hydrolysis degree of hydrolyzed polyacrylamide grafted carboxymethyl cellulose on dye removal efficiency. *Cellulose* 20:2605–2614.
121. S. Machida, H. Narita, T. Katsura. 1971. Flocculation properties of cellulose-acrylamide graft copolymers. *Macromolecular Materials and Engineering* 20(1):47–56.
122. R. Rodriguez, C. Alvarez-Lorenzo, A. Concheiro. 2003. Cationic cellulose hydrogels: Kinetics of the cross-linking process and characterization as pH-/ion-sensitive drug delivery systems. *Journal of Controlled Release* 86:253–265.
123. X. Zhang, Y. Yang, T. Chung. 2002. The influence of cold treatment on properties of temperature sensitive poly (N-isopropylacrylamide) hydrogels. *Journal of Colloid and Interface Science* 246:105–111.
124. A. Dabrowski, Z. Hubicki, P. Podkoscielny, E. Robens. 2004. Selective removal of the heavy metal ions from waters and industrial wastewaters by ion-exchange method. *Chemosphere* 56:91–106.
125. S.M. Ibrahim, K.M. El Salmawi, A.H. Zahran. 2007. Synthesis of crosslinked superabsorbent carboxymethylcellulose/acrylamide hydrogels through electron-beam irradiation. *Journal of Applied Polymer Science* 104:2003–2008.
126. P.S.K. Murthy, Y.M. Mohan, K. Varaprasad, B. Sreedhar, K.M. Raju. 2008. First successful design of semi-IPN hydrogel–silver nanocomposites: A facile approach for antibacterial application. *Journal of Colloid and Interface Science* 318:217–224.
127. J. Kim, K. Lee, T. Hefferan, B. Currier, M. Yaszemski, L. Lu. 2008. Synthesis and evaluation of novel biodegradable hydrogels based on poly(ethyleneglycol) and sebacic acid as tissue engineering scaffolds. *Biomacromolecules* 9:149–157.
128. B. Adhikari, S. Majumdar. 2004. Polymers in sensor applications. *Progress in Polymer Science* 29:699–766.
129. A. Pourjavadi, H. Ghasemzadeh, R. Soleyman. 2007. Synthesis, characterization, and swelling behavior of alginate-*g*-poly(sodium acrylate)/kaolin superabsorbent hydrogel composites. *Journal of Applied and Polymer Science* 105:2631–2639.
130. M.R. Guilherme, A.V. Reis, A.T. Paulino, A.R. Fajardo, E.C. Muniz, E.B. Tambourgi. 2007. Superabsorbent hydrogel based on modified polysaccharide for removal of Pb^{2+} and Cu^{2+} from water with excellent performance. *Journal of Applied and Polymer Science* 105:2903–2909.
131. R. Rodriguez, C. Alvarez-Lorenzo, A. Concheiro. 2003. Cationic cellulose hydrogels: Kinetics of the cross-linking process and characterization as pH-/ion-sensitive drug delivery systems. *Journal of Controlled Release* 86:253–265.

132. X. Zhang, Y. Yang, T. Chung. 2002. The influence of cold treatment on properties of temperature sensitive poly(N-isopropylacrylamide) hydrogels. *Journal of Colloid and Interface Science* 246:105–111.
133. M. Chanda, G.L. Rempel. 1997. Chromium(III) removal by poly(ethyleneimine) granular sorbents made by a new process of templated gel filling. *Reactive and Functional Polymers* 35:197–207.
134. A. Saglam, S. Bektas, S. Patir, O. Genc, A. Denizli. 2001. Novel metal complexing ligand: Thiazolidine carrying poly(hydroxyethylmethacrylate) microbeads for removal of cadmium(II) and lead(II) ions from aqueous solutions. *Reactive and Functional Polymers* 47:185–192.
135. S.T. Lee, F.L. Mi, Y.J. Shen, S. Shyu. 2001. Equilibrium and kinetic studies of copper(II) ion uptake by chitosan-tripolyphosphate chelating resin. *Polymer* 42:1879–1892.
136. M.S. Mohy Eldin, H.M.E. Sherif, E.A. Soliman, A.A. Elzatahry, A.M. Omer. 2011. Polyacrylamide-grafted carboxymethyl cellulose: Smart pH-sensitive hydrogel for protein concentration. *Journal of Applied Polymer Science* 122:469–479.
137. M.S. Mohy Eldin, A.M. Omer, E.A. Soliman, E.A. Hassanb. 2013. Superabsorbent polyacrylamide grafted carboxymethyl cellulose pH sensitive hydrogel: I. Preparation and characterization. *Desalination and Water Treatment* 51:3196–3206.
138. R.V. Kulkarni, B. Sa. 2008. Novel pH-sensitive interpenetrating network hydrogel beads of carboxymethylcellulose-(polyacrylamide-grafted-alginate) for controlled release of ketoprofen: Preparation and characterization. *Current Drug Delivery* 5(4):256–264.
139. A.W.M. El-Naggar, S.G.A. Alla, H.M. Said. 2006. Temperature and pH responsive behaviours of CMC/AAc hydrogels prepared by electron beam irradiation. *Materials Chemistry and Physics* 95(1):158–163.
140. C. Chang, B. Duan, J. Cai, L. Zhang. 2010. Superabsorbent hydrogels based on cellulose for smart swelling and controllable delivery. *European Polymer Journal* 46(1):92–100.
141. P.D. Kartick, D. Kundu, M. Chatterjee, M.K. Naskar. 2013. Preparation of NaA zeolite membranes using poly(ethyleneimine) as buffer layer, and study of their permeation behavior. *Journal of the American Ceramic Society* 96(1):68–72.
142. A. Bhattacharya, B.N. Misra. 2004. Grafting: A versatile means to modify polymers techniques, factors and applications. *Progress in Polymer Science* 29:767–814.
143. J.P. Chowdhury, G. Ghosh, B.K. Guha. 1988. Styrene grafted cellulose acetate reverse osmosis membrane for ethanol separation. *Journal of Membrane Science* 35:301–310.
144. S.P. Vyas, R.K. Khar. 2002. *Controlled Drug Delivery Concepts and Advances*. Vallabh Prakashan, New Delhi, India.
145. S. Pal, G. Sen, S. Mishra, R.K. Dey, U. Jha. 2008. Carboxymethyl tamarind: Synthesis, characterization and its application as novel drug-delivery agent. *Journal of Applied Polymer Science* 110:392–400.
146. J. Herman, J.P. Remon, J.D. Vilder. 1989. Modified starches as hydrophilic matrices for controlled oral delivery. I. Production and characterisation of thermally modified starches. *International Journal of Pharmaceutics* 56:51–63.
147. V. Lenaerts, Y. Dumoulin, M.A. Mateescu. 1991. Controlled release of theophylline from cross-linked amylose tablets. *Journal of Controlled Release* 15:39–46.
148. Y. Wen, J. Kwon Oh. 2014. Dual-stimuli reduction and acidic pH-responsive bionanogels: Intracellular delivery nanocarriers with enhanced release. *RSC Advances* 4:229–237.
149. Q. Yan, J. Yuan, F. Zhang, X. Sui, X. Xie, Y. Yin, S. Wang, Y. Wei. 2009. Cellulose-based dual graft molecular brushes as potential drug nanocarriers: Stimulus-responsive micelles, self-assembled phase transition behavior, and tunable crystalline morphologies. *Biomacromolecules* 10(8):2033–2042.
150. M. Sadeghi, M. Yarahmadi. 2011. Synthesis and properties of carboxymethyl cellulose (CMC) graft copolymer with on-off switching properties for controlled release of drug. *African Journal of Biotechnology* 10(56):12085–12093.

22 Surface Grafting of Cellulose Nanowhisker

Hou-Yong Yu, Jin Huang, and Peter R. Chang

CONTENTS

22.1 INTRODUCTION

Cellulose nanowhiskers (CNWs), an acid-hydrolyzed form of native cellulose, have attracted much attention due to their inherent mechanical properties, high surface area–volume ratio, plentiful active hydroxyl groups, and especially their potential for application as a reinforcing agent in nanocomposites [1–4]. The hydrophilic character of CNWs means they can easily be used as nanofillers to reinforce hydrophilic polymers; however, the dispersion of CNWs in organic solvents and hydrophobic polymer matrices is greatly restricted. In addition, surface sulfate groups on CNWs prepared by sulfuric acid hydrolysis usually result in a mismatch between the thermal stability of CNWs and the thermoprocessing temperature. On the other hand, the reactive hydroxyl groups on CNWs are able to participate in the formation of covalent bonds and/or physical interactions with many polymer matrices.

Recently, chemical modification (mainly surface grafting based on the "graft onto" and "graft from" strategies) has been carried out in order to regulate the physicochemical and hydrophilic/hydrophobic properties of CNWs [3–6]. Moreover, the introduction of a hydrophobic species with a structure similar to that of the polymer matrix facilitates interaction, and as a result, the compatibility and interfacial interaction between CNWs and the polymer matrix are improved by chemical modification. In general, strong interfacial interaction is beneficial for stress transfer from the polymer matrix to the rigid CNWs, contributing to the reinforcing effect of CNWs. At the same time, the change in the surface hydrophilic/hydrophobic properties due to surface grafting of different molecules or polymers contributes to better dispersion of CNWs in various solvents. Further, the shielding of sulfate groups after surface grafting effectively enhances the thermal stability of CNWs to meet the requirements for thermal processing. In this chapter, "graft onto" and "graft from" surface grafting strategies for the development of CNW nanocomposites are illustrated, and the effects of surface grafting of CNWs on thermal processability and miscibility of CNWs with the matrix are reviewed. The perspective and current challenges in surface grafting of CNWs for the development of high-performance and functional nanocomposites are also outlined.

22.2 "GRAFT ONTO" STRATEGY

22.2.1 Grafting via Silylation

The "graft onto" strategy involves a reaction between hydroxyl groups on the CNW surface and functional end groups of polymer chains, and generally abides by the same reaction mechanism as conjugation of small molecules. Silylation is a common reaction for surface grafting alkyl chlorosilanes to CNWs to improve dispersibility in hydrophobic polymers [7–9]. For example, a series

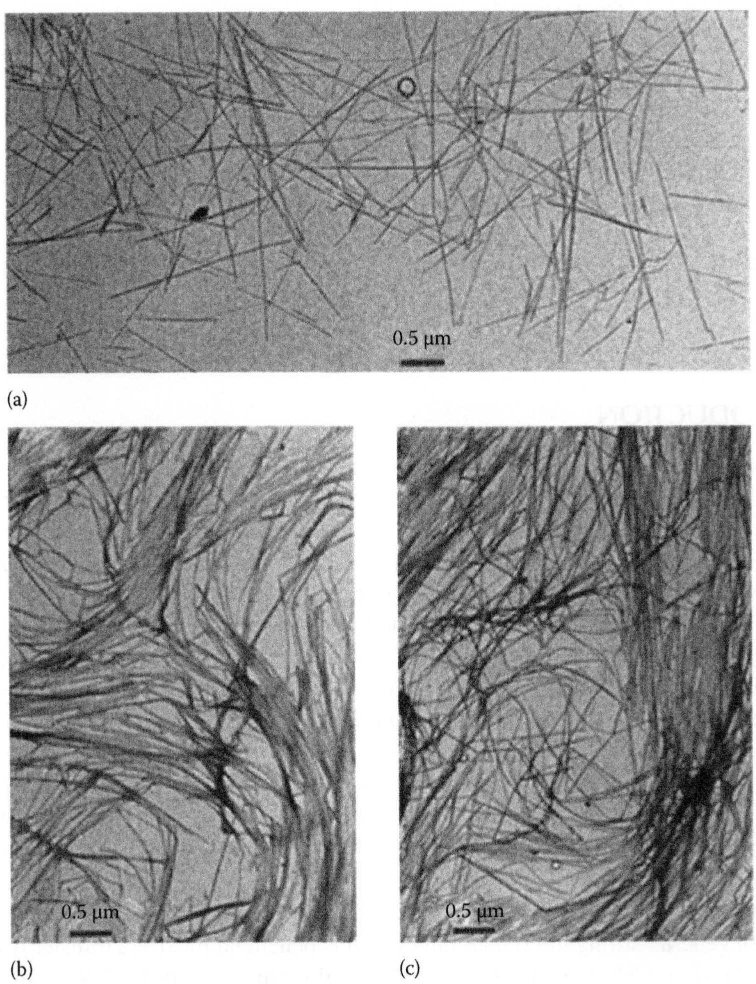

FIGURE 22.1 (a) TEM images of underivatized CNWs, (b) silylated CNWs with isopropyl-DMSiCl and a molar ratio SiCl/anhydroglucopyranose unit (AGU) of 8/1, (c) with *n*-octyl-DMSiCl and a molar ratio SiCl/AGU of 6/1. *(Continued)*

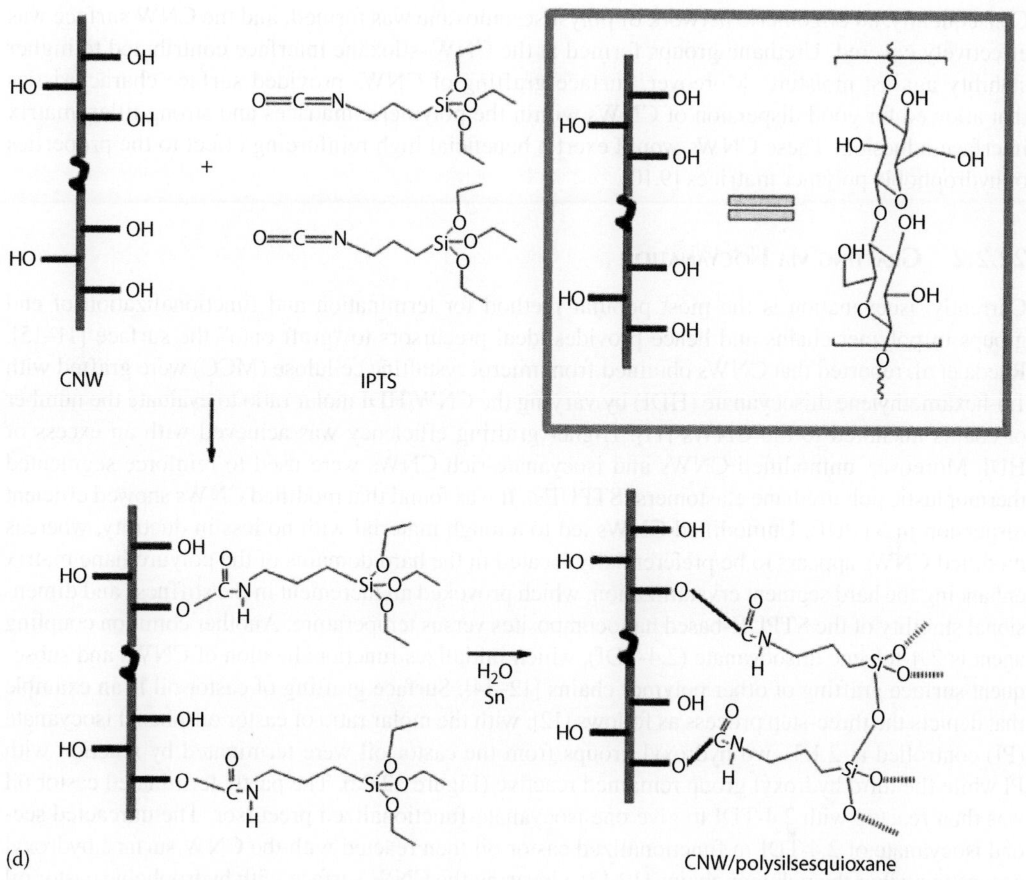

FIGURE 22.1 (Continued) (d) Proposed reaction between CNW surface and IPTS. (Reprinted from Goussé, C. et al., *Polymer*, 43, 2645, 2002; de Oliveira de Oliveira Taipina, M.O. et al., *Cellulose*, 20, 217, 2013. With permission.)

of alkyl dimethylchlorosilanes (alkyl-DMSiCl) with alkyl moieties of isopropyl (C3), *n*-butyl (C4), *n*-octyl (C8), and *n*-dodecyl (C12), respectively, were reacted with CNWs derived from tunicin. The surface of CNWs was only partially silylated and gave different degrees of surface substitution (DSs). Figure 22.1 shows TEM images of underivatized and partially silylated CNWs. It was found that the moderate extent of silylation kept the integrity and slender morphology of the CNWs, but they stuck together and swelled slightly thus showing a wavy contour. Furthermore, surface silylation also resulted in CNWs that were readily dispersible in low-polarity solvents such as THF. Suspensions of CNWs modified with isopropyl-DMSiCl in THF that had a *DS* of 0.4 appeared flocculated, while when the DS was 0.6, the suspension was in a stable/cloudy state. The solution with a DS of 0.6 was birefringent when observed between crossed polarizers, which indicated that the dispersibility of silylated CNWs increased as the DS of surface silylation increased [7]. It should be pointed out that when silylation conditions were too harsh, partial solubilization of CNWs and loss of nanostructure occurred. The nanocomposite films with silylated CNWs made by solution casting exhibited high water contact angles (117°–146°) ascribed to decreased surface energy and higher surface roughness after surface grafting [8]. de Oliveira Taipina et al. described a new approach for CNW-based polysilsesquioxane by surface grafting of CNWs with 3-isocyanatepropyltriethoxysilane (IPTS) [9] in which isocyanate groups were highly reactive to hydroxyl groups of CNWs through hydrolysis-condensation of ethoxysilane groups (Figure 22.1d).

Consequently, an oligomeric network of polysilsesquioxane was formed, and the CNW surface was effectively covered. Urethane groups formed at the CNW–siloxane interface contributed to higher stability against moisture. Moreover, surface grafting of CNWs provided surface characteristics that allowed for good dispersion of CNWs within the polymeric matrices and strong filler–matrix interface adhesion. These CNWs would exert a beneficial high reinforcing effect to the properties of hydrophobic polymer matrices [9,10].

22.2.2 Grafting via Isocyanation

Currently, isocyanation is the most popular method for termination and functionalization of end groups in polymer chains and hence provides ideal precursors to "graft onto" the surface [11–15]. Rueda et al. reported that CNWs obtained from microcrystalline cellulose (MCC) were grafted with 1,6-hexamethylene diisocyanate (HDI) by varying the CNW/HDI molar ratio to evaluate the number of chains anchored to the CNWs [11]. Higher grafting efficiency was achieved with an excess of HDI. Moreover, unmodified CNWs and isocyanate-rich CNWs were used to reinforce segmented thermoplastic polyurethane elastomers (STPUEs). It was found that modified CNWs showed efficient dispersion in STPUE. Unmodified CNWs led to a tough material with no loss in ductility, whereas modified CNWs appears to be preferentially located in the hard domains of the polyurethane matrix enhancing the hard segment crystallization, which provoked an increment in the stiffness and dimensional stability of the STPUE-based nanocomposites versus temperature. Another common coupling agent is 2,4-toluene diisocyanate (2,4-TDI), which initializes functionalization of CNWs and subsequent surface grafting of other polymer chains [12–14]. Surface grafting of castor oil is an example that depicts the three-step process as follows [12]: with the molar ratio of castor oil/phenyl isocyanate (PI) controlled at 2.1:3, two hydroxyl groups from the castor oil were terminated by reaction with PI while the third hydroxyl group remained reactive (Figure 22.2a). The partly terminated castor oil was then reacted with 2,4-TDI to give one isocyanate-functionalized precursor. The unreacted second isocyanate of 2,4-TDI in functionalized castor oil then reacted with the CNW surface hydroxyl groups to anchor the polymer chains [12,13]. Covering the CNW surface with hydrophobic castor oil resulted in a significant decrease in surface energy. The weight fraction of castor oil in the grafted CNWs was determined by elemental analysis to be 17.7 wt%. The change in surface energy after grafting contributed to a significant increase in the water contact angle (Figure 22.2b) and showed high dispersion stability in ethyl ether, toluene, acetone, DMF, and THF.

The concepts and method mentioned earlier have also been applied to surface grafting of polycaprolactone (PCL) [14] to CNWs. PCLs with molecular weights of 10,000 and 42,500 were grafted onto the CNW surface. The lower-molecular-weight PCL resulted in a higher grafting efficiency. The grafting process did not change the initial morphological integrity and native crystallinity, while the grafted PCL chains organized in a semicrystalline shell on the CNW surface. The shielding by hydrophobic PCL chains significantly increased the water contact angle for PCL-grafted CNWs, and the higher grafting efficiency contributed by the 10,000 molecular weight PCL resulted in the highest water contact angle value [14].

22.2.3 Grafting via Esterification

Esterification is an important reaction for the surface modification of CNWs with organic acid chloride or anhydride [16–20]. A series of organic acid chlorides with different aliphatic chains (C_6, C_{12}, and C_{18}) were grafted onto the surface of CNW in toluene using triethylamine as a catalyst [18]. The organic acid chloride was successfully anchored to hydroxyl groups on the CNW surface as proven by FTIR results. It was found that the initial crystalline structure of CNWs was retained after esterification and that a new ill-defined peak located at approximately 21° for the modified CNWs indicated that the aliphatic chains on the CNW surface tended to self-crystallize. In addition, surface coverage by large alkane chains was determined by x-ray photoelectron spectroscopy

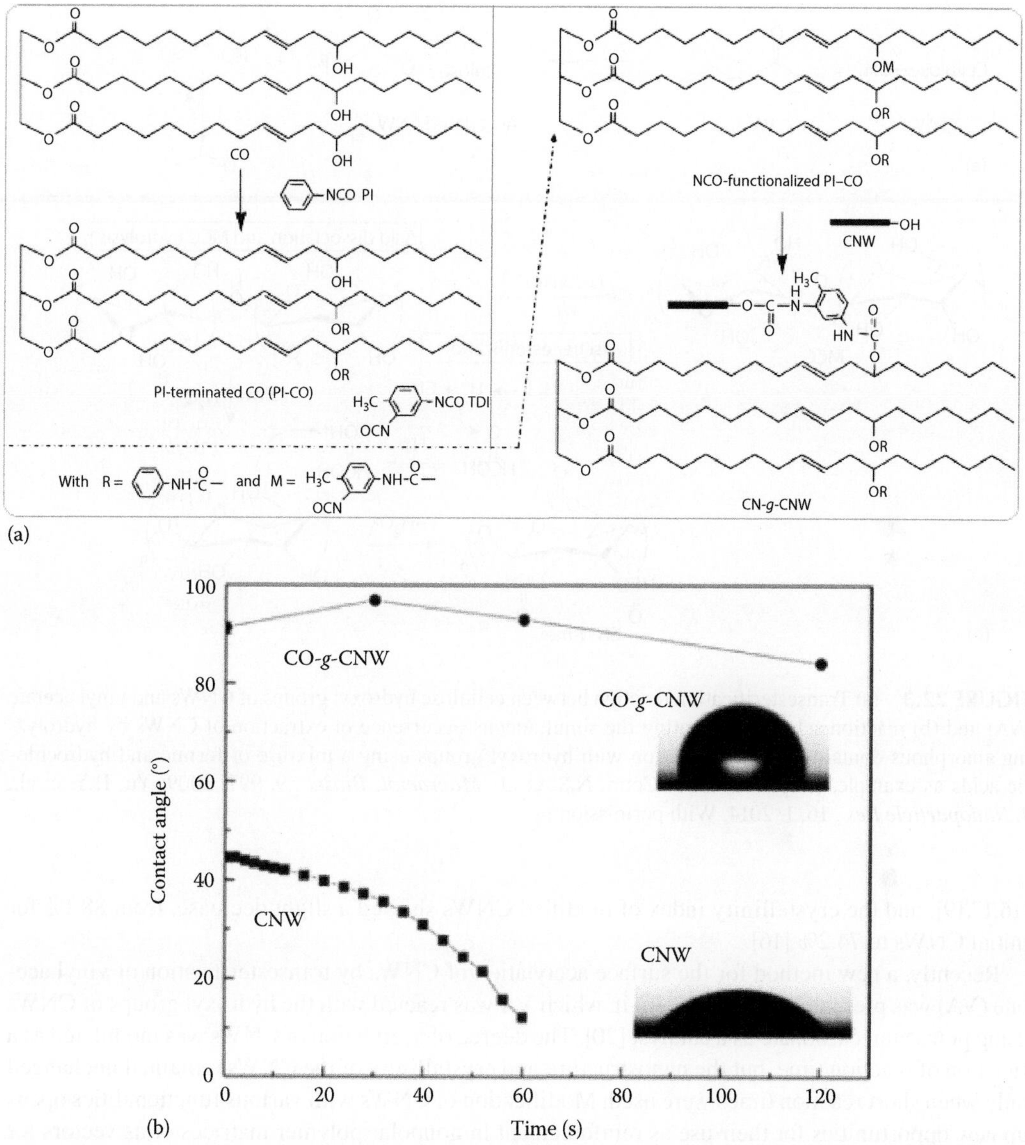

FIGURE 22.2 (a) Schematic illustration of the reaction process and (b) dependence of contact angle to water upon time for the CNW and castor oil-grafted CNW (CO-*g*-CNW) with photographs of a water drop on the surface of CNW and CO-*g*-CNW at the moment of depositing the drop. (Reprinted from Shang, W. et al., *Cellulose*, 20, 179, 2013. With permission.)

(XPS) to be 7.1, 17.6, and 23.0 for hexanoyl chloride, lauroyl chloride, and stearoyl chloride, respectively, showing an increasing tendency with an increase in the carbon number of the organic acid chloride. The DSs for hexanoyl chloride, lauroyl chloride, and stearoyl chloride were 0.68, 0.32, and 0.31, respectively. The water contact angle also increased due to the coverage of CNWs with hydrophobic aliphatic chains. Thus, after grafting aliphatic chains, the polar contribution to surface energy obviously declined, and there was a significant decrease in total surface energy [18]. Reacting CNW surface hydroxyl groups with acetic anhydride and alkenyl succinic anhydride also resulted in a significant decrease in the surface energy [16,17,19]. Furthermore, these chemical modifications had almost no effect on the rod-like morphology and crystalline structure of CNWs

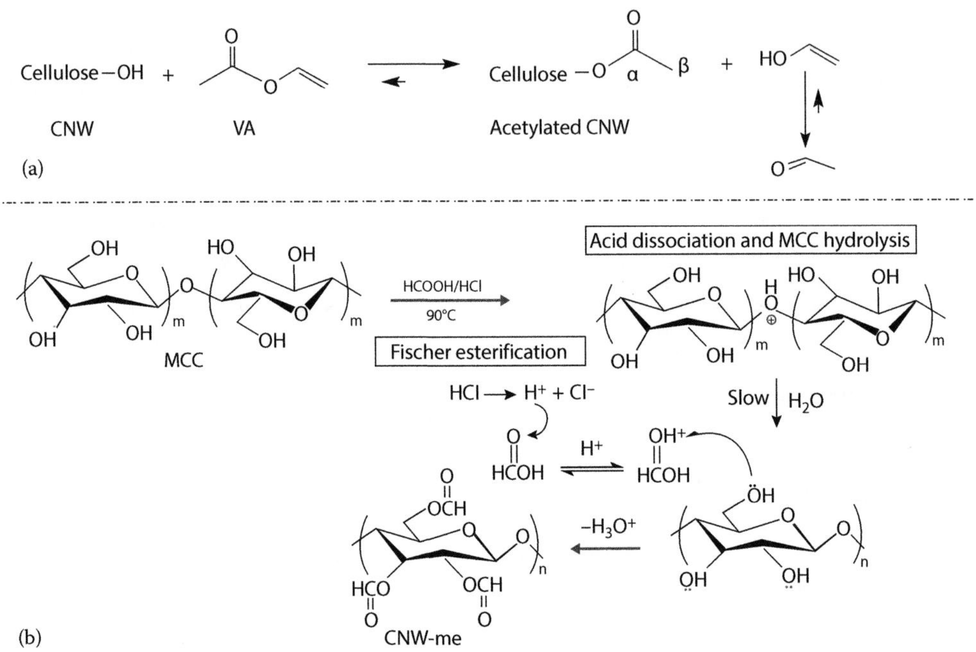

FIGURE 22.3 (a) Transesterification reaction between cellulose hydroxyl groups of CNWs and vinyl acetate (VA) and (b) reaction scheme illustrating the simultaneous occurrence of extraction of CNWs by hydrolyzing amorphous domains and esterification with hydroxyl groups using a mixture of formic and hydrochloric acids as example. (Reprinted from Cetin, N.S. et al., *Macromol. Biosci.*, 9, 997, 2009; Yu, H.Y. et al., *J. Nanoparticle Res.*, 16, 1, 2014. With permission.)

[16,17,19], and the crystallinity index of modified CNWs showed a slight decrease, from 88.1% for initial CNWs to 74.2% [16].

Recently, a new method for the surface acetylation of CNWs by transesterification of vinyl acetate (VA) was presented (Figure 22.3a) in which VA was reacted with the hydroxyl groups of CNWs using potassium carbonate as a catalyst [20]. The degree of acetylation of CNWs was modulated as a function of reaction time, but the nanostructure and crystallinity of the CNWs remained unchanged only when short reaction times were used. Modification of CNWs with various functionalities opens up new opportunities for their use as reinforcement in nonpolar polymer matrices or as vectors for the improvement of optical, electronic, or selective permeation properties [20].

Fischer esterification of hydroxyl groups simultaneous with the hydrolysis of amorphous cellulose chains using organic acids (such as formic, acetic and butyric acid) mixed with hydrochloric acid to extract CNWs has become a viable one-pot reaction methodology that allows isolation of functionalized CNWs in a single-step process [21,22]. Figure 22.3b schematically illustrates the reaction during extraction and esterification of CNWs using a mixture of formic and hydrochloric acids. The hydronium ions of hydrochloric acid dissociation digest amorphous cellulose regions and catalyze the esterification of hydroxyl groups on the exposed cellulose chains to obtain modified CNWs (CNW-me) with many ester groups. Moreover, the crystallinity and thermal stability of the modified CNWs were improved as compared to neat MCC. In addition, modified CNWs prepared by mixed acetic and hydrochloric acid hydrolysis showed no change in thermal stability, and their onset of degradation remained at around 300°C. Moreover, these modified CNWs had increased hydrophobicity and good dispersion in many organic solvents. Consequently, this simultaneous extraction and functionalization method can provide surface-functionalized CNWs that are compatible with a hydrophobic matrix and suitable for thermoprocessing [21,22].

Recently, long chain aliphatics were grafted onto CNWs by heterogeneous esterification with hexanoyl chloride (C6), lauroyl chloride (C12), and stearoyl chloride (C18) [23] and by gas-phase esterification with palmitoyl chloride (C16) [24]. Modified CNWs were found to be hydrophobic and thus dispersed in nonpolar solvents. It should be pointed out that preconditioning of dry CNWs into aerogels was required (so more surface was accessible to palmitoyl chloride vapors) prior to gas-phase palmitoylation. Thus, the modified CNWs exhibited high DS values, high viscosity, and no birefringence in a stirred toluene suspension [24].

22.2.4 Grafting via Click Chemistry

Click chemistry is a new method that has been used for surface grafting of amine-terminated monomers onto CNWs to obtain nanomaterials with novel and stimuli-responsive characteristics [25–27]. Filpponen et al. and Sadeghifar et al. synthesized novel nanoplatelet gel-like nanomaterials using CNWs as the starting material [25,26]. The surface modification contained three steps, as follows: hydroxyl groups on the CNW surfaces were selectively activated to convert them to carboxylic groups by 2,2,6,6-tetramethyl-1-piperidinyloxy (TEMPO)-mediated hypohalite oxidation. Terminal amine functionalities of molecules were then grafted on TEMPO-oxidized CNWs, which were used to prepare surface-functionalized CNWs with terminal alkyne or azide functionalities as essential precursors. Finally, they were brought together via click chemistry to obtain unique nanoplatelet gels. Pahimanolis et al. prepared terminal azide-functionalized CNWs via etherification of 1-azido-2,3-epoxypropane in NaOH water/isopropanol at ambient temperature, avoiding the TEMPO-mediated hypohalite oxidation. The azide groups in CNWs were reacted with propargylamine and 5-(dimethylamino)-*N*-(2-propyl)-1-naphthalenesulfonamide using copper-catalyzed azide–alkyne cycloaddition (CuAAC) (Figure 22.3), yielding pH-responsive 1,2,3-triazole-4-methanamine-decorated CNWs and highly fluorescent CNWs, respectively [27] (Figure 22.4).

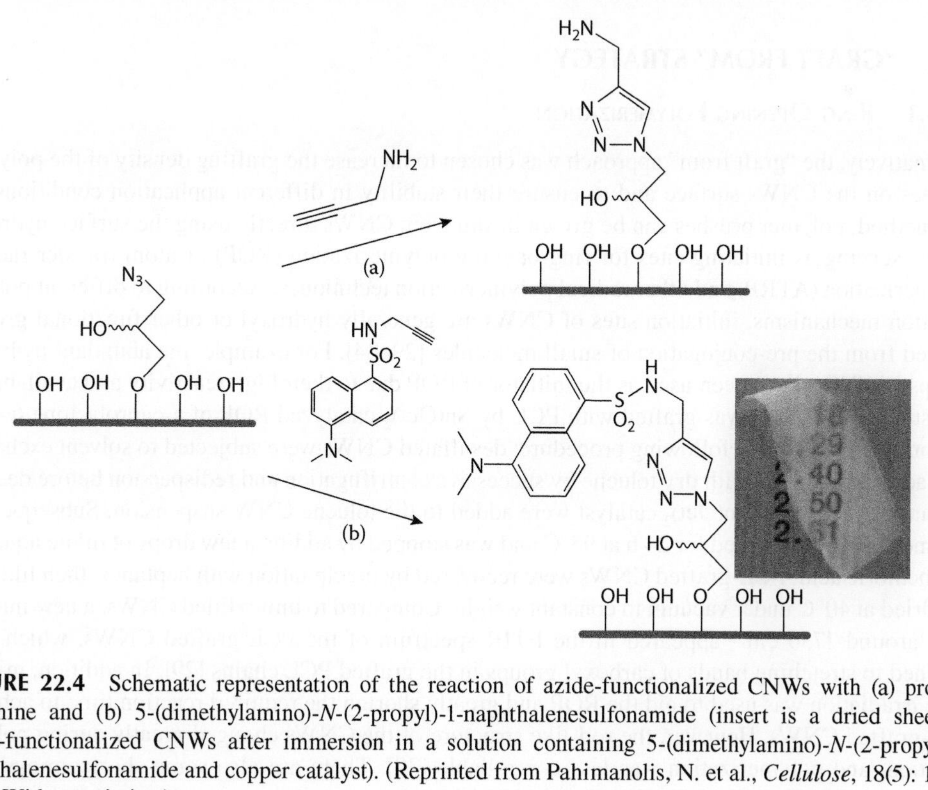

FIGURE 22.4 Schematic representation of the reaction of azide-functionalized CNWs with (a) propargylamine and (b) 5-(dimethylamino)-*N*-(2-propyl)-1-naphthalenesulfonamide (insert is a dried sheet of azide-functionalized CNWs after immersion in a solution containing 5-(dimethylamino)-*N*-(2-propyl)-1-naphthalenesulfonamide and copper catalyst). (Reprinted from Pahimanolis, N. et al., *Cellulose*, 18(5): 1201, 2011. With permission.)

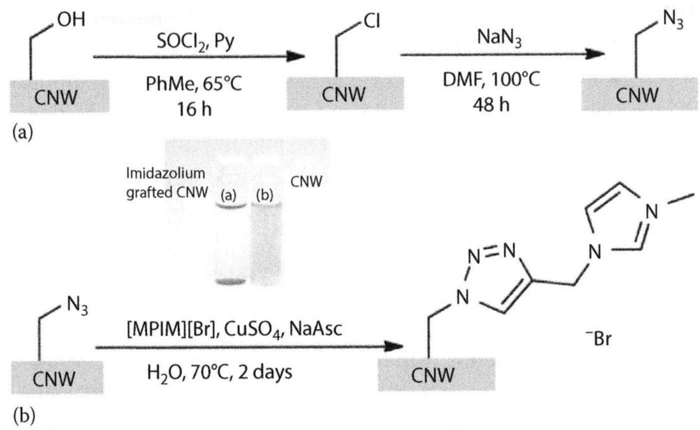

FIGURE 22.5 (a) Synthetic route for azidation of CNWs. (b) Grafting [MPIM][Br] on the CNWs using heterogeneous click chemistry (photo showing adsorption of Orange II dye by (a) the modified CNWs and (b) CNWs). (Reprinted from Eyley, S. and Thielemans, W., *Chem. Commun.*, 47, 4177, 2011. With permission.)

It is believed that successful grafting of azide groups onto CNWs is a prerequisite to perform the azide–alkyne cycloaddition "click" reaction. Eyley and Thielemans synthesized ionic liquid 1-methyl-3-propargylimidazolium bromide ([MPIM][Br])-*graft*-azido CNWs in an aqueous solution via "click" chemistry using copper sulfate as a pre-catalyst and sodium ascorbate as a reductant (Figure 22.5). It was demonstrated that modified CNWs were successfully exchanged for bistriflimide and an anionic dye, which provided an opportunity for the synthesis of a wide variety of ion exchange systems or catalysts using CNWs as a support material [28].

22.3 "GRAFT FROM" STRATEGY

22.3.1 Ring-Opening Polymerization

Alternatively, the "graft from" approach was chosen to increase the grafting density of the polymer brushes on the CNWs surface and to ensure their stability in different application conditions. In this method, polymer brushes can be grown in situ from CNWs directly using the surface hydroxyl groups serving as initiating sites for ring-opening polymerization (ROP) or atom transfer radical polymerization (ATRP) and other radical polymerization techniques. According to different polymerization mechanisms, initiation sites of CNWs are generally hydroxyl or other functional groups derived from the pre-conjugation of small molecules [29–34]. For example, the abundant hydroxyl groups of CNWs have been used as the initiator of ROP due to their high reactivity and availability. The surface of CNWs was grafted with PCL by $Sn(Oct)_2$-catalyzed ROP of ε-caprolactone (ε-CL) monomer [29] using the following procedure: desulfated CNWs were subjected to solvent exchange with acetone and then with dry toluene by successive centrifugation and redispersion before desired amounts of ε-CL and $Sn(Oct)_2$ catalyst were added to the toluene CNW suspension. Subsequently, polymerization proceeded for 24 h at 95°C and was stopped by adding a few drops of dilute aqueous hydrochloric acid. PCL-grafted CNWs were recovered by precipitation with heptanes, then filtered, and dried at 40°C under vacuum to constant weight. Compared to unmodified CNWs, a new intense peak around 1730 cm^{-1} appeared in the FTIR spectrum of the PCL-grafted CNWs, which was assigned to stretching bands of carboxyl groups in the grafted PCL chains [29]. In addition, microwave irradiation was used to aid the ROP and greatly shorten the required reaction time to achieve PCL-grafted CNWs. However, the rod-like structure of the CNWs changed greatly during polymerization, and polymerization was less controllable [30]. There are also some shortcomings that restrict the reproducibility of ROP. Labet and Thielemans reported that many low-molecular-weight organic compounds were adsorbed on the surface of fresh CNWs prepared by acid hydrolysis [33]. They found that Soxhlet extraction with different solvents (dichloromethane, ethanol, ethyl acetate, heptane, methanol, isopropanol) could remove these adsorbed species of freeze-dried CNWs, and the effect of these extractions on the chemical structure and surface composition of the CNWs was investigated by FTIR, elemental analysis, and XPS. It was found that Soxhlet extraction with ethanol before reaction was the most effective way to remove adsorbed low-molecular-weight organic compounds, leading to improved reproducibility between reactions using CNWs from different batches. In addition, the resulting PCL-grafted CNWs made good reinforcing agents for bionanocomposites due to their improved dispersibility in organic solvent or the PCL matrix [34]. It was also found that PCL-grafted CNWs had better mechanical strength in comparison to ungrafted CNWs. The PCL graft chain length played an important role in the mechanical properties, and the strongest bionanocomposites were achieved after reinforcement by CNWs grafted with chains of the longest length.

The process for grafting polymer chains onto the surface of CNWs was as follows: CNWs were prepared by acid hydrolysis of MCC or other raw materials and modified by ROP of L-lactide, initiated from the active hydroxyl groups of the CNWs [31,32]. Graft effectiveness was determined by the presence of the C=O peak in the FTIR spectra of modified CNWs and evidenced by the long-term stability of a suspension of poly(lactic acid) (PLA)-grafted CNWs in chloroform. Moreover, the rod-like shape was maintained after modification, and the modified CNWs showed good dispersion in many nonpolar solvents. Therefore, "grafting from" CNWs with L-lactide is a very promising way to achieve good dispersion of CNWs within hydrophobic polymer matrices, which inevitably contributes to the enhanced/improved properties of the resultant bionanocomposites. Novel CNW-*graft*-PCL-block-PLA graft-block copolymers have been prepared using sequential ROP of ε-CL and L-lactide (L-LA) [35]. The thus-modified CNWs are interesting/useful nanofillers (due to their related microstructures) in PCL- or PLA-based nanocomposites.

22.3.2 Radical Polymerization

Surface grafting of CNWs with polymer chains or monomers via "graft onto" and ROP methods are generally performed in organic media where tedious and time-consuming solvent exchange processes are required. CNWs are often partially agglomerated, and grafting density and graft chain length are difficult to control. It is difficult for "graft onto" methods to diffuse the grafted polymer chains through the grafted "brushes" to reach the reactive sites due to steric hindrance between the long graft chains, and as a result, grafting density is low. Recently, radical polymerization as a method for novel surface modification of CNWs has attracted attention [36–44]. Acrylic monomers and poly (4-vinylpyridine) were grafted on the surface of CNWs in an aqueous medium by a redox-initiated free radical copolymerization method with cerium ammonium nitrate (CAN) as initiator [36,37]. The reaction began via a ceric–cerous redox reaction as the cerium ion chelated with two adjacent hydroxyl groups in a cellulose chain, resulting in radical formation on an opened glucose ring. The radical then reacted with carbon–carbon double bonds to form CNW graft copolymers (Figure 22.6a). After surface modification, the nanostructure of the cellulose was preserved, and the hydrophilic/hydrophobic properties of the modified CNWs could be modulated by different grafted polymer chains [36,37]. Kan et al. synthesized novel pH-responsive nanocomposites by surface-initiated graft polymerization of 4-vinylpyridine on the CNW surface with the initiator ceric (IV) ammonium nitrate [37].

It is well known that ATRP has been used extensively as a versatile technique for the synthesis of well-defined polymers with novel macromolecular structures. ATRP has also been used to synthesize graft copolymers with controllable graft length and composition [38–44]. Generally, ATRP has many advantages including simplicity, cost, and robustness [39,40]. Inexpensive copper-mediated surface-initiated ATRP (SI-ATRP) is considered to be one of the most efficient ways to "graft from" polymer chains or brushes exhibiting high grafting density and low polydispersity [40].

Before surface grafting polymer chains on CNWs via ATRP, the hydroxyl groups on CNWs were esterified with 2-bromoisobutyryl bromide using pyridine and 4-dimethylaminopyridine as catalysts to yield 2-bromoisobutyryloxy groups (Figure 22.6b). The initiator-modified CNW is an essential precursor for ATRP-initiated polymerization of polymers such as poly(acrylic acid) (PAA) [38], poly(styrene) (PS) [39,42], poly(*N*-isopropylacrylamide) [40], poly(6-[4-(4-methoxyphenylazo) phenoxy]hexyl methacrylate) (PMMAZO) [41], and poly(*N*,*N*-dimethylaminoethyl methacrylate) (PDMAEMA) [43]. Majoinen et al. reported that pH-responsive hybrid nanoparticles consisting of crystalline CNWs tethered with PAA polyelectrolyte brushes were successfully prepared by SI-ATRP, as shown in Figure 22.6b [38]. Individually dispersed rod-like nanoparticles with PAA brushes were clearly observed, despite high grafting densities (0.3 chains/nm^2) and dense polymer brush formation on the CNWs. Yi et al. used the SI-ATRP technique to graft PS, PMMAZO, and PDMAEMA chains on the CNW surface and investigated the liquid crystalline phase behavior of CNW-based copolymers [41–43]; however, the effects of reaction conditions were not studied in detail. The influence of grafting conditions on the control of graft density of PS brushes on CNWs using excess initiator was presented by Morandi et al. [39]. Freeze-dried CNWs were used as the raw material for the preparation of the initiator-modified CNW precursor, although it was well known that dry CNWs often aggregate and thus surface modification of CNWs was limited.

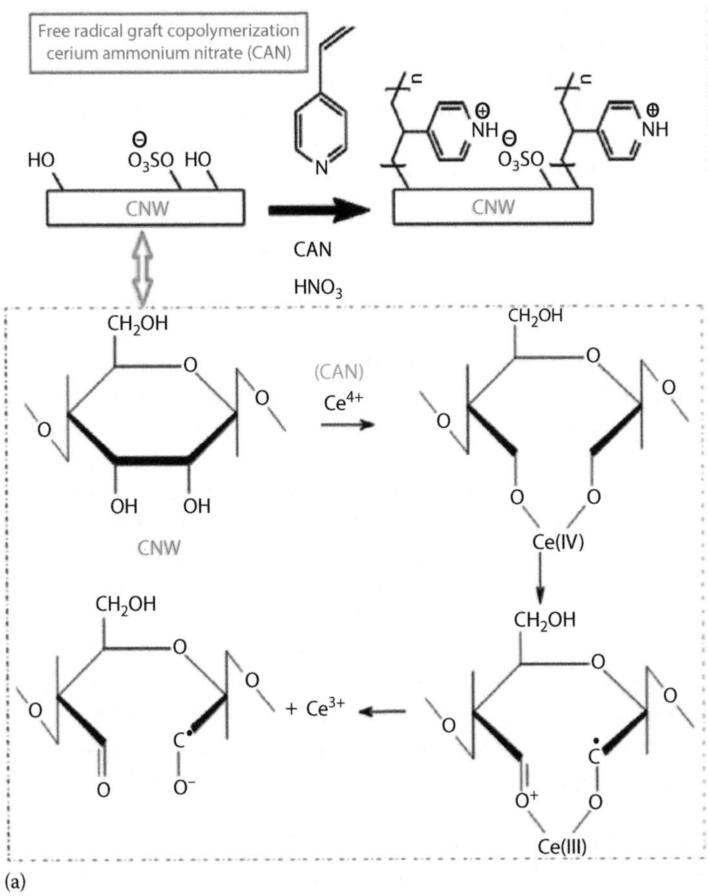

FIGURE 22.6 (a) Graft polymerization of poly(4-vinylpyridine) with CAN initiator from the surface of sulfuric acid–hydrolyzed CNWs, and the generally accepted mechanism for the formation of a radical site on cellulose through ceric ion reduction. (*Continued*)

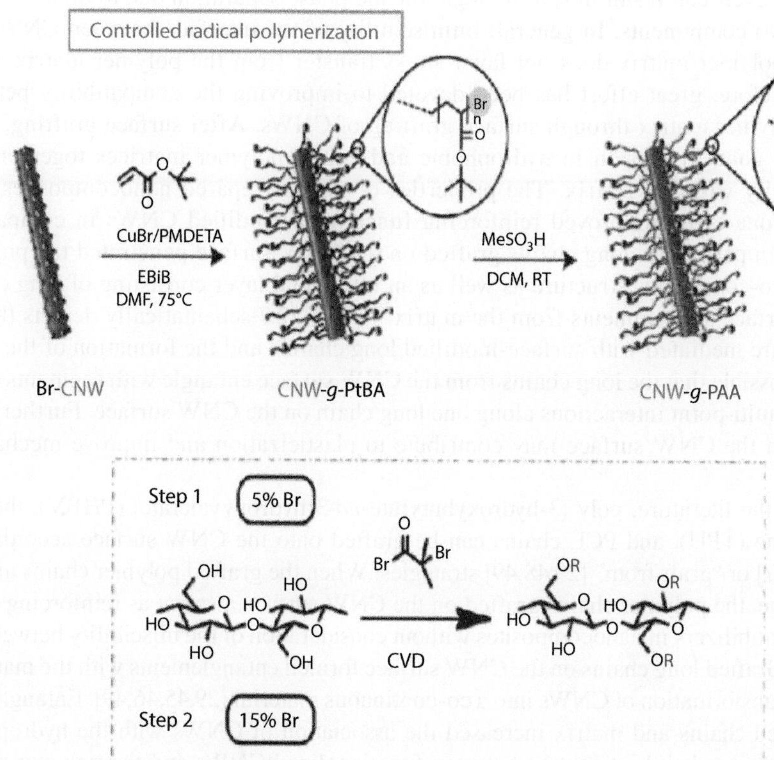

FIGURE 22.6 (Continued) (b) Reaction scheme for Cu-mediated ATRP of tBA, followed by acid hydrolysis of the tertiary alkyl functionality to yield PAA brushes grafted from the CNW surface. (Reprinted from Labet, M. and Thielemans, W., *Cellulose*, 18, 607, 2011; Majoinen, J. et al., *Biomacromolecules*, 12, 2997, 2011. With permission.)

Zoppe et al. provided a new method for grafting from never-dried CNWs with SI-ATRP in which a solvent exchange process was employed to redisperse CNWs in dry THF using successive centrifugation [40]. It was found that increased initiator or monomer loading led to increased molecular mass of polymer brushes. This could be ascribed to local heterogeneities shifting the SI-ATRP equilibrium to the active state. This work also provided the basis for preparation of temperature-responsive materials based on CNWs as the matrix.

22.4 SURFACE GRAFTING FOR NANOCOMPOSITES

22.4.1 Improving Miscibility with Polymer Matrix

The reinforcing effect of CNWs in nanocomposites depends mainly on good dispersion and interfacial interaction (hydrogen bonding) that originate from good compatibility between CNWs and the polymer matrix. It is well known that hydrogen bonding among unmodified CNWs together

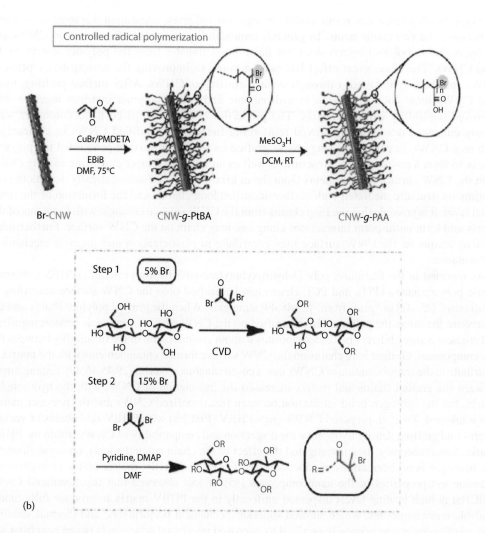

with high loading levels can result in self-aggregation and phase separation due to poor miscibility between the two components. In general, immiscibility of the interface between CNWs and the hydrophobic polymer matrix does not favor stress transfer from the polymer matrix to the rigid CNWs. Therefore, great effort has been devoted to improving the compatibility between CNWs and the polymer matrix through surface grafting of CNWs. After surface grafting, modified CNWs show good dispersion in hydrophobic and apolar polymer matrices together with improved miscibility with the matrix. The properties of the as-prepared nanocomposites were greatly enhanced due to the improved reinforcing function of modified CNWs in comparison with neat CNWs. In particular, long chains grafted on the CNW surface penetrated the polymer matrix to form a co-continuous structure as well as an interfacial layer consisting of long chains from the CNW surface and segments from the matrix. Figure 22.7 schematically depicts the co-continuous structure mediated with surface-modified long chains, and the formation of the interfacial layer. It is possible that the long chains from the CNW surface entangle with segments of the matrix and form multi-point interactions along one long chain on the CNW surface. Furthermore, the long chains on the CNW surface may contribute to plasticization and improve mechanical performance.

As reported in the literature, poly (3-hydroxybutyrate-*co*-3-hydroxyvalerate) (PHBV), thermoplastic polyurethane (TPU), and PCL chains can be grafted onto the CNW surface according to "graft onto" [45–47] or "graft from" [29,48,49] strategies. When the grafted polymer chains and the matrix are the same, the polymer chains grafted on the CNW surface also act as reinforcing fillers and efficient compatibilizers in nanocomposites without consideration of the miscibility between the two components. Grafted long chains on the CNW surface formed entanglements with the matrix to contribute to the transformation of CNWs into a co-continuous material [29,45,46,49]. Entanglement between the grafted chains and matrix increased the association of CNWs with the hydrophobic matrix, but the hydrogen bond interaction between functionalized CNWs and the polymer matrix was weakened. Yu et al. prepared CNWs-*graft*-PHBV (PHCNs) with PHBV side chains of various lengths and grafting density to improve the dispersion and compatibility of CNWs within the PHBV matrix. Simultaneously, they investigated the effect of the chain entanglements, co-crystallization, and hydrogen bond interactions of functionalized CNWs and PHBV matrix on the crystallization behavior and properties of the nanocomposites [45]. It was observed that functionalized CNWs (PHCNs) at high loading levels dispersed uniformly in the PHBV matrix to produce fully biodegradable nanocomposites, which showed superior mechanical performance and thermal stability. This reinforcement was primarily ascribed to improved interfacial adhesion between nanofiller and

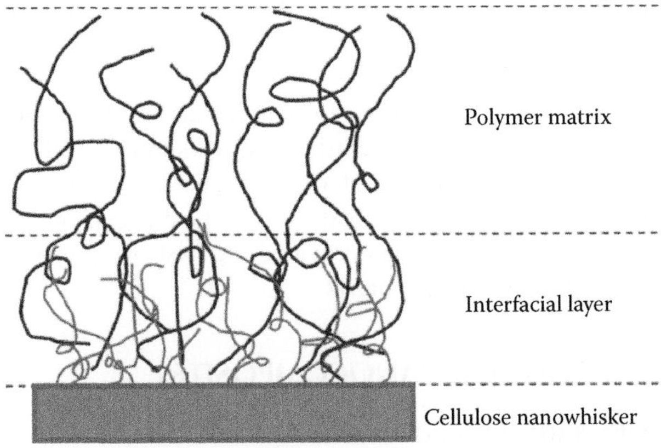

FIGURE 22.7 Schematic diagram of co-continuous structure mediated with surface-modified long chains and the formation of an interfacial layer between long chain–modified CNWs and the polymer matrix (black line: matrix segments; gray line: long chains grafted on the CNW surface).

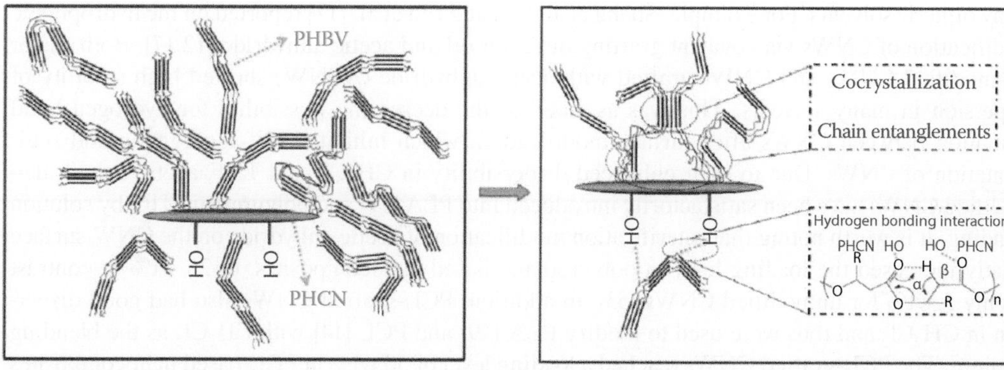

FIGURE 22.8 Sketch for the formation of hydrogen bond interactions and the evolution of polymer aggregate structure and crystal structure in PHBV/modified CNW (PHCN) nanocomposites. (Reprinted from Yu, H.Y. et al., *ACS Sustain. Chem. Eng.*, 2, 875, 2014. With permission.)

matrix due to chain entanglements, co-crystallization, and hydrogen bond interactions between the hydroxyl groups of PHCNs and the carboxyl groups of PHBV (Figure 22.8). In addition, the nanocomposites were nontoxic to human MG-63 cells and showed great potential in bioplastic and biomedical materials. Based on the same reinforcing mechanism, TPU chains were covalently grafted onto CNWs by particular association with hard segments [46]. Due to covalent attachment of TPU molecules to the stiff surface of CNWs and the web-like structure, pullout of CNWs from the TPU matrix required more energy even at a low content, which contributed to better mechanical properties. Also, the network structure of CNWs with a large aspect ratio can slow the propagation speed of cracks during tensile fracture.

Another strategy has been used to develop co-continuous nanocomposites by in situ formation of a chemical linkage between the matrix segments and the CNW surface with grafted polymer chains. For example, in nanocomposites of waterborne polyurethane (WPU) with PCL soft segments and CNWs, segments of the WPU matrix were grafted in situ on the CNW surface through a reaction between isocyanate and hydroxyl groups. The PCL segments in grafted WPU chains were able to form a crystalline structure on the CNW surface and thus induced co-crystallization with the PCL segments in the WPU matrix to construct a co-continuous structure due to improved miscibility. The formation of a co-continuous structure allowed for good dispersion of the CNWs and strong interfacial adhesion between the CNWs and matrix. Moreover, this co-continuous structure acted as a network fulcrum point to transfer stress evenly to other WPU chains and rigid CNWs, enhancing the mechanical properties of the nanocomposites [47]. In conclusion, affinity between the grafted chains and matrix segments is a prerequisite for enhancing compatibilization and thus mechanical properties of the resulting nanocomposites [45–49].

22.4.2 Enhancing Processability of Nanocomposites

Good dispersion of CNWs within the polymer matrix is a prerequisite for obtaining high-performance nanocomposites [50–52]. And in solution blending, good dispersion of CNWs in aqueous or organic solvent blending media was essential. Because of the hydrophilic character of CNWs, they homogenously disperse in water and are thus usually used to reinforce hydrophilic polymers; however, most polymers are hydrophobic. Surface coating amphiphilic compounds on CNWs reduces surface energy and promotes dispersion in organic solvents in which unmodified CNWs tend to sediment [52]; however, this physical interaction can be cleaved by highly polar solvent or be affected by solidification of the blending solution [16]. Surface grafting of CNWs with small molecules and polymer chains is considered to be a useful method for achieving high dispersibility in many organic solvents. For example, Shang et al. [12] and Lin et al. [17] reported on the hydrophobic modification of CNWs via covalent grafting of castor oil and acetic anhydride [12,17]. Both castor oil–modified CNWs and CNWs grafted with acetic anhydride (ACNW) showed high stability of dispersion in many solvents. This was ascribed to the decreasing possibility for hydrogen bond formation between CNWs after surface modification, which inhibited self-aggregation and sedimentation of CNWs. Due to their enhanced dispersibility in CH_2Cl_2 and THF, acetic anhydride–modified CNWs have been satisfactorily introduced into PLA [17] and polyurethane [16] by solution blending. It is worth noting that esterification modification of acetic anhydride on the CNW surface greatly increased the loading level in polyurethane-based nanocomposites, to 25 wt% in contrast to only 5 wt% for unmodified CNWs [53]. In addition, PCL-grafted CNWs also had good dispersion in CH_2Cl_2 and thus were used to modify PLA [49] and PCL [14] with CH_2Cl_2 as the blending medium. The PCL-grafted CNWs reached a loading level of 50 wt% in PCL-based nanocomposites in contrast to a 30 wt% loading level for ungrafted CNWs. Moreover, PCL-based nanocomposites filled with PCL-grafted CNWs showed better mechanical performance than those filled with ungrafted CNWs. Figure 22.9 shows PHBV nanocomposites with CNWs (unmodified or modified) using different solution casting procedures. It was found that agglomeration of CNWs occurred in the PHBV matrix when 4.6 wt% unmodified CNWs was introduced during direct solution casting [54]. Use of polyethylene glycol (PEG) as a compatibilizer [55] or combining a solvent exchange

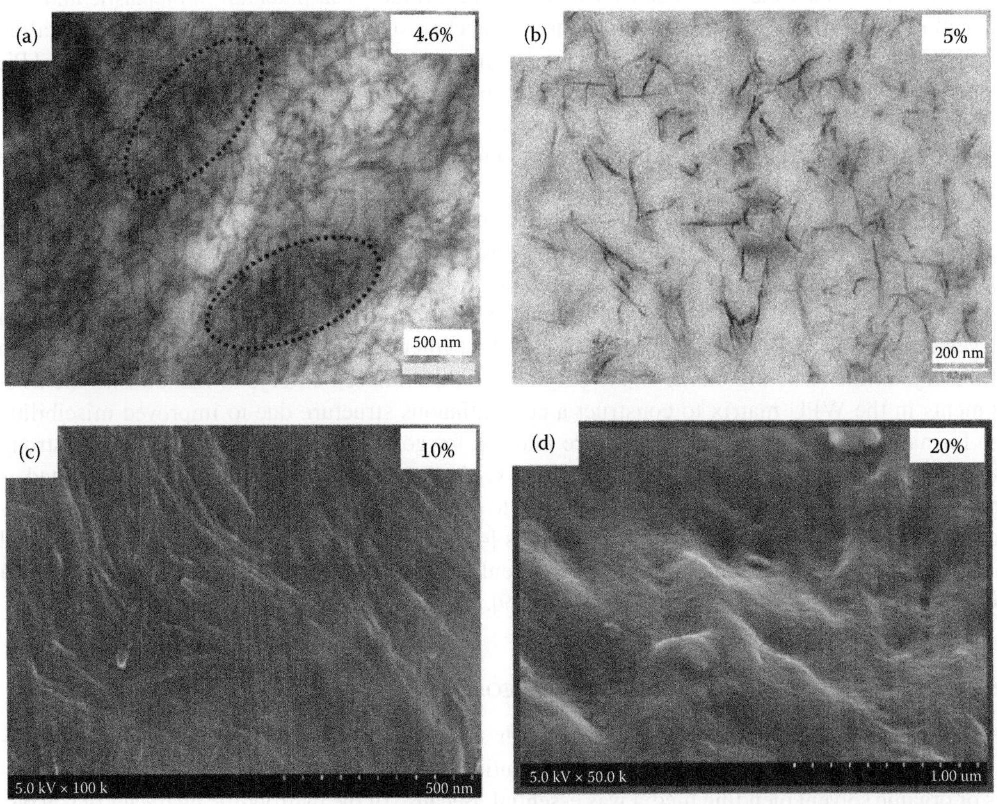

FIGURE 22.9 TEM images of (a) PHBV/unmodified CNW nanocomposites prepared by direct solution casting and (b) solution casting with a compatibilizer. FE-SEM images of fracture morphology of (c) PHBV/unmodified CNW nanocomposites produced by solution casting combined with solvent exchange and (d) PHBV/modified CNW nanocomposites produced by direct solution casting. (Reprinted from Yu, H.Y. et al., *ACS Sustain. Chem. Eng.*, 2, 875, 2014; Yu, H.Y. et al., *Carbohydr. Polym.*, 89, 971, 2012; Ten, E. et al., *Ind. Eng. Chem. Res.*, 51, 2941, 2012; Ten, E. et al., *Polymer*, 51, 2652, 2010. With permission.)

procedure [51] during fabrication of the nanocomposite improved the dispersion of CNWs in the PHBV matrix. Once the dosage of CNWs exceeded 5 wt%, agglomeration of CNWs inevitably occurred. When PHBV-grafted CNWs were incorporated into a PHBV matrix, even high loading levels (i.e., 20 wt%) of the modified CNWs dispersed well, significantly improving the mechanical and thermal stability [45]. In essence, the addition of thus-modified CNWs could enhance processability of nanocomposites.

Large-scale manufacturing and wider application of CNW-filled nanocomposites prepared using thermoprocessing methods is expected to be realized soon. However, CNWs prepared through conventional sulfuric acid hydrolysis present not only poor miscibility with the hydrophobic polymer matrix, but also low thermal stability, thereby preventing the application of thermoprocessing technologies in the production of CNW-filled nanocomposites [56,60]. It has been proven that small amounts of sulfate groups cause a considerable decrease in the degradation temperatures of CNWs. Generally, those sulfate groups induced the rapid degradation of CNWs at 180°C, but neutralization by aqueous NaOH greatly enhanced the thermal stability of CNWs [57]. Therefore, an alternative method using hydrochloric acid instead of sulfuric acid can be used to extract CNWs from raw cellulose materials, which avoids the formation of sulfate groups on the CNW surface as the factor causing thermal instability. Using HCl hydrolysis, the as-prepared CNWs have an obvious tendency toward aggregation and do not favor dispersion and distribution in the matrix [57]. Although physical modification of the CNW surface with homopolymers as compatibilizer and amphiphilic surfactants is beneficial for enhancing thermal stability and compatibility with the hydrophobic matrix, these effects usually fail under the shear of thermoprocessing due to cleavage of the association between CNWs and the modified species. Furthermore, excess strong affinity between the matrix and the species used in physical modification may destroy the association between the CNW and modified species, while immiscibility between the matrix and the physically modified species on the CNW surface may form separate phases assigned to the matrix and modified species [58,59]. Therefore, surface grafting of CNWs has been considered to be a good way to enhance thermal stability by shielding sulfate groups and simultaneously improving miscibility with the matrix and dispersion in the matrix.

Surface grafting of CNWs with the silane coupling agent stearoyl chloride and long chain polymers showed improved thermal stability and miscibility with the matrix when introduced to the polymer matrix via melt processing [18,31,60]. For example, PLA-grafted [31] and PCL-grafted [60] CNWs were melt-compounded with the corresponding PCL and PLA matrices using extrusion technology. Polymer grafting enhanced the thermal stability of the CNWs and hence matched the temperature of the extrusion process. It was observed that PLA-grafted CNWs eliminated the dark color resulting from thermal degradation of CNWs, and the resultant nanocomposites appeared colorless and transparent [31]. The enhanced thermal stability was ascribed to the protection of grafted PLA and its mediated entanglement with the matrix, like a shell for the sulfate groups on the CNW surface [31]. In these two nanocomposite systems, improved miscibility between the CNWs and matrix depended not only on the affinity of the molecular structure of the grafted chain and matrix, but also on entanglement with the matrix and formation of a physical chain network between these grafted long chains, which was absent in systems containing CNWs modified by small molecules and short chains. The effects of the co-continuous structure induced by grafted long chains will be discussed in a later section. In addition to the reinforcing effect, polymer-grafted CNWs could act as plasticization and nucleation agents to facilitate crystallization of the nanocomposites [31].

The cooperative effect of physical and chemical modification of CNWs has been verified to be very predominant for compatibilization with the hydrophobic matrix and enhanced thermal stability [61]. A series of surface-modified CNWs involving PEO-attaching, PEG-grafting, and a combination of the two were prepared. It was observed that modification by both PEO-attaching and PEG-grafting showed the highest thermal stability and the highest contact angle. Furthermore, PEG-grafted CNWs displayed a roughly two times higher PEO-adsorbing capability than pristine CNW due to the possibility of entanglement formation between grafted PEG chains and attached

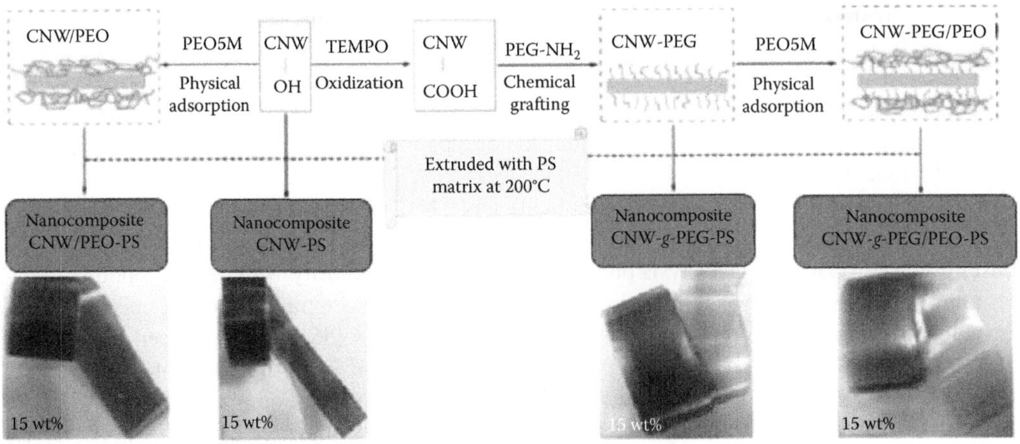

FIGURE 22.10 Schematic illustration of physical attaching and/or chemical grafting of the CNW surface with PEO and PEG, respectively, and photographs of the corresponding PS-based nanocomposites containing 15 wt% pristine or modified CNWs. (Reprinted from Lin, N. and Dufresne, A., *Macromolecules*, 46, 5570, 2013. With permission.)

PEO chains. These surface-modified CNWs were respectively melt-compounded with PS by twin-screw extrusion at 200°C. As shown in Figure 22.10, in contrast with the dark PS filled with pristine CNWs, the PS filled with modified CNWs was transparent due to enhanced thermal stability of the surface physical/chemical modification and cooperation between surface grafting and subsequent attaching that gave optimal light transmittance. This indicated that surface physical/chemical modification resulted in the matching of thermal stability to thermoprocessing temperature. Moreover, surface modification contributed to good dispersion of CNWs in the matrix and to compatibility with the hydrophobic PS matrix; hence, mechanical reinforcement and improved barrier properties were achieved. A combination of surface grafting and subsequent attaching showed optimal effects [61].

22.4.3 Developing Functional Materials

Recently, new diversified functional nanomaterials based on CNWs have been developed through a facile grafting reaction between terminal OH groups on the CNW surface and special functional groups of polymers. Dong and Roman reported that fluorescent modification of CNWs was carried out using a three-step reaction to covalently graft fluorescent molecules to the surface of CNWs. Fluorescently labeled cellulose nanocrystals were studied by using fluorescence techniques (such as spectrofluorometry, fluorescence microscopy, and flow cytometry), for example, the interaction of cellulose nanocrystals with cells and the biodistribution of CNWs in vivo [62]. Nielsen et al. developed novel sensing nanomaterials using two versatile synthetic strategies for dual fluorescent labeling of CNWs (one reaction with the isothiocyanates and the other with the thiol–ene click reaction). The dual fluorescent labeling of modified CNWs was effectively sensitive to pH change, showing great potential in biosensors [63]. Edwards et al. synthesized peptide-conjugated CNWs through covalent grafting of *n*-succinyl-alanine–alanine-valine-paranitroanilide (Suc-Ala–Ala-Val-pNA) onto glycine-esterified CNWs, which can be used as human neutrophil elastase biosensors [64].

Yu et al. prepared CNWs/silver (Ag) nanocomposites by formic acid/hydrochloric acid hydrolysis of commercial MCC and redox reaction with silver ammonia aqueous solution ($Ag(NH_3)_2(OH)$) in a one-pot green synthesis. This CNW/Ag nanocomposite was incorporated into PHBV and PLA as a bifunctional nanofiller to produce multifunctional packaging materials with improved thermal stability, mechanical properties, and antibacterial activity [21].

Hasani et al. found that thixotropic hydrogels formed in CNW suspensions after surface functionalization where epoxypropyltrimethylammonium chloride was reacted with CNWs. The cationic functionalization process reversed the surface charge and led to a reduction in the total surface charge density [65]. Jasmani et al. also reported on cationic CNWs prepared by a simple one-pot reaction using 4-(1-bromoethyl/bromomethyl) benzoic acid, pyridine, and CNWs. Grafting consisted of an esterification reaction between 4-(1-bromoethyl/bromomethyl) benzoic acid and CNWs and a nucleophilic attack on the C–Br bond of 4-(1-bromoethyl/bromomethyl)benzoic acid by pyridine [1]. It was found that the cationic pyridinium CNWs exhibited a stable aqueous suspension with the ability to exchange anions, which could potentially be used in many related applications.

22.5 CONCLUSION AND PROSPECTS

Surface grafting of CNWs based on the "graft onto" and "graft from" strategies has been considered as an efficient way to overcome the hydrophilic nature and poor thermal stability of CNWs, and poor miscibility between CNWs and the hydrophobic polymer matrix. Grafting functional end groups of macromolecules or polymer chains to hydroxyl groups on the CNW surface can be carried out using the "graft onto" strategy that includes silylation, isocyanation, esterification, and click chemistry. One cannot expect high grafting densities with this method because of steric hindrance and blocking of reactive sites by the already grafted polymer chains. The "graft from" strategy refers to the fact that polymer brushes can be grown in situ from CNWs directly using the surface hydroxyl groups acting as initiating sites to react with reactive monomers via ROP and radical polymerization reactions (including ATRP). This has been proven to be a very effective method for creating high-density grafting and well-controlled polymer structures on the CNW surface.

Surface grafting of CNWs shows significant positive effects on the processing and properties of nanocomposites. After surface grafting, the miscibility between CNWs and the polymer matrix and the processability of nanocomposites were improved because CNWs showed not only better dispersibility in many kinds of aqueous and organic solvents, but also better shielding of surface-modified species on the sulfate groups formed during acid hydrolysis. This improved the dispersion and loading levels of CNWs in the matrix for solution casting. It also improved the thermal stability of CNWs so that it matched the thermoprocessing temperatures for large-scale production of CNW-filled nanocomposites through melt compounding, extrusion, compression, and injection molding. Moreover, surface grafting can also change the structure and properties (such as reduced surface energy and increased hydrophobicity) of the CNW surface and hence provide new functionality to attach to, or interact with, the polymer matrix. Also, interfacial structure and interaction of nanocomposites including chain entanglements, co-crystallization, and hydrogen bond interactions between functionalized CNWs and the polymer matrix could be tailored by different lengths and grafting densities of grafted chains. When long chain polymers with structures similar to the matrix are grafted on the CNW surface, the stretching long chains may penetrate and entangle with matrix segments and together with multisite interactions form a co-continuous structure. This would improve interfacial adhesion and induce better compatibility between CNWs and polymer matrix, enhancing the mechanical performance of nanocomposites due to efficient stress transfer from the matrix to rigid CNWs. In addition, surface grafting of CNWs with polymers with special functional groups has been developed for various applications in medical materials, biosensors, ion exchange, and multifunctional packaging materials.

Overall, surface grafting of CNWs is a good way to promote the development of CNW-filled nanocomposites and extend the application of CNWs. To the best of our knowledge, however, there are three main challenges to surface grafting of CNWs and preparation of nanocomposites. The two strategies of "graft onto" and "graft from" that have been studied have, for the most part, focused on improved compatibilization and processability of nanocomposite systems. Compatibilization of

CNWs with matrix materials is still mostly unsolved because, in addition to miscibility between CNW and polymer matrix, the effects of various other parameters on the performance of CNW nanocomposites are quite complicated. The first major challenge is to improve strength and stiffness of nanocomposites without sacrificing toughness. The second challenge is to control CNW properties, that is, to develop methods for the preparation of CNWs with controlled size and aspect ratio, minimized crystal defects, and controlled surface chemistry. The last but not least major challenge is the cost reduction that ranging from the initial production and subsequent surface grafting of CNWs. Concurrently, environmentally-friendly processing and scalable/practical manufacturing must be sought and/or developed in order to meet competiveness, commercialization, safety, sustainability and environmental requirements.

ACKNOWLEDGMENTS

This work was supported by the National Natural Science Foundation of China (51373131, 51403187), Program of New Century Excellent Talents, Ministry of Education of China (NCET-11-0686), Fundamental Research Funds for the Central Universities (Self-Determined and Innovative Research Funds of WUT2012-Ia-006), Foundation of State Key Laboratory of Pulp and Paper Engineering (201212), ecoENERGY Innovation Initiative of Canada, Program of Energy Research and Development (PERD) of Canada, the Young Researchers Foundation of Key Laboratory of Advanced Textile Materials and Manufacturing Technology, Ministry of Education, Zhejiang Sci-Tech University (2013QN06), and Top Priority Discipline of Zhejiang Province in Zhejiang Sci-Tech University (2013YBZX01), Zhejiang Provincial Natural Science Foundation of China under Grant No. LQ14E030007, and the Scientific Research Foundation of Zhejiang Sci-Tech University (ZSTU) under Grant. No. 13012115-Y.

REFERENCES

1. Jasmani, L., Eyley, S., Wallbridge, R., and Thielemans, W. (2013). A facile one-pot route to cationic cellulose nanocrystals. *Nanoscale*, *5*(21), 10207–10211.
2. Chen, D., Lawton, D., Thompson, M. R., and Liu, Q. (2012). Biocomposites reinforced with cellulose nanocrystals derived from potato peel waste. *Carbohydrate Polymers*, *90*(1), 709–716.
3. Lin, N., Huang, J., and Dufresne, A. (2012). Preparation, properties and applications of polysaccharide nanocrystals in advanced functional nanomaterials: A review. *Nanoscale*, *4*(11), 3274–3294.
4. Habibi, Y., Lucia, L. A., and Rojas, O. J. (2010). Cellulose nanocrystals: Chemistry, self-assembly, and applications. *Chemical Reviews*, *110*(6), 3479–3500.
5. Kalia, S., Boufi, S., Celli, A., and Kango, S. (2014). Nanofibrillated cellulose: Surface modification and potential applications. *Colloid and Polymer Science*, *292*(1), 5–31.
6. Abdul Khalil, H. P. S., Bhat, A. H., and Ireana Yusra, A. F. (2012). Green composites from sustainable cellulose nanofibrils: A review. *Carbohydrate Polymers*, *87*(2), 963–979.
7. Goussé, C., Chanzy, H., Excoffier, G., Soubeyrand, L., and Fleury, E. (2002). Stable suspensions of partially silylated cellulose whiskers dispersed in organic solvents. *Polymer*, *43*(9), 2645–2651.
8. Andresen, M., Johansson, L. S., Tanem, B. S., and Stenius, P. (2006). Properties and characterization of hydrophobized microfibrillated cellulose. *Cellulose*, *13*(6), 665–677.
9. de Oliveira Taipina, M. O., Ferrarezi, M. M. F., Yoshida, I. V. P., and Gonçalves, M. C. (2013). Surface modification of cotton nanocrystals with a silane agent. *Cellulose*, *20*(1), 217–226.
10. Pei, A., Zhou, Q., and Berglund, L. A. (2010). Functionalized cellulose nanocrystals as biobased nucleation agents in poly (L-lactide) (PLLA)—Crystallization and mechanical property effects. *Composites Science and Technology*, *70*(5), 815–821.
11. Rueda, L., Fernández d'Arlas, B., Zhou, Q., Berglund, L. A., Corcuera, M. A., Mondragon, I., and Eceiza, A. (2011). Isocyanate-rich cellulose nanocrystals and their selective insertion in elastomeric polyurethane. *Composites Science and Technology*, *71*(16), 1953–1960.
12. Shang, W., Huang, J., Luo, H., Chang, P. R., Feng, J., and Xie, G. (2013). Hydrophobic modification of cellulose nanocrystal via covalently grafting of castor oil. *Cellulose*, *20*(1), 179–190.

13. Kloser, E. and Gray, D. G. (2010). Surface grafting of cellulose nanocrystals with poly (ethylene oxide) in aqueous media. *Langmuir*, *26*(16), 13450–13456.
14. Habibi, Y. and Dufresne, A. (2008). Highly filled bionanocomposites from functionalized polysaccharide nanocrystals. *Biomacromolecules*, *9*(7), 1974–1980.
15. Yu, H. Y. and Qin, Z. Y. (2014). Surface grafting of cellulose nanocrystals with poly (3-hydroxybutyrate-*co*-3-hydroxyvalerate). *Carbohydrate Polymers*, *101*, 471–478.
16. Lin, S., Huang, J., Chang, P. R., Wei, S., Xu, Y., and Zhang, Q. (2013). Structure and mechanical properties of new biomass-based nanocomposite: Castor oil-based polyurethane reinforced with acetylated cellulose nanocrystal. *Carbohydrate Polymers*, *95*(1), 91–99.
17. Lin, N., Huang, J., Chang, P. R., Feng, J., and Yu, J. (2011). Surface acetylation of cellulose nanocrystal and its reinforcing function in poly (lactic acid). *Carbohydrate Polymers*, *83*(4), 1834–1842.
18. Junior de Menezes, A., Siqueira, G., Curvelo, A. A. S., and Dufresne, A. (2009). Extrusion and characterization of functionalized cellulose whiskers reinforced polyethylene nanocomposites. *Polymer*, *50*(19), 4552–4563.
19. Yuan, H., Nishiyama, Y., Wada, M., and Kuga, S. (2006). Surface acylation of cellulose whiskers by drying aqueous emulsion. *Biomacromolecules*, *7*(3), 696–700.
20. Cetin, N. S., Tingaut, P., Özmen, N., Henry, N., Harper, D., Dadmun, M., and Sebe, G. (2009). Acetylation of cellulose nanowhiskers with vinyl acetate under moderate conditions. *Macromolecular Bioscience*, *9*(10), 997–1003.
21. Yu, H. Y., Qin, Z. Y., Sun, B., Yan, C. F., and Yao, J. M. (2014). One-pot green fabrication and antibacterial activity of thermally stable corn-like CNC/Ag nanocomposites. *Journal of Nanoparticle Research*, *16*(1), 1–12.
22. Braun, B. and Dorgan, J. R. (2009). Single-step method for the isolation and surface functionalization of cellulosic nanowhiskers. *Biomacromolecules*, *10*(2), 334–341.
23. Bendahou, A., Hajlane, A., Dufresne, A., Boufi, S., and Kaddami, H. (2014). Esterification and amidation for grafting long aliphatic chains on to cellulose nanocrystals: A comparative study. *Research on Chemical Intermediates*, *40*(1), 1–18.
24. Fumagalli, M., Sanchez, F., Boisseau, S. M., and Heux, L. (2013). Gas-phase esterification of cellulose nanocrystal aerogels for colloidal dispersion in apolar solvents. *Soft Matter*, *9*(47), 11309–11317.
25. Filpponen, I. and Argyropoulos, D. S. (2010). Regular linking of cellulose nanocrystals via click chemistry: Synthesis and formation of cellulose nanoplatelet gels. *Biomacromolecules*, *11*(4), 1060–1066.
26. Sadeghifar, H., Filpponen, I., Clarke, S. P., Brougham, D. F., and Argyropoulos, D. S. (2011). Production of cellulose nanocrystals using hydrobromic acid and click reactions on their surface. *Journal of Materials Science*, *46*(22), 7344–7355.
27. Pahimanolis, N., Hippi, U., Johansson, L. S., Saarinen, T., Houbenov, N., Ruokolainen, J., and Seppälä, J. (2011). Surface functionalization of nanofibrillated cellulose using click-chemistry approach in aqueous media. *Cellulose*, *18*(5), 1201–1212.
28. Eyley, S. and Thielemans, W. (2011). Imidazolium grafted cellulose nanocrystals for ion exchange applications. *Chemical Communications*, *47*(14), 4177–4179.
29. Habibi, Y., Goffin, A. L., Schiltz, N., Duquesne, E., Dubois, P., and Dufresne, A. (2008). Bionanocomposites based on poly (ε-caprolactone)-grafted cellulose nanocrystals by ring-opening polymerization. *Journal of Materials Chemistry*, *18*(41), 5002–5010.
30. Chen, G., Dufresne, A., Huang, J., and Chang, P. R. (2009). A novel thermoformable bionanocomposite based on cellulose nanocrystal-*graft*-poly (ε-caprolactone). *Macromolecular Materials and Engineering*, *294*(1), 59–67.
31. Goffin, A. L., Raquez, J. M., Duquesne, E., Siqueira, G., Habibi, Y., Dufresne, A., and Dubois, P. (2011). From interfacial ring-opening polymerization to melt processing of cellulose nanowhisker-filled polylactide-based nanocomposites. *Biomacromolecules*, *12*(7), 2456–2465.
32. Peltzer, M., Pei, A., Zhou, Q., Berglund, L., and Jiménez, A. (2013). Surface modification of cellulose nanocrystals by grafting with poly (lactic acid). *Polymer International*, *63*(6), 1056–1062. doi: 10.1002/pi.4610.
33. Labet, M. and Thielemans, W. (2011). Improving the reproducibility of chemical reactions on the surface of cellulose nanocrystals: ROP of ε-caprolactone as a case study. *Cellulose*, *18*(3), 607–617.
34. Lonnberg, H., Larsson, K., Lindstrom, T., Hult, A., and Malmstrom, E. (2011). Synthesis of polycaprolactone-grafted microfibrillated cellulose for use in novel bionanocomposites—Influence of the graft length on the mechanical properties. *ACS Applied Materials and Interfaces*, *3*(5), 1426–1433.

35. Goffin, A. L., Habibi, Y., Raquez, J. M., and Dubois, P. (2012). Polyester-grafted cellulose nanowhiskers: A new approach for tuning the microstructure of immiscible polyester blends. *ACS Applied Materials and Interfaces*, *4*(7), 3364–3371.
36. Littunen, K., Hippi, U., Johansson, L. S., Österberg, M., Tammelin, T., Laine, J., and Seppälä, J. (2011). Free radical graft copolymerization of nanofibrillated cellulose with acrylic monomers. *Carbohydrate Polymers*, *84*(3), 1039–1047.
37. Kan, K. H. M., Li, J., Wijesekera, K., and Cranston, E. D. (2013). Polymer-grafted cellulose nanocrystals as pH-responsive reversible flocculants. *Biomacromolecules*, *14*(9), 3130–3139.
38. Majoinen, J., Walther, A., McKee, J. R., Kontturi, E., Aseyev, V., Malho, J. M., Ruokolainen, J., and Ikkala, O. (2011). Polyelectrolyte brushes grafted from cellulose nanocrystals using Cu-mediated surface-initiated controlled radical polymerization. *Biomacromolecules*, *12*(8), 2997–3006.
39. Morandi, G., Heath, L., and Thielemans, W. (2009). Cellulose nanocrystals grafted with polystyrene chains through surface-initiated atom transfer radical polymerization (SI-ATRP). *Langmuir*, *25*(14), 8280–8286.
40. Zoppe, J. O., Habibi, Y., Rojas, O. J., Venditti, R. A., Johansson, L. S., Efimenko, K., Österberg, M., and Laine, J. (2010). Poly (N-isopropylacrylamide) brushes grafted from cellulose nanocrystals via surface-initiated single-electron transfer living radical polymerization. *Biomacromolecules*, *11*(10), 2683–2691.
41. Xu, Q., Yi, J., Zhang, X., and Zhang, H. (2008). A novel amphotropic polymer based on cellulose nanocrystals grafted with azo polymers. *European Polymer Journal*, *44*(9), 2830–2837.
42. Yi, J., Xu, Q., Zhang, X., and Zhang, H. (2008). Chiral-nematic self-ordering of rodlike cellulose nanocrystals grafted with poly (styrene) in both thermotropic and lyotropic states. *Polymer*, *49*(20), 4406–4412.
43. Yi, J., Xu, Q., Zhang, X., and Zhang, H. (2009). Temperature-induced chiral nematic phase changes of suspensions of poly (N,N-dimethylaminoethyl methacrylate)-grafted cellulose nanocrystals. *Cellulose*, *16*(6), 989–997.
44. Morandi, G. and Thielemans, W. (2012). Synthesis of cellulose nanocrystals bearing photocleavable grafts by ATRP. *Polymer Chemistry*, *3*(6), 1402–1407.
45. Yu, H. Y., Qin, Z. Y., Yan, C. F., and Yao, J. M. (2014). Green nanocomposites based on functionalized cellulose nanocrystals: A study on the relationship between interfacial interaction and property enhancement. *ACS Sustainable Chemistry and Engineering*, *2*(4), 875–886. dx.doi.org/10.1021/sc400499g.
46. Yao, X., Qi, X., He, Y., Tan, D., Chen, F., and Fu, Q. (2014). Simultaneous reinforcing and toughening of polyurethane via grafting on the surface of microfibrillated cellulose. *ACS Applied Materials and Interfaces*, *6*(4), 2497–2507.
47. Cao, X., Habibi, Y., and Lucia, L. A. (2009). One-pot polymerization, surface grafting, and processing of waterborne polyurethane-cellulose nanocrystal nanocomposites. *Journal of Materials Chemistry*, *19*(38), 7137–7145.
48. Raquez, J. M., Murena, Y., Goffin, A. L., Habibi, Y., Ruelle, B., DeBuyl, F., and Dubois, P. (2012). Surface-modification of cellulose nanowhiskers and their use as nanoreinforcers into polylactide: A sustainably-integrated approach. *Composites Science and Technology*, *72*(5), 544–549.
49. Lin, N., Chen, G., Huang, J., Dufresne, A., and Chang, P. R. (2009). Effects of polymer-grafted natural nanocrystals on the structure and mechanical properties of poly (lactic acid): A case of cellulose whisker-*graft*-polycaprolactone. *Journal of Applied Polymer Science*, *113*(5), 3417–3425.
50. Yu, H. Y., Qin, Z. Y., Liu, L., Yang, X. G., Zhou, Y., and Yao, J. M. (2013). Comparison of the reinforcing effects for cellulose nanocrystals obtained by sulfuric and hydrochloric acid hydrolysis on the mechanical and thermal properties of bacterial polyester. *Composites Science and Technology*, *87*, 22–28.
51. Yu, H. Y., Qin, Z. Y., Liu, Y. N., Chen, L., Liu, N., and Zhou, Z. (2012). Simultaneous improvement of mechanical properties and thermal stability of bacterial polyester by cellulose nanocrystals. *Carbohydrate Polymers*, *89*(3), 971–978.
52. Zhou, Q., Brumer, H., and Teeri, T. T. (2009). Self-organization of cellulose nanocrystals adsorbed with xyloglucan oligosaccharide–poly (ethylene glycol)–polystyrene triblock copolymer. *Macromolecules*, *42*(15), 5430–5432.
53. Pei, A., Malho, J. M., Ruokolainen, J., Zhou, Q., and Berglund, L. A. (2011). Strong nanocomposite reinforcement effects in polyurethane elastomer with low volume fraction of cellulose nanocrystals. *Macromolecules*, *44*(11), 4422–4427.
54. Ten, E., Bahr, D. F., Li, B., Jiang, L., and Wolcott, M. P. (2012). Effects of cellulose nanowhiskers on mechanical, dielectric, and rheological properties of poly (3-hydroxybutyrate-*co*-3-hydroxyvalerate)/cellulose nanowhisker composites. *Industrial and Engineering Chemistry Research*, *51*(7), 2941–2951.

55. Ten, E., Turtle, J., Bahr, D., Jiang, L., and Wolcott, M. (2010). Thermal and mechanical properties of poly (3-hydroxybutyrate-*co*-3-hydroxyvalerate)/cellulose nanowhiskers composites. *Polymer*, *51*(12), 2652–2660.
56. Petersson, L. and Oksman, K. (2006). Biopolymer based nanocomposites: Comparing layered silicates and microcrystalline cellulose as nanoreinforcement. *Composites Science and Technology*, *66*(13), 2187–2196.
57. Yu, H., Qin, Z., Liang, B., Liu, N., Zhou, Z., and Chen, L. (2013). Facile extraction of thermally stable cellulose nanocrystals with a high yield of 93% through hydrochloric acid hydrolysis under hydrothermal conditions. *Journal of Materials Chemistry A*, *1*(12), 3938–3944.
58. Jiang, L., Morelius, E., Zhang, J., Wolcott, M., and Holbery, J. (2008). Study of the poly (3-hydroxybutyrate-*co*-3-hydroxyvalerate)/cellulose nanowhisker composites prepared by solution casting and melt processing. *Journal of Composite Materials*, *42*(24), 2629–2645.
59. Bondeson, D. and Oksman, K. (2007). Dispersion and characteristics of surfactant modified cellulose whiskers nanocomposites. *Composite Interfaces*, *14*(7–9), 617–630.
60. Goffin, A. L., Raquez, J. M., Duquesne, E., Siqueira, G., Habibi, Y., Dufresne, A., and Dubois, P. (2011). Poly (ε-caprolactone) based nanocomposites reinforced by surface-grafted cellulose nanowhiskers via extrusion processing: Morphology, rheology, and thermo-mechanical properties. *Polymer*, *52*(7), 1532–1538.
61. Lin, N. and Dufresne, A. (2013). Physical and/or chemical compatibilization of extruded cellulose nanocrystal reinforced polystyrene nanocomposites. *Macromolecules*, *46*(14), 5570–5583.
62. Dong, S. and Roman, M. (2007). Fluorescently labeled cellulose nanocrystals for bioimaging applications. *Journal of the American Chemical Society*, *129*(45), 13810–13811.
63. Nielsen, L. J., Eyley, S., Thielemans, W., and Aylott, J. W. (2010). Dual fluorescent labelling of cellulose nanocrystals for pH sensing. *Chemical Communications*, *46*(47), 8929–8931.
64. Edwards, J. V., Prevost, N., Sethumadhavan, K., Ullah, A., and Condon, B. (2013). Peptide conjugated cellulose nanocrystals with sensitive human neutrophil elastase sensor activity. *Cellulose*, *20*(3), 1223–1235.
65. Hasani, M., Cranston, E. D., Westman, G., and Gray, D. G. (2008). Cationic surface functionalization of cellulose nanocrystals. *Soft Matter*, *4*(11), 2238–2244.

23 Nanocellulose Preparation, Surface Chemical Modification, and Its Application

Abbas Dadkhah Tehrani and Mohammad Hossein Babaabbasi

CONTENTS

23.1 INTRODUCTION

Currently, biobased materials are an important global research topic as there is a genuine interest and need to decrease society's dependency on petroleum-based products. Cellulose as the most abundant natural polymer available in earth is produced in nature at an annual rate of 7.5×10^{10} tons and is present in natural fibers such as wood, cotton, or hemp, as well as in a wide variety of living species, such as animals, plants, and bacteria (Habibi et al., 2010). Extensive interest has been recently focused on finding new material applications for this biopolymer. One of these applications has been the development of cellulose nanoparticles. Cellulose is a linear polymer consisting of β-D-glucopyranose units linked together by β-1,4-linkages. Hierarchy levels in wood fibers are presented in Figure 23.1 (Rowland and Roberts, 1972). The cellulosic components of a wood fiber wall structure are the cellulose molecule, the elementary fibril or microfibrils, the fibril and

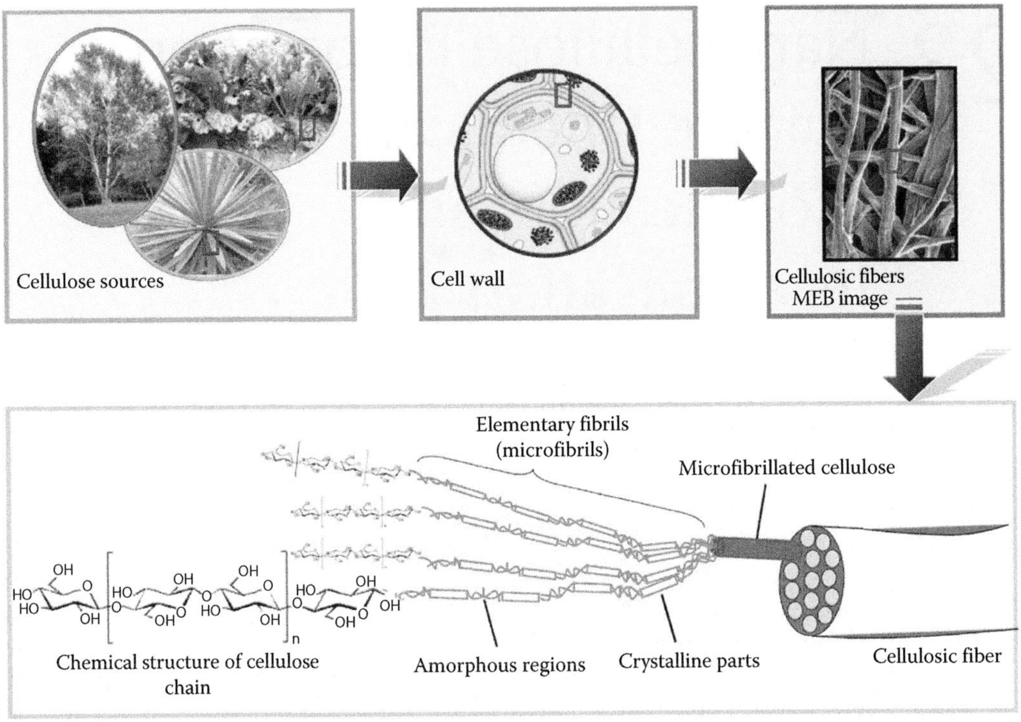

FIGURE 23.1 Organization of the cellulose chains into microfibrils and fibril aggregates. (From Lavoine, N. et al., *Carbohydr. Polym.*, 90, 735, 2012.)

the lamellar membrane. The term "elementary fibril" refers to a component with a diameter of 3.5 nm that is composed of about 36 individual cellulose chains (Frey-Wyssling, 1954; Somerville, 2006; Mutwil et al., 2008). It seems that elementary fibrils are universal structural units of natural cellulose in all kinds of cellulose sources. Elementary fibrils assembled into larger units known as microfibrillated cellulose (MFC) to reduce the free energy of the surface. Therefore, MFC has diameters in multiples of 3.5 nm (30–50 nm). Each microfibril can also be considered as a flexible semicrystalline strand with cellulose crystals linked along the microfibrils axis by disordered amorphous domains. Microfibrils then in turn are assembled into fibers. Ultimately, fiber aggregates form a lamellar structure in wood fibers (Meier, 1962; Nj Heyn, 1969; Blackwell and Kolpak, 1975; Chinga-Carrasco, 2011; Chinga-Carrasco et al., 2011).

23.2 KINDS OF NANOCELLULOSE

Cellulose nanowhiskers (CNWs), MFC, and bacterial cellulose (BC) are three main types of nanocellulose (NC); each type has its own characteristics, functions, and preparation methods (Andresen et al., 2006). Typical structures of these cellulose types on the nanoscale can be seen in the electron micrographs in Figure 23.2.

23.2.1 Cellulose Nanowhisker

In essence, CNWs refer to elongated rigid needle-shaped, single-crystalline particles with diameter in the range of 3–30 nm and lengths of a few hundred nanometers to few micrometers, mainly prepared through acid hydrolysis process (Brinchi et al., 2013). Also several terminologies have been used in the literature for CNWs (Petersson and Oksman, 2006; Petersson et al., 2007;

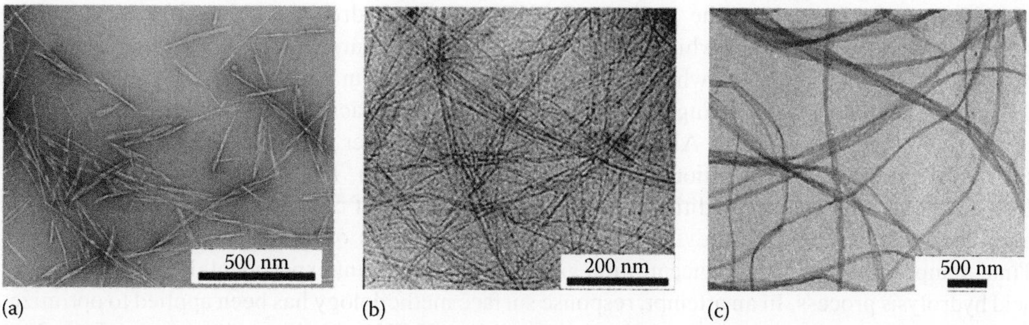

FIGURE 23.2 Transmission electron micrographs of (a) cellulose nanowhisker of unmodified sisal. (Reprinted with permission from Siqueira, G., Bras, J., and Dufresne, A., New process of chemical grafting of cellulose nanoparticles with a long chain isocyanate, *Langmuir*, 26, 402–411, 2009. Copyright 2009 American Chemical Society.) (b) Microfibrillated cellulose. (Reprinted with permission from Pääkkö, M., Ankerfors, M., Kosonen, H. et al., Enzymatic hydrolysis combined with mechanical shearing and high-pressure homogenization for nanoscale cellulose fibrils and strong gels, *Biomacromolecules*, 8, 1934–1941, 2007. Copyright 2007 American Chemical Society.) (c) Scanning electron micrograph of BNC. (Reprinted with permission from Rodríguez, K., Renneckar, S., and Gatenholm, P., Biomimetic calcium phosphate crystal mineralization on electrospun cellulose-based scaffolds, *ACS Appl. Mater. Interfaces*, 3, 681–689, 2011. Copyright 2011 American Chemical Society.)

John and Thomas, 2008), such as cellulose nanocrystals (CNCs) and cellulose nanofibers. The development of CNWs was addressed by Rånby et al. for first time in 1951. They applied controlled acid hydrolysis to the cellulose and obtained a colloidal suspension; morphological investigation of these suspensions by transmission electron microscopy (TEM) revealed the presence of needle-shaped nanoparticles. Further studies demonstrated that the crystalline structure of this rod-like particle and the original fibers are the same (Rånby, 1951).

23.2.1.1 Cellulose Nanowhiskers Preparation

Nanocrystalline cellulose or CNWs can be manufactured through several methods: acid hydrolysis, enzymatic hydrolysis, and mechanical disintegration (Siqueira et al., 2010b). However, fabrication of CNCs through acid hydrolysis process is most common reported method (Pan et al., 2013). As previously discussed, cellulose is a linear, high-molecular-weight homopolysaccharide composed of repeating β-D-glucopyranose unit whose chains aggregate to form microfibrils. Each microfibril can be considered as cellulose crystals linked along the microfibril axis by disordered amorphous domains that randomly orient in a spaghetti-like arrangement. Amorphous domains have lower density compared to the nanocrystalline regions, and therefore, they are subjected to acid or enzyme attacks. Under controlled hydrolysis conditions, the amorphous regions release individual crystallites; because of their size and shape, these rod particles are generally called "CNWs" (Siqueira et al., 2010a; Mittal et al., 2011).

Sulfuric acid and hydrochloric acid hydrolysis processes are two main processes used to produce nanocrystalline cellulose. However, preparation of nanowhiskers in the presence of other acids, such as hydrobromic acid (Filpponen, 2009) and phosphoric acid (Koshizawa, 1960; Usuda et al., 1967; Okano et al., 1999; CamareroEspinosa et al., 2013), has also been reported. Recently, increased attention has been paid to the CNW as a promising material for advanced applications, and they have been produced from different sources. Also, the effect of various parameters, such as the reaction time, reaction temperature, and types of acid used for hydrolysis process, on the properties of resulting CNWs has been extensively developed (Grossman et al., 2013).

Types of acid used for hydrolysis process have a critical effect on the properties of CNCs. For example, CNW prepared by sulfuric acid and HCl are different in several properties because of sulfate esters formed on the surface of CNWs during hydrolysis with sulfuric acid. The sulfuric-acid-hydrolyzed nanowhiskers are negative surface charged, which lead to their better dispersion in aqueous solution, while nanowhiskers obtained from HCl agglomerate and therefore do not display the same birefringent character as the sulfuric-acid-hydrolyzed whiskers (Araki et al., 1998; Peng et al., 2011). Also, they decompose at a lower temperature. It seems that the sulfate esters catalyze degradation reaction (Wang et al., 2007). The size and yield of produced CNWs depend on reaction condition, type, and concentration of cellulose and acid. Some works have been oriented toward studying the effect of these factors on the final product properties. Time, temperature, and acid concentration are the most important experimental factors affecting acid hydrolysis process. In an attempt, response surface methodology has been applied to optimize the reaction condition and in optimal reaction condition, CNWs with dimension ranging from 200 to 400 nm in length were obtained by using 63.5 wt% sulfuric treatment of microcrystalline cellulose (MCC) over a period of 2 h and with a yield of 30% optimal condition (Bondeson et al., 2006). Very recently, Espinosa et al. reported successful fabrication of CNWs by using phosphoric acid. The produced CNW through this approach was readily dispersible in polar solvents such as water, dimethyl sulfoxide (DMSO), and dimethylformamide (DMF). Furthermore, obtained nanowhiskers showed a much higher thermal stability than sulfuric acid nanowhiskers and do not suffer from limited thermal stability, which restricts the processing of sulfuric acid nanowhisker nanocomposites. As the phosphate ester groups are well known to promote the nucleation of hydroxyapatite, authors proposed that phosphoric acid nanowhiskers may also be useful in the context of scaffolds for bone regeneration (CamareroEspinosa et al., 2013).

Also, fabrication of cellulose particles with different shape through acid hydrolysis was reported. Li et al. (2001) preswelled the fibers prior to acid hydrolysis and investigated the potential of preparing nanospherical cellulose structures from short-staple cotton, and Zhang et al. developed a procedure for preparation of cellulose nanospheres with sizes ranging from 60 to over 570 nm. They found a near-linear relationship between cellulose nanoparticle size and treatment time (Zhang et al., 2007). Haafiz et al. successfully isolated regular spherical particles from MCC using acid hydrolysis method (MohamadHaafiz et al., 2013). Ultimately, as presented in Figure 23.3, rectangular- and square-shaped NC crystals were observed by Maiti et al. They applied acid hydrolysis route to China cotton, South African cotton, and waste tissue papers without any chemical pretreatment and prepared cellulose nanoparticles, which was completely different from conventional NC like nanofibrils, nanowhiskers, and MFC. The approximate ranges of diameter of NC obtained from cotton and waste tissue paper were 30–60 nm and 10–90 nm, respectively (Maiti et al., 2013).

23.2.2 Microfibrillated Cellulose

Long and flexible cellulosic material with diameters in the order of 1–100 nm, and length in the micrometer scale are generally prepared through mechanical disintegration process called MFC (Chakraborty et al., 2006). It is also known as nanofibrillar cellulose (Ahola et al., 2008; Stenstad et al., 2008). MFC consists of alternating crystalline and amorphous domains, and cellulose microfibril is the main component of MFC. Mechanical disintegration process was the first approach used by Herrick et al. (1983) and Turbak et al. (1983) for the extraction of cellulose microfibrils from wood cell. They used a high-pressure homogenizer for this purpose and successfully prepared a gel-like material, which they named as MFC. Currently, it is produced at a pilot plant scale, with ongoing efforts for commercial scale production. In addition, there are upcoming related cellulose whiskers and nanocrystalline cellulose pilot plants (Release, 2011; Lavoine et al., 2012).

23.2.2.1 MFC Production Processes

MFC is typically produced by mechanical approaches. Fabrication of MFC from various sources and by using different equipment has been reported, with each having advantages and disadvantages

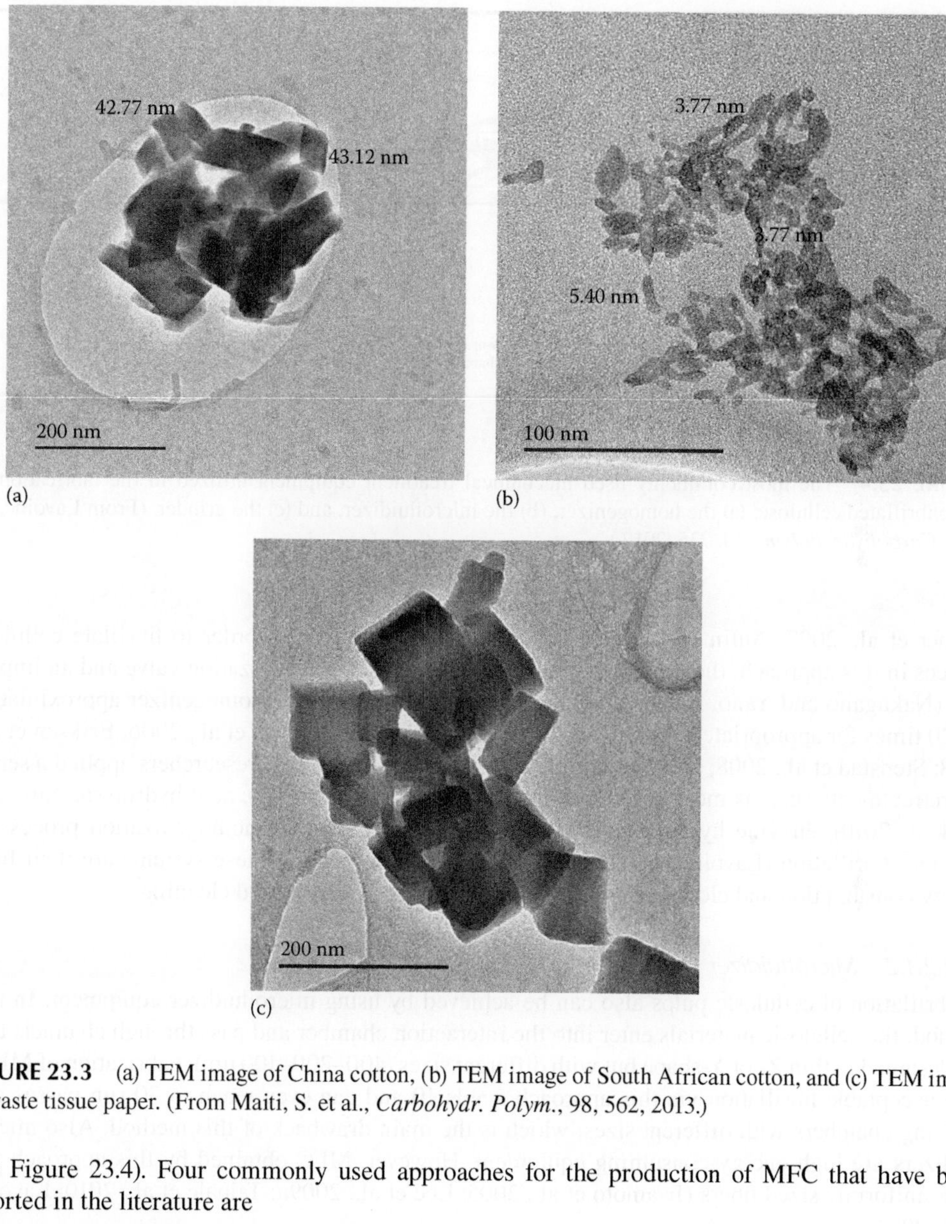

FIGURE 23.3 (a) TEM image of China cotton, (b) TEM image of South African cotton, and (c) TEM image of waste tissue paper. (From Maiti, S. et al., *Carbohydr. Polym.*, 98, 562, 2013.)

(see Figure 23.4). Four commonly used approaches for the production of MFC that have been reported in the literature are

1. MFC production using homogenizer
2. MFC production by utilizing microfluidizers
3. Cryocrushing approach
4. Microgrinding process

Recently published books and reviews also provide extensive information on the topic (Lavoine et al., 2012; Szczęsna-Antczak et al., 2012; Missoum et al., 2013; Grossman et al., 2013; AbdulKhalil et al., 2014).

23.2.2.1.1 Homogenizer Systems

The first mechanical treatment apparatus utilized for fibrillation of cellulose was the homogenizer system. This system is still used for this purpose (Nakagaito and Yano, 2004; Iwamoto et al., 2005;

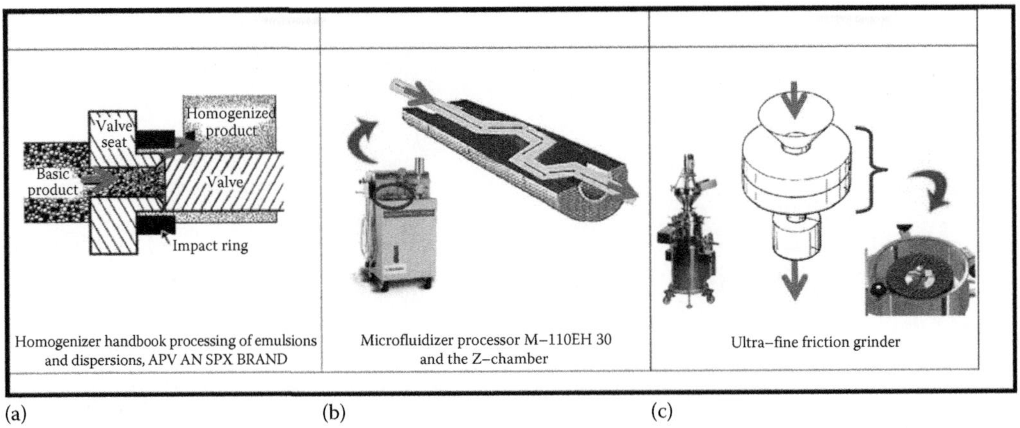

FIGURE 23.4 The most commonly used mechanical treatment equipment utilized in the fabrication of microfibrillated cellulose: (a) the homogenizer, (b) the microfluidizer, and (c) the grinder. (From Lavoine, N. et al., *Carbohydr. Polym.*, 90, 735, 2012.)

Leitner et al., 2007; Aulin et al., 2010; Uetani and Yano, 2011). In order to fibrillate cellulose sources in this approach, the pulp fibers are forced against a homogenization valve and an impact ring (Nakagaito and Yano, 2004). The fibers are passed through the homogenizer approximately 10–20 times for appropriate fibrillation (Herrick et al., 1983; Andresen et al., 2006; Eriksen et al., 2008; Stenstad et al., 2008; Syverud and Stenius, 2009). Also, several researchers applied a series of pretreatments such as mechanical cutting (Henriksson et al., 2008), acid hydrolysis (Siró and Plackett, 2010), enzyme hydrolysis, grinding, and refining prior to homogenization process to facilitate fibrillation (Lavoine et al., 2012). The main drawbacks of these systems are their high energy consumption and clogging the system by long fibers, which need cleaning.

23.2.2.1.2 Microfluidizer

Defibrillation of cellulosic pulps also can be achieved by using microfluidizer equipment. In this method, the cellulosic materials enter into the interaction chamber and pass through channels that are designed in thin Z- or Y-shape but with different sizes (400–200–100 μm). Fabrication of MFCs with acceptable fibrillation via this approach needs 10 and can even reach to 30 run passes and applying chambers with different sizes, which is the main drawback of this method. Also microfluidizers are high-energy-consuming equipment. However, MFC obtained by this approach has more uniformly sized fibers (Iwamoto et al., 2005; Lee et al., 2009a; Taipale et al., 2010; Lavoine et al., 2012).

23.2.2.1.3 Microgrinding Process

Through this process, wood fibers are passed through a gap between two disks. These disks have bursts and grooves that contact the fibers to split them up and lead to defibrillation (Nakagaito and Yano, 2004). Masuko was the first to build and sell apparatus using this approach. Production of MFC through other mechanical process often needs the mechanical fiber shortening pretreatment; however, grinding process does not require such pretreatments. Also it needs fewer passes to obtain MFC rather than homogenizer process, for example, Iwamoto et al. (2007) reported that nanosized fibers of pulp fibers from *Pinus radiata* could be obtained with a grinder only at five passes. The disadvantage of this process is the degradation of fibers during process, which affects the physical properties of resulting MFC (Hassan et al., 2012; Wang and Drzal, 2012).

23.2.2.1.4 Cryocrushing Approach

Cryocrushing is another approach for fabrication of MFC, which is very rarely used. This method was first developed by Dufresne et al. (1997) for the production of MFC from sugar beet pulp. In this method, at first the water in the wood pulp freezes by liquid nitrogen and then fibrillation process is carried out by applying high-impact forces (Chakraborty et al., 2005; Janardhnan et al., 2006; Janardhnan and Sain, 2007). This method is not appropriate for large-scale production, and the diameter of resulting MFC in this procedure ranges between 50 and 100 nm.

In fact, the high-energy consumption of MFC production limits their commercial scale production. Therefore, much research has focused on the development of pretreatments and posttreatments, which leads to the reduction in energy consumption of the processes. Different pretreatment strategies such as enzyme (Henriksson et al., 2007; Pääkkö et al., 2007), alkaline-acid (Wang and Sain, 2007; Alemdar and Sain, 2008), and 2,2,6,6-tetramethylpiperidine 1-oxyl(TEMPO) oxidation (Isogai et al., 2011a,b) have been reported. Also, in some cases, a combination of two or more methods have been applied. As reported by Siró and Plackett, these treatments can reduce energy consumption to the extent of 1000 kWh/ton from 20,000 to 30,000 kWh/ton for cellulosic fibers (Siró and Plackett, 2010). Generally, these treatments strategies facilitate the microfibrillation of fibers and reduce energy consumption by limiting the hydrogen bonds, and or add a repulsive charge, and or decrease the degree of polymerization (DP) or the amorphous link between individual MFCs. However, these strategies are outside the scope of this chapter, and an exhaustive list of pretreatment and posttreatment used for this purpose has been presented by Lavoine et al. (2012).

23.2.3 Bacterial Cellulose

As the earth's most abundant polymer, cellulose can be classified into plant cellulose and BC, both of which are naturally occurring. BC, sometimes called microbial cellulose, is a form of cellulose that is produced by a bottom–up method from glucose by several living organisms, of which *Acetobacter* strains are best known. Extensive research on BC revealed that it is chemically identical to plant cellulose, but its macromolecular structure and properties differ from the latter. For example, BC because of its ultrafine network architecture has higher water holding capacity and hydrophilicity and greater tensile strength. Furthermore, it is chemically pure, containing no hemicellulose or lignin (Karande et al., 2011). Also, BC because of its high purity and high biocompatibility has received increased attention especially for biomedical and biological applications. Scanning electron microscopy image of BC is shown in Figure 23.1. As shown in Figure 23.1, BC has a network architecture consisting of fibrils with diameter about 3–4 nm (Brown et al., 1976; Zaar, 1977), and length ranging from 1 to 9, which form a dense reticulated structure, stabilized by extensive hydrogen bonding, whereas the width of cellulose fibers produced by pulping of birch or pine wood is two orders of magnitude larger. As these thin microfibrils are significantly smaller than those in plant cellulose, they make BC much more porous. Also, BC has a higher degree of crystallinity than plant cellulose, which extensively affects its properties (Iguchi et al., 2000; Grossman et al., 2013).

23.3 CHEMICAL MODIFICATION OF CELLULOSE NANOPARTICLES

Cellulose nanoparticles generally are obtained as aqueous suspensions or gel-like structures, which agglomerate in aqueous and organic suspensions. Also, due to their hydrophilic nature, cellulose nanoparticles are not compatible with nonpolar polymeric matrixes. Therefore, most investigations have focused on surface modification of cellulose nanoparticles to prevent their agglomeration and make them compatible with hydrophobic polymers matrixes. Various modification approaches have been reported in literature such as physical and chemical polymer grafting and molecular grafting.

However, the following section highlights some recent studies on the modifications through chemical grafting of polymers.

Cellulose nanoparticles contain a large number of surface hydroxyl groups available for surface modification, which play a critical role in graft polymerization reactions. There are two main polymer grafting methods including grafting-from and grafting-to approaches. The "grafting-to" approach involves the attachment of presynthesized and characterized polymer chains to the hydroxyl groups of the cellulose nanoparticles surfaces. Conversely, "grafting-from" involves the surface-initiated, in situ polymerization from initiators immobilized on the surface. Also ranges of polymers through various mechanisms have been grafted on the surface of cellulose nanoparticles, which are detailed in the following text and classified based on the polymerization mechanism.

23.3.1 Ring Opening Polymerization Method

This method broadly has been used for grafting cyclic monomers such as caprolactone, lactide, and oxazolines on the surface of cellulose nanoparticles. PCL [poly(ε-caprolactone)] is a semicrystalline, hydrophobic polyester with a low glass transition temperature around −60°C and a melting temperature around 60°C. However, PCL is a ductile polymer and is, therefore, commonly used in combination with other polymers or with different reinforcing fillers. "Grafting-from" of PCL polymers to various substrates has been extensively considered, and the ring-opening polymerization (ROP) of cyclic caprolactone monomer by cationic, anionic, or coordination–insertion mechanisms has been used successfully to graft PCL from cellulose (Lönnberg et al., 2011b), starch (Namazi and Dadkhah, 2008), silica nanoparticles (Joubert et al., 2004, 2005), and recently carbon nanotubes (Zeng et al., 2006; Lee et al., 2011a).

The "grafting-from approach" applied to CNWs was first reported by Habibi et al. (2008), who grafted PCL on the surface of CNWs by stannous octoate (Sn(Oct)2)-catalyzed ROP. TEM results showed that initial morphological integrity and native crystallinity of CNCs have not been affected by surface grafting. It is worth noting that prior to the ROP reaction, some precautions were taken by the authors because of acidity of the CNWs. Actually, the preparation of CNW with sulfuric acid leads to the formation of sulfate ester groups on the surface of CNWs that may cause complete destruction of the CNW during the polymerization reaction at high temperature (95°C). As the authors state, neutralization of the CNW solution by NaOH can improve the CNW thermal stability.

Other authors, Lönnberg et al. (2008), reported modification of MFC with PCL, via similar approach and investigated the thermal behavior of MFC grafted with different amounts of PCL using thermal gravimetric analysis (TGA) and differential scanning calorimetry (DSC). Pure MFC can only be dispersed in polar solvents; however, as shown in Figure 23.5, the grafted MFCs were well dispersed in nonpolar solvents such as THF after grafting with PCL.

Also, PCL is a suitable candidate for the preparation of thermoformable bionanocomposite based on natural nanocrystals. Chang and coworkers developed thermoformable bionanocomposite based on CNCs by ROP of ε-caprolactone monomer onto MCC powder under microwave irradiation (Chen et al., 2009a). The MCC particles showed needle-like nanoparticles, with mean length and diameter of about several hundred nanometers and 30 nm, respectively. Interestingly after the grafting process, the resultant nanoparticles showed different shapes. They have a spherical shape with a diameter of less than 40 nm. It seems that the structure of MCC could be destroyed by the graft polymerization process itself. Labet and Thielemans (2011) during surface chemical modification of CNCs via ROP of caprolactone have encountered reproducibility issues when the same reactions were carried out on nanocrystals from different hydrolysis batches, indicating a variable surface composition. Given the inherent purity of the nanoparticles themselves, it was believed that the presence of adsorbed species at the surface of the nanocrystals blocking reactive sites may cause reproducibility issues. In order to investigate the adsorbed species at the surface of the nanocrystals, they extracted nanocrystals from several batches with different solvents such as ethanol, heptane,

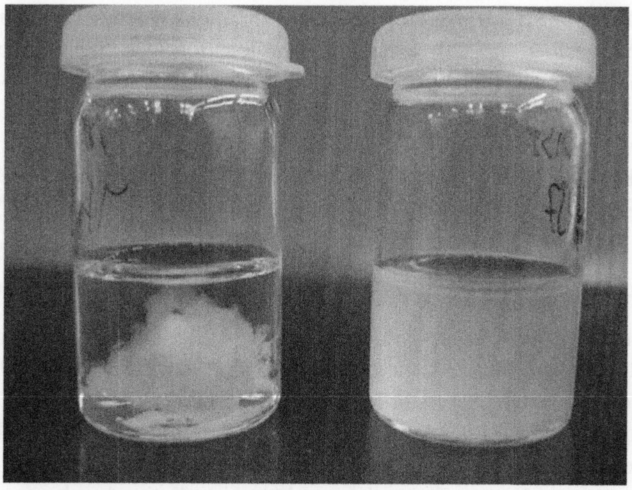

FIGURE 23.5 Unmodified MFC (left vial) and MFC-*g*-PCL (right vial) in THF, after sonication. (From Lönnberg, H. et al., *Eur. Polym. J.*, 44, 2991, 2008.)

and ethylacetate and then analyzed the extracted impurities using both mass spectrometry and NMR spectroscopy. Results showed a high number of peaks, suggesting that a large number of impurities were removed, which were identified as xylobiose, 1,6-anhydroglucose, vanillic acid, and 3,4,5-trimethoxyphenol. The authors also reported successful grafting of ε-caprolactone using citric acid as a benign catalyst.

Poor interfacial adhesion in immiscible cellulose–polymer interfaces is one of the major issues that limit NC applications. To tailor the interfacial adhesion, the grafting of polymers from cellulose films was investigated using ROP of ε-caprolactone (Lönnberg et al., 2011a) with various graft lengths. Films of MFC were hot-pressed together with a PCL-film to form a bilayer laminate. It was observed that interfacial peeling toughness correlates very strongly with PCL DP, indicating PCL grafts form physical entanglements in the PCL matrix and promotes significant plastic deformation in the PCL bulk, thus increasing interfacial peeling energy. ROP approach also may be used for graft polymerization of other cyclic monomers on the surface of cellulose particles. Synthesis of CNW-*g*-PLA nanohybrids was reported following similar conditions used for the surface modification of CNW by PCL chains. In this procedure, CNWs were included in polylactide (PLA)-based composites. In order to improve the compatibility between CNW and the hydrophobic polyester matrix, prior to the blending, PLA chains were chemically grafted onto the surface of CNW. The authors demonstrated that the chemical grafting of CNW with hydrophobic PLA enhances their compatibility with the polymeric matrix and thus improves the final properties of the nanocomposites (Goffin et al., 2011a). Modified cellulose and starch nanoparticles with PCL can be ingredients of choice for bionanocomposites. As previously mentioned, great efforts have been devoted to improve the interfacial adhesion between natural nanocrystals and polymeric matrices by grafting of the hydrophobic polyester onto the surface of CNWs. Mechanical performance of obtained CNW-*g*-PCL and starch nanocrystal-*g*-PCL, which was incorporated into a PLA matrix to produce new nanocomposites, has been compared. It seems that the rod structure of cellulose whiskers (CWs), which are distinctly different from platelet-like starch nanocrystals (StNs), enhanced the mechanical performance of PLA-based materials in comparison with platelet-like nanoparticles of starch nanocrystal-*g*-PCL. This better enhancement of the mechanical performance of PLA-based materials is attributed to the ability of rigid CW nanoparticles to endure higher stress as well as the essential associations of the facile transfer of the stress to the CW nanoparticles mediated with grafted PCL chains (Lin et al., 2009).

Finally, Dadkhah Tehrani et al. have developed a chemical strategy following different routes implicating cationic ring opening graft polymerization reaction of 2-ethyl oxazoline to chemically modify CNW. In this procedure, a tosylate group was introduced on the CNW via tosylation reaction followed by cationic ROP of oxazoline. In the next step, the side chains of obtained graft copolymer (CNW-*g*-POX) were hydrolyzed in acidic condition and converted to polyethyleneimine. Briefly, in this work, water-soluble modified CNW (CNW-*g*-PEI) has been prepared from water-insoluble unmodified CNW (Dadkhah Tehrani and Neysi, 2013).

23.3.2 Grafting of Vinyl Monomers through Free Radical Polymerization

Methods for "grafting-from" cellulose-based material, including radical polymerization of vinyl monomers (Geacintov et al., 1960; Zahran and Mahmoud, 2003; Roy et al., 2009), via free radical polymerization have been extensively studied since the 1960s. However, most studies have been done with macroscopic cellulose fibers and only a few with cellulose nanoparticles.

Various monomers and initiating systems were utilized for modification of cellulose nanoparticles through this approach. For example, electron beam irradiation has been used for the polymerization of acrylic acid on the surface of microsized and nanosized BC particles extracted from Nata de coco and hydrogels with different sizes of cellulose particles. The cellulose nanoparticles were prepared by acid hydrolysis and expected to alter several physicochemical properties of the hydrogel. As the nanocellulose has more surfaces available for reaction, the crosslink density and swelling degree was also expected to be modified. Although similar in chemical structure to cellulose, cellulose whiskers formed hydrogels with higher glass transition temperature and SEM observations revealed that swollen nanocellulose hydrogel has smaller and homogenous pores arrangement while microcellulose has bigger and irregular pores, thus affecting their swelling degree (Johari et al., 2012). In a similar study, Anirudhan et al. addressed graft polymerization of a nanocellulose-based hydrogel by graft copolymerization reaction of glycidylmethacrylate onto NC. They applied ethyleneglycoldimethacrylate as cross-linker and benzoyl peroxide as initiator. They obtained graft copolymer immobilized with poly(acrylic acid). Poly(acrylic acid)-modified poly(glycidylmethacrylate)-grafted NC (PAPGNC) was used for the adsorption of a small globular enzyme lysozyme (LYZ) from aqueous solutions. The presence of a cross-linking agent in this system led to the creation of an interpenetrating polymer network with free COOH groups at the chain end (Anirudhan and Rejeena, 2012).

Littunen et al. selected ammonium cerium (IV) nitrate as initiator for free radical copolymerization reaction on the surface of NC. It is a selective method for grafting of polysaccharides (Okieimen, 2003; O'Connell et al., 2006). Most importantly, through this method, aqueous medium as a green environmental-friendly medium can be used, without the tedious solvent exchange required by many controlled copolymerization methods (Jenkins and Hudson, 2001). Cerium ion chelates with two adjacent hydroxyl groups in a cellulose chain and initiation occurs via a redox reaction, resulting in radical formation on an opened glucose ring. This mechanism is illustrated in Figure 23.6 (Mishra et al., 2003). Acrylic monomers used in the grafting were glycidyl methacrylate, ethyl acrylate, methyl methacrylate, butyl acrylate, and 2-hydroxyethyl methacrylate. Also, the researchers pointed out that graft yields were higher than those reported in studies with macroscopic cellulose but surprisingly independent of the water solubility of each monomer (Littunen et al., 2011).

Similarly, Per Stenstad and coworkers grafted a series of glycidyl methacrylate with various lengths of the polymer chains by regulating the amount of glycidyl methacrylate added. Using this procedure, epoxy functionality has been introduced onto the MFC surface. They used both aqueous and organic solvents as media for MFC modification (Stenstad et al., 2008).

$K_2S_2O_8$ is one of the most commonly used initiators for this purpose. It is applied as a free radical initiator for preparation poly(methacrylic acid-*co*-vinyl sulfonic acid)-grafted-NC Poly(MAA-*co*-VSA)-*g*-MNC) via graft copolymerization technique. Poly(MAA-*co*-VSA)-*g*-MNCC was used to adsorb the IgG from aqueous solutions. In this case, the easy separation of IgG from aqueous

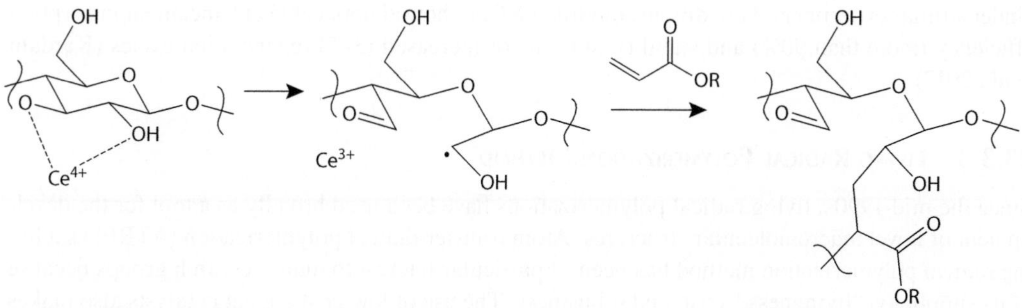

FIGURE 23.6 Mechanism of cerium-initiated copolymerization. (From Littunen, K. et al., *Carbohydr. Polym.*, 84, 1039, 2011.)

solutions via adsorption is followed by the application of magnetic field, for the rapid development of biotechnology (Anirudhan and Rejeena, 2013). In a different work, Zhou et al. manufactured rod-shaped CNCs and used to reinforce polyacrylamide (PAM) hydrogels through in situ free-radical polymerization in the presence of cross-linker N,N_0-methylenebisacrylamide (NMBA) and by utilizing potassium persulfate as the initiator. They found that the CNCs accelerated the formation of hydrogels and improved the crosslink density of hydrogels. Thus, the authors concluded CNCs were not only a reinforcing agent for hydrogel but also operated as a multifunctional cross-linker and the polymer has been grafted onto the surface of CNWs. The following scheme (see Figure 23.7) is proposed for mechanism of formation of nanocomposite hydrogels.

The pure PAM gel had a relatively smooth porous structure, whereas composite gels showed rough porous network structure with many nanocrystals in the cavities of the pores. This supported the presence of strong interactions of PAM chains with the nanocrystals in composite gels (Zhou et al., 2011b). Likewise, Yang et al. conducted similar grafting reactions. AM-*g*-NCW was found to self-assemble in a lyotropic state (Yang and Ye, 2012). The AM-*g*-NCW aqueous suspension exhibited an anisotropic zone with fingerprint patterns. Although a large number of studies have been carried out with grafting of acidic monomers such as acrylic and itaconic acid containing weak acid group (COOH), only limited work has been conducted with grafting of vinyl sulfonic acid having strong acid group (SO_3H). Recently, graft copolymerization of vinyl sulfonic acid onto NCFs led to improved decontamination of toxic metals from water bodies. The modified NCFs were examined for removal of Cd(II), Pb(II), Ni(II), and Cr(III) ions in single and multimetal solutions.

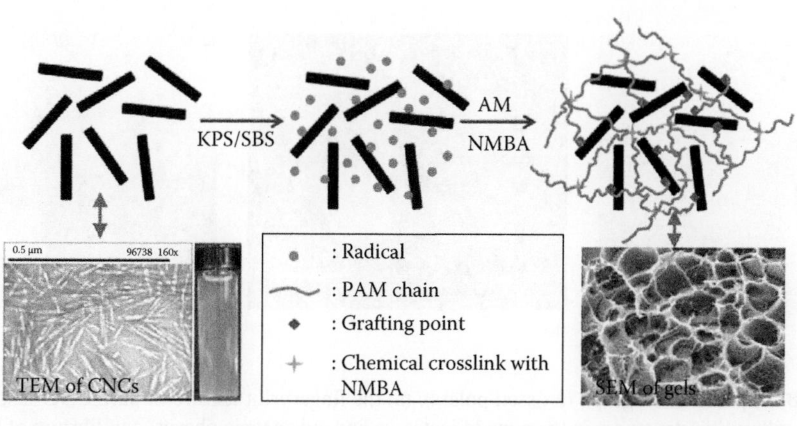

FIGURE 23.7 Scheme of the gelation mechanisms of PAM–CNC nanocomposite hydrogels. (From Zhou et al., *Biomacromolecules*, 12, 2617, 2011a.)

Under similar experimental conditions, modified NCFs showed noticeable enhancement in sorption efficiency (more than 90%) and stability in terms of increased (3–5) regeneration cycles (Kardam et al., 2012).

23.3.3 Living Radical Polymerization Method

Since the mid-1990s, living radical polymerizations have been used broadly as a tool for the development of novel macromolecular structures. Atom transfer radical polymerization (ATRP) as a living radical polymerization method has been of particular interest to many research groups because of its simplicity, "livingness," cost, and robustness. The use of low-cost copper catalysts also makes it a remarkable option for surface modification. Surface-initiated ATRP (SI-ATRP) is one of the most efficient approaches to "graft from" polymer chains, which leads to high surface grafting density and low polydispersity. ATRP can be applied to a wide range of monomers with different chemical structures and architectures, which should allow modification of the surface properties of the cellulose-based nanoparticles while keeping the primary rod-shaped morphology of nanoparticles. This approach is employed for the preparation of an amphotropic polymer based on cellulose nanoparticles, which could exhibit liquid-crystalline behavior both in the solvent and in the heating process. This graft copolymer has been successfully synthesized through grafting of poly{6-[4-(4-methoxyphenylazo)phenoxy] hexyl methacrylate} (PMMAZO), as a liquid-crystalline polymers from CNCs using ATRP. The PMMAZO-grafted CNC shows smectic-to-nematic transition at 95°C and nematic-to-isotropic transition at 135°C, and exhibits analogous lyotropic liquid-crystalline phase behavior above 135°C (Xu et al., 2008). Yi et al. recently used this approach to manufacture cellulose nanoparticle graft-PS, involving use of ATRP. In this procedure, the hydroxyl groups on CNC were esterified with 2-bromoisobutyrylbromide to produce a macroinitiator for polymerization of styrene on the surface of CNWs. The CNC is not a thermotropic material. Surprisingly, the authors observed the fingerprint texture for PSt-grafted CNC when the PSt grafted CNC is cooled to 163°C. The optical micrographs of pure CNC and PSt-grafted CNC are shown in Figure 23.8. They concluded that PSt side chains act as a solvent above the melting temperature of the side chains and the PSt-grafted CNC orients spontaneously in isotropic melt. This is the first report of spontaneous chiral nematic phase of CNC at thermotropic state. According to the obtained results, researchers pointed out that observation of liquid crystal phase behavior of the PSt-grafted CNC is a chiral interaction arising from the shape of the rods and not from the chiral character of the cellulose chain (Yi et al., 2008).

An interesting aspect is the influence of PS chain length on NC-*g*-PS properties. This question has been studied by Morandi et al., who fabricated a range of nanocrystals-*g*-polystyrene with different

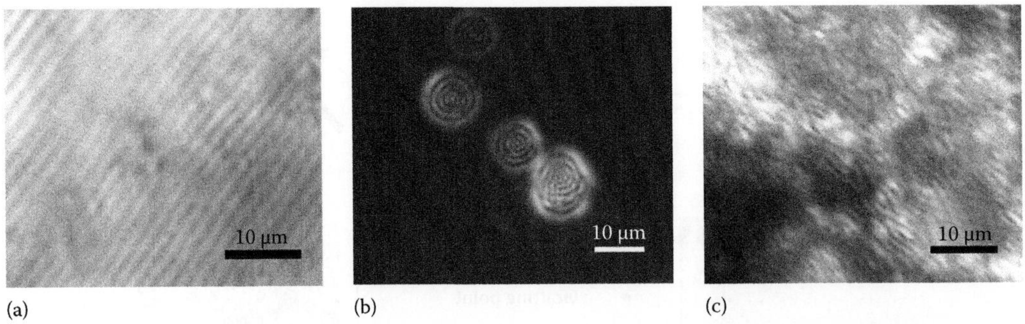

FIGURE 23.8 Optical micrograph (crossed polars): (a) the fingerprint texture of pure CNC suspension (3.1 wt%), (b) the spherulitic structures in the zone of isotropic and anisotropic phases; equilibrium of PSt-grafted CNC suspension (5.7 wt%), and (c) the fingerprint texture in the zone of anisotropic phase of PSt-grafted CNC suspension (5.7 wt%). (From Yi, J. et al., *Polymer*, 49, 4406, 2008.)

graft lengths by polystyrene chains via surface-initiated ATRP. The nanocrystals-*g*-polystyrene (NC-*g*-PS) particles were compared with pure CNCs for their capacity to absorb 1,2,4-trichlorobenzene from water. The results showed that modified CNCs have higher adsorption capacity, while none of the modified nanocrystals also displayed faster absorption kinetics (Morandi et al., 2009). A further approach to modification of NC via free radical living polymerization involves surface-initiated single-electron transfer living radical polymerization, which was used for design of smart materials. The discovery of a Cu(0)-mediated single-electron transfer living radical polymerization (SET-LRP) process has led to great advances in ultrafast polymerizations. Unlike ATRP, latter techniques are derived from the low activation energy in an outer-sphere electron transfer mechanism and the rapid disproportionation of Cu(I) with N-containing ligands in polar solvents (Zoppe et al., 2010). "Smart" materials are responsive polymers that can respond to changes in their environment, such as light, heat, ionic strength, and pH. Such materials are mainly interesting for drug-delivery and sensing applications. As one of the most studied thermoresponsive polymers, poly(*N*-isopropylacrylamide) (poly(NiPAAm)) has been grafted onto the surface of nanocellulose via this approach by Zoppe et al., who reported on the grafting poly(NiPAAm) from CNCs to develop brushes with various surface densities and degrees of polymerization. In this case, never-dried CNCs have been utilized as the substrate for surface modification, because drying of the CNCs can lead to aggregation (Zoppe et al., 2010). In contrast with poly(NiPAAm)-*g*-CNCs, unmodified CNCs showed no thermoresponsive behavior. The aggregation and thermoresponsive behavior of poly(NiPAAm)-*g*-CNCs was further demonstrated by light transmittance, which indicated the possibility of a precise control over aggregation following the lower critical solution temperature (LCST) of the poly(NiPAAm) brushes (Zoppe et al., 2011) Poly(*N*,*N*-dimethylaminoethyl methacrylate) (PDMAEMA) is other valuable thermosensitive polymer, which exhibits a temperature-dependent solubility (Zhang et al., 2006). PDMAEMA is a potential candidate for biomaterials and gene delivery systems (Van de Wetering et al., 1998) because of its ability to interact with DNA, enzyme, and polyanion drugs by means of electrostatic attraction. Yi et al. have been introduced PDMAEMA polymers onto CNC surface to investigate the temperature-induced liquid-crystalline phase behaviors of PDMAEMA-grafted CNC suspensions. Obtained copolymer exhibited fingerprint texture in lyotropic state. Researchers analyzed the effect of temperature and found that the temperature-induced changes of PDMAEMA polymer chains result in changes of fingerprint texture. On the other hand, with increasing temperature, the spacing of the fingerprint lines decreases (Yi et al., 2009).

23.3.4 Graft Modification through Coupling Reaction

Typically, graft copolymerization on the surface of NC has been focused on grafting-from method, because it can be difficult to gain sufficient graft density using a grafting-to approach. However, Harrisson et al. obtained composites comprised 60%–64% grafted polymer by mass through grafting-to strategy. Amine-terminated poly(styrene) and poly(*tert*-butyl acrylate) are used for graft reaction on the surface of rigid nanoscale rods of oxidized cellulose microcrystals (Harrisson et al., 2011). As shown in Figure 23.9, the synthetic strategy for fabrication of the polymer-grafted cellulose microcrystals involves (1) the production of cellulose nanoparticles, (2) the oxidation of the cellulose (formation of carboxylic acid group on the surface), (3) preparation of amine-functionalized polymers, and (4) grafting of the polymers to the cellulose surface via amidation reaction by using carbodiimide.

Also, isocyanates are reactive functional groups and suitable candidates for coupling reaction that are widely used in grafting polymers on the surface of biopolymers. Cellulose and starch nanocrystals obtained from the acid hydrolysis were subjected to isocyanate-mediated reaction to graft polycaprolactone (PCL) chains with various molecular weights on their surface. Using a casting/evaporation technique, their nanocomposite films are produced from both unmodified and PCL-grafted nanoparticles and PCL as matrix. Mechanical properties of resulting films of modified particles were notably different compared to unmodified nanoparticles. The grafting of PCL chains

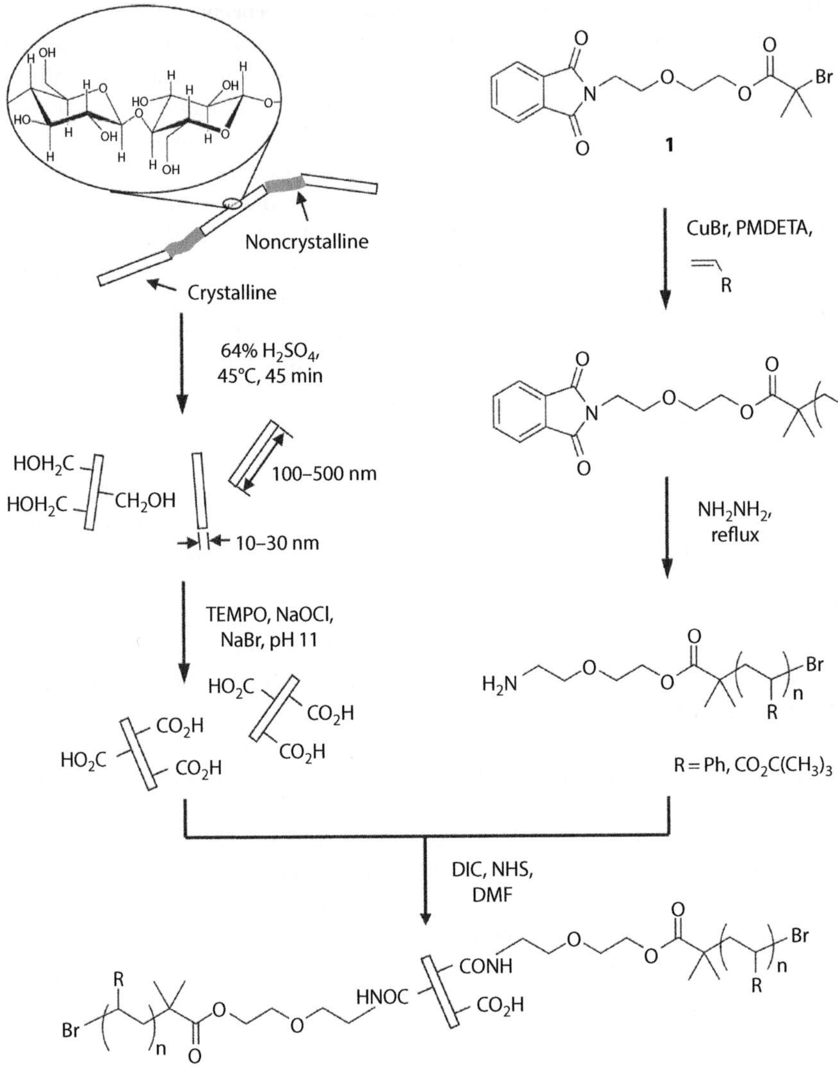

FIGURE 23.9 Preparation of polymer-grafted cellulose microcrystals. (Reprinted with permission from Harrisson, S., Drisko, G.L., Malmström, E., Hult, A., and Wooley, K.L., Hybrid rigid/soft and biologic/synthetic materials: Polymers grafted onto cellulose microcrystals, *Biomacromolecules*, 12, 1214–1223, 2011. Copyright 2011 American Chemical Society.)

on the surface results in lower modulus values but extensively higher strain at break. This unusual behavior clearly reflects the originality of the reinforcing phenomenon of polysaccharide nanocrystals resulting from the formation of a percolating network, thanks to chain entanglements and cocrystallization (Habibi and Dufresne, 2008).

As against nano cellulose crystal (NCC) suspensions derived from sulfuric acid that often stabilize by electrostatic repulsion forces, NCC suspensions obtained from hydrochloric acid hydrolysis show limited dispersibility in water and the resulting agglomerates precipitate or flocculate. An approach for modifying NCC surfaces is to achieve steric colloidal stabilization. Steric stabilization refers to the stability imparted to colloids by the adsorption or grafting of polymers onto their surfaces. The advantage of sterically stabilized systems is that they tend to remain dispersed well even at high salt concentrations, whereas shielding will cause electrostatic systems to destabilize at high ionic strengths. For example, a two-step process was employed for this purpose by grafting PEG onto the surface of NCC: in the first step, NCC suspensions prepared by sulfuric acid hydrolysis were desulfated with sodium hydroxide, and in the second step, the surfaces of the crystals were functionalized with epoxy-terminated poly(ethylene oxide) (PEO epoxide) under alkaline conditions. Upon concentration of the aqueous suspensions of poly(ethylene oxide)-grafted nanocrystalline cellulose, a chiral nematic phase was observed (Kloser and Gray, 2010). In this work, epoxy group was used for the coupling of polymer surface grafting. Azzam et al. have also addressed graft reaction of thermosensitive amine-terminated statistical polymers (Jeffamines) onto the surface of CNCs by a peptidic coupling reaction. Commercial statistical copolymers of ethylene oxide (EO) and propylene oxide (PO) are known as Jeffamines. The modified nanocellulose showed unusual properties like colloidal stability at high ionic strength, surface activity, and thermoreversible aggregation. Using a range of experimental techniques, these researchers found that a high grafting density could be achieved when the reaction was performed in DMF rather than water. Peptidic coupling reaction has already been successfully used for the grafting of PEG or DNA oligonucleotides (Araki et al., 2001; Mangalam et al., 2009) onto the surface of CNCs (Azzam et al., 2010). A Japanese research group also used water-soluble carbodiimide for grafting of poly(ethylene glycol) having a terminal amino group on one end (PEG-NH_2) on the surface of oxidized cellulose nanoparticle that contained carboxylic acid functional group in its surface through peptidic coupling reaction. The freeze-dried PEG-grafted cellulose microcrystals exhibited significantly enhanced dispersion stability and ability to redisperse into either water or chloroform. It is to be noted in this case that PEG-grafted microcrystals formed a chiral nematic mesophase similar to that of the ungrafted sample, but with a reduced spacing of the fingerprint pattern. There are two proposed mechanisms in literature for the formation of the chiral nematic phase of the cellulose microcrystal suspension: one is based on the spiral arrangement of charge groups on cellulose microcrystals, and the other is the mechanism with twisting of microcrystals together with charge envelopes. In this work, authors rejected the former mechanism (Araki et al., 2001). Benkaddour et al. recently used a new approach to manufacture CNC-*g*-PCL, involving use of click reactions in the "grafting-from" approach. The advantage of this method was ascribed to high molecular weight grafting of PCL on the surface of cellulose nanoparticles. In the case of the "grafting-to" approach, PCL (Mw = 80,000 or more) cannot diffuse into the fiber, because of its large molecular weight, and only surface grafting may occur. In this context, the oxidized NCs bearing propargyl groups (ONC-PR) were produced through reacting amino groups of propargylamine (PR) with carboxyl groups of ONC. In parallel, azido-polycaprolactone (PCL-N_3) was prepared from PCL-diol in two steps: (1) tosylation of PCL (PCL-OTs) and (2) nucleophilic displacement of tosyl group using sodium azide. Ultimately, ONC-PR was reacted with PCL-N_3 through click chemistry and ONC-*g*-PCL prepared (Benkaddour et al., 2013).

23.3.5 Other Methods

Pranger et al. have produced a biobased polymer nanocomposite (PNC) by using nanoparticles CW as the reinforcer through in situ polymerization techniques in a thermosetting furfuryl alcohol matrix. In situ polymerization with CW offers an attractive processing route for producing poly (furfuryl alcohol) (PFA) matrix nanocomposites without the use of solvents or surfactants. CW plays a key role in this in situ polymerization process, catalyzing the polymerization, thus eliminating the use of strong mineral acid catalysts. Thermal analysis showed that PNC was characterized by extensively higher temperature at the onset of degradation compared to unmodified PFA. Therefore, it suggested that CW can also improve the thermal stability of the consolidated PNCs (Pranger and Tannenbaum, 2008). Cellulose particles also have been used for fabrication of electrically conductive nanofibrils. In producing nanofibrils from conducting polymers, the production of the fibers that possess dimensions in the nanoscale while maintaining the mechanical strength at the macroscale has become a critical issue. In this sense, different attempts have been made to develop electrically conductive polymer fibers using various physical, chemical, and electrochemical methods, which have potential applications as sensors, electrostatic and radar shielding, antistatic and anticorrosive coatings, and shape-memory conductive composites. The flexible and shining films could be obtained through the oxidative polymerization of aniline using ammonium peroxydisulfate as initiator and nanofibrils as matrix. Bulk polyaniline (PANi) as well as other conducting polymers cannot form films from aqueous solutions as they do not resuspend to create uniform and flexible films. Interestingly, cellulose nanoparticle/PA nanocomposite aqueous solutions can form flexible film, in an easier way by using casting method from aqueous solution. These films may be the precursor for the production of cellulose-based electrically conductive nanocomposites with superior mechanical properties and have found interesting applications in sensors antistatic and anticorrosive nanocoatings (Mattoso et al., 2009). Subsequently, a similar procedure was followed by Auad et al who added the PA-modified nanocrystals using this technique to the segmented polyurethane. Segmented polyurethanes exhibited shape-memory properties, and hence the shape-memory behavior was also observed for the composites that contain only up to 4 wt% of fibrils at about the same level as that of the unfilled polyurethane (PU). The researchers demonstrated that two-phase structure of the polymer led to the material's ability to "remember" and autonomously recover its original shape after being deformed in response to an external thermal stimulus (Auad et al., 2011). Very recently, Finnish researchers reported a facile approach for fabrication of highly processable NFC/PANi suspensions containing various PANi loading. They successfully produced NFC/PANi composite papers that exhibited high electrical conductivity and good mechanical characteristics. In this case, the suspension of nanofibrillated cellulose (NFC), which was prepared by combining an enzymatic hydrolysis and mechanical shearing, acted as platform, stabilizer, and reinforcement for PANi deposition during the in situ synthesis (Luong et al., 2013) (Figure 23.10).

Through a similar strategy, highly flexible paper-like materials of PPy/T-CNs nanocomposites were produced, which exhibited good mechanical properties and high electrical conductivity values. Polypyrrole (PPy), one of the most prominent types of conjugated polymers, has been grafted onto the surface of CNCs (T-CNs) via the in situ oxidative chemical polymerization by using ammonium persulfate (APS) as oxidant. Tunicate CNC (T-CNs) plays the role as a dopant and template for tuning the morphologies of PPy nanoparticles (Zhang et al., 2013). Müller et al. used $FeCl_3$ and BC instead of APS and CNCs, respectively. They successfully produced BC/PPy composites that displayed electrical resistivity similar to the PPy alone (0.33 cm). Detailed analyses revealed the thickness and the electrical resistivity of the composite were dependent on the pyrrole (Py) concentration in the reaction medium (Müller et al., 2011).

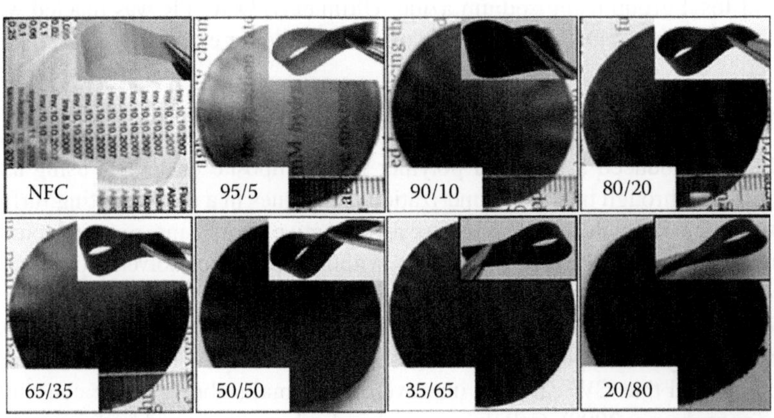

FIGURE 23.10 Photographs of NFC and NFC/PANi composite papers containing different concentrations of PANi between 5 and 80 wt%, prepared by vacuum filtration; the corresponding insets demonstrate the high flexibility of pure NFC and the composite papers. (From Luong, N.D. et al., *European Polymer Journal*, 49, 335, 2013.)

23.4 CELLULOSE NANOPARTICLE APPLICATIONS

Cellulose nanoparticles because of their unique properties such as superior mechanical properties, biodegradability, high aspect ratio, and nontoxicity have gained a significant amount of attention in various applications. Several potential applications have already been demonstrated including biosensors and bioimaging, drug delivery, catalysis, antimicrobial and medical applications, enzyme immobilization, supercapacitors, batteries, antistatic coating, corrosion protection, and electrical devices (Virji et al., 2006; Rodriguez et al., 2009; John et al., 2010; Kim et al., 2010; Liew et al., 2010; Lam et al., 2012). The most researched application of cellulose nanoparticles is their utility as a reinforcement material in nanocomposite materials and their biomedical applications; in this chapter, the focus has been on these applications. Therefore, Chapter 24 will briefly describe only the application of cellulose nanoparticles as reinforcement in nanocomposites and their biomedical applications are their most important applications.

23.4.1 Nanocomposites

The potential of nanocomposites in various parts of research and application is promising and is attracting growing investments. In the nanocomposite industry, reinforcing particles are particles whose at least one of their dimensions is smaller than 100 nm (Dufresne, 2010). The properties of nanocomposites are strongly influenced by nanoparticle size and filler fraction, nanoparticle shape, nanoparticle distribution, polymer molecular weight, and the nature of the interactions between the nanoparticle and the polymer matrix (Smith et al., 2003). Nanoparticles from natural polysaccharides, such as cellulose nanoparticles and starch nanocrystals, are potential reinforcements where the nanosized fillers impart enhanced mechanical and barrier properties. The main advantages of these natural nanofillers are their renewable nature, availability, biodegradability, and specially their relatively reactive surfaces, which can be modified accordingly (Namazi and Dadkhah, 2010; Grossman et al., 2013). As polymer fillers, they have a greater impact on mechanical properties, permeability to gases and water, thermal stability and heat distortion temperature, surface appearance, and optical clarity than conventional polymer fillers. They are an attractive nanomaterial for a multitude of potential applications in a diverse range of fields (Dufresne, 2008). As a result of their unique properties, cellulose nanoparticles have become an important class of renewable nanomaterials; one of their most important applications is the reinforcement of polymeric matrices in nanocomposite materials. Favier et al. (1995) were the first to address the use of NCC as reinforcing fillers in poly(styrene *co*-butyl acrylate) (poly(*S*-*co*-BuA))-based nanocomposites. Cellulose fibrils have attracted more interest as reinforcing components in different polymer matrices. They have approximately a two times higher modulus of elasticity, a higher aspect ratio, and a better compatibility with matrix materials compared to fibers (Oksman et al., 2006; Oksman and Sain, 2006). Chemical compatibility between the filler material and the continuous matrix can be expected to play a vital role, both in the dispersion of the filler in the matrix material and in the development of suitable adhesion between the two phases (Hubbe et al., 2008). However, the poor interfacial adhesion between natural fibers and polymeric matrix is the key issue that dictates the overall performance of the composites. Interaction of two or more different materials with each other depends on the nature and strengths of the intermolecular forces of the components involved. CNCs have a weak interaction with hydrophobic matrix materials due to their inherent hydrophilicity; and therefore, the surface of cellulosic materials tends to be incompatible with many plastic materials that are most commonly considered in the production of composites, for example, polyethylene, polypropylene, styrene, etc. In addition, the property of cellulosic fibers to absorb water can be considered to be undesirable in many potential applications of composites (Hubbe et al., 2008; Eichhorn, 2011). In order to prevent CNCs from aggregating, and to improve dispersion and compatibility in the matrix material, modification of the CNC surface is required. Some methods of CNC surface modification include graft polymerization, silylation, and the use of surfactants (Heux et al., 2000;

Araki et al., 2001; Goussé et al., 2002). One of the most notable among them is polymerization from the surface of CNWs (Eichhorn, 2011; Kalia et al., 2011; Grossman et al., 2013). Up to now, many nanocomposite materials have been reported by utilizing cellulose nanoparticles in the production of a wide range of natural and synthetic polymeric matrices (Grossman et al., 2013); some of them are mentioned in Table 23.1.

23.4.2 Biomedical Application

Indeed, cellulose nanoparticles promises to be a very versatile material with a wide range of biomedical applications and biotechnological applications, such as tissue engineering, drug delivery, wound dressings, and medical implants (Cherian et al., 2010; Thakur, 2013). In fact, biomedical devices recently have gained a significant amount of attention because of an increased interest in tissue-engineered products for both wound care and the regeneration of damaged or diseased organs. NC, particularly BC, because of its biocompatibility, high hydrophilicity, high liquid loading capacity, high aspect ratio, transparency, and non-toxicity, is an attractive candidate for a wide range of applications in various fields, especially those related to biomedical and biotechnology applications. Much work has already focused on designing ideal biomedical devices from BC, such as artificial skin, artificial blood vessels, artificial cornea, heart valve prosthesis, artificial urethra, artificial bone, artificial cartilage, artificial porcine knee menisci, and deliveries of drug, hormone, and protein. The potential various biomedical applications of BC-based materials are shown in Figure 23.11 (Fu et al., 2013). In recent years, bacterial NFC has been the most widely studied form of NFC in the biomedical applications. However, several studies have also explored possible applications of plant-based NFC for these purposes. For example, recently, the uses of nanocrystalline cellulose and MFC as a drug delivery excipient have been reported. Furthermore, NCC has been used to bind the ionizable drugs such as tetracycline and doxorubicin. Tagging cetyl trimethylammonium bromide (CTAB) to the surface of NCC has made it possible to bind significant quantities of hydrophobic anticancer drugs such as paclitaxel, etoposide, and docetaxel (Lam et al., 2012). It has been shown that even though the cellulose materials were chemically fairly similar, their use as drug nanoparticle matrices led to very different release profiles. Using nanofibrillar celluloses from different sources could lead to either immediate or sustained release. The use of these versatile biomaterials is envisioned to be very useful in many pharmaceutical nanoparticle applications and in controlled drug delivery (Valo et al., 2013).

23.5 CONCLUSION

Cellulose is a nature-based polymer that is a suitable semicrystalline polymer for preparing renewable and potentially biodegradable nanoparticles. Recently, there has been a growing interest in the developing application of NC not only because of its origin from an abundant, renewable resource and is biodegradable, but also because of its specific properties such as high aspect ratio, high tensile strength, and a specific Young's modulus comparable to steel and Kevlar. Consequently, several techniques have been used for preparing, and rendering different types of, cellulose nanoparticles over the years (CNW, MFC and BC). On the one hand, nanocrystalline particles (CNW) are prepared by hydrolysis and , MFC is prepared by mechanical treatment. Moreover, cellulose nanoparticles have several advantages. They are renewable, biodegradable, nanoscaled, crystalline, and present needle-like or fibrillar morphology favorable for a broad range of applications. However, the industrial-scale production of MFC is still a challenge, and some progress is necessary before it can be used in industrial applications. Also, some drawbacks limit its use, such as aggregation, low concentration suspension, and incompatibility with hydrophobic polymeric matrices for instance. One solution to overcome these problems is their chemical modification. The main chemical modifications of NC through chemical grafting of

TABLE 23.1
Some of the Cellulose Nanoparticle–Based Nanocomposites in Various Polymeric Matrixes Reported in the Literature

Reinforcer	Matrix	References
Cellulose nanocrystals (CNCs)	Polyvinyl alcohol (PVA)	Peresin et al. (2010), Paralikar et al. (2008), Zimmermann et al. (2004, 2005), Roohani et al. (2008), Lu et al. (2008), Lee et al. (2009b), Jalaluddin et al. (2011), Li et al. (2012), Hossain et al. (2012), Fortunati et al. (2013), Lee and Deng (2012), Endo et al. (2013), Virtanen and Vartiainen (2014), Zhang et al. (2014), Cho and Park (2011)
Microfibrillated cellulose	PVA	Qiu and Netravali (2012), Frone et al. (2011), Srithep et al. (2012), Bertolla et al. (2014)
Bacterial cellulose nanowhiskers (BCNWs)	Ethylene vinyl alcohol (EVOH)	Martínez-Sanz et al. (2011, 2012, 2013)
CNCs	Poly(acrylic acid) (PAA)	Lu and Hsieh (2009)
CNWs	Polystyrene (PS)	Rojas et al. (2009)
Bacterial cellulose microfibrils	Poly(methyl methacrylate) (PMMA)	Olsson et al. (2010), Fahma et al. (2013)
CNCs	PMMA	Dong et al. (2012)
CNCs	Ethylene vinyl acetate	Mahi and Rodrigue (2012)
Cellulose nanofibril	Poly(acrylamide)	Kurihara and Isogai (2014)
Cellulose whiskers modified by grafting organic acid chlorides	Polyethylene	Junior de Menezes et al. (2009)
CNCs	Polyurethane	Marcovich et al. (2006), Cao et al. (2009), Pei et al. (2011), Li and Ragauskas (2011, 2012), Liu et al. (2012b, 2013), Aranguren et al. (2013), Rueda et al. (2013), Li et al. (2011), Lin et al. (2013), Saralegi et al. (2013), Park et al. (2013), Floros et al. (2012), Zhao et al. (2013), Wu et al. (2014)
Bacterial cellulose	Polyurethane	Juntaro et al. (2012), Seydibeyoğlu et al. (2013), Pinto et al. (2013)
CNCs	Starch-based plastics	Lin et al. (2009), Liu et al. (2010), Chen et al. (2009b), Angles and Dufresne (2000, 2001), Cao et al. (2008a,b), Kvien et al. (2007), Mathew and Dufresne (2002), Orts et al. (2005), Mathew et al. (2008), Svagan et al. (2009), Nasri-Nasrabadi et al. (2014)
Cellulose whiskers	Chitosan	Li et al. (2009), Khan et al. (2012)
Microfibrillated cellulose	Chitosan	Hassan et al. (2011), O'Kelly (2014)
CNWs	Glucomannan	Mikkonen et al. (2010)
CNWs	Regenerated cellulose	Qi et al. (2009), Magalhaes et al. (2009), Ma et al. (2011)
CNWs	Poly(3-hydroxybutyrate-*co*-3-hydroxyvalerate) (PHBV)	Jiang et al. (2008), Ten et al. (2010, 2012a,b, 2013), Yu et al. (2011)
Nanofibrillated cellulose	PHBV	Srithep et al. (2013)
Cellulose nanocrystalline whiskers	Plasticized poly(vinyl chloride) (PVC)	Chazeau et al. (1999a–c, 2000)

(Continued)

TABLE 23.1 (*Continued*)
Some of the Cellulose Nanoparticle–Based Nanocomposites in Various Polymeric Matrixes Reported in the Literature

Reinforcer	Matrix	References
Cellulose nanocrystals (CNCs)	Poly(lactic acid) (PLA)	Xiang et al. (2009), Ramirez (2010), Bondeson and Oksman (2007a), Oksman et al. (2006), Pei et al. (2010), Braun et al. (2012), Petersson et al. (2007), Lin et al. (2011), Fortunati et al. (2012a,b), Shi et al. (2012), Liu et al. (2012a), Ali and Noori (2014), Cacciotti et al. (2014), Wang et al. (2014a)
Cellulose whisker modified by polyvinyl alcohol	PLA	Bondeson and Oksman (2007b)
Microfibrillated cellulose	PLA	Suryanegara et al. (2009, 2010), Iwatake et al. (2008), Jonoobi et al. (2010, 2012), Nakagaito et al. (2009), Tingaut et al. (2009), Wang and Drzal (2012), Tanpichai et al. (2012), Boissard et al. (2011)
CNCs	Polypropylene	Gray (2008)
Microfibrillated cellulose	Polypropylene	Iwamoto et al. (2014)
CNCs	Carboxymethyl cellulose (CMC)	Choi and Simonsen (2006)
Cellulose whiskers	Soy protein isolate (SPI)	Wang et al. (2006)
Cellulose nanofillers	Waterborne epoxy	Ruiz et al. (2001), Xu et al. (2013)
Cellulose whiskers	Natural rubber (NR)	Bendahou et al. (2009, 2010), Rosa et al. (2009), Siqueira et al. (2011b), Visakh et al. (2012b), Xu et al. (2012)
Cellulose nanofiber (CNF)	NR	Abraham et al. (2013), Visakh et al. (2012a,c)
Cellulose whiskers	Poly(styrene-*co*-hexylacrylate)	Elmabrouk et al. (2009)
Cellulose whiskers	Latex	Favier et al. (1995), Dubief et al. (1999), Dufresne et al. (1999), Dufresne (2000)
Cellulose nanofiber	Hydroxypropyl cellulose (HPC)	Zimmermann et al. (2004, 2005)
Microfibrillated cellulose (MFC)	Melamine formaldehyde (MF)	Henriksson and Berglund (2007)
CNCs	Poly(ε-caprolactone) (PCL)	Zoppe et al. (2009), Habibi et al. (2008), Lin et al. (2009), Habibi and Dufresne (2008), Chen et al. (2009a), Goffin et al. (2011b), Siqueira et al. (2011a), Sheng et al. (2013)
CNF	Polycaprolactone/polypropylene hybrid	Lee et al. (2011b)
Cellulose nanocrystals (CNCs)	Polyethylene oxide (PEO)	Zhou et al. (2011a)
Bacterial cellulose whiskers	PEO	Park et al. (2007), Zhou et al. (2012)
CNWs	PEO	Changsarn et al. (2011)
Cellulose nanoparticles	Hydroxypropylmethylcellulose (HPMC)	Bilbao-Sainz et al. (2011)
CNFs	Poly(ethylene glycol) (PEG)	Wang et al. (2014b)
CNWs	Silk fibroin (SF)	Huang et al. (2011), Noishiki et al. (2002)
Tunicate cellulose whiskers	Epoxy resin	Šturcová et al. (2005), Rusli and Eichhorn (2008), Matos Ruiz et al. (2000)
CNWs	Poly(vinyl acetate) (PVAc)	Capadona et al. (2008), Rusli et al. (2010), De Rodriguez et al. (2006), Kaboorani et al. (2012), Gong et al. (2011)
CNCs	POE	AziziSamir et al. (2004a,b, 2005, 2006)

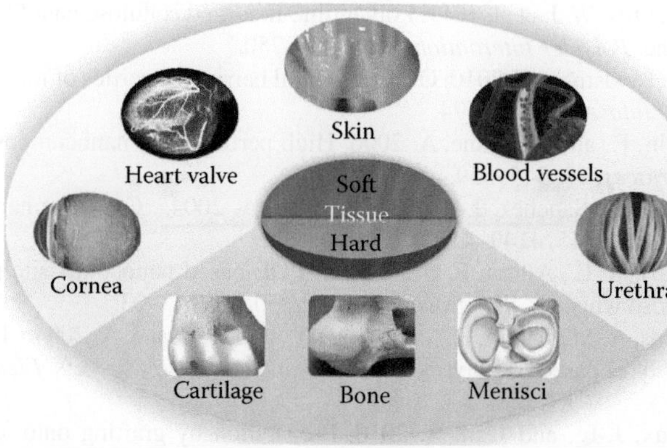

FIGURE 23.11 Prospects for the various biomedical applications of BC-based materials. (From Fu, L. et al., *Carbohydr. Polym.*, 92, 1432, 2013.)

synthetic polymers that have been proposed in the literature are reviewed in this chapter. Recent and relevant examples of the distinct applications, with particular emphasis on nanocomposites and biomedical application, are also presented.

REFERENCES

Abdul Khalil, H., Davoudpour, Y., Islam, M. N. et al. 2014. Production and modification of nanofibrillated cellulose using various mechanical processes: A review. *Carbohydrate Polymers*, 99, 649–665.

Abraham, E., Deepa, B., Pothan, L. et al. 2013. Physicomechanical properties of nanocomposites based on cellulose nanofibre and natural rubber latex. *Cellulose*, 20, 417–427.

Ahola, S., Österberg, M., and Laine, J. 2008. Cellulose nanofibrils—Adsorption with poly(amideamine) epichlorohydrin studied by QCM-D and application as a paper strength additive. *Cellulose*, 15, 303–314.

Alemdar, A. and Sain, M. 2008. Isolation and characterization of nanofibers from agricultural residues—Wheat straw and soy hulls. *Bioresource Technology*, 99, 1664–1671.

Ali, N. A. and Noori, F. T. M. 2014. Crystallinity, mechanical, and antimicrobial properties of polylactic acid/microcrystalline cellulose/silver nanocomposites. *International Journal of Application or Innovation in Engineering and Management*, 3, 77–81.

Andresen, M., Johansson, L.-S., Tanem, B. S., and Stenius, P. 2006. Properties and characterization of hydrophobized microfibrillated cellulose. *Cellulose*, 13, 665–677.

Angles, M. N. and Dufresne, A. 2000. Plasticized starch/tunicin whiskers nanocomposites. 1. Structural analysis. *Macromolecules*, 33, 8344–8353.

Angles, M. N. and Dufresne, A. 2001. Plasticized starch/tunicin whiskers nanocomposite materials. 2. Mechanical behavior. *Macromolecules*, 34, 2921–2931.

Anirudhan, T. and Rejeena, S. 2012. Poly(acrylic acid)-modified poly(glycidylmethacrylate)-grafted nanocellulose as matrices for the adsorption of lysozyme from aqueous solutions. *Chemical Engineering Journal*, 187, 150–159.

Anirudhan, T. and Rejeena, S. 2013. Poly(methacrylic acid-*co*-vinyl sulfonic acid)-grafted-magnetite/nanocellulose superabsorbent composite for the selective recovery and separation of immunoglobulin from aqueous solutions. *Separation and Purification Technology*, 119, 82–93.

Araki, J., Wada, M., and Kuga, S. 2001. Steric stabilization of a cellulose microcrystal suspension by poly(ethylene glycol) grafting. *Langmuir*, 17, 21–27.

Araki, J., Wada, M., Kuga, S., and Okano, T. 1998. Flow properties of microcrystalline cellulose suspension prepared by acid treatment of native cellulose. *Colloids and Surfaces A: Physicochemical and Engineering Aspects*, 142, 75–82.

Aranguren, M. I., Marcovich, N. E., Salgueiro, W., and Somoza, A. 2013. Effect of the nano-cellulose content on the properties of reinforced polyurethanes. A study using mechanical tests and positron anihilation spectroscopy. *Polymer Testing*, 32, 115–122.

Auad, M. L., Richardson, T., Orts, W. J. et al. 2011. Polyaniline-modified cellulose nanofibrils as reinforcement of a smart polyurethane. *Polymer International*, 60, 743–750.

Aulin, C., Gällstedt, M., and Lindström, T. 2010. Oxygen and oil barrier properties of microfibrillated cellulose films and coatings. *Cellulose*, 17, 559–574.

Azizi Samir, M. A. S., Alloin, F., and Dufresne, A. 2006. High performance nanocomposite polymer electrolytes. *Composite Interfaces*, 13, 545–559.

Azizi Samir, M. A. S., Alloin, F., Sanchez, J.-Y., and Dufresne, A. 2004a. Cellulose nanocrystals reinforced poly(oxyethylene). *Polymer*, 45, 4149–4157.

Azizi Samir, M. A. S., Chazeau, L., Alloin, F. et al. 2005. POE-based nanocomposite polymer electrolytes reinforced with cellulose whiskers. *Electrochimica Acta*, 50, 3897–3903.

Azizi Samir, M. A. S., Mateos, A. M., Alloin, F., Sanchez, J.-Y., and Dufresne, A. 2004b. Plasticized nanocomposite polymer electrolytes based on poly(oxyethylene) and cellulose whiskers. *Electrochimica Acta*, 49, 4667–4677.

Azzam, F., Heux, L., Putaux, J.-L., and Jean, B. 2010. Preparation by grafting onto, characterization, and properties of thermally responsive polymer-decorated cellulose nanocrystals. *Biomacromolecules*, 11, 3652–3659.

Bendahou, A., Habibi, Y., Kaddami, H., and Dufresne, A. 2009. Physico-chemical characterization of palm from *Phoenix dactylifera*-L, preparation of cellulose whiskers and natural rubber-based nanocomposites. *Journal of Biobased Materials and Bioenergy*, 3, 81–90.

Bendahou, A., Kaddami, H., and Dufresne, A. 2010. Investigation on the effect of cellulosic nanoparticles' morphology on the properties of natural rubber based nanocomposites. *European Polymer Journal*, 46, 609–620.

Benkaddour, A., Jradi, K., Robert, S., and Daneault, C. 2013. Grafting of polycaprolactone on oxidized nanocelluloses by click chemistry. *Nanomaterials*, 3, 141–157.

Bertolla, L., Dlouhý, I., Philippart, A., and Boccaccini, A. R. 2014. Mechanical reinforcement of Bioglass®-based scaffolds by novel polyvinyl-alcohol/microfibrillated cellulose composite coating. *Materials Letters*, 118, 204–207.

Bilbao-Sainz, C., Bras, J., Williams, T., Senechal, T., and Orts, W. 2011. HPMC reinforced with different cellulose nano-particles. *Carbohydrate Polymers*, 86, 1549–1557.

Blackwell, J. and Kolpak, F. J. 1975. The cellulose microfibril as an imperfect array of elementary fibrils. *Macromolecules*, 8, 322–326.

Boissard, C. I., Bourban, P.-E., Tingaut, P., Zimmermann, T., and Månson, J.-A. E. 2011. Water of functionalized microfibrillated cellulose as foaming agent for the elaboration of poly(lactic acid) biocomposites. *Journal of Reinforced Plastics and Composites*, 30, 709–719.

Bondeson, D., Mathew, A., and Oksman, K. 2006. Optimization of the isolation of nanocrystals from microcrystalline cellulose by acid hydrolysis. *Cellulose*, 13, 171–180.

Bondeson, D. and Oksman, K. 2007a. Dispersion and characteristics of surfactant modified cellulose whiskers nanocomposites. *Composite Interfaces*, 14, 617–630.

Bondeson, D. and Oksman, K. 2007b. Polylactic acid/cellulose whisker nanocomposites modified by polyvinyl alcohol. *Composites Part A: Applied Science and Manufacturing*, 38, 2486–2492.

Braun, B., Dorgan, J. R., and Hollingsworth, L. O. 2012. Supra-molecular ecobionanocomposites based on polylactide and cellulosic nanowhiskers: Synthesis and properties. *Biomacromolecules*, 13, 2013–2019.

Brinchi, L., Cotana, F., Fortunati, E., and Kenny, J. 2013. Production of nanocrystalline cellulose from lignocellulosic biomass: Technology and applications. *Carbohydrate polymers*, 94, 154–169.

Brown, R. M., Willison, J., and Richardson, C. L. 1976. Cellulose biosynthesis in *Acetobacter xylinum*: Visualization of the site of synthesis and direct measurement of the in vivo process. *Proceedings of the National Academy of Sciences*, 73, 4565–4569.

Cacciotti, I., Fortunati, E., Puglia, D., Kenny, J. M., and Nanni, F. 2014. Effect of silver nanoparticles and cellulose nanocrystals on electrospun poly(lactic) acid mats: Morphology, thermal properties and mechanical behavior. *Carbohydrate Polymers*, 103, 22–31.

Camarero Espinosa, S., Kuhnt, T., Foster, E. J., and Weder, C. 2013. Isolation of thermally stable cellulose nanocrystals by phosphoric acid hydrolysis. *Biomacromolecules*, 14, 1223–1230.

Cao, X., Chen, Y., Chang, P., Muir, A., and Falk, G. 2008a. Starch-based nanocomposites reinforced with flax cellulose nanocrystals. *Express Polymer Letters*, 2, 502–510.

Cao, X., Chen, Y., Chang, P. R., Stumborg, M., and Huneault, M. A. 2008b. Green composites reinforced with hemp nanocrystals in plasticized starch. *Journal of Applied Polymer Science*, 109, 3804–3810.

Cao, X., Habibi, Y., and Lucia, L. A. 2009. One-pot polymerization, surface grafting, and processing of waterborne polyurethane-cellulose nanocrystal nanocomposites. *Journal of Materials Chemistry*, 19, 7137–7145.

Capadona, J. R., Shanmuganathan, K., Tyler, D. J., Rowan, S. J., and Weder, C. 2008. Stimuli-responsive polymer nanocomposites inspired by the sea cucumber dermis. *Science*, 319, 1370–1374.

Chakraborty, A., Sain, M., and Kortschot, M. 2005. Cellulose microfibrils: A novel method of preparation using high shear refining and cryocrushing. *Holzforschung*, 59, 102–107.

Chakraborty, A., Sain, M., and Kortschot, M. 2006. Reinforcing potential of wood pulp-derived microfibres in a PVA matrix. *Holzforschung*, 60, 53–58.

Changsarn, S., Mendez, J. D., Shanmuganathan, K. et al. 2011. Biologically inspired hierarchical design of nanocomposites based on poly(ethylene oxide) and cellulose nanofibers. *Macromolecular Rapid Communications*, 32, 1367–1372.

Chazeau, L., Cavaille, J., Canova, G., Dendievel, R., and Boutherin, B. 1999a. Viscoelastic properties of plasticized PVC reinforced with cellulose whiskers. *Journal of Applied Polymer Science*, 71, 1797–1808.

Chazeau, L., Cavaille, J., and Perez, J. 2000. Plasticized PVC reinforced with cellulose whiskers. II. Plastic behavior. *Journal of Polymer Science Part B: Polymer Physics*, 38, 383–392.

Chazeau, L., Cavaille, J. Y., and Terech, P. 1999b. Mechanical behaviour above Tg of a plasticised PVC reinforced with cellulose whiskers; a SANS structural study. *Polymer*, 40, 5333–5344.

Chazeau, L., Paillet, M., and Cavaille, J. 1999c. Plasticized PVC reinforced with cellulose whiskers. I. Linear viscoelastic behavior analyzed through the quasi—Point defect theory. *Journal of Polymer Science Part B: Polymer Physics*, 37, 2151–2164.

Chen, G., Dufresne, A., Huang, J., and Chang, P. R. 2009a. A novel thermoformable bionanocomposite based on cellulose nanocrystal-graft—Poly(ε-caprolactone). *Macromolecular Materials and Engineering*, 294, 59–67.

Chen, Y., Liu, C., Chang, P. R., Cao, X., and Anderson, D. P. 2009b. Bionanocomposites based on pea starch and cellulose nanowhiskers hydrolyzed from pea hull fibre: Effect of hydrolysis time. *Carbohydrate Polymers*, 76, 607–615.

Cherian, B. M., Leão, A. L., De Souza, S. F. et al. 2010. Isolation of nanocellulose from pineapple leaf fibres by steam explosion. *Carbohydrate Polymers*, 81, 720–725.

Chinga-Carrasco, G. 2011. Cellulose fibres, nanofibrils and microfibrils: The morphological sequence of MFC components from a plant physiology and fibre technology point of view. *Nanoscale Research Letters*, 6, 1–7.

Chinga-Carrasco, G., Yu, Y., and Diserud, O. 2011. Quantitative electron microscopy of cellulose nanofibril structures from *Eucalyptus* and *Pinus radiata* kraft pulp fibres. *Microscopy and Microanalysis*, 17, 563–571.

Cho, M.-J. and Park, B.-D. 2011. Tensile and thermal properties of nanocellulose-reinforced poly(vinyl alcohol) nanocomposites. *Journal of Industrial and Engineering Chemistry*, 17, 36–40.

Choi, Y. and Simonsen, J. 2006. Cellulose nanocrystal-filled carboxymethyl cellulose nanocomposites. *Journal of Nanoscience and Nanotechnology*, 6, 633–639.

Dadkhah Tehrani, A. and Neysi, E. 2013. Surface modification of cellulose nanowhisker throughout graft polymerization of 2-ethyl-2-oxazoline. *Carbohydrate Polymers*, 97, 98–104.

De Rodriguez, N. L. G., Thielemans, W., and Dufresne, A. 2006. Sisal cellulose whiskers reinforced polyvinyl acetate nanocomposites. *Cellulose*, 13, 261–270.

Dong, H., Strawhecker, K. E., Snyder, J. F. et al. 2012. Cellulose nanocrystals as a reinforcing material for electrospun poly(methyl methacrylate) fibers: Formation, properties and nanomechanical characterization. *Carbohydrate Polymers*, 87, 2488–2495.

Dubief, D., Samain, E., and Dufresne, A. 1999. Polysaccharide microcrystals reinforced amorphous poly(β-hydroxyoctanoate) nanocomposite materials. *Macromolecules*, 32, 5765–5771.

Dufresne, A. 2000. Dynamic mechanical analysis of the interphase in bacterial polyester/cellulose whiskers natural composites. *Composite Interfaces*, 7, 53–67.

Dufresne, A. 2008. Polysaccharide nano crystal reinforced nanocomposites. *Canadian Journal of Chemistry*, 86, 484–494.

Dufresne, A. 2010. Processing of polymer nanocomposites reinforced with polysaccharide nanocrystals. *Molecules*, 15, 4111–4128.

Dufresne, A., Cavaille, J. Y., and Vignon, M. R. 1997. Mechanical behavior of sheets prepared from sugar beet cellulose microfibrils. *Journal of Applied Polymer Science*, 64, 1185–1194.

Dufresne, A., Kellerhals, M. B., and Witholt, B. 1999. Transcrystallization in Mcl-PHAs/cellulose whiskers composites. *Macromolecules*, 32, 7396–7401.

Eichhorn, S. J. 2011. Cellulose nanowhiskers: Promising materials for advanced applications. *Soft Matter*, 7, 303–315.

Elmabrouk, A. B., Wim, T., Dufresne, A., and Boufi, S. 2009. Preparation of poly(styrene-*co*-hexylacrylate)/cellulose whiskers nanocomposites via miniemulsion polymerization. *Journal of Applied Polymer Science*, 114, 2946–2955.

Endo, R., Saito, T., and Isogai, A. 2013. TEMPO-oxidized cellulose nanofibril/poly(vinyl alcohol) composite drawn fibers. *Polymer*, 54, 935–941.

Eriksen, O., Syverud, K., and Gregersen, O. 2008. The use of microfibrillated cellulose produced from kraft pulp as strength enhancer in TMP paper. *Nordic Pulp and Paper Research Journal*, 23, 299–304.

Fahma, F., Hori, N., Iwata, T., and Takemura, A. 2013. The morphology and properties of poly(methyl methacrylate)-cellulose nanocomposites prepared by immersion precipitation method. *Journal of Applied Polymer Science*, 128, 1563–1568.

Favier, V., Canova, G., Cavaille, J. et al. 1995. Nanocomposite materials from latex and cellulose whiskers. *Polymers for Advanced Technologies*, 6, 351–355.

Filpponen, E. I. 2009. The synthetic strategies for unique properties in cellulose nanocrystal materials. *Ph.D. thesis*, North Carolina State University.

Floros, M., Hojabri, L., Abraham, E. et al. 2012. Enhancement of thermal stability, strength and extensibility of lipid-based polyurethanes with cellulose-based nanofibers. *Polymer Degradation and Stability*, 97, 1970–1978.

Fortunati, E., Armentano, I., Zhou, Q. et al. 2012a. Multifunctional bionanocomposite films of poly(lactic acid), cellulose nanocrystals and silver nanoparticles. *Carbohydrate Polymers*, 87, 1596–1605.

Fortunati, E., Peltzer, M., Armentano, I. et al. 2012b. Effects of modified cellulose nanocrystals on the barrier and migration properties of PLA nano-biocomposites. *Carbohydrate Polymers*, 90, 948–956.

Fortunati, E., Puglia, D., Monti, M. et al. 2013. Cellulose nanocrystals extracted from okra fibers in PVA nanocomposites. *Journal of Applied Polymer Science*, 128, 3220–3230.

Frey-Wyssling, A. 1954. The fine structure of cellulose microfibrils. *Science*, 119, 80–82.

Frone, A. N., Panaitescu, D. M., Donescu, D. et al. 2011. Preparation and characterization of PVA composites with cellulose nanofibers obtained by ultrasonication. *BioResources*, 6, 487–512.

Fu, L., Zhang, J., and Yang, G. 2013. Present status and applications of bacterial cellulose-based materials for skin tissue repair. *Carbohydrate Polymers*, 92, 1432–1442.

Geacintov, N., Stannett, V., Abrahamson, E., and Hermans, J. 1960. Grafting onto cellulose and cellulose derivatives using ultraviolet irradiation. *Journal of Applied Polymer Science*, 3, 54–60.

Goffin, A.-L., Raquez, J.-M., Duquesne, E. et al. 2011a. From interfacial ring-opening polymerization to melt processing of cellulose nanowhisker-filled polylactide-based nanocomposites. *Biomacromolecules*, 12, 2456–2465.

Goffin, A.-L., Raquez, J.-M., Duquesne, E. et al. 2011b. Poly(ε-caprolactone) based nanocomposites reinforced by surface-grafted cellulose nanowhiskers via extrusion processing: Morphology, rheology, and thermo-mechanical properties. *Polymer*, 52, 1532–1538.

Gong, G., Pyo, J., Mathew, A. P., and Oksman, K. 2011. Tensile behavior, morphology and viscoelastic analysis of cellulose nanofiber-reinforced (CNF) polyvinyl acetate (PVAc). *Composites Part A: Applied Science and Manufacturing*, 42, 1275–1282.

Gousse, C., Chanzy, H., Excoffier, G., Soubeyrand, L., and Fleury, E. 2002. Stable suspensions of partially silylated cellulose whiskers dispersed in organic solvents. *Polymer*, 43, 2645–2651.

Gray, D. G. 2008. Transcrystallization of polypropylene at cellulose nanocrystal surfaces. *Cellulose*, 15, 297–301.

Grossman, R. F., Nwabunma, D., Dufresne, A., Thomas, S., and Pothan, L. A. 2013. *Biopolymer Nanocomposites: Processing, Properties, and Applications*. John Wiley & Sons, Hoboken, NJ.

Habibi, Y. and Dufresne, A. 2008. Highly filled bionanocomposites from functionalized polysaccharide nanocrystals. *Biomacromolecules*, 9, 1974–1980.

Habibi, Y., Goffin, A.-L., Schiltz, N. et al. 2008. Bionanocomposites based on poly(ε-caprolactone)-grafted cellulose nanocrystals by ring-opening polymerization. *Journal of Materials Chemistry*, 18, 5002–5010.

Habibi, Y., Lucia, L. A., and Rojas, O. J. 2010. Cellulose nanocrystals: Chemistry, self-assembly, and applications. *Chemical Reviews*, 110, 3479–3500.

Harrisson, S., Drisko, G. L., Malmström, E., Hult, A., and Wooley, K. L. 2011. Hybrid rigid/soft and biologic/synthetic materials: Polymers grafted onto cellulose microcrystals. *Biomacromolecules*, 12, 1214–1223.

Hassan, M. L., Hassan, E. A., and Oksman, K. N. 2011. Effect of pretreatment of bagasse fibers on the properties of chitosan/microfibrillated cellulose nanocomposites. *Journal of Materials Science*, 46, 1732–1740.

Hassan, M. L., Mathew, A. P., Hassan, E. A., El-Wakil, N. A., and Oksman, K. 2012. Nanofibers from bagasse and rice straw: Process optimization and properties. *Wood Science and Technology*, 46, 193–205.

Henriksson, M. and Berglund, L. A. 2007. Structure and properties of cellulose nanocomposite films containing melamine formaldehyde. *Journal of Applied Polymer Science*, 106, 2817–2824.

Henriksson, M., Berglund, L. A., Isaksson, P., Lindström, T., and Nishino, T. 2008. Cellulose nanopaper structures of high toughness. *Biomacromolecules*, 9, 1579–1585.

Henriksson, M., Henriksson, G., Berglund, L., and Lindström, T. 2007. An environmentally friendly method for enzyme-assisted preparation of microfibrillated cellulose (MFC) nanofibers. *European Polymer Journal*, 43, 3434–3441.

Herrick, F. W., Casebier, R. L., Hamilton, J. K., and Sandberg, K. R. 1983. Microfibrillated cellulose: Morphology and accessibility. *Journal of Applied Polymer Science: Applied Polymer Symposium*, ITT Rayonier Inc., Shelton, WA.

Heux, L., Chauve, G., and Bonini, C. 2000. Nonflocculating and chiral-nematic self-ordering of cellulose microcrystals suspensions in nonpolar solvents. *Langmuir*, 16, 8210–8212.

Hossain, K. M. Z., Ahmed, I., Parsons, A. J. et al. 2012. Physico-chemical and mechanical properties of nanocomposites prepared using cellulose nanowhiskers and poly(lactic acid). *Journal of Materials Science*, 47, 2675–2686.

Huang, J., Liu, L., and Yao, J. 2011. Electrospinning of *Bombyx mori* silk fibroin nanofiber mats reinforced by cellulose nanowhiskers. *Fibers and Polymers*, 12, 1002–1006.

Hubbe, M. A., Rojas, O. J., Lucia, L. A., and Sain, M. 2008. Cellulosic nanocomposites: A review. *BioResources*, 3, 929–980.

Iguchi, M., Yamanaka, S., and Budhiono, A. 2000. Bacterial cellulose—A masterpiece of nature's arts. *Journal of Materials Science*, 35, 261–270.

Isogai, A., Saito, T., and Fukuzumi, H. 2011a. TEMPO-oxidized cellulose nanofibers. *Nanoscale*, 3, 71–85.

Isogai, T., Saito, T., and Isogai, A. 2011b. Wood cellulose nanofibrils prepared by TEMPO electro-mediated oxidation. *Cellulose*, 18, 421–431.

Iwamoto, S., Nakagaito, A. N., and Yano, H. 2007. Nano-fibrillation of pulp fibers for the processing of transparent nanocomposites. *Applied Physics A*, 89, 461–466.

Iwamoto, S., Nakagaito, A., Yano, H., and Nogi, M. 2005. Optically transparent composites reinforced with plant fiber-based nanofibers. *Applied Physics A*, 81, 1109–1112.

Iwamoto, S., Yamamoto, S., Lee, S.-H., and Endo, T. 2014. Mechanical properties of polypropylene composites reinforced by surface-coated microfibrillated cellulose. *Composites Part A: Applied Science and Manufacturing*, 59, 26–29.

Iwatake, A., Nogi, M., and Yano, H. 2008. Cellulose nanofiber-reinforced polylactic acid. *Composites Science and Technology*, 68, 2103–2106.

Jalaluddin, A., Araki, J., and Gotoh, Y. 2011. Toward "strong" green nanocomposites: Polyvinyl alcohol reinforced with extremely oriented cellulose whiskers. *Biomacromolecules*, 12, 617–624.

Janardhnan, S. and Sain, M. M. 2007. Isolation of cellulose microfibrils—An enzymatic approach. *Bioresources*, 1, 176–188.

Janardhnan, S., Sain, M., Pervaiz, M., and Dougherty, W. 2006. Novel SMA chemistries in surface sizing of paper and boards. *Annual Meeting-Pulp and Paper Technical Association of Canada*, Pulp and Paper Technical Association of Canada, Montreal, Quebec, Canada, 1999, p. 283.

Jenkins, D. W. and Hudson, S. M. 2001. Review of vinyl graft copolymerization featuring recent advances toward controlled radical-based reactions and illustrated with chitin/chitosan trunk polymers. *Chemical Reviews*, 101, 3245–3274.

Jiang, L., Morelius, E., Zhang, J., Wolcott, M., and Holbery, J. 2008. Study of the poly(3-hydroxybutyrate-*co*-3-hydroxyvalerate)/cellulose nanowhisker composites prepared by solution casting and melt processing. *Journal of Composite Materials*, 42, 2629–2645.

Johari, N., Ahmad, I., and Halib, N. 2012. Comparison study of hydrogels properties synthesized with micro- and nano-size bacterial cellulose particles extracted from Nata de coco. *Chemical and Biochemical Engineering Quarterly*, 26, 399–404.

John, A., Mahadeva, S. K., and Kim, J. 2010. The preparation, characterization and actuation behavior of polyaniline and cellulose blended electro-active paper. *Smart Materials and Structures*, 19, 045011.

John, M. J. and Thomas, S. 2008. Biofibres and biocomposites. *Carbohydrate Polymers*, 71, 343–364.

Jonoobi, M., Harun, J., Mathew, A. P., and Oksman, K. 2010. Mechanical properties of cellulose nanofiber (CNF) reinforced polylactic acid (PLA) prepared by twin screw extrusion. *Composites Science and Technology*, 70, 1742–1747.

Jonoobi, M., Mathew, A. P., Abdi, M. M., Makinejad, M. D., and Oksman, K. 2012. A comparison of modified and unmodified cellulose nanofiber reinforced polylactic acid (PLA) prepared by twin screw extrusion. *Journal of Polymers and the Environment*, 20, 991–997.

Joubert, M., Delaite, C., Bourgeat-Lami, E., and Dumas, P. 2004. Ring-opening polymerization of ε-caprolactone and L-lactide from silica nanoparticles surface. *Journal of Polymer Science Part A: Polymer Chemistry*, 42, 1976–1984.

Joubert, M., Delaite, C., Lami, E. B., and Dumas, P. 2005. Synthesis of poly(ε-caprolactone)–silica nanocomposites: From hairy colloids to core–shell nanoparticles. *New Journal of Chemistry*, 29, 1601–1609.

Junior de Menezes, A., Siqueira, G., Curvelo, A. A., and Dufresne, A. 2009. Extrusion and characterization of functionalized cellulose whiskers reinforced polyethylene nanocomposites. *Polymer*, 50, 4552–4563.

Juntaro, J., Ummartyotin, S., Sain, M., and Manuspiya, H. 2012. Bacterial cellulose reinforced polyurethane-based resin nanocomposite: A study of how ethanol and processing pressure affect physical, mechanical and dielectric properties. *Carbohydrate Polymers*, 87, 2464–2469.

Kaboorani, A., Riedl, B., Blanchet, P. et al. 2012. Nanocrystalline cellulose (NCC): A renewable nano-material for polyvinyl acetate (PVA) adhesive. *European Polymer Journal*, 48, 1829–1837.

Kalia, S., Dufresne, A., Cherian, B. M. et al. 2011. Cellulose-based bio-and nanocomposites: A review. *International Journal of Polymer Science*, 2011, 1–35.

Karande, V., Bharimalla, A., Hadge, G., Mhaske, S., and Vigneshwaran, N. 2011. Nanofibrillation of cotton fibers by disc refiner and its characterization. *Fibers and Polymers*, 12, 399–404.

Kardam, A., Raj, K. R., and Srivastava, S. 2012. Novel nano cellulosic fibers for remediation of heavy metals from synthetic water. *International Journal of Nano Dimension*, 3, 155–162.

Khan, A., Khan, R. A., Salmieri, S. et al. 2012. Mechanical and barrier properties of nanocrystalline cellulose reinforced chitosan based nanocomposite films. *Carbohydrate Polymers*, 90, 1601–1608.

Kim, J., Yun, S., Mahadeva, S. K. et al. 2010. Paper actuators made with cellulose and hybrid materials. *Sensors*, 10, 1473–1485.

Kloser, E. and Gray, D. G. 2010. Surface grafting of cellulose nanocrystals with poly(ethylene oxide) in aqueous media. *Langmuir*, 26, 13450–13456.

Koshizawa, T. 1960. Degradation of wood cellulose and cotton linters in phosphoric acid. *Kami Pa Gikyoshi*, 14, 455.

Kurihara, T. and Isogai, A. 2014. Properties of poly(acrylamide)/TEMPO-oxidized cellulose nanofibril composite films. *Cellulose*, 21, 291–299.

Kvien, I., Sugiyama, J., Votrubec, M., and Oksman, K. 2007. Characterization of starch based nanocomposites. *Journal of Materials Science*, 42, 8163–8171.

Labet, M. and Thielemans, W. 2011. Improving the reproducibility of chemical reactions on the surface of cellulose nanocrystals: ROP of ε-caprolactone as a case study. *Cellulose*, 18, 607–617.

Lam, E., Male, K. B., Chong, J. H., Leung, A. C., and Luong, J. H. 2012. Applications of functionalized and nanoparticle-modified nanocrystalline cellulose. *Trends in Biotechnology*, 30, 283–290.

Lavoine, N., Desloges, I., Dufresne, A., and Bras, J. 2012. Microfibrillated cellulose—Its barrier properties and applications in cellulosic materials: A review. *Carbohydrate Polymers*, 90, 735–764.

Lee, J. and Deng, Y. 2012. Increased mechanical properties of aligned and isotropic electrospun PVA nanofiber webs by cellulose nanowhisker reinforcement. *Macromolecular Research*, 20, 76–83.

Lee, R.-S., Chen, W.-H., and Lin, J.-H. 2011a. Polymer-grafted multi-walled carbon nanotubes through surface-initiated ring-opening polymerization and click reaction. *Polymer*, 52, 2180–2188.

Lee, S.-H., Teramoto, Y., and Endo, T. 2011b. Cellulose nanofiber-reinforced polycaprolactone/polypropylene hybrid nanocomposite. *Composites Part A: Applied Science and Manufacturing*, 42, 151–156.

Lee, S.-Y., Chun, S.-J., Kang, I.-A., and Park, J.-Y. 2009a. Preparation of cellulose nanofibrils by high-pressure homogenizer and cellulose-based composite films. *Journal of Industrial and Engineering Chemistry*, 15, 50–55.

Lee, S.-Y., Mohan, D. J., Kang, I.-A. et al. 2009b. Nanocellulose reinforced PVA composite films: Effects of acid treatment and filler loading. *Fibers and Polymers*, 10, 77–82.

Leitner, J., Hinterstoisser, B., Wastyn, M., Keckes, J., and Gindl, W. 2007. Sugar beet cellulose nanofibril-reinforced composites. *Cellulose*, 14, 419–425.

Li, Q., Zhou, J., and Zhang, L. 2009. Structure and properties of the nanocomposite films of chitosan reinforced with cellulose whiskers. *Journal of Polymer Science Part B: Polymer Physics*, 47, 1069–1077.

Li, W., Yue, J., and Liu, S. 2012. Preparation of nanocrystalline cellulose via ultrasound and its reinforcement capability for poly(vinyl alcohol) composites. *Ultrasonics Sonochemistry*, 19, 479–485.

Li, X.-F., Ding, E., and Li, G. 2001. A method of preparing spherical nano-crystal cellulose with mixed crystalline forms of cellulose I and II. *Chinese Journal of Polymer Science*, 19, 291–296.

Li, Y. and Ragauskas, A. J. 2011. Cellulose nano whiskers as a reinforcing filler in polyurethanes. *Algae*, 75, 10–15.

Li, Y. and Ragauskas, A. J. 2012. Ethanol organosolv lignin-based rigid polyurethane foam reinforced with cellulose nanowhiskers. *RSC Advances*, 2, 3347–3351.

Li, Y., Ren, H., and Ragauskas, A. J. 2011. Rigid polyurethane foam/cellulose whisker nanocomposites: Preparation, characterization, and properties. *Journal of Nanoscience and Nanotechnology*, 11, 6904–6911.

Liew, S. Y., Thielemans, W., and Walsh, D. A. 2010. Electrochemical capacitance of nanocomposite polypyrrole/cellulose films. *The Journal of Physical Chemistry C*, 114, 17926–17933.

Lin, N., Chen, G., Huang, J., Dufresne, A., and Chang, P. R. 2009. Effects of polymer-grafted natural nanocrystals on the structure and mechanical properties of poly(lactic acid): A case of cellulose whisker-*graft*-polycaprolactone. *Journal of Applied Polymer Science*, 113, 3417–3425.

Lin, N., Huang, J., Chang, P. R., Feng, J., and Yu, J. 2011. Surface acetylation of cellulose nanocrystal and its reinforcing function in poly(lactic acid). *Carbohydrate Polymers*, 83, 1834–1842.

Lin, S., Huang, J., Chang, P. R. et al. 2013. Structure and mechanical properties of new biomass-based nanocomposite: Castor oil-based polyurethane reinforced with acetylated cellulose nanocrystal. *Carbohydrate Polymers*, 95, 91–99.

Littunen, K., Hippi, U., Johansson, L.-S. et al. 2011. Free radical graft copolymerization of nanofibrillated cellulose with acrylic monomers. *Carbohydrate Polymers*, 84, 1039–1047.

Liu, D., Yuan, X., and Bhattacharyya, D. 2012a. The effects of cellulose nanowhiskers on electrospun poly(lactic acid) nanofibres. *Journal of Materials Science*, 47, 3159–3165.

Liu, D. G., Zhong, T. H., Chang, P. R., Li, K. F., and Wu, Q. L. 2010. Starch composites reinforced by bamboo cellulosic crystals. *Bioresource Technology*, 101, 2529–2536.

Liu, H., Cui, S., Shang, S., Wang, D., and Song, J. 2013. Properties of rosin-based waterborne polyurethanes/cellulose nanocrystals composites. *Carbohydrate Polymers*, 96, 510–515.

Liu, H., Song, J., Shang, S., Song, Z., and Wang, D. 2012b. Cellulose nanocrystal/silver nanoparticle composites as bifunctional nanofillers within waterborne polyurethane. *ACS Applied Materials and Interfaces*, 4, 2413–2419.

Lönnberg, H., Fogelström, L., Berglund, L., Malmström, E., and Hult, A. 2008. Surface grafting of microfibrillated cellulose with poly(ε-caprolactone)—Synthesis and characterization. *European Polymer Journal*, 44, 2991–2997.

Lönnberg, H., Fogelström, L., Zhou, Q. et al. 2011a. Investigation of the graft length impact on the interfacial toughness in a cellulose/poly(ε-caprolactone) bilayer laminate. *Composites Science and Technology*, 71, 9–12.

Lönnberg, H., Larsson, K., Lindstrom, T., Hult, A., and Malmström, E. 2011b. Synthesis of polycaprolactone-grafted microfibrillated cellulose for use in novel bionanocomposites—Influence of the graft length on the mechanical properties. *ACS Applied Materials and Interfaces*, 3, 1426–1433.

Lu, J., Wang, T., and Drzal, L. T. 2008. Preparation and properties of microfibrillated cellulose polyvinyl alcohol composite materials. *Composites Part A: Applied Science and Manufacturing*, 39, 738–746.

Lu, P. and Hsieh, Y.-L. 2009. Cellulose nanocrystal-filled poly(acrylic acid) nanocomposite fibrous membranes. *Nanotechnology*, 20, 415–604.

Luong, N. D., Korhonen, J. T., Soininen, A. J. et al. 2013. Processable polyaniline suspensions through in situ polymerization onto nanocellulose. *European Polymer Journal*, 49, 335–344.

Ma, H., Zhou, B., Li, H.-S., Li, Y.-Q., and Ou, S.-Y. 2011. Green composite films composed of nanocrystalline cellulose and a cellulose matrix regenerated from functionalized ionic liquid solution. *Carbohydrate Polymers*, 84, 383–389.

Magalhaes, W. L. E., Cao, X., and Lucia, L. A. 2009. Cellulose nanocrystals/cellulose core-in-shell nanocomposite assemblies. *Langmuir*, 25, 13250–13257.

Mahi, H. and Rodrigue, D. 2012. Linear and non-linear viscoelastic properties of ethylene vinyl acetate/nanocrystalline cellulose composites. *Rheologica Acta*, 51, 127–142.

Maiti, S., Jayaramudu, J., Das, K. et al. 2013. Preparation and characterization of nano-cellulose with new shape from different precursor. *Carbohydrate Polymers*, 98, 562–567.

Mangalam, A. P., Simonsen, J., and Benight, A. S. 2009. Cellulose/DNA hybrid nanomaterials. *Biomacromolecules*, 10, 497–504.

Marcovich, N., Auad, M., Bellesi, N., Nutt, S., and Aranguren, M. 2006. Cellulose micro/nanocrystals reinforced polyurethane. *Journal of Materials Research*, 21, 870–881.

Martínez-Sanz, M., Lopez-Rubio, A., and Lagaron, J. M. 2013. Nanocomposites of ethylene vinyl alcohol copolymer with thermally resistant cellulose nanowhiskers by melt compounding (II): Water barrier and mechanical properties. *Journal of Applied Polymer Science*, 128, 2197–2207.

Martínez-Sanz, M., Olsson, R. T., Lopez-Rubio, A., and Lagaron, J. M. 2011. Development of electrospun EVOH fibres reinforced with bacterial cellulose nanowhiskers. Part I: Characterization and method optimization. *Cellulose*, 18, 335–347.

Martínez-Sanz, M., Olsson, R. T., Lopez-Rubio, A., and Lagaron, J. M. 2012. Development of bacterial cellulose nanowhiskers reinforced EVOH composites by electrospinning. *Journal of Applied Polymer Science*, 124, 1398–1408.

Mathew, A. P. and Dufresne, A. 2002. Morphological investigation of nanocomposites from sorbitol plasticized starch and tunicin whiskers. *Biomacromolecules*, 3, 609–617.

Mathew, A. P., Thielemans, W., and Dufresne, A. 2008. Mechanical properties of nanocomposites from sorbitol plasticized starch and tunicin whiskers. *Journal of Applied Polymer Science*, 109, 4065–4074.

Matos Ruiz, M., Cavaille, J., Dufresne, A., Gerard, J., and Graillat, C. 2000. Processing and characterization of new thermoset nanocomposites based on cellulose whiskers. *Composite Interfaces*, 7, 117–131.

Mattoso, L., Medeiros, E., Baker, D. et al. 2009. Electrically conductive nanocomposites made from cellulose nanofibrils and polyaniline. *Journal of Nanoscience and Nanotechnology*, 9, 2917–2922.

Meier, H. 1962. Chemical and morphological aspects of the fine structure of wood. *Pure and Applied Chemistry*, 5, 37–52.

Mikkonen, K. S., Mathew, A. P., Pirkkalainen, K. et al. 2010. Glucomannan composite films with cellulose nanowhiskers. *Cellulose*, 17, 69–81.

Mishra, A., Srinivasan, R., and Gupta, R. 2003. *P. psyllium*-g-polyacrylonitrile: Synthesis and characterization. *Colloid and Polymer Science*, 281, 187–189.

Missoum, K., Belgacem, M., and Bras, J. 2013. Nanofibrillated cellulose surface modification: A review. *Materials*, 6, 1745–1766.

Mittal, A., Katahira, R., Himmel, M. E., and Johnson, D. K. 2011. Effects of alkaline or liquid-ammonia treatment on crystalline cellulose: Changes in crystalline structure and effects on enzymatic digestibility. *Biotechnology for Biofuels*, 4, 1–16.

Mohamad Haafiz, M., Eichhorn, S., Hassan, A., and Jawaid, M. 2013. Isolation and characterization of microcrystalline cellulose from oil palm biomass residue. *Carbohydrate Polymers*, 93, 628–634.

Morandi, G., Heath, L., and Thielemans, W. 2009. Cellulose nanocrystals grafted with polystyrene chains through surface-initiated atom transfer radical polymerization (SI-ATRP). *Langmuir*, 25, 8280–8286.

Müller, D., Rambo, C. R., D.O.S. Recouvreux, Porto, L. M., and Barra, G. M. O. 2011. Chemical in situ polymerization of polypyrrole on bacterial cellulose nanofibers. *Synthetic Metals*, 161, 106–111.

Mutwil, M., Debolt, S., and Persson, S. 2008. Cellulose synthesis: A complex complex. *Current Opinion in Plant Biology*, 11, 252–257.

Nakagaito, A. N., Fujimura, A., Sakai, T., Hama, Y., and Yano, H. 2009. Production of microfibrillated cellulose (MFC)-reinforced polylactic acid (PLA) nanocomposites from sheets obtained by a papermaking-like process. *Composites Science and Technology*, 69, 1293–1297.

Nakagaito, A. N. and Yano, H. 2004. The effect of morphological changes from pulp fiber towards nano-scale fibrillated cellulose on the mechanical properties of high-strength plant fiber based composites. *Applied Physics A*, 78, 547–552.

Namazi, H. and Dadkhah, A. 2008. Surface modification of starch nanocrystals through ring-opening polymerization of ε-caprolactone and investigation of their microstructures. *Journal of Applied Polymer Science*, 110, 2405–2412.

Namazi, H. and Dadkhah, A. 2010. Convenient method for preparation of hydrophobically modified starch nanocrystals with using fatty acids. *Carbohydrate Polymers*, 79, 731–737.

Nasri-Nasrabadi, B., Behzad, T., and Bagheri, R. 2014. Preparation and characterization of cellulose nanofiber reinforced thermoplastic starch composites. *Fibers and Polymers*, 15, 347–354.

Nj Heyn, A. 1969. The elementary fibril and supermolecular structure of cellulose in soft wood fiber. *Journal of Ultrastructure Research*, 26, 52–68.

Noishiki, Y., Nishiyama, Y., Wada, M., Kuga, S., and Magoshi, J. 2002. Mechanical properties of silk fibroin—Microcrystalline cellulose composite films. *Journal of Applied Polymer Science*, 86, 3425–3429.

O'Connell, D., Birkinshaw, C., and O'Dwyer, T. 2006. A chelating cellulose adsorbent for the removal of Cu(II) from aqueous solutions. *Journal of Applied Polymer Science*, 99, 2888–2897.

Okano, T., Kuga, S., Wada, M., Araki, J., and Ikuina, J. 1999. A fine cellulose particle and its production, Nisshin Oil Mills Ltd., Japan. JP Patent, 98–151052.

Okieimen, F. 2003. Preparation, characterization, and properties of cellulose—Polyacrylamide graft copolymers. *Journal of Applied Polymer Science*, 89, 913–923.

Oksman, K., Mathew, A., Bondeson, D., and Kvien, I. 2006. Manufacturing process of cellulose whiskers/polylactic acid nanocomposites. *Composites Science and Technology*, 66, 2776–2784.

Oksman, K. and Sain, M. 2006. *Cellulose Nanocomposites: Processing, Characterization, and Properties.* American Chemical Society, Washington, DC.

Olsson, R. T., Kraemer, R., Lopez-Rubio, A. et al. 2010. Extraction of microfibrils from bacterial cellulose networks for electrospinning of anisotropic biohybrid fiber yarns. *Macromolecules*, 43, 4201–4209.

Orts, W. J., Shey, J., Imam, S. H. et al. 2005. Application of cellulose microfibrils in polymer nanocomposites. *Journal of Polymers and the Environment*, 13, 301–306.

Pääkkö, M., Ankerfors, M., Kosonen, H. et al. 2007. Enzymatic hydrolysis combined with mechanical shearing and high-pressure homogenization for nanoscale cellulose fibrils and strong gels. *Biomacromolecules*, 8, 1934–1941.

Pan, M., Zhou, X., and Chen, M. 2013. Cellulose nanowhiskers isolation and properties from acid hydrolysis combined with high pressure homogenization. *BioResources*, 8, 933–943.

Paralikar, S. A., Simonsen, J., and Lombardi, J. 2008. Poly(vinyl alcohol)/cellulose nanocrystal barrier membranes. *Journal of Membrane Science*, 320, 248–258.

Park, S. H., Oh, K. W., and Kim, S. H. 2013. Reinforcement effect of cellulose nanowhisker on bio-based polyurethane. *Composites Science and Technology*, 86, 82–88.

Park, W. I., Kang, M., Kim, H. S., and Jin, H. J. 2007. Electrospinning of poly(ethylene oxide) with bacterial cellulose whiskers. *Macromolecular Symposia*, 249–250, 289–294.

Pei, A., Malho, J.-M., Ruokolainen, J., Zhou, Q., and Berglund, L. A. 2011. Strong nanocomposite reinforcement effects in polyurethane elastomer with low volume fraction of cellulose nanocrystals. *Macromolecules*, 44, 4422–4427.

Pei, A., Zhou, Q., and Berglund, L. A. 2010. Functionalized cellulose nanocrystals as biobased nucleation agents in poly(L-lactide)(PLLA)—Crystallization and mechanical property effects. *Composites Science and Technology*, 70, 815–821.

Peng, B., Dhar, N., Liu, H., and Tam, K. 2011. Chemistry and applications of nanocrystalline cellulose and its derivatives: A nanotechnology perspective. *The Canadian Journal of Chemical Engineering*, 89, 1191–1206.

Peresin, M. S., Habibi, Y., Zoppe, J. O., Pawlak, J. J., and Rojas, O. J. 2010. Nanofiber composites of polyvinyl alcohol and cellulose nanocrystals: Manufacture and characterization. *Biomacromolecules*, 11, 674–681.

Petersson, L., Kvien, I., and Oksman, K. 2007. Structure and thermal properties of poly(lactic acid)/cellulose whiskers nanocomposite materials. *Composites Science and Technology*, 67, 2535–2544.

Petersson, L. and Oksman, K. 2006. Biopolymer based nanocomposites: Comparing layered silicates and microcrystalline cellulose as nanoreinforcement. *Composites Science and Technology*, 66, 2187–2196.

Pinto, E. R., Barud, H. S., Polito, W. L., Ribeiro, S. J., and Messaddeq, Y. 2013. Preparation and characterization of the bacterial cellulose/polyurethane nanocomposites. *Journal of Thermal Analysis and Calorimetry*, 114, 549–555.

Pranger, L. and Tannenbaum, R. 2008. Biobased nanocomposites prepared by in situ polymerization of furfuryl alcohol with cellulose whiskers or montmorillonite clay. *Macromolecules*, 41, 8682–8687.

Press release. 2011. Nanocellulose-for the first time on a large scale-Innventia [Online]. *Innventia*. http://www.innventia.com/en/About-us/News1/Press-Release-Nanocellulose-for-the-first-time-on-a-large-scale/ (accessed March 26, 2014).

Qi, H., Cai, J., Zhang, L., and Kuga, S. 2009. Properties of films composed of cellulose nanowhiskers and a cellulose matrix regenerated from alkali/urea solution. *Biomacromolecules*, 10, 1597–1602.

Qiu, K. and Netravali, A. N. 2012. Fabrication and characterization of biodegradable composites based on microfibrillated cellulose and polyvinyl alcohol. *Composites Science and Technology*, 72, 1588–1594.

Ramirez, M. A. 2010. Cellulose nanocrystals reinforced electrospun poly(lactic acid) fbers as potential scaffold for bone tissure engineering. *MS thesis*, North Carolina State University.

Rånby, B. G. 1951. Fibrous macromolecular systems. Cellulose and muscle. The colloidal properties of cellulose micelles. *Discussions of the Faraday Society*, 11, 158–164.

Rodriguez, F., Castillo-Ortega, M., Encinas, J. et al. 2009. Preparation, characterization, and adsorption properties of cellulose acetate-polyaniline membranes. *Journal of Applied Polymer Science*, 111, 1216–1224.

Rodríguez, K., Renneckar, S., and Gatenholm, P. 2011. Biomimetic calcium phosphate crystal mineralization on electrospun cellulose-based scaffolds. *ACS Applied Materials and Interfaces*, 3, 681–689.

Rojas, O. J., Montero, G. A., and Habibi, Y. 2009. Electrospun nanocomposites from polystyrene loaded with cellulose nanowhiskers. *Journal of Applied Polymer Science*, 113, 927–935.

Roohani, M., Habibi, Y., Belgacem, N. M. et al. 2008. Cellulose whiskers reinforced polyvinyl alcohol copolymers nanocomposites. *European Polymer Journal*, 44, 2489–2498.

Rosa, M. F., Medeiros, E. S., Imam, S. H., Malmonge, J. A., and Mattoso, L. H. C. 2009. Nanocompósitos de borracha natural reforçados com nanowhiskers de fbra de coco imaturo. *Embrapa Agroindústria Tropical-Artigo em anais de congresso (ALICE)*. São Carlos-SP, pp 222–224.

Rowland, S. P. and Roberts, E. J. 1972. The nature of accessible surfaces in the microstructure of cotton cellulose. *Journal of Polymer Science Part A-1: Polymer Chemistry*, 10, 2447–2461.

Roy, D., Semsarilar, M., Guthrie, J. T., and Perrier, S. 2009. Cellulose modification by polymer grafting: A review. *Chemical Society Reviews*, 38, 2046–2064.

Rueda, L., Saralegui, A., Fernández D'arlas, B. et al. 2013. Cellulose nanocrystals/polyurethane nanocomposites. Study from the viewpoint of microphase separated structure. *Carbohydrate Polymers*, 92, 751–757.

Ruiz, M. M., Cavaille, J. Y., Dufresne, A., Graillat, C., and Gerard, J. F. 2001. New waterborne epoxy coatings based on cellulose nanofillers. *Macromolecular Symposia*, 169, 211–222.

Rusli, R. and Eichhorn, S. J. 2008. Determination of the stiffness of cellulose nanowhiskers and the fiber-matrix interface in a nanocomposite using Raman spectroscopy. *Applied Physics Letters*, 93, 033111.

Rusli, R., Shanmuganathan, K., Rowan, S. J., Weder, C., and Eichhorn, S. J. 2010. Stress-transfer in anisotropic and environmentally adaptive cellulose whisker nanocomposites. *Biomacromolecules*, 11, 762–768.

Saralegi, A., Rueda, L., Martin, L. et al. 2013. From elastomeric to rigid polyurethane/cellulose nanocrystal bionanocomposites. *Composites Science and Technology*, 88, 39–47.

Seydibeyoğlu, M. Ö., Misra, M., Mohanty, A. et al. 2013. Green polyurethane nanocomposites from soy polyol and bacterial cellulose. *Journal of Materials Science*, 48, 2167–2175.

Shi, Q., Zhou, C., Yue, Y. et al. 2012. Mechanical properties and in vitro degradation of electrospun bionanocomposite mats from PLA and cellulose nanocrystals. *Carbohydrate Polymers*, 90, 301–308.

Shng, L., Jiang, R., Zhu, Y., and Ji, Y. 2013. Electrospun cellulose nanocrystals/polycaprolactone nanocomposite fiber mats. *Journal of Macromolecular Science, Part B*, 53, 820–828.

Siqueira, G., Bras, J., and Dufresne, A. 2009. New process of chemical grafting of cellulose nanoparticles with a long chain isocyanate. *Langmuir*, 26, 402–411.

Siqueira, G., Bras, J., and Dufresne, A. 2010a. Cellulosic bionanocomposites: A review of preparation, properties and applications. *Polymers*, 2, 728–765.

Siqueira, G., Fraschini, C., Bras, J. et al. 2011a. Impact of the nature and shape of cellulosic nanoparticles on the isothermal crystallization kinetics of poly(ε-caprolactone). *European Polymer Journal*, 47, 2216–2227.

Siqueira, G., Tapin-Lingua, S., Bras, J., Da Silva Perez, D., and Dufresne, A. 2010b. Morphological investigation of nanoparticles obtained from combined mechanical shearing, and enzymatic and acid hydrolysis of sisal fibers. *Cellulose*, 17, 1147–1158.

Siqueira, G., Tapin-Lingua, S., Bras, J., Da Silva Perez, D., and Dufresne, A. 2011b. Mechanical properties of natural rubber nanocomposites reinforced with cellulosic nanoparticles obtained from combined mechanical shearing, and enzymatic and acid hydrolysis of sisal fibers. *Cellulose*, 18, 57–65.

Siró, I. and Plackett, D. 2010. Microfibrillated cellulose and new nanocomposite materials: A review. *Cellulose*, 17, 459–494.

Smith, J. S., Bedrov, D., and Smith, G. D. 2003. A molecular dynamics simulation study of nanoparticle interactions in a model polymer-nanoparticle composite. *Composites Science and Technology*, 63, 1599–1605.

Somerville, C. 2006. Cellulose synthesis in higher plants. *Annual Review of Cell and Developmental Biology*, 22, 53–78.

Srithep, Y., Ellingham, T., Peng, J. et al. 2013. Melt compounding of poly(3-hydroxybutyrate-*co*-3-hydroxyvalerate)/nanofibrillated cellulose nanocomposites. *Polymer Degradation and Stability*, 98, 1439–1449.

Srithep, Y., Turng, L.-S., Sabo, R., and Clemons, C. 2012. Nanofibrillated cellulose (NFC) reinforced polyvinyl alcohol (PVOH) nanocomposites: Properties, solubility of carbon dioxide, and foaming. *Cellulose*, 19, 1209–1223.

Stenstad, P., Andresen, M., Tanem, B. S., and Stenius, P. 2008. Chemical surface modifications of microfibrillated cellulose. *Cellulose*, 15, 35–45.

Šturcová, A., Davies, G. R., and Eichhorn, S. J. 2005. Elastic modulus and stress-transfer properties of tunicate cellulose whiskers. *Biomacromolecules*, 6, 1055–1061.

Suryanegara, L., Nakagaito, A. N., and Yano, H. 2009. The effect of crystallization of PLA on the thermal and mechanical properties of microfibrillated cellulose-reinforced PLA composites. *Composites Science and Technology*, 69, 1187–1192.

Suryanegara, L., Nakagaito, A. N., and Yano, H. 2010. Thermo-mechanical properties of microfibrillated cellulose-reinforced partially crystallized PLA composites. *Cellulose*, 17, 771–778.

Svagan, A. J., Hedenqvist, M. S., and Berglund, L. 2009. Reduced water vapour sorption in cellulose nanocomposites with starch matrix. *Composites Science and Technology*, 69, 500–506.

Syverud, K. and Stenius, P. 2009. Strength and barrier properties of MFC films. *Cellulose*, 16, 75–85.

Szczęsna-Antczak, M., Kazimierczak, J., Antczak, T. et al. 2012. Nanotechnology–Methods of Manufacturing Cellulose Nanofibers. *Fibres and textiles in Eastern Europe*, 20, 8–12.

Taipale, T., Österberg, M., Nykänen, A., Ruokolainen, J., and Laine, J. 2010. Effect of microfibrillated cellulose and fines on the drainage of kraft pulp suspension and paper strength. *Cellulose*, 17, 1005–1020.

Tanpichai, S., Sampson, W., and Eichhorn, S. 2012. Stress-transfer in microfibrillated cellulose reinforced poly(lactic acid) composites using Raman spectroscopy. *Composites Part A: Applied Science and Manufacturing*, 43, 1145–1152.

Ten, E., Bahr, D. F., Li, B., Jiang, L., and Wolcott, M. P. 2012a. Effects of cellulose nanowhiskers on mechanical, dielectric, and rheological properties of poly(3-hydroxybutyrate-*co*-3-hydroxyvalerate)/cellulose nanowhisker composites. *Industrial and Engineering Chemistry Research*, 51, 2941–2951.

Ten, E., Jiang, L., and Wolcott, M. P. 2012b. Crystallization kinetics of poly(3-hydroxybutyrate-*co*-3-hydroxyvalerate)/cellulose nanowhiskers composites. *Carbohydrate Polymers*, 90, 541–550.

Ten, E., Jiang, L., and Wolcott, M. P. 2013. Preparation and properties of aligned poly(3-hydroxybutyrate-*co*-3-hydroxyvalerate)/cellulose nanowhiskers composites. *Carbohydrate Polymers*, 92, 206–213.

Ten, E., Turtle, J., Bahr, D., Jiang, L., and Wolcott, M. 2010. Thermal and mechanical properties of poly(3-hydroxybutyrate-*co*-3-hydroxyvalerate)/cellulose nanowhiskers composites. *Polymer*, 51, 2652–2660.

Thakur, V. K. 2013. *Green Composites from Natural Resources*. CRC Press, Boca Raton, FL.

Tingaut, P., Zimmermann, T., and Lopez-Suevos, F. 2009. Synthesis and characterization of bionanocomposites with tunable properties from poly(lactic acid) and acetylated microfibrillated cellulose. *Biomacromolecules*, 11, 454–464.

Turbak, A. F., Snyder, F. W., and Sandberg, K. R. 1983. Microfibrillated cellulose, a new cellulose product: Properties, uses, and commercial potential. *Journal of Applied Polymer Science Applied Polymer Symposium*, 37, 815–827.

Uetani, K. and Yano, H. 2011. Zeta potential time dependence reveals the swelling dynamics of wood cellulose nanofibrils. *Langmuir*, 28, 818–827.

Usuda, M., Suzuki, O., Nakano, J., and Migita, N. 1967. Acid hydrolysis of cellulose in concentrated phosphoric acid: Effects of modified groups of cellulose on the rate of hydrolysis. *Kogyo Kagaku Zasshi*, 70, 349–352.

Valo, H., Arola, S., Laaksonen, P. et al. 2013. Drug release from nanoparticles embedded in four different nanofibrillar cellulose aerogels. *European Journal of Pharmaceutical Sciences*, 50, 69–77.

Van De Wetering, P., Cherng, J.-Y., Talsma, H., Crommelin, D., and Hennink, W. 1998. 2-(Dimethylamino) ethyl methacrylate based (co) polymers as gene transfer agents. *Journal of Controlled Release*, 53, 145–153.

Virji, S., Kaner, R. B., and Weiller, B. H. 2006. Hydrogen sensors based on conductivity changes in polyaniline nanofibers. *The Journal of Physical Chemistry B*, 110, 22266–22270.

Virtanen, S., Vartiainen, J., Setälä, H., Tammelin, T., and Vuoti, S. 2014. Modified nanofibrillated cellulose-polyvinyl alcohol films with improved mechanical performance. *RSC Advances*, 4, 11343–11350.

Visakh, P., Thomas, S., Oksman, K., and Mathew, A. P. 2012a. Cellulose nanofibres and cellulose nanowhiskers based natural rubber composites: Diffusion, sorption, and permeation of aromatic organic solvents. *Journal of Applied Polymer Science*, 124, 1614–1623.

Visakh, P., Thomas, S., Oksman, K., and Mathew, A. P. 2012b. Crosslinked natural rubber nanocomposites reinforced with cellulose whiskers isolated from bamboo waste: Processing and mechanical/thermal properties. *Composites Part A: Applied Science and Manufacturing*, 43, 735–741.

Visakh, P., Thomas, S., Oksman, K., and Mathewa, A. P. 2012c. Effect of cellulose nanofibers isolated from bamboo pulp residue on vulcanized natural rubber. *BioResources*, 7, 2156–2168.

Wang, B. and Sain, M. 2007. The effect of chemically coated nanofiber reinforcement on biopolymer based nanocomposites. *BioResources*, 2, 371–388.

Wang, N., Ding, E., and Cheng, R. 2007. Thermal degradation behaviors of spherical cellulose nanocrystals with sulfate groups. *Polymer*, 48, 3486–3493.

Wang, T. and Drzal, L. T. 2012. Cellulose-nanofiber-reinforced poly(lactic acid) composites prepared by a water-based approach. *ACS Applied Materials and Interfaces*, 4, 5079–5085.

Wang, X., Qu, P., and Zhang, L. 2014a. Thermal and structure properties of biobased cellulose nanowhiskers/poly(lactic acid) nanocomposites. *Fibers and Polymers*, 15, 302–306.
Wang, Y., Cao, X., and Zhang, L. 2006. Effects of cellulose whiskers on properties of soy protein thermoplastics. *Macromolecular Bioscience*, 6, 524–531.
Wang, Z., Ma, H., Hsiao, B. S., and Chu, B. 2014b. Nanofibrous ultrafiltration membranes containing cross-linked poly(ethylene glycol) and cellulose nanofiber composite barrier layer. *Polymer*, 55, 366–372.
Wu, G.-M., Chen, J., Huo, S.-P., Liu, G.-F., and Kong, Z.-W. 2014. Thermoset nanocomposites from two-component waterborne polyurethanes and cellulose whiskers. *Carbohydrate Polymers*, 105, 207–213.
Wu, T., Fanwood, R., O'Kelly, K., and Chen, B. 2014. Mechanical behavior of transparent nano fibrillar cellulose-chitosan nano composite films in dry and wet conditions. *Journal of Mechanical Behavior of Biomedical Materials*, 32, 279–286.
Xiang, C., Joo, Y. L., and Frey, M. W. 2009. Nanocomposite fibers electrospun from poly(lactic acid)/cellulose nanocrystals. *Journal of Biobased Materials and Bioenergy*, 3, 147–155.
Xu, Q., Yi, J., Zhang, X., and Zhang, H. 2008. A novel amphotropic polymer based on cellulose nanocrystals grafted with azo polymers. *European Polymer Journal*, 44, 2830–2837.
Xu, S., Girouard, N., Schueneman, G., Shofner, M. L., and Meredith, J. C. 2013. Mechanical and thermal properties of waterborne epoxy composites containing cellulose nanocrystals. *Polymer*, 54, 6589–6598.
Xu, S., Gu, J., Luo, Y., and Jia, D. 2012. Effects of partial replacement of silica with surface modified nanocrystalline cellulose on properties of natural rubber nanocomposites. *Express Polymer Letters*, 6, 14–25.
Yang, J. and Ye, D. Y. 2012. Liquid crystal of nanocellulose whiskers' grafted with acrylamide. *Chinese Chemical Letters*, 23, 367–370.
Yi, J., Xu, Q., Zhang, X., and Zhang, H. 2008. Chiral-nematic self-ordering of rodlike cellulose nanocrystals grafted with poly(styrene) in both thermotropic and lyotropic states. *Polymer*, 49, 4406–4412.
Yi, J., Xu, Q., Zhang, X., and Zhang, H. 2009. Temperature-induced chiral nematic phase changes of suspensions of poly(N,N-dimethylaminoethyl methacrylate)-grafted cellulose nanocrystals. *Cellulose*, 16, 989–997.
Yu, H.-Y., Qin, Z.-Y., and Zhou, Z. 2011. Cellulose nanocrystals as green fillers to improve crystallization and hydrophilic property of poly(3-hydroxybutyrate-*co*-3-hydroxyvalerate). *Progress in Natural Science: Materials International*, 21, 478–484.
Zaar, K. 1977. Biogenesis of cellulose by *Acetobacter xylinum*. *Cytobiologie*, 16, 1–15.
Zahran, M. and Mahmoud, R. 2003. Peroxydiphosphate–metal ion–cellulose thiocarbonate redox system-induced graft copolymerization of vinyl monomers onto cotton fabric. *Journal of Applied Polymer Science*, 87, 1879–1889.
Zeng, H. L., Gao, C., and Yan, D. Y. 2006. Poly(ε-caprolactone)—Functionalized carbon nanotubes and their biodegradation properties. *Advanced Functional Materials*, 16, 812–818.
Zhang, D., Zhang, Q., Gao, X., and Piao, G. 2013. A nanocellulose polypyrrole composite based on tunicate cellulose. *International Journal of Polymer Science*, 2013, 1–6.
Zhang, J., Elder, T. J., Pu, Y., and Ragauskas, A. J. 2007. Facile synthesis of spherical cellulose nanoparticles. *Carbohydrate Polymers*, 69, 607–611.
Zhang, M., Liu, L., Zhao, H. et al. 2006. Double-responsive polymer brushes on the surface of colloid particles. *Journal of Colloid and Interface Science*, 301, 85–91.
Zhang, W., He, X., Li, C. et al. 2014. High performance poly(vinyl alcohol)/cellulose nanocrystals nanocomposites manufactured by injection molding. *Cellulose*, 21, 485–494.
Zhao, Q., Sun, G., Yan, K., Zhou, A., and Chen, Y. 2013. Novel bio-antifelting agent based on waterborne polyurethane and cellulose nanocrystals. *Carbohydrate Polymers*, 91, 169–174.
Zhou, C., Chu, R., Wu, R., and Wu, Q. 2011a. Electrospun polyethylene oxide/cellulose nanocrystal composite nanofibrous mats with homogeneous and heterogeneous microstructures. *Biomacromolecules*, 12, 2617–2625.
Zhou, C., Wang, Q., and Wu, Q. 2012. UV-initiated crosslinking of electrospun poly(ethylene oxide) nanofibers with pentaerythritol triacrylate: Effect of irradiation time and incorporated cellulose nanocrystals. *Carbohydrate Polymers*, 87, 1779–1786.
Zhou, C., Wu, Q., Yue, Y., and Zhang, Q. 2011b. Application of rod-shaped cellulose nanocrystals in polyacrylamide hydrogels. *Journal of Colloid and Interface Science*, 353, 116–123.
Zimmermann, T., Pöhler, E., and Geiger, T. 2004. Cellulose fibrils for polymer reinforcement. *Advanced Engineering Materials*, 6, 754–761.
Zimmermann, T., Pöhler, E., and Schwaller, P. 2005. Mechanical and morphological properties of cellulose fibril reinforced nanocomposites. *Advanced Engineering Materials*, 7, 1156–1161.

Zoppe, J. O., Habibi, Y., Rojas, O. J. et al. 2010. Poly(N-isopropylacrylamide) brushes grafted from cellulose nanocrystals via surface-initiated single-electron transfer living radical polymerization. *Biomacromolecules*, 11, 2683–2691.

Zoppe, J. O., Osterberg, M., Venditti, R. A., Laine, J., and Rojas, O. J. 2011. Surface interaction forces of cellulose nanocrystals grafted with thermoresponsive polymer brushes. *Biomacromolecules*, 12, 2788–2796.

Zoppe, J. O., Peresin, M. S., Habibi, Y., Venditti, R. A., and Rojas, O. J. 2009. Reinforcing poly(ε-caprolactone) nanofibers with cellulose nanocrystals. *ACS Applied Materials and Interfaces*, 1, 1996–2004.

24 Synthesis and Characterization of Sulfonyl-Terminated Polymer-Grafted Magnetic Nanocellulose and Its Application as a pH-Responsive Antibiotic Drug Carrier for the Controlled Delivery of Ciprofloxacin

T.S. Anirudhan, J. Nima, and P.L. Divya

CONTENTS

24.1 INTRODUCTION

Polysaccharides are ubiquitous biopolymers built from monosaccharides. Due to the presence of various derivable groups on molecular chains, polysaccharides can be easily modified chemically and biochemically, resulting in many kinds of polysaccharide derivatives. Polysaccharides are gaining increasing attention as components of stimuli-responsive drug delivery systems (DDSs), particularly since they can be obtained in a well-characterized and reproducible way from natural sources [1]. They are usually renewable, nontoxic, and biocompatible, and show a number of specific physicochemical properties that make them advantageous for different applications in DDS. Hydrogels are three-dimensional, hydrophilic, polymeric networks capable of imbibing large amounts of water or biological fluids and have a wide variety of biomedical applications [2]. Polysaccharide-based hydrogels have potential application as DDS, as the issues of safety, toxicity, and availability are greatly simplified. Drug delivery is an intriguing field of research that has captured the interest of researchers because delivering a medicine to its site of therapeutic action is one of the main limitations of pharmaceutical and biotechnology industries [3]. DDSs have the advantage of increasing the residence time of a drug within a patient, reducing dosing frequency and toxic effects, and improving patient compliance and consequently efficacy with most dosage requirements. The ideal drug delivery carriers will ensure that the drug is released at the right site, in the right dose, and for the required time. They will also be biocompatible or biodegradable [3]. Recent efforts in drug development resulted in a number of controlled DDS consisting of a drug encapsulated within a suitable polymer carrier that enables drugs to be delivered either via novel routes or in a sustainable fashion or both. By selecting a biocompatible carrier, drugs could be made available at various locations in the body [4]. Stimuli-responsive smart materials such as thermo-responsive, pH-responsive, and electrical-responsive polymer and magnetic materials as DDS have achieved increasing attention for controlled release under specific conditions.

A large number of polysaccharides have been studied and exploited in several fields related to pharmaceutics. Among all biopolymers used in the formulation of DDS, cellulose and its derivatives are the most widely used. The individualization of cellulose nanofiber (nanocellulose, NC) from renewable sources has gained more attention in recent years because of their exceptional mechanical properties, large specific area, low coefficient of thermal expansion, high aspect ratio, environmental benefits, and low cost [5]. Magnetic iron nanoparticles (MNPs) can be used in cellular labeling, detoxification of biological fluids, targeted drug delivery, magnetic resonance imaging, hyperthermia, tissue repair, and magnetofection [6,7]. Due to their small size, MNPs can efficiently penetrate across barriers through small capillaries into individual cells, thus allowing efficient drug accumulation at the target site. Hence, the unwanted side effects of the therapeutic agent are reduced, and the therapeutic efficacy is enhanced [8]. The present chapter focuses on the synthesis and characterization of a novel cellulose-based hydrogel, poly(hydroxyethyl methacrylate-copolymerized 2-acrylamido-2-methylpropane sulfonic acid)-glycidyl methacrylate grafted-magnetic NC [p(HEMA-*co*-AMPS)-GMA-MNC]. The drug chosen for the present investigation is ciprofloxacin (CP), an antibiotic (Figure 24.1). CP is a fluoroquinolone and has been widely used against urinary tract infections, bacterial prostatitis, sexually transmitted diseases, and joint, skin and soft tissue, respiratory tract, and gastrointestinal infections. This antibiotic drug is unique in that it provides many advantages over other antibiotic classes, including a low

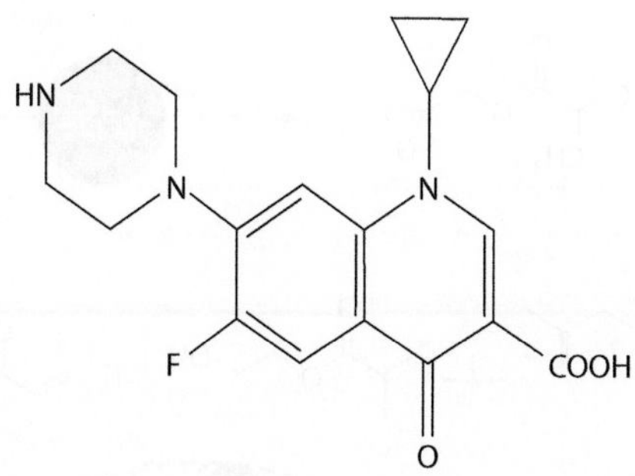

FIGURE 24.1 Chemical structure of ciprofloxacin.

working concentration, a low contamination recurrence rate, a long half-life, wide distribution within body tissue and fluids, and a lack of cytotoxicity on mammalian cells [9]. Grafting is an effective method of chemical modification of cellulosic fibers. During grafting, the side chains are covalently bonded to the main polymer backbone or substrate to form a copolymer with branched structure. In the present work, NC coated on magnetic surface is further modified by graft polymerization using GMA and further polymerized using HEMA and AMPS. Monomers are grafted using $K_2S_2O_8$ as radical initiator and ethylene glycol dimethacrylate (EGDMA) as cross-linker. The loading characteristics and release behavior of the drugs were studied, and the effect of pH and temperature on the release was determined.

24.2 EXPERIMENTAL

24.2.1 Materials

Analytical-grade chemicals were used throughout the investigation. Cellulose was obtained from Central Drug House Ltd., New Delhi. Ferric chloride hexahydrate, $FeCl_3 \cdot 6H_2O$ (98%) and ferrous sulfate heptahydrate, $FeSO_4 \cdot 7H_2O$ (99%) were obtained from Fischer, United States. GMA, EGDMA, and hydroquinone were purchased from Sigma Aldrich (Milwaukee, United States). $K_2S_2O_8$, ammonia solution, triethylamine, and AMPS were procured from E. Merck (Worli, Mumbai, India). Double-distilled water with specific conductivity less than 1 μ ohm/cm was used throughout the study.

24.2.2 Preparation of the DDS p(HEMA-*co*-AMPS)-GMA-MNC

Figure 24.2 illustrates the general procedure for the preparation of p(HEMA-*co*-AMPS)-GMA-MNC. This reaction procedure consists of the following steps:

Preparation of nanocellulose (NC) from cellulose: About 5.0 g of cellulose was dispersed in 250 mL distilled water under magnetic stirring (20 min). To the homogenized mixture, 140 mL 98.0% H_2SO_4 was added dropwise, without cause heating. After complete addition, the mixture was heated at 50°C for 2 h. The hot mixture was diluted 10 times with ice-cooled distilled water. The obtained white colloid was centrifuged, washed many times with water, and freeze-dried.

Preparation of magnetic nanocellulose (MNC): Magnetic nanocellulose (MNC) was prepared by co-precipitating Fe(II) and Fe(III) ions in aqueous solution containing NC with ammonia. About 1.50 g of NC was added to 200 mL of distilled water and stirred well for 10 min. An amount of 1.49 g of $FeCl_3 \cdot 6H_2O$ and 0.765 g of $FeSO_4 \cdot 7H_2O$ were added to the solution, which acts as a source of iron present in MNC. Chemical precipitation was achieved by adding $NH_3 \cdot H_2O$ dropwise under

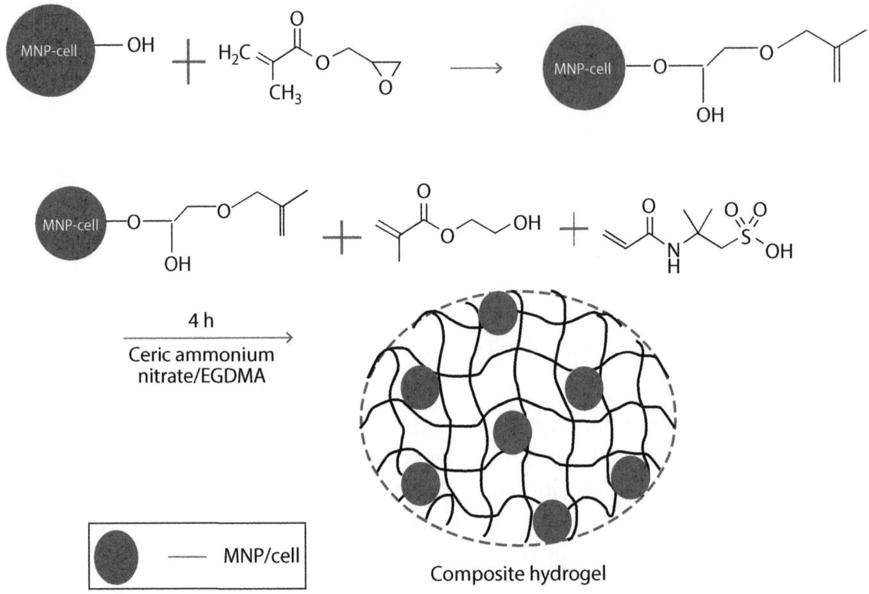

FIGURE 24.2 Proposed reaction mechanism for the synthesis of p(HEMA-*co*-AMPS)-GMA-MNC.

vigorous stirring at a constant pH of 10.0, upon which an orange color suspension obtained was changed to a black precipitate. After incubation for 4 h at 60°C, the mixture was cooled to room temperature with stirring, and the resulting MNC particles were separated magnetically and washed several times with distilled water and finally with ethanol. The product thus obtained was dried.

Synthesis of GMA-grafted MNC (GMA-MNC): MNC of 3 g was treated with 4.5 mL GMA and 10.5 mL triethylamine at 90°C under mechanical stirring for 2 h. To the mixture, 0.09 g hydroquinone was added in order to minimize the effect of free radical reaction at the unsaturated end of GMA molecule. After reaction, the samples were separated by filtration and refluxed with acetone for 3 h.

Synthesis of p(HEMA-co-AMPS)-GMA-MNC: GMA-MNC was dispersed in 100 mL distilled water under magnetic stirring for 1 h at 70°C and then $K_2S_2O_8$ (0.16 g; initiator) was added and kept at 60°C for 10 min. Then a mixture of AMPS (6.67 mL) and HEMA (4.2 mL) was added to this after cooling it to 40°C. EGDMA of 1.1 mL was added, and the temperature was raised to 70°C, for 2 h to complete the reaction. The obtained product was filtered and washed with distilled water and ethanol to remove homopolymers.

24.2.3 Equipments and Methods of Characterization

The x-ray diffraction (XRD) patterns of the samples were recorded using an X'Pert Pro x-ray diffractometer using Cu Kα radiations at a scanning speed of 2°/min and at a wavelength of 1.5406 Å. Scanning electron microscopy (SEM) analysis was done using a Philips XL 30 CP scanning electron microscope. The Fourier transform infrared (FTIR) spectra were recorded using a Shimadzu FTIR spectrometer in the wavelength range 400–4000 cm^{-1} using a KBr window at a resolution of 4 cm^{-1}. Concentration of drug in solution was determined spectrophotometrically on a JASCO UV-vis (model V-530, India) spectrophotometer. A Systronic model μ pH system 361-pH meter was used for measuring and adjusting the pH of the solutions. A temperature-controlled water bath shaker (Labline, India) with a temperature variation of ±1°C was used for the equilibrium studies. Borosil glasswares were used throughout the experiment.

24.2.4 Experimental

24.2.4.1 Effect of pH on Binding CP

Experiments were performed using two different concentrations of CP (10, 25 mg/L) to determine the optimum pH for the effective encapsulation of CP onto p(HEMA-*co*-AMPS)-GMA-MNC. CP solution of 50 mL was treated with 0.1 g of p(HEMA-*co*-AMPS)-GMA-MNC at different pH values ranging from 2.0 to 12.0 at constant temperature (30°C) and time (150 min). The concentration of CP present in the solution after binding experiments was measured by UV–visible spectrophotometer at 270 nm. The optimum pH selected was used for further studies.

24.2.4.2 Binding Kinetics

The effect of equilibrium time and initial concentration for the binding of Cp was performed by using four different initial concentrations of CP (100, 150, 200, 250 mg/L). Briefly 0.1 g of p(HEMA-*co*-AMPS)-GMA-MNC was placed in a 100 mL stoppered flask containing 50 mL of the solution. The pH was adjusted to the optimum value. The samples were shaken in a temperature (30°C)-controlled water bath shaker. Samples were then drawn from the flask at predetermined time intervals, and residual CP concentration was determined using spectrophotometric method. The data obtained from the experiment were used for calculating various kinetic parameters by using kinetic equations.

24.2.4.3 Swelling Study of p(HEMA-*co*-AMPS)-GMA-MNC

Time (at two different pHs 7.4 and 1.8), and temperature (20°C, 37°C) in which a dry weight of the polymer (0.1 g, W_d) was put into a weighed teabag, and immersed in 100 mL of solutions of desired pH for different time intervals at room temperature. After each interval, the sample containing teabag was withdrawn and blotted on filter paper to remove excess water and weighed to determine the weight of the swollen polymer particles (W_s). The degree of swelling is calculated as follows:

$$\text{Swelling (\%)} = \frac{(W_s - W_d)}{W_d} \times 100 \tag{24.1}$$

24.2.4.4 In Vitro Release of the Drug

The in vitro drug release studies of the entrapped drug were performed by placing 0.1 g of drug-loaded DDS into 50 mL KCl–HCl solution with pH 1.8 (simulative gastric pH) in a water bath shaker. The amount of drug released was determined by collecting aliquots of the solution at fixed time intervals. The temperature was maintained at 37°C throughout the study. Absorbance was measured by spectrophotometric method. The release studies were continued until no more change in the concentration of drug in the solution occurred. The experiments were repeated using Na_2HPO_4–KH_2PO_4 solution at pH 7.4 (simulated intestinal pH). The percentage of drug released in both cases was calculated by following the equation:

$$\text{Drug released (\%)} = \frac{C_t}{C_\infty} \times 100 \tag{24.2}$$

where C_t and C_∞ are the concentration of drug released at time t and that of drug released completely, respectively.

24.2.5 Antibacterial Studies

Antibacterial activities of bare drug, sample, and drug-loaded sample were analyzed using two different bacteria by disk diffusion method. The study was carried out by using zone of inhibition methodology.

24.3 RESULTS AND DISCUSSION

24.3.1 Characterization

24.3.1.1 FTIR Spectra

The FTIR spectra of cellulose, NC, MNC, GMA-MNC, p(HEMA-*co*-AMPS)-GMA-MNC are presented in Figure 24.3. The spectrum of cellulose shows the characteristic broad peak related to hydrogen-bonded O–H stretching vibration at 3443 cm^{-1}, and the peaks at 2930 and 1033 cm^{-1} could be attributed to the C–H stretching and C–H bending of the CH_2 group. The peaks at 1630

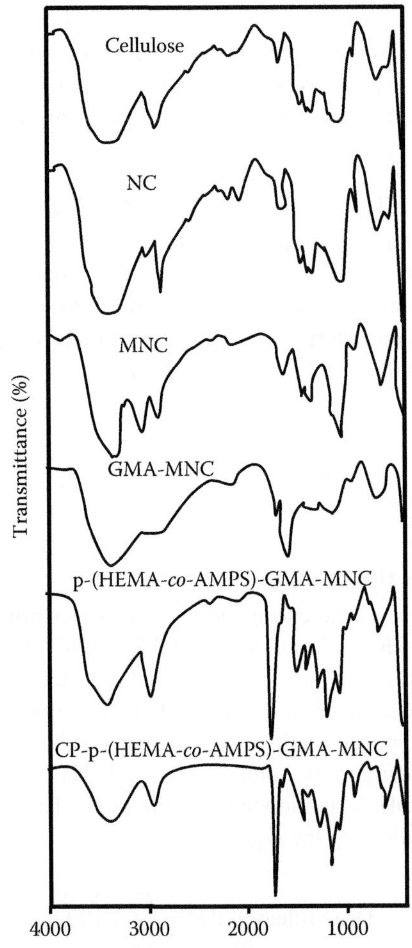

FIGURE 24.3 FTIR spectra of cellulose, NC, MNC, GMA-MNC, p(HEMA-*co*-AMPS)-GMA-MNC, and CP-p(HEMA-*co*-AMPS)-GMA-MNC.

and 663 cm^{-1} are due to the C=O stretching of hemicelluloses and β-glycosidic linkage in cellulose, respectively. The band at 890 cm^{-1} is characteristic of glycosidic ring in cellulose structure. All the characteristic peaks of cellulose are retained in NC with slight shift in its position, which may be due to the removal of intramolecular H-bonding during acid hydrolysis. In the spectrum of MNC, a characteristic absorption band of Fe–O in the tetrahedral sites was observed at 564 cm^{-1} [10]. The interaction between cellulose and magnetic core is indicated by a small shift in the stretching peaks of O–H (3260 cm^{-1}). O–H bending vibration is shown by a strong peak at 1250 cm^{-1}. In the spectrum of GMA–MNC, the absence of characteristic absorption peaks of epoxide ring at 2997, 1270, and 846 cm^{-1} and the presence of intense carbonyl stretching peak at 1720 cm^{-1} support the reaction between epoxide group of GMA and cellulose [11]. A small shift in the peak of Fe–O and O–H of MNC clearly confirms the existence of grafting [12–14]. In the spectrum of p(HEMA-*co*-AMPS)-GMA-MNC, the characteristic absorption peaks at 1034, 1245, and 751 cm^{-1} correspond to SO_3H of AMPS. The presence of HEMA is evident from the observed bands at 1725 (C–O stretching), 1170 (O–C–C stretching), 3520 (O–H stretching), 2949 (asymmetric stretching of methylene group), and 1450 cm^{-1} (O–H bending). In the IR spectrum of CP-p(HEMA-*co*-AMPS)-GMA-MNC, all the characteristic peaks of polymer were retained with smaller shift indicating the interaction between CP and p(HEMA-*co*-AMPS)-GMA-MNC. The spectrum also marked the presence of drug as evident from the observed band of C–N stretching (1250 cm^{-1}) and C–F stretching (943 cm^{-1}). Similarly, C–H out-of-plane bending (900–690 cm^{-1}) also indicates the presence of CP in p(HEMA-*co*-AMPS)-GMA-MNC. The peak at 1250–1600 cm^{-1} can be assigned to quinoline group of CP.

24.3.1.2 XRD Analysis

XRD method can be used to determine the degree of crystallinity of polymers. The XRD patterns of cellulose, NC, MNC, GMA-MNC, p(HEMA-*co*-AMPS)-GMA-MNC, and CP-p(HEMA-*co*-AMPS)-GMA-MNC are shown in Figure 24.4. The XRD pattern of cellulose shows peaks at $2\theta = 22.8°$ and 34.5°, which correspond to the crystalline nature of cellulose. Also a broad hump at $2\theta = 15.5°$ is observed, which indicates the amorphous nature. The XRD spectrum of NC retained its position as that of cellulose; however, they appeared even sharper indicating more crystalline nature, which occurred due to the partial removal of amorphous regions because of acid hydrolysis treatment of cellulose [15]. MNC showed peaks at $2\theta = 18.50°$, 30.0°, 42.58°, 55.25°, and 62.65°, which reveals that the magnetic particle has pure Fe_3O_4 with spinel structure. The spectrum showed a small shift in the typical cellulose peaks indicating the successful coating of NC on the surface of Fe_3O_4. XRD pattern of GMA–MNC shows that, upon graft polymerization, a significant decrease in crystallinity occurs. Also there was a decrease in reflection sharpness and decrease in scattering angle compared to cellulose. Absence of characteristic peaks of cellulose and decreased crystallinity in p(HEMA-*co*-AMPS)-GMA-MNC suggests that polymerization had occurred during modification. The diffraction pattern of CP-p(HEMA-*co*-AMPS)-GMA-MNC possesses new peaks at $2\theta = 19.25°$, 26.82°, and 29.32°, which clearly indicates the loading of CP onto p(HEMA-*co*-AMPS)-GMA-MNC.

24.3.1.3 SEM Analysis

Figure 24.5 shows the SEM images of cellulose, NC, MNC, GMA-MNC, p(HEMA-*co*-AMPS)-GMA-MNC. From the images, it is clear that the morphology of each of them is quite different. Cellulose displayed a spindle-like structure because of strong intramolecular hydrogen bonding, while the surface of NC looks fluffy and is very small compared to cellulose. Due to the small particle size, the surface area is increased, which in turn increases the grafting efficiency. The surface of MNC appears to be irregular and highly porous in nature with microscale interstitial spaces. The surface of GMA-MNC shows aggregated structure with some porous nature, which may be due to the presence of organic functional groups on the surface of MNC. The surface

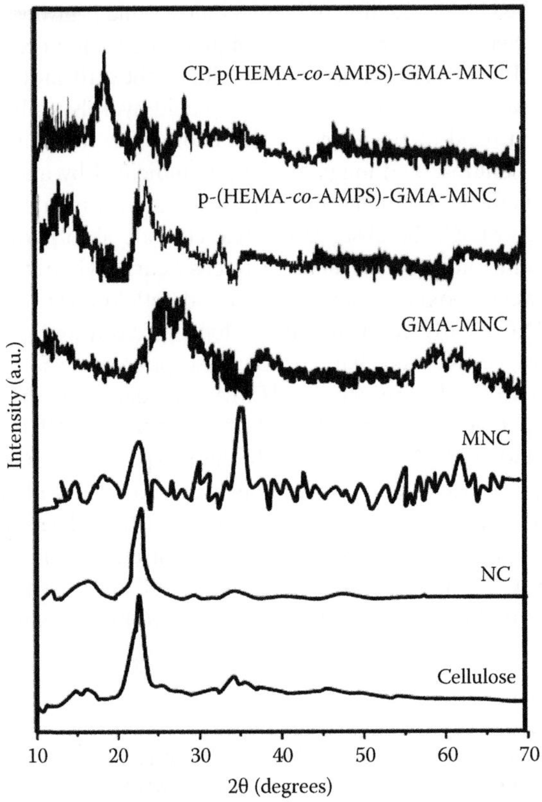

FIGURE 24.4 XRD spectra of cellulose, NC, MNC, GMA-MNC, p(HEMA-*co*-AMPS)-GMA-MNC, and CP-p(HEMA-*co*-AMPS)-GMA-MNC.

of p(HEMA-*co*-AMPS)-GMA-MNC shows small grain-like appearance with some aggregation. The surface was found to be porous in nature. Surface morphology of CP-p(HEMA-*co*-AMPS)-GMA-MNC was found to be rigid, compact, and smooth, which clearly indicates the drug loading.

24.3.2 Effect of pH on Encapsulation of CP

The effect of pH on the encapsulation of CP onto p(HEMA-*co*-AMPS)-GMA-MNC was studied in the pH range 2.0–12. In the DDS, the predominant surface functional groups for the effective encapsulation of drug are SO_3^- and O–H. As seen in Figure 24.6, the amount of CP loaded was remarkably affected by the solution pH and was found maximum at 5.0. At this pH, CP exists as CP^+ ions so that both electrostatic interaction and hydrogen bonding are possible between the DDS and CP. As the solution pH increased above 6.0, the percentage of encapsulation began to decrease. This can be explained as follows: the pKa_1 and pKa_2 values of CP are 6.1 and 8.7, respectively. The cationic form of CP exists due to protonation of the amine group and piperazine moiety when solution pH is above 6.1. Between pH 6.1 and 8.7, the CP exists as zwitterionic species, so that effective interaction between the side chain groups of the DDS and CP is prevented. This happens as a result of repulsion between the COO^- groups of CP and SO_3^- groups present on the side chain of the DDS, thereby effectively reducing the H-bonding interaction.

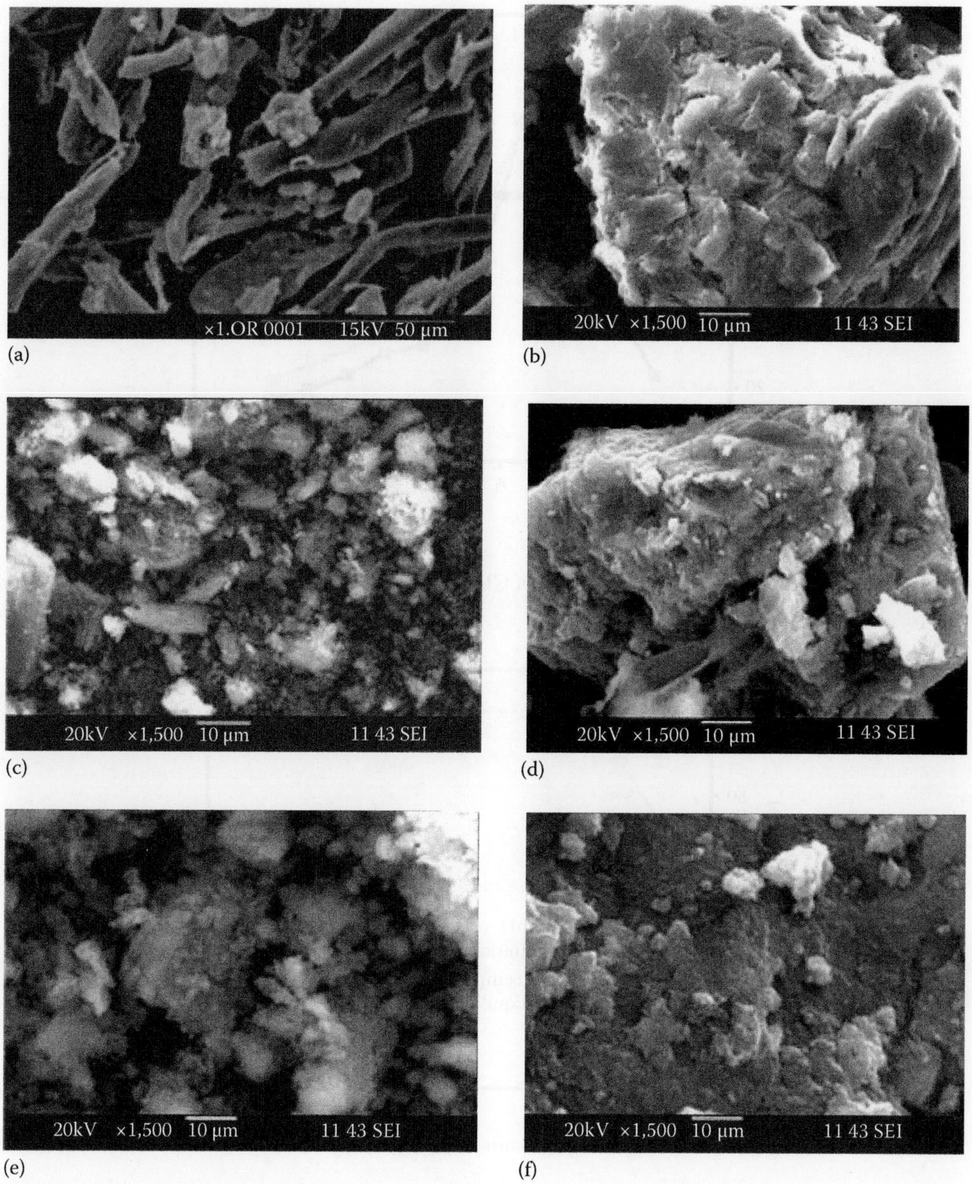

FIGURE 24.5 SEM photographs of (a) cellulose, (b) NC, (c) MNC, (d) GMA-MNC, (e) p(HEMA-*co*-AMPS)-GMA-MNC, and (f) CP-p(HEMA-*co*-AMPS)-GMA-MNC.

As the pH is increased above 8.7, CP exists only as negative ions, which caused electrostatic repulsion between anionic DDS and the drug so that encapsulation decreased further.

24.3.3 Effect of Adsorbent Dose on Encapsulation

Experiments were conducted using different amounts of adsorbent dose to study the variation in the encapsulation of drug with respect to the dosage of DDS. From Figure 24.7, it is clear that as dosage of DDS increased, encapsulation percentage also increased and found to be maximum when 2.0 g/L

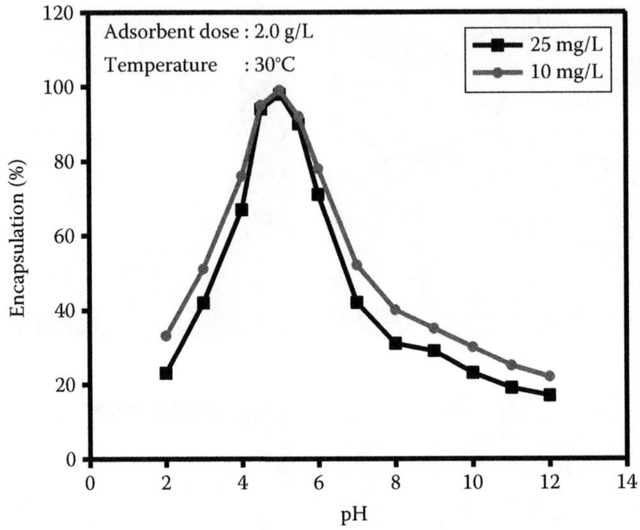

FIGURE 24.6 Effect of pH on the encapsulation of CP.

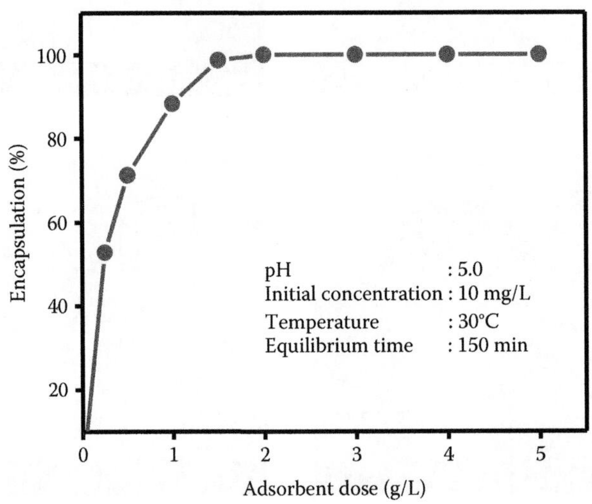

FIGURE 24.7 Effect of adsorbent dose on the encapsulation of CP.

of the DDS is used. The increase in encapsulation percentage with respect to increase in adsorbent dosage can be explained on the basis of the increase in adsorption sites for the drug molecules. The DDS of 2.0 g/L contains sufficient reaction sites for the encapsulation of 99.0% of drug molecules. Further experiments were conducted using 2.0 g/L of the adsorbent.

24.3.4 Kinetic Studies

Kinetic studies were employed in order to evaluate the binding efficiency of CP onto p(HEMA-*co*-AMPS)-GMA-MNC. The kinetic data obtained at different time intervals were analyzed using pseudo-first-order and pseudo-second-order kinetic models [16] as shown in Equations 24.3 and 24.4, respectively.

$$q_t = q_e(1 - e^{(-k_1)t}) \quad (24.3)$$

$$\frac{t}{q_t} = \frac{1}{k_2 q_e^2} + \frac{t}{q_e} \quad (24.4)$$

where

- q_e and q_t (mg/g) are the amount of CP adsorbed on p(HEMA-*co*-AMPS)-GMA-MNC at equilibrium and time t (min), respectively
- k_1 (min^{-1}) is the rate constant for the pseudo-first-order kinetics
- k_2 (g/mg/min) is the rate constant for pseudo-second-order kinetics

The kinetic parameters were determined from the slope and intercept of the plots (Figure 24.8) and are given in Table 24.1. From the results, it can be seen that the correlated q_e values are very close to the experimental q_e values in the case of pseudo-second-order kinetics rather than pseudo-first-order kinetics. Also R^2 values closer to unity and low χ^2 values were obtained for this model. This suggests the chemisorption mechanism between p(HEMA-*co*-AMPS)-GMA-MNC and CP during binding process.

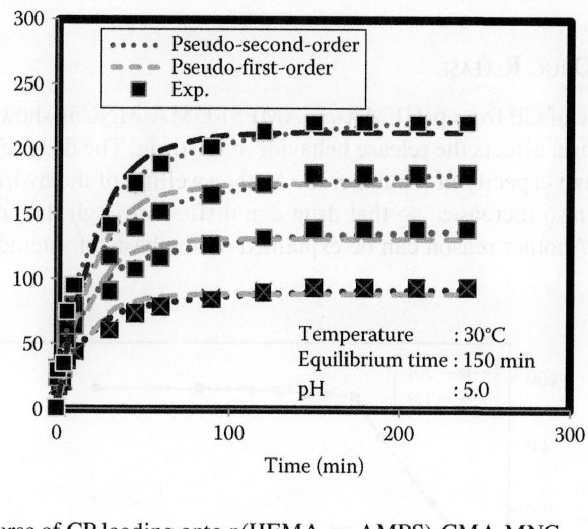

FIGURE 24.8 Time course of CP loading onto p(HEMA-*co*-AMPS)-GMA-MNC.

TABLE 24.1
Kinetic Parameters for the Binding of CP onto p(HEMA-*co*-AMPS)-GMA-MNC

		Pseudo First Order				Pseudo Second Order			
C_0 (g/L)	q_e, exp (mg/g)	k_1 (min^{-1})	q_e, cal (mg/g)	R^2	χ^2	k_2 (g/mg/min)	q_e, cal (mg/g)	R^2	χ^2
100	94.00	6.12×10^{-2}	88.47	0.935	7.5	0.92×10^{-3}	93.83	0.984	2.67
150	138.15	5.53×10^{-2}	131.37	0.945	13.4	0.56×10^{-3}	137.06	0.999	4.34
200	180.80	4.98×10^{-2}	173.22	0.965	19.2	0.38×10^{-3}	179.64	0.999	6.12
250	220.75	4.62×10^{-2}	213.19	0.982	22.3	0.29×10^{-3}	218.74	0.999	6.83

24.3.5 Swelling Characteristics

24.3.5.1 Swelling Behavior of p(HEMA-*co*-AMPS)-GMA-MNC at pH 1.8 and 7.4

The swelling capacity of the hydrogel was studied as a function of time at two different pH values, 1.8 and 7.4. The swelling capacity of the material can be explained on the basis of hydrophilicity and pH dependence of AMPS and HEMA groups. From Figure 24.9, it is clear that as time increases, swelling percentage also increases. Maximum swelling percentage was reached at 90 min followed by slow increase up to 240 min. Comparing the swelling at two pH values, it was found that maximum swelling is obtained at 7.4. This is because at acidic pH, the sulfonate group (AMPS) is in unionized state so that a hydrogen bond interaction exists between the OH groups (HEMA) and SO_3H groups. But when pH is increased to 7.4, sulfonic acid groups get ionized to give SO_3^- groups. So the hydrogel becomes anionic, and there occurs electrostatic repulsion between similarly charged groups. As a result, swelling of the hydrogel increases.

24.3.5.2 Effect of Temperature on Swelling

The temperature dependence of swelling profile can be tested by conducting the experiment at two different temperatures, 20°C and 37°C. From the graph (Figure 24.10), it is clear that as temperature increases, swelling percentage also increases. This increase in swelling percentage with respect to temperature indicates the occurrence of upper critical solution temperature behavior of anionic hydrogels [17].

24.3.6 In Vitro Drug Release

In vitro release profile of CP from p(HEMA-*co*-AMPS)-GMA-MNC is shown in Figure 24.11. The structure of the hydrogel affects the release behavior of the drug. The drug release can be explained in terms of the swelling capacity of the material. As the swelling of the hydrogel increases, surface area of the material also increases, so that drug can diffuse through the aqueous pathway to the surface of the DDS. Another reason can be explained on the basis of interaction between the drug

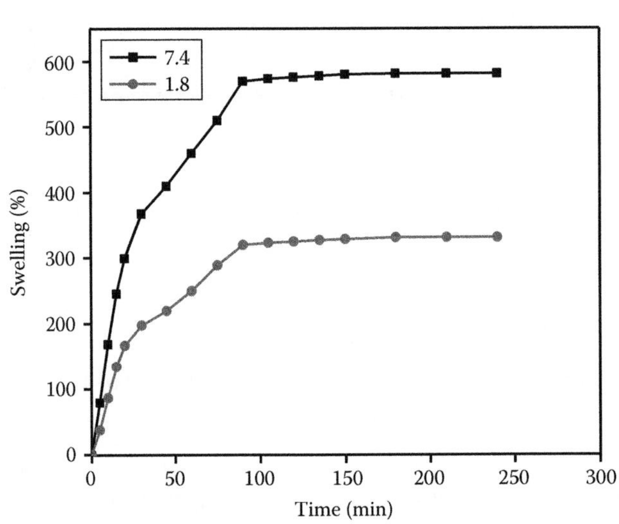

FIGURE 24.9 Swelling kinetic profiles of p(HEMA-*co*-AMPS)-GMA-MNC with time at pH 1.8 and 7.4.

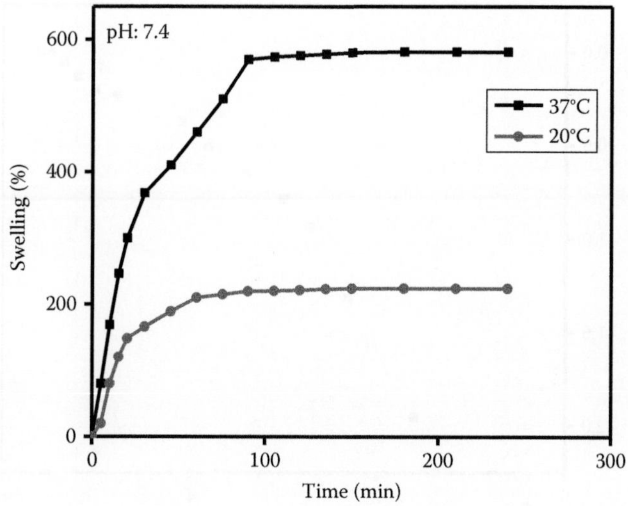

FIGURE 24.10 Swelling (%) of p(HEMA-*co*-AMPS)-GMA-MNC as a function of temperatures.

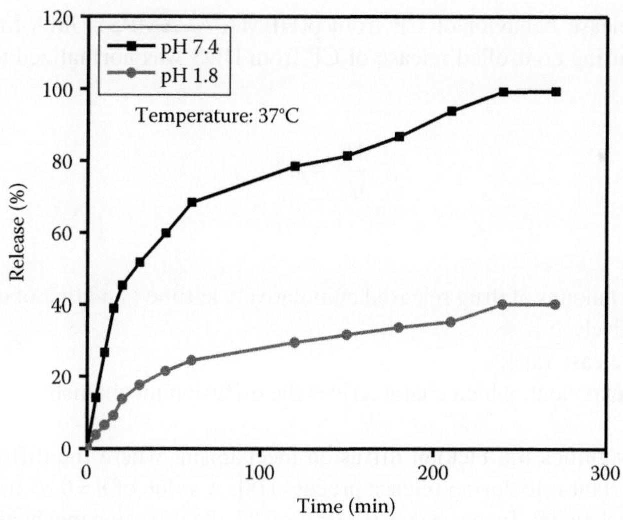

FIGURE 24.11 In vitro release profile of CP from p(HEMA-*co*-AMPS)-GMA-MNC at pH 1.8 and 7.4.

and DDS at two different pH values. At lower pH (1.8), there is the possibility of hydrogen bonding interaction between the drug and the carrier. But at pH 7.4, CP is present in zwitterionic form, and the hydrogel is present in the anionic form, so that hydrogen bonding is decreased, and there occurs anion–anion repulsion between the DDS and CP, which also favors the release of CP at 7.4. The CP release percentage was increased with increase in time, and a maximum was achieved at 4 h. Maximum release was found at pH of 7.4 (99.2%) than 1.8 (40.1%).

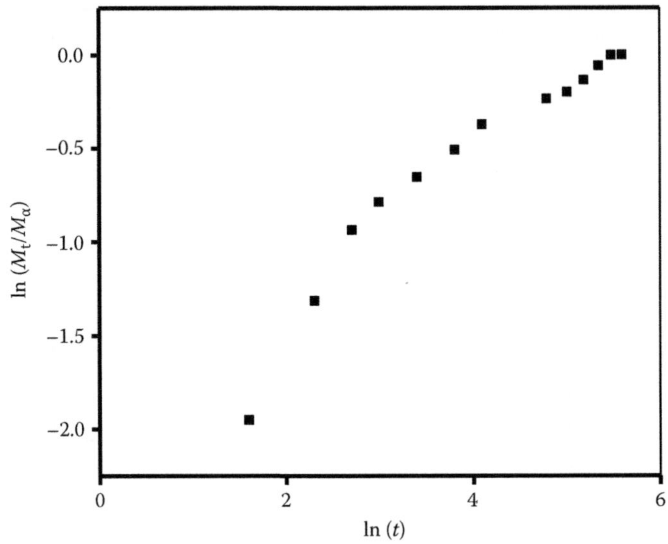

FIGURE 24.12 $\ln(M_t/M_\alpha)$ versus $\ln(t)$ plot for p(HEMA-*co*-AMPS)-GMA-MNC.

24.3.6.1 Drug Release Mechanism

To investigate the release behavior of CP from p(HEMA-*co*-AMPS)-GMA-MNC, a fraction of drug released data during controlled release of CP from DDS was normalized to fit to the Peppas potential equation:

$$\frac{M_t}{M_\alpha} = kt^n \tag{24.5}$$

where

M_t and M_α are the amount of drug released cumulatively at time t and that of drug released completely, respectively
k is the apparent release rate
n is the diffusion exponent, which characterizes the diffusion mechanism

A value of $n=0.43$ signifies the Fickian diffusion mechanism, where the diffusion of drug molecules plays an important role during release process [18]. A value of $n=0.85$ indicates a swelling-controlled release mechanism. In the case of $0.43<n<0.85$, the diffusion mechanism is non-Fickian, where both drug diffusion and polymer relaxation control the overall rate of drug release. Plots of ln (M_t/M_α) against $\ln(t)$ are shown in Figure 24.12 for p(HEMA-*co*-AMPS)-GMA-MNC obtained under optimum conditions. The profile is linear in the early stages of release with $n=0.54$ and $R^2=0.994$. Since the value of "n" lies between 0.43 and 0.85, the diffusion of drug and swelling of the polymer play an important role in the release mechanism.

24.3.7 Antibacterial Activity

The in vitro activities of CP, p(HEMA-*co*-AMPS)-GMA-MNC, and CP-p(HEMA-*co*-AMPS)-GMA-MNC against gram-negative bacterium *Escherichia coli* and the gram-positive bacterium *Bacillus* were tested using the disk diffusion method. The results, depicted in Figure 24.13, clearly support the experiment and thus validate the action of the samples in vitro against gram-negative and gram-positive bacteria.

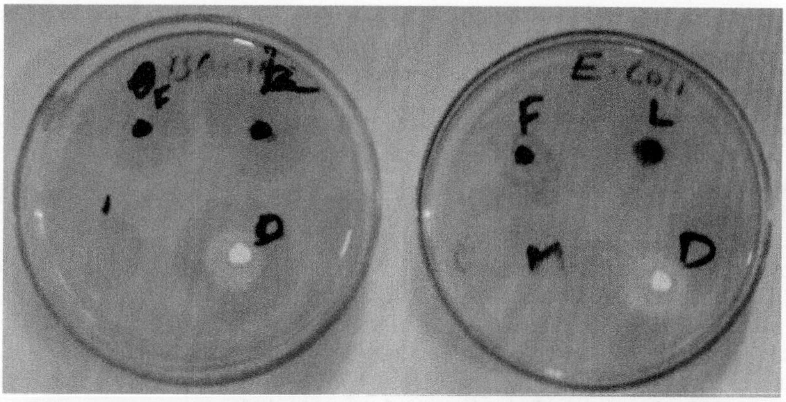

FIGURE 24.13 In vitro antibacterial activities of CP (D), p(HEMA-*co*-AMPS)-GMA-MNC (F), and CP-p(HEMA-*co*-AMPS)-GMA-MNC (L). Left, gram-positive bacteria (*Bacillus*); right, gram-negative bacteria (*Escherichia coli*).

24.4 CONCLUSIONS

In the present chapter, we have described the synthesis and characterization of a novel drug carrier, poly(hydroxyl ethyl methacrylate-copolymerized 2-acrylamido-2-methylpropane sulfonic acid)-glycidyl methacrylate-grafted-MNC, [p(HEMA-*co*-AMPS)-GMA-MNC], in which GMA-grafted MNC is polymerized using two hydrophilic functional monomers HEMA and AMPS using EGDMA as cross-linker and $K_2S_2O_8$ as initiator. Here, the SO_3H groups (of AMPS) and OH group (HEMA) are the main functional moieties that can interact with positively charged drug, CP, through electrostatic and hydrogen bonding interactions. The prepared samples were characterized using FTIR, XRD, and SEM techniques. The optimum pH was found to be 5.0, which can be explained on the basis of complementary charges of CP and the functional moieties present on the DDS. Binding mechanism was well explained by pseudo-second-order kinetic model. From the swelling studies, it was found that the swelling rate was maximum at pH 7.4 compared to 1.8, which further explains the release mechanism. The release rate was also found to be higher at pH 7.4 (99.2% at 4 h). By using Peppas equation, release profile was found to follow non-Fickian diffusion model. Antibacterial activities clearly depicted the action of drug and the samples against gram-negative and gram-positive bacteria.

REFERENCES

1. Carmen, A.L., Barbara, B.F., Ana, M.P., Angel, C., Cross-linked ionic polysaccharides for stimuli-sensitive drug delivery, *Advanced Drug Delivery Reviews*, 65, 2013, 1148–1171.
2. Hoffman, A.S., Hydrogels for biomedical applications, *Advanced Drug Delivery Reviews*, 54, 2002, 3–12.
3. Orive, G., Hernandez, R.M., Rodriguez, G.A., Dominguez, G.A., Pedraz, J.L., Drug delivery in biotechnology: Present and future, *Current Opinion in Biotechnology*, 14, 2003, 659–664.
4. Dusan, R., Branka, K.R., The effects of irradiation on controlled drug delivery/controlled drug release systems, *Radiation Physics and Chemistry*, 77, 2008, 288–344.
5. Nishino, T., Matsuda, I., Hirao, K., All cellulose composite, *Macromolecules*, 37, 2004, 7683–7687.
6. Arun, K., Jena, P.K., Behera, S., Lockey, R.F., Mohapatra, S., Multifunctional magnetic nanoparticles for targeted delivery, *Nanomedicine: Nanotechnology, Biology and Medicine*, 6, 2010, 64–69.
7. Yuan, G., Venkatasubramanian, R., Hein, S., Misra, R.D.K., A stimulus-responsive magnetic nanoparticle drug carrier: Magnetite encapsulated by chitosan-grafted-copolymer, *Acta Biomaterialia*, 4, 2008, 1024–1037.
8. Yih, T.C., Al-Fandi, M., Engineered nanoparticles as precise drug delivery systems, *Journal of Cellular Biochemistry*, 97, 2006, 1184–1190.

9. Marzo, A., Bal, D., Liquid chromatography as an analytical tool for selected antibiotic classes: A reappraisal addressed to pharmacokinetic applications, *Journal of Chromatography A*, B-12, 2002, 17–34.
10. Nyquist, R.A., Kagel, R.O., *Infrared Spectra of Inorganic Compounds (3800–45 cm^{-1})*. Academic Press, New York, 1971, ix, 495pp.
11. Mariano, P., Md. Minhaz-Ul, H., Vera, A., Functionalization, compatibilization and properties of polyolefin composites with natural fibres, *Polymers*, 2, 2010, 554–574.
12. Anirudhan, T.S., Priya S., Adsorption potential of sulfonated poly(glycidylmethacrylate)-grafted cellulose for separation of lysozyme from aqueous phase: Mass transfer analysis, kinetic and equilibrium profiles, *Colloids and Surfaces A*, 377, 2011, 156–166.
13. Silverstein, R.M., Bassler, G.C., Terrence, C.M., *Spectroscopic Identification of Organic Compounds*. John Wiley & Sons, Inc., New York, 1991.
14. Xie, J., Riley, C., Kumar, M., Chittur, K., FTIR-ATR study of protein adsorption and brushite transformation to hydroxyapatite, *Biomaterials*, 23, 2002, 3609–3616.
15. Alemdar, A., Sain, M., Isolation and characterization of nanofibres from agricultural residues-wheat straw and soy hulls, *Bioresource Technology*, 99, 2008, 1664–1671.
16. Ho, Y.S., Mckay, G., Pseudo-second-order model for sorption processes, *Process Biochemistry*, 34, 1999, 451–465.
17. Ekici, S., Saraydin, D., Interpenetrating polymeric network hydrogels for potential gastrointestinal drug release, *Polymer International*, 56, 2007, 1371–1377.
18. Falk, B., Garramone, S., Shivkumar, S., Diffusion coefficient of paracetamol in a chitosan hydrogel, *Materials Letters*, 58, 2004, 3261–3265.

25 Grafting of Cellulose and Cellulose Derivatives by CuAAC Click Chemistry

Faten Hassan Hassan Abdellatif, Jérôme Babin, Carole Arnal-Herault, and Anne Jonquieres

CONTENTS

25.1 INTRODUCTION

Cellulose is one of the most abundant and inexpensive polysaccharides. Nevertheless, its supramolecular structure, its insolubility in water and most organic solvents, and its poor processability have been limiting for several applications. Chemical modification of cellulose has led to a variety of cellulosic derivatives with a broad property diversity and has opened new scopes to cellulose-based materials. Chemical modifications have also offered new functionalities to cellulose-based materials such as water or oil repellency, antibacterial properties, or stimuli-responsive behaviors.

Recently, important progress has been made for cellulose and its derivatives with new modification strategies based on the copper(I)-catalyzed Huisgen 1,3-dipolar cycloaddition of azide and alkyne (CuAAC) click chemistry (Figure 25.1). Since the pioneering work of Sharpless and coworkers on CuAAC click chemistry[1,2] and its first application to polymer chemistry in 2004,[3] CuAAC

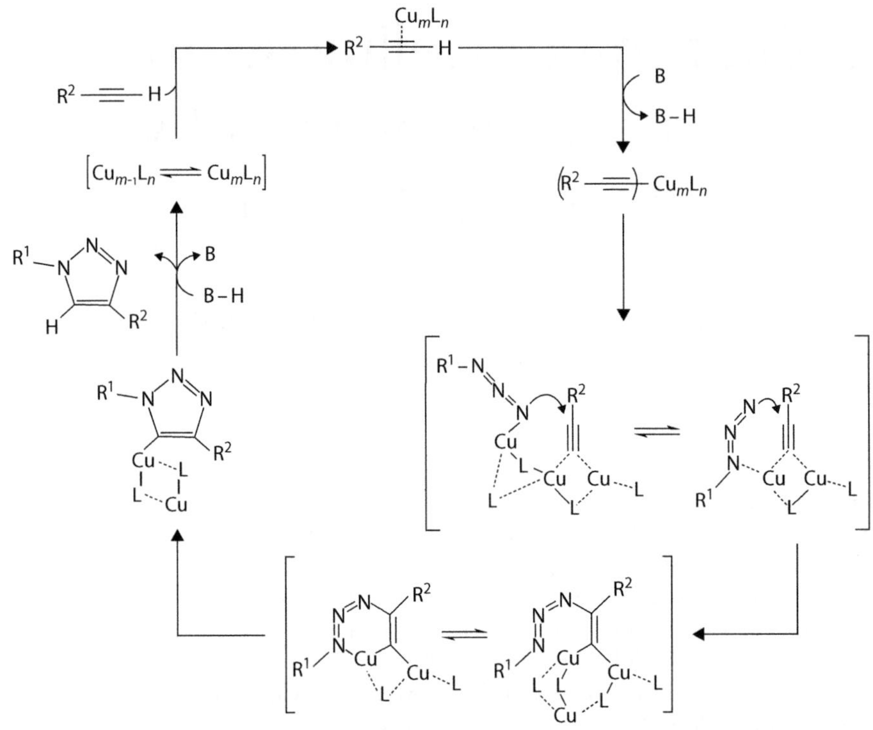

FIGURE 25.1 Copper(I)-catalyzed Huisgen 1,3-dipolar cycloaddition of alkynes and azides (CuAAC). (Binder, W.H. and Sachsenhofer, R.: 'Click' Chemistry in polymer and material science: An update. *Macromol. Rapid Commun.* 2008. 29. 952–981, Figure 1, p. 954, Copyright Wiley-VCH Verlag GmbH & Co. KGaA. Reproduced with permission.)

click chemistry has become one of the best approaches to complex macromolecular architectures and polymer modification.[4–10]

Over the past few years, CuAAC click chemistry has offered new ways of modifying cellulose and its derivatives in particular mild conditions and with hydrolytically stable triazole linkers. Its high reliability, efficiency, and tolerance of different functional groups have contributed to developing great structural and functional variety for cellulosic materials. According to the work of Liebert et al. on the first modification of cellulose by CuAAC click chemistry[11] and to related recent reviews on polysaccharides,[10,12,13] CuAAC click chemistry still offers opportunities for polysaccharide modification with great potential for a wide range of applications in smart packaging, advanced food, health care, drug delivery, biomaterials, biosensors, bactericidal and antifouling materials, biofunctional films, etc.

This chapter focuses on the emerging field of cellulose/cellulose derivative grafting by CuAAC click chemistry for the synthesis of advanced materials and gels. The first part reports on cellulose pre-click modification for introducing azide or alkyne groups, which are necessary for CuAAC click chemistry. The chapter then reviews the use of CuAAC click chemistry for the preparation of different cellulose-based macromolecular architectures: (1) cross-linked networks for structural materials and hydrogels, (2) block and graft copolymers, and (3) dendronized celluloses. Recent works on cellulose-based polyelectrolytes obtained by CuAAC click chemistry are also reviewed before addressing the particular issue of advanced cellulose (nano)materials by CuAAC surface modification.

25.2 PRECLICK MODIFICATION OF CELLULOSE AND CELLULOSE DERIVATIVES FOR CuAAC CLICK CHEMISTRY

Preclick modification of cellulose and cellulose derivatives is an essential step for CuAAC click chemistry, which consists of introducing azide or alkyne groups onto the anhydroglucose rings (Figure 25.2).[10,14]

This functionalization is mainly achieved after activation of the cellulose hydroxyl groups by tosylation. The resulting *p*-toluene sulfonic ester of cellulose (tosyl cellulose) is one of the most widely used intermediates in cellulose chemistry due to its high reactivity and its solubility in a wide range of organic solvents.[15] Tosylation of cellulose can be carried out by homogeneous reaction of cellulose with *p*-toluene sulfonic acid in DMAc/LiCl. A wide range of substitution degrees for the tosyl group (DS_{tosyl}) can be obtained by varying the molar ratio of *p*-toluene sulfonic acid to the cellulose hydroxyl groups. Furthermore, cellulose tosylation takes place preferably at position 6, as expected from the better reactivity of the corresponding primary hydroxyl groups. Consequently,

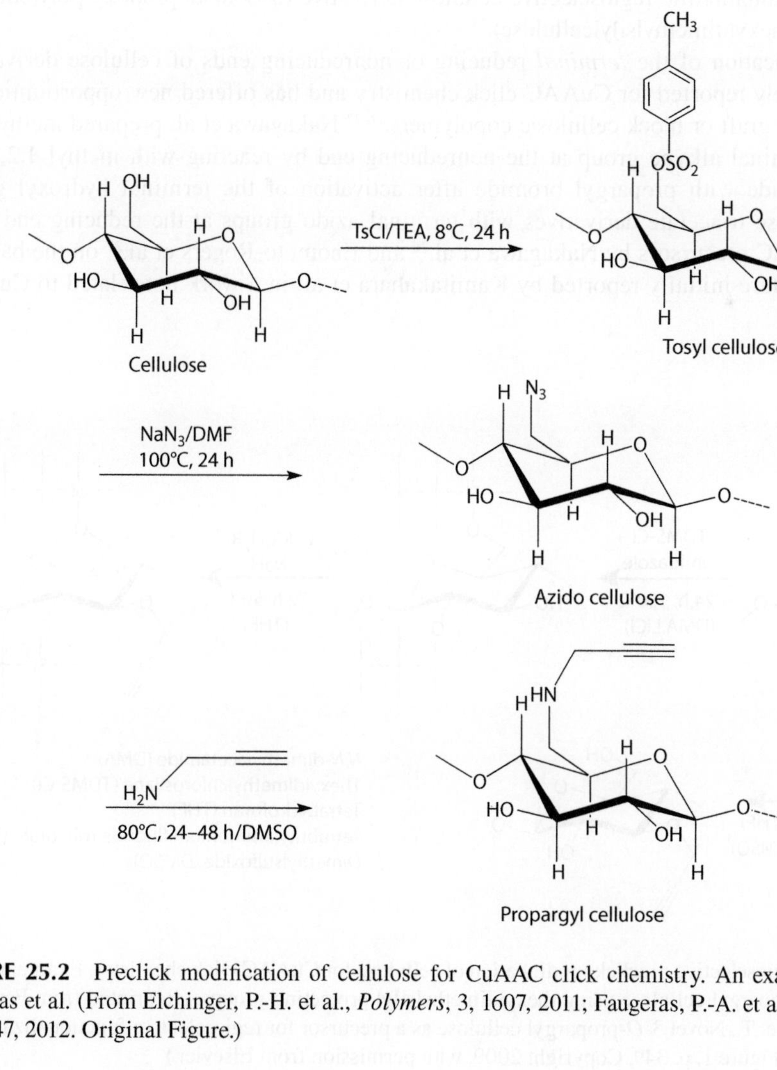

FIGURE 25.2 Preclick modification of cellulose for CuAAC click chemistry. An example according to Faugeras et al. (From Elchinger, P.-H. et al., *Polymers*, 3, 1607, 2011; Faugeras, P.-A. et al., *Carbohydr. Res.*, 356, 247, 2012. Original Figure.)

cellulose tosylation has been shown to be regioselective for $DS_{tosyl} < 1$.[14,16] In addition, the tosyl group is an excellent leaving group to perform nucleophilic substitutions with, for example, sodium azide or propargyl amine and introduce azido or propargyl groups, respectively. Other miscellaneous techniques have been reported to a much less extent for cellulose random premodification for the CuAAC click chemistry.[14,17–20]

The properties of cellulose derivatives generally differ for random or regioselective substitution of the hydroxyl groups of the anhydroglucose rings. Regioselectivity is thus an important issue in cellulose chemistry. The introduction of the azido or propargyl groups at positions 2 and 3 requires regioselective cellulose modification as initially reported by Koschella et al. for propargyl groups.[21,22] Regioselective modification involves protecting group chemistry and additional synthetic steps, which are justified only when specific positions are targeted for the azido or propargyl groups.[23] As an example, Figure 25.3 shows the regioselective cellulose modification for introducing propargyl groups at position 3 according to Fenn et al.[24] In the later work, thexyldimethylsilyl protecting groups were chosen due to their high selectivity for positions 2 and 6 in homogeneous conditions. 2,6-Di-*O*-thexyldimethylsilyl cellulose was then treated with allyl halide (e.g., propargyl bromide) to produce 3-*O*-propargyl cellulose regioselectively. Xu et al. reported the same strategy to prepare an azido amphiphilic regioselective cellulose derivative (3-*O*-azidopropoxy poly(ethylene glycol)-2,6-di-*O*-thexyldimethylsilylcellulose).[25]

Preclick modification of the *terminal* reducing or nonreducing ends of cellulose derivatives has been very rarely reported for CuAAC click chemistry and has offered new opportunities for designing original graft or block cellulosic copolymers.[26,27] Nakagawa et al. prepared methyl cellulose with a terminal alkyne group at the nonreducing end by reacting with methyl 1,2,3-tri-*O*-methyl celluloside with propargyl bromide after activation of the terminal hydroxyl group by NaH.[26] Cellulose triacetate derivatives with terminal azido groups at the reducing end were obtained as CuAAC precursors by Nakagawa et al.[26] and Enomoto-Rogers et al.[27] on the basis of a multistep procedure initially reported by Kamitakahara et al. in a work not related to CuAAC click chemistry.[28]

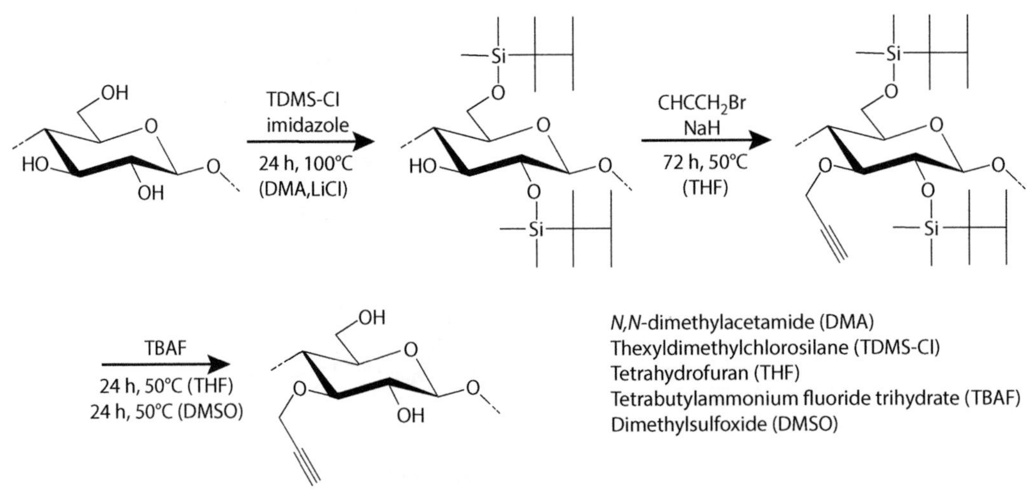

FIGURE 25.3 Regioselective preclick modification of cellulose for CuAAC click chemistry. Example of the synthesis of 3-*O*-propargyl cellulose using thexyldimethylsilyl protecting groups. (Reprinted from Fenn, D., Pohl, M., and Heinze, T., Novel 3-*O*-propargyl cellulose as a precursor for regioselective functionalization of cellulose, 347–352, Figure 1, p. 349, Copyright 2009, with permission from Elsevier.)

25.3 ADVANCED CROSS-LINKED CELLULOSE-BASED NETWORKS BY CuAAC CLICK CHEMISTRY

CuAAC click chemistry has brought new simple ways of cross-linking cellulose and cellulose derivatives on the basis of azido or propargyl cellulose. Compared to former cross-linking strategies using difunctional agents, the new approaches based on CuAAC click chemistry offered specific advantages for designing cross-linked cellulose-based newtorks.[14] The chemical stability of the triazole ring formed by reaction of azido with alkyne groups was one of the important advantages compared to the weakness of former ester-containing cross-linking bridges toward hydrolysis. The new strategy also allowed a much better control of network formation by avoiding intramolecular reactions of the azido or alkyne groups. In this new strategy, the azido or alkyne side groups had to react with complementary groups on other polysaccharide chains to form the cross-linking bridges, leading to improved three-dimensional networks.

25.3.1 Cross-Linked Cellulose-Based Structural Materials

Over the past few years, new strategies based on CuAAC click chemistry have led to original advanced cross-linked structural materials from cellulose alone or cellulose combined with other polysaccharides. A nice example was reported by Faugeras et al. with a simple approach for cellulose cross-linking (Figure 25.4).[14] In this work, azido cellulose with a DS_{azide} of 1.5 was reacted with propargyl cellulose with a DS_{alkyne} of 1.3. CuAAC click chemistry was performed in $DMSO/H_2O$ with $CuSO_4$, $5H_2O$ in the presence of sodium ascorbate (reducing agent) for 7 days at room temperature or activated by microwave irradiation. Scanning electron microscopy (SEM) revealed very significant differences between the azido or propargyl celluloses, and the resulting cross-linked porous networks.

This promising approach was then extended to the cross-linking of azido cellulose with propargylated starch.[29] In the later four-step strategy, 6-azido 6-deoxy cellulose with a DS_{azide} of 0.4 obtained under microwave irradiation was reacted with propargylated starch with a DS_{alkyne} of 2.2. The cross-linked cellulose/starch networks were obtained in high yield (83%). SEM characterization

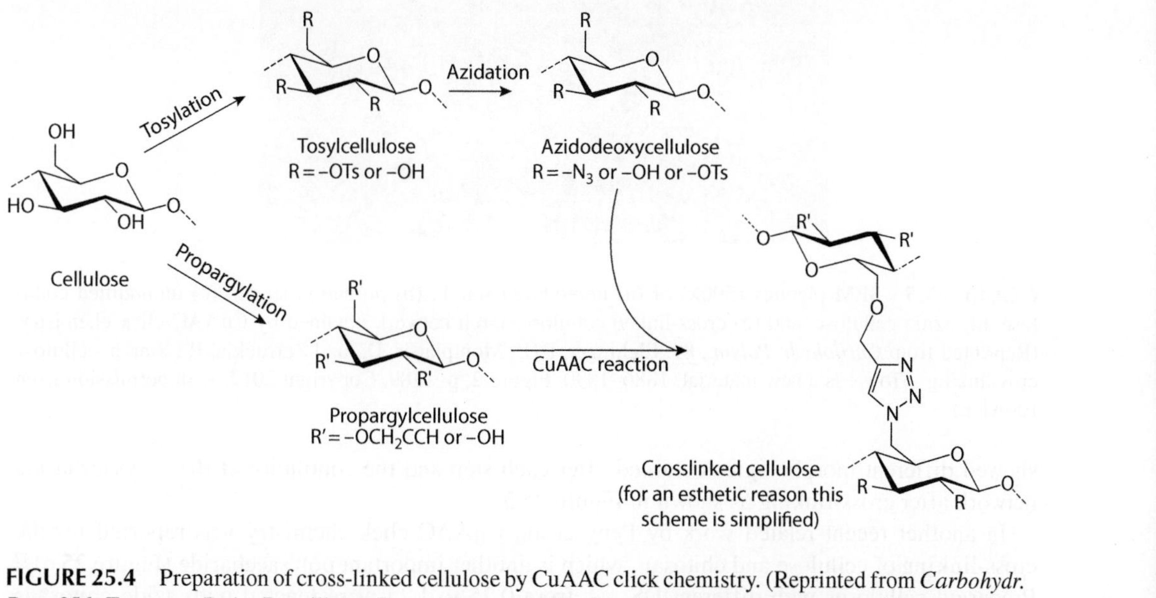

FIGURE 25.4 Preparation of cross-linked cellulose by CuAAC click chemistry. (Reprinted from *Carbohydr. Res.*, 356, Faugeras, P.-A., Brouillette, F., and Zerrouki, R., Crosslinked cellulose developed by CuAAC, a route to new materials, 247–251, Figure 1, p. 248, Copyright 2012, with permission from Elsevier.)

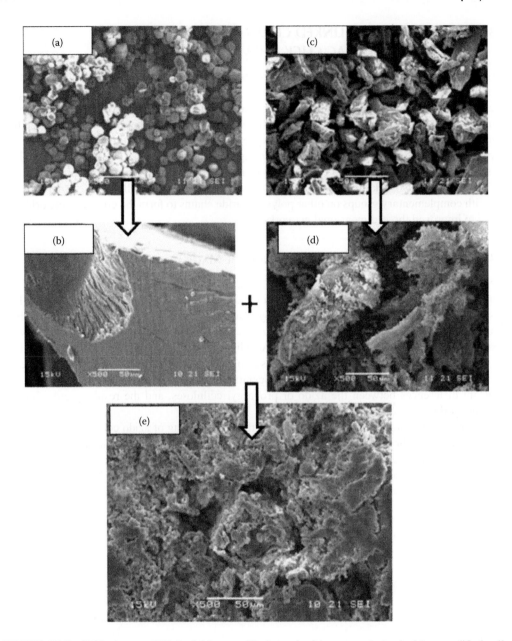

FIGURE 25.5 SEM pictures (500×) of (a) unmodified starch, (b) propargyl starch, (c) unmodified cellulose, (d) azido cellulose, and (e) cross-linked cellulose/starch network obtained by CuAAC click chemistry. (Reprinted from *Carbohydr. Polym.*, 89, Elchinger, P.H., Montplaisir, D., and Zerroukia, R., Starch–cellulose crosslinking—Towards a new material, 1886–1890, Figure 2, p. 1889, Copyright 2012, with permission from Elsevier.)

showed different morphologies obtained after each step and the continuity of the polysaccharide network after cross-linking as shown in Figure 25.5.

In another recent related work by Peng et al., CuAAC click chemistry was reported for the cross-linking of cellulose and chitosan, which is another important polysaccharide (Figure 25.6).[17] Propargyl celluloses with different DS_{alkyne} from 0.25 to 1.24 were reacted with azido chitosans with DS_{azide} from 0.02 to 0.46 in $DMSO/H_2O$ with $CuSO_4$, $5H_2O$ in the presence of sodium ascorbate at room temperature for 48 h. FTIR characterization showed the significant decrease in the

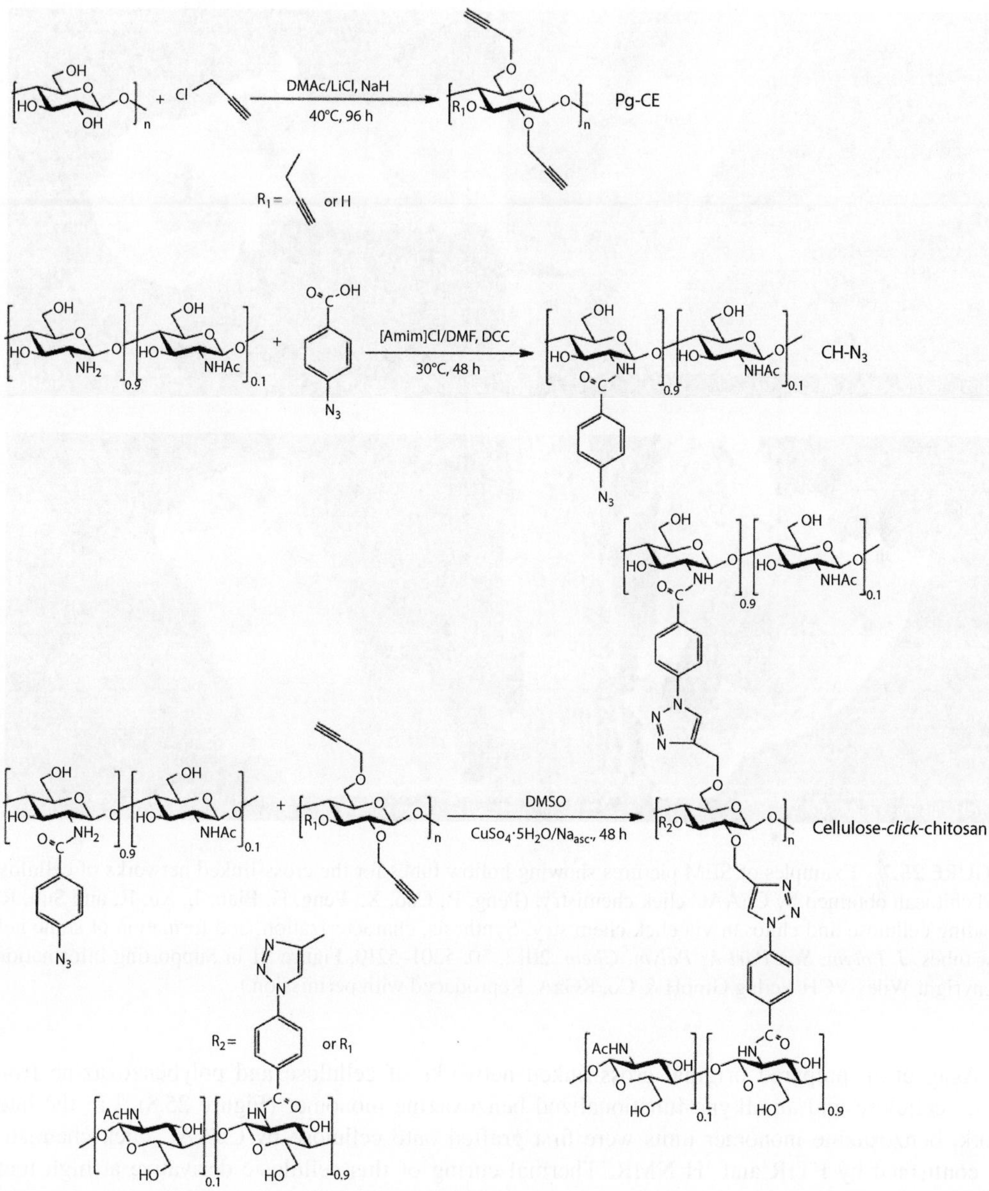

FIGURE 25.6 Preparation of cross-linked networks of cellulose and chitosan by CuAAC click chemistry. (Peng, P., Cao, X., Peng, F., Bian, J., Xu, F., and Sun, R.: Binding cellulose and chitosan via click chemistry: Synthesis, characterization, and formation of some hollow tubes. *J. Polym. Sci. Part A: Polym. Chem.* 2012. 50. 5201–5210, Scheme 1, p. 5202, Copyright Wiley-VCH Verlag GmbH & Co. KGaA. Reproduced with permission.)

alkyne and azido bands after click chemistry. Complementary CP/MAS ^{13}C NMR experiments proved the formation of triazole rings. The cross-linked cellulose/chitosan networks had improved thermal stability compared to cellulose, chitosan, and even cellulose/chitosan complex. SEM pictures obtained after the fracture of the cross-linked networks revealed the striking presence of hollow tubes of millimeter size, which were not observed for the corresponding cellulose/chitosan complex (Figure 25.7).

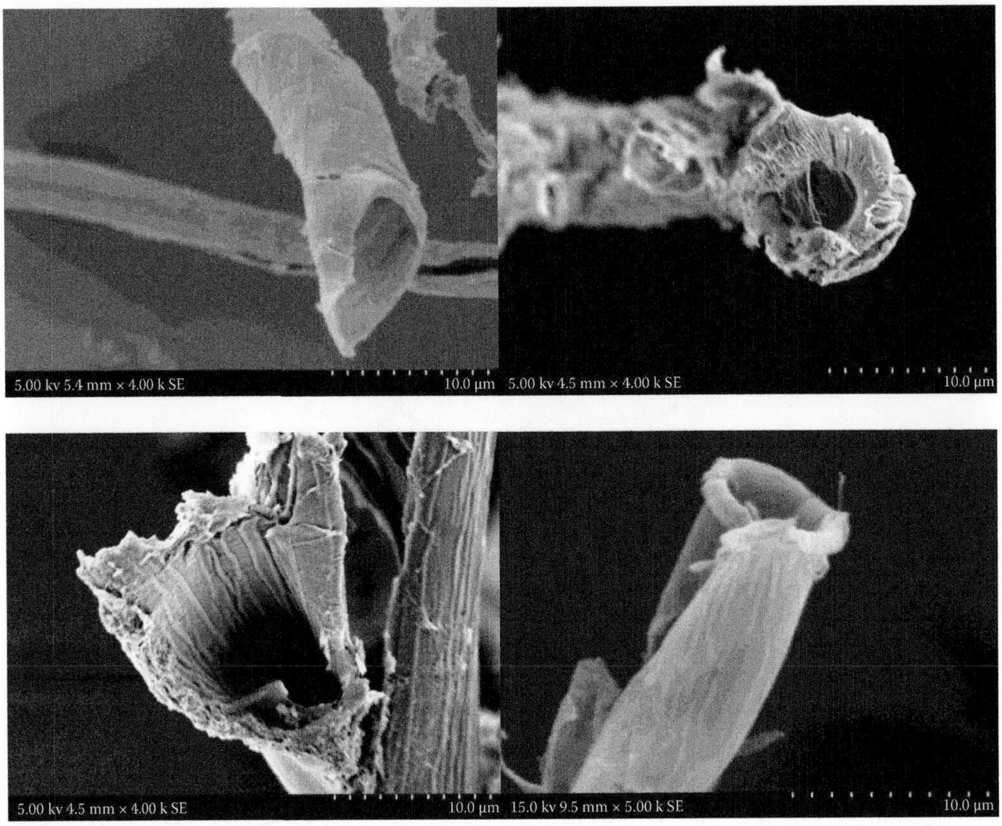

FIGURE 25.7 Examples of SEM pictures showing hollow tubes for the cross-linked networks of cellulose and chitosan obtained by CuAAC click chemistry. (Peng, P., Cao, X., Peng, F., Bian, J., Xu, F., and Sun, R.: Binding cellulose and chitosan via click chemistry: Synthesis, characterization, and formation of some hollow tubes. *J. Polym. Sci. Part A: Polym. Chem.* 2012. 50. 5201–5210, Figure S1 in Supporting information, Copyright Wiley-VCH Verlag GmbH & Co. KGaA. Reproduced with permission.)

Agag et al. prepared original cross-linked networks of cellulose and polybenzoxazine from azido cellulose and an alkyne-functionalized benzoxazine monomer (Figure 25.8).[30] In the later work, benzoxazine monomer units were first grafted onto cellulose by CuAAC click chemistry as confirmed by FTIR and ^{1}H NMR. Thermal curing of this cellulosic derivative at high temperature (200°C/1 h) led to the ring-opening polymerization of the benzoxazine monomer units. Thermogravimetric analysis showed that the resulting cross-linked cellulose/polybenzoxazine networks were much more resistant to heat than virgin cellulose, with a residual weight increased by one order of magnitude at 800°C.

25.3.2 Cross-Linked Cellulose-Based Hydrogels

CuAAC click chemistry has also offered innovative pathways to cross-linked polysaccharide-based hydrogels, which have been recently reviewed by Elchinger et al. and Uliniuc et al.[10,13] Among them, cellulose-based hydrogels have remained really scarce so far, despite their high potential as cross-linked bio-based hydrogels.

In this respect, Koschella et al. have reported the carboxymethylation of azido and alkyne celluloses leading to water-soluble cellulose derivatives for CuAAC click chemistry.[31] Transparent hydrogels were then readily obtained by adding $CuSO_4$, $5H_2O$ and ascorbic acid to aqueous solutions

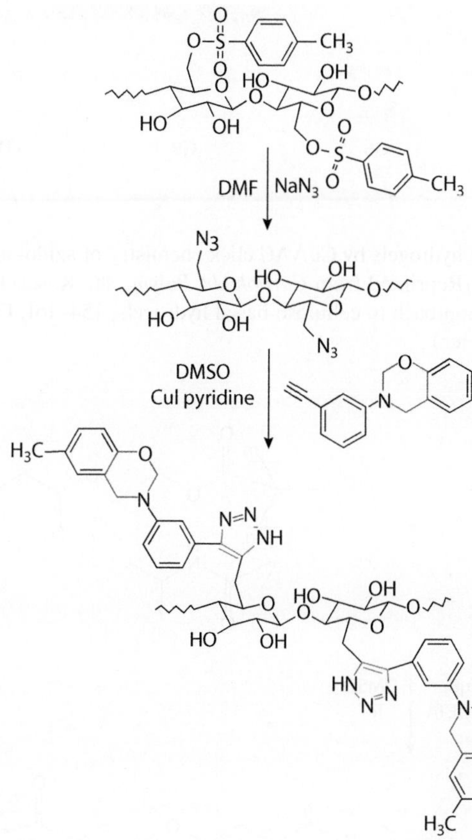

FIGURE 25.8 Synthesis of benzoxazine-functional cellulose by CuAAC click chemistry, considered as an interesting intermediate for preparing cross-linked cellulose/polybenzoxazine networks. (Agag, T., Vietmeier, K., Chernykh, A., and Ishida, H.: Side-chain type benzoxazine-functional cellulose via click chemistry. *J. Appl. Polym. Sci.* 2012. 125. 1346–1351, Figure 2, p. 1348, Copyright Wiley-VCH Verlag GmbH & Co. KGaA. Reproduced with permission.)

containing both cellulose derivatives with equimolar ratio of azido and alkyne groups (Figure 25.9). Rheologic measurements showed that the gelation time strongly decreased with increasing DS_{azide}, DS_{alkyne}, and copper catalyst concentration. Some of the freshly prepared hydrogels could further swell in water up to a water content of approximately 100%. However, in these challenging conditions, these hydrogels lost their mechanical withstanding and disintegrated. According to the authors, improving click chemistry for these systems could lead to advanced stimuli-responsive cellulose-based hydrogels.

Following another interesting synthetic pathway combining classical radical polymerization, polymer modification, and CuAAC click chemistry, Zhang et al. synthesized a series of original temperature-responsive hydrogels from an azido cellulose with a DS_{azide} of 0.95 and an alkyne-functionalized thermo-responsive copolymer (poly(*N*-isopropyl acrylamide-*co*-hydroxyl ethyl methacrylate) P(NIPAM-*co*-HEMA)).[32] The grafting of the alkyne-functionalized P(NIPAM-*co*-HEMA) onto the azido cellulose was carried out in DMSO in the presence of CuBr and *N*,*N*,*N*′,*N*″,*N*″-pentamethyldiethylenetriamine (PMDETA) at room temperature with different amounts of the thermo-responsive grafts (Figure 25.10). After freeze-drying and cryo-fracture of the cross-linked hydrogels, SEM pictures revealed discontinuous porous inner structures. The average pore sizes decreased from 40 and 10 μm when the amount of the thermo-responsive grafts increased from 50 to 80 wt%, leading to higher cross-linking degrees.

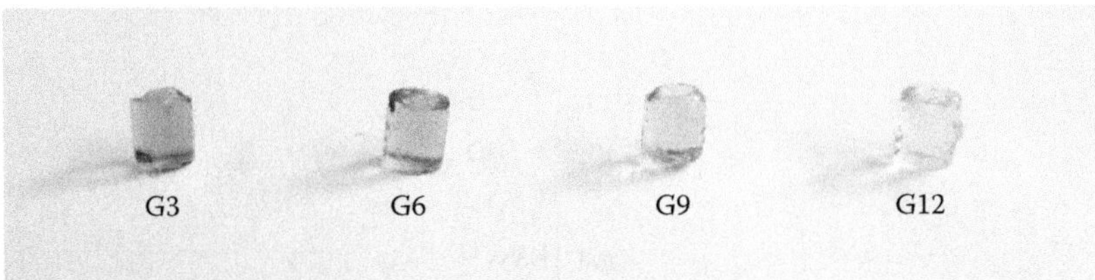

FIGURE 25.9 Freshly prepared hydrogels by CuAAC click chemistry of azido- and alkyne-carboxymethyl celluloses in various conditions. (Reprinted from *Carbohydr. Polym.*, 86, Koschella, A., Hartlieba, M., and Heinze, T., A "click-chemistry" approach to cellulose-based hydrogels, 154–161, Figure 3, p. 160, Copyright 2011, with permission from Elsevier.)

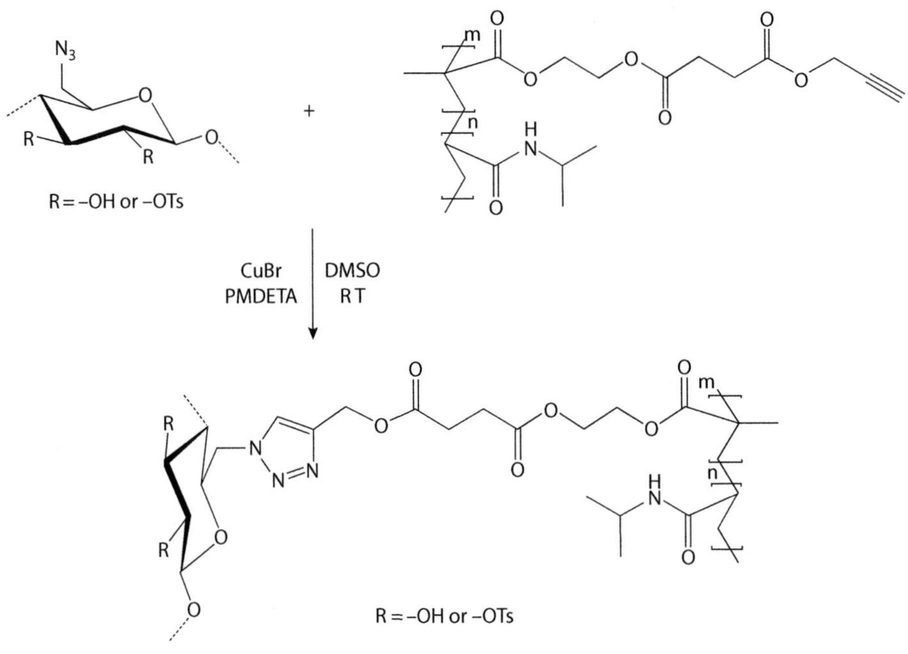

FIGURE 25.10 Preparation of thermo-responsive cross-linked hydrogels from an azido cellulose and an alkyne-functionalized copolymer P(NIPAM-*co*-HEMA) by CuAAC click chemistry. (Reprinted from Elchinger, P.-H. et al., *Polymers*, 3, 1617, 2011, Figure 12. Copyright 2011, with permission from MDPI AG; Zhang, J. et al., *Carbohydr. Polym.*, 77, 583, 2009.)

25.4 BLOCK AND GRAFT CELLULOSIC COPOLYMERS BY CuAAC CLICK CHEMISTRY

To the best of our knowledge, the synthesis of *block copolymers* from cellulose or its derivatives by CuAAC click chemistry has been reported only once so far. In 2012, Nakagawa et al. prepared amphiphilic diblock copolymers from cellulose triacetate with a terminal azido group at position 1 and methyl cellulose with a terminal alkyne group at position 4 (Figure 25.11).[26] CuAAC click chemistry in the presence of CuBr, sodium ascorbate, and PMDETA initially led to diblock copolymers with two *hydrophobic* blocks made of low-molecular-weight cellulose triacetate and methyl cellulose. After cleavage of the acetate groups by sodium methanolate in the organic medium, the cellulose triacetate block was converted into a hydrophilic cellulose

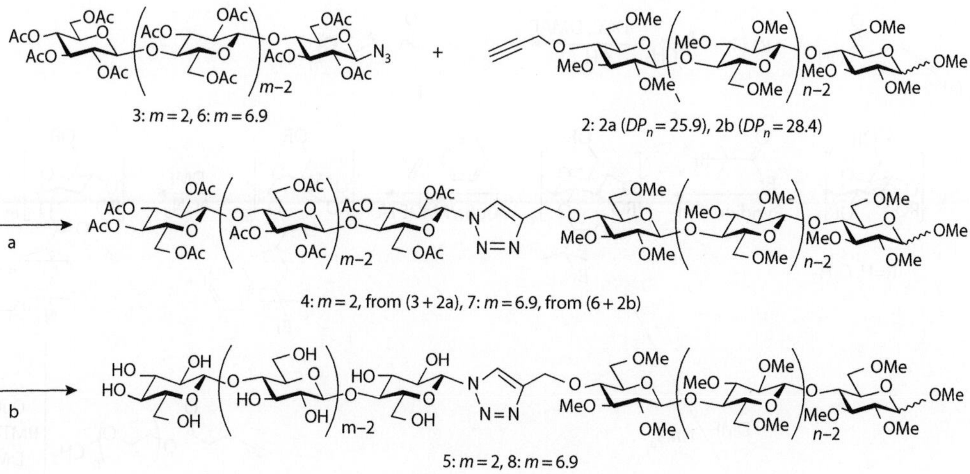

FIGURE 25.11 Preparation of amphiphilic cellulose-based diblock copolymers by CuAAC click chemistry. (With kind permission from Springer Science+Business Media: *Cellulose*, Synthesis and thermoreversible gelation of diblock methylcellulose analogues via Huisgen 1,3-dipolar cycloaddition, 19, 2012, 1315–1326, Nakagawa, A., Kamitakahara, H., and Takano, T., Figure 3, p. 1318, Copyright 2012.)

block. An amphiphilic diblock copolymer was finally obtained with thermoreversible gelation properties.

The preparation of *graft copolymers* from cellulose or cellulose derivatives has been widely investigated, and over the past few years, a few bibliographic reviews have pointed out the recent progress made for controlling this grafting by various techniques.[10,12,33–35] Nevertheless, CuAAC click chemistry has been rarely reported for the preparation of graft copolymers from cellulose and its derivatives so far. This click chemistry is currently emerging as a promising method for cellulose grafting and designing original materials with very different properties. Graft cellulosic copolymers are obtained by the grafting of cellulosic derivatives in homogeneous solution. The grafting of (nano)cellulose surfaces is considered in Section 25.7.2 of this chapter.

By combining controlled radical polymerization (ATRP) with CuAAC click chemistry, Li et al. prepared two closely related series of ethyl cellulose (EC) graft copolymers. For the first series of graft copolymers, an EC macroinitiator with brominated side groups was used for the "grafting from" of polystyrene (PS) grafts with controlled lengths (Figure 25.12).[19] The bromine terminal atoms of the PS grafts were then substituted for azido groups. These azido groups were further reacted with an alkyne-monomethoxy poly(ethylene glycol) by CuAAC click chemistry, leading to EC derivatives with diblock grafts PS-*b*-PEG. For the second series of copolymers, the bromine atoms of the EC macroinitiator were partially converted into azide groups. The resulting "clickable" macroinitiator was then used for the one-pot "grafting from" of styrene by ATRP and "grafting onto" of ω-alkyne monomethoxy-PEG by CuAAC click chemistry. This second smart strategy took advantage of the orthogonality of ATRP and CuAAC click chemistry for obtaining EC copolymers grafted by both PS and PEG grafts in a *single* synthesis step.

Amphiphilic cellulosic graft copolymers were obtained by Xu et al. with PEG grafts bearing azido terminal groups for click chemistry.[25] The multistep synthesis allowed the regioselective grafting of PEG with allyl terminal groups at position 3 with thexyldimethylsilyl protecting groups at positions 2 and 6. The allyl terminal groups of the PEG grafts were then converted into azido groups in three steps. Honeycomb films were then prepared by the breathing figures method, and their pore sizes were controlled by the X_n of the functional PEG grafts. The honeycomb films were grafted by biotin by CuAAC click chemistry, leading to advanced functional porous films for bio-applications. Very recently, further studies showed the availability of the grafted biotin for conjugation with

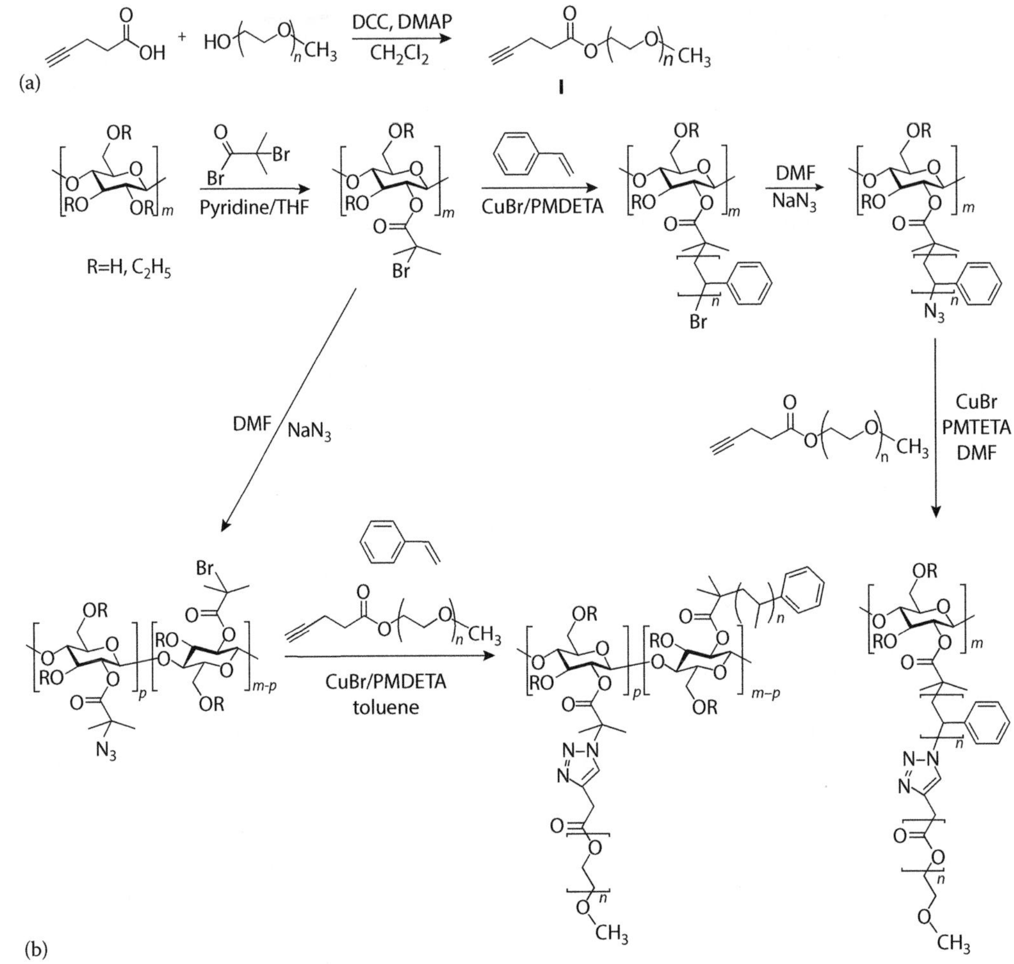

FIGURE 25.12 Two strategies for the synthesis of ethyl cellulose graft copolymers (a) with diblock PS-b-PEG grafts or (b) with both PS and PEG grafts by CuAAC click chemistry in homogeneous solution. (Li, Q., Kang, H., and Liu, R.: Block and hetero ethyl cellulose graft copolymers synthesized via sequent and one-pot ATRP and "Click" reactions. *Chinese J. Chem.* 2012. 30. 2169–2175, Figure 1, p. 2170, Copyright Wiley-VCH Verlag GmbH & Co. KGaA. Reproduced with permission.)

fluorescent avidin inside the pores of the honeycomb films (Figure 25.13).[20] CuAAC click chemistry also enabled to functionalize the honeycomb films with quantum dots, which were again located inside the pores as shown by confocal fluorescence microscopy. In another related work by the same team, the grafting of an alkynated quaternary ammonium compound led to honeycomb films with antifouling and antibacterial properties for *Escherichia coli*.[36]

Negishi et al. reported the regioselective grafting of different alkyne-functionalized maltoside (Mal) and lactoside (Lac) oligosaccharides onto azido cellulose at position 6.[37] The grafting was carried out by CuAAC click chemistry in DMSO in the presence of $CuBr_2$, ascorbic acid, and propylamine at room temperature for 12 h with yields ranging from 65% to 79%. Water solubility of the grafted copolymers was strongly influenced by the nature of the space between cellulose and the grafted oligosaccharides. The water solubility was much lower in case of a hydrophobic spacer although molecular dynamics simulations showed that hydrophilic and hydrophobic spacers led to the same type of sheet-like structures for the grafted copolymers.

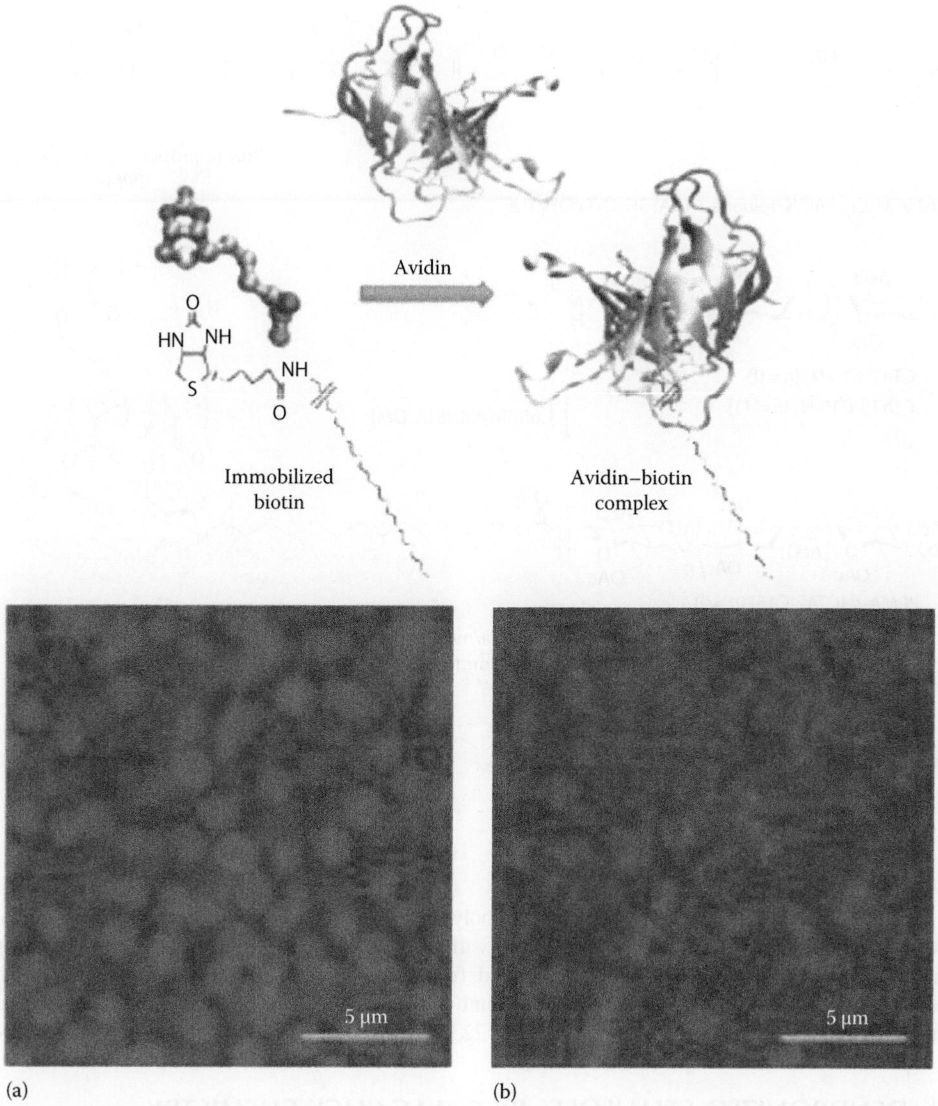

FIGURE 25.13 Biofunctional honeycomb films made of an amphiphilic cellulosic graft copolymer with PEG-biotin grafts obtained by CuAAC click chemistry. Comparison of the combined confocal fluorescent (gray) and optical (dark) images (a) before and (b) after conjugation with avidin. (Reprinted with permission from Xu, W.Z. and Kadla, J.F., Honeycomb films of cellulose azide: Molecular structure and formation of porous films, *Langmuir*, 29, 727–733, 2013, Figure 6, p. 731. Copyright 2013 American Chemical Society.)

Compared with the former works on cellulosic copolymers grafted by CuAAC click chemistry, another originality of the recent work of Enomoto-Rogers et al. was to consider grafted copolymers with *cellulosic grafts* rather than cellulosic main chains (Figure 25.14).[27] In this new work, an amorphous polymethacrylate with alkyne side groups was initially prepared in three steps using protecting group chemistry. The "grafting onto" of cellulose triacetate grafts with azido groups at the reducing end was then carried out by CuAAC click chemistry. After cleavage of the acetate groups by sodium methanolate, a polymethacrylate comb copolymer was obtained with cellulosic grafts. An analysis by wide-angle X-ray diffraction showed that a film of this grafted copolymer was semicrystalline with a diffraction pattern corresponding to that of regenerated cellulose.

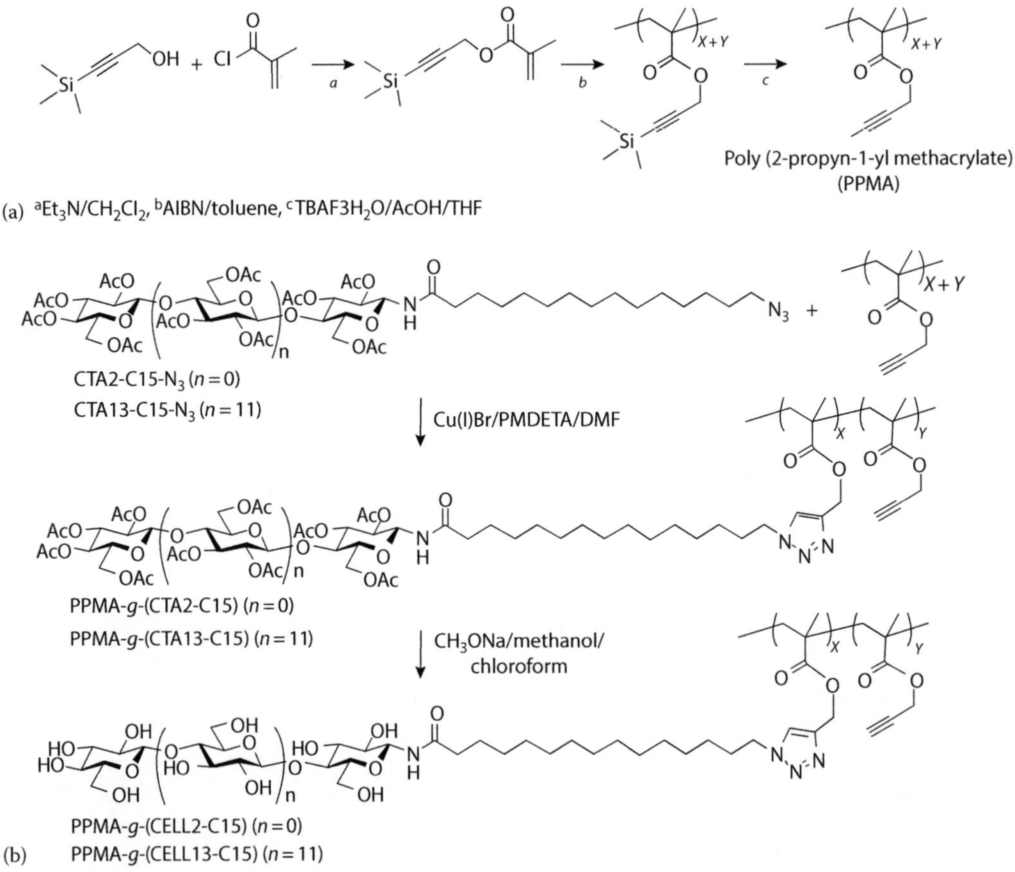

FIGURE 25.14 Preparation of polymethacrylate copolymers grafted with cellulosic side chains by CuAAC click chemistry (a) Synthesis of a polymethacrylate with alkyne side groups and (b) grafting of this polymethacrylate with cellulosic side chains. (Reprinted from *Carbohydr. Polym.*, 87, Enomoto-Rogers, Y., Kamitakahara, H., Yoshinaga, A., and Takano, T., Comb-shaped graft copolymers with cellulose side-chains prepared via click chemistry, 2237–2245, Figure 1, p. 2239, Copyright 2012, with permission from Elsevier.)

25.5 DENDRONIZED CELLULOSES BY CuAAC CLICK CHEMISTRY

The grafting of dendrons onto cellulose by CuAAC click chemistry has led to a variety of biofunctional materials over the past few years. Dendrons are fractal structures with increasing number of functional groups from one generation to the next one. Dendronization of cellulose can thus increase its chemical functionality tremendously and offer interesting prospects for a wide range of bio-applications (e.g., biosensors, drug delivery systems, and biocatalysts).

In their first attempt to prepare dendronized cellulose, Pohl and Heinze regioselectively grafted polyamido amine (PAMAM) dendrons of first and second generations, with an azido moiety at their focal point, onto an alkyne cellulose with a DS_{alkyne} of 0.48 at position 6 (Figure 25.15).[16] The grafting rate decreased from 70% to 50% for the dendrons of first and second generations, respectively, most likely due to strong steric hindrance. All the dendronized cellulose derivatives were soluble in aprotic dipolar solvents (DMSO, DMF, and DMAc).

Pohl et al. also investigated the reverse strategy consisting in grafting PAMAM dendrons with an alkyne moiety at their focal point onto an azido cellulose with a DS_{azido} of 0.75 at position 6. In homogeneous conditions in DMSO, grafting rates of 89%, 75%, and 41% were obtained for the dendrons of first, second, and third generations, respectively. Here again, steric hindrance limited

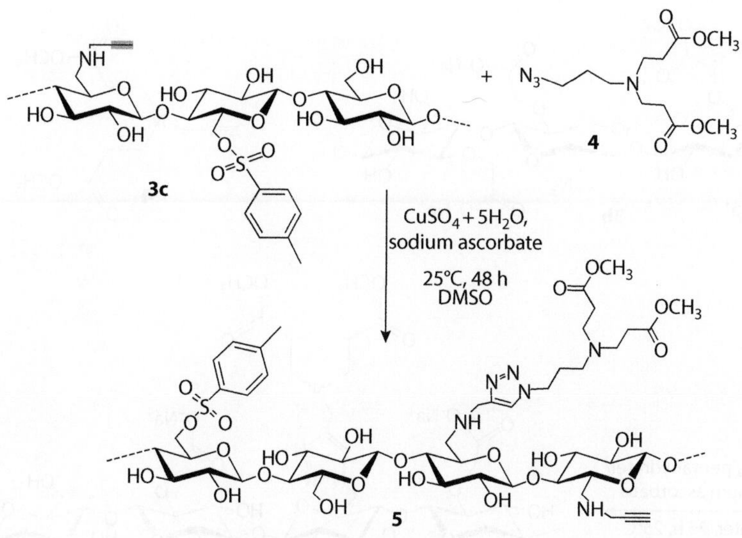

FIGURE 25.15 Preparation of dendronized cellulose with PAMAM dendrons of first generation from an alkyne-functionalized cellulose at position 6 by CuAAC click chemistry. (Pohl, M. and Heinze, T.: Novel biopolymer structures synthesized by dendronization of 6-deoxy-6-aminopropargyl cellulose. *Macromol. Rapid Commun.* 2008. 29. 1739–1745, Figure 2, p. 1743, Copyright Wiley-VCH Verlag GmbH & Co. KGaA. Reproduced with permission.)

the grafting rate of the bulkiest dendrons, but, overall, the new work greatly improved the number of grafted dendrons and the functionality of the dendronized celluloses. Heterogeneous grafting in MeOH was also remarkably well achieved with comparable grafting rates as those obtained in homogeneous conditions.[38]

The regioselective grafting of PAMAM dendrons onto cellulose at position 3 required more demanding protecting group chemistry.[24] Thexyldimethylsilyl groups were chosen as protective groups due to their high selectivity for positions 2 and 6, leaving position 3 available for introducing alkyne side groups with a DS_{alkyne} of 1. After deprotection, alkyne cellulose was successfully grafted with azido-functionalized PAMAM dendrons of first and second generations, but the grafting rates were fairly low (≤25%).

Water-soluble dendronized celluloses were also prepared by Pohl et al. from a carboxymethylated azido cellulose with a DS_{azide} of 0.81 by CuAAC click chemistry in water at ambient temperature (Figure 25.16).[39] The grafting of alkyne-functionalized PAMAM dendrons proceeded mainly at position 6 with grafting rates varying from 63% to 48% from the first to third generations of dendrons. A thorough physical chemical investigation showed that the grafting of dendrons had no or a weak influence on the cellulosic chain stiffness or conformation in solution.

Novel biofunctional cellulosic films were also developed by the same team from dendronized cellulose containing a high number of amino groups, which are particularly appropriate for further modification with biomolecules.[40] In the first approach, azido cellulose was first grafted with alkyne dendrons containing terminal amine groups in homogeneous solution, and the resulting dendronized cellulose was then simply blended with cellulose acetate. The second approach considered simple surface grafting of an azido cellulose film with the same dendrons in mild conditions. After careful removal of the residual copper ions by complexation with diethyldithiocarbamate trihydrate to avoid any detrimental interference with the targeted biomolecules, the cellulosic films were successfully biofunctionalized with a glucose oxidase enzyme in two steps (Figure 25.17).

Highly versatile dendronized cellulosic surfaces were also developed by Montanez et al.[41] After its functionalization by azido groups, cellulose paper was grafted with functional dendrons of

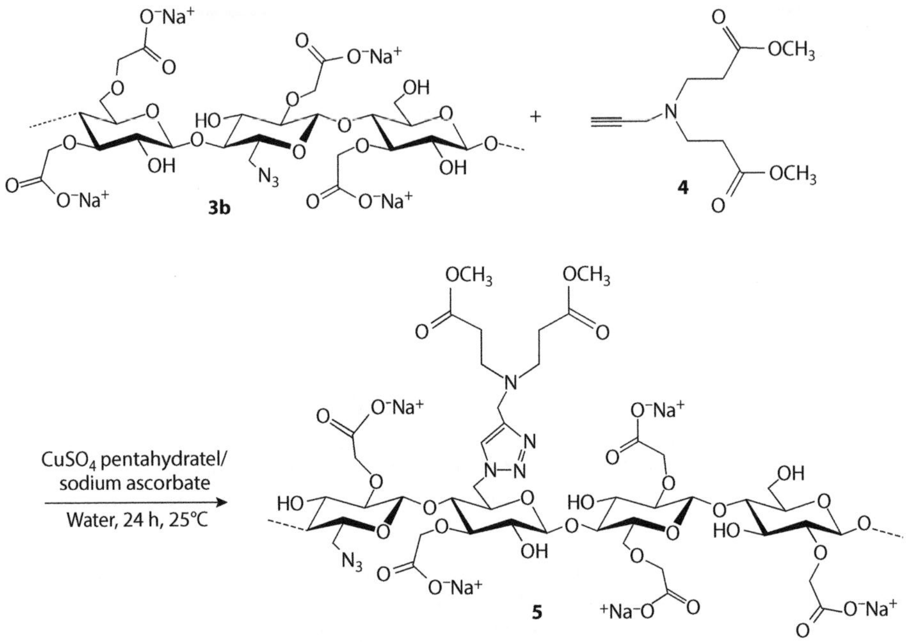

FIGURE 25.16 Preparation of dendronized carboxymethyl cellulose with PAMAM dendrons of first generation from an azido-functionalized cellulose at position 6 by CuAAC click chemistry. (Reprinted from *Eur. Polym. J.*, 45, Pohl, M., Morris, G.A., Harding, S.E., and Heinze, T., Studies on the molecular flexibility of novel dendronized carboxymethyl cellulose derivatives, 1098–1110, Figure 2 p. 1103, Copyright 2009, with permission from Elsevier.)

first to fifth generations by CuAAC click chemistry in mild conditions (Figure 25.18). The dendron terminal groups were then chemically modified to obtain a very high number of orthogonal chemical functions at the periphery. By this high precision multistep strategy, each hydroxyl group initially present at cellulose surface eventually led to 64 dendritic OH and 32 dendritic azido groups. Biofunctionalization was then successfully achieved with different alkyne-functionalized molecules including amoxicillin and mannose. In the latter case, the biofunctional surface allowed the detection of lectin protein at a concentration as low as 5 nM. This dendronized cellulosic platform is particularly promising for bio and chemical sensors, with respect to the high number of the orthogonal functions present at the periphery and its versatility to address a wide range of sensing applications.

25.6 CELLULOSIC POLYELECTROLYTES BY CuAAC CLICK CHEMISTRY

Polysaccharide-based polyelectrolytes have become very important in the formulation of aqueous solutions for a wide range of applications. Today, food and health-care industries largely rely on their particular properties in solution and in particular on their strong thickening effect at very low polymer concentration owing to the polyelectrolyte effect.

As first shown by Liebert et al., CuAAC click chemistry offered new pathways to original cellulosic polyelectrolytes.[11] Unlike cellulosic ester polyelectrolytes, these new polyelectrolytes were stable toward hydrolysis owing to the high stability of the triazole linkers between cellulose and the ionic side groups.

In the first work, 6-azido-6-deoxycelluloses with DS_{azide} ranging from 0.88 to 0.99 were grafted with an alkyne-functionalized carboxylic acid methyl ester and 2-ethynylaniline (Figure 25.19).[11]

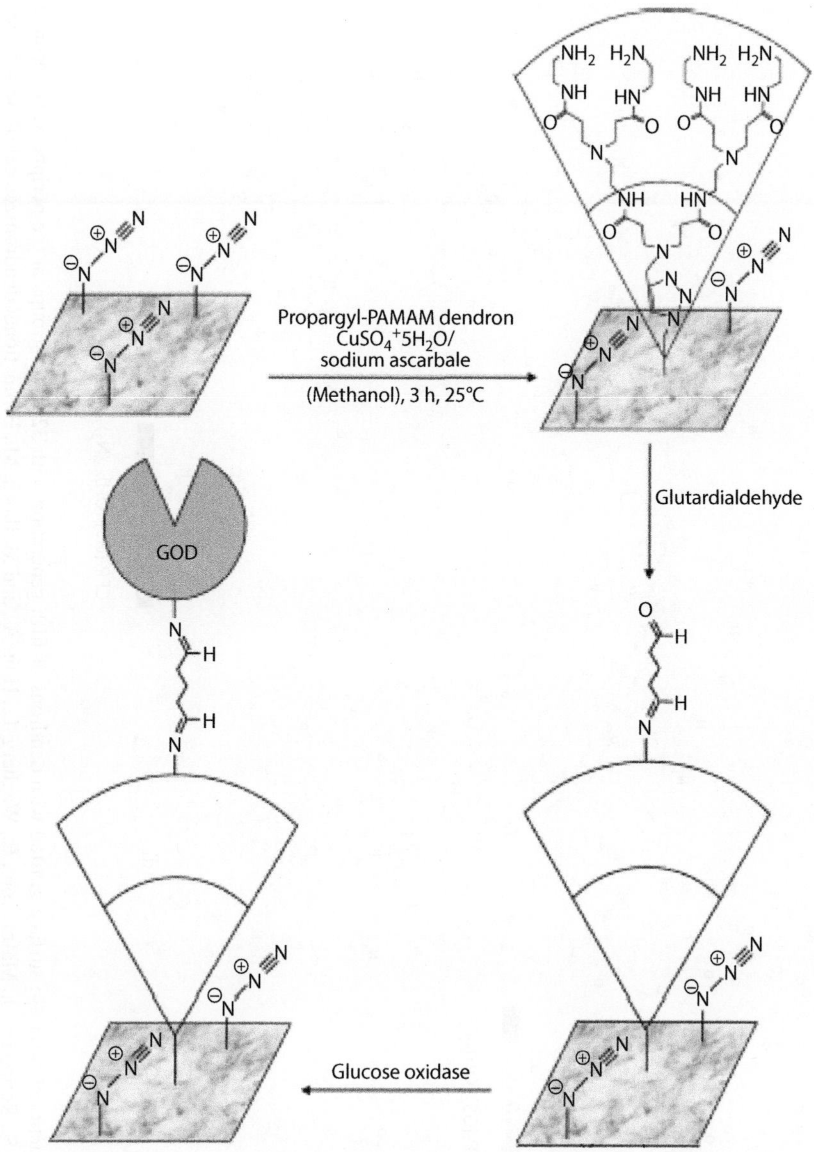

FIGURE 25.17 Two-step biofunctionalization of an azido cellulose film grafted by alkyne dendrons containing terminal amino groups, with a glucose oxidase enzyme. (Reprinted with permission from Pohl, M., Michaelis, N., Meister, F., and Heinze, T., Biofunctional surfaces based on dendronized cellulose, *Biomacromolecules*, 10, 382–389, 2009, Figure 6, p. 387. Copyright 2009 American Chemical Society.)

Both molecular reagents were considered as precursors for anionic and cationic groups, respectively, after appropriate modification of the grafted cellulose derivatives. High degree of substitution (0.86) was obtained for the carboxylic acid methyl ester in very mild conditions (25°C/molar ratio of 1 with respect to the azido groups). The efficient grafting of 2-ethynylaniline required much higher temperature (70°C) and a large excess in molecular reagent (3 equiv.). Both cellulosic derivatives were soluble in DMF or DMSO. Their modification with strong base or acid led to anionic and cationic cellulosic polyelectrolytes, respectively.

In another work by the same team, this approach was transposed to the grafting of acetylenedicarboxylic acid dimethyl ester by means of click chemistry followed by saponification of the

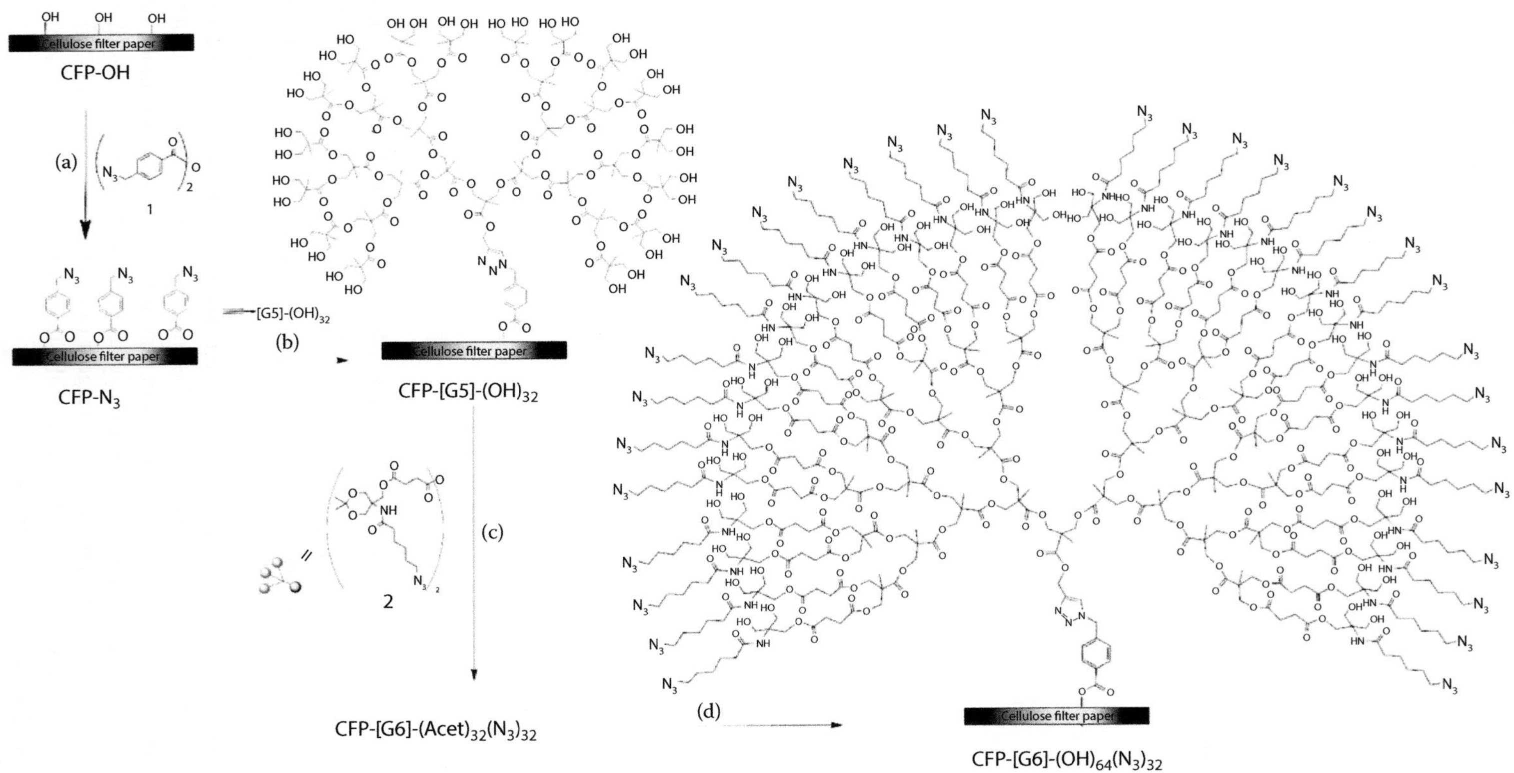

FIGURE 25.18 Schematic drawing of a biofunctional cellulose surface grafted with dendrons of fifth generation with 32 azido groups at the periphery. (Reprinted permission from Montanez, M.I., Hed, Y., Utsel, S., Ropponen, J., Malmstrom, E., Wagberg, L., Hult, A., and Malkoch, M., Bifunctional dendronized cellulose surfaces as biosensors, *Biomacromolecules*, 12, 2114–2125, 2011, Figure 1, p. 2216. Copyright 2011 American Chemical Society.)

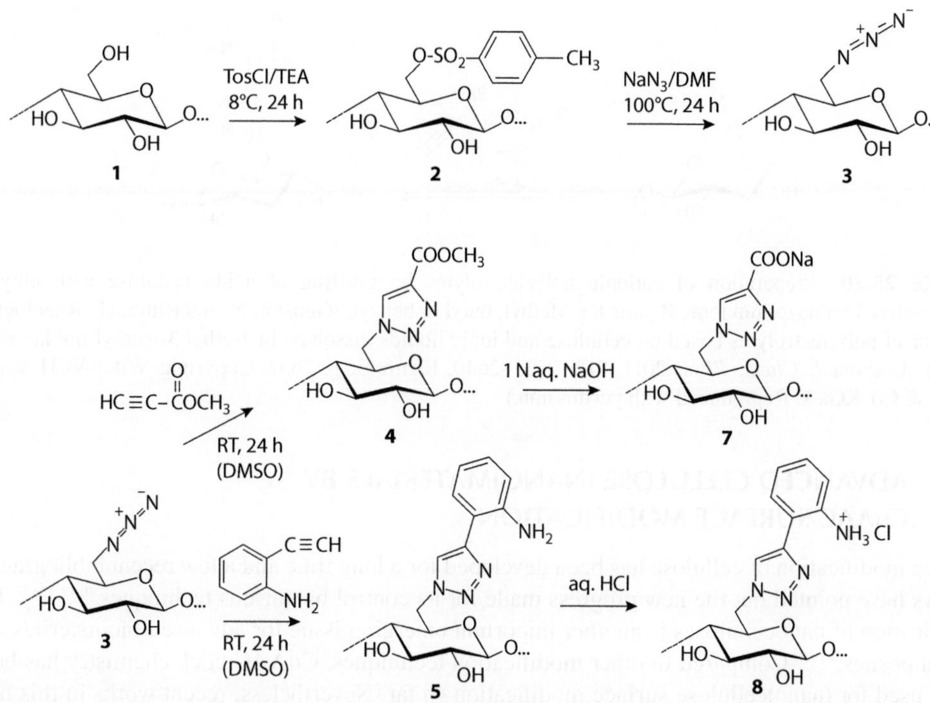

FIGURE 25.19 Preparation of anionic and cationic cellulosic polyelectrolytes by CuAAC click chemistry and further modification by strong base or acid. (Liebert, T., Hänsch, C., and Heinze, T.: Click chemistry with polysaccharides. *Macromol. Rapid Commun.* 2006. 27. 208–213, Figure 1, p. 210, Copyright Wiley-VCH Verlag GmbH & Co. KGaA. Reproduced with permission.)

ester side groups.[42] The CuAAC click reaction of 6-azido-6-deoxycellulose with the alkyne-functionalized diester was performed with a grafting rate of 62% and enabled to greatly increase the number of anionic groups obtained after saponification compared to that of the first work. Furthermore, the later anionic cellulosic polyelectrolytes displayed tensioactive properties and formed interesting ionotropic gels by precipitation in aqueous solutions containing multivalent ions (Ca^{2+}, Al^{3+}) or a cationic polyelectrolyte (poly(diallyldimethyl ammonium) chloride (polyDADMAC)).

Another interesting approach to novel cationic cellulosic polyelectrolytes based on azido cellulose and alkyne-functionalized ionic liquids was reported by Gonsior and Ritter.[43] Cellulose is known to be soluble in a few ionic liquids including 1-ethyl-3-methyl imidazolium acetate (emim)(ac), but its viscosity is fairly high in these particular solvents. In the later work, 6-azido 6-deoxy cellulose with a DS_{azido} of approximately 1 was grafted with three different alkyne-functionalized ionic liquids (i.e., 1-methyl, 1-butyl, and 1-benzyl 3-propargyl imidazolium bromides) in DMSO/H_2O by CuAAC click chemistry at 25°C for 48 h (Figure 25.20). Almost quantitative grafting was reached in these conditions with very high degrees of substitution for the grafted ionic liquids. Rheology experiments were carried out for virgin cellulose and the corresponding cationic polyelectrolytes in the ionic liquid 1-ethyl-3-methyl imidazolium acetate used as a solvent. The results showed that cellulose grafting with ionic liquids decreased solution viscosity by at least one order of magnitude compared to that of virgin cellulose. Furthermore, the solution viscosity decreased with the size of the alkyl substituent on the imidazolium ionic liquids, the methyl substituent thus providing the lowest solution viscosity.

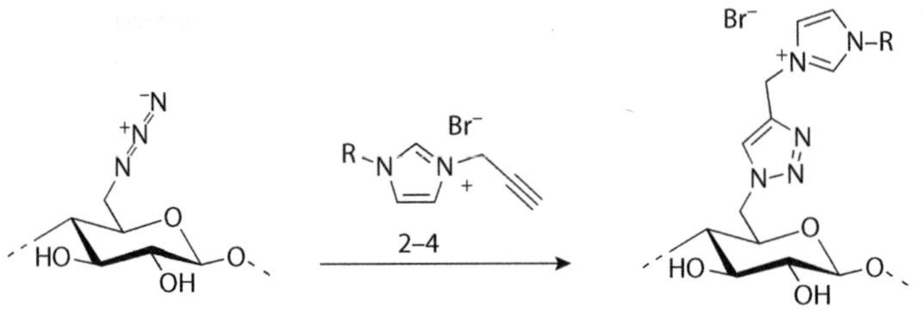

FIGURE 25.20 Preparation of cationic polyelectrolytes by grafting of azido cellulose with alkyne-functionalized imidazolium ionic liquids R = Methyl, butyl or benzyl. (Gonsior, N. and Ritter, H.: Rheological behavior of polyelectrolytes based on cellulose and ionic liquids dissolved in 1-ethyl-3-methyl imidazolium acetate. *Macromol. Chem. Phys.* 2011. 212. 2633–2640, Figure 3, p. 2637, Copyright Wiley-VCH Verlag GmbH & Co. KGaA. Reproduced with permission.)

25.7 ADVANCED CELLULOSE (NANO)MATERIALS BY CuAAC SURFACE MODIFICATION

Surface modification of cellulose has been developed for a long time and a few recent bibliographic reviews have pointed out the new progress made for its control by various techniques.[10,12,33–35] The modification of nanocelluloses is another important emerging issue for advanced biomaterials and biocomposites.[44–48] Compared to other modification techniques, CuAAC click chemistry has been rarely used for (nano)cellulose surface modification so far. Nevertheless, recent works in this field show that this click chemistry offers a tremendous potential for designing original materials with very different properties and functionalities from nano- to macroscales.

25.7.1 Advanced Materials by Cellulose Surface Modification

Adapting a procedure reported by Hafrén et al. for cellulose paper grafting with a fluorescent probe,[49] Krouit et al. grafted cellulose Avicel powder by an aliphatic polyester in heterogeneous conditions.[50] The cellulosic powder was first functionalized with alkyne side groups with relatively long spacers in C_{11} for improving grafting efficiency. The "grafting onto" was then performed with an α,ω-diazido-polycaprolactone (PCL) by CuAAC click chemistry in mild conditions. In addition to surface grafting, the PCL difunctionality may have also led to limited surface cross-linking. These grafted cellulosic powders were considered as interesting precursors for the development of fully biodegradable cellulosic composites.[51]

A combination of controlled radical polymerization with CuAAC click chemistry was another interesting approach for the *controlled* surface grafting of cellulose. In a first work by Haddleton and coworkers,[52] an azide-functionalized fluorescent polymethacrylate (PMMA) oligomer with controlled molecular weight was obtained by controlled radical copolymerization (ATRP) of methyl methacrylate (MMA) and a fluorescent methacrylate comonomer. This fluorescent oligomer with an azido terminal group was then grafted onto an alkyne-functionalized cotton by CuAAC click chemistry. An azido-monomethoxy poly(ethylene glycol) was also grafted onto the same cotton derivative.

A thorough comparison of the methods of "grafting from" and "grafting onto" by CuAAC click chemistry has been recently reported by Hansson et al. for the cellulose surface grafting with PMMA grafts of different lengths.[53] In this work, PMMA was first "grafted from" a cellulose paper bearing initiator groups by controlled radical polymerization (ARGET ATRP) (Figure 25.21). Following a procedure well known for the control of the graft molecular weight by the "grafting from" method, the use of an alkyne-functional sacrificial initiator enabled to obtain free alkyne-functionalized PMMA oligomers with the same molecular weights as those of the PMMA grafts.

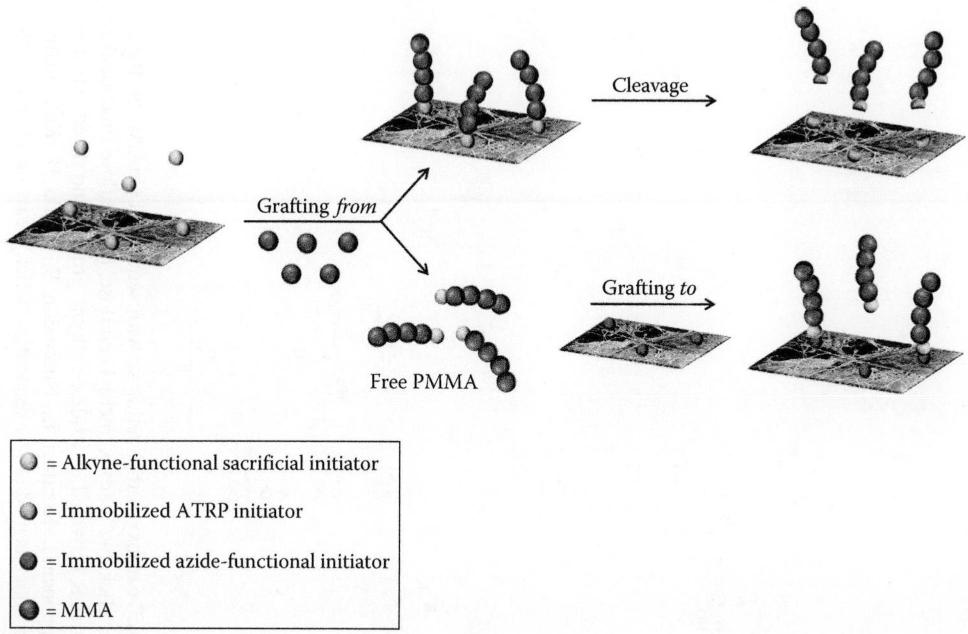

FIGURE 25.21 Cellulose surface modification by the methods of "grafting from" and "grafting onto" by CuAAC click chemistry with free alkyne-functional PMMA oligomers obtained during "grafting from" in the presence of an alkyne-functional sacrificial initiator. (Reprinted with permission from Hansson, S., Trouillet, V., Tischer, T., Goldmann, A.S., Carlmark, A., Barner-Kowollik, C., and Malmström, E., Grafting efficiency of synthetic polymers onto biomaterials: A comparative study of grafting-from versus grafting-to, *Biomacromolecules*, 14, 64–74, 2013, Figure 1, p. 65. Copyright 2013 American Chemical Society.)

These alkyne-functional PMMA oligomers were then "grafted onto" an azide-functionalized cellulose paper. A comparison of both surface grafting methods with identical grafts showed that the grafting density on the cellulosic surface was higher for the method of "grafting from," which also enabled a better control of the graft content. The method of "grafting onto" was limited by lower grafting density and efficiency for the longest grafts, mainly owing to the limited accessibility of the alkyne terminal groups of the corresponding PMMA oligomers.

Recently, Filpponen et al. have proposed a very different strategy for cellulose surface modification based on a combination of adsorption of a "clickable" carboxymethyl cellulose (CMC) on cellulose surface with sequential CuAAC grafting in mild conditions (Figure 25.22).[18,54] In the first step, a CMC modified with azido or alkyne groups was adsorbed on various cellulosic surfaces (i.e., regenerated cellulose, cellulose paper, cellulose nanofibrils [CNFs]) by simple coating or dipping in a functionalized CMC aqueous solution. Low CMC degree of substitution (DS_{azide} or DS_{alkyne}) and the presence of electrolytes in the aqueous solution were both important for a good adsorption of the functionalized CMC onto cellulosic surfaces.[54] The grafting of alkyne-functionalized bovine serum albumin, azido-functionalized fluorescent probe, and monomethoxy PEG was then performed in mild conditions by CuAAC click chemistry. The versatility of this approach appears particularly interesting for modifying a variety of cellulosic surfaces.

25.7.2 Advanced Materials by Nanocellulose Surface Modification

Cellulose nanomaterials represent a new class of cellulosic materials (e.g., cellulose nanocrystals [CNCs] and nanofibrils [CNFs]) with one dimension in the nanometer scale, which offer particularly high prospects for a wide range of applications.[44–47] Taking advantage of their high aspect ratio and

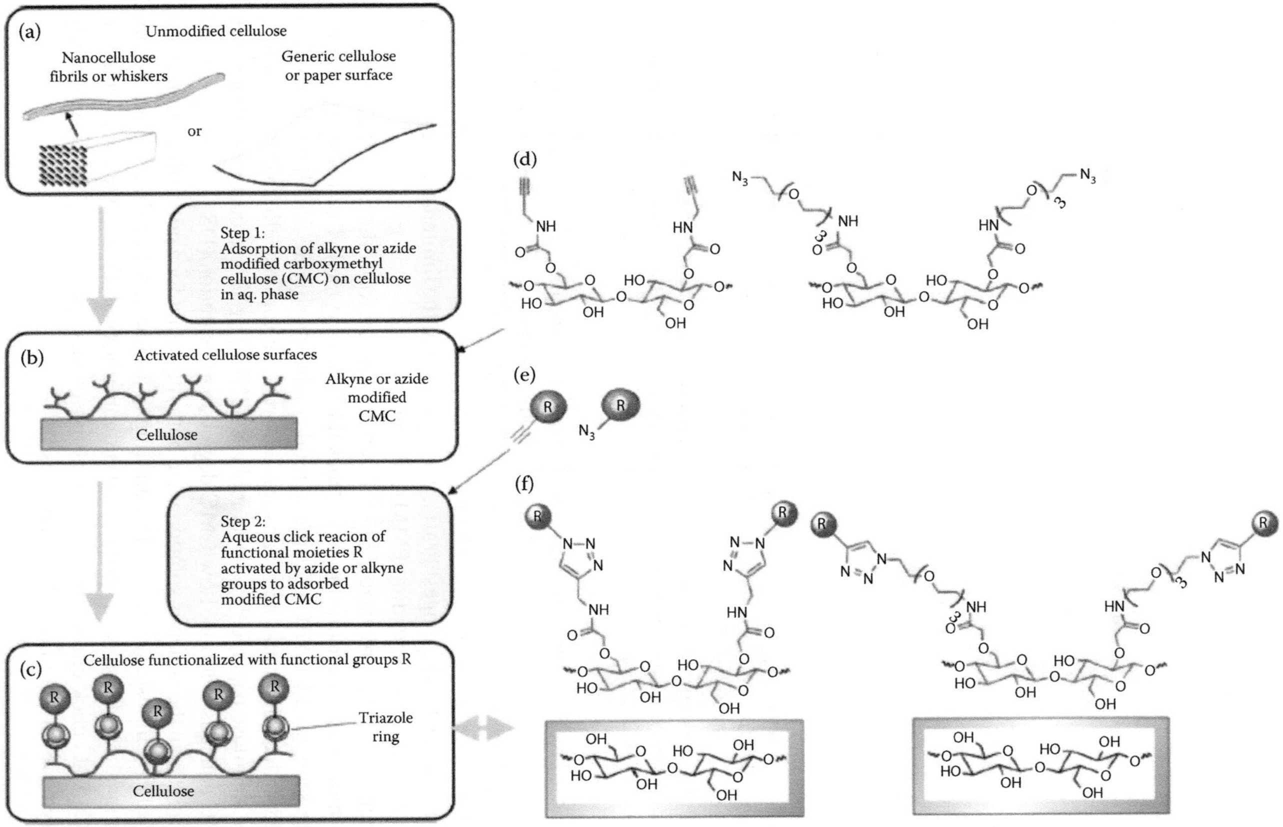

FIGURE 25.22 Cellulose surface modification based on a combination of adsorption of a "clickable" carboxymethyl cellulose with sequential CuAAC grafting in mild conditions. (a) Unmodified cellulose, (b) activated cellulose surfaces obtained by adsorption of a "clickable" carboxymethyl cellulose, (c) cellulose functionalized with functional groups R, (d) alkyne or azide modified carboxymethyl cellulose, (e) functional moieties R activated by azide or alkyne groups, and (f) adsorbed carboxymethyl cellulose after functionalization by click chemistry. (Reprinted with permission from Filpponen, I., Kontturi, E., Nummelin, S., Rosilo, H., Kolehmainen, E., Ikkala, O., and Laine, J., Generic method for modular surface modification of cellulosic materials in aqueous medium by sequential "Click" reaction and adsorption, *Biomacromolecules*, 13, 736–742, 2012, Figure 1, p. 737. Copyright 2012 American Chemical Society.)

outstanding mechanical properties, these renewable cellulosic materials have been mainly used as fillers to reinforce polymer materials in composites. In particular, their incorporation in biopolymers has led to original biocomposites for a sustainable composite industry.[51] Cellulose nanomaterials have also brought new functionalities to cellulose and offered new pathways to advanced materials for the paper, food, health-care, cosmetics, and pharmaceutical industries.

So far, chemical modification of cellulose nanomaterials has been investigated mainly for improving their compatibility with polymer matrices in composite materials and has been the subject for a few recent reviews.[44,45,47,48] Nevertheless, chemical modification of cellulose nanomaterials by CuAAC click chemistry has been rarely reported so far and has not been reviewed yet.

25.7.2.1 Advanced Nanomaterials by Cellulose Nanocrystal Modification

CNCs are rod-like or whisker nanoparticles with high aspect ratio (typically 3–5 nm in width, 50–500 nm in length) obtained by cellulose acid hydrolysis. Filpponen and Argyropoulos described their surface functionalization with azido and alkyne groups in two steps.[55] In the first step, hydroxyl groups on the CNC surface were converted into carboxylic acid groups by TEMPO-mediated hypohalite oxidation. In the second step, these carboxylic acid groups were reacted with azido- or alkyne-functionalized amines by ethylcarbodiimide coupling in the presence of *N*-hydroxysuccinimide. CuAAC click chemistry of the azide- and alkyne-surface functionalized CNCs led to the formation of nanoplatelet gels. TEM analysis showed that the nanoplatelets formed after click chemistry retained the rectangular shape of virgin CNCs and that they were the result of a highly regular CNC packing. The same team further investigated the CuAAC coupling of other azide- and alkyne-surface functionalized CNCs for new nanoplatelet gels.[56] TEM analysis showed the importance of solvent polarity for the CNC packing during nanocellulose gelification induced by CuAAC click chemistry. The CNCs were uniformly oriented in the nanoplatelets prepared in water, while they were rather randomly oriented for those prepared in organic solvent (DMF).

Filpponen et al. also reported smart photoresponsive CNCs obtained by CuAAC grafting with coumarin and anthracene fluorescent probes (Figure 25.23).[57] Fluorescence microscopy confirmed the fluorescence of the grafted CNCs. Furthermore, UV-photoinduced reversible cycloadditions of coumarin and anthracene resulted in the formation of photoresponsive cellulosic nano-arrays.

Taking advantage of another photoresponsive character, Feese et al. developed photobactericidal cellulose nanoparticles by CuAAC grafting of azide CNCs with an alkyne-functionalized porphyrin.[58] The porphyrin photosensitizer was then activated upon illumination and generated cytotoxic species including singlet oxygen. The resulting photobactericidal effect was the most intense for the bacteria *Staphylococcus aureus*, which represent one of the most dangerous threats to human health. In another work by Eyley and Thielemans, an alkyne-functionalized imidazolium ionic liquid was grafted onto azide-functionalized CNCs for anion exchange applications.[59] These cellulose nanoparticles grafted with imidazolium species could also have interesting bactericidal properties.

Original hybrid CNC–protein nanoparticles have also been reported by Karaaslan et al. recently.[60] In this work, CNCs alkyne-functionalized at their reducing ends were coupled with azido-functionalized β-casein micelles by CuAAC click chemistry in water. AFM and TEM imaging showed a variety of shapes for the CNC/β-casein conjugates obtained in these conditions. Such hybrid polysaccharide–protein nanoparticles could be interesting building blocks for new biomaterials.

25.7.2.2 Advanced Nanomaterials by Cellulose Nanofibril Modification

CNFs can be prepared from a variety of cellulose sources.[44,45] These nano-objects have outstanding mechanical properties with a Young modulus similar to that of Kevlar. Owing to their original

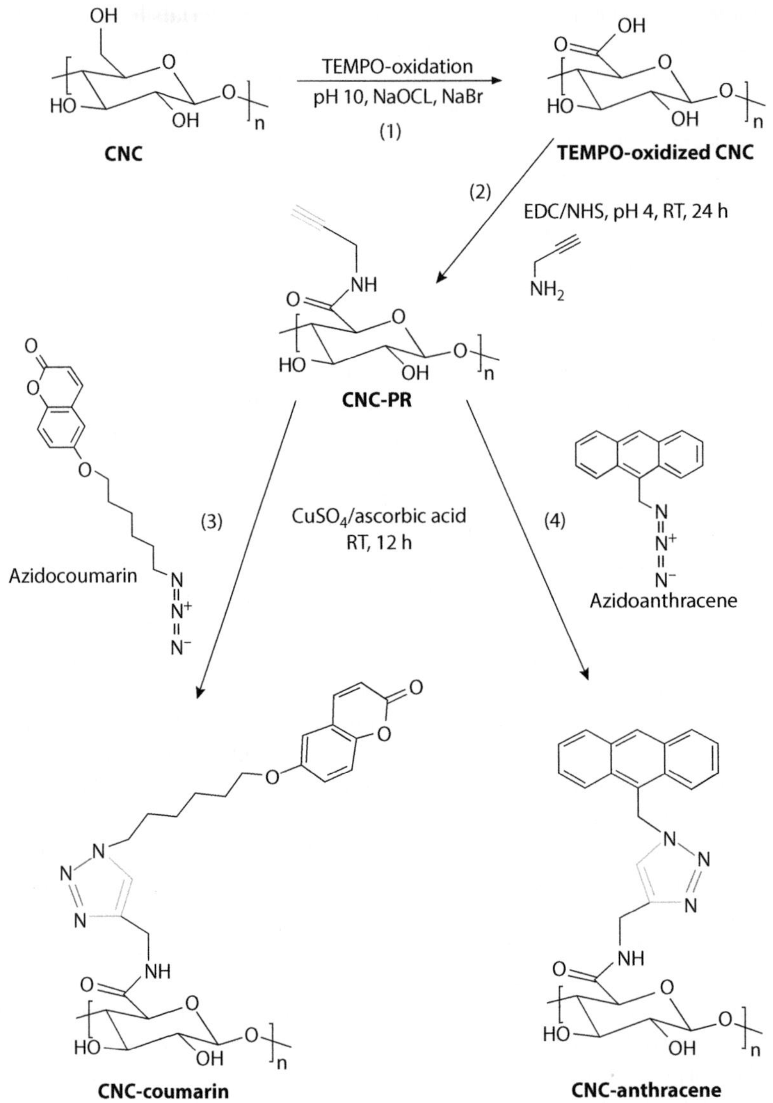

FIGURE 25.23 Photoresponsive CNCs obtained by CNCs grafting with coumarin and anthracene fluorescent moieties by CuAAC click chemistry. (From Filpponen, I. et al., *Nanomater. Nanotechnol.*, 1, 36, 2011, Figure 1. Copyright 2011, with permission from Open Access CC BY.)

properties, CNFs can also, in particular conditions, lead to optically transparent cellulosic paper very different from the white paper obtained from common cellulose (Figure 25.24).

Smart pH-responsive or fluorescent CNFs have been obtained by CNF surface modification by CuAAC click chemistry in mild conditions in aqueous media.[61] The CNF surface was first functionalized with azido groups by reaction with 1-azido-2,3-epoxypropane in the presence of sodium hydroxide. The azido-CNFs were then used as a nano-platform for introducing amino or fluorescent side groups. Figure 25.25 showed an image for a fluorescent pale yellow-green CNF film obtained after grafting of a fluorescent probe. AFM images confirmed that the nanofibrillated structure was well maintained after surface functionalization. Furthermore, the CNFs with amine side groups displayed pH-responsive rheological properties. The addition of acetic acid to their aqueous suspension led to lower viscosity and a very strong decrease in the storage and loss

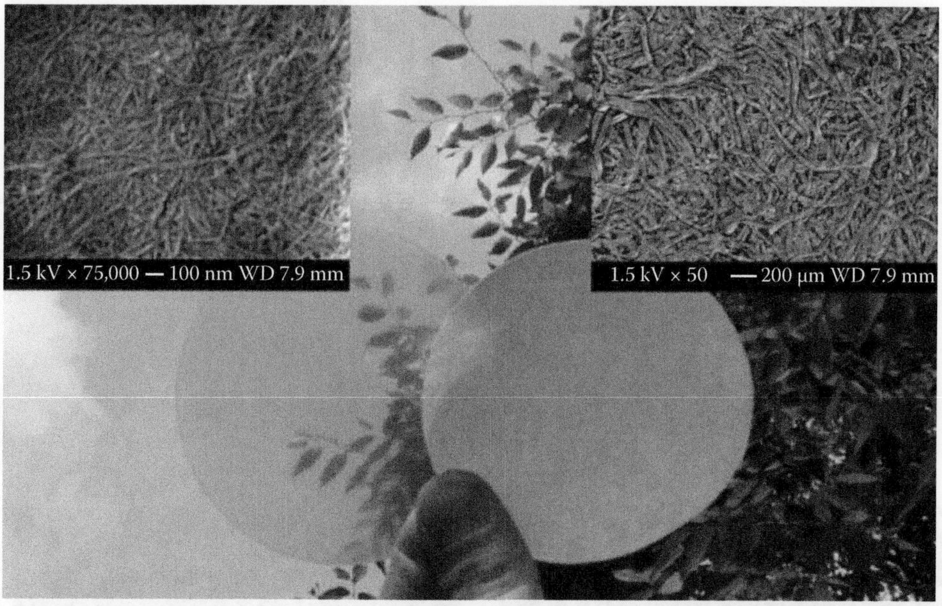

FIGURE 25.24 Optically transparent nanofiber paper (left) composed of 15 nm cellulose nanofibers (upper left, scale bar in inset: 100 nm) and conventional cellulose paper (right) composed of 30 μm pulp fibers (upper right, scale bar in inset: 200 μm). (Nogi, M., Iwamoto, S., Nakagaito, A.N., and Yano, H.: Optically transparent nanofiber paper. *Adv. Mater.* 2009. 21. 1595–1598, Figure 1, p. 1595, Copyright Wiley-VCH Verlag GmbH & Co. KGaA. Reproduced with permission.)

moduli. In that case, amine protonation was responsible for strong ionic repulsions and a collapse of the CNF network.

CNFs functionalized by amine groups by CuAAC click chemistry were also reported by Luong et al. for the development of graphene/cellulose nanocomposite papers with high electrical and mechanical performance.[62] These nanocomposites were obtained by filtering stable dispersions of reduced graphite oxide and amine-functionalized CNFs. The very good dispersion of graphene obtained in this work was partially due to the nucleophilic addition of the CNF amine groups with epoxy groups present on graphene. CNF functionalization by CuAAC click chemistry provided an efficient compatibilization system for graphene contents up to 10 wt%. A strong enhancement of the mechanical properties was already observed after addition of graphene in very low amount (0.3 wt%). Furthermore, the electrical conductivity of the graphene/CNF nanocomposite papers strongly increased from 4.79×10^{-4} to 71.8 S m^{-1} with their graphene content from 0.3 to 10 wt%. The high flexibility, stability, and mechanical and electrical conductivity performance of the new graphene/CNF nanocomposites offer interesting prospects for portable electronics and electromagnetic shielding devices.

25.8 CONCLUSION

Over the past few years, CuAAC click chemistry has offered new ways of modifying cellulose and its derivatives in particular mild conditions and with hydrolytically stable triazole linkers. Its high reliability, efficiency, and tolerance of different functional groups have contributed to developing great structural and functional varieties for cellulosic materials.

A wide range of copolymer architectures have been easily obtained from azido- or alkyne-functionalized cellulosic derivatives: structural or hydrogel cross-linked networks, block and graft copolymers, and dendronized celluloses. New cationic and anionic polyelectrolytes have also been easily prepared with greatly improved hydrolytic stability compared to former polyelectrolyte

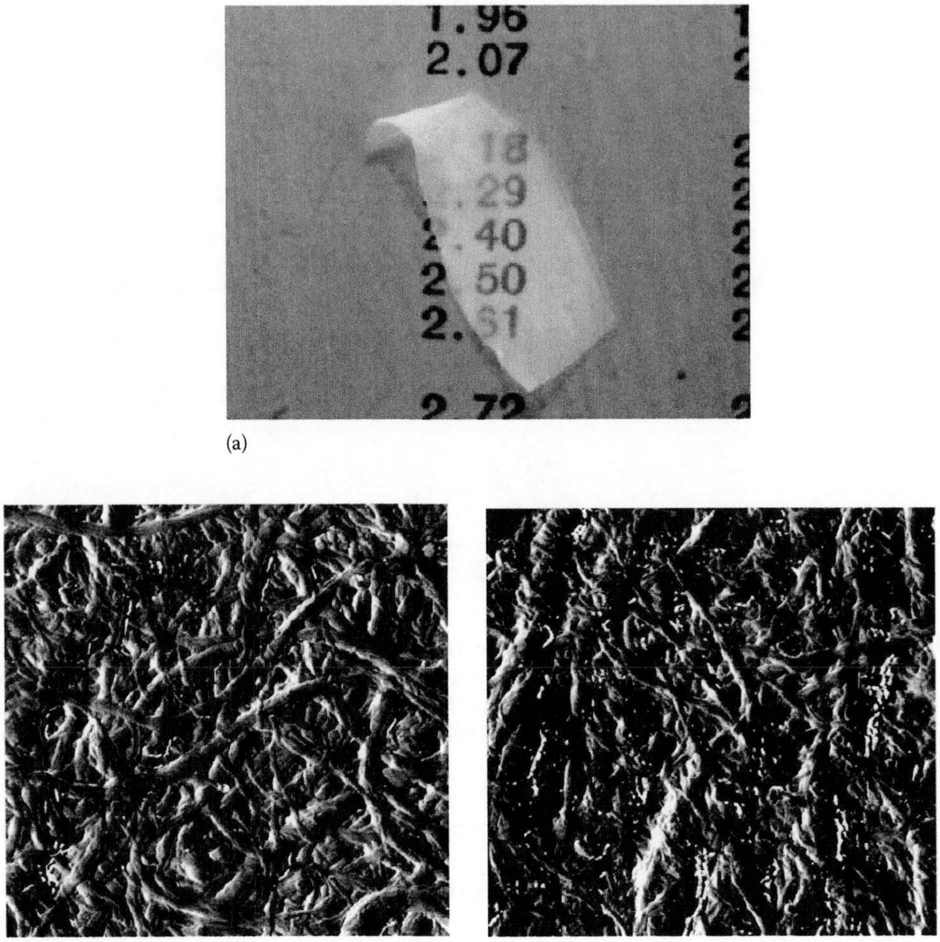

(a)

(b) (c)

FIGURE 25.25 (a) Image of a fluorescent pale CNF film obtained after surface grafting of a fluorescent dye by CuAAC click chemistry. AFM phase images of (b) unmodified and (c) azide-functionalized NFC with a scan size of 2 μm. (With kind permission from Springer Science+Business Media *Cellulose*, Surface functionalization of nanofibrillated cellulose using click-chemistry approach in aqueous media, 18, 2011, 1201–1212, Pahimanolis, N., Hippi, U., Johansson, L.-S., Saarinen, T., Houbenov, N., Ruokolainen, J., and Seppälä, J., Figure 2, p. 1206.)

cellulosic esters. The recent progress made on cellulose nanomaterial modification has shown another great potential for the development of new cellulosic materials for advanced applications from nano- to macroscale.

CuAAC click chemistry has also brought a new range of functionalities to cellulose and its derivatives. Thermo-, pH-, and photo-responsive cellulosic (nano)materials have been obtained by simple grafting of responsive moieties in homogeneous or heterogeneous conditions. Fluorescent and (photo)bactericidal properties were also easily provided to cellulosic (nano)materials by CuAAC click chemistry.

Within the frame of sustainable chemistry, CuAAC click chemistry will certainly contribute to greatly extend the scope and functionality of cellulose-based materials for a wide range of applications in smart packaging, advanced food, health care, drug delivery, biomaterials, biocomposites, biosensors, bactericidal materials, and biofunctional films.

ACKNOWLEDGMENT

The authors would like to thank the ELEMENT Erasmus Mundus Programme for the PhD scholarship awarded to Faten Hassan Hassan Abdellatif.

REFERENCES

1. Kolb, H. C., M. G. Finn, and K. Barry Sharpless. 2001. Click chemistry: Diverse chemical function from a few good reactions. *Angewandte Chemie International Edition* 40:2004–2021.
2. Rostovtsev, V. V., L. G. Green, V. V. Fokin, and K. B. Sharpless. 2002. A stepwise Huisgen cycloaddition process: Copper(I)-catalyzed regioselective "Ligation" of azides and terminal alkynes. *Angewandte Chemie International Edition* 41:2596–2599.
3. Wu, P., A. K. Feldman, A. K. Nugent, C. J. Hawker, A. Scheel, B. Voit, J. Pyun, J. M. J. Fréchet, K. B. Sharpless, and V. V. Fokin. 2004. Efficiency and fidelity in a click-chemistry route to triazole dendrimers by the copper(I)-catalyzed ligation of azides and alkynes. *Angewandte Chemie International Edition* 43:3928–3932.
4. Fournier, D., R. Hoogenboom, and U. S. Schubert. 2007. Clicking polymers: A straightforward approach to novel macromolecular architectures. *Chemical Society Reviews* 36:1369–1380.
5. Moses, J. and A. Moorhouse. 2007. The growing applications of click chemistry. *Chemical Society Reviews* 2007:1249–1262.
6. Binder, W. H. and R. Sachsenhofer. 2008. 'Click' Chemistry in polymer and material science: An update. *Macromolecular Rapid Communications* 29:952–981.
7. Lutz, J.F. and Z. Zarafshani. 2008. Efficient construction of therapeutics, bioconjugates, biomaterials and bioactive surfaces using azide–alkyne "click" chemistry. *Advanced Drug Delivery Reviews* 60:958–970.
8. Meldal, M. and C. W. Tornoe. 2008. Cu-catalyzed azide-alkyne cycloaddition. *Chemical Reviews* 108:2952–3015.
9. Barner-Kowollik, C., F. E. Du Prez, P. Espeel, C. J. Hawker, T. Junkers, H. Schlaad, and W. Van Camp. 2011. "Clicking" polymers or just efficient linking: What is the difference. *Angewandte Chemie International Edition* 50:60–62.
10. Elchinger, P.-H., P.-A. Faugeras, B. Boens, F. Brouillette, D. Montplaisir, R. Zerrouki, and R. Lucas. 2011. Polysaccharides: The "Click" chemistry impact. *Polymers* 3:1607–1651.
11. Liebert, T., C. Hänsch, and T. Heinze. 2006. Click chemistry with polysaccharides. *Macromolecular Rapid Communications* 27:208–213.
12. Tizzotti, M., A. Charlot, E. Fleury, M. Stenzel, and J. Bernard. 2010. Modification of polysaccharides through controlled/living radical polymerization grafting—Towards the generation of high performance hybrids. *Macromolecular Rapid Communications* 31:1751–1772.
13. Uliniuc, A., M. Popa, T. Hamaide, and M. Dobromir. 2012. New approaches in hydrogel synthesis—Click chemistry: A review. *Cellulose Chemistry and Technology* 46:1–11.
14. Faugeras, P.-A., F. Brouillette, and R. Zerrouki. 2012. Crosslinked cellulose developed by CuAAC, a route to new materials. *Carbohydrate Research* 356:247–251.
15. Heinze, T., T. Liebert, and A. Koschella. 2006. Sulphonic acid esters. In *Esterification of Polysaccharides*, Berlin, Germany: Springer, 117–128.
16. Pohl, M. and T. Heinze. 2008. Novel biopolymer structures synthesized by dendronization of 6-deoxy-6-aminopropargyl cellulose. *Macromolecular Rapid Communications* 29:1739–1745.
17. Peng, P., X. Cao, F. Peng, J. Bian, F. Xu, and R. Sun. 2012. Binding cellulose and chitosan via click chemistry: Synthesis, characterization, and formation of some hollow tubes. *Journal of Polymer Science Part A: Polymer Chemistry* 50:5201–5210.
18. Filpponen, I., E. Kontturi, S. Nummelin, H. Rosilo, E. Kolehmainen, O. Ikkala, and J. Laine. 2012. Generic method for modular surface modification of cellulosic materials in aqueous medium by sequential "Click" reaction and adsorption. *Biomacromolecules* 13:736–742.
19. Li, Q., H. Kang, and R. Liu. 2012. Block and hetero ethyl cellulose graft copolymers synthesized via sequent and one-pot ATRP and "Click" reactions. *Chinese Journal of Chemistry* 30:2169–2175.
20. Xu, W. Z. and J. F. Kadla. 2013. Honeycomb films of cellulose azide: Molecular structure and formation of porous films. *Langmuir* 29:727–733.
21. Koschella, A. and D. Klemm. 1997. Silylation of cellulose regiocontrolled by bulky reagents and dispersity in the reaction media. *Macromolecular Symposia* 120:115–125.

22. Koschella, A., T. Heinze, and D. Klemm. 2001. First synthesis of 3-*O*-functionalized cellulose ethers via 2,6-di-*O*-protected silyl cellulose. *Macromolecular Bioscience* 1:49–54.
23. Fox, S. C., B. Li, D. Xu, and K. J. Edgar. 2011. Regioselective esterification and etherification of cellulose: A review. *Biomacromolecules* 12:1956–1972.
24. Fenn, D., M. Pohl, and T. Heinze. 2009. Novel 3-*O*-propargyl cellulose as a precursor for regioselective functionalization of cellulose. *Reactive and Functional Polymers* 69:347–352.
25. Xu, W. Z., X. Zhang, and J. F. Kadla. 2012. Design of functionalized cellulosic honeycomb films: Site-specific biomolecule modification via "Click Chemistry". *Biomacromolecules* 13:350–357.
26. Nakagawa, A., H. Kamitakahara, and T. Takano. 2012. Synthesis and thermoreversible gelation of diblock methylcellulose analogues via Huisgen 1,3-dipolar cycloaddition. *Cellulose* 19:1315–1326.
27. Enomoto-Rogers, Y., H. Kamitakahara, A. Yoshinaga, and T. Takano. 2012. Comb-shaped graft copolymers with cellulose side-chains prepared via click chemistry. *Carbohydrate Polymers* 87:2237–2245.
28. Kamitakahara, H., Y. Enomoto, C. Hasegawa, and F. Nakatsubo. 2005. Synthesis of diblock copolymers with cellulose derivatives. 2. Characterization and thermal properties of cellulose triacetate-block-oligoamide 15. *Cellulose* 12:527–541.
29. Elchinger, P. H., D. Montplaisir, and R. Zerroukia. 2012. Starch–cellulose crosslinking—Towards a new material. *Carbohydrate Polymers* 87:1886–1890.
30. Agag, T., K. Vietmeier, A. Chernykh, and H. Ishida. 2012. Side-chain type benzoxazine-functional cellulose via click chemistry. *Journal of Applied Polymer Science* 125:1346–1351.
31. Koschella, A., M. Hartlieba, and T. Heinze. 2011. A "click-chemistry" approach to cellulose-based hydrogels. *Carbohydrate Polymers* 86:154–161.
32. Zhang, J., X. D. Xu, D. Q. Wu, X. Z. Zhang, and R. X. Zhuo. 2009. Synthesis of thermosensitive P(NIPAAm-co-HEMA)/cellulose hydrogels via "click" chemistry. *Carbohydrate Polymers* 77:583–589.
33. Billy, M., A. Ranzani Da Costa, P. Lochon, R. Clément, M. Dresch, S. Etienne, J. M. Hiver, L. David, and A. Jonquières. 2010. Cellulose acetate graft copolymers with nano-structured architectures: Synthesis and characterization. *European Polymer Journal* 46:944–957.
34. Malmström, E. and A. Carlmark. 2012. Controlled grafting of cellulose fibres—An outlook beyond paper and cardboard. *Polymer Chemistry* 3:1702–1713.
35. Carlmark, A. 2013. Tailoring cellulose surfaces by controlled radical polymerization methods. *Macromolecular Chemistry and Physics* 214:1539–1544.
36. Xu, W. Z., G. Z. Gao, and J. F. Kadla. 2013. Synthesis of antibacterial cellulose materials using a clickable quaternary ammonium compound. *Cellulose* 20:1187–1199.
37. Negishi, K., Y. Mashiko, E. Yamashita, A. Otsuka, and T. Hasegawa. 2011. Cellulose chemistry meets click chemistry: Syntheses and properties of cellulose-based glycoclusters with high structural homogeneity. *Polymers* 3:489–508.
38. Pohl, M., J. Schaller, F. Meister, and T. Heinze. 2008. Selectively dendronized cellulose: Synthesis and characterization. *Macromolecular Rapid Communications* 29:142–148.
39. Pohl, M., G. A. Morris, S. E. Harding, and T. Heinze. 2009. Studies on the molecular flexibility of novel dendronized carboxymethyl cellulose derivatives. *European Polymer Journal* 45:1098–1110.
40. Pohl, M., N. Michaelis, F. Meister, and T. Heinze. 2009. Biofunctional surfaces based on dendronized cellulose. *Biomacromolecules* 10:382–389.
41. Montanez, M. I., Y. Hed, S. Utsel, J. Ropponen, E. Malmstrom, L. Wagberg, A. Hult, and M. Malkoch. 2011. Bifunctional dendronized cellulose surfaces as biosensors. *Biomacromolecules* 12:2114–2125.
42. Koschella, A., M. Richter, and T. Heinze. 2010. Novel cellulose-based polyelectrolytes synthesized via the click reaction. *Carbohydrate Research* 345:1028–1033.
43. Gonsior, N. and H. Ritter. 2011. Rheological behavior of polyelectrolytes based on cellulose and ionic liquids dissolved in 1-ethyl-3-methyl imidazolium acetate. *Macromolecular Chemistry and Physics* 212:2633–2640.
44. Siro, I. and D. Plackett. 2010. Microfibrillated cellulose and new nanocomposite materials: A review. *Cellulose* 17:459–494.
45. Moon, R. J., A. Martini, J. Nairn, J. Simonsen, and J. Youngblood. 2011. Cellulose nanomaterials review: Structure, properties and nanocomposites. *Chemical Society Reviews* 40:3941–3994.
46. Seppälä, J. 2012. Editorial corner—A personal view, nanocellulose—A renewable polymer of bright future. *eXPRESS Polymer Letters* 6:257.
47. Silva, J. P., F. K. Andrade, and F. M. Gama. 2013. Bacterial cellulose surface modifications. In *Perspectives in Nanotechnology. Bacterial Nano Cellulose: A Sophisticated Multifunctional Material*, M. Gama, P. Gatenholm, and K. D. Paul (eds.), Boca Raton, FL: CRC Press, Taylor & Francis Group.

48. Habibi, Y. 2014. Key advances in the chemical modification of nanocelluloses. *Chemical Society Reviews* 43:1519–1542.
49. Hafrén, J., W. Zou, and A. Cordova. 2006. Heteregeneous "Organoclick" derivatization of polysaccharides. *Macromolecular Rapid Communications* 27:1362–1366.
50. Krouit, M., J. Bras, and M. N. Belgacem. 2008. Cellulose surface grafting with polycaprolactone by heterogeneous click-chemistry. *European Polymer Journal* 44:4074–4081.
51. Dufresne, A. and M. N. Belgacem. 2013. Cellulose-reinforced composites: From micro-to nanoscale. *Polimeros-Ciencia E Tecnologia* 23:277–286.
52. Chen, G., L. Tao, G. Mantovani, V. Ladmiral, D. P. Burt, J. V. Macpherson, and D. M. Haddleton. 2007. Synthesis of azide/alkyne-terminal polymers and application for surface functionalisation through a [2+3] Huisgen cycloaddition process, "click chemistry". *Soft Matter* 3:732–739.
53. Hansson, S., V. Trouillet, T. Tischer, A. S. Goldmann, A. Carlmark, C. Barner-Kowollik, and E. Malmström. 2013. Grafting efficiency of synthetic polymers onto biomaterials: A comparative study of grafting-from versus grafting-to. *Biomacromolecules* 14:64–74.
54. Junka, K., I. Filpponen, L. S. Johansson, E. Kontturi, O. J. Rojas, and J. Laine. 2014. A method for the heterogeneous modification of nanofibrillar cellulose in aqueous media. *Carbohydrate Polymers* 100:107–115.
55. Filpponen, I. and D. S. Argyropoulos. 2010. Regular linking of cellulose nanocrystals via click chemistry: Synthesis and formation of cellulose nanoplatelet gels. *Biomacromolecules* 11:1060–1066.
56. Sadeghifar, H., I. Filpponen, S. P. Clarke, D. F. Brougham, and D. S. Argyropoulos. 2011. Production of cellulose nanocrystals using hydrobromic acid and click reactions on their surface. *Journal of Materials Science* 46:7344–7355.
57. Filpponen, I., H. Sadeghifar, and D. S. Argyropoulos. 2011. Photoresponsive cellulose nanocrystals. *Nanomaterials and Nanotechnology* 1:34–43.
58. Feese, E., H. Sadeghifar, H. S. Gracz, D. S. Argyropoulos, and R. A. Ghiladi. 2011. Photobactericidal porphyrin-cellulose nanocrystals: Synthesis, characterization, and antimicrobial properties. *Biomacromolecules* 12:4177–4179.
59. Eyley, S. and W. Thielemans. 2011. Imidazolium grafted cellulose nanocrystals for ion exchange applications. *Chemical Communications* 47:4177–4179.
60. Karaaslan, M. A., G. Z. Gao, and J. F. Kadla. 2013. Nanocrystalline cellulose/beta-casein conjugated nanoparticles prepared by click chemistry. *Cellulose* 20:2655–2665.
61. Pahimanolis, N., U. Hippi, L.-S. Johansson, T. Saarinen, N. Houbenov, J. Ruokolainen, and J. Seppälä. 2011. Surface functionalization of nanofibrillated cellulose using click-chemistry approach in aqueous media. *Cellulose* 18:1201–1212.
62. Luong, N. D., N. Pahimanolis, U. Hippi, J. T. Korhonen, J. Ruokolainen, L.-S. Johansson, J.-D. Nam, and J. Seppala. 2011. Graphene/cellulose nanocomposite paper with high electrical and mechanical performances. *Journal of Materials Chemistry* 21:13991–13998.
63. Nogi, M., S. Iwamoto, A. N. Nakagaito, and H. Yano. 2009. Optically transparent nanofiber paper. *Advanced Materials* 21:1595–1598.

Index

C

D

E

F

I

J

L

M

N

O

For Product Safety Concerns and Information please contact our EU
representative GPSR@taylorandfrancis.com Taylor & Francis Verlag GmbH,
Kaufingerstraße 24, 80331 München, Germany

Printed and bound by CPI Group (UK) Ltd, Croydon, CR0 4YY
01/05/2025
01858524-0001